QUICK REFERENCE FOR PROTOCOL FOR ALL NURSING INTERVENTIONS

All nursing skills must include certain basic steps for the safety and well-being of the patient and the nurse. To prevent repetition, these steps are referred to at the beginning and end of each skill as standard protocols. The complete Standard Protocol includes the essential steps that must be done consistently with each patient contact to deliver responsible and safe nursing care.

BEFORE THE SKILL

1. **Verify health care provider's orders if the skill is a dependent or collaborative nursing intervention.** Independent nursing interventions are verified with the nursing care plan or primary nurse. *Dependent and collaborative interventions include invasive procedures and medically determined therapies, such as medication administration, wound care applications, and urinary catheterization.*
2. **Gather equipment/supplies and complete necessary charges according to agency policy.** Some equipment is reusable and is kept at the bedside. Some equipment is disposable and charged to the patient as used. *Check agency policy.*

   SUPPL
   - Arm
   - Con
   - Clea non- pate
3. **Perforn the Han** solution use. The
4. **Introdu** both yo used in domesti *right to care.*
5. **Explain can exp**

done relieves patient's level of anxiety and enhances his or her ability to cooperate.

6. **Adjust the bed to appropriate height and lower side rail on the side nearest you.** Check locks on the bed wheel. *Minimizes caregivers muscle strain and prevents injury. Prevents bed from moving.*
7. **Provide adequate lighting for procedure.** Ensures adequate illumination of patient's body and equipment.
8. **Provide privacy for patient. Position and drape patient as needed.**

DURING THE SKILL

9. **Promote patient independence, decision making, and involvement if possible.** *Participation enhances patient motivation and cooperation.*
10. **Assess patient tolerance, being alert for signs of discomfort and fatigue.** *Ability to tolerate interventions varies depending on severity of illness or pain. Use nursing judgment to provide rest and comfort measures.*

COMPLETION PROTOCOL (END OF SKILL)

11. **Assist patient to a position of comfort, and organize needed toiletry or personal items within reach.**
12. **Be certain patient has a way to call for help with call-light or alarm in easy reach, and be sure patient knows how to use it.** *Minimizes risk of falls.*
13. **Raise the appropriate number of side rails and lower the bed to the lowest position. Side rails are considered a restraint and cannot be used to prevent a patient from getting into and out of bed.** *Nursing judgment may allow alert, cooperative patients to have side rails down.*
14. **Dispose of used supplies and equipment.** Leave patient room tidy. *(See CDC Guidelines, Chapter 5).*
15. **Remove and dispose of gloves, if used. Perform hand hygiene for at least 15 seconds.** *Wearing gloves does not eliminate the need for hand hygiene.*
16. **Document and report patient's response and expected or unexpected outcomes.** *Enhances continuity of nursing care.*

NURSING INTERVENTIONS & CLINICAL SKILLS

5th EDITION

Anne Griffin Perry, RN, EdD, FAAN
Professor and Associate Dean
School of Nursing
Southern Illinois University Edwardsville
Edwardsville, Illinois

Patricia A. Potter, RN, MSN, PhD, FAAN
Research Scientist
Siteman Cancer Center at Barnes-Jewish Hospital
Washington University School of Medicine
St. Louis, Missouri

Martha Keene Elkin, RN, MSN
Nursing Educator for Associate Degree Nursing
Sumner, Maine

Section Editor:
Wendy Ostendorf, RN, MS, EdD, CNE
Associate Professor of Nursing
Neumann University
Aston, Pennsylvania

ELSEVIER
MOSBY

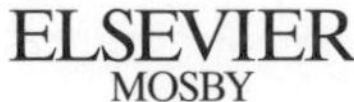

3251 Riverport Lane
St. Louis, Missouri 63043

NURSING INTERVENTIONS AND CLINICAL SKILLS ISBN: 978-0-323-06968-7

Notices

Knowledge and best practice in this field are constantly changing. As new research and experience broaden our understanding, changes in research methods, professional practices, or medical treatment may become necessary.

Practitioners and researchers must always rely on their own experience and knowledge in evaluating and using any information, methods, compounds, or experiments described herein. In using such information or methods they should be mindful of their own safety and the safety of others, including parties for whom they have a professional responsibility.

With respect to any drug or pharmaceutical products identified, readers are advised to check the most current information provided (i) on procedures featured or (ii) by the manufacturer of each product to be administered, to verify the recommended dose or formula, the method and duration of administration, and contraindications. It is the responsibility of practitioners, relying on their own experience and knowledge of their patients, to make diagnoses, to determine dosages and the best treatment for each individual patient, and to take all appropriate safety precautions.

To the fullest extent of the law, neither the Publisher nor the authors, contributors, or editors, assume any liability for any injury and/or damage to persons or property as a matter of products liability, negligence or otherwise, or from any use or operation of any methods, products, instructions, or ideas contained in the material herein.

ISBN: 978-0-323-06968-7

Managing Editor: Jean Sims Fornango
Editorial Assistant: Sarah Graddy
Publishing Services Manager: Deborah L. Vogel
Senior Project Managers: Deon Lee; Jodi M. Willard
Design Direction: Margaret Reid

Printed in United States of America

Last digit is the print number: 9 8 7 6 5 4 3 2 1

CONTRIBUTORS

Aurelie Chinn, RN, MSN
Academic Nursing Skills Specialist/ Simulation Coordinator/Instructor
ADN Program
Cabrillo College
Aptos, California

Janice C. Colwell, RN, MS, CWOCN, FAAN
Clinical Nursing Specialist
University of Chicago Medical Center
Chicago, Illinois

Kelly Jo Cone, PhD, RN, CNE
Professor, Graduate Program
Saint Francis Medical Center College of Nursing
Peoria, Illinois

Ruth Curchoe, RN, MSN, CIC
Director, Infection Prevention and Control
Unity Health Systems
Rochester, New York

Wanda Cleveland Dubuisson, PhD, RN
Associate Professor
School of Nursing
The University of Southern Mississippi
Hattiesburg, Mississippi

Jane Fellows, RN, MSN, CWOCN
Ostomy Clinical Nurse Specialist
Duke University Health System
Durham, North Carolina

Susan Jane Fetzer, RN, BA, BSN, MSN, MBA, PhD
Associate Professor
College of Health and Human Services
University of New Hampshire
Durham, New Hampshire

Nancy Laplante, PhD, RN
Assistant Professor
Neumann University
Aston, Pennsylvania

Catherine Limbaugh, RN, BSN, MSN, ACNS-BC, OCN
Coordinator, Oncology Nursing Fellowship Program
Siteman Cancer Center at Barnes-Jewish Hospital
St. Louis, Missouri

Nelda K. Martin, RN, ANP-BC, CCNS
Critical Care Clinical Nurse Specialist/ Adult Nurse Practitioner
Barnes-Jewish Hospital
St. Louis, Missouri

Barbara Maxwell, MS, RN, LNC
Associate Professor of Nursing
SUNY Ulster Nursing Department
Stone Ridge, New York

Peter R. Miller, RN, MSN, ONC
Instructor
Central Maine Medical Center School of Nursing
Lewiston, Maine

Kim Campbell Olivieri, RN, MS, CS
Clinical Nurse Educator
Beth Israel Deaconess Medical Center
Boston, Massachusetts

Jacqueline Raybuck Saleeby, PhD, RN, MSN
Associate Professor
Maryville University
Town and Country, Missouri

Virginia Strootman, RN, MSN, CRNI
Quintiles Health Management Services
Clinical Resource Nurse
Parsippany, New Jersey

Donna L. Thompson, MSN, CRNP, FNP-BC, CCCN
Nurse Practitioner/Continence Specialist
Urology Health Specialists
Drexel Hill, Pennsylvania;
Adjunct Faculty
Neumann University
Aston, Pennsylvania

Terry L. Wood, PhD, RN, CNE
Clinical Assistant Professor
Southern Illinois University Edwardsville
Edwardsville, Illinois

Rita Wunderlich, MSN, PhD
Director, Baccalaureate Nursing Program;
Associate Professor
St. Louis University School of Nursing
St. Louis, Missouri

Rhonda Yancey, BSN, RN
Senior Practice Specialist
Barnes-Jewish Hospital
St. Louis, Missouri

Valerie J. Yancey, PhD, RN, HNC, CHPN
Associate Professor
School of Nursing
Southern Illinois University Edwardsville
Edwardsville, Illinois

REVIEWERS

Colleen Andreoni, MSN, DNP(c), ANP-BC, CEN
Assistant Professor/Nurse Practitioner
Loyola University—Chicago
Niehoff School of Nursing
Maywood, Illinois

Marty Bachman, PhD, RN, CNS, CNE
Nursing Department Chair, Program Director
Front Range Community College—Larimer Campus
Fort Collins, Colorado

Korbi Berryhill, RN, MSN, CRRN
Assistant Professor and Vocational Nursing Program Director
South Plains College, Reese
Lubbock, Texas

Joanne Bonesteel, MS, RN
Nursing Faculty
Excelsior College School of Nursing
Albany, New York

Jeanie Burt, MSN, MA, RN, CNE
Assistant Professor
College of Nursing
Harding University
Searcy, Arkansas

Norma Butler, RN, BSEd
ACT Manager
Tennessee Technology Center at Nashville
ACT Center
Nashville, Tennessee

Susan Caro-Dupre, MN, RN, CNOR
Assistant Professor
Nicholls State University
Thibodaux, Louisiana

Shari L. Clarke, BSN, MA, MSN
Advance Practice RN/Clinical Faculty
Kennesaw State University
Kennesaw, Georgia

Lauren G. Cline, BSN, MN, RN
Clinical Nurse Educator
University of Washington Medical Center;
Clinical Faculty
University of Washington School of Nursing
Seattle, Washington

Diane K. Daddario, MSN, ACNS-BC, RN, BC, CMSRN
Nursing Instructor
Pennsylvania College of Technology, Williamsport
Urology Nurse Specialist
Geisinger Medical Center
Danville, Pennsylvania

Susan S. Erue, PhD, MSN, RN-BC
Chair, Division of Nursing, and Associate Professor
Iowa Wesleyan College
Mount Pleasant, Iowa

Teresa N. Gore, RN, DNP, FNP
Assistant Clinical Professor
Simulation Learning Coordinator
Auburn University School of Nursing
Auburn, Alabama

Bridget Miller Guidry, MSN, APRN-C, CCRN
Assistant Professor in Nursing
Nicholls State University
Thibodaux, Louisiana

Sally Hartman, MSN, RN-BC, IBCLC
Assistant Clinical Professor
Nursing Department
Indiana University–Purdue University
Fort Wayne, Indiana

Jennifer Ann Hassloch, RN, BN, ADip. Crit Care, MN
Nursing Instructor
Walton Career Development Center
Defuniak Springs, Florida

Patricia Hutchison, RN, MSN, CDE
Education Coordinator
Grove City Medical Center
Grove City, Pennsylvania

Jamie L. Jones, BSN, RN
Faculty Instructor
Department of Nursing
University of Arkansas at Little Rock
Little Rock, Arkansas

Amy Karioris, RN, BSN
Faculty Associate
College of Nursing
University of Wisconsin
Milwaukee, Wisconsin

Linda L. Kerby, RN-C-R, BSN, MA, BA
Mastery Educational Consultations
Leawood, Kansas

Patricia Ketcham, RN, MSN
Director of Nursing Laboratories
School of Nursing
Oakland University
Rochester, Michigan

Penny Killian, MSN, RN, MHPNP
Assistant Clinical Professor
Drexel University
Philadelphia, Pennsylvania

Susan M. Koos, MS, RN, CNE
Professor
Heartland Community College
Normal, Illinois

Nancy Laplante, PhD, RN
Assistant Professor of Nursing
Neumann University
Aston, Pennsylvania

Sue Engman Lazear, RN, MN
Director
Specialists in Medical Education
Woodinville, Washington

Laura Logan, CNS, MSN, RN
Clinical Instructor
DeWitt School of Nursing
Stephen F. Austin State University
Nacogdoches, Texas

Barbara Maxwell, MS, RN, LNC
Associate Professor of Nursing
SUNY Ulster Nursing Department
Stone Ridge, New York

Lesia D. McBride, BSN, RN
Director Quality Resources
Community Hospital of Anderson
Anderson, Indiana

Susie McGregor-Huyer, RN, MSN, CHPN, CLNC
MH Consultants
Mahtomedi, Minnesota;
Faculty
University of Phoenix
Phoenix, Arizona/Minneapolis-St. Paul, Minnesota

Trecia Meadows, RN, BSN
Nursing Instructor
Walton Career Development Center
Practical Nursing Program
DeFuniak Springs, Florida

Virginia F. Ostermeier, MSN, APRN-BC
Associate Professor
Richland Community College
Decatur, Illinois

Shirley E. Otto, MSN, RN, AOCN
Instructor
National American University
Wichita, Kansas

Catherine J. Pagel, MSN, RN
Assistant Professor of Nursing
Associate Degree Nursing Department
Mercy College of Health Science
Des Moines, Iowa

Nancy E. Pea, RN, MSN
Assistant Professor/Nursing Program Coordinator
St. Louis Community College at Florissant Valley
St. Louis, Missouri

Elaine T. Princevalli, RN, BSN, MS
Instructor, LPN Program
Stone Academy
Hamden, Connecticut

Pat Recek, MSN, RN
Assistant Dean, Health Sciences
Professor Vocational Nursing
Austin Community College
Austin, Texas

Anita K. Reed, MSN, RN
Associate Professor of Nursing
St. Elizabeth School of Nursing/St. Joseph College
Lafayette/Rensselaer, Indiana

Diane Saleska, RN, MSN
Associate Professor
University of Missouri—St. Louis
St. Louis, Missouri

Maura C. Schlairet, EdD, MSN, RN, CNL
Associate Professor, College of Nursing
Valdosta State University
Valdosta, Georgia

Susan Parnell Scholtz, PhD, RN
Associate Professor of Nursing
Moravian College
Bethlehem, Pennsylvania

Kathleen Lloren Shea, RN, MSN
Clinical Faculty
San Francisco State University
San Francisco, California

E. Bradley Strecker, RN, BSN, MA, MS(N), CRRN
Associate Professor
Director, Accelerated BSN Program
Mid-America Nazarene University
Olathe, Kansas

Linda M. Stubblefield, BSN, RN
Nursing Program Faculty
Gavilan College Allied Health
Gilroy, California

Marianne Swihart, RN, BSN, MSN, MEd
Associate ADN Professor
Pasco Hernando Community College
New Port Richey, Florida

Mary Tedesco-Schneck, MSN, CPND
Assistant Professor Department of Nursing
Husson University
Bangor, Maine

Holly A. Thiercof, MSN, RN, ACNP
Nursing Program Faculty
Health Sciences Department
Santa Monica College
Santa Monica, California

Kathleen S. Whalen, PhD, RN, CNE
Associate Professor
Loretto Heights School of Nursing
Regis University
Denver, Colorado

CONTRIBUTORS TO PREVIOUS EDITIONS

Elizabeth A. Ayello, RN, BSN, MS, PhD, CS, CETN
Margaret R. Benz, RN, MSN(R), BC, APN
Barbara J. Berger, MSN, RN
V. Christine Champagne, APRN, BC
Janice C. Colwell, Rn, MS, CWOCN
Kelly Jo Cone, PhD, RN, CNE
Karen S. Conners, RNC, MSN
Eileen Costantinou, MSN, RN
Deborah Crump, RN, MS, CHPN
Sheila A. Cunningham, BSN, MSN
Wanda Cleveland Dubuisson, PhD, RN
Julie Eddins, RN, BSN, MSN, CRNI
Deborah Oldenburg Erickson, RN, BSN, MSN
Joan O. Ervin, RN, BSN, MN, CCRN
Sue Fetzer, BA, BSN, MSN, MBA, PhD
Melba J. Figgins, MSN, BSN
Janet B. Fox-Moatz, RN, BSN, MSN
Lynn C. Hadaway, MEd, RNC, CRNI
Amy Hall, RN, PhD
Susan A. Hauser, RN, BSN, BA, MS
Mimi Hirshberg, RN, MSN
Carolyn Chaney Hoskins, RN, BSN, MSN
Maureen B. Huhmann, MS, RD
Meredith Hunt, MSN, RNC, NP
Nancy Jackson, RN, BSN, MSN(R), CCRN
Linda L. Kerby, RN-C-R, BSN, MA, BA
Marilee Kuhrik, BSN, MSN, PhD
Nancy Kuhrik, BSN, MSN, PhD
Amy Lawn, BSN, MS, CIC
Kristine M. L'Ecuyer, RN, MSN, CCNS
Antoinette Kanne Ledbetter, RN, BSN, MS, TNS
Mary MacDonald, RN, MSN
Mary Kay Knight Macheca, MSN(R), RN, CS, ANP, CDE
Cynthia L. Maskey, RN, MS
Constance C. Maxey, RN-BC, MSN
Barbara McGeever, RN, RSM, BSN, MSN, DNS(c)
Mary "Dee" Miller, RN, BSN, MS, CIC
Peter R. Miller, RN, MSN, ONC
Rose M. Miller, RN, BSN, MSN, MPA, ACLS
Karen Montalto, RN, DNSc
Kathleen Mulryan, RN, BSN, MSN
Elaine K. Neel, RN, BSN, MSN
Kim Campbell Oliveri, RN, MS, CS
Marsha Evans Orr, RN, MS
Wendy Ostendorf, RN, MS, EdD, CNE
Shirley E. Otto, MSN, RN, AOCN
Deborah Paul-Cheadle, RN
Roberta J. Richmond, MSN, RN, CCRN
Paulette D. Rollant, RN, BSN, MSN, PhD, CCRN
Jacqueline Raybuck Salleby, PhD, RN, MSN
Linette M. Sarti, RN, BSN, CNOR
Lynn Schallom, RN, MSN, CCRN, CCNS
Kelly Schwartz, RN, BSN
Julie Snyder, RN, MSN, BC
Phyllis G. Stallard, BSN, MSN, ACCE
Victoria Steelman, PhD, RN, CNOR
Patricia A. Stockert, RN, PhD
Sue G. Thacker, RNC, BSN, MS, PhD
Donna L. Thompson, MSN, CRNP, FNP-BC, CCCN
Nancy Tomaselli, RN, MSN, CS, CRNP, CWOCN, CLNC
Stephanie Trinkl, BSN, MSN
Kathryn Tripp, BSN
Paula Vehlow, RN, MS
Pamela Becker Weilitz, MSN(R), RN, CN, ANP
Jana L. Weindel-Dees, RN, BSN, MSN
Joan Domigan Wentz, MSN, RN
Trudie Wierda, RN, MSN
Laurel A. Wiersema-Bryant, MSN, RN, CS
Terry L. Wood, PhD, RN, CNE
Rita Wunderlich, MSN, PhD
Rhonda Yancey, BSN, RN
Valerie J. Yancey, PhD, RN, HNC, CHPN

ACKNOWLEDGMENTS

We appreciate the talents and expertise of Wendy Ostendorf, our section editor. Wendy's insight and creativity helped take this text to the next level. Her knowledge of the nursing literature and clinical practice, her commitment to excellence, and her attention to detail were important from the beginning of this revision to the publication of the newest edition.

We also wish to acknowledge the many clinical nurses, educators, and students who provided valuable feedback for the revision of this text. Clinical nurses and nurse educators offered their comments and recommendations on the accuracy and clarity of the content. Students provided valuable insight into the needs of those struggling to learn the art and science of nursing. Our contributors shared their clinical wisdom and expertise in writing a state-of-the-art textbook. Our reviewers helped refine and polish the material to provide the best possible information for teaching clinical nursing skills.

Thanks to the talented and dedicated professionals at Elsevier. Tamara Myers, Executive Editor, provided support, leadership, enthusiasm, and a healthy sense of humor during the revision process. Jean Sims Fornango, Managing Editor, spent countless hours tracking the progress of this text. Her organizational skills, commitment to accuracy, and dedication to quality kept the project on target. Sarah Graddy, Editorial Assistant, cheerfully assisted with countless details. Karen Edwards, Assistant Director, Debbie Vogel, Book Production Manager, and Jodi Willard, Senior Project Manager, helped ensure an accurate, consistent book through their organization, careful editing, and guidance of the project through the production process. The creativity of Margaret Reid, Book Designer, provides an attractive and unique visual appeal to the text. These contributions significantly enhance the learning process.

Finally, thanks to our friends, families, and colleagues for their understanding, patience, and encouragement.

Anne Griffin Perry
Patricia A. Potter

PREFACE TO THE STUDENT

You will find a number of features built in to this book to help you identify key pieces of information and study more efficiently:

- **Quick Reference to Standard Protocols** in the front of the text reminds you of steps to be consistently taken before, during, and after every care interaction with a patient. Each skill and procedure will remind you to review these steps.
- **Clean glove logo** reminds you when it is essential to apply clean gloves to protect yourself and your patient from transmission of microorganisms.
- **Safety Alert** helps you identify important safety issues for each skill and procedure.
- **Video clips, checklists,** and **audio glossary** are available for your use on the companion Evolve site: http://evolve.elsevier.com/Perry/nursinginterventions

Video clip icon alerts you to related videos on the Evolve site for the text.

Delegation and Collaboration section provides guidelines for assigning a skill to nursing assistive personnel.

SKILL 22.1 ADMINISTERING ORAL MEDICATIONS

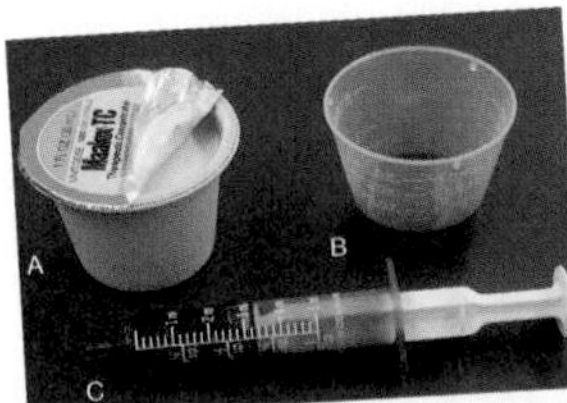

FIG 22-1 **A,** Liquid medication in a single-dose package. **B,** Liquid measured in a medicine cup. **C,** Oral medicine in syringe.

SKILL 30.2 USING AN AUTOMATED EXTERNAL DEFIBRILLATOR

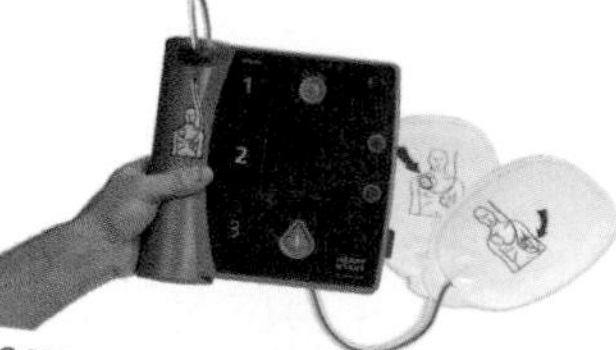

FIG 30-3 Automated external defibrillator device. (Courtesy Philips Medical Systems.)

Safety Alerts identify important safety issues.

STEPS	RATIONALE
i. To prepare tablets or capsules from a floor stock bottle, pour required number into bottle cap and transfer medication to medication cup. Do not touch medication with fingers. Return extra tablets or capsules to bottle.	Avoids contamination of medications and avoids waste. Floor stock bottles are common in long-term care settings for over-the-counter (OTC) drugs such as laxatives and nonopioid analgesics.
j. When using a blister pack, "pop" medications through foil or paper backing into a medication cup.	Long-term care agencies use blister packs, which provide about a 1-month supply of prescription drugs for a patient. Each "blister" usually contains a single dose. Blister packs are prepared by a pharmacist or pharmaceutical company.
k. If it is necessary to break a medication to give half the dose, use a clean, gloved hand to break the tablet or cut with a clean pill-cutting device (see illustration). Only break tablets prescored by the manufacturer (line transverses the center of the tablet).	Reduces contamination of the tablet. Tablets that are not prescored cannot be broken into equal halves, resulting in an inaccurate dose. A cutting device results in a more even split of a tablet (ISMP, 2006).
l. Place all tablets or capsules that patient will receive in one medicine cup, except for those requiring preadministration assessments (e.g., pulse rate, blood pressure).	Serves as a reminder to complete appropriate assessment and facilitates withholding drugs (if necessary).

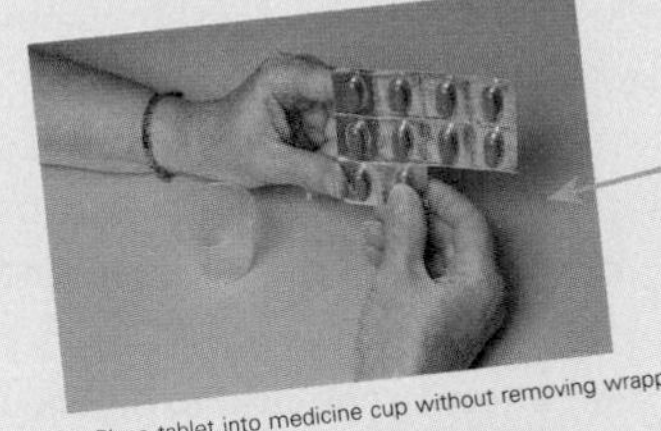

STEP 2h Place tablet into medicine cup without removing wrapper.

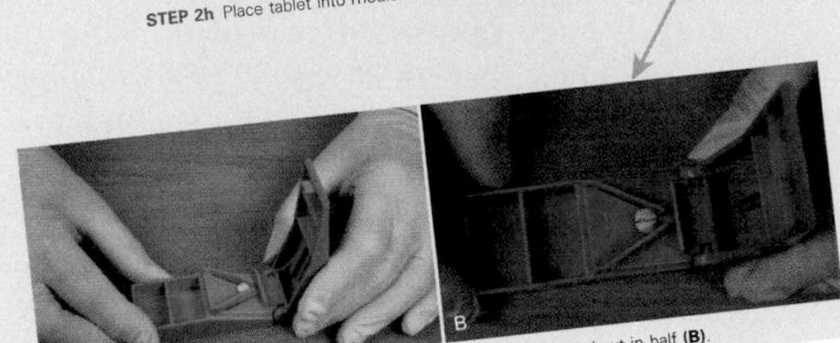

STEP 2k Tablet is placed in pill-cutting device (A) and cut in half (B).

Continued

Glove logo reminds you to apply clean gloves when appropriate.

Extensive illustrations demonstrate key step-by-step procedures.

...head of the bed and stay with the patient. ...r staff member notify the patient's health ...

...ns, oxygen saturation, and breath sounds. ...dverse effects (side effect, toxic effect, ...

...r doses and assess vital signs. ...e provider and pharmacy. ...possible administration of emergency med-...ications for allergic reaction.

Recording and Reporting

- Record in nurses' notes check for tube placement, GRV, and pH of aspirate.
- Record drug, dose, route, and time administered on MAR immediately *after* administration, not before. Include initials or signature. Record patient teaching and validation of understanding in nurses' notes.
- Record total amount of water used for medication administration on proper intake/output (I&O) form.
- Report adverse effects, patient response, and/or withheld drugs to nurse in charge or health care provider.

Sample Documentation

NOTE: Documentation for medications via feeding tube is usually done on the MAR. Fluids given without medications must be recorded as intake on I&O. Other documentation occurs only if a problem is noted.

1300 Unable to administer medication because of clogged feeding tube, despite attempts to irrigate with 60 mL of tap water. Health care provider notified; medications and tube feeding held pending placement of new tube.

Special Considerations

Geriatric

- Assess patient for use of medications that may affect the pH of gastric secretions such as H_2-receptor antagonists or antacids. H_2-receptor antagonists reduce volume of gastric acid secretion and the acid content of secretions, thus causing the pH value to be higher or more basic (Metheny, 2006).

Home Care

Teach patient or family caregiver:

- How to store medications and tube feeding supplements.
- How to check placement of tube before administering any medication.
- Importance of not giving medication and to notify the health care provider if there is any doubt concerning the placement of the tube.
- About importance of consistent irrigation of feeding tube before, during, and after medications are given.
- Provide the patient or primary caregiver with resources to determine which medications can be crushed, which medications should not be crushed, and how to obtain liquid formulations of the medications.

SKILL 22.3 APPLYING TOPICAL MEDICATIONS TO THE SKIN

- *Nursing Skills Online: Nonparenteral Medication Administration, Lesson 2* — *Video Clips*

Topical administration of medications involves applying drugs locally to skin, mucous membranes, or tissues. Topical drugs such as lotions, patches, pastes, and ointments primarily produce local effects; but they can also create systemic effects if absorbed through the skin. Systemic effects are more likely to occur if the skin is thin, drug concentration is high, contact with the skin is prolonged, or the drug is applied to broken skin. To protect from accidental exposure, apply topical drugs using gloves and applicators. Skin encrustations and dead tissue harbor microorganisms and block contact of medications with the affected tissue or membrane. Simply applying new medications over previously applied drugs does little to prevent infection or provide a therapeutic benefit. Always cleanse the skin or a wound thoroughly before applying a dose of a topical drug. Apply each type of medication, whether an ointment, lotion, or patch, in a specific way to ensure proper penetration and absorption.

ASSESSMENT

1. Check accuracy and completeness of each MAR with health care provider's medication order. Check patient's name, drug name and dosage, route of administration, and time for administration. Recopy or reprint any portion of printed MAR that is difficult to read. *Rationale: The health care provider's order is the most reliable source and only legal record of drugs patient is to receive. Ensures that patient receives the right medications (Eisenhauer and others, 2007; Furukawa and others, 2008).*
2. Review pertinent information related to medication, including action, purpose, normal dose and route, time of onset and peak action, side effects, and nursing implications. *Rationale: Allows you to anticipate effects of drug and observe patient's response.*
3. Assess condition of skin or membrane where medication is to be applied (see Chapter 7). You can do this just before applying the medication. If there is an open wound, apply clean gloves. First wash site thoroughly with mild, nondrying soap and warm water; rinse; and dry. Remove any previously applied medication or debris. Also remove any blood, secretions, excretions, or other body fluids. Assess for symptoms of skin irritation such as pruritus or burning. *Rationale: Provides baseline to determine change in condition of skin after therapy. Topical agents can lessen or aggravate these symptoms.*

Recording and Reporting clarifies what information should be recorded in which record for correct documentation of patient care.

Special Considerations indicates modifications needed for pediatric, geriatric, or home care performance of a skill.

Sample Documentation shows you how to record a nurse's narrative note with proper terminology and phrasing.

PREFACE TO THE INSTRUCTOR

The evolution of technology and knowledge influences the way we teach clinical skills to nursing students and improves the quality of care possible for every patient. However, the foundation for success in performing nursing skills remains a competent and well-informed nurse who thinks critically and asks the right questions at the right time to provide appropriate nursing care. This edition of *Nursing Interventions & Clinical Skills* retains the successful elements of previous editions but incorporates material key to this shift in how nurses practice. We have retained the concise format, clear language, and streamlined approach that were hallmarks of previous editions. New photos and line drawings update the generous illustration program. All skills and procedures are presented within the framework of the nursing process.

In this 5th edition, we've reorganized topics to make it easier to locate related information. For example, you will now find all skills related to Urinary Elimination in one chapter (Chapter 18). Information related to the *Quality and Safety Education for Nurses* (QSEN) initiative is highlighted by headings that coordinate with key competencies. You will now find sections on *Patient-Centered Care*, *Safety*, and *Evidence-Based Practice Trends* at the beginning of each chapter. Information on *Delegation and Collaboration*, *Safety Alerts*, and *Documentation* is included with the procedure-specific information.

KEY FEATURES

- Comprehensive coverage of nursing skills—from basic skills such as measuring temperature to complex advance skills such as intravenous therapy and management of endotracheal tubes
- Extensive full-color art program, including dozens of new photographs
- Standard and Completion Protocols
- Glove Logos to visually highlight circumstances in which the use of clean gloves is recommended
- Safety Alerts in the flow of the skill to alert the student to special precautions and specific risks
- Delegation and Collaboration guidelines in the planning section for each skill and procedure
- Step-by-step presentation of steps of each skill, with supporting rationales that are often evidence based
- Recording and Reporting sections to provide a concise, bulleted list of information to be documented and reported
- Sample Documentation sections to provide examples of clear variance notes or narrative documentation
- Special Considerations sections to provide information on adaptation of skills in specific circumstances, such as in the home care setting or when caring for a child or older adult

NEW TO THIS EDITION

- A new Chapter 1, Using Evidence in Nursing Practice, prepares students to implement evidence-based practice.
- New Skills and Procedural Guidelines prepare the students for practice:
  - Hand-Off Communications
  - SBAR Communication
  - Assessing the Genitalia and Rectum
  - Eye Care for the Comatose Patient
  - Site Care of Enteral Feeding Tubes
  - Selection of a Pressure-Reducing Support Surface
  - Catheterizing a Urinary Diversion
  - Administering Nasal Medications
  - Performing a Wound Assessment
  - Wound Irrigation
- Completely revamped and expanded end-of-chapter exercises include case-based critical thinking questions and review items that use a variety of formats. Answers with rationales are available in the back of the text.

ANCILLARIES

Evolve Instructor Resources:
- *Instructor Resource Manual* provides teaching strategies, clinical activities, and answers to end-of-chapter review questions with rationales
- *Test Bank* includes 750 testing items in a variety of testing formats
- *PowerPoint* slide sets for each chapter
- Answer keys to *Nursing Skills Online 2.0* quizzes and exams
- Answer key to review questions in *Mosby's Nursing Video Skills* video set

Evolve Student Resources:
- 50 video clips from the recently revised *Mosby's Nursing Video Skills: Basic, Intermediate, Advanced* set.
- Skills Performance Checklists for every skill and procedure in PDF format

Also available:
- **Nursing Skills Online 2.0** contains 18 modules rich with animations, videos, interactive activities, and exercises to help students prepare for their clinical lab experience. The instructionally designed lessons focus on topics that are difficult to master and pose a high risk to the patient if done incorrectly. Lesson quizzes allow students to check their learning curve and review as needed, and the module exams feed out to an instructor grade book. Modules cover Airway Management, Blood Therapy, Bowel Elimination/Ostomy Care, Chest Tubes, Enteral Nutrition, Infection Control, Injections, IV Fluid Administration, IV Fluid Therapy

Management, IV Medication Administration, Nonparenteral Medication Administration, Safe Medication Administration, Safety, Specimen Collection, Urinary Catheterization, Vascular Access, Vital Signs, and Wound Care. Available alone or packaged with the text.

- **Mosby's Nursing Video Skills: Basic, Intermediate, Advanced version 3.0** provides 126 skills with overview information covering skill purpose, safety, and delegation guides; equipment lists; preparation procedures; procedure videos with printable step-by-step guidelines; appropriate follow-up care; documentation guidelines; and interactive review questions. Available online, as a student DVD set, or as a networkable DVD set for the institution.

CONTENTS

UNIT 3 BASIC HUMAN NEEDS

UNIT 4 ACTIVITY AND MOBILITY

UNIT 5 PROMOTING ELIMINATION

UNIT 6 MEDICATION ADMINISTRATION

UNIT 7 DRESSINGS AND WOUND CARE

UNIT 8 COMPLEX NURSING INTERVENTIONS

UNIT 9 SUPPORTIVE NURSING INTERVENTIONS

APPENDIXES

CHAPTER

1

Using Evidence in Nursing Practice

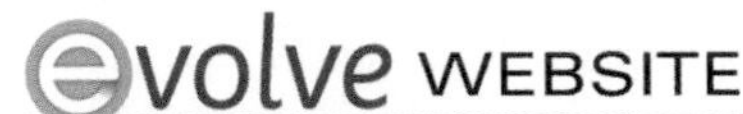

http://evolve.elsevier.com/Perry/nursinginterventions

The general public is more informed about their own health and health care issues than ever before. In 1999 the Institute of Medicine (IOM) published a classic report, *To Err is Human: Building a Safer Health System* (IOM, 2000), which contained information on the occurrence of medical errors within the United States and how they could be prevented. Basically health care in the United States reportedly was not as safe as it should and can be. This report, along with initiatives from groups such as The Joint Commission and the National Quality Forum, led to greater scrutiny as to why certain health care approaches are used. As a result, evidence-based practice (EBP) became a response to the broad societal forces that nurses and other health care professionals face.

Simply stated, EBP is the use of the current best evidence in making patient care decisions. EBP applies to all types of health care professionals. A clinician works with colleagues from other disciplines to update a policy and procedure that pertains to intravenous (IV) site care. A nurse educator wants to use current evidence to improve a simulated laboratory teaching technique. A nurse manager studies the evidence and works with physicians on his or her unit to find ways to improve nurse and physician communication. In each case nurses and other health care colleagues use a problem-solving approach that integrates use of the best available scientific evidence rather than making decisions on intuition, past policy, or experience alone.

New evidence in the scientific literature is reported every day. Although the scientific basis of nursing practice has grown, some practices are still not research based (i.e., based on findings from well-designed research studies) because findings are nonconclusive or researchers have not yet studied the specific practices (Titler and others, 2001). However, use of evidence does change practice. For example, in the past nurses applied antibiotic ointment routinely to IV sites, assuming that this would reduce infection at the site. However, research has shown that topical antibiotics offer no benefit; thus the current standard of care is simply to apply a sterile transparent or gauze dressing to an IV site (Infusion Nurses Society, 2006). The challenge is to obtain the very best, most current information when you need it in your practice.

The best evidence comes from well-designed, systematically conducted research studies found in scientific journals. The journals come from nursing and all related health care disciplines. Yet there are sources of evidence that do not originate from research. They include quality or performance improvement data, risk management and infection control information, medical record audits, and clinicians' expertise. Nonresearch-based data offer valuable information about practice trends and the nature of problems in a specific setting. For example, expert clinicians are an invaluable resource because of their experience and their familiarity with the current literature. However, it is important to never rely on nonresearch-based information alone. Research-based evidence is more likely to be timely and relevant to current practice conditions. When you face a practice problem, always seek the best sources of evidence that help you find the best solution in caring for your patients.

STEPS OF EVIDENCE-BASED PRACTICE

Evidence-based practice (EBP) is a problem-solving approach to clinical practice that integrates the conscientious use of best evidence along with a clinician's expertise and patient preferences and values in making decisions about patient care (Melnyk and Fineout-Overholt, 2011; Sackett and others, 2000). Using a step-by-step approach ensures that you will obtain the strongest available evidence to apply in patient care. There are six steps of EBP:

1. Ask a clinical question.
2. Collect the most relevant and best evidence.
3. Critically appraise the evidence you gather.
4. Integrate all the evidence along with your clinical expertise, patient preferences, and values in making a practice decision or change.
5. Evaluate the practice change or decision.
6. Share the outcomes with others.

Ask a Clinical Question

EBP begins with forming a relevant and meaningful clinical question. Nurses and other health care providers face questions in their practice each day. Make it a habit to always question what does not make sense to you such as a recurring problem in the care of patients or a problem or area of interest that is time consuming, costly, or not logical (Callister and others, 2005). Titler and others (2001) suggest using either problem-focused or knowledge-focused triggers to identify clinical questions.

Problem-Focused Trigger

A problem-focused trigger is a question faced while caring for a patient or a trend seen in a practice setting.

Examples:

- "How can we reduce the rate of pressure ulcers since it has been increasing over the last 3 months on our surgical unit?"
- "What approaches can be used to reduce the fall rate on the neurology floor?"

Knowledge-Focused Trigger

A knowledge-focused trigger is a question regarding new information about a topic.

Examples:

- "What is the current evidence for reducing phlebitis in peripheral IV catheters?"
- "What is known about ways to enhance learning in older adults?"

Typically practice questions begin to form as health care professionals talk more about patient care. EBP becomes an easier process when you and your colleagues can agree on a relevant clinical question. Once you ask a question, the next step is to search for evidence. You ask a question that is focused and specific enough that it leads you to the most relevant scientific articles in the literature and evidence that you have on your nursing unit (e.g., quality improvement reviews). Melnyk and Fineout-Overholt (2011) suggest using a PICO format to state your questions. Box 1-1 summarizes the four elements of a PICO question. Let's use this example: You are a staff nurse working on a general surgery unit. You are meeting with colleagues on the EBP committee to review monthly performance measures for the unit. One measure is patient satisfaction with pain relief measures. The scores for the unit have dropped over the last 2 months. As your colleagues discuss the issue, one nurse mentions caring for a patient who had an epidural catheter for analgesia. The patient progressed very well during hospitalization. Your colleagues wonder if epidural analgesia is a good option for more patients. Typically patients on the unit receive patient-controlled analgesia. As a result, you ask this PICO question, "*In abdominal surgery patients (P), is epidural analgesia (I) compared with patient-controlled analgesia (C) more effective in pain relief (O)?*"

A clearly stated PICO question will lead you to the most relevant research and clinical articles that apply to your clinical situation. The question should identify knowledge gaps and reveal the type of evidence that you lack for your clinical practice. A well-designed PICO question does not have to include all four elements. However, the goal is to ask a question that contains as many of the PICO elements as possible in a logically framed question. Sometimes nurses ask meaningful questions that do not require all four elements. For example, "How do oncology nurses cope with the death of a cancer patient?"

Incomplete PICO questions do not lead you to a well-defined set of scientific articles. For example, background questions such as "What are best practices for pain management?" or "What approaches can be used to assess health literacy?" lead you to the scientific literature, but the articles are too numerous and diverse. What you want to be able to gather after stating a question are a few very good, current scientific articles. A complete PICO question provides this focus.

> **BOX 1-1 DEVELOPING A PICO QUESTION**
>
> **P = Patient Population**
> Identify your patients by age, gender, ethnicity, disease or type of health problem.
>
> **I = Intervention or Area of Interest**
> Identify the intervention that you want to use in practice and that you believe is worthwhile (e.g., a treatment, diagnostic test, an educational approach).
>
> **C = Comparison Intervention or Area of Interest**
> What is the usual standard of care or current intervention that you want to compare against the intervention of interest?
>
> **O = Outcome**
> What result do you wish to achieve or observe as a result of an intervention (e.g., change in patient's behavior, physical status, or perception)?

Collect the Best Evidence

After you identify a clear and concise PICO question, your next step is to search for the available evidence, both external and internal. External evidence consists of the scientific literature (computerized bibliographical databases), national guidelines, and national benchmarking. Internal evidence includes agency policy and procedure manuals, quality improvement data, and clinical practice guidelines. One rule to follow: do not rely on nonscientific evidence. Always go to the scientific literature for the most current evidence about your question. Generally it is wise to focus your article search on those written within the last 5 years unless your search includes a "classic" research article.

When searching the scientific literature for evidence, seek the help of a medical librarian when possible. A medical librarian knows the relevant databases (Box 1-2).

A database is an electronic library of published scientific studies, including peer-reviewed research. A peer-reviewed article has been evaluated by a panel of experts familiar with

BOX 1-2 SEARCHABLE SCIENTIFIC LITERATURE DATABASES AND SOURCES

CINAHL: Cumulative Index of Nursing and Allied Health Literature; Includes studies in nursing, allied health, and biomedicine (http://www.cinahl.com)
MEDLINE: Includes studies in medicine, nursing, dentistry, psychiatry, veterinary medicine, and allied health (http://www.ncbi.nim.nih.gov)
EMBASE: Biomedical and pharmaceutical studies (http://www.embase.com)
PsycINFO: Psychology and related health care disciplines (http://www.apa.org/psycinfo)
Cochrane Database of Systematic Reviews: Full text of regularly updated systematic reviews prepared by the Cochrane Collaboration; includes completed reviews and protocols (http://www.cochrane.org/reviews)
National Guidelines Clearinghouse: Repository for structured abstracts (summaries) about clinical guidelines and their development; also includes condensed version of guideline for viewing (http://www.guideline.gov)
PubMed: Health science library at the National Library of Medicine; offers free access to journal articles (http://www.nlm.nih.gov)
On-Line Journal of Knowledge Synthesis for Nursing: Electronic journal containing articles that provide a synthesis of research and an annotated bibliography for selected references (http://nursingsociety.org/publications/journals)

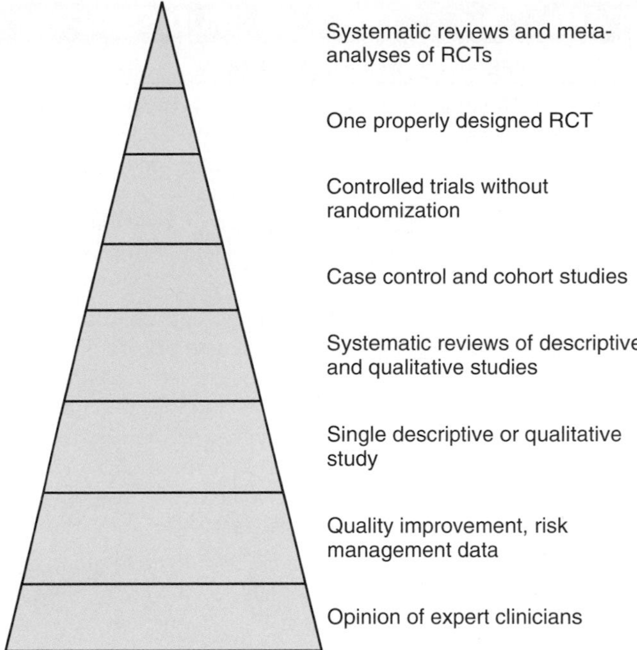

FIG 1-1 The evidence hierarchy pyramid. *RCT,* Randomized controlled trials. (Modified from Guyatt G, Rennie D: *User's guide to the medical literature,* Chicago, 2002, American Medical Association: AMA Press. Harris RP and others: Current methods of the U.S. Preventive Services Task Force: a review of the process, *Am J Prev Med* 20:21, 2001.)

the topic of the article. The librarian helps translate elements of your PICO question into the language or key words that yield the most relevant articles you want to read. For example, in the PICO question, *In abdominal surgery patients, is epidural analgesia more effective in pain relief than patient-controlled analgesia?,* the key words are *abdominal surgery, epidural analgesia, patient-controlled analgesia,* and *pain.* When conducting a search, it is necessary to enter and manipulate the different key words until you get the combination that gives you the articles you want to read about your topic. Sometimes when you enter a key word to search, you get results for articles that seem unrelated to your topic. The word(s) you select sometimes has one meaning to one author and a very different meaning to another. For example, you might choose a key word *oncology* when use of the key word *cancer* might be more successful. Another example is using two terms such as *infection* and *incidence* instead of the term *infection rate.* A medical librarian helps you learn how to choose alternative words or terms that identify your PICO question.

MEDLINE, CINAHL, and PubMed are among the most comprehensive databases and represent the scientific knowledge base of health care (Melnyk and Fineout-Overholt, 2011). PubMed is a free resource on the Internet. You can only access MEDLINE and CINAHL through vendors, which are usually available through academic institutions by subscription. The Cochrane Database of Systematic Reviews is a valuable source of synthesized or preappraised evidence. The database includes the full text of regularly updated systematic reviews and protocols for reviews currently in progress. The National Guidelines Clearinghouse (NGC) is a database supported by the Agency for Healthcare Research and Quality (AHRQ). It contains clinical guidelines, which are systematically developed statements about a plan of care for a specific set of clinical circumstances involving a specific patient population. The NGC is valuable when you are developing a plan of care for a patient.

When you search the literature, you will get a list of many different types of scientific articles. You might ask, "Which articles are the best to read?" The pyramid in Fig. 1-1 is one example of a hierarchy for ordering the strength of available evidence.

At the top of the pyramid are systematic reviews, the strongest source of scientific evidence. At the bottom is the opinion of expert clinicians. At this point in your nursing career you are probably not an expert on the different types of scientific studies. However, you can learn enough about the types of studies to help you decide which articles to read. Table 1-1 describes types of studies in the evidence hierarchy.

If your PICO question yields an article on your topic that is a systematic review, celebrate! It provides an excellent summary of the evidence available. In a systematic review a researcher has asked the same PICO question that you have asked and then examined all of the well-designed experimental research questions on that topic. The review then

TABLE 1-1 TYPES OF STUDIES IN THE EVIDENCE HIERARCHY

STUDY TYPE	DESCRIPTION	EXAMPLE
Systematic review or meta-analysis	A panel of experts reviews the evidence from randomized controlled trials about a specific clinical question and summarizes the state of the science. In a meta-analysis there is the addition of a statistical analysis that combines data from all studies.	Nine studies examined the use of continuous epidural analgesia (CEA) compared with intravenous opioid patient-controlled analgesia in relieving postoperative abdominal pain. The review revealed that CEA is superior in relieving pain for up to 72 hours (Werawatganon and Charuluxanun, 2005)
Randomized controlled trial	A researcher tests an intervention against the usual standard of care. Participants are randomly assigned to either a control group (receives standard care) or a treatment group (receives the experimental intervention), with both measured on the same outcomes to see if there is a difference.	Researchers randomly assigned 107 critical care patients to receive intermittent nasogastric feedings (treatment group) or continuous feedings (control group). Patients in the intermittent feeding group had a higher total intake at day 7, earlier extubation, and a lower risk of aspiration pneumonia (Chen and others, 2006).
Case control study	Researchers study one group of subjects with a certain condition (e.g., obesity) at the same time as another group of subjects who do not have the condition to determine if there is an association between the condition and predictor variables (e.g., exercise pattern, family history, history of depression).	Researchers from Singapore compared 61 patients with known ocular keratitis with 188 population-based and 178 hospitalized patients to determine what contact lens cleaning methods contributed to keratitis. The use of a specific contact lens cleaning solution was found to increase the risk for keratitis (Saw and others, 2007).
Descriptive study	The study describes the concepts under study. It sometimes examines the prevalence, magnitude, and/or characteristics of a concept.	Researchers explored nurses' and doctors' perceptions of infection control practices in relation to management of infectious disease (Watkins and others, 2006).
Qualitative study	Studies explore phenomena such as individuals' experiences with health problems and the contexts in which the experiences occur.	Researchers asked 392 nurses to discuss a care episode from their practice. Cases describing cancer patients involved nurses' use of powerful emotive language. The influence of patients' cancer experience affects nurses personally and professionally (Kendall, 2007).
Quality improvement data, risk management information	Data collected within a health care agency offers important trending information about clinical conditions and problems. Staff in the agency review the data periodically to identify problem areas and then seek solutions.	Article reviews use of quality improvement process in a nursing home setting, where staff adopted best practices for pressure ulcer care for residents (Berlowitz and Frantz, 2007).
Clinical experts	Accessing clinical experts on a nursing unit is an excellent way to learn about current evidence. Clinical experts often write clinical articles on topics that require application of evidence in the literature.	Clinical article describes an evidence-based practice project, in which a team of nurses applied evidence from the literature to change their hospital's approach to intravenous (IV) site care and IV catheter stabilization (Winfield and others, 2007).

determines whether the evidence for which you are searching exists and whether it is strong enough for you to change practice.

Individual randomized controlled trials (RCTs) are the gold standard for research (Titler and others, 2001). An RCT is an experimental study that establishes cause and effect and is the best way for testing a therapy or intervention. Historically there have been few RCTs conducted in nursing. The nature of nursing causes researchers to ask questions that are not easily answered by an RCT or are difficult to conduct in a clinical setting. Nurses care for patients' responses to health problems in busy clinical settings. For example, a nurse might be interested in studying a new approach for managing a patient symptom such as pain. He or she wants to try the use of massage and analgesics compared with analgesics alone. To conduct an RCT the nurse would have to refrain from offering the new approach (massage and analgesia) to a subgroup of patients (control group). In busy clinical settings there are often barriers that make conducting RCTs difficult. Therefore nurse researchers often rely on quasi-experimental, descriptive, and qualitative studies to conduct their research.

The use of clinical experts is at the bottom of the evidence pyramid, but do not consider clinical experts a poor source of evidence. Expert clinicians often use evidence as they build their practice, and they are rich sources of information for clinical problems. The use of experts coupled with scientific literature will give you a strong source of evidence.

Critique the Evidence

Once you conduct a literature search and gather any data you might have about your question, it becomes time to critique the evidence. A critique tells you if there is sufficient evidence to answer your PICO question and change practice. In most settings nurses and other health care providers collaborate in critiquing the evidence. Each member of an EBP committee shares in reading articles and using specific criteria in each article review.

The critique of evidence determines the value, feasibility, and use of evidence for making a practice change. During the critique you evaluate the scientific merit and clinical applicability of each of the studies from the literature. Then together you review findings from the group of studies and determine if there is a strong enough basis for use of the evidence in practice. In the example of the PICO question described earlier, a critique answers if there is strong evidence to use epidural analgesia instead of patient-controlled analgesia for pain control in patients who undergo abdominal surgery.

It takes time to acquire the skills to critique evidence from the literature. Hopefully a member of an EBP committee has experience in this area. When you read an article, do not let the statistics or technical wording cause you to put it down and walk away. Know the elements of an article and use a careful approach when reviewing each one. Evidence-based articles include the following elements:

Abstract: A brief summary of the article that quickly tells you if it is research or clinically based. An abstract summarizes the purpose of the study or clinical topic, the major themes or findings, and the implications for nursing practice.

Introduction: Contains information about the purpose of the article and the importance of the topic for the audience who reads the article. It contains brief supporting evidence as to why the topic is important from the author's point of view.

Together, the abstract and introduction determine if you want to continue to read an entire article. You will know if the topic of the article is similar to your PICO question or related closely enough to provide you with useful information. If so, continue reading the next elements of the article:

Literature review or background: A good author offers a detailed background of the level of scientific or clinical information that exists about the topic of the article. The background is a discussion about what led the author to conduct a study or report on a clinical topic. Perhaps the article does not address your PICO question the way you hope, but possibly it leads you to other more useful articles. The literature review of a research article usually gives you a good idea of how past research led to the researcher's question.

Narrative: The "middle section" or narrative of an article differs according to the type of evidence-based article it is, either clinical or research (Melnyk and Fineout-Overholt, 2011). A clinical article describes a clinical topic, which often includes a description of a patient population, the nature of a certain disease or health problem, how it affects patients, and the appropriate nursing therapies. Clinical articles often describe how to use a therapy or new technology. A research article describes the research study, including its purpose, the study design, and the results. The narrative of a research article includes these subsections:

- *Purpose statement:* Explains the focus or intent of a study. It identifies what concepts will be researched, including research questions or hypotheses, predictions made about the relationship, or difference between study variables (a concept, characteristic, or trait that varies within subjects in the study.)
- *Methods or design:* Explains how a research study is organized and conducted to answer the research question or test hypotheses. This is where you learn about the type of study (e.g., RCT, case control) (see Table 1-1). You also learn how many subjects or persons were in the study. In health care studies subjects sometimes include patients, family members, or health care staff. The language in the methods section is sometimes confusing if it explains details about how the researcher designs the study to minimize bias to obtain the most accurate results possible.
- *Results or conclusions:* Clinical and research articles have a summary section. In a clinical article the author explains the clinical implications for the topic presented. In a research article the author details the results of the study and explains whether a hypothesis is supported or how a research question is answered. A qualitative study presents a thorough summary of the descriptive themes and ideas that arise from the researcher's analysis of data. A quantitative study includes a statistical analysis section. It is important to learn common statistical terms, especially in clinical trial studies. Statistics reveal if a tested intervention had a significant effect or if the effect size was large enough to adopt the intervention in practice. When reading statistical analysis, ask these questions: Does the researcher describe the results? Were the results significant statistically? What was the size of the effect of the intervention? What was the sample size? A good author discusses any limitations or weaknesses to a study in the results section. The information on limitations further helps you to decide if you want to use the evidence with your patients.

- *Clinical implications:* A research article includes a section that explains if the findings from the study have clinical implications. The researcher explains how to apply findings in a practice setting for the type of subjects studied.

After you critique each article, synthesize or combine the findings from all of the articles to determine the strength of evidence. Remember, depending on the type of articles you read, evidence will range from rigorous or strong to weak. It is a challenge for members of an EBP committee to weigh each article and then collectively judge the level of evidence available. Are findings from the studies valid, reliable, and relevant to the patient population or area of interest? Use critical thinking to consider the accuracy of the evidence and how well the evidence addresses the question. Also consider the evidence in light of the concerns, values, and preferences of your patient population. Ethically it is important to consider evidence that will benefit patients and do no harm. You decide to use the evidence in your practice when it is relevant, is easily applicable in your setting of practice (e.g. resources and support are available), and has the potential for improving patient outcomes.

Apply the Evidence

Once you decide that evidence is strong and applicable to your patients, you decide how to incorporate it into practice. One way you may choose to use evidence is by directly applying it in the care of a patient. For example, you may find evidence in the literature for the use of an alternative pain therapy (e.g., music therapy) for cancer patients. You then try the therapy the next time you care for a patient who is receptive to its use.

Most practice changes involve a group such as the members of an EBP committee. In this case it is always wise to pilot a practice change. This means implementing the change for a small group of patients over a limited time frame. Piloting a practice change allows you to identify any issues with implementation and determine if the change resulted in beneficial patient outcomes. When a pilot is successful, it becomes easier to make a change on a larger scale and then evaluate the outcome.

In the example of the staff nurses who are exploring the use of epidural analgesia compared with patient-controlled analgesia, the evidence shows that epidural analgesia is consistently more effective in relieving pain. The staff now must decide how to make changes in the use of analgesia on their nursing unit. In this step of EBP it becomes important to know your resources and understand how change is made in your organization and how to gain consensus for a practice change. It is important to involve all of the health care disciplines that the change will affect. For example, physicians and pharmacists would participate in decisions about changing use of analgesia after surgery.

There are various options for integrating evidence such as through a new policy and procedure, a clinical practice guideline, or new assessment and teaching tools. When choosing a way to integrate evidence, always consider how the staff who are affected by the change will most likely accept it. For example, the nurses reviewing epidural and patient-controlled analgesia choose to meet with the physician who participates in their quality improvement committee. They present the results of their literature critique in a professional manner and emphasize how the evidence shows that patients will benefit through better pain relief and a shorter length of stay. The physician agrees to talk with his fellow surgeons and trial the use of epidural analgesia over the next 3 months.

Evaluate the Practice Change

When you apply evidence in your practice, you want to be able to evaluate the effect or outcome. Collecting initial baseline data and identifying the outcomes you choose to measure before implementing a change gives you a basis for evaluating the effects of any change. This approach is often called a predata and postdata collection method.

Outcome measurement tells you how an intervention worked. It is important to be precise in identifying the outcomes you want to measure before you begin implementation. This allows you to collect outcomes before you begin and then during implementation.

Sometimes evaluation is as simple as determining if the expected outcomes you set for an intervention are met. For example, after using a new transparent IV dressing, does the IV line dislodge, or does the patient develop the complication of phlebitis? When using a new approach to preoperative teaching, does the patient learn what to expect after surgery?

Selecting appropriate outcomes requires careful thinking. Box 1-3 outlines the features of a desirable outcome. The surgical nurses collaborate with the physicians in identifying the outcomes for their project. The staff decide to measure pain severity, a nondirectional measure. This means that they are not just measuring increased or decreased pain; they choose to simply measure pain severity scores. The use of a pain scale (see Chapter 13) to measure pain severity is a reliable and valid method for consistently measuring patients' perceptions of pain each time it is used. It is a simple and inexpensive tool to use in a clinical area. The scale is appropriate to use in an acute care setting because it is easy for patients to complete. A pain scale shows the change in a patient's pain over time.

BOX 1-3 FEATURES OF OUTCOME MEASURES

- Reliable
- Valid
- Measurable
- Suited to population
- Not overly costly to collect
- Sensitive to change in the individual
- Nondirectional—defined as the desired behavior or response

Data from Melnyk BM and Fineout-Overholt E: *Evidence-based practice in nursing & healthcare: a guide to best practice,* Philadelphia, 2005, Lippincott Williams & Wilkins.

When selecting outcomes, consider how you will measure them. Observations, physical measurements, surveys, and questionnaires are just a few examples of how you can measure outcomes. For example, if your outcome is a change in weight, the obvious measurement approach is use of a scale. If your outcome is a patient's adherence to a treatment plan, you might choose to use self-report or have the patient complete a diary.

When an EBP change occurs on a large scale, an evaluation is more formal. For example, after the physician team implements epidural analgesia for abdominal surgery patients, nurses on the surgical unit collect information about patients' pain severity, doses of epidural and patient-controlled analgesia used, and the patients' length of stay. The nurses are able to take the information and compute the average pain severity, epidural and patient-controlled dosages, and length of stay for all patients over a 4-week time frame. With the analysis the nurses can present data to the surgeons to determine if the use of epidural analgesia will continue. In this example the patients who received epidural analgesia had lower average pain scores and used a lower analgesic dosage on average than patient-controlled patients. The length of stay for the two groups was about the same. Outcome data tell you if the practice change was beneficial. Sometimes evaluation data show the need to modify a practice change or even discontinue it.

Share the Outcomes with Others

After applying evidence it is important to share outcomes from the change in practice to nursing and other health care colleagues. This is true whether the results are successful or unsuccessful. There are many ways to communicate the outcomes of EBP: talking with a colleague, sharing results in staff meetings or a committee, presenting in workshops or seminars, submitting an abstract for a poster presentation, and publishing an article. In the case example the lead nurse on the EBP committee and a surgeon decide to make a joint presentation at a nursing grand rounds session.

As a professional you are responsible for communicating important information about nursing practice. Sharing evidence and the effects of any practice change motivates others and makes them excited about practice improvements.

EVIDENCE IN NURSING SKILLS

Nurses who work in clinical settings must use the current best evidence to guide their practice and improve patient outcomes. One way is through the use of policies and procedures that provide direction for implementing procedures such as the skills in this text (Long and others, 2009). Nurses rely on policies and procedures to contain the most current information regarding safe and effective practices.

More and more nursing organizations are adopting an approach for ensuring evidence-based policies and procedures (Husbands, 2008; Oman and others, 2008).

It is common for nurses to raise questions about day-to-day clinical issues such as why procedures are performed the way they are. Thus implementing EBP into policy and procedure (P&P) review makes sense. Nurses on P&P committees are adopting formal processes for the routine review of P&Ps to ensure that new evidence is integrated into organizational policy. An EBP approach to P&P review and development demonstrates how an organization integrates EBP into practice, an important consideration for The Joint Commission and Magnet Hospital review (Oman and others, 2008).

REVIEW QUESTIONS

Case Study for Questions 1 and 2

The nurses on a medical oncology unit are discussing problems in teaching their patients about the side effects of oral chemotherapy and the proper way to take the drugs at home. One nurse has just attended a 1-day workshop on cancer survivorship and has told the manager about the group's interest in developing a program for cancer patients. Currently the nurses use a teaching booklet that some patients complain as being difficult to read. The next meeting clinicians talk about developing an informational program on side effects of chemotherapy. One of the clinicians asks, "Do we think a DVD program is something that would work?"

1. Write a PICO question for the clinical case study.
2. What would be an outcome that the nurses would measure in a study designed to educate their patients, and how would they measure it?
3. When you conduct a scientific literature review, your aim is to gather articles about studies that involved scientific rigor. Order the sources of scientific evidence, beginning with the most rigorous. Use all options.
   a. Single descriptive study
   b. Controlled trial without randomization
   c. Systematic review
   d. Case control study
   e. One randomized controlled trial
   f. Systematic review of qualitative study
4. A committee of nurses have collected a set of six articles about approaches for preventing falls. They have read each article, reviewed the relevance of the articles to their practice, and discussed the strength of evidence available. This is an example of which step of evidence-based practice?
   1. Ask a clinical question.
   2. Collect the most relevant and best evidence.
   3. Critically appraise the evidence you gather.
   4. Apply the evidence along with your clinical expertise, patient preferences, and values.

5. A group of staff nurses are meeting to discuss evidence-based practice issues. Which of the following clinical questions is an example of a knowledge-focused trigger?
    1. The unit has seen an increased rate of falls, and staff wonder if it is related to patients receiving opioid analgesics.
    2. The nurses on the unit have seen an increase in wound infections.
    3. The nurses anticipate that physicians will be using more local anesthesia for surgical procedures.
    4. During the last 3 months the unit has had more medication errors.
6. When attempting to identify a PICO question, what are the limitations of asking a background question? Select all that apply.
    1. The background question will lead you to too many articles to read.
    2. The background question will limit your search to only systematic review articles.
    3. The background question will lead you to a set of articles on diverse topics.
    4. The background question limits the focus of your search.
7. Nurses on an evidence-based practice committee find an article that describes a research study that examined nurses' perceptions of communication with physicians. This is an example of which of the following type of studies?
    1. Descriptive study
    2. Case control study
    3. Randomized controlled trial
    4. Systematic review
8. Which of the following are characteristics of a randomized controlled trial research study? Select all that apply.
    1. The study examines the subjective context in which persons' experiences occur.
    2. The study includes two groups, both measured on the same outcomes, to see if there are differences.
    3. The study tests a new intervention against the usual standard of care.
    4. The study examines subjects with a certain condition at the same time as another group of subjects who do not have the condition.
9. When reading a scientific article, what information will the nurse learn after reading the literature review or background section?
    1. A discussion about what led the author to conduct a study or report on a clinical topic
    2. Information about the purpose of the article and the importance of the topic for the audience who reads it
    3. Identification of the concepts that will be researched
    4. Explanation of whether a hypothesis is correct or how a research question is answered
10. In the following PICO question, identify the four elements. Does the use of hourly rounds compared with standard observations reduce the number of falls in medical inpatients? Fill in the elements.

    P:

    I:

    C:

    O:

REFERENCES

Berlowitz DR, Frantz RA: Implementing best practices in pressure ulcer care: the role of continuous quality improvement, *J Am Med Directors Assoc* Mar; 8(3 Suppl 1):S37, 2007.

Callister LC and others: Inquiry in baccalaureate nursing education: Fostering evidence-based practice, *J Nurs Educ* 44(2):59, 2005.

Chen YC and others: The effect of intermittent nasogastric feeding on preventing aspiration pneumonia in ventilated critically ill patients, *J Nurs Res* 14(3):167, 2006.

Husbands D: Policy and procedure development: a novel approach, *ORL Head Neck Nurs* 26(2):18-22, 2008.

Infusion Nurses Society: Infusion Nursing Standards of Practice, *J Intraven Nurs* 29(Suppl 1):S1, 2006.

Institute of Medicine: *To err is human: building a safer health system*, Washington, DC, 2000, National Academy Press.

Kendall S: Witnessing tragedy: nurses' perception of caring for patients with cancer, *Int J Nurs Pract* 13(2):111, 2007.

Long EL and others: Promotion of safe outcomes: Incorporating evidence into policies and procedures, *Nurs Clin North Am* 44(1):57, 2009.

Melnyk BM, Fineout-Overholt E: *Evidence-based practice in nursing & healthcare: a guide to best practice*, ed 2, Philadelphia, 2011, Lippincott Williams & Wilkins.

Oman K and others: Evidence-based policy and procedures: an algorithm for success, *JONA* 38(1):47, 2008.

Sackett DL and others: *Evidence-based medicine: how to practice and teach EBM*, London, 2000, Churchill Livingstone.

Saw SM and others: Risk factors for contact lens related fusarium keratitis: a case control study in Singapore, *Arch Ophthalmol* 125(5):611, 2007.

Titler MG and others: The Iowa model of evidence-based practice to promote quality care, *Crit Care Clin North Am* 13(4):497, 2001.

Watkins RE and others: Perceptions of infection control practice among health professionals, *Contemp Nurse* 22(1):109, 2006.

Werawatganon T, Charuluxanum S: Patient controlled intravenous opioid analgesia versus continuous epidural analgesia for pain after intra-abdominal surgery, *The Cochrane Database Rev* 1, 2005.

Winfield C and others: Evidence the first word in safe IV practice, *Am Nurs Today* 2(5):31, 2007.

CHAPTER 2

Communication and Collaboration

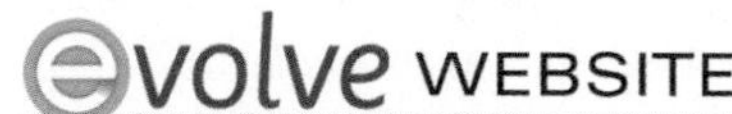

http://evolve.elsevier.com/Perry/nursinginterventions

Communication is a basic human need and the foundation for establishing a caring relationship between the nurse and patient. It involves the expression of emotions, ideas, and thoughts through verbal (words or written language) and nonverbal (e.g., behaviors) exchanges. Verbal communication includes both the spoken and written word. Nonverbal communication includes body movement, physical appearance, personal space, touch, and facial expression. The interaction between the skilled nurse and patient progresses to a therapeutic level in which you offer goal-directed activities to help the patient share thoughts and feelings. With time and practice, you develop therapeutic communication skills and maintain a congenial and warm style that helps patients feel comfortable in sharing their feelings.

Multiple essential interpersonal skills are necessary to communicate therapeutically with patients. These skills include having empathy and a nonjudgmental attitude, being aware of both verbal and nonverbal communication, using appropriate body language, being patient and sensitive to patients' cues, and giving feedback appropriately. Many factors influence the complex process of communication (Box 2-1).

The basic elements of communication include a message, a sender, a receiver, and feedback (Fig. 2-1). The message is the information expressed which can be motivated by experience, emotions, ideas, or actions. The message may be sent through different channels, including visual, auditory, and tactile senses. For communication to be effective the receiver must be aware of the sender's message. The message received is understood as filtered through perceptions shaped from previous experiences. People tend to interpret life experiences through general assumptions and values they hold; in essence, this is the concept of filtering. The more aware people are of how these assumptions influence how they perceive the world and others, the more open they can be when interacting with others. Feedback, verbal or nonverbal, is a response to the sender that can indicate if the meaning of the message sent was received. Because communication is a two-way process, you give feedback to and seek feedback from patients to validate patients' understanding of the messages sent.

Silence is a therapeutic technique, and it gives the nurse and patient time to think. It is important for the nurse to be aware of the patient's inner feelings and nonverbal behavior that provides cues to the patient's feelings. Reflecting the nurse's impressions can validate what the patient is experiencing. If silence lasts too long or becomes uncomfortable for the patient, it can be helpful to say, "You seem very quiet," or "Could you tell me what you need right now?" or "How are you feeling?"

Barriers to effective therapeutic communication techniques exist in the form of ineffective responses and behaviors (Box 2-2). The use of these nontherapeutic techniques can hinder the therapeutic relationship between the patient and the nurse.

Nurses learn effective communication, but it requires practice as does any other skill. An attitude of acceptance is helpful to promote open communication. To listen effectively, face the patient, maintain eye contact, pay attention to what patient is conveying, and give feedback to verify accurate understanding. Even though you may not agree with a patient response, you can accept his or her right to an opinion. It is best to avoid arguing with patients. Instead simply reflect understanding of what they are communicating without agreeing or disagreeing.

Preoccupation with the techniques of communication can interfere with rather than enhance the communication process. Ineffective communication may not halt conversation, but it often tends to inhibit patients' willingness to express concerns openly. Find an appropriate environment, allow for sufficient time, and facilitate communication according to patients' circumstances and needs. Be aware

BOX 2-1 FACTORS THAT INFLUENCE COMMUNICATION

Perceptions: Personal views based on past experiences
Values: Beliefs that a person considers important in life
Emotions: Subjective feelings about a situation (e.g., anger, fear, frustration, pain, anxiety, personal appearance)
Sociocultural background: Language, gestures, and attitudes common for a specific group of people relating to family origin, occupation, or lifestyle
Knowledge level: Level of education and experience influences a person's knowledge base.
Roles and relationships: Conversation between two nurses differs from conversation between the nurse and patient.
Environment: Noise, lack of privacy, and distractions influence effectiveness.
Space and territoriality: Distance of 18 inches to 4 feet is ideal for sitting with a patient for an interaction. Patients from different cultures may have different needs for personal space.

BOX 2-2 INEFFECTIVE RESPONSES AND BEHAVIORS

- Not listening
- Talking too much
- Appearing too busy
- Using clichés
- Seeming uncomfortable with silence
- Laughing nervously
- Not paying attention
- Smiling inappropriately
- Being opinionated
- Showing disapproval
- Avoiding sensitive topics
- Belittling feelings
- Arguing
- Minimizing problems
- Being superficial
- Being defensive
- Changing the subject
- Focusing on personal problems of the nurse
- Having a closed posture
- Making flippant remarks
- Ignoring the patient
- Lying/being insincere
- Making false promises
- Making sarcastic remarks

From Keltner N and others: *Psychiatric nursing: a psychotherapeutic management approach,* ed 5, St Louis, 2007, Mosby.

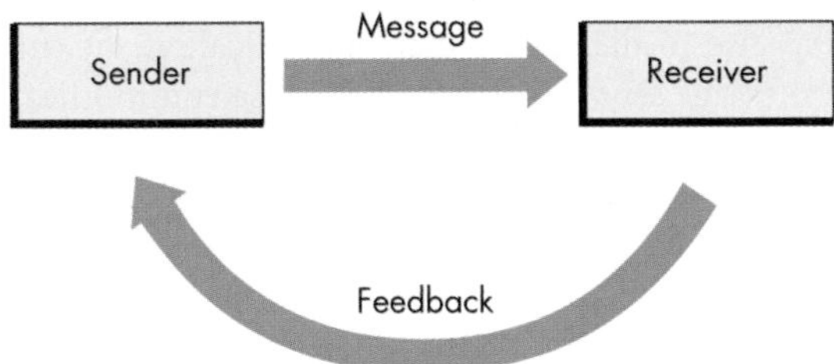

FIG 2-1 Communication is a two-way process.

of techniques that facilitate or inhibit communication (Table 2-1).

PATIENT-CENTERED CARE

Patient-centered care involves an awareness of patient's needs, preferences, and values. Patient-centered communication facilitates the development of a positive nurse-patient relationship in which the patient is an active partner. You need to actively listen to your patients rather than focus on nursing tasks. Providing privacy is important; ideally communication between you and your patient should take place in a quiet place with minimal external distraction. Often the curtain is drawn, especially when patients are immobile or alternative rooms are unavailable (Jasmine, 2009).

It is important to recognize cultural diversity and demonstrate respect for people as unique individuals. Culture is just one factor that influences communication between two persons. Awareness of cultural norms or values enhances understanding of nonverbal cues. Consider any potential communication barriers with persons from other cultures, including cultural perspective, heritage, and health traditions of both the patient and the nurse. Questions to consider include the following: Who is the nurse from a cultural perspective? Who is the patient from a cultural perspective? What is the nurse's heritage? What is the patient's heritage?

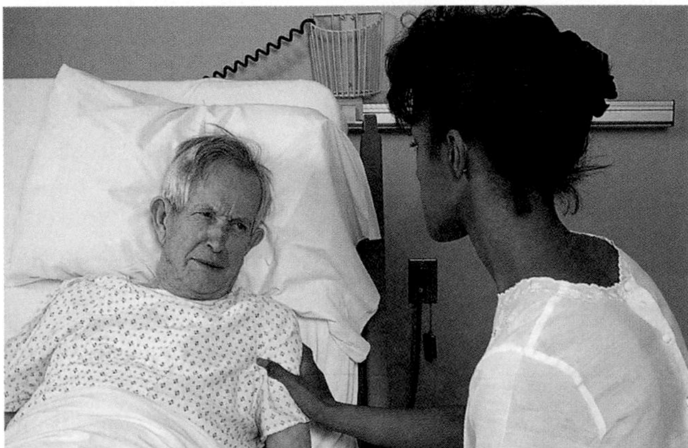

FIG 2-2 Therapeutic use of touch needs to take cultural factors into considerations.

What are the health traditions of the nurse's heritage? What are the health traditions of the patient's heritage? Transcultural communication is most effective when each person attempts to understand the other's point of view from that person's cultural heritage. Adopt an attitude of flexibility, respect, and interest to bridge any communication barriers imposed by cultural differences.

- *Use of language, gestures, and vocal emphasis of words:* Taking care to determine if understanding was achieved is important. Overly technical jargon or terms unique to a culture should be avoided.
- *Eye contact:* Direct eye contact is valued in some cultures, whereas other cultures find it improper and intrusive (e.g., it may be improper to make eye contact with authority figure).
- *Use of touch/personal space:* Some cultures are "noncontact" cultures and have needs for clear boundaries; other cultures value close contact, handshakes, and embracing (Fig. 2-2).

TABLE 2-1 FACILITATING AND INHIBITING COMMUNICATION

TECHNIQUE	EXAMPLES	RATIONALE
Initiating and Encouraging Interaction		
Giving information	"It is time for me to …" "I will be here until …"	Informs patient of facts needed to understand situation Provides a means to build trust and develop a knowledge base for patients to make decisions
Stating observations	"You're smiling." "I see you're up already."	By calling patient's attention to what is observed, nurse encourages patient to be aware of behavior
Open questions/ comments	"What is your biggest concern?" "Tell me about your health."	Allows patient to choose the topic of discussion according to circumstances and needs
General leads	"And then?" "Go on …" "Say more …"	Encourages patient to continue talking
Focused questions/ comments	"Tell me about your pain or comfort." "What did your doctor say?" "How has your family reacted?" "What is your biggest fear?"	Encourages patient to give more information about specific topic of concern
Helping Patient Identify and Express Feelings		
Sharing observations	"You look tense." "You seem uncomfortable when …"	Promotes patient's awareness of nonverbal behavior and feelings underlying the behavior; helps clarify meaning of the behavior
Paraphrasing	Patient: "I couldn't sleep last night." Nurse: "You've had trouble sleeping?"	Encourages patient to describe the situation more fully; demonstrates that nurse is listening and concerned
Reflecting feelings	"You were angry when that happened?" "You seem upset …"	Focuses patient on identified feelings based on verbal or nonverbal cues
Focused comments	"That seems worth talking about more." "Tell me more about …"	Encourages patient to think about and describe a particular concern in more detail
Ensuring Mutual Understanding		
Seeking clarification	"I don't quite follow you …" "Do you mean …?" "Are you saying that …?"	Encourages patient to expand on a topic that is not yet clear or that seems contradictory
Summarizing	"So there are three things that you're upset about: your family being too busy, your diet, and being in the hospital so long."	Reduces the interaction to three or four points identified by nurse as significant; allows patient to agree or add other concerns
Validation	"Did I understand you correctly that …?" "What made you decide to eat that when you know it gives you stomach pain?"	Allows clarification of ideas that nurse may have interpreted differently than intended by patient
Inhibiting Communication		
"Why" questions	"Why did you go back to bed?"	Asks patient to justify reasons; implies criticism and makes patient feel defensive; better to state what happened and encourage telling the whole story (e.g., "I noticed you went back to bed.")
Sidestepping or changing subject	Patient: "I'm having a hard time with my family." Nurse: "Do you have any grandchildren?"	Eases nurse's own discomfort and avoids exploring topic identified by patient
False reassurance	"Everything will be okay." "Surgery is no big deal."	Vague and simplistic and tends to belittle patient's concerns; does not invite a response
Giving advice	"You really should exercise more." "You shouldn't eat fast food every day."	Keeps patient from actively engaging in finding a solution; often patient knows what should/should not be done and needs to explore alternative ways of dealing with issue
Stereotyped responses	"You have the best doctor in town." "All patients with cancer worry about that."	Does not invite patient to respond
Defensiveness	"The nurses here work very hard." "Your doctor is extremely busy."	Moves focus away from patient's feelings without acknowledging concerns

BOX 2-3 SPECIAL APPROACHES FOR PATIENT WHO SPEAKS A DIFFERENT LANGUAGE

- Use a caring tone of voice and facial expression to help alleviate the patient's fears.
- Speak slowly and distinctly but not loudly.
- Use gestures, pictures, and role playing to help the patient understand.
- Repeat the message in different ways if necessary.
- Be alert to words the patient seems to understand and use them frequently.
- Keep messages simple and repeat them frequently.
- Avoid using medical terms that the patient may not understand.
- Use an appropriate language dictionary or have interpreter or family make flash cards to communicate key phrases.

Modified from Giger J, Davidhizar R: *Transcultural nursing: assessment and intervention,* ed 5, St Louis, 2008, Mosby.

- *Time orientation:* Many cultures are oriented to the present; some cultures value planning for the future.
- *Nonverbal behaviors:* Use gestures with shared meaning.

The United States is culturally and ethnically diverse, reflecting a mixture of health care beliefs and practices. As society becomes more diverse, it is essential for health care providers, including nurses, to learn about cultural and ethnic differences. This process begins with self-awareness and involves getting to know oneself: one's personality, values, beliefs, and ethics when caring for patients who are different from oneself (Purnell and Paulanka, 2008).

Patients with limited English proficiency may not possess adequate vocabulary skills to communicate effectively. You often need a translator or interpreter when a patient does not speak the nurse's language (Giger and Davidhizar, 2008). Interpreters serve to decode the patient's words and provide meaning behind the message, whereas translators just restate the words from one language to another. Often the patient speaks the same language with limited ability or uses language with a meaning different from the nurse's meaning. For example, the patient may know customary greetings such as "How are you?" and not understand "pain" or "nausea." When communication fails, avoid the tendency to speak louder, stop talking, concentrate on the tasks, or begin doing things for rather than with the patient. Inappropriate responses may result in painful isolation, anger, or misunderstanding for the patient and his or her inability to cooperate. Box 2-3 describes special approaches to communicate to patients who speak different languages.

Patients with sensory losses require communication techniques that maximize existing sensory and motor functions. Some patients are unable to speak because of physical or neurological alterations such as paralysis; a tube in the trachea to facilitate breathing (Fig. 2-3); or a stroke resulting in aphasia, difficulty understanding, or verbalizing. When a patient experiences receptive aphasia, there is impaired comprehension of both written and spoken language. Expressive aphasia affects the motor function of speech so the patient has difficulty speaking and writing but is able to hear and understand. For patients with speech difficulties, speech pathologists are helpful.

BOX 2-4 COMMUNICATION AIDS

- Pad and felt-tipped pen or magic slate
- Board with words, letters, or pictures denoting basic needs (e.g., water, bedpan, pain medication)
- Call bells or alarms
- Sign language
- Use of eye blinks or movement of fingers for simple responses (e.g., "yes" or "no")
- Flash cards with pictures rather than words
- Computer/electronic devices

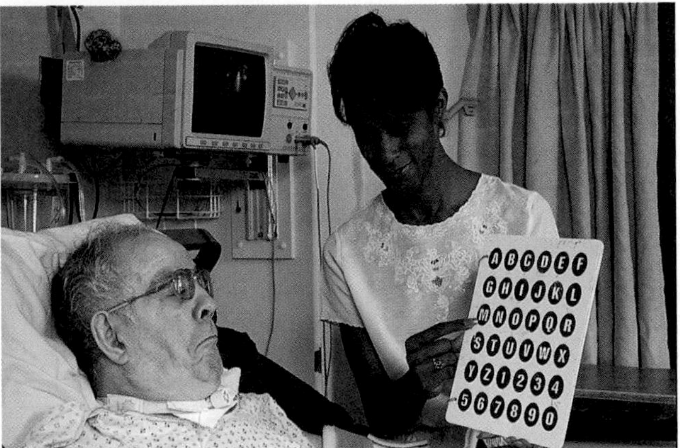

FIG 2-3 Communication tools for patients who cannot speak because of a tracheostomy.

Hearing impairment affects one's quality of life and may be easily overlooked by health care providers. Communication is impaired when a message is lost or misinterpreted because the patient did not hear correctly. Aids such as pictures, electronic communication, two-way text messaging, and communication software can be used to communicate with patients successfully (Box 2-4).

SAFETY

Miscommunication, both between health care providers and between provider and patient, can adversely affect patient safety. You should consider personal safety when interacting with patients who are potentially violent. Patients who are angry and frustrated and believe that no one is listening may be more likely to behave in a violent manner.

The illness experience is a stressor, and some patients have trouble coping. Do not be offended by challenging and difficult patients but rather approach them with patience, acknowledging their distress. The nurse-patient connection is enhanced when you display empathy and genuineness (Mitchell, 2007).

EVIDENCE-BASED PRACTICE TRENDS

Kluge MA, Glick L: Teaching therapeutic communication VIA camera cues and clues: the video inter-active (VIA) method, *J Nurs Educ* 45(11):463-468, 2006.

McNeill C and others: Relationship skills building with older adults, *J Nurs Educ* 47(6):269-271, 2008.

Nursing students need experience in practicing therapeutic communication skills with a diverse group of patients in a variety of settings. Research demonstrates that practicing these skills in a controlled setting before interacting with patients is beneficial. One study used prerecorded video footage of simulated patients to present students real-world situations that they may encounter in the clinical setting; students engaged in scripted therapeutic interactions with these video patients. Students' communication techniques, both verbal and nonverbal, were evaluated; the students reported positively to this type of communication skills building. In addition to video-interactive methods, students have been studied during their one-on-one interaction with geriatric patients (Kluge and Glick, 2006). One study examined nursing students and their interactions with older adult patients; students were assigned four visits to a continual-care community. Three of these visits involved a 1-hour session focusing on therapeutic communication techniques and establishing a therapeutic nurse-patient relationship (McNeill and others, 2008). The fourth hour involved observing older adults with cognitive impairments interact with each other. Students wrote about the importance of patience and listening when communicating with older adults.

SKILL 2.1 ESTABLISHING THE NURSE-PATIENT RELATIONSHIP

A therapeutic nurse-patient relationship is the foundation of nursing care and involves patient-centered, goal-directed interactions using therapeutic communication skills. Therapeutic communication empowers patients to make decisions. Factors that influence communication include the patient's perceptions, values, sociocultural background, and knowledge level. Therapeutic communication differs from social communication because it is patient centered and goal directed with limited disclosure from the professional. However, an important aspect of therapeutic communication is the nurse's ability to show caring for the patient. Caring establishes trust and openness and facilitates patient communication.

Usually nurses avoid sharing details of their personal lives with patients. Sometimes personal self-disclosure is effective if it helps the patient to focus on key issues. However, social communication that involves equal opportunity for personal disclosure and in which both participants seek to have personal needs met is not appropriate between nurses and patients (Keltner and others, 2007).

The nurse-patient relationship is characterized by three overlapping phases: orientation, working, and termination. The orientation phase involves learning about the patient and any initial concerns and needs. During the orientation phase, clarify your role and the roles of other health care professionals, collect information, establish goals, correct misunderstandings, and establish rapport between yourself and the patient. It is quite common to encounter a patient who needs comfort and support while experiencing threatening situations. A newly diagnosed illness, separation from family and friends, the discomfort of surgery or diagnostic and treatment procedures, grief, and loss are just a few examples of health-related situations that require the skill of comforting.

A variety of communication techniques facilitate or inhibit communication during the working phase (see Table 2-1). Active listening and empathy are two of the most effective ways to facilitate communication. Active listening conveys interest in the patient's needs, concerns, and problems and requires complete attention to understand the entire verbal and nonverbal message. Empathy is the act of effectively communicating to other persons that their feelings are understood. After they know that their feelings have been accepted, they do not have to struggle to explain or justify their reactions (Fortinash and Holoday-Worret, 2008).

Listening techniques are learned behaviors. At first they seem awkward and time consuming. However, as with any skill, they become more comfortable with practice. It is essential that you appear natural, relaxed, and at ease while listening.

Prepare for the termination phase at the beginning of the interaction by indicating the purpose of the communication session and the amount of time available. The termination phase consists of evaluation and summary of progress toward identified goals.

ASSESSMENT

1. Determine patient's need to communicate (e.g., patient who constantly uses call light, is crying, does not understand an illness, has just been admitted to the hospital or nursing home).
2. Assess reason patient needs health care.
3. Assess factors about self and patient that influence communication: perceptions, values and beliefs, emotions, sociocultural background, severity of illness, knowledge, age level, verbal ability, roles and relationships, environmental setting, physical comfort, and discomfort. *Rationale: Facilitates accurate assessment of the experiences of the patient.*
4. Assess patient's language and ability to speak. Does the patient have difficulty finding words or associating ideas with accurate word symbols? Does the patient have difficulty with expression of language and/or reception of messages? *Rationale: Identifies the appropriate communication aids to be used (e.g., use of an interpreter, use of communication board).*

5. Observe patient's pattern of communication and verbal or nonverbal behavior (e.g., gestures, tone of voice, eye contact). *Rationale: Patterns of communication may influence the type and manner of communication used by the nurse.*
6. Encourage the patient to ask for clarification at any time during the communication. *Rationale: Gives the patient a sense of control and keeps the channels of communication open.*
7. Identify cultural influences that affect communication. What language does the patient predominantly use in thinking? Does he or she need an interpreter or translator? Is he or she able to read and/or write in English? What verbal or nonverbal communication shows respect (e.g., tempo, eye/body contact, topic restrictions)? *Rationale: Knowledge of cultural factors facilitates communication.*

PLANNING

Expected Outcomes focus on using therapeutic communication skills to obtain information about the patient's ideas, needs, and concerns.

1. Patient expresses ability to communicate with the nurse without feeling threatened or defensive.
2. Patient expresses thoughts and feelings to the nurse through verbal and nonverbal communication.
3. Patient identifies factors that provide support and comfort.
4. Patient verbalizes feeling understood.

Delegation and Collaboration

The skill of establishing a therapeutic nurse-patient relationship is a professional nursing skill and may not be delegated. Nursing assistive personnel (NAP) may observe and receive a lot of important information because of the length of time they are with the patient. Instruct the NAP about the following:

- All information discussed is confidential.
- Patient concerns, including anger and anxiety, are communicated to the nurse to determine if additional nursing interventions are needed.
- All interactions are respectful and kind, including special considerations for patients who have cognitive or sensory impairment.
- Be aware of nonverbal behaviors, both of self and patient.

IMPLEMENTATION *for* ESTABLISHING THE NURSE-PATIENT RELATIONSHIP

STEPS	RATIONALE
Orientation Phase	
1. Create a climate of warmth and acceptance. Consider the need to alter the environment by lowering noise level and providing privacy and comfort. Also consider timing in relation to visitors or personal routines.	Environmental factors can promote open communication.
2. Be aware of cultural and gender differences. Plan for identified difficulties associated with culture, language, age, and gender. Consider inability to read or write English.	These factors can influence expression of discomfort, anxiety, or confusion.
3. Acknowledge and respond to physical discomforts, if any, by positioning, administering medication, or other comfort measures. Consider individual preferences and expressed needs.	Physical discomfort, difficulty breathing, and pain interfere with communication.
4. Provide an introduction by addressing the patient by name and introducing self and role. For example, "Hello, my name is Jane Jones, and I am the student nurse who will take care of you today."	
5. Be aware of nonverbal cues that are both sent and received (e.g., eye contact, facial expression, posture, body language). Be particularly alert to behaviors that are incongruent with the patient's verbal message.	Incongruence is an indication that something may be interfering with open communication. Behaviors are often more accurate than words, and clarification may be necessary before proceeding.
6. Explain purpose of the interaction when information is to be shared.	Confidentiality is maintained when patient information is shared only with members of the health care team.
7. Encourage the patient to ask for clarification at any time during the communication.	
Working Phase	
8. Ask one question at a time and allow sufficient time to answer. Use direct and open-ended questions. Avoid asking questions about information that the patient may not know yet (e.g., medical diagnosis).	This encourages patient to tell a more complete story.

STEPS	RATIONALE
9. Use clear and concise statements with a patient who experiences altered levels of consciousness and cognition; repeat information.	This helps patient receive your message correctly.
10. Focus on understanding the patient, providing feedback, encouraging problem solving, and providing an atmosphere of warmth and acceptance.	Patients' misinterpretations need to be clarified because patients experiencing emotionally charged situations may not comprehend the message (Keltner and others, 2007).
11. Adjust the amount and quality of time for communicating, depending on patient's needs.	Flexibility and adaptation of techniques may be necessary to encourage patient's self-expression.
12. Provide empathy, which involves a sensitive and accurate awareness of patient's feelings.	Empathy helps patients explain and explore their feelings so problem solving may occur.
13. Remain centered on any current patient concern. Avoid introducing new information.	Patients may be overwhelmed by additional information. Talking about self or other people or events shifts the focus away from patients (Fortinash and Holoday-Worret, 2008).
14. Communicate understanding by repeating what you understand the message to be (e.g., "I understand you … ," "I hear you saying … ," "I sense that …"). Offer feedback to clarify message.	Communicating understanding tends to decrease the intensity of feelings and conveys empathy (Keltner and others, 2007).
15. Offer honest reassurance to the extent possible (e.g., that someone cares, that there is hope, that patient is not alone).	This shows interest and concern for patient (Keltner and others, 2007).
16. Allow silence, which can be an effective means of allowing organization of thoughts and processing of information. When patient becomes emotionally upset or cries, a quiet period can be helpful.	This provides acceptance and willingness to wait for patient to be ready to continue.
17. Avoid communication barriers (see Table 2-1).	Barriers may not halt interaction, but they tend to divert conversation to less meaningful topics.
Termination Phase	
18. Explore support services available and what services the patient has previously used. Refer to other health professionals as appropriate.	
19. Summarize with patients what you discussed during the interaction. Ask patients to state their understanding of the information shared or conclusion reached.	This interaction encourages the patient to compare perceptions with the nurse and helps to determine if the nurse needs to clarify anything.

EVALUATION

1. Observe patient's verbal and nonverbal responses (e.g., body language, verbal statements) after discussion of feelings and circumstances that have been identified.

2. Ask patient for feedback regarding message communicated. Was communication accurately interpreted by caregivers?

3. Verify if information obtained from patient is accurate regarding his or her thoughts, needs, and concerns.

Unexpected Outcomes and Related Interventions

1. Patient continues to verbally and nonverbally express feelings of anxiety, fear, anger, confusion, distrust, and helplessness.
   a. Assess patient's level of anxiety, fear, and distrust.
   b. Come back at another time to repeat the message.
   c. Determine influences affecting clear communication (e.g., cultural issues, literacy issues, physical limits).
2. Feedback between nurse and patient reveals a lack of understanding.
   a. Assess for and remove barriers to communication.
   b. Repeat the message using another approach if possible.
3. Nurse is unable to acquire information about patient's ideas, fears, and concerns.
   a. Try alternative communication techniques to promote the patient's willingness to communicate openly.
   b. Rephrase question after there has been time for understanding and response.
   c. Offer another professional for the patient to talk with to obtain the necessary information.

Recording and Reporting

- Record information-related interventions and patient responses.
- Report pertinent information, subjective data, and nonverbal cues, including response to illness, response to therapy, and questions or concerns.

Sample Documentation

1345 Patient expresses anxiety about current hospitalization. Is fidgeting in the bed, wringing his hands. Expresses much concern about fears of cancer with recent diagnostic tests. Encouraged to talk with his wife and the physician about concerns and questions.

Special Considerations

Pediatric

- Use vocabulary that is familiar to the child based on his or her level of understanding and usual patterns of communication.
- Consider the child's developmental level to select the most appropriate communication techniques (e.g., storytelling and drawing). Be sure to include parent and child (Hockenberry and Wilson, 2009).

Geriatric

- Be aware of any cognitive or sensory impairment.
- Avoid stereotyping older adults as having cognitive or sensory impairments.
- Speak face-to-face with the hard-of-hearing patient, articulate clearly in a moderate tone of voice, and assess whether the patient hears and understands the words.
- Make sure that older patients with visual impairments have any necessary assistive devices such as eyeglasses and large-print reading material.

Home Care

- Identify a primary caregiver for the patient. This individual may be a family member, friend, or neighbor.
- Assess the patient's and primary caregiver's level of understanding regarding the patient's condition.
- Incorporate the patient's usual daily habits and routines into the communication event (e.g., bathing and dressing patient).

SKILL 2.2 INTERVIEWING

The interview involves communication initiated for a specific purpose and focused on a specific content area such as the initial assessment of newly admitted patients or obtaining a health history in a health care provider's office. In nursing the interviewer obtains information about the patient's health state, lifestyle, support systems, patterns of illness, patterns of adaptation, strengths and limitations, and resources. This information can be used for an admission database or health history and provides data for identifying the patient's expectations and for responding appropriately to individualized patient needs.

The interview facilitates a positive nurse-patient relationship, which makes it easier for patients to ask questions about the health care environment and expectations regarding daily routines and procedures. It is important to encourage patients to ask questions at any time. They also have the right not to answer questions. Indicating the purpose of the interview helps to establish trust and put the patient at ease.

The interview is best scheduled at a time when there are minimal interruptions and visitors are not present. In some cases it is beneficial to include family members in the interview while the focus is clearly kept on identifying the patient's needs. Before beginning tell the patient about the purpose of the interview and the types of data to be obtained. Then spend time becoming acquainted with the patient. Establish a time frame for the interview and honor this commitment to the patient. Ask questions to form a database from which you can develop a care plan (Box 2-5). Carefully observe for evidence of discomfort and be willing to stop the interview when appropriate.

A direct-question technique is a structured format requiring one- or two-word answers and is frequently used to clarify previous information or obtain basic routine information (e.g., allergies, marital status). The open-ended question technique promotes a more complete description of identified areas of concern. Examples of open-ended questions/comments include "What are your health concerns?" "How have you been feeling?" and "Tell me about your problem."

ASSESSMENT

1. Review available information, which may include admission information such as name, address, age, marital status, employment, and reason for admission or reason for office visit.
2. Consider factors that may influence ability or willingness of patient or significant other to respond to questions such as physical pain, nausea, or anxiety. *Rationale: These factors may need to be alleviated before the interview.*

BOX 2-5 INTERVIEW DATABASE

- Health-related concerns
- Perception of health status
- Past health problems and therapies
- Effect of health status on role; influence on relationship with members of household
- Influence on occupation
- Ability to complete activities of daily living

3. Determine if patient is alert and oriented. Assess for hearing and speech difficulties. *Rationale: These factors may interfere with the interview, and another source of information will be needed.*
4. Consider factors that may influence ability of patient to communicate such as cultural or language barriers.

PLANNING

Expected Outcomes focus on gathering information through the interview process for a database to develop an appropriate plan of care.

1. Patient (or significant other) is able to describe health concerns.
2. Verbal and nonverbal messages are congruent.

Delegation and Collaboration

The skill of interviewing is a professional nursing skill and may not be delegated.

IMPLEMENTATION *for* INTERVIEWING

STEPS	RATIONALE
1. Greet patient and significant others and introduce yourself by name and job title. Tell patient the reason for the interview and how long you expect it to last. Assure patient that this information will be kept confidential.	This relieves anxiety about giving information to a stranger and encourages participation. The nurse may need to modify communication approaches to accommodate the patient's culture and practices.
2. Provide privacy and eliminate distractions, unnecessary noise, and interruptions by going to a quiet unoccupied room and/or closing the door. If others are present, ask patient if they should stay.	Distractions and interruptions may interfere with therapeutic interactions between nurse and patient.
3. Sit facing patient at approximately the same eye level (see illustration).	This facilitates active listening and places patient more at ease. It may be necessary to avoid direct eye contact with a patient whose culture views it as inappropriate.

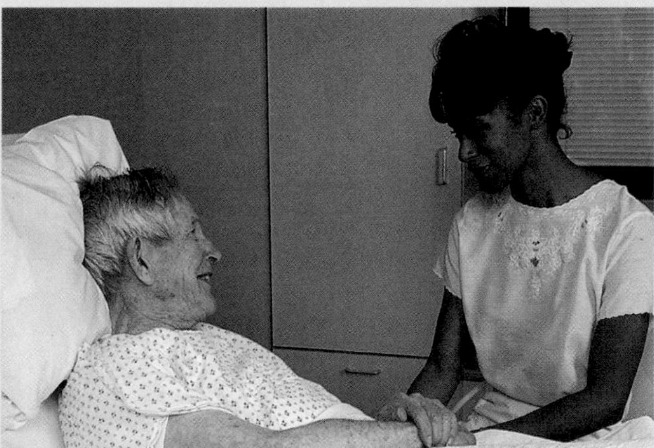

STEP 3 Sitting facing the patient may facilitate communication.

STEPS	RATIONALE
4. If patient is alert enough to state name, where he or she is, and what day it is, proceed with the interview. Confirm information obtained from patient with other caregivers or family members if patient is disoriented or confused or does not seem reliable.	An alert and oriented patient is a reliable source of information.
5. If patient is talkative, refocus the interview when patient strays from the topic.	
6. Ask what led patient to seek health care. Attempt to obtain a descriptive account of all the events in the order in which they occurred. Ask open-ended questions and listen to patient's story.	Active listening encourages the exchange of information. Conducting an interview by only asking questions may make patient feel like a subject of interrogation.

Continued

STEPS	RATIONALE
7. Observe and clarify nonverbal behaviors. Validate with patient the emotions or messages conveyed.	This provides a focus for collecting more specific and accurate data related to the primary areas of concern.
8. For each symptom that patient reports, determine when, where, and under what circumstances it occurred. Also determine location; quality; quantity; duration; and aggravating, alleviating, and associated factors (Table 2-2).	
9. For each symptom, also clarify the absence of other related symptoms.	
10. Identify past hospitalizations, past surgical procedures and complications, and previous major health problems.	
11. Determine whether patient regularly takes medications and, if so, for what period of time. Ask the name, reason for taking, dosage, and frequency. Specifically ask about dietary supplements or over-the-counter (OTC) medications such as aspirin, acetaminophen, ibuprofen, laxatives, sleeping pills, diet pills, herbal supplements/remedies, or other types of alternative therapies.	Patients may not think of dietary supplements or OTC medications because these do not require prescriptions. However, both of these classifications of medications may have interactive effects with current or future prescribed medications.
12. Clarify if patient takes narcotics, insulin, digitalis, contraceptives, steroids, or hormone replacements.	Patients may not mention these if such drugs seem unrelated to the reason for admission or when they think that the physician would have previously conveyed this information.
13. Identify risk factors related to lifestyle that influence the patient's health, knowledge level, and awareness of the risk.	Risk factors include smoking, alcohol use, drug abuse, lack of exercise, stress, nutritional factors (e.g., fluids, cholesterol, carbohydrates, fiber, and salt), exposure to violence, and unprotected sexual activity.
14. Continue with additional areas of interest or concern according to the focus of the interview.	
15. Give information that tells patients you are nearly finished.	This offers patient a chance to ask final questions.
16. Summarize your understanding of patient's health concerns.	

TABLE 2-2 DIMENSIONS OF A SYMPTOM

DIMENSIONS	QUESTIONS TO ASK
Location	"Where do you feel it?" "Does it move around?" "Show me where."
Quality or character	"What is it like? Sharp, dull, stabbing, aching?"
Severity	"On a scale of 0 to 10, with 10 the worst, how would you rate what you feel right now?" "What is the worst it has been?" "In what ways does this interfere with your usual activities?"
Timing	"When did you first notice it?" "How long does it last?" "How often does it happen?"
Setting	"Does it occur in a particular place or under certain circumstances?"
Aggravating or alleviating factors	"What makes it better?" "What makes it worse?" "When does it change?" "Have you noticed other changes associated with this?"

EVALUATION

1. Ask if patient or significant other has had an adequate opportunity to describe health concerns.
2. Observe patient's nonverbal expressions during interview. Do they match verbal statements?

Unexpected Outcomes and Related Interventions

1. Family or significant other answers for patient, even when patient is capable of answering.
   a. Direct the question to patient, using patient's name.
   b. Acknowledge the answer given by a family member, then state that you are interested specifically in what the patient has to say about it.
   c. Conclude the interview and resume again after the family members are gone. If necessary, you may suggest that family take a break for a while, get coffee or a meal, or walk outside briefly for some fresh air.
2. Patient is unable to communicate, and family members are present.
   a. Interview family member as you would patient.
   b. Explore the needs of family and patient.

Recording and Reporting

- Complete the information included in the admission profile: reason for admission; medical-surgical history; family history; allergies; health habits, including cultural beliefs about health, current prescribed therapies (include all OTC medications and supplements), and any current unprescribed therapies/alternative treatments.

Sample Documentation

Complete standardized assessment form according to agency policy.

Special Considerations

Pediatric

- Evaluate the child's usual pattern of communication, including use of age-appropriate language.
- Consider the child's developmental level when interviewing the child.
- Include parents in the interviewing process when appropriate.

Geriatric

- Be aware of any cognitive or sensory impairment.
- Encourage patients with auditory and/or visual impairments to use assistive devices to aid in communication.

Home Care

- Assess for the presence of any cognitive or physical impairments that may hinder communication.
- Identify the patient's primary caregiver and include in interviewing process.
- Assess patient's and caregiver's level of understanding regarding patient's condition.

SKILL 2.3 COMMUNICATING WITH ANXIOUS, ANGRY, DEPRESSED, AND COGNITIVELY IMPAIRED PATIENTS

Anxiety can result from many factors. A newly diagnosed illness, separation from loved ones, the threat of pending diagnostic tests or surgical procedures, a language barrier, and expectations of life changes are just a few factors that can cause anxiety. How successfully a patient copes with anxiety depends in part on previous experiences, the presence of other stressors, the significance of the event causing anxiety, and the availability of supportive resources. You can help to decrease anxiety through effective communication. Communication methods reviewed in this skill may help an anxious patient clarify factors causing anxiety and cope more effectively. There are stages of anxiety with corresponding behavioral manifestations: mild, moderate, severe, and panic (Box 2-6).

The degree and frequency of anger range from everyday mild annoyance to anger related to feelings of helplessness and powerlessness. It is important to understand that in many cases the patient's ability to express anger is sometimes necessary for recovery. When a patient experiences a significant loss, anger becomes a means to help cope with grief. A patient may express anger toward a health care professional, but often the anger hides a specific problem or concern. A patient with a new diagnosis of cancer may voice anger with the nurse's care instead of expressing a fear of dying.

It is stressful to deal with an angry patient. Anger can represent rejection or disapproval of the nurse's care. Satisfying the needs of one angry patient often can result in a failure to meet the priorities of other patients. Create a safe and private environment for your patients to express some anger and frustration.

However, remember that anger is the common underlying factor associated with a potential for violence. In the health care setting health care professionals may become the target of the patient's anger when the patient cannot express it toward a significant other. Deescalation skills are useful techniques for managing the potentially violent patient. These skills range from using nonthreatening verbal and nonverbal messages to safely disengaging and controlling the aggressor physically (Fortinash and Holoday-Worret, 2008).

Depression is a mood disorder that may have many causes. Persons with mild depression describe themselves as feeling sad, blue, downcast, and tearful. They commonly feel apathetic, hopeless, helpless, worthless, guilty, and angry. Other symptoms include difficulty sleeping or sleeping too much, irritability, weight loss or gain, headaches, and feelings of fatigue regardless of the amount of sleep. In some cases there is a high level of anxiety, physical complaints, and social isolation. Thoughts of death and decreased libido may also occur

BOX 2-6 BEHAVIORAL MANIFESTATIONS OF ANXIETY: STAGES OF ANXIETY

Mild Anxiety
Increased auditory and visual perception
Increased awareness of relationships
Increased alertness
Able to problem solve

Moderate Anxiety
Selective inattention
Decreased perceptual field
Focus only on relevant information
Muscle tension; diaphoresis

Severe Anxiety
Focus on fragmented details
Headache, nausea, dizziness
Unable to see connections between details
Inability to recall events

Panic State of Anxiety
Does not notice surroundings
Feeling of terror
Unable to cope with any problem

(Keltner and others, 2007). Many patients in acute care settings who suffer from either acute or chronic health conditions have symptoms of depression. Some patients have been formally diagnosed and are treated with medication and/or psychotherapy. Others may not have been diagnosed and therefore have not been treated.

Cognitive impairment among patients can be either short term or long term. These patients pose a challenge for all caregivers. Often patients cannot think, speak, or understand what they have been told. Memory loss and confusion may be present in patients who suffer from some form of dementia or brain injury. Persons with mental illness or developmental disabilities may have some degree of cognitive impairment. Other causes of cognitive impairment include fatigue and effects of medications. Use a normal tone of voice and simple words and speak slowly when communicating with patients who are cognitively impaired.

ASSESSMENT

1. Observe for physical, behavioral, and verbal cues of anxiety such as dry mouth, sweaty palms, tone of voice, frequent use of call light, difficulty concentrating, wringing of hands, and statements such as "I'm scared." *Rationale: Certain behaviors indicate anxiety.*
2. Assess for possible factors causing patient anxiety (e.g., hospitalization, fatigue, fear, pain).
3. Assess factors influencing communication with the patient (e.g., environment, timing, presence of others, values, experiences, need for personal space because of heightened anxiety).
4. Assess own level of anxiety as nurse and make a conscious effort to remain calm. *Rationale: Anxiety is highly contagious, and one's own anxiety can worsen the patient's anxiety.*
5. Observe for behaviors that indicate that the patient is angry (e.g., pacing, clenched fists, loud voice, throwing objects) and/or patient expression that indicates anger (e.g., repeated questioning of the nurse, irrational complaints about care, no adherence to requests, belligerent outbursts, threats).
6. Assess factors that influence the angry patient's communication such as refusal to comply with treatment goals, use of sarcasm or hostile behavior, having a low frustration level, or being emotionally immature.
7. Consider resources available to assist in communicating with the potentially violent patient such as other members of the health care team and family members.
8. Assess for physical, behavioral, and verbal cues that indicate that the patient is depressed such as feelings of sadness, tearfulness, difficulty concentrating, increase in reports of physical complaints, and statements such as "I'm sad/depressed."
9. Assess for possible factors causing patient's depression (e.g., acute or chronic illness, personal vulnerability, past history).
10. Nurse may need to confer with family members about possible causes of patient's depression, including past history of the illness.
11. Assess the level of cognitive impairment of the patient.
12. Ascertain the most effective means of communication with the cognitively impaired patient (i.e., verbal or written communication or nonverbal communication).

PLANNING

Expected Outcomes focus on reducing the patient's anxiety and/or depression through the use of effective communication techniques, focus on promoting effective and socially appropriate verbal and nonverbal expressions of anger, and focus on recognizing symptoms of cognitive impairments in patients and using effective communication skills.

1. Patient establishes rapport, achieves a sense of calm, and discusses coping and decision making about current situation.
2. Patient's physical and emotional discomforts are acknowledged.
3. Patient discusses factors causing anxiety, anger, and/or depression.
4. Patient's anger is diffused, and problem solving is initiated.
5. Patient states that coping strategies improve well-being.
6. Patient engages in a meaningful exchange with the nurse.

Delegation and Collaboration

Therapeutic communication is a goal of all patient interactions. Communicating for the purpose of reducing anxiety and therapeutic communication with a depressed patient cannot be delegated to nursing assistive personnel (NAP). The NAP may interact with anxious and/or depressed patients and must know what to observe and report to the nurse. All NAP who have contact with angry or cognitively impaired patients must be able to communicate effectively with those patients.

IMPLEMENTATION *for* COMMUNICATING WITH ANXIOUS, ANGRY, DEPRESSED, AND COGNITIVELY IMPAIRED PATIENTS

STEPS	RATIONALE
1. Provide brief, simple introduction; introduce self; and explain purpose of interaction.	Brief reintroductions help to continually orient patients.
2. Use appropriate nonverbal behaviors (e.g., relaxed posture, eye contact). Stay with the patient at the bedside.	Patients experiencing emotionally charged situations may not comprehend the verbally delivered message. Focus on understanding the patient, providing feedback, assisting in problem solving, and providing an atmosphere of warmth and acceptance.
3. Use appropriate responses that are clear and concise.	This promotes effective communication so the patient can explore causes of anxiety and steps to alleviate anxious feelings. It conveys empathy.
4. Help patient acquire alternative coping strategies such as progressive relaxation, slow deep-breathing exercises, and visual imagery.	Stress-reduction techniques are nonpharmacological strategies that patient can use to reduce anxiety.
5. Minimize noise in physical setting.	Decreasing environmental stimuli may reduce patient's anxiety.
6. Adjust the amount and quality of time for communicating depending on patient's needs.	Flexibility and adaptation of techniques may be necessary based on patient's ability to communicate, level of anxiety, and need for more time to establish trust.
7. Create a climate of patient acceptance. Maintain a nonthreatening verbal approach using a calm tone of voice. Try to determine the source of the anger. Use an open body language with a concerned nonthreatening facial expression, open arms (not folded), hands not in pockets, relaxed posture, and a safe distance (e.g., not invading the patient's personal space).	A relaxed atmosphere may prevent further escalation.
8. Respond to the potentially violent patient with therapeutic silence and allow patient to ventilate feelings. Use active listening for understanding. Do not argue with patient. Avoid defensiveness with patient.	These techniques often deescalate anger because anger expends emotional and physical energy; patient runs out of momentum and energy to maintain anger at a high level. Arguing escalates anger.
9. Answer questions calmly and honestly. If patient presents a power-struggle type of question (e.g., "Who said you were in charge; I don't have to listen to you"), set limits using clear, concise language Inform patient of potential consequences, and follow through with consequences if behaviors are not altered.	Setting limits on power-struggle questions provides structure and diffuses anger (Fortinash and Holoday-Worret, 2008).
10. Maintain personal space. It may be necessary to have someone with you and to keep the door open. Position self between the patient and the exit.	Steps promote nurses' safety when patient becomes violent.
11. If the patient is making verbal threats to harm others, remain calm yet professional and continue to set limits with inappropriate behavior. If a distinct likelihood of imminent harm to others is present, notify the proper authorities (e.g., nurse manager, security).	Angry patients lose the ability to process information rationally and therefore may impulsively express themselves through intimidation.

SAFETY ALERT The potentially violent patient can be impulsive and explosive; therefore it is imperative that the nurse keep personal safety skills in mind. In this case avoid touch.

Continued

STEPS	RATIONALE
12. Encourage safe coping behaviors (e.g., physical exercise as a means of directing energy in an acceptable way, writing about negative thoughts).	
13. Use open-ended questions such as, "Tell me about how you are feeling."	Encourages the patient to continue talking, facilitating a discussion of symptoms and circumstances.
14. Encourage small decisions and independent actions. When necessary, make decisions that patients are not ready to make.	Depressed patients may be overly dependent and indecisive.
15. Spend time and provide honest affirmation with patient who is withdrawn.	Communicates the patient's worth.
16. Ask, "Are you having thoughts of suicide?" If the answer is yes, ask, "Have you thought about how you would do it?" (plan); "Do you have what you need?" (means); "Have you thought about when you would do it?" (time set).	Depressed patients are at increased risk for suicide. Ninety-five percent of all suicide hotline callers answer no at some point in this series of questions or indicate that the time is set for some date in the future. The more developed the plan, the greater the risk of suicide (Keltner and others, 2007). Referral is needed.
17. Speak slowly and calmly to a cognitively impaired patient, using simple words.	Have realistic expectations of the abilities of the patient.
18. Address patient by name and maintain eye contact.	Helps to keep patient's attention.
19. Ask one question at a time and give patient time to respond. Repeat and rephrase if necessary.	Rushing the patient increases level of confusion.
20. Break down tasks into small steps.	
21. Use nonverbal gestures when communicating what to do (e.g., demonstrate action such as brushing your teeth).	Patients who cannot follow verbal commands may understand nonverbal gestures.
22. Maintain consistent routine.	Minimizes confusion and frustration.

EVALUATION

1. Have patient discuss ways to cope with anxiety in the future and make decisions about current situation.
2. Observe for continuing presence of physical signs and symptoms or behaviors reflecting anxiety and/or depression.
3. Ask patient to discuss factors causing anxiety and/or depression.
4. Ask patient if feelings of anger have subsided.
5. Determine patient's ability to answer questions and solve problems.

Unexpected Outcomes and Related Interventions

1. Physical signs and symptoms of anxiety, anger, and/or depression continue.
   a. Use refocusing or distraction skills such as relaxation and imagery to reduce anxiety.
   b. Be direct and clear when communicating with patient to avoid misunderstanding.
   c. When used appropriately, touch may help control feelings of panic or confusion.
   d. Administering medication as prescribed may be necessary.
   e. Provide security measures (see agency protocol).
   f. Evaluate support system.
   g. Refer patient to mental health professional for consultation.
   h. Use distraction techniques or redirection with cognitively impaired patients.

Recording and Reporting

- Record factors/actions that cause the patient's anxiety, anger, and/or depression.
- Document nonverbal behaviors; methods used to relieve anxiety, anger, and/or depression (pharmacological and nonpharmacological methods); and patient response (verbal and nonverbal).
- Record and report threats of violence made and who was notified.

Sample Documentation

1800 Patient expressed extreme anger toward staff related to food served cold and no-smoking policy. Stated, "I just can't take this abuse any more. I have to get out of here now." Threatened to leave the hospital against medical advice. The nurse manager and the patient's doctor were notified. Encouraged to write about his feelings; family plans to stay with patient until he is calmer.

Special Considerations

Pediatric

- Evaluate the child's usual pattern of communication, including use of age-appropriate language.
- Anxiety and/or depression may be expressed through restless behavior, physical complaints, or behavioral regression.
- Children tend to have less internal control over their behaviors; immediately setting limits for inappropriate behaviors exhibited by the child is effective (Hockenberry and Wilson, 2009).

Geriatric

- Be aware of any cognitive or sensory impairment; patients who have cognitive impairments may exhibit tantrum-like behaviors in response to real or perceived frustration.
- Anxiety is often the result of change in usual patterns and environment.
- Depression among older adults is a major health concern; suicide risk is increased in older adults (Keltner and others, 2007).

Home Care Considerations

- Personal safety for the nurse against potentially violent patients or family members extends to all health care settings, including the patient's home. The nurse may be in a potentially dangerous situation while giving care to the patient at home; you may give care to the patient without support from other staff members.
- Be aware of physical surroundings, including possible exits. Maintain nonthreatening position, including body language, position, and rate of speech, when interacting with an angry or potentially violent patient. The nurse should attempt to deescalate the patient. If deescalation does not occur and the nurse thinks that safety may be threatened, the nurse should call for assistance or remove staff from situation.
- Have numbers for emergency use posted near phone (e.g., mental health provider, emergency response units, neighbors).

IMPROVING INTERDISCIPLINARY COMMUNICATION

According to research, factors such as hospital working conditions and ineffective communication between physicians and nurses negatively affect patient outcomes and contribute to interprofessional conflict (Boone and others, 2008; Manojilovich and DeCicco, 2007). In addition, poor communication results in fragmented care and increases the risk of patient care errors. Skillful communication between nurses and nurses and other health care professions improves the continuity of care, prevents or resolves conflict, increases collaboration between health care professionals, and helps increase patient satisfaction. When critical information is not communicated clearly, the patient is adversely affected. Recently The Joint Commission published the National Patient Safety Goals and identified as one of its goals to improve the effectiveness of communication among caregivers (TJC, 2010). Hand-off communications (see Procedural Guideline 2.1) and *S*ituation, *B*ackground, *A*ssessment, and *R*ecommendation (SBAR) communication (see Procedural Guideline 2.2) are two techniques to improve interdisciplinary communication in health care settings.

PROCEDURAL GUIDELINE 2.1
Hand-Off Communications

The quality of patient care is improved when transferring information from one health care provider to another, called a *hand-off*. Hand-off communication uses clear language and effective communication techniques. These hand-offs are interactive, providing the opportunity for all health care personnel involved to ask questions or seek clarification (Amato-Vealey and others, 2008; Chard, 2008).

Delegation and Collaboration

The skill of hand-off communications cannot be delegated to nursing assistive personnel (NAP). Instruct the NAP about the following:

- Patient information received during the transfer of care
- Pertinent information or change in clinical status to report to the nurse such as changes in the patient's vital signs, level of comfort, or clinical condition

Procedural Steps

1. Be interactive in your communication with health care personnel during patient hand-off.
2. Use clear language and avoid confusing abbreviation and jargon.
3. Use effective communication techniques.
4. Use standardized reporting tool/checklists during patient hand-off.
5. Use up-to-date information regarding patient's condition and treatment.
6. Limit interruptions during the hand-off process.
7. Verify information received, including a read-back or repeat-back process.
8. The hand-off process should include a clear transfer of responsibility.

PROCEDURAL GUIDELINE 2.2
SBAR Communication

The *Situation*, *Background*, *Assessment*, and *Recommendation* (SBAR) communication technique provides a predictable structure for communication among health care personnel. This is a hand-off model that includes four components: *Situation*—state what is happening at the present time; *Background*—explain circumstances leading up to situation; *Assessment*—what you think the problem is; and *Recommendation*—what to do to correct the problem. You can use the SBAR tool as a checklist to improve patient safety during hand-offs from one health care personnel to another (Haig and others, 2006).

Delegation and Collaboration

The skill of SBAR communications cannot be delegated to nursing assistive personnel (NAP). Instruct the NAP about the following:

- Patient information received during the transfer of care
- Pertinent information or change in clinical status to report to the nurse such as changes in the patient's vital signs, level of comfort, or clinical condition

Procedural Steps

1. Identify self, unit, and patient's name and room number when initiating transfer of care.
2. State patient's condition and severity.
3. Provide background information related to situation.
4. Include the following information: admitting diagnosis, date of admission, list of current medications, allergies, laboratory/test results, vital signs, code status, and any other pertinent clinical information.
5. Give assessment of the situation during the transfer of care.
6. Give any recommendations regarding the patient during the transfer of care.
7. Read back and/or repeat back any physician's orders.

REVIEW QUESTIONS

Case Study for Questions 1 and 2

1. An 84-year-old cognitively impaired older adult patient was transferred from a nursing home to an acute care facility. The patient has a history of vascular dementia from a series of strokes. According to the nursing home staff, the patient has become increasingly agitated and combative in the last few days; this behavior is unusual for the patient. Laboratory tests revealed a urinary tract infection. The patient began receiving antibiotics for the infection. You are the nurse caring for this patient. Which of the following is an example of ineffective communication techniques to use with this cognitively impaired patient?
   1. Address patient by name.
   2. Challenge patient if patient is confused.
   3. Ask one question at a time.
   4. Speak slowly and use simple words.
2. How would you handle communicating with the nursing home staff during the transfer of care when you discharge this patient? Select the appropriate order of the components of the communication hand-off:
   1. RSAB
   2. ABSR
   3. SBAR
   4. RABS
3. What should the nurse know when observing and interpreting a patient's nonverbal communication?
   1. Patients are usually very aware of their nonverbal cues.
   2. Verbal responses are more important than nonverbal cues.
   3. Nonverbal cues have obvious meaning and are easily interpreted.
   4. Nonverbal cues provide significant information and need to be validated.
4. A patient has been withdrawn, suspicious, and explosive since admission. He is wary of staff and other patients. Which approach by the nurse is most appropriate?
   1. Refraining from touch
   2. Patting his arm when he seems frightened
   3. Reaching out to shake his hand as an initial greeting
   4. Placing an arm around his shoulders while walking down the hall
5. The nurse in the mental health unit reviews therapeutic and nontherapeutic communication techniques with a nursing student. Which of the following are therapeutic communication techniques? Select all that apply.
   1. Restating
   2. Listening
   3. Asking the patient "Why?"
   4. Maintaining neutral responses
   5. Giving advice or approval or disapproval
   6. Providing acknowledgement
6. Which of the following approaches creates a barrier to communication?
   1. Using too many different skills during a single interaction
   2. Giving advice rather than encouraging the patient to problem solve
   3. Allowing the patient to become too anxious before changing the subject
   4. Focusing on what the patient is saying rather than on the skill used

7. The patient states, "I get pretty discouraged when I realize I have been struggling with these issues for over a year." The nurse responds, "Yes you have, but lots of other people take even longer to resolve their problems; don't be so hard on yourself." What does this interaction represent?
   1. The patient is expressing a lack of willingness to collaborate with the nurse.
   2. The patient is offering the opportunity for the nurse to revise the plan of care.
   3. The nurse has responded ineffectively to the patient's concerns.
   4. The nurse is using techniques consistent with the evaluation phase of the nurse-patient relationship.
8. Which of the following techniques are examples of non-therapeutic communication? Select all that apply.
   1. Paraphrasing
   2. Challenging
   3. Asking "what" questions
   4. Asking "why" questions
9. Which of the following factors has documented negative effects on patient outcomes?
   1. Interprofessional conflict
   2. Ineffective communication between health care personnel
   3. Stressful working environment for nurses
   4. All of the above
10. Which of the following methods would you use when communicating with an angry patient: (a) maintain personal space, (b) encourage safe coping behaviors, (c) use therapeutic silence, and (d) use touch as a therapeutic technique.
   1. A, B, D
   2. A, C, D
   3. A, B, C
   4. B, C, D

REFERENCES

Amato-Vealey EJ and others: Hand-off communication: a requisite for perioperative patient safety, *AORN J* 88(5):763, 2008.

Boone BN and others: Conflict management training and nurse-physician collaborative behaviors, *J Nurs Staff Dev* 24(4):168, 2008.

Chard R: Implementing a process for hand-off communication, *AORN J* 88(6):1005, 2008.

Fortinash K, Holoday-Worret P: *Psychiatric-mental health nursing*, ed 4, St Louis, 2008, Mosby.

Giger J, Davidhizar R: *Transcultural nursing: assessment and intervention*, ed 5, St Louis, 2008, Mosby.

Haig KM and others: SBAR: a shared mental model for improving communication between clinicians, *J Qual Patient Saf* 32(3):167, 2006.

Hockenberry MJ, Wilson D: *Wong's essentials of pediatric nursing*, ed 8, St Louis, 2009, Mosby.

Jasmine TJX: The use of effective therapeutic communication skills in nursing practice, *Singapore Nurs J* 36(1):35, 2009.

Keltner N and others: *Psychiatric nursing: a psychotherapeutic management approach*, ed 5, St Louis, 2007, Mosby.

Kluge MA, Glick L: Teaching therapeutic communication VIA camera cues and clues: the video-interactive (VIA) model, *J Nurs Educ* 45(11):463, 2006.

Manojilovich M, DeCicco B: Healthy work environments, nurse-physician collaboration, and patients' outcomes, *Am J Crit Care* 16(6):536, 2007.

McNeill C and others: Relationship skills building with older adults, *J Nurs Educ* 47(6):269, 2008.

Mitchell J: Enhancing patient connectedness: understanding the nurse-patient relationship, *Int J Hum Caring* 11(4):79-82, 2007.

Purnell L, Paulanka B: *Transcultural health care: a culturally competent approach*, ed 3, Philadelphia, 2008, FA Davis.

The Joint Commission: *2010 National patient safety goals hospital program*, http://www.jointcommission.org, accessed May 25, 2010, 2010, Oakbrook Terrace, Ill, The Commission.

CHAPTER

3

Documentation and Informatics

evolve WEBSITE

http://evolve.elsevier.com/Perry/nursinginterventions

Health care documentation is anything written or printed in a patient's medical record. It is an essential component of health care delivery because, when done correctly and appropriately, documentation ensures better continuity of care to patients, increases communication between care providers, and improves patient safety (Barthold, 2009). Although some health care agencies still use printed records, electronic documentation continues to become more of a standard. An electronic record is intended to integrate all relevant patient information into one record that is accessible each time a patient enters a health care system. The design of any documentation system should maintain health care standards and reduce errors (McGeehan, 2007). The Joint Commission (TJC, 2010a) sets standards for documentation of health care.

Informatics refers to the property and structure of information or data. It is important that nurses know how to record and report data and then apply the information for patient care. Nursing informatics is a specialty that integrates nursing science, computer science, and information science to manage and communicate data, information, and knowledge in nursing practice. The application of informatics results in an efficient and effective nursing information system that better manages and communicates data to improve patient outcomes and promote patient safety (Roux and Halstead, 2009).

PATIENT-CENTERED CARE

Patient-centered care involves nurses individualizing their care to patients and being responsive in meeting patient needs (Radwin and others, 2009). Thorough documentation is central to patient-centered care. A nurse is responsible for documenting detailed information about the care that he or she provides to patients, including aspects of care that are individualized. When you provide a level of detail, the medical record becomes a valuable resource for all health care providers. Communication among members of the health care team by way of documentation is essential for accurate and timely delivery of therapies. When you record an entry into a patient record, it must convey information about the patient's status, the specific type of interventions delivered, patient responses to care, and critical information that allows all care providers to deliver an organized and comprehensive plan of care.

SAFETY

The patient's medical record is a legal document that reflects all aspects of a patient's care while in a health care setting. As a result, there are standards that all health care organizations integrate into a documentation system to ensure that the care delivered represents safe practices.

Information entered into the medical record must be accurate, thorough, and current because all care providers rely on the information to deliver and coordinate patient care. Inaccurate or incomplete documentation or falsification of information in a medical record can result in medical or nursing therapies that are unnecessary, inappropriate, and delayed, all resulting potentially in negative patient outcomes.

EVIDENCE-BASED PRACTICE

Cheevakasemsook A and others: The study of nursing documentation complexities, *Int J Nurs Pract* 12(6):366, 2006.

Elfering A and others: Work stress and patient safety: observer-rated work stressors as predictors of characteristics of safety-related events reported by young nurses, *Ergonomics* 49(5-6):457, 2006.

Documentation system designs, both printed and electronic, challenge nurses to know when and how to enter information correctly. A good percentage of nursing time in an acute care setting is documenting information. A study by Elfering and others (2006) showed that the most frequent safety-related stressful events for young nurses working in hospitals included incomplete or incorrect documentation (40.3%) and delays in delivery of patient care (9.7%). Nursing documentation complexities may contribute to this stress. Research suggests that complexities in documentation include disruption, incompleteness, and inappropriate charting (Cheevakasemsook and others, 2006). Following good standards of practice in documentation is essential. This begins with attending to documentation and avoiding interruptions so complete, timely, relevant, and informative information is entered in the patient record.

ELECTRONIC HEALTH RECORD

The traditional paper medical record is episode oriented, with a separate record for each patient visit to a health care agency. Key information such as patient allergies, current medications, and complications from treatment may be lost from one episode of care to the next. The Electronic Health Record (EHR) is a longitudinal electronic record of patient health information generated by one or more encounters in any care delivery setting (HIMSS, 2010). It automates and streamlines the clinician's workflow. It has the ability to generate a complete record of a clinical patient encounter and support other care-related activities directly or indirectly via interface, including evidence-based decision support, quality management, and outcomes reporting. Electronic forms and flow sheets are designed by nursing and other health care providers. They incorporate professional nursing standards, regulatory requirements, and evidence-based practice into the content of the forms. Designing forms that collect the pertinent information ensures improved communication among health care providers and ultimately safer patient care.

You must obtain patient consent before information in the EHR is transferred or shared with another institution. Use precautions to protect the patient's information, and institutions need to develop guidelines and policies to ensure privacy and confidentiality of the information consistent with federal and state regulations such as the Health Insurance Portability and Accountability Act (HIPAA).

CONFIDENTIALITY

Nurses are legally and ethically obligated to keep information about patients confidential. Do not disclose information about a patient's status to other patients, family members (unless the patient grants permission), or health care staff not involved in the patient's care. In 1996 legislation to protect patient privacy for health information in the form of HIPAA was proposed; the Act was finalized in 2003 with specific guidelines for communication of patients' personal health information (United States Department of Health and Human Services, [USDHHS], 2003). Under HIPAA patients have access to their medical records, and providers must obtain consent from the patient before information is released for health-related purposes. These standards require the USDHHS to establish national standards for electronic health care transactions and national identifiers for providers, health plans, and employers. HIPAA also addresses the security and privacy of health data. Adopting these standards will improve the efficiency and effectiveness of the nation's health care system by encouraging the widespread use of electronic data interchange in health care.

Only health care providers directly involved in a specific patient's care have legitimate access to the medical record. Other professionals may use records for data gathering, research, or education only with permission and according to established agency, state, and federal guidelines. Many states require reporting of certain infectious or communicable diseases through the public health department, which must be done through proper channels.

Computerized documentation poses risks to patient confidentiality. Most security mechanisms for information systems use a combination of logical and physical restrictions to protect information such as firewalls and antivirus spyware. However, there are also guidelines for clinicians to use to protect patient information. They include proper use of passwords and being sure not to leave a computer terminal unattended when patient information is still displayed (see Procedural Guideline 3.2). It is important to follow agency policy if backup files are accidentally deleted. Also follow confidentiality procedures for documenting sensitive patient information.

LEGAL GUIDELINES IN DOCUMENTATION

Accurate documentation is one of the best defenses for legal claims associated with nursing care. To limit nursing liability, documentation must clearly indicate that individualized, goal-directed nursing care was provided to a patient based on a nursing assessment. The record needs to describe exactly what happens to a patient. This is best achieved by charting immediately after providing care to a patient. Even though nursing care may have been excellent, in a court of law "care not documented is care not provided." Know your agency policies for documenting, either in paper format or electronically.

The Nurses Service Organization (a medical malpractice, professional liability, and risk management company) (2006) has identified common charting mistakes that result in malpractice: (1) failing to record pertinent health or drug information, (2) failing to record nursing actions, (3) failing to record that medications have been given, (4) failing to record drug reactions or changes in patient's condition, (5) writing illegible or incomplete records, and (6) failing to document discontinued medications.

STANDARDS

Current TJC (2010a) standards require that all patients who are admitted to a health care institution have an assessment of physical, psychosocial, environmental, self-care, patient education, and discharge planning needs. The standards also require documentation to be within the context of the nursing process. The nursing process shapes your approach and direction of care and how you report and document:

- Record assessments that offer a database from which health care team members can draw conclusions about the patient's problems.
- Record information about the patient's concerns or condition to assist caregivers in problem identification, planning, and setting priorities.
- Describe care activities in detail to reflect the implementation of the plan of care.
- Evaluate patient responses to nursing care to show the patient's success in achieving expected outcomes of care.

GUIDELINES FOR QUALITY DOCUMENTATION

Nurses practice in a variety of settings and use a variety of forms and formats to communicate specific information about a patient's health care. The use of standard documentation guidelines ensures more efficient, safe, individualized patient care. Ideally forms are designed to make data easy to enter, find, and interpret and to avoid unnecessary duplication. For example, most nursing forms have a place for patient identification, date and times, and a key to indicate the meaning of abbreviations or entries used and the type of information required. Because of legal requirements, you must follow agency documentation standards. Regardless of the documentation method, all nurses must follow certain basic guidelines.

Factual

A factual record or report contains descriptive and objective information about what a nurse sees, hears, feels, or smells. An example of an objective description is "pulse 54, strong, and irregular." Avoid using words such as *good, adequate, fair,* or *poor* that are subject to interpretation. Inferences are conclusions based on factual data. An example of an inference is "The patient has a poor appetite," which would be based on factual data, including the amount of food the patient ate during a meal and his or her fluid intake. For example, "The patient ate only two bites of toast for breakfast, with 180 mL of apple juice."

The only subjective data included in a record or report are what the patient actually verbalizes. Subjective information is documented using the patient's words in quotes; for example, Patient states, "I feel sick to my stomach" or Patient states, "I do not like the food choices here." In both cases document the actual food intake and the subjective data.

Accurate

The use of exact, precise measurements is a means to make comparisons and determine when a patient's condition has changed. Charting that an "abdominal wound is 5 cm in length, without redness or edema" is more accurate than the statement "large abdominal wound is healing well." Accurate charting requires you to use only approved TJC (2010b) or health care agency abbreviations and write out all terms that may be confusing. TJC has published an official "Do Not Use" list because of potential errors occurring in the area of medication administration (see Chapter 21). Correct spelling is essential because terms are easy to misinterpret (e.g., *accept* or *except, dysphagia* or *dysphasia*).

Records need to reflect your accountability during the time frame that you care for a patient. Thus you must chart your own observations and actions. Your signature holds you accountable for any information recorded. When you report observations to another caregiver and interventions are performed by someone else, that fact must be clearly indicated (e.g., "Surgical dressings removed by Dr. Kline. Pulse of 104 reported to J. Kemp, RN"). Each written entry must end with your first name or first initial, last name, and title. Nursing students sign off using the approved abbreviation for the school and the program level on any signature.

Complete

The information within a recorded entry must be complete, containing appropriate and essential information. There are criteria for thorough communication for certain health situations. For example, when recording discharge planning, measurable patient goals or expected outcomes, progress toward goals, and need for referrals are always included. When documenting patient behavior, onset, behaviors exhibited, and precipitating factors are included. The following is an example of what may occur when a note has not been recorded completely.

A nurse explains and demonstrates a teaching session about giving insulin injections. The patient eagerly expresses a desire to give the next injection when it is due. Documentation is as follows: "Discussed learning about insulin injection technique." During the next shift another nurse spends time demonstrating the injection technique and assessing the patient's readiness to give the injection because the previous teaching was not communicated. As a result, time is wasted repeating information that the patient learned previously instead of coaching the patient through a self-injection.

Concise

Concise documentation facilitates efficient retrieval of pertinent information. When you learn to write concisely, less time is needed for documentation. A comparison of a concise and lengthy note follows.

Concise, Factual Entry	Lengthy Entry Using Vague Terms
0900 Left toes cool and pale, without inflammation, capillary return >5 sec; left pedal pulse 1+; right pedal pulse 4+. Patient responds to tactile stimulation and is able to wiggle toes on left foot. Describes pain in left foot as dull, aching 4 (scale 0-10).	0900 The patient's left toes are cool, with pale color. There is no inflammation. There is slow capillary return present greater than 5 seconds. Dorsalis pedis pulse in left foot is weak, and the patient complains of some discomfort. The pain in left foot is described as aching.

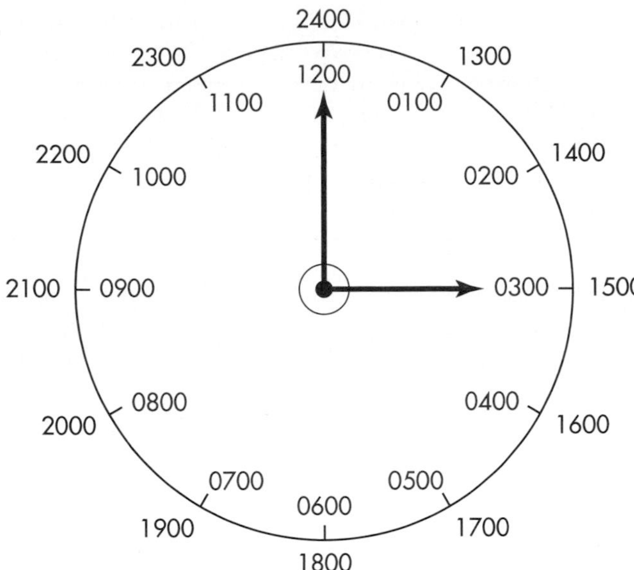

FIG 3-1 Comparison of military time and standard time.

Current

Effective documentation includes making timely entries in a patient's record, which avoids omissions and delay in patient care. Many health care agencies keep records and computers near the patient's bedside to facilitate immediate documentation of care activities. Document the following activities or findings at the time of occurrence:

- Changes from baseline vital signs
- Pain assessment
- Administration of medications and treatments
- Preparation for diagnostic tests or surgery
- Change in patient status and who was notified
- Patient response to an intervention
- Admission, transfer, discharge, or death of a patient

Writing notes on a work pad at the time of an event helps to ensure accuracy when you later complete your formal documentation. Often nurses on a care unit design worksheets that incorporate their standards of care.

Many agencies use military time, a 24-hour time system, to avoid misinterpretation of AM and PM times. The military clock ends with midnight at 2400 and begins at 1 minute after midnight at 0001. The following examples compare standard with military time: 10:22 AM is 1022 military time; 3:15 PM is 1515 military time (Fig. 3-1).

Organized

Organized notes are written in a logical order. For example, an organized note follows the nursing process to describe the assessment, interventions, and patient's response in a sequence. Communication is also more effective when it is organized. When making a record entry, make a list of what to include before beginning to write in the permanent legal record. Identifying relevant content is helpful in deleting unnecessary words. The following compares a well-organized note with a disorganized note:

Organized Note	Disorganized Note
7/17 0630 Patient reports sharp pain 9 (scale 0-10) in left lower quadrant of abdomen, worsened by turning onto right side. Positioning on left side decreases pain to 8 (scale 0-10). Abdomen is tender to touch and rigid. Bowel sounds are absent. Dr. Phillips notified. To x-ray for CT scan of abdomen. T. Reis, RN	7/17 0630 Patient experiencing sharp pain in lower quadrant of abdomen. MD notified. Abdomen tender to touch, rigid, with bowel sounds absent. Positioning on left side offers minimal relief of pain. CT scan ordered of the abdomen. J. Adams, RN

Methods of Recording

The method of recording selected by a nursing administration reflects the philosophy of the department. Staff use the same method of recording throughout an agency. There are several acceptable methods for recording health care data.

The problem-oriented medical record (POMR) is a structured method of documentation that emphasizes a patient's problems. It is organized using the nursing process. Organization of data is by problem or diagnosis. Ideally each member of the health care team contributes to a single list of identified patient problems. Each recording includes a database, problem list, care plan, and progress notes.

A source record is a way to organize chart information by each discipline instead of by patient problems. The advantage of a source record is that caregivers can easily locate the section of the chart to make entries. Members of each discipline can go to sections such as nurse's notes, physician or health care provider's notes, or laboratory results. A disadvantage of the source record is fragmented data.

Charting by exception (CBE) is a method of recording that aims to eliminate redundancy and make documentation of routine care more concise. The emphasis is on recording abnormal findings and trends in clinical care. It is a shorthand method for documenting based on defined standards for normal nursing assessments and interventions. CBE simply involves completing a flow sheet that incorporates these standards, thus minimizing the need for lengthy narrative notes. However, the CBE system can be used inappropriately when nurses fail to enter notes that describe abnormal findings or unexpected changes in a patient's condition.

Structure communication using the SBAR approach is a technique that provides a framework for communication among members of the health care team. SBAR is a mnemonic for the following:

S: Situation (state what is happening at the present time)
B: Background (explain the circumstances leading up to the situation)
A: Assessment (what you think the problem is)
R: Recommendation (what you would do to correct the problem)

SBAR promotes the provision of safe, efficient, timely, and patient-centered communication (Haig and others, 2006).

PROCEDURAL GUIDELINE 3.1
Documenting Nurses' Progress Notes

Nurses practice in a variety of settings and use a variety of forms and formats to communicate information about a patient's health care. Ideally forms are designed to make data easy to find and interpret and reduce duplication. Medical record forms that nurses traditionally have used for documentation include nursing admission history, physical assessment and vital signs graphic, medication administration records, nurses' notes, and nursing care flow sheets (Box 3-1). Many agencies have a variety of worksheets that are useful for routine patient care and are not a permanent part of the record.

Progress notes are a format for documenting a record of a patient's progress. A variety of formats for progress notes, including SOAP (*S*ubjective data, *O*bjective data, *A*ssessment or *A*nalysis, and *P*lan), SOAPE (SOAP plus *E*valuation), PIE (*P*roblem, *I*ntervention, and *E*valuation), APIE (*A*ssessment, *P*lan, *I*ntervention, and *E*valuation), and DAR (*D*ata, *A*ction, and patient *R*esponse) are used in focus charting. Any caregiver needs to be able to read a progress note and understand what type of problem a patient has, the level of care provided, and the results of the interventions. The nurse who is responsible for the patient care provided signs each entry.

Delegation and Collaboration

The skill of documenting nurse progress notes can be delegated to nursing assistive personnel (NAP) for aspects of care that the NAP provides, such as hygiene measures and patient activity. Instruct the NAP about the following:

- Which information needs to be entered within a set time frame

Equipment

- Patient care profile
- Multidisciplinary treatment plan or progress note form

Steps

1. Review assessment data, problems identified (nursing diagnoses), goals and expected outcomes, interventions, and patient responses during contact with each patient before documentation.
2. After each patient contact, identify information that needs to be documented to ensure quality, accuracy, timeliness, and continuity of information. Consider abnormal findings, changes in patient's status, and new problem identification.
3. Obtain necessary forms or access appropriate computer screens for documentation.
4. Record date and time for each entry and do not leave open spaces between notes.
5. Use agency format (e.g., SOAP, PIE, DAR) and document in chronological order the following:
   a. Pertinent, factual objective data
   b. Selected subjective data that validate and clarify
   c. Nursing actions taken
   d. Evaluation of patient responses to nursing actions
   e. Any additional nursing actions
   f. To whom information has been reported, including name and status
6. Make progress note entries:
   a. Use a SOAP format: *S*ubjective data, *O*bjective data, *A*ssessment or *A*nalysis, and *P*lan. Usually based on a

BOX 3-1 NURSING DOCUMENTATION FORMS AND WORKSHEETS

Nursing History Forms

Complete an assessment for each patient at the time of admission to a health care agency. The history includes basic biographical data (e.g., age, method of admission, physician or health care provider), admitting medical diagnosis or chief complaint, and a brief medical-surgical history (e.g., previous surgeries or illnesses, allergies, medication history, patient's perceptions about illness or hospitalization, physical assessment of all body systems). The nursing history form provides for a systematic and complete patient assessment and the identification of relevant nursing diagnoses. The nursing history provides baseline data to compare with changes in the patient's condition throughout the hospitalization.

Graphic Sheets and Flow Sheets

Forms include routine observations made on a repeated basis using a check mark (e.g., when bath is given, patient is turned) or by entering data (e.g., vital signs and input and output). When completing a flow sheet, review previous entries to identify changes.

Computerized Patient Care Summary

Includes pertinent information about patients and their ongoing care plans such as basic demographic data (e.g., age, religion), physician or health care provider's name, primary medical diagnosis, current physician's orders, nursing orders or interventions, scheduled tests or procedures, safety precautions to use in the patient's care, and factors related to activities of daily living (ADLs).

Nursing Kardex (Worksheet)

The Kardex includes information needed for daily care on a flip card or in a notebook and is usually kept at the nurses' station. Information can be used for change-of-shift report and facilitates access to information without referring to the patient record. The worksheet includes demographic data, tests ordered, therapies, and information related to ADLs. It may include standardized or individualized nursing care plans.

PROCEDURAL GUIDELINE 3.1
Documenting Nurses' Progress Notes—cont'd

numbered list of problems or nursing diagnoses such as "Anxiety related to preparation for surgery":

S: *Subjective data*—The patient's statements regarding the problem (e.g., Patient stated, "I am dreading this surgery because last time I had a terrible reaction to the anesthesia and such terrible pain when they made me get out of bed.")

O: *Objective data*—Observations that support or are related to subjective data (e.g., frequent turning in bed and loud, agitated voice)

A: *Assessment/Analysis*—Conclusions reached based on data (e.g., fear related to pain/anesthesia)

P: *Plan*—The plan for dealing with the situation (e.g., "Notified anesthesiologist, Dr. Moore, of experience. Discussed alternatives for anesthesia and pain-control options. Stressed importance of activity for circulation and healing. Encouraged to keep nurses informed of pain level and need for medication and told patient that pain usually is present but manageable.")

b. Make progress note entry using a PIE format: *P*roblem, *I*ntervention, and *E*valuation. Problem-oriented system in which progress notes are written based on a list of numbered or labeled patient problems such as "Anxiety related to preparation for surgery":

P: *Problem*—Preoperative anxiety (e.g., Patient stated, "I am dreading this surgery because last time I had a terrible reaction to the anesthesia and such terrible pain when they made me get out of bed."). Observed frequent turning in bed and loud, agitated voice.

I: *Intervention*—Notified anesthesiologist, Dr. Moore, of experience. Discussed with patient alternatives for anesthesia and pain-control options. Stressed importance of activity for circulation and healing. Told to keep nurses informed of pain level and need for medication. Told patient that pain usually is present but manageable.

E: *Evaluation*—Patient stated that she was "very relieved." Stated she would tell the nurses about pain.

c. Make progress note entries using a DAR format: *D*ata, *A*ction, and patient *R*esponse. Used in focus charting; a way to organize progress notes to make them clearer and more organized

D: *Data*—Patient states, "I am dreading this surgery because last time I had a terrible reaction to the anesthesia and such terrible pain when they made me get out of bed." Observed frequent turning in bed and loud, agitated voice.

A: *Action*—Notified anesthesiologist, Dr. Moore, of experience. Discussed alternatives for anesthesia and pain-control options. Stressed importance of activity for circulation and healing. Encouraged to keep nurses informed of pain level and need for medication and told patient that pain usually is present but manageable.

R: *Response*—Patient stated that she was "very relieved." Stated she would tell the nurses about pain.

d. Make a progress note entry using a *basic narrative note format.* Usually not based on a problem list:

Patient states, "I am dreading this surgery because last time I had a terrible reaction to the anesthesia and such terrible pain when they made me get out of bed." Observed frequent turning in bed and loud, agitated voice. Notified anesthesiologist, Dr. Moore, of experience. Discussed alternatives for anesthesia and pain-control options. Stressed importance of activity for circulation and healing. Encouraged to keep nurses informed of pain level and need for medication and told patient that pain usually is present but manageable.

e. Progress note entry using a CBE: Charting *by Exception* system. A progress note describes deviations from the patient's normal assessment findings; nurse uses standardized flow sheets and assessment forms to document normal findings. Variance note is a narrative that describes exceptions to the norm:

"Patient reports sharp pain in right great toe, rated as a 10 on pain scale of 0 to 10. States the pain began 30 minutes ago. Right great toe is red, warm to touch. Pedal pulses palpable. Unable to assess capillary refill of right great toe because of patient's complaint of pain in toe."

7. Sign progress note with full name or first initial and last name and status according to agency policy. Students are usually required to indicate their level of education and school affiliation.

8. Review previously documented entries with those that you enter, noting if there is significant change in the patient's status. Report any changes to the patient's health care provider.

PROCEDURAL GUIDELINE 3.2
Use of Electronic Health Records

Electronic Health Records (EHRs) organize data in a standardized format and allow members of the patient's health care team to document care immediately and track the patient's progress. Policies and procedures to ensure confidentiality of the patient's information must be maintained at all times.

Delegation and Collaboration

Authorized members of the health care team have access to all parts of the patient's electronic record. The skill of charting patient information may be delegated to nursing assistive personnel (NAP) for certain aspects of care such as vital signs, intake and output, or other content areas as defined by the institution.

Procedural Steps

1. Sign on to the EHR using only your password.
2. Never share passwords and keep your password private.
3. Do not leave patient information on the monitor where others can view it.
4. Review assessment data, problems identified (nursing diagnoses), goals and expected outcomes, and interventions and patient responses during contact with each patient before data entry.
5. Follow procedures for entering information in all appropriate program functions.
6. Review previously documented entries with those you enter, noting if there is significant change in the patient's status. Report changes to the patient's health care provider.
7. Know and implement procedures to correct documentation errors.
8. Save information as documentation is completed.
9. Sign off when you leave the computer.

PROCEDURAL GUIDELINE 3.3
Documenting an Incident Occurrence

Health care errors do occur. There is no national reporting of such occurrences, but individual health care agencies have their staff complete occurrence reports when deviations in standards of care and adverse events occur. The National Quality Forum (2002) identified a standardized list of preventable, serious adverse events that facilitate the reporting of such events (Box 3-2). An incident or occurrence report is a risk management tool that enables health care providers to identify risks within an agency, analyze them, act to reduce the risks, and evaluate the results. The incident report is completed by any member of the health care or hospital staff when a patient experiences an adverse event while in the hospital. The incident report alerts hospital administration of the event and provides an opportunity to monitor trends and patterns in care and identify ways to improve existing care.

Delegation and Collaboration

The nurse instructs the nursing assistive personnel (NAP) to report any incident in which they are involved and complete the document in a timely manner (see agency policy).

Equipment

- An incident or occurrence report form

Procedural Steps

1. When you witness an adverse event or find a patient who has just experienced an adverse event, assess the patient's condition and observe the environmental setting.
2. Protect the patient from further injury by calling for assistance immediately or taking action to create a safe environment (e.g., if patient is having an allergic reaction

BOX 3-2 EXAMPLES OF SERIOUS REPORTABLE EVENTS OCCURRING WITHIN A HEALTH CARE FACILITY

- Surgery performed on wrong patient
- Patient death or injury associated with use of restraints or bedrails
- Patient death or injury associated with use or function of a device in patient care in which device is used for function other than intended
- Patient death or injury associated with a fall
- Patient death or injury associated with hypoglycemia, onset of which occurs in a health care facility
- Retention of a foreign object in a patient after surgery
- Patient elopement for more than 4 hours
- Patient death or injury associated with medication error
- Patient death or injury associated with a hemolytic reaction to a blood product
- Stage 3 or 4 pressure ulcer acquired after admission to a health care facility
- Patient death or injury associated with electrical shock

Data from National Quality Forum: *Serious reportable events in healthcare: a consensus report,* Washington, DC, 2002, National Quality Forum.

PROCEDURAL GUIDELINE 3.3
Documenting an Incident Occurrence—cont'd

to blood, stop infusion and instill normal saline intravenously; if patient has fallen, call for assistance and be sure that patient is in safe alignment).

3. Obtain agency reporting form.
4. Objectively and accurately document what you observed or heard related to the incident.
5. If someone witnessed the event with you, record their information. Identify them as the source of information.
6. Record details in chronological order.
7. Do not document in the medical record "incident report filed." The incident report is a facility report and not part of the medical record. However, do document your assessment findings of the patient's condition.
8. File the report properly with the risk management department or designated person.

REVIEW QUESTIONS

1. A nurse manager reviews the nurses' notes in a patient's medical record and finds the following entry, "Patient is difficult to care for, refuses suggestions for improving appetite." Which of the following directions should the manager give to the staff nurse who entered the note?
   1. Avoid rushing when charting an entry.
   2. Use correction fluid to correct a mistake.
   3. Enter only objective and factual information about the patient.
   4. Use a black marker to cover over the mistaken entry.
2. The nurse observes the patient quickly pacing back and forth in the room and asks the patient what is wrong. The patient states, "I don't know what is going to happen to me. I am afraid I will be put in a nursing home." How does the nurse document this interaction with the patient?
   1. "Patient observed to be agitated and confused."
   2. "The patient appears to be anxious."
   3. "The patient is disoriented and paranoid."
   4. "The patient stated, 'I don't know what is going to happen to me.'"
3. The nurse is caring for a patient over a 12-hour shift. She conducts her routine assessment at the beginning of the shift and assists the patient to the bathroom to void. During that time the nurse administers medications at 0900 and at 1500. At 1400 the patient receives 1 unit of packed red blood cells (PRBCs) intravenously. At 1530 the physical therapist visits with the patient to discuss discharge. Which of the activities performed by the nurse should be recorded immediately? Select all that apply.
   1. Visit by the physical therapist
   2. Medication administration
   3. Urine output
   4. Patient's ability to ambulate to bathroom
   5. Administration of blood product
4. Match the correct entry with the appropriate SOAP category
   1. Repositioned patient on right side
   2. "The pain increases every time I turn on my left side."
   3. Acute pain related to surgical incision
   4. Left lower surgical incision sutures intact; no drainage noted
5. List two ways that the nurse as caregiver can maintain confidentiality of patient data when using electronic medical record keeping.
6. Which of the following information is included in an occurrence report? Select all that apply.
   1. Information about the person involved in the incident
   2. Data from individuals who witnessed the event
   3. Information received from nurses from another unit
   4. Your opinion of what happened and how the incident could have been prevented
7. According to HIPAA regulations, patients do not have the right to access their medical records.
   True/False
8. Military time is frequently used to document care. A patient was ambulated in the hall at 5:30 PM. What time would it be if documented according to military time?
   1. 0530
   2. 1530
   3. 1730
   4. 1630
9. Which of the following is/are an example(s) of objective data? Select all that apply.
   1. "The skin is warm to the touch."
   2. "Patient is demanding."
   3. "The patient reports having abdominal cramping."
   4. "The patient is wringing her hands while pacing in the room."
10. Which of the following information would not be included in a patient's record?
    1. Patient's report of pain not relieved by analgesic medication
    2. Assessment of patient's surgical wound
    3. Incident report filed after patient fell out of bed
    4. Patient's response to a PRN medication

REFERENCES

Barthold M: Standardizing electronic nursing documentation, *Nurs Manage* 40(5):15, 2009.

Cheevakasemsook A and others: The study of nursing documentation complexities, *Int J Nurs Pract* 12(6):366, 2006.

Elfering A and others: Work stress and patient safety: observer-rated work stressors as predictors of characteristics of safety-related events reported by young nurses, *Ergonomics* 49(5-6):457-469, 2006.

Haig K and others: SBAR: a shared mental model for improving communication between clinicians, *J Qual Patient Saf* 32(3):168, 2006.

Healthcare Information and Management Systems Society: *The electronic health record,* 2010, http://himss.org/asp/topics_ehr.asp, accessed February 7, 2010.

National Quality Forum: *Serious reportable events in healthcare: a consensus report*, Washington, DC, 2002, National Quality Forum.

McGeehan R: Best practice in record keeping, *Nurs Stand* 21(17):51, 2007.

Nurses Service Organization: *8 Common charting mistakes to avoid,* 2006, http://www.nso.com/nursing-resources/article/16.jsp, accessed February 9, 2010.

Radwin LE and others: Relationships between patient-centered cancer nursing interventions and desired health outcomes in the context of the health care system, *Res Nurs Health* 32(1):4, 2009.

Roux G, Halstead J: *Issues and trends in nursing: essential knowledge for today and tomorrow*, Sudbury, 2009, Jones and Bartlett.

The Joint Commission: *Comprehensive accreditation manual for hospitals (CAMH): The official handbook*, Chicago, 2010a, Joint Commission Resources.

The Joint Commission: *National patient safety goals: 2010 critical access hospital and hospital national patient safety goals,* 2010, http://www.jointcommission.org/PatientSafety, accessed January 18, 2010b.

US Department of Health and Human Services: Standards for privacy of individually identifiable health information, Health Insurance Portability and Accountability Act of 1996, *Fed Regist* 64:60053, 1999, http://www.hhs.gov/ocr/HIPAA, revised 2003, accessed January 18, 2010.

CHAPTER

4

Patient Safety and Quality Improvement

evolve WEBSITE

http://evolve.elsevier.com/Perry/nursinginterventions

Video Clips

Nursing Skills Online

Safety is freedom from physical and psychological injury. It is a standard that affects all nursing work. Nurses in all health care settings are responsible for identifying and eliminating safety hazards. Following agency policy and procedures and providing ongoing communication with co-workers are two key ways to maintain the safety of patients. Communication failures are the number one root cause of all sentinel events reported to The Joint Commission (TJC) (Rossi, 2009). TJC annually lists National Patient Safety Goals (NPSGs) to reduce risks for medical errors and the potentially serious consequences known as sentinel events (TJC, 2010a). A sentinel event is defined by TJC (2009a) as an unexpected occurrence involving death, serious physical or psychological injury, or risk thereof. These events include any process variation (e.g., medication administration, restraint application) for which a recurrence would carry a significant chance of a serious adverse outcome. They are "sentinel" because they signal the need for immediate investigation and response. Each goal has a set of evidence-based recommendations on which health care agencies focus their attention. Box 4-1 cites TJC 2010 NPSGs for hospitals (TJC, 2010a).

PATIENT-CENTERED CARE

Being hospitalized puts patients at risk for injury in an unfamiliar and confusing environment. The experience is usually at least minimally frightening. Normal life cues such as a bed without side rails and the direction one usually takes to the bathroom are absent. Thought processes and coping mechanisms are affected by illness and its accompanying emotions. Thus patients are more vulnerable to injury. For patients of diverse backgrounds this vulnerability may be intensified. It is a nurse's responsibility to diligently protect all patients regardless of their socio-economic status, disease state, or cultural background. Most untoward events are related to failures of communication. Health care providers must be particularly attentive regarding communication with persons of diverse backgrounds. This is especially important during assessment, when a nurse must use an approach that recognizes a patient's cultural background so appropriate questions can be raised to clearly reveal health behaviors and risks. Safety is enhanced when patients are considered in light of the whole person, including their cultural background.

SAFETY

Safety begins with the patient's immediate environment. Nurses are responsible for making patients' bedside areas safe. Fig. 4-1 shows a variety of environmental interventions for patient safety. The call light/bed control system allows patients to adjust the position of the bed and signal caregivers when they need assistance. A full set of side rails (two or four to a bed) is a physical restraint. Recent research shows that having side rails raised increases the occurrence of falls (Krauss and others, 2005). Raising only one of two, or three of four, side rails gives patients room to exit a bed safely and move around within the bed. It is also important to keep a bed in low position with wheels locked when stationary. ALWAYS CHECK a bed for structural risks (e.g., wobbly or damaged rails or soft mattresses). Electronic bed and chair alarms are available to warn nurses when a patient who needs assistance tries to leave the bed or chair on his or her own. One example is pressure-sensitive strips placed beneath a patient on a bed or chair. Additional devices to use at a patient's bedside are a bedside commode, a nonskid floor mat, an overhead trapeze, and a movable hand rail.

Strategies for patient safety include encouraging patients to be active participants in their care and improving communication between caregivers and patients. It is imperative that an institution support a "culture of safety" in which a safety concern can be voiced by anyone without fear. For example, if a patient observes a health care provider not washing hands before a dressing change, the patient should be encouraged and comfortable to point out such omissions. The same applies to health care staff.

Accurate patient identification is a crucial key to safety, whether at the bedside before a procedure, before surgery, when entering documentation, or when discussing patient care with colleagues. Safe practice means that the identification process is followed so patients get the right medications and treatments at the right times and do not suffer from injury associated with health care interventions. Nurses must be conscientious in the patient identification process and other safety practices at all times.

BOX 4-1 THE JOINT COMMISSION 2010: NATIONAL PATIENT SAFETY GOALS FOR HOSPITALS

- Improve the accuracy of patient identification.
- Improve the effectiveness of communication among caregivers.
- Improve the safety of using medications.
- Reduce the risk of health care–associated infections.
- Accurately and completely reconcile medications across the continuum of care.
- The organization identifies safety risks inherent in its patient population.
- Universal Protocol for Preventing Wrong-Site, Wrong-Procedure, and Wrong-Person Surgery.

EVIDENCE-BASED PRACTICE TRENDS

Currie L: Fall and injury prevention. In Hughes R, editor: *Patient safety and quality: an evidence-based handbook for nurses,* Rockville, Md, 2008, Agency for Healthcare Research and Quality.

Zijlstra GA and others: Interventions to reduce fear of falling in community-living older people: a systematic review, *J Am Geriatr Soc* 55(4):603, 2007.

All of the National Patient Safety Goals are sensitive to nursing interventions. Like TJC, the Agency for Healthcare Research and Quality (AHRQ) reviews ongoing research and recommends evidence-based nursing interventions for safety problems. There continues to be significant research in the area of fall prevention. Evidence supports multifactorial approaches to fall prevention in the acute care setting. A multifactorial program uses multiple interventions because individuals are at risk for falls for a variety of reasons. These interventions include the use of a fall risk assessment tool, assessment and collaboration for the adjustment of medications, changes in the environment, staff education, use of alarm devices, and interventions for disorders contributing to the risk. In the community setting home-based exercise, environmental adaptations, and community-based tai chi delivered in a group format are effective in reducing the risk for falls.

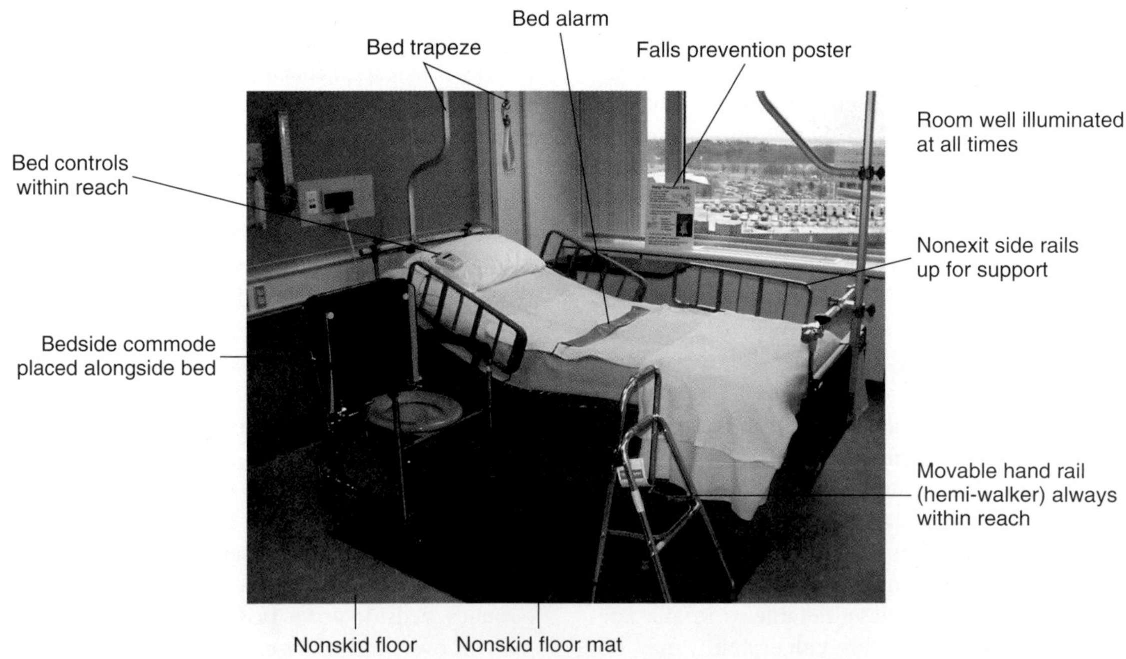

FIG 4-1 Making the hospital patient's environment safe. (From U.S. Department of Veterans Affairs, National Center for Patient Safety: *2004 Falls toolkit, falls notebook interventions,* 2004, http://www.patientsafety/gov/Safetytopics/fallstoolkit/index.html, accessed March 2010.)

SKILL 4.1 FALL PREVENTION

- **Nursing Skills Online: Safety Module, Lesson 1**

Patient falls are frequently reported adverse events in the adult inpatient setting. They are the most common cause of nonfatal injury in adults over the age of 65 in the United States. Falls are costly. Injuries related to falls are responsible for about 15% of hospital readmissions within the first month after discharge (Currie, 2008). Medicare and many state Medicaid agencies no longer reimburse hospital costs associated with fall-related injuries (Krauss and others, 2008). In adults over the age of 65, injuries related to falls are the most common cause of accidental death. Even when one considers the underlying factors that contribute to one's potential for falling, the trauma related to a fall is the most common cause of morbidity (Currie, 2008).

It is likely that falls are generally underreported, except when an injury occurs. For this reason injury rates are considered more informative and a more consistent quality measure. Overall data indicate that the risk for fall in the acute care setting in the United States is about 1.9% to 3% of all hospitalizations, thus approximating more than 1 million falls a year (Currie, 2008).

There are many strategies for fall and injury prevention. Prevention programs work best within the context of strong organizational support and broad interdisciplinary cooperation. A consistent approach to evaluate risk must be developed. A number of fall risk assessment tools are available (ICSI, 2008). Most of these tools identify levels of risk such as low and high. One such tool is the Johns Hopkins Fall Risk Assessment Tool (Poe and others, 2007). Once a patient's risk is assessed, it is important to communicate the risk for a fall clearly through the care continuum with which the patient will interact. Assessment findings associated with an increased risk for fall and injury direct the development of fall prevention interventions. Patients and situations change. The actual prevention of falls and injuries requires diligent ongoing nursing assessment and the engagement of the whole health care team in the implementation of planned patient-specific interventions (ICSI, 2008).

ASSESSMENT

1. Assess the patient's age and motor, sensory, balance, and cognitive status (see Chapter 7), including ability to follow directions and cooperate. Focus on fall risks such as age greater than 65 years, confusion, decreased hearing, decreased night vision, orthostatic hypotension or dizziness, impaired gait, decreased energy or fatigue, and decreased peripheral sensation. *Rationale: Physiological factors predispose patients to fall.*
2. Use the agency's fall risk assessment tool. All tools include a fall history. Be specific and follow the acronym SPLATT (Meiner and Lueckenotte, 2006):
   Symptoms at time of fall
   Previous fall
   Location of fall
   Activity at time of fall
   Time of fall
   Trauma after fall
3. Assess elimination patterns. *Rationale: Incontinence or urgency and the attempt to rush to a bathroom or find a urinal may predispose a patient to falls.*
4. Assess patient's medications (including over-the-counter [OTC] medications and herbal products) for use of antidepressants, antipsychotics, hypnotics (especially benzodiazepines), anxiolytics, diuretics, antihypertensives, antihistamines, anti-Parkinson drugs, hypoglycemics, muscle relaxants, analgesics, and laxatives. *Rationale: Certain medications may increase risk for falls and injury (*Levy, 2008*).*
5. If applicable, confer with health care provider on possibility of reducing or adjusting number of medications. *Rationale: Polypharmacy is a fall risk. Number of medications can be reduced safely if a balance is achieved between benefits of medications and risk of adverse events (*Tinetti, 2003*).*
6. Assess patient's risk for a fall injury such as osteoporosis, being on anticoagulants, history of previous fracture, cancer, and recent chest or abdominal surgery. *Rationale: Factors increase likelihood of injury from a fall.*
7. Assess risk factors in the health care facility that pose a threat to patient's safety (Poe and others, 2007) (e.g., being attached to equipment such as sequential compression hose or intravenous [IV] tubing, improperly lighted room, clutter, obstructed walkway to bathroom, and proximity of frequently needed items such as a urinal or eyeglasses).
8. Assess condition of equipment. *Rationale: Equipment in poor repair (such as uneven legs on a bedside commode) increases the risk for fall.*
9. Assess patient's fear of falling: consider patients over age 80, female, perceived in poor general health, history of multiple falls. *Rationale: These factors correlate with fear of falling, increasing risk for falls (*Zijlstra and others, 2007*).*

PLANNING

Expected Outcomes focus on fall and injury prevention and appropriate use of safety equipment.

1. The patient's environment is as free of hazards as possible.
2. The patient and/or family member is able to identify safety risks.
3. The patient and/or family member verbalizes understanding of fall prevention interventions.
4. The patient does not suffer a fall or injury.

Delegation and Collaboration

The skill of assessing and communicating a patient's risk for fall cannot be delegated, neither can the education of the patient/family regarding the risk for fall. Skills used to prevent falls can be delegated. Instruct the nursing assistive personnel (NAP) by:

- Explaining the patient's mobility limitations and any specific measures to reduce risks.
- Teaching specific environmental safety precautions to use (e.g., bed locked in low position, call light within reach, nonskid footwear).

Equipment

- Hospital bed with side rails
- Wheelchair
- Call light/intercom system

IMPLEMENTATION *for* FALL PREVENTION

STEPS	RATIONALE
1. See Standard Protocol (inside front cover).	
SAFETY ALERT Before using any equipment for the first time, know the safety features and proper method of operation.	
2. Introduce yourself to patient, including your name and title.	Reduces patient uncertainty.
3. Identify patient by using two identifiers (e.g., name and birthday or name and account number, according to facility policy).	Ensures correct patient. Complies with The Joint Commission standards and improves patient safety (TJC, 2010a).
4. Adjust bed to proper height.	Enhances patient's ability to move in bed and transfer out of bed safely.
5. Encourage the use of properly fitted skid-proof footwear. Option: place nonslip padded floor mat on exit side of bed.	Prevents falls from slipping on floor.
6. Orient patient to surroundings and call light/bed control system.	
a. Provide patient's hearing aid and glasses.	Enables patient to remain alert to conditions in environment.
b. Explain and demonstrate how to use call light/intercom system.	Knowledge of location and use of call light is essential to patient safety.
c. Explain to patient/family when and why to use call system (e.g., report pain, get out of bed, go to bathroom). Provide clear instructions to patient/family regarding mobility restrictions.	Increases likelihood of nurse being able to respond.
d. Consistently secure call light/bed control system to an accessible location within patient's reach.	Ensures that patient is able to reach device immediately when needed.
7. Provide environmental interventions.	
a. Remove excess equipment, supplies, and furniture from rooms and halls.	Reduces likelihood of falling or tripping over objects.
b. Keep floors clutter and obstacle free, particularly the path to the bathroom.	Reduces likelihood of falling or tripping over objects.
c. Coil and secure excess electrical, telephone, and any other cords or tubing.	Reduces the risk of entanglement.
d. Clean all spills promptly. Post a sign indicating a wet floor. Remove the sign when the floor is dry.	Reduces the risk of falling on slippery, wet surfaces.
e. Ensure adequate glare-free lighting; use a night light at night.	Glare may be a problem for older adults because of vision changes.
f. Have assistive devices (e.g., cane, walker, bedside commode) on exit side of bed.	Provides added support when transferring out of bed.
g. Arrange necessary items (e.g., water pitcher, telephone, reading materials, dentures) within patient's easy reach and in a logical way.	Facilitates independence and self-care; prevents falls related to reaching for hard-to-reach items.
h. Secure locks on beds, stretchers, and wheelchairs.	Prevents accidental movement of devices during patient transfer.

STEPS	RATIONALE
8. When ambulating a patient, have patient wear a gait belt and walk along patient's side (see Chapter 16).	Gait belt gives nurse a secure hold on patient during ambulation.
9. Use a wheelchair to transport safely.	
a. Determine level of assistance needed to transfer patient to wheelchair (see Chapter 15).	Patient's condition may require more than a one-person assist.
10. Use of hospital bed side rails	
a. Explain to patient/family the reasons for using side rails: preventing falls and turning self in bed.	Promotes patient and family cooperation.
b. Check agency policies regarding side rail use. In a four–side rail bed, keep the top two side rails up and the lower two rails down. In a two–side rail bed, keep one rail down. Place bed in low position with bed wheels locked (see illustration).	Side rails are considered a restraint device when used to prevent the patient from getting out of bed voluntarily (National Guidelines Clearinghouse, 2005). Minimizes risk of patient falling out of bed. With bed in low position, if patient climbs out of bed and falls, trauma may be reduced.

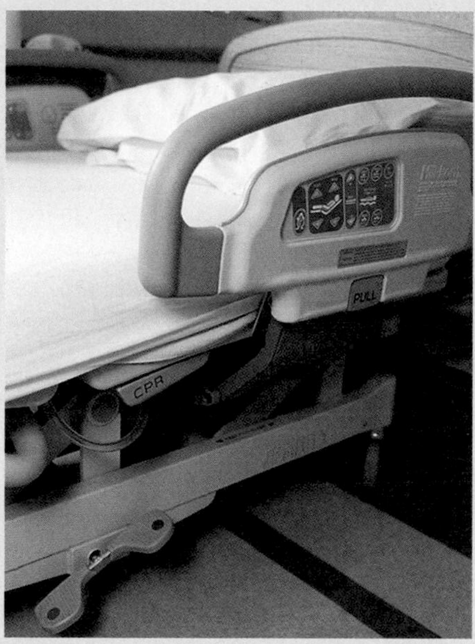

STEP 10b Hospital bed should be kept in lowest position with wheels locked and upper side rails up (as appropriate).

STEPS	RATIONALE
c. In a four–side rail bed, leave one upper side rail up and one down when patient is oriented and able to get out of bed independently.	

> **SAFETY ALERT** Side rails may cause entrapment of the head and body. Assess for excessive gaps and openings between bed frame and mattress. Use side rail netting or protective padding to prevent mattress from being pushed to one side.

STEPS	RATIONALE
11. Additional interventions for patients at *moderate risk* for fall:	Level of risk defined by fall risk assessment tool.
a. Institute agency-specific flagging system (e.g., yellow sign on door indicating risk for fall, yellow sticker on chart, yellow fall risk armband, yellow dot on assignment board).	Communicates patients at highest risk for fall to all health care team members. Color-coded bands are easily recognizable. A national effort aimed at standardizing patient wristband colors has gained support in several states within the United States.
b. Prioritize call light responses to patients at risk for fall, using a team approach.	Ensures rapid response to calls from patients at risk for fall.
c. Monitor and assist patient in following daily schedules.	Patients are less likely to attempt some activity on their own when they know what to expect.

Continued

STEPS	RATIONALE
d. Establish elimination schedule, using bedside commode with assistance if appropriate.	Proactive toileting helps keep patient from being unattended with a sudden need to use the toilet.
e. Confer with physical therapy on feasibility of gait training and muscle-strengthening exercises.	Single intervention strategies that are shown to reduce risk of falls among older adults include gait and exercise training (Tinetti, 2003).
f. Place patients in Geri chair or wheelchair with a wedge cushion. Use wheelchair only for transport, not for sitting for an extended period of time.	Designed to maintain alignment and comfort.
g. Consider use of slip-resistant mat for patient sitting in recliner.	Helps prevent patient from sliding down and out of chair.
12. Interventions for patients at *high risk* for fall (implement strategies for moderate risk).	
a. Remain with patient during toileting.	Prevents patient from trying to get up while waiting for assistance.
b. Be cautious with overlay mattresses that may raise the patient near level of side rails; remove mattress or use side-rail protectors.	Prevents patient from rolling out of the bed over the overlay. Prevents patient from getting snarled in side rails.
c. Use a low bed, which has a very low height above the floor, and floor mats.	Bed that is low to the ground is designed to reduce risk of fall and injury from a fall. Floor mats reduce slipping.
d. Consider restraint alternatives (see Skill 4.2).	May help safely avoid the need to restrain the patient.
e. Accompany patient during transport. Alert receiving area to patient's risk for fall.	Provides safety during transport/transfer.
f. Use restraints only when alternatives are exhausted (see Skill 4.3).	Provides least restrictive environment.
13. See Completion Protocol (inside front cover).	

EVALUATION

1. Conduct hourly rounds.
2. Observe patient's immediate environment for presence of hazards.
3. Evaluate patient's ability to use assistive devices such as walker or bedside commode.
4. Ask patient/family to identify safety risks.
5. Determine patient's response to safety modifications and that no falls or injuries have occurred.

Unexpected Outcomes and Related Interventions

1. Patient starts to fall while ambulating with a caregiver.
   a. Assist patient safely to the floor (See Chapter 16, Skill 16.2)
2. Patient suffers a fall.
   a. Call for assistance.
   b. Assess patient for injury and stay with patient until assistance arrives to help lift patient to bed or wheelchair.
   c. Notify health care provider and family.
   d. Note pertinent events related to fall and treatment provided in medical record.
   e. Follow sentinel event reporting policy of institution.
   f. Evaluate patient and environment to determine whether fall could have been prevented.
   g. Reinforce identified risks with patient and review safety measures needed to prevent a fall.
   h. Monitor patient closely after the fall since injuries are not always immediately apparent.

Recording and Reporting

- Record in nursing notes specific interventions to prevent falls and promote safety.
- Report patient's fall risks and measures taken to reduce risks to all health care personnel.
- Report immediately to physician or health care provider if the patient sustains a fall or an injury.

Sample Documentation

0900 Fall risk assessment completed. Patient placed on high-risk fall precautions because of history of falls, weakness, and urinary frequency. Call light within reach, top side rails up, hourly room checks, night-light on at all times, bedside commode in place. Instructed to call for help to ambulate. Patient voiced understanding. Patient demonstrated correct use of call light.

1615 Found patient on floor in bathroom after responding to emergency call light. Patient stated, "I slipped on the wet floor." Alert and oriented × 3. No apparent injury from fall. BP 110/74, P 82 and regular, R 20. Assisted to bed and instructed to call for help before getting out of bed. Voiced understanding. Demonstrated use of call light. Call light placed within patient's reach. Side rails up × 2. Dr. Justine and family notified of fall.

Special Considerations

Pediatric

- Never leave a child of any age unattended on a raised surface (Hockenberry and Wilson, 2007).
- Place hoods or tents over an infant's or child's crib to prevent accidental falls.

Geriatric

- Older patients with short-term memory loss or cognitive dysfunction may be unable to follow directions and may attempt to climb out of bed or get up from a chair unassisted.
- Older adults, especially postmenopausal women, are at risk for fractured hips. Fractures can cause independent patients to become more dependent or immobilized (Meiner and Lueckenotte, 2006).

Home Care

- Assess home environment and institute safety measures as appropriate (see Chapter 32)
- Items should be kept in their familiar positions and within easy reach.
- Place gates at both ends of stairs to prevent toddlers from falling.
- If patient has a history of falls and lives alone, recommend that he or she wear an electronic safety alert device. The device is turned on by the wearer to alert a monitoring site to call emergency services for help.

SKILL 4.2 DESIGNING A RESTRAINT-FREE ENVIRONMENT

Video Clips

Physical and chemical restraints restrict a patient's physical activity or normal access to the body and are not a usual part of treatment indicated by a patient's condition or symptoms. Serious and often fatal complications can develop from the use of restraints. Because of the risks associated with restraint use, current legislation emphasizes reducing the use of restraints. A restraint-free environment is the first goal of care for all patients.

Patients at risk for fall or wandering present special safety challenges when trying to create a restraint-free environment. Wandering is the meandering, aimless, or repetitive locomotion that exposes a patient to harm and is frequently in conflict with boundaries, limits, or obstacles (NANDA, 2009). This is a common problem in patients who are confused or disoriented. Interrupting a wandering patient can increase distress. The Department of Veteran Affairs has many suggestions for managing the wandering patient, most of which are environmental adaptations. Some of these include hobbies, social interaction, regular exercise, and a circular unit design (VA, 2010). Modifications of the environment are effective alternatives to restraints. More frequent observation of patients, involvement of family during visitation, and frequent reorientation are also helpful measures. Introduction of meaningful and familiar stimuli within a patient's environment can reduce the types of behaviors (e.g., wandering, restlessness, confusion) that may lead to restraint use.

ASSESSMENT

Assess patient's risk for fall as in Skill 4.1.

PLANNING

Expected Outcomes focus on maintaining patient safety while avoiding the need for physical restraints.

1. Patient is injury free and/or does not inflict injury on others.
2. Patient displays cooperative behavior toward staff, visitors, and other patients.

Delegation and Collaboration

The skills of assessing a patient's behavior, orientation to the environment, and the decision for safety measures cannot by delegated. Actions for promoting a safe environment can be delegated to nursing assistive personnel (NAP). Instructs the NAP about the following:

- Using specific diversional or activity measures for making the environment safe
- Placing alarm devices
- Reporting patient behaviors and actions (e.g., confusion, combativeness) to the nurse

Equipment

- Visual or auditory stimuli (e.g., calendar, clock, radio, television)
- Diversional activities (e.g., puzzles, games, audio books, music, DVDs)
- Wedge pillow
- Ambularm, pressure-sensitive bed, or chair alarm

IMPLEMENTATION *for* DESIGNING A RESTRAINT-FREE ENVIRONMENT

STEPS	RATIONALE
1. See Standard Protocol (inside front cover).	
2. Orient patient and family to surroundings, introduce to staff, and explain all treatments and procedures. Frequent reorientation in a calm manner may be needed.	Promotes patient understanding and cooperation.

Continued

STEPS	RATIONALE
3. Provide the same caregivers to the extent possible. Encourage family and friends to stay with the patient. Companions can be helpful. In some institutions volunteers can be good companions.	Reduces anxiety and increases safety when one person provides care and supervision is constant.
4. Place patient in a room that is easily accessible to caregivers.	Facilitates close observation. Watching the activities on the unit distracts patient (VA, 2010).
5. Be sure that patient has glasses, hearing aid, or other sensory-aid devices on and functioning. Then provide visual and auditory stimuli meaningful to specific patient (e.g., calendar, radio/MP3 player [patient's choice of music], family pictures).	Sensory deficit increases risk of confusion and disorientation. Meaningful stimuli orient patient to day, time, and physical surroundings.
6. Anticipate patient's basic needs (e.g., toileting, relief of pain or hunger) as soon as possible.	Meeting basic needs in a timely fashion decreases patients' discomfort, anxiety, and risk for fall and injury.

SAFETY ALERT Getting out of bed for toileting is a common event leading to a patient's fall (Tzeng, 2010), especially during evening or night hours when a room is darkened.

STEPS	RATIONALE
7. Provide scheduled ambulation, chair activity, and toileting (e.g., ask patient every 1 to 2 hours if needing to void). Organize treatments so patient has some uninterrupted periods throughout the day.	Regular voiding decreases risk of patient trying to reach bathroom alone. Provide time for sleep and rest. Constant activity may overstimulate patient.
8. Position intravenous (IV) catheters, urinary catheters, and tubes/drains out of patient view. Camouflage by wrapping IV site with bandage or stockinette and placing undergarments on patient with urinary catheter.	Maintains medical treatment by reducing visibility of and access to tubes/lines.
9. Use stress reduction techniques such as back rub, massage, and guided imagery (see Chapter 13).	Reducing anxiety may reduce the urge to wander.
10. Use diversional activities such as puzzles, games, books, folding towels, drawing, or offering an object to hold. Be sure that it is an activity in which patient expresses interest.	Meaningful diversional activities provide distraction, help to reduce boredom, and provide tactile stimulation. Minimize wandering.
11. Position patient on a wedge cushion and apply a wrap-around belt (see illustration). (NOTE: this is not a restraint if patient is able to self-release.)	Wedge cushion prevents slipping out of a chair and makes it difficult for patient to get out of chair without assistance. The wrap-around belt helps remind patient to call for help and allows patient to lift flap for self-release.

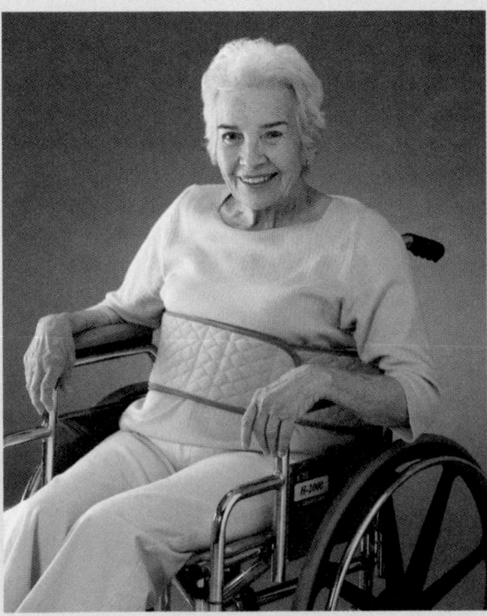

STEP 11 Wrap-around belt.(Courtesy Posey Company, Arcadia, Calif.)

STEPS	RATIONALE
12. *To use Ambularm monitoring device:*	
a. Explain use of device to patient and family.	Alarm alerts staff to patient who is standing or rising up without help.
b. Measure patient's thigh circumference just above knee to determine appropriate size. For leg circumference less than 18 inches, use regular size; use large size for 18 inches or greater.	Band that is too loose may slip off; band that is too tight may interfere with circulation or cause skin irritation.
c. Test battery and alarm by touching snaps to corresponding snaps on leg band.	
d. Apply leg band just above knee and snap battery securely in place (see illustration).	
e. Instruct patient that alarm will sound unless leg is kept in horizontal position (see illustration).	
f. To assist patient to ambulate, deactivate alarm by unsnapping device from leg band.	

> **SAFETY ALERT** Use of Ambularm is contraindicated in the presence of impaired circulation, swelling, skin irritation, or breaks in the skin.

STEPS	RATIONALE
13. *To use a pressure-sensitive bed or chair pad with alarms:*	
a. Explain use of device to patient and family.	Alarm activates sooner if placed under back. By the time the buttocks are off the sensor, the patient may be nearly out of the bed.
b. When using in the bed, position device so that it is under the patient's mid-to-low back or under the buttocks.	
c. Test alarm by applying and releasing pressure.	Ensures that alarm is audible through call light system.
14. Consult with family, physical therapy, speech therapy, and occupational therapy for appropriate activities to provide stimulation and exercise.	Involvement in meaningful and purposeful activities reduces tendency to wander.
15. Reduce/eliminate invasive treatments as much as possible (e.g., tube feedings, blood sampling).	Stimuli increase patient's restlessness.
16. See Completion Protocol (inside front cover).	

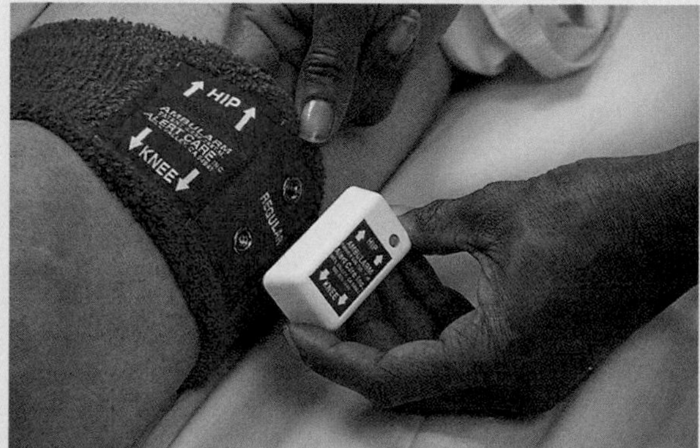

STEP 12d Snap battery in place to activate alarm.(Courtesy Alert-Care Mill Valley, Calif.)

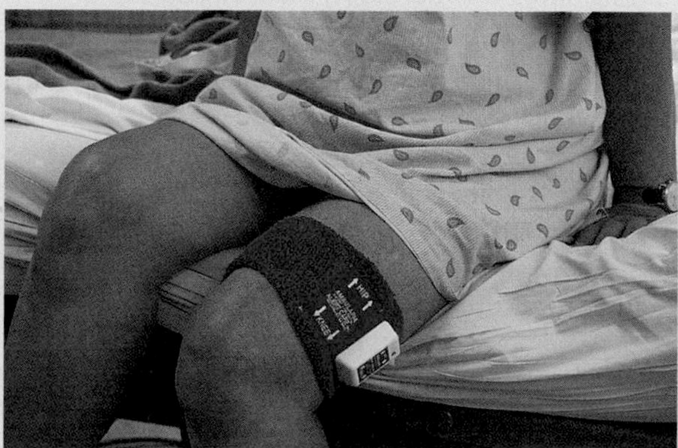

STEP 12e Audio alarm sounds when patient approaches near-vertical position.(Courtesy Alert-Care Mill Valley, Calif.)

EVALUATION

1. Observe patient for any injuries.
2. Observe patient's behavior toward staff, visitors, and other patients.

Unexpected Outcomes and Related Interventions

1. Patient displays behaviors that increase risk for injury to self or others.
   a. Review episodes for a pattern (e.g., activity, time of day) that indicates alternatives that could eliminate the behavior.
   b. Discuss with all caregivers and support service personnel alternative interventions to promote safe, consistent care.
2. Patient sustains an injury or is out of control, placing others at risk for injury.
   a. Notify health care provider and complete a safety event report according to agency policy.
   b. Identify alternative measures to promote safety without a restraint.
   c. As a last resort, identify appropriate restraint to use (see Skill 4.3).

Recording and Reporting

Document all behaviors that relate to cognitive status and ability to maintain safety: orientation to time, place, and person; ability to follow directions; mood and emotional status; understanding of condition and treatment plan; medication effects related to behaviors; restraint alternatives used; and patient response.

Sample Documentation

0900 Up and dressed; oriented to person but not time or place. Patient became tearful when unable to reach wife by telephone. Pacing in room. Reoriented to place. Explained to patient wife is due to visit later in afternoon. Set radio to favorite talk show.

1000 Participated for 15 minutes with ball toss to music at OT; then resting in rocking chair, smiling, and interacting socially with roommate.

Special Considerations

Pediatric

- Distraction techniques can decrease the need for restraints. Examples include having a child hold a stuffed animal while an IV line is being inserted or blowing bubbles while a drain is being removed.

Geriatric

- A sudden onset of confusion, weakness, and functional decline in a previously oriented patient may indicate the presence of an underlying illness in the older adult.
- Assess for physical causes of behavior changes such as urinary or respiratory infection, hypoxia, fever, fluid and electrolyte imbalance, side effects of multiple drug administration, depression, anemia, hypothyroidism, or fecal impaction (Ebersole and others, 2008).

Home Care

- Patients at risk for self-injury or violence toward others need intensive supervision. Family and/or caregiver must recognize this need and be willing and able to provide it.

SKILL 4.3 APPLYING PHYSICAL RESTRAINTS

- **Nursing Skills Online: Safety Module, Lesson 2**

Video Clips

A physical restraint is any manual method or physical device that immobilizes or reduces the ability of a person to move their extremities, body, or head freely. A drug may be considered a chemical restraint when it is given to manage behavior or restrict freedom of movement and is not part of the standard treatment for a patient's condition (NAPHS, 2007). Physical or chemical restraints should be the last resort and used only when all other reasonable alternatives fail. Restraints are a temporary means to maintain patient safety. Restraints do not prevent falls. Research has shown that patients suffer fewer injuries if left unrestrained (Park and Tang, 2007). A health care provider's order is required and must be based on a face-to-face assessment of the patient. The order must be current and specify the duration and circumstances under which the restraint is to be used. Orders should be renewed according to agency policy (usually every calendar day) and based on reassessment and reevaluation of the restrained patient. Regulatory agencies such as TJC and the CMS offer guidelines regarding safe use of restraints (HCPro, Inc., 2009). Long-term settings require informed consent from family members before using restraints on a patient.

Patients who need temporary restraints include those at risk for falls and confused or combative patients at risk for self-injury or violence to self or others. In addition, health care providers apply restraints to prevent interruption of therapy such as an intravenous (IV) catheter, urinary or surgical drains, or life-support equipment.

The use of restraints is associated with serious complications, including pressure ulcers, constipation, urinary and fecal incontinence, urinary retention, and functional deficits. In some cases restricted breathing or circulation has resulted in death. Loss of self-esteem, humiliation, fear, and anger are additional serious concerns. The Food and Drug Administration, which regulates restraints as medical devices, requires manufacturers to label restraints as "prescription only." Many patients do not easily accept use of restraints. Cultural values affect how patients and family members perceive their use. Before using restraints, assess the meaning of restraints for both the patient and family. Culturally sensitive care may include removing restraints when family members are present.

ASSESSMENT

1. Assess patient's behavior (e.g., confusion, disorientation, agitation, restlessness, combativeness, or inability to follow directions). *Rationale: If patient's behavior continues despite the use of restraint alternative, the use of physical restraint may be needed.*
2. Review agency policies regarding restraints. Check health care provider's order for purpose, type, location, and time or duration of restraint. Determine if a signed consent for use of restraint is needed. *Rationale: Health care provider's order for the least restrictive type of restraint is required.*
3. Review manufacturer's instructions for restraint application and determine the most appropriate size restraint. *Rationale: Correct application of appropriate-size restraint reduces risk of injury.*
4. Inspect the area where the restraint is to be placed. Note any nearby tubing or devices. Assess condition of the skin; sensation, including color; adequacy of circulation; and range of joint motion. *Rationale: Provides baseline assessment to monitor patient's response to restraint.*

PLANNING

Expected Outcomes focus on protecting the patient from injury and maintaining prescribed therapy.

1. Patient maintains intact skin integrity, perfusion, and function of restrained body part.
2. Patient is free of injury.
3. Patient's therapies are uninterrupted.
4. Restraint is discontinued as soon as possible.
5. Patient's self-esteem and dignity are maintained.

Delegation and Collaboration

The skills of assessing patient's behavior, orientation to the environment, need for restraints, and appropriate use cannot be delegated. Patient/family education cannot be delegated. The application and routine checking of a restraint can be delegated to nursing assistive personnel (NAP). TJC (2009b) requires training on first aid for anyone who monitors patients in restraints. Instruct the NAP about the following:

- The appropriate type of restraint to use
- How to routinely check the patient's circulation, skin integrity, and breathing
- When and how to change the patient's position and provide range-of-motion (ROM) exercises, toileting, and skin care
- When to report signs and symptoms of patient not tolerating restraint (e.g., increased agitation, constricted circulation, change in skin integrity, changes in breathing) and what to do

Equipment

- Proper restraint
- Padding (if needed)

IMPLEMENTATION *for* APPLYING PHYSICAL RESTRAINTS

STEPS	RATIONALE
1. **See Standard Protocol (inside front cover).**	
2. Identify patient using two identifiers (e.g., name and birthday or name and account number, according to facility policy).	Ensure that the right intervention is being done to the right patient.
3. Educate patient and family about need for restraint. Talk with patient in a calm, confident manner and explain what you are going to do.	Reduces anxiety and may promote cooperation.
4. Be sure that patient is comfortable and in proper body alignment.	Promotes comfort, prevents contractures, and prevents neurovascular injury.
5. If necessary, pad skin and bony prominences that will be under restraint.	Protects skin from irritation.
6. Apply proper-size restraint; *follow manufacturer's directions.*	

Continued

STEPS	RATIONALE
a. *Belt restraint* Have patient in a sitting position. Apply belt over clothes, gown, or pajamas. Make sure to place restraint at the waist, not the chest or abdomen. Remove wrinkles or creases in clothing. Bring ties through slots in belt. Help patient lie down if in bed. Avoid applying belt too tightly (see illustrations). However, ensure that straps secured to bed are snug so belt does not slide to sides of bed.	Restrains center of gravity and prevents patient from rolling off stretcher or falling out of bed. Tight application or misplacement can interfere with breathing.
b. *Extremity (ankle or wrist) restraint* Commercially available limb restraints are often made of sheepskin with foam padding. Wrap limb restraint around wrist or ankle with soft part toward skin and secured snugly (but not tightly) in place by Velcro strap. Insert two fingers under secured restraint (see illustration).	Maintains immobilization of extremity to protect patient from fall or accidental removal of device (e.g., IV tube, Foley catheter). Tight restraint constricts circulation and causes neurovascular injury or causes occlusion of therapeutic devices. Checking for constriction prevents neurovascular injury.

SAFETY ALERT Patient with extremity restraint is at risk for aspiration if positioned supine. Place patient in lateral position or with head of bed elevated rather than supine.

STEPS	RATIONALE
c. *Mitten restraint* A thumbless mitten device restrains patient's hands. Place hand in mitten, being sure that Velcro strap(s) are around wrist rather than forearm (see illustration).	Prevents patient from dislodging invasive equipment, removing dressings, or scratching. May be considered a restraint alternative if untethered and patient is physically and cognitively able to remove the mitten.

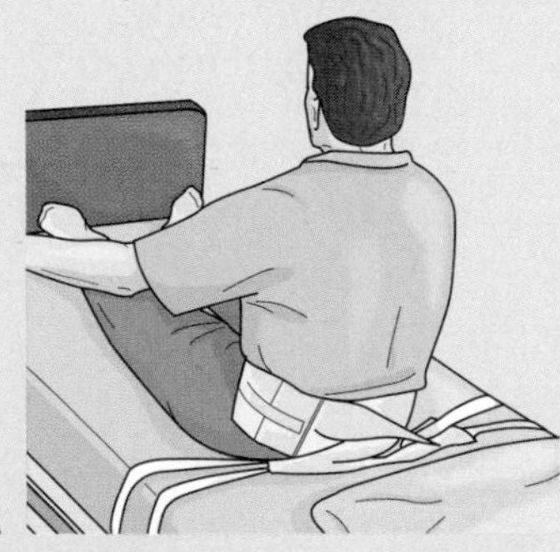

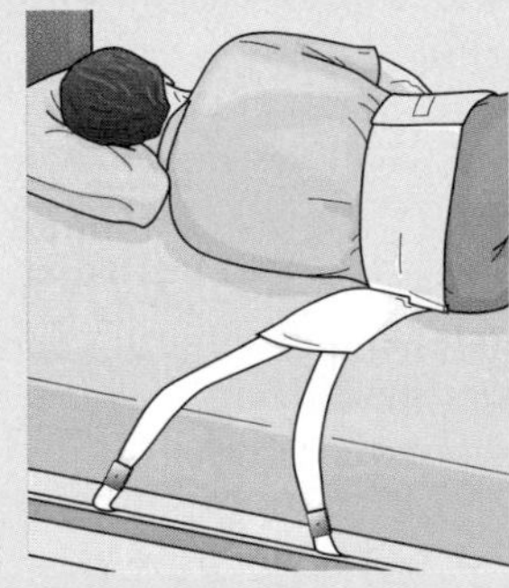

STEP 6a A, Apply belt restraint with patient sitting. **B,** A properly applied belt restraint allows patient to turn in bed. (**A** and **B** from Sorrentino SA: *Mosby's textbook for nursing assistants*, ed 7, St Louis, 2008, Mosby.)

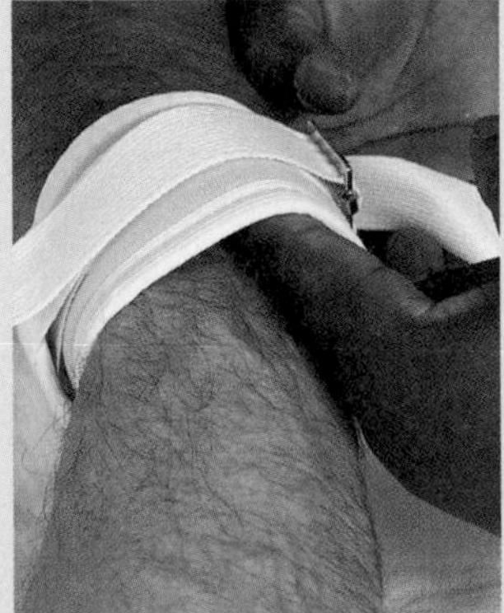

STEP 6b Securing an extremity restraint. Check restraint for constriction by inserting two fingers under restraint. (From Sorrentino SA: *Mosby's textbook for nursing assistants,* ed 7, St Louis, 2008, Mosby.

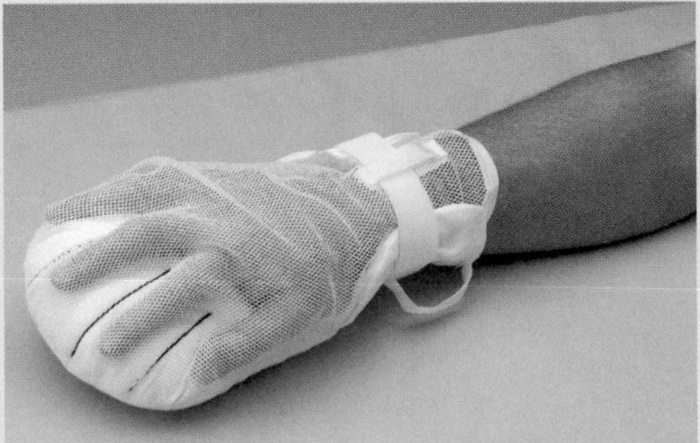

STEP 6c Mitten restraint. (Courtesy Posey Company, Arcadia, Calif.)

STEPS	RATIONALE
d. *Elbow restraint (freedom splint)* Restraint consists of rigidly padded fabric that wraps around the arm. It is closed with Velcro similar to a child's sneaker. The upper end has a clamp that hooks to the sleeve of the patient's gown or shirt (see illustration).	Commonly used with infants and children to prevent elbow flexion. May also be used for adults. Keeps elbow joint rigid. May be considered a restraint alternative if patient is cognitively and physically able to remove it.
7. Attach restraint straps to portion of bed frame that moves when head of bed is raised or lowered. *Do not attach to side rails.* Can also attach restraint to chair frame for patient in chair or wheelchair.	Strap does not tighten and restrict circulation when bed is raised or lowered. Attaching to side rail could cause serious injury when lowered.
8. Secure restraint with a quick-release tie (see illustration), a buckle, or an adjustable seat belt–like locking device. *Do not tie in a knot.*	Allows for quick release in an emergency.
9. Insert two fingers under secured restraint.	Checking for constriction prevents neurovascular injury.

SAFETY ALERT Restraints should not interfere with equipment such as IV tubes. They are not placed over access devices such as an arteriovenous dialysis shunt.

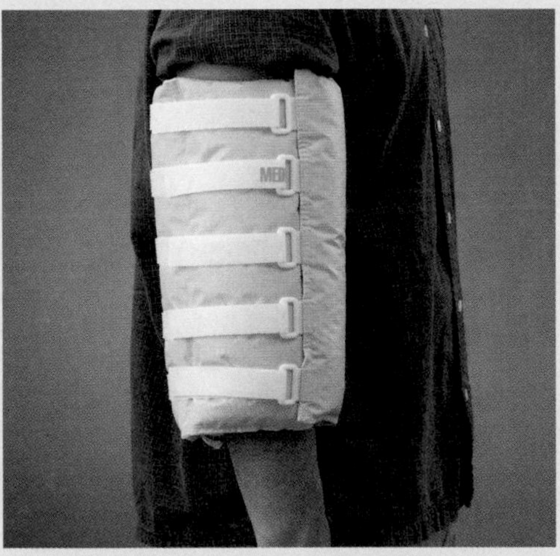

STEP 6d Freedom Elbow Restraint. (Courtesy Posey Company, Arcadia, Calif.)

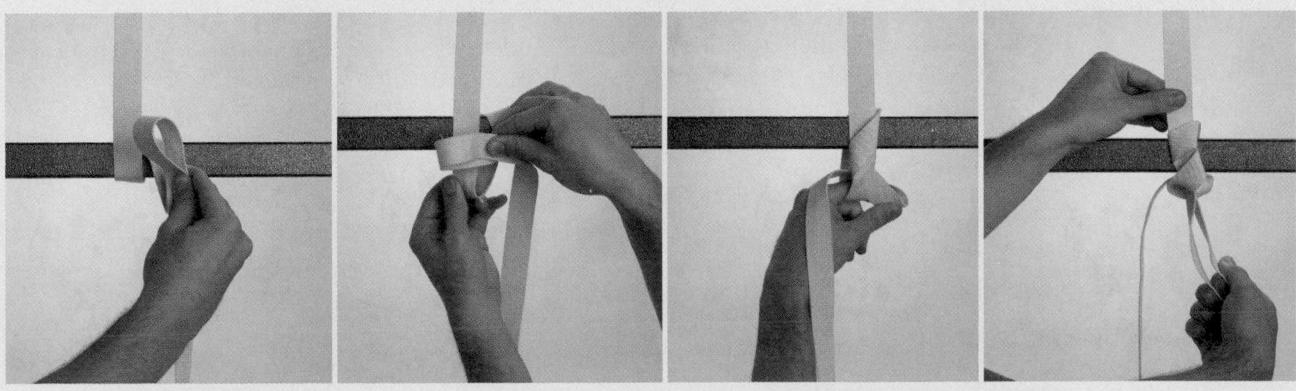

STEP 8 The Posey quick release tie. (Courtesy Posey Company, Arcadia, Calif.)

Continued

STEPS	RATIONALE
10. Assess proper placement of restraint, including skin integrity, pulses, temperature, color, and sensation of the restrained body part. Remove restraints at least every 2 hours (or according to agency policy) and evaluate patient each time. Perform ROM exercises. If patient is violent or noncompliant, remove one restraint at a time and/or have staff assist while removing the restraints.	Provides baseline to later determine if injury develops from restraint. Provides opportunity to change patient's position, perform full ROM, toileting, and exercise and to provide food or fluids.

SAFETY ALERT Violent or aggressive patient must never be left unattended while restraints are off.

STEPS	RATIONALE
11. Secure call light within reach.	Allows patient, family, or caregiver to obtain assistance quickly.

SAFETY ALERT Restraints restrict movement, making patients unable to perform activities of daily living without assistance. Providing food/fluids and assisting with toileting and other activities is essential.

STEPS	RATIONALE
12. Leave bed or chair with wheels locked. Keep bed in lowest position.	Locked wheels prevent bed or chair from moving if patient tries to get out. If patient falls when bed is in lowest position, this reduces chance of injury.
13. See Completion Protocol (inside front cover).	

EVALUATION

1. Following application, evaluate patient's condition for signs of injury routinely (see agency policy). Visual checks can be used if the patient is too agitated to approach. Evaluate for proper placement of restraint, skin integrity, pulses, temperature, color, and sensation of restrained body part.
2. Evaluate patient's need for toileting and fluids and release restraint to provide ROM when an extremity is restrained, at least every 2 hours (see agency policy).
3. Inspect patient for any complications of immobility.
4. Observe IV catheters, urinary catheters, and drainage tubes to determine that they are positioned correctly and that therapy remains uninterrupted.
5. Evaluate patient's need for restraint use on an ongoing basis (see agency policy). When a restraint is used for violent or self-destructive behavior, a physician or licensed independent practitioner must evaluate the patient in person within 1 hour of the initiation of the restraints. Orders may be renewed within the following limits: 4 hours for adults 18 years of age or older, 2 hours for children and adolescents 9 to 17 years of age, 1 hour for children under 9 years of age (TJC, 2009b).
6. Observe patient's behavior and reaction to the presence of restraints.

Unexpected Outcomes and Related Interventions

1. Skin underlying restraint becomes reddened or damaged.
   a. Provide appropriate skin therapy (see Chapter 25).
   b. Notify health care provider and reassess the need for continued use of restraint.
   c. Use a different type of restraint or additional padding.
   d. Remove restraints more frequently. Change wet or soiled restraints.
2. Patient has altered neurovascular status to an extremity (cyanosis; pallor; coldness of the skin; or complaints of tingling, pain, or numbness).
   a. Remove restraint immediately; stay with patient.
   b. Notify health care provider.
3. Patient becomes confused, disoriented, or agitated.
   a. Identify reason for change in behavior and attempt to eliminate cause.
   b. Use restraint alternatives such as companionship or supervision, pain relief, other comfort measures, changing or eliminating bothersome treatments, reality orientation, music therapy, therapeutic touch, reminiscence, behavior modification, companionship, crafts, or active listening (Park and others, 2010).
   c. Determine the need for more or less sensory stimulation.
4. Patient becomes deconditioned related to restraint use.
   a. Remove restraint if at all possible.
   b. Notify health care provider.
   c. Implement strict schedule of ROM (refer to Chapter 16) and consider seeking physical therapy consult.

Recording and Reporting

- Record nursing interventions, including restraint alternatives tried in nurses' notes.
- Record patient's behavior before restraints applied, level of orientation, and patient or family member's statement of understanding of the purpose of restraint and consent for application (if required by agency).

- Record type and location of restraint applied, time applied, and specific initial and ongoing (see agency policy) assessments related to breathing, circulation, skin integrity, and musculoskeletal system integrity in nurses' notes or flow sheet.
- Record patient's behavior after restraint application. Record times patient was assessed, attempts to use alternatives to restraint and patient's response, times restraint was released (temporarily and permanently), and patient's response when restraints were removed.

Sample Documentation

2020 Patient has repeatedly attempted to get out of bed. Remains disoriented to name, date, and location. Provided sitter and attempted to reorient repeatedly without success. Conferred with Dr. Lynch. Patient must remain on bed rest following spinal surgery. Dr. Lynch here to assess patient; ordered belt restraint for next 24 hours.

2030 Belt restraint applied around waist, able to breathe deeply without restriction. Skin under restraint is intact, without redness. Patient able to move extremities. Initiating hourly observations of patient. Instructed patient and family on purpose of device. Family at bedside.

Special Considerations

Pediatric

- When a child needs to be restrained for a procedure, it is best that the person applying the restraint not be the child's parent or guardian.
- When an infant or child requires short-term restraint for treatment or examination that involves the head and neck, a mummy wrap can be effective (Hockenberry and Wilson, 2007).
- Remain with the infant while restrained and remove the restraint immediately after treatment is complete.

Geriatric

- Advanced age is an independent risk factor for fall. When combined with other potential risks associated with aging (e.g., a history of falls, cognitive impairment, visual impairment, gait and balance disorders, musculoskeletal disorders, use of assistive devices for mobility, polypharmacy, incontinence or need for assistance with toileting, and depression), the risk is exacerbated (Ferris, 2008).
- Consider the risks associated with restraints (e.g., increased risk for pressure ulcers, impaired muscular strength and balance, decreased cardiovascular endurance) for the older adult (Gastmans and Milisen, 2006). All the complications of immobility are amplified, leading to an overall increased risk for functional decline.
- Consider the psychological impact. Older adults in restraints are prone to feel shame, a loss of dignity, anxiety, anger, apathy, depression, isolation and disillusionment (Gastmans and Milisen, 2006).

Home Care

- If a restraint is needed for use at home, a health care provider's order is required, and clear instructions should be given to the family caregiver. Clearly document instructions given.

SKILL 4.4 SEIZURE PRECAUTIONS

A seizure involves a sudden, violent, involuntary series of muscle contractions that occur rhythmically such as during acute or chronic seizure disorders, during febrile episodes (especially in children), and after a head injury. Status epilepticus, characterized by prolonged seizures lasting more than 10 minutes or a series of seizures that occur in rapid succession over 30 minutes, is a medical emergency (Eliahu and others, 2008). Observation during a seizure is critical. Observe a patient carefully before, during, and after the seizure so the episode can be documented accurately. Careful observation may help to determine the type of seizure.

The role of the nurse is to protect the patient from harm, assess cardiopulmonary effects, assist with airway management if indicated, and administer antiseizure medications as ordered. Tongue blades are no longer used to maintain an airway. Forcing something into the patient's mouth could result in injury to the jaw, tongue, or teeth and cause stimulation of the gag reflex, thus causing vomiting, aspiration, and respiratory distress. Insert an airway only when there is clear access for insertion, possibly after seizure activity has resolved and if the patient needs airway support. Padded tongue blades do not belong at the bedside and are NOT indicated for use during seizures (South Carolina Department of Disabilities and Special Needs, 2006).

ASSESSMENT

1. Assess patient's seizure history and knowledge of precipitating factors, noting frequency of seizures, presence of aura, body parts affected, and sequence of events if known. Confer with family. *Rationale: Information about seizure enables nurse to anticipate onset of seizure activity.*
2. Assess for medical and surgical conditions that may lead to seizures or worsen existing seizure condition (e.g., electrolyte disturbances, heart disease, excessive fatigue, alcohol or caffeine use). *Rationale: These factors are common conditions that precipitate seizures.*
3. Assess medication history and patient's adherence. Note therapeutic drug levels of anticonvulsants if available. *Rationale: Seizure medications must be taken as prescribed and not stopped suddenly. This may precipitate a seizure.*

4. Assess patient's cultural perspective about the meaning of seizures and their treatment. *Rationale: Some cultures follow different caring practices for a person with seizures.*

PLANNING

Expected Outcomes focus on maintenance of self-esteem and prevention of injury, airway obstruction, and aspiration.

1. Patient does not suffer traumatic physical injury during a seizure.
2. Patient's airway is patent during seizure activity.
3. Patient verbalizes positive self-feelings after a seizure episode.

Delegation and Collaboration

Assessment of patient's risk for seizures cannot be delegated. Care of patients on seizure precautions can be delegated to nursing assistive personnel (NAP). Instruct the NAP about the following:

- Taking immediate action in the event of seizure by protecting patient from falling or injury, not attempting to restrain patient, and not placing anything in patient's mouth
- Informing the registered nurse immediately when seizure activity develops
- Observing the patient's seizure pattern

Equipment

- Padding for side rails and headboard
- Suction machine and Yankauer suction catheter
- Oral airway
- Oxygen via nasal cannula or face mask
- Intravenous (IV) insertion equipment: 0.9% normal saline (NS) infusion
- Emergency medications: IV diazepam (Valium), lorazepam (Ativan), phenytoin (Dilantin), valproate (Depacon)
- Clean gloves
- Equipment for vital signs

IMPLEMENTATION *for* SEIZURE PRECAUTIONS

STEPS	RATIONALE
1. See Standard Protocol (inside front cover).	
2. For patients with known risk, keep bed in lowest position with side rails up. Have oral suction equipment ready at bedside.	Modifications to environment minimize risk of injury during seizure activity. Oral suctioning may be required after a seizure to prevent aspiration of secretions.
3. Provide or encourage use of bracelet or identification card noting existing seizure disorder and medications taken.	Communicates patient's risk for seizure activity to emergency health care providers.
4. *Seizure response*	
a. Position patient safely (1) If standing or sitting, guide patient to floor and protect head by cradling in your lap or placing pillow under head. Turn patient onto side. (2) If patient is in bed, turn patient to side and raise side rails.	Position protects patient from aspiration and traumatic injury, especially head injury.
b. Stay with patient.	
c. Clear surrounding area of furniture.	Ensures that emergency response staff can access patient.
d. Keep patient in side-lying position, supporting head flexed slightly forward.	Position prevents tongue from blocking airway and promotes drainage of secretions, reducing risk of aspiration.
e. Do not restrain. If patient is flailing limbs, hold them loosely. Loosen restrictive clothing/gown.	Prevents musculoskeletal injury and airway obstruction.
f. Do not force any objects into patient's mouth such as fingers, medicine, tongue depressor, or airway when teeth are clenched.	Prevents injury to mouth and nurse's hands.
g. Maintain patient's airway; suction as needed. Provide oxygen if ordered. *Use oral airway only if easy access to oral cavity is possible.*	Prevents hypoxia during seizure activity.
h. Observe sequence and timing of seizure activity. Note type of seizure activity (tonic, clonic, staring, blinking), whether more than one type of seizure occurs, sequence of seizure progression, level of consciousness, nature of breathing, presence of incontinence.	Assists in accurate documentation, diagnosis, and eventual treatment of seizure.

STEPS	RATIONALE
i. Provide patient privacy if possible. Have staff control flow of visitors in area.	Embarrassment is common after a seizure.
5. Status epilepticus is a medical emergency.	Airway occlusion and aspiration are potential complications of this medical emergency.
a. Call health care provider and response team immediately.	
b. Insert an oral airway (see Chapter 30) when jaw is relaxed between seizure activity. Hold airway with curved side up, insert downward until airway reaches back of throat, and then rotate downward and follow natural curve of tongue.	

SAFETY ALERT Do not place fingers in patient's mouth. Patient may accidentally bite nurse's fingers during seizure. Do not force airway into patient's mouth.

STEPS	RATIONALE
c. Access oxygen and suction equipment, keeping airway patent.	Intensive monitoring and treatment are required for this medical emergency.
d. Prepare for IV insertion if saline lock or catheter is not in place. Patient usually receives 0.9% sodium chloride.	Provides route for IV medication.
6. After seizure, assist patient to side-lying position of comfort in bed with side rails up and bed in lowest position (see illustration). Place call light in reach.	Provides for continued safety.

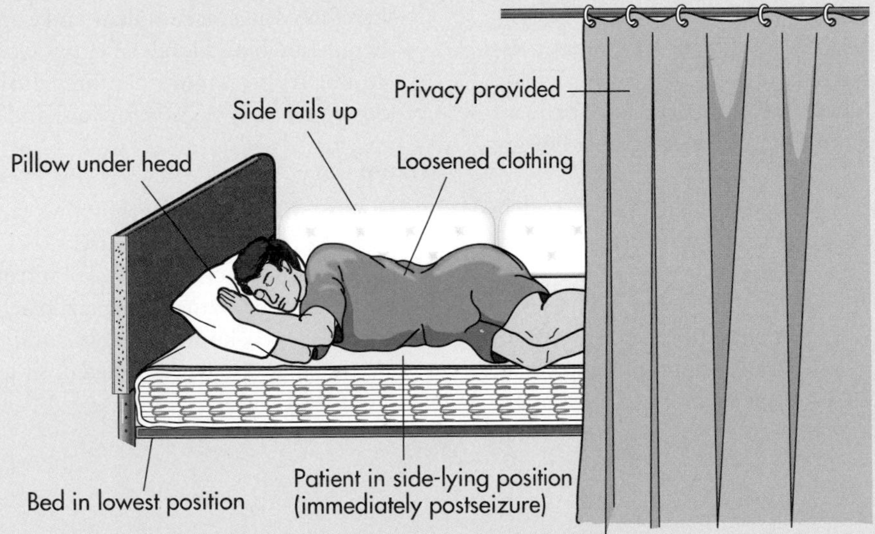

STEP 6 Position of patient following seizure and when on seizure precautions.

STEPS	RATIONALE
7. As patient regains consciousness, reorient and reassure. Explain what happened and provide a quiet, nonstimulating environment. Patient may be confused and experiencing postictal drowsiness. Foster an atmosphere of acceptance and give time for patient to express feelings.	Patients who accept the reality of a disease and integrate this into their own self-concept have higher levels of self-esteem.
8. Pad side rails and headboard if indicated.	Reduces risk for traumatic injury from future seizures. Do not use pillows to pad side rails because they pose a suffocation risk.
9. **See Completion Protocol (inside front cover).**	

EVALUATION

1. Examine patient to determine presence of any traumatic injuries (including oral cavity, extremities) resulting from seizure.
2. Evaluate airway and oxygenation status (oxygen saturation, vital signs), mental status, and orientation after seizure.
3. Ask patient to verbalize feelings after the seizure.

Unexpected Outcomes and Related Interventions

1. Patient suffers traumatic injury.
   a. Continue to protect patient from further injury.
   b. Notify health care provider immediately.
   c. Administer treatments for injury.
   d. Ensure that environment is free of additional safety hazards.
2. Patient verbalizes feelings of embarrassment and humiliation.
   a. Offer support and allow patient to verbalize feelings.
   b. Encourage patient and family to participate in decision making and planning care.

Recording and Reporting

- Record timing of seizure activity, sequence of events, presence of aura (if any), level of consciousness, posture, color, movements of extremities, incontinence, and patient's status (physical and emotional) immediately following seizure.
- Report to physician or health care provider immediately as seizure begins. Status epilepticus is an emergency.

Sample Documentation

1000 Observed patient sitting in chair in room. Cry heard; patient observed sliding to floor, not responding to verbal stimuli. Patient assisted to floor with head supported. Pillow placed under head. Tonic and clonic movements of all four extremities noted, lasting 2 minutes. No cyanosis noted; respiratory pattern slightly irregular. No incontinence noted. At conclusion of tonic and clonic movements, patient slept for 20 minutes; respirations 16 per minute and regular, O_2 saturation 95%.

1020 Patient awake and alert. Requested nurse describe sequence of events. Stated that this was his "usual type of seizure."

Special Considerations

Pediatric

- Teach parents what to observe for in seizures because many times they are present at onset.
- Encourage children with severe atonic seizures to wear helmets.

Geriatric

- Older adults may have symptoms that block the recognition of a seizure disorder such as confusion lasting several days, unusual behaviors, or receptive and expressive language problems (Ettinger, 2007).
- Older adults metabolize anticonvulsants more slowly; therefore drugs accumulate and cause toxicity. Monitor therapeutic blood levels of drugs closely.
- Do not try to remove dentures during a seizure. If they loosen, tilt head slightly forward and remove after seizure.

Home Care

- Discuss with family precipitating factors and care of the patient experiencing a seizure.
- Unless seizure activity is well controlled, instruct patient to not take tub baths or engage in activities such as swimming unless a knowledgeable family member is present. Driving may also be restricted until seizures are controlled for at least 1 year.

PROCEDURAL GUIDELINE 4.1
Fire, Electrical, and Chemical Safety

Fires in health care settings are typically electrical or anesthetic related. Although smoking is not allowed in facilities, smoking-related fires continue to pose a significant risk because of unauthorized smoking. For fire safety the best intervention is prevention. If a fire occurs, health care personnel report the exact location of the fire, contain it, and extinguish it only if safe and possible. All personnel are then mobilized to evacuate patients if necessary. Nursing measures also include complying with agency smoking policies and keeping combustible materials away from heat sources. Most agencies have fire doors that are held open by magnets and close automatically when a fire alarm sounds. Fire doors should never be blocked.

All electrical devices are routinely checked and maintained by health care agency engineering departments. Each biomedical device (e.g., suction machine, intravenous [IV] pump) must have a current safety inspection sticker. All devices must be properly grounded, using a three-prong electrical plug. Generally patients are discouraged from bringing electrical devices to health care agencies. If a patient brings a device, it must be inspected for safe wiring and function before use through the process established by the institution.

Chemicals in medications (e.g., chemotherapy drugs), anesthetic gases, and cleaning solutions are toxic. Chemicals cause injury to the body after skin or mucous membrane contact or ingestion or when vapors are inhaled. Health care facilities provide employees access to material safety data sheets (MSDSs) for each hazardous chemical in the workplace. An MSDS form contains information about

PROCEDURAL GUIDELINE 4.1
Fire, Electrical, and Chemical Safety—cont'd

properties of the chemical and information on safe handling, disposal, and protective equipment to use.

Delegation and Collaboration

The skill of fire, electrical, radiation, and chemical safety can be delegated to nursing assistive personnel (NAP). When an event occurs, a nurse leads the health care team in an emergency response. In the event of fire, this is done in collaboration with the fire department. In the event of a radioactive or chemical event, it is done in collaboration with the appropriate Safety Officer.

Equipment

Fire

- Appropriate fire extinguisher for fire: Type A, B, C, or ABC.

Chemical

- Appropriate personal protective equipment
- MSDS form

Procedural Steps

1. Review agency policies regularly for rapid response to fire, electrical, radiation, and chemical emergency.
2. Know the location of fire alarms, emergency equipment (e.g., fire extinguishers), MSDS forms, exit routes.
3. Assess a patient's mental status and ability to ambulate, transfer, or move to anticipate procedure that will be needed to evacuate patient.
4. Be alert to situations that increase the risk for fire. For example, a patient on oxygen is charging his cell phone in the bed.
5. Know which patients are on oxygen. O_2 delivery may be shut off in the event of a severe fire.
6. Know who keeps a complete current list of patients on the division and patients currently off the unit.
7. Inspect equipment for current maintenance sticker. Check electrical equipment for basic safety features: intact cords and plugs, intact casing. Know agency process for tagging and reporting broken or unsafe equipment.
8. For patients receiving radioactive implants, assess their knowledge of risks of radiation exposure, purpose of safety precautions, and whether they are pregnant or may have visitors who are pregnant.
9. Assess patient and staff understanding of radiation risks and precautions appropriate to the specific situation.
10. *Fire safety (follow the acronym* RACE*)*
    a. *R*escue the patient from immediate injury by removing from area or shielding from fire to avoid burns.
    b. *A*ctivate the fire alarm immediately. Follow agency policy for alerting staff to respond. (In many situations perform Steps a and b simultaneously by using the call system to alert staff while you help patients at risk.)
    c. *C*ontain the fire by (1) closing all doors and windows, (2) turning off oxygen and electrical equipment, and (3) placing wet towels along base of doors.
    d. *E*vacuate patients.
        (1) Direct ambulatory patients to walk by themselves to a safe area. Know the fire exits and emergency evacuation route.
        (2) Move bedridden patients by stretcher, bed, or wheelchair.
        (3) If patient is on life support, maintain respiratory status manually until he or she is removed from fire area.
        (4) For patients who cannot walk or ambulate:
            (a) Place on blanket and drag out of area.
            (b) Use two-person swing: Place patient in sitting position and have two staff members form a seat by clasping forearms together (see illustration). Lift patient into "seat" and carry out of area of danger (see illustration).

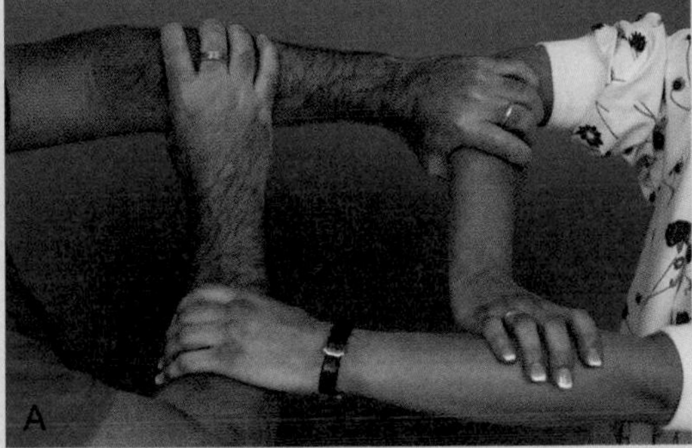

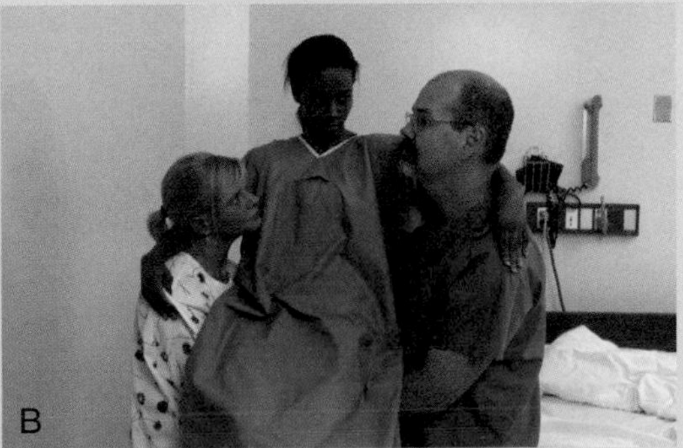

STEP 10d(4)(b) A, Hands positioned to form two-person evacuation swing. **B,** Patient is seated firmly on swing and holds nurses by shoulders for emergency evacuation.

Continued

PROCEDURAL GUIDELINE 4.1
Fire, Electrical, and Chemical Safety—cont'd

(5) Use a "back-strap" method: Stand in front of patient and place patient's arms around your neck. Grasp patient's wrists firmly against your chest. Pull patient onto your back and carry out of danger.

> **SAFETY ALERT** Consider the patient's weight and size when choosing an evacuation carry. Have a staff member assist to avoid injury.

e. *E*xtinguish fire using appropriate fire extinguisher: type A for ordinary combustibles (e.g., wood, cloth, paper, most plastics), type B for flammable liquids (e.g., gasoline, grease, anesthetic gas); type C for electrical equipment, and type ABC for any type of fire.
   (1) To use extinguisher follow the acronym PASS:
      (a) *P*ull the pin (see illustration).
      (b) *A*im nozzle at base of fire.
      (c) *S*queeze extinguisher handles (see illustration).
      (d) *S*weep from side to side to coat area evenly.

11. *Electrical safety*
   a. If a person receives an electrical shock, immediately unplug electrical source and then assess for presence of a pulse.

> **SAFETY ALERT** Do not touch a person who is being shocked while he or she is still engaged with the source of electricity. If unable to disconnect source, call emergency number for assistance.

   b. Once the source of electricity is disconnected, intervene on the person's behalf. If patient is pulseless, institute emergency resuscitation (see Skill 30.3).
   c. Notify emergency personnel and patient's health care provider.
   d. If patient has a pulse and remains alert and oriented, obtain vital signs and assess the skin for signs of thermal injury.

12. *Chemical safety*
   a. Attend to any person exposed to a chemical. Treat chemical splashes to eyes immediately; flush eyes with water and use clean, lukewarm tap water for at least 20 minutes; stand under a shower or place head under running faucet. Remove contact lenses if flushing does not remove them.
   b. Notify persons in the immediate spill area and evacuate all nonessential personnel from area.
   c. Refer to MSDS and, if spilled material is flammable, turn off electric and heat sources.
   d. Avoid breathing vapors of spilled material; apply appropriate respirator.
   e. Use appropriate personal protective equipment to clean up spill.
   f. Dispose of any materials used in cleanup as hazardous waste.

13. Follow agency policy for reporting a sentinel event. Documentation will likely be made as a sentinel event report and not in nurses' notes.

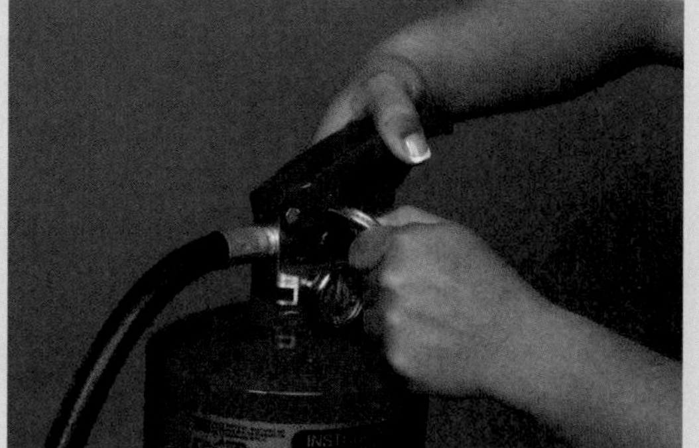

STEP 10e(1)(a) Remove safety pin from fire extinguisher.

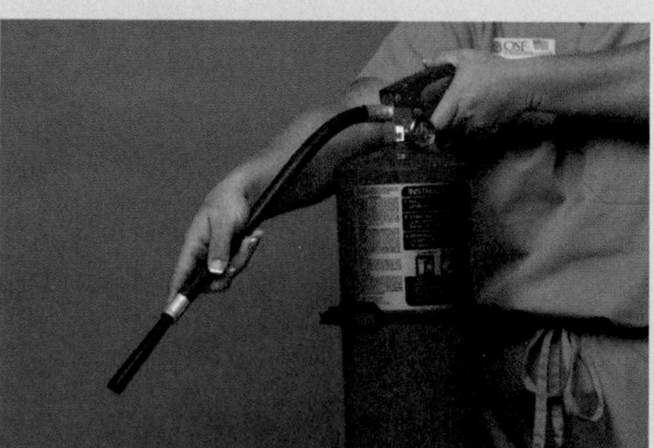

STEP 10e(1)(c) Aim hose at base of fire and squeeze handles, sweeping from side to side.

PROCEDURAL GUIDELINE 4.2
Conducting a Root Cause Analysis

Root cause analysis (RCA) is a process of responding to sentinel events with the purpose of discovering the causes of the event and developing an effective plan for preventing future events. Examples of these events are death of a patient while in restraints or death of a patient related to receiving the wrong chemotherapy. TJC (2010b) requires an RCA of sentinel events with a resultant action plan. An RCA needs to be thorough and credible. RCA is not about placing blame or relieving accountability; it is about looking at all the details that may have contributed to the error. Most facilities have a dedicated safety department that includes a specially trained team to lead all RCAs. The persons closest to the error and persons close to any system processes that may have contributed to the error must participate. This gives the process value for genuine practice improvement and the prevention of similar events in the future. Box 4-2 offers an example of an RCA for a patient fall.

Procedural Steps

1. In response to a sentinel event, ensure that immediate needs of patient/family are met. Report the event according to agency policy.
2. The designated safety team reviews the event such as an error in the patient identification process, a medication error, a patient fall, a treatment delay, or a complication from a procedure and identifies professionals involved in the sentinel event.
3. The team analyzes factors leading to and associated with the sentinel event by asking these questions (TJC, 2010b):
   a. What happened? Describe details of event, when it occurred, and area within hospital affected.
   b. Why did it happen? Describe process or activity in which the event occurred. Use a flow chart to show steps in the process.
   c. What were the factors contributing to the event? Describe steps contributing to the event, the people involved, equipment performance, environmental factors, and factors beyond organization control.
4. For each of the previous questions the team decides if any element was a root cause and whether action should be taken.
5. Further analysis asks why the event happened and the proximate factors contributing to the event. Examples are:
   a. Human resource issues—staffing, competence, staff performance
   b. Educational issues—can orientation and training be improved?
   c. Information management issues—to what degree was all necessary information available, accurate, and complete? Was communication among all participants adequate?
   d. Leadership issues—does the unit culture support risk identification and reduction? What barriers exist for communicating need to prevent adverse events?
6. A number of additional approaches can be used to analyze data in an RCA; for example:
   a. "Ask why five times" (Williams, 2001)
      (1) Use a brainstorming method to identify factors contributing to the event.
      (2) Ask "Why" at least five times to get to as many answers as possible.
   b. Change analysis: Process that follows the following six steps (Williams, 2001).
      (1) Describes the event
      (2) Redescribes the same situation but without the event
      (3) Compares the two situations
      (4) Considers all the differences
      (5) Analyzes the differences
      (6) Identifies the consequences of the differences.
      (7) For example, a patient gets the wrong dose of insulin. The steps leading to the event are detailed. The steps that would have led to the patient receiving the right dose are detailed. The

BOX 4-2 PATIENT FALL

A female patient falls in the bathroom and sustains a serious head injury. In the analysis several proximal events were identified. After returning from x-ray, the transporter left the patient in the room without handing the patient off to a caregiver, even though there was a specific hand-off process. In addition, nurses in the procedure area did not call to alert the registered nurses (RNs) on the unit that the patient was returning. The patient's spouse thought that he could safely walk his wife to the bathroom. The patient thought that it would be OK. The nursing unit was very busy at the time; several patients were returning from surgery. There was little staff education and poor enforcement of the transporter hand-off process. Transporters may not have felt supported when they stayed and waited for the nurse to accept the patient. Therefore the hand off was not a well established practice, even though it was hospital policy. The RN who found the patient on the floor was able to get emergency response quickly. Action plan includes steps to in-service all transporters and nursing staff in procedure area and nursing division about the hand-off process. Charge nurses on division are designated to take phone calls from the procedure area when the patient is returning to the division.

Continued

PROCEDURAL GUIDELINE 4.2
Conducting a Root Cause Analysis—cont'd

differences are reviewed to see if a root cause can be identified.

c. Fish Diagrams (Fig. 4-2) (Gano, 2007)
   (1) Arrange a list of causal factors in a fish diagram. Depending on the model used, there are predetermined categories (e.g., People, Equipment, Environment) into which causes for events should be able to be identified.

7. Develop an action plan for risk reduction—For each factor in the analysis that needs an action, develop a plan.
8. Implement the plan—Consider if pilot testing the planned improvement is needed.
9. Evaluate results.

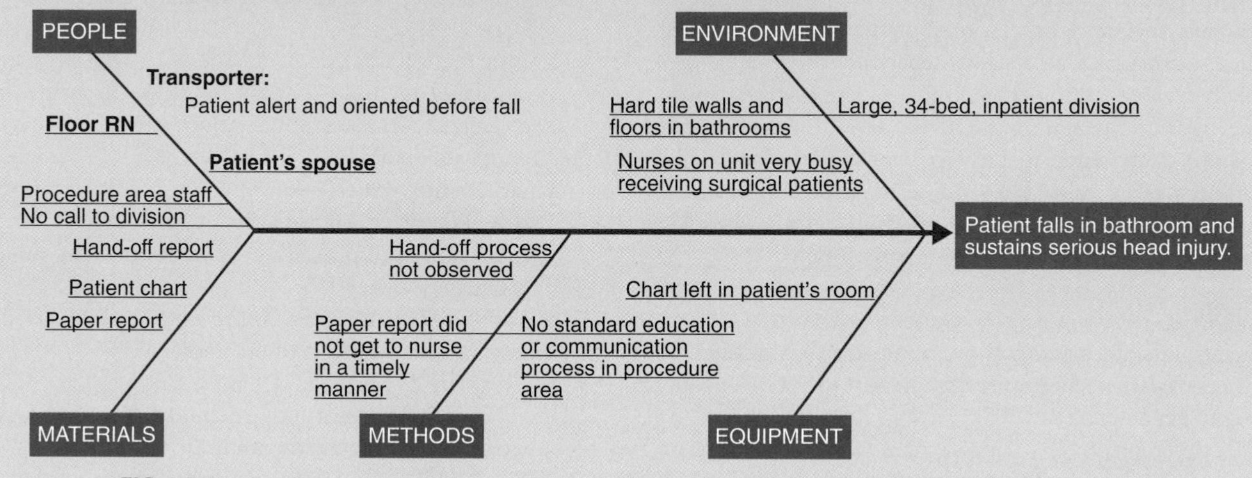

FIG 4-2 Root cause analysis for a patient fall. (Adapted from the Institute for Healthcare Improvement, IHI, 2004.)

REVIEW QUESTIONS

Case Study for Questions 1 and 2

Mrs. Smith is 85 years old. She has severe pneumonia and is slightly confused. Her family states that she usually has a clear mind. She is on many medications, including omeprazole (Prilosec), furosemide (Lasix), and metformin (Glucophage). She is receiving intravenous (IV) antibiotics. You've reminded her several times not to pull on her IV line, but she has pulled out three IV lines in the last 24 hours. Her family is staying with her, but she is too quick for them. The nurse has decided to try a restraint alternative next.

1. Which of the following is the best approach to prevent removal of Mrs. Smith's IV line?
   1. Obtain a health care provider's order for a restraint.
   2. Place a tethered mitten on the hand opposite the extremity with the IV line.
   3. Camouflage the IV site with a stockinette.
   4. Place a soft wrist restraint on the extremity opposite the extremity with the IV line.
2. Mrs. Smith becomes agitated and keeps trying to get out of bed. The nurse assesses her risk for fall. Which of the following factors increase her risk for fall? Select all that apply.
   1. Her age
   2. Multiple medications
   3. Patient care equipment
   4. History of pneumonia
   5. Altered cognition
3. The nurse's co-worker is standing in some spilled water holding the refrigerator door. He is being electrocuted. What is the first thing that the nurse is going to do?
   1. Take his vital signs.
   2. Call the rapid response team.
   3. Unplug the refrigerator.
   4. Wipe up the water from the floor.
4. The nurse enters a patient's room to find him actively seizing. What is the nurse's primary responsibility?
   1. Insert an airway.
   2. Call the physician.
   3. Protect the patient from harm.
   4. Put up the side rails.
5. The nurse is asked to participate in a root cause analysis related to a serious medical error that occurred on her nursing unit. Why should the nurse be pleased to participate in this project?
   1. The nurse gets off of the division for several hours.
   2. This is a problem-solving approach to preventing future similar errors.
   3. The nurse wants to be sure that the person who committed the error is punished.
   4. It will provide the nurse with a chance to network.

6. The nurse is giving Mr. Jones his morning medications. When she says, "Here is your warfarin," he responds, "I don't take warfarin." Which response is best in this situation?
   1. Tell him the doctor ordered it for him and he should take it.
   2. Tell him that he probably calls it by a different name at home.
   3. Ignore him because he doesn't understand his medications.
   4. Hold the medication until the nurse is able to verify that the patient should take it.
7. Mr. Macalister threw his cigarette in the trash as the nurse walked into his room. Now the trash is smoldering. What is the first thing that the nurse should do?
   1. Activate the fire alarm.
   2. Contain the fire with a blanket.
   3. Move Mr. Macalister into the hall.
   4. Tell Mr. Macalister that he cannot smoke in the hospital.
8. The nurse is rounding on a patient with wrist restraints. It has been 2 hours since the last rounds for this patient. Which of the following will she do? Select all that apply.
   1. Release the restraints for range of motion (ROM).
   2. Assess the extremity for perfusion and skin integrity.
   3. Offer toileting.
   4. Offer a drink of water.
9. Mrs. Jones tends to wander. Sometimes she forgets where she is. She likes to go down the stairs and outside. What can the nurse do to avoid restraining her? Select all that apply.
   1. Schedule walks into her day.
   2. Offer a diversional activity.
   3. Move her to a room close to the nurses' station.
   4. Notify the police that she may be found wandering outside.

REFERENCES

Currie L: Fall and injury prevention. In Hughes R, editor: *Patient safety and quality: an evidence-based handbook for nurses*, Rockville, Md, 2008, Agency for Healthcare Research and Quality.

Ebersole P and others: *Toward healthy aging: human needs and nursing response*, ed 7, St Louis, 2008, Mosby.

Eliahu SF and others: I. Status epilepticus, *South Med J* 101(4), April 2008.

Ettinger AB: *Diagnosing and treating epilepsy in the elderly—US Neurological Disease 1*, October 2007, at http://www.touchneurology.com/files/article_pdfs/neuro_7343, accessed February 14, 2010.

Ferris M: Protecting hospitalized elders from falling, *Topics Adv Pract Nurs eJournal* 8(4), 2008, http://www.medscape.com/viewarticle/585961, accessed February 14, 2010.

Gano DL: *Apollo root cause analysis—a new way of thinking: comparison of common root cause analysis tools and methods*, 2007, http://www.apollorca.com/_public/site/files/ARCA_Appendix.pdf, accessed August 18, 2010.

Gastmans C, Milisen K: Use of physical restraint in nursing homes: clinical-ethical considerations, *J Med Ethics* 32(3), 2006, http://www.ncbi.nlm.nih.gov/pmc/articles/PMC2564468/, accessed February 14, 2010.

HCPro, Inc: Joint Commission and CMS alignment: restraint management, Accreditation Monthly, June 9, 2009, http://www.hcpro.com/ACC-234182-1000/Joint-Commission-and-CMS-Alignment-Restraint-Management.html, accessed February 12, 2010.

Hockenberry MJ, Wilson D: *Wong's nursing care of infants and children*, ed 8, St Louis, 2007, Mosby.

Institute for Clinical Systems Improvement (ICSI): *Prevention of falls (acute care)*, 2008, http://www.guideline.gov/summary/summary.aspx?ss=15&doc_id=13697&nbr=007031&string=patient+AND+falls#s23, accessed through National Guidelines Clearinghouse (NGC) February 7, 2010.

Krauss MJ and others: A case-control study of patient, medication, and care-related risk factors for inpatient falls, *J Gen Intern Med* 20:116, 2005.

Krauss MJ and others: Intervention to prevent falls on the medical service in a teaching hospital, *Infect Control Hosp Epidemiol* 29(6), 2008.

Levy HD: Pharmacological therapy and the impact on falls in the elderly, *Expert Rev Clin Pharmacol* 1(6), 2008, http://www.expert-reviews.com/doi/pdf/10.1586/17512433.1.6.721, accessed February 13, 2009.

Meiner SE, Lueckenotte AG: *Gerontologic nursing*, ed 3, St Louis, 2006, Mosby.

National Association of Psychiatric Health Systems (NAPHS) Restraint and Seclusion: Implementing the CMS Hospital Patients' Rights Conditions of Participation Final Rule 2007, http://www.naphs.org/documents/patientrightsfinalrule_000.ppt, accessed February 11, 2010.

National Guidelines Clearinghouse, U.S. Department of Health and Human Services: *Prevention of falls and fall injuries in the older adult*, 2005, http://www.guideline.gov/, accessed September 27, 2010.

North American Nursing Diagnosis Association (NANDA) International: *Nursing diagnoses: definitions and classification 2009-2011*, United Kingdom, 2009, Wiley-Blackwell.

Park M, Tang J: Changing the practice of physical restraint use in acute care, *J Gerontol Nurs* 33(2):9, 2007.

Park M and others: *Changing the practice of physical restraint use in acute care*, Iowa City, Ia, 2010, University of Iowa Gerontological Nursing Interventions Research Center, Research Translation and Dissemination Core, http://www.guideline.gov/summary/summary.aspx?ss=15&doc_id=8626&nbr=&string=, accessed through National Guidelines Clearinghouse on February 13, 2010.

Poe SS and others: The Johns Hopkins fall risk assessment tool post implementation evaluation, *J Nurs Care Qual* 22(4), 2007.

Rossi SM: Tips for improving manager hand-off communication, *Nurs Manage* 40(12), 2009.

South Carolina Department of Disabilities and Special Needs: *Nursing management of seizures*, 2006, http://ddsn.sc.gov/providers/manualsandguidelines/Documents/HealthCareGuidelines/NursingMgmtSeizures.pdf, accessed February 14, 2010.

The Joint Commission: *Facts about patient safety*, 2009a, accessed January 10, 2010 at http://www.jointcommission.org/GeneralPublic/PatientSafety/.

The Joint Commission: *Provision of care, treatment, and services: restraint/seclusion for hospitals that use the JC for deemed status purposes*, 2009b. http://www.jointcommission.org/accreditationprograms/Hospitals/Standards/09_FAQs, accessed March, 2010.

The Joint Commission, National Patient Safety Goals (NPSGs): Chapter outline and overview: hospital, 2010a, http://www.jointcommission.org/NR/rdonlyres/CEE2A577-BC61-4338-8780-43F132729610/0/NPSGChapterOutline_FINAL_HAP_2010.pdf, accessed January 31, 2010.

The Joint Commission: *A framework for a root cause analysis and action plan in response to a sentinel event, Sentinel Event Forms and Tools*, 2010b, http://www.jointcommission.org/sentinelevents/forms, accessed February 22, 2010.

Tinetti ME: Preventing falls in elderly persons, *N Engl J Med* 348(1):42, 2003.

Tzeng HM: Understanding the prevalence of inpatient falls associated with toileting in adult acute care settings, *J Nurs Care Qual* 25(1):22-30, 2010.

VA National Center for Patient Safety: *VHA NCPS escape and elopement management*, 2010, http://www4.va.gov/ncps/CogAids/EscapeElope/index.html#page=page-13, accessed February 11, 2010.

Williams PM: Techniques for root cause analysis, *Baylor University Medical Center Proc* 12:154-157, 2001, http://www.pubmedcentral.nih.gov/articlerender.fcgi?artid=1292997, accessed January 31, 2009.

Zijlstra GA and others: Interventions to reduce fear of falling in community-living older people: a systematic review, *J Am Geriatr Soc* 55(4):603, 2007.

CHAPTER

5

Infection Control

evolve WEBSITE

http://evolve.elsevier.com/Perry/nursinginterventions
Video Clips
Nursing Skills Online

Infection prevention practices that reduce or eliminate sources and transmission of infection help to protect patients and health care providers from disease. The nurse's role is vital in the prevention and control of infection. As a nurse, you are responsible for teaching patients and their families about the signs and symptoms of infections, modes of transmission, and methods of prevention.

Health care–associated infections (HAIs), formerly called *nosocomial infections,* are those that result from delivery of health services in a health care setting and were not present on admission (CDC, 2007). In hospitals, HAIs account for an estimated 2 million infections, 90,000 deaths, and $4.5 billion in excess health care costs annually (CDC, 2006a). Such infections are more likely to develop in patients with chronic illnesses; immunosuppressed, poorly nourished older adults; and patients on broad-spectrum antibiotics (Fardo, 2009; Stricof, 2009).

PATIENT-CENTERED CARE

The presence of a pathogen does not mean that an infection will begin. An infection develops in a cyclical process called the *chain of infection,* which includes the following six elements: (1) an infectious agent or pathogen, (2) a reservoir or source for pathogen growth, (3) a portal of exit from the reservoir, (4) a method or mode of transmission, (5) a portal of entrance into the host, and (6) a susceptible host. An infection develops if the chain remains intact (Fig. 5-1). Nurses use infection-control practices to break an element of the chain so infection will not be transmitted. The nurse's efforts to minimize the onset and spread of infection are based on asepsis and the principles of aseptic technique. Asepsis is defined as the absence of disease-producing (pathogenic) organisms that involves the purposeful prevention of transfer of microorganisms (Iwamoto, 2009). The two types of aseptic techniques that a nurse practices are medical and surgical asepsis.

Medical asepsis, or clean technique, includes procedures used to reduce the number of and prevent the spread of microorganisms (Box 5-1). Hand hygiene, barrier techniques (e.g., use of gloves and gown), and routine environmental cleaning are examples of medical asepsis. Surgical asepsis, or sterile technique, includes procedures used to eliminate all microorganisms from an area (Box 5-2). Sterilization destroys all microorganisms and their spores (Rutala, 2009). Nurses in the operating room (OR), labor and delivery, and procedural areas practice sterile technique. Nurses also use surgical aseptic techniques at the patient's bedside in three situations:

1. During procedures that require intentional perforation of a patient's skin such as insertion of an intravenous (IV) catheter
2. When the integrity of the skin is broken such as with a surgical incision or burn
3. During procedures that involve insertion of devices or surgical instruments into normally sterile body cavities (e.g., insertion of a urinary catheter).

SAFETY

In 2007 the Centers for Disease Control and Prevention (CDC) updated guidelines for the set of precautions known as *Standard Precautions* (CDC, 2007). Part of the rationale for the development of standard precautions is that any patient may be a source for infection. Most microorganisms causing infections or disease are in colonized body substances of patients, regardless of whether a culture confirmed an infection and a diagnosis was made.

Body substances such as feces, urine, mucus, and wound drainage can contain potentially infectious organisms. All

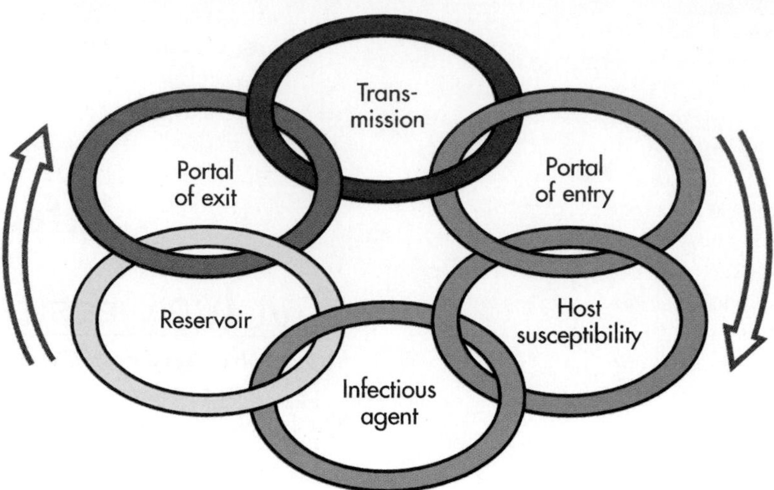

FIG 5-1 Chain of infection.

BOX 5-1 MEDICAL ASEPSIS PRINCIPLES

- Use hand hygiene with an appropriate alcohol-based instant hand antiseptic or soap and water as an essential part of patient care and infection prevention.
- Always know a patient's susceptibility to infection. Age, nutritional status, stress, disease processes, and forms of medical therapy place patients at risk.
- Recognize the elements of the chain of infection and initiate measures to prevent the onset and spread of infection.
- Consistently incorporate the basic principles of asepsis into patient care.
- Protect fellow health care workers from exposure to infectious agents through proper use and disposal of equipment.
- Be aware of body sites where nosocomial infections are most likely to develop (e.g., urinary or respiratory tract). This enables you to direct preventive measures.

BOX 5-2 SURGICAL ASEPSIS PRINCIPLES

- All items used within a sterile field must be sterile.
- A sterile barrier that has been permeated by punctures, tears, or moisture must be considered contaminated.
- Once a sterile package is opened, a 2.5 cm (1 inch) border around the edges is considered unsterile.
- Tables draped as part of a sterile field are considered sterile only at table level.
- If there is any question or doubt about the sterility of an item, the item is considered unsterile.
- Sterile persons or items contact only sterile items; unsterile persons or items contact only unsterile items.
- Movement around and in the sterile field must not compromise or contaminate the sterile field.
- A sterile object or field out of the range of vision or an object held below a person's waist is contaminated.
- A sterile object or field becomes contaminated by prolonged exposure to air; stay organized and complete any procedure as soon as possible.

patients are at risk for carrying an infection, which requires health care workers to use standard precautions to prevent exposure. Fundamental to standard precautions is the use of barrier protection. Barrier protection includes the appropriate use of personal protective equipment (PPE) such as gloves, masks or respirators, eyewear, and gowns to protect health care providers from exposure to blood and body fluids (CDC, 2005b).

Barrier protection protects the health care worker from the patient's blood and body fluids and helps prevent the transfer of organisms to other patients, health care workers, and the environment. It is also an important technique for protecting patients who are immunosuppressed (e.g., patients receiving chemotherapy). The use of some form of PPE is indicated for all patients who potentially have an infection that can be transmitted to others. The CDC (2005a) and the Occupational Safety and Health Administration (OSHA, 2001) have stressed the importance of barrier protection to prevent the transmission of diseases such as hepatitis B, acquired immunodeficiency syndrome, and tuberculosis (TB).

As a nurse, you help to ensure that all health care providers (e.g., respiratory therapists, physicians, other nurses) working with patients and support staff (e.g., housekeepers) maintain infection prevention practices at all times. This applies to family members as well. When a hospitalized patient has an infection, the nurse decides on the optimal room placement to minimize the chances of infection spreading to other patients. In addition, two patients with "like" infections can be placed in the same room. This is called *cohorting*. The knowledgeable and judicious use of infection prevention practices can make a difference as to whether a patient recovers from an illness or develops serious or even fatal complications.

EVIDENCE-BASED PRACTICE TRENDS

Herud T and others: Association between use of hand hygiene products and rates of healthcare-associated infections in a large university hospital in Norway, *Am J Infect Control* 37(4):311-317, 2009.

Herud and others (2009) conducted a study comparing the amount of hand-hygiene products used within a hospital with infection rates. They observed a decline in infections from 8% to 6% with increased use of hand-hygiene products. Handwashing continues to be an important and effective infection prevention measure, but compliance is often low. Deterrents to handwashing compliance include the amount of time required for soap-and-water handwashing with heavy workloads, skin irritation and dryness from frequent handwashing, inconvenient access to sinks, and inadequate knowledge of hand-hygiene protocols (CDC, 2002). The development of alcohol-based hand antiseptics for reducing bacterial counts on the hands offers an alternative to traditional handwashing that is highly effective. Hand hygiene effectively reduces HAIs when performed correctly (WHO, 2009).

SKILL 5.1 HAND HYGIENE

- **Nursing Skills Online: Infection Control, Lesson 2**

Video Clips

Hand hygiene is a general term that applies to handwashing, antiseptic handwash, antiseptic hand rub, or surgical hand antisepsis. Handwashing refers to washing hands thoroughly with plain soap and water. An antiseptic handwash is defined as washing hands with water and soap containing an antiseptic agent. The use of antimicrobial soap (antiseptic) is recommended in certain health care settings. Antimicrobials effectively reduce bacterial counts on the hands and often have residual antimicrobial effects that last for several hours. An antiseptic hand rub is an alcohol-based waterless product that, when applied to all surfaces of the hands, reduces the number of microorganisms on the hands. These alcohol-based foams or gels contain cosmetic emollients to prevent skin dryness. Surgical hand antisepsis is an antiseptic handwash or antiseptic hand rub that surgical personnel use before performing a surgical procedure (see Chapter 29).

The decision to perform hand hygiene depends on four factors: (1) the intensity or degree of contact with patients or contaminated objects, (2) the amount of contamination that may occur with the contact, (3) the patient's or health care worker's susceptibility to infection, and (4) the procedure or activity to be performed (Haas, 2009). *Hand hygiene is not an option.* It is a critical responsibility of all health care workers. Follow these guidelines for hand hygiene (WHO, 2009; CDC, 2008):

1. When hands are visibly dirty, when soiled with blood or other body fluids, before eating, and after using the toilet, wash hands with either plain soap and water or an antimicrobial soap and water.
2. Wash hands if exposed to spore-forming organisms such as *Clostridium difficile* or *Bacillus anthracis.*
3. If hands are not visibly soiled, use an alcohol-based hand rub for routinely decontaminating hands in the following clinical situations:
   a. Before and after having direct contact with patients
   b. Before applying sterile gloves and inserting an invasive device such as indwelling urinary catheters and peripheral vascular catheters
   c. After contact with body fluids or excretions, mucous membranes, or nonintact skin
   d. After contact with wound dressings (if hands are not visibly soiled)
   e. When moving from a contaminated body site to a clean body site during patient care
   f. After contact with inanimate objects (e.g., medical equipment) in the immediate vicinity of the patient
   g. After removing gloves

ASSESSMENT

1. Inspect surface of hands for breaks or cuts in skin or cuticles. Cover any skin lesions with a dressing before providing patient care. If lesions are too large to cover, you may be restricted from direct patient care. *Rationale: Open cuts or wounds can harbor high concentrations of microorganisms. Agency policy often prevents nurses from caring for high-risk patients if open lesions are present on hands.*
2. Inspect hands for visible soiling. *Rationale: Visible soiling requires handwashing with soap and water.*
3. Note condition of nails. Avoid artificial nails, extenders, and long or unkempt nails. Natural nail tips should be less than ¼ inch long. See agency policy. *Rationale: Subungual areas of hand harbor high concentrations of bacteria. Long nails and chipped or old polish increase number of bacteria residing on nails, requiring more vigorous hand hygiene. Artificial nails increase the microbial load on hands* (CDC, 2008).
4. Consider the type of nursing activity being performed. The decision whether to use an antiseptic or not depends on the procedure that you will perform and the patient's immune status. *Rationale: Determines hand hygiene technique to use.*

PLANNING

Expected Outcomes focus on preventing the transmission of infection.

1. Hands and areas under fingernails are clean and free of debris.

Delegation and Collaboration

The skill of hand hygiene is performed by all caregivers. Hand hygiene is not optional.

Equipment

Handwashing

- Easy-to-reach sink with warm running water
- Antimicrobial or nonantimicrobial soap
- Paper towels or air dryer
- Disposable nail cleaner (optional)

Antiseptic Hand Rub

- Alcohol-based waterless antiseptic containing emollient

IMPLEMENTATION *for* HAND HYGIENE

STEPS	RATIONALE
1. Be sure fingernails are short, filed, and smooth.	Many microorganisms on hands come from beneath the fingernails.
2. Push wristwatch and long uniform sleeves above wrists. Avoid wearing rings during surgical scrubs.	Provides complete access to fingers, hands, and wrists (CDC, 2002; WHO, 2009).
3. *Antiseptic hand rub*	
a. Dispense ample amount of product into palm of one hand (see illustration).	Use enough product to thoroughly cover hands.
b. Rub hands together, covering all surfaces of hands and fingers with antiseptic (see illustration).	Provides enough time for antimicrobial solution to work.
c. Rub hands together until the alcohol is dry. Allow hands to dry completely before applying gloves.	Removes transient organisms. Drying ensures complete antimicrobial action.
4. *Handwashing using regular or antimicrobial soap*	
a. Stand in front of sink, keeping hands and uniform away from sink surface. (If hands touch sink during handwashing, repeat steps.)	Inside of sink is a contaminated area. Reaching over sink increases risk of touching edge, which is contaminated.
b. Turn on water. Turn faucet on or push knee pedals laterally to regulate flow and temperature.	Knee pedals within the OR and treatment areas are preferred to prevent hand contact with faucet. Faucet handles have been found likely to be contaminated with organic debris and microorganisms (AORN, 2007).
c. Avoid splashing water against uniform.	Microorganisms travel and grow in moisture.
d. Regulate flow of water so temperature is warm.	Warm water removes less of the protective oils.
e. Wet hands and wrists thoroughly under running water. Keep hands and forearms lower than elbows during washing.	Hands are the most contaminated parts to be washed. Water flows from least to most contaminated area, rinsing microorganisms into sink.

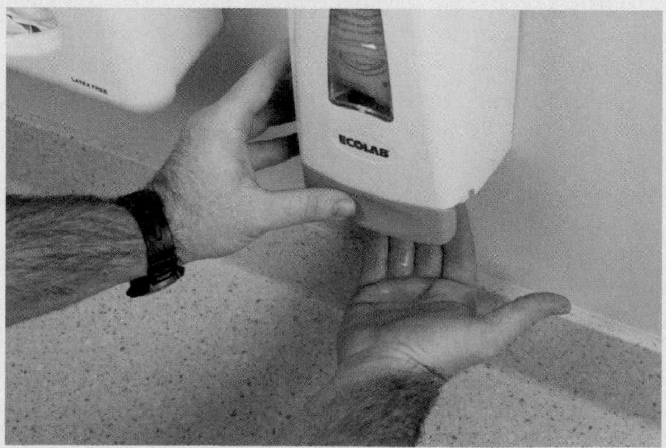

STEP 3a Apply waterless antiseptic to hands.

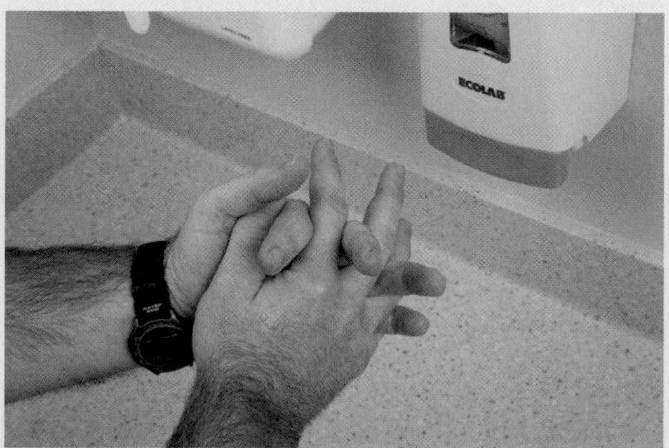

STEP 3b Rub hands thoroughly.

STEPS	RATIONALE
f. Apply 3 to 5 mL of soap and rub hands together vigorously, lathering thoroughly (see illustration). Soap granules and leaflet preparations may be used.	Necessary to ensure that all surfaces of hands and fingers are covered and cleansed.
g. Perform hand hygiene using plenty of lather and friction *for at least 15 seconds.* Interlace fingers and rub palms and backs of hands with circular motion at least 5 times each. Keep fingertips down to facilitate removal of microorganisms.	Soap cleanses by emulsifying fat and oil and lowering surface tension. Friction and rubbing mechanically loosen and remove dirt and transient bacteria. Interlacing fingers and thumbs ensures that you cleanse all surfaces.
h. Areas underlying fingernails are often soiled. Clean with fingernails of other hand and additional soap or with an orangewood stick *(optional).*	Area under nails can be highly contaminated, which increases risk for transmission of infection from nurse to patient.

SAFETY ALERT Do not tear or cut skin under or around nail.

STEPS	RATIONALE
i. Rinse hands and wrists thoroughly, keeping hands down and elbows up (see illustration).	Rinsing mechanically washes away dirt and microorganisms.
j. Dry hands thoroughly from fingers to wrists and forearms with paper towel or warm air dryer.	Drying from cleanest (fingertips) to least clean (forearms) area avoids contamination. Drying prevents chapping and roughened skin.

SAFETY ALERT Paper towels should dispense cleanly without hand or paper-towel contact with other surfaces.

STEPS	RATIONALE
k. If used, discard paper towel in proper container.	Prevents transfer of microorganisms.
l. Use clean, dry paper towel to turn off hand faucet. Avoiding touching handles with hands. Turn off water with knee pedals (if applicable).	Prevents transfer of pathogens from faucet to hands (Haas, 2009).
m. If hands are dry or chapped at end of shift, use a small amount of lotion or barrier cream dispensed from an individual-use container.	There is a risk of organism growth in lotion; thus it should not be applied during patient care activities.

SAFETY ALERT Large, refillable containers of lotion have been associated with HAIs and should not be used.

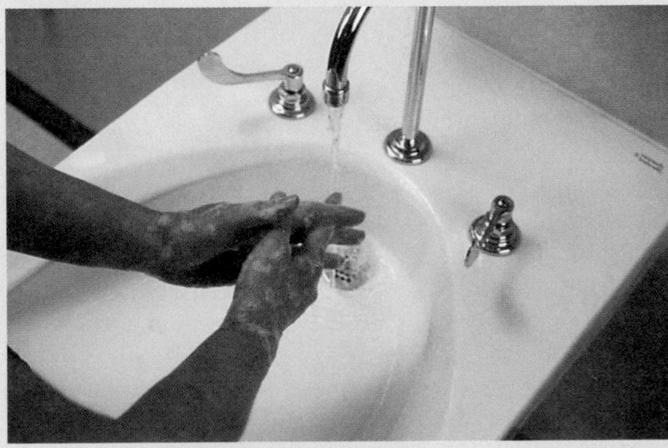

STEP 4f Lather hands thoroughly.

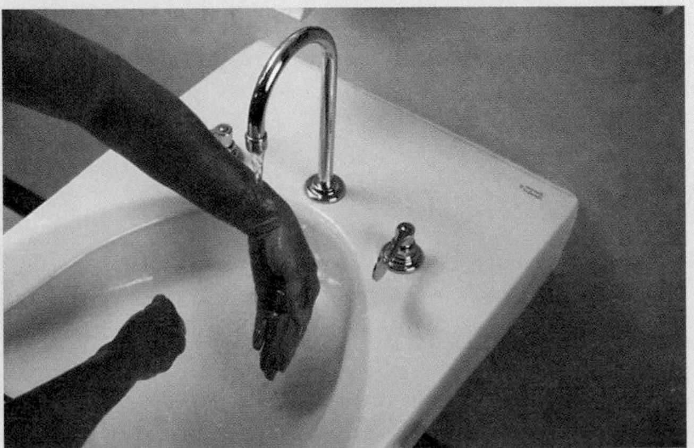

STEP 4i Rinse hands.

EVALUATION

1. Inspect surfaces of hands for obvious signs of soil or other contaminants.
2. Inspect hands for dermatitis or cracked skin.

Unexpected Outcomes and Related Interventions

1. Hands or areas under fingernails remain soiled.
   a. Repeat hand hygiene.
2. Repeated use of soaps or antiseptics cause dermatitis or cracked skin.
   a. Rinse and dry hands thoroughly; avoid excessive amounts of soap; try various products; use hand lotions or barrier creams. Small containers are preferred because large containers have been found to harbor pathogens.

Recording and Reporting

- It is unnecessary to document handwashing.
- Report dermatitis, psoriasis, and cuts to agency employee health and/or infection-control department.

Special Considerations

Gerontological

- Older adults are at greater risk for infection.
- The impact of infection is greater for older adults. Hand hygiene by staff is essential.

SKILL 5.2 APPLYING PERSONAL PROTECTIVE EQUIPMENT

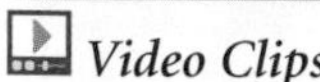 *Video Clips*

Certain procedures performed at a patient's bedside require the application of PPE such as a mask, cap, eyewear, gown, or gloves. Standard precautions require nurses to wear clean gloves before coming in contact with mucous membranes, nonintact skin, blood, body fluids, or other infectious material. Nurses wear gloves routinely when performing a variety of procedures (e.g., nasogastric tube insertion, perineal care, enema administration). Masks are worn when nurses work over sterile areas or equipment, such as changing a central line dressing. Protective eyewear becomes important when there is the risk of the eyes being exposed to the splattering of blood or other body fluids.

Always assess a patient's potential for acquiring an infection before applying a mask or other PPE (e.g., does the patient have a large open wound, or do you, as the nurse, have a respiratory infection?). If you wear a mask, change it when it becomes moist or soiled (e.g., splattered with blood). Consider wearing a surgical cap to secure loose hair that might contaminate a sterile field. Follow standard precautions whenever using PPE.

ASSESSMENT

1. Review type of procedure to be performed and consult agency policy regarding use of PPE. *Rationale: Not all procedures require PPE. Ensures that nurse and patient are properly protected.*
2. If you have symptoms of a respiratory infection, either avoid performing the procedure or apply a mask. *Rationale: A greater number of pathogenic microorganisms reside within the respiratory tract when infection is present.*
3. Assess the patient's risk for infection (e.g., older adult, neonate, immunocompromised patient). *Rationale: Some patients are at greater risk for acquiring an infection; thus you must use additional protective barriers.*

PLANNING

Expected Outcomes focus on prevention of localized or systemic infection.

1. Patient remains afebrile 24 to 48 hours after the procedure or during course of repeated procedures.
2. Patient displays no signs of localized infection (e.g., redness, tenderness, edema, drainage) or systemic infection (e.g., fever, change in white blood cell [WBC] count) 24 hours after the procedure.

Delegation and Collaboration

All health care providers use clean gloves. The skill of applying PPE can be delegated to nursing assistive personnel (NAP). Instruct the NAP to:

- Be available to hand off equipment or assist with patient positioning during a sterile procedure.
- Perform hand hygiene after glove removal.

Equipment

- Clean gloves
- Gown (Gowns may be either disposable or reusable depending on facility protocol.)
- Mask
- Surgical cap (Note: Use if required by agency policy or to secure hair to prevent contamination of sterile field.)
- Hairpins, rubber bands, or both
- Protective eyewear (e.g., goggles or glasses with appropriate side shields)

IMPLEMENTATION *for* APPLYING PERSONAL PROTECTIVE EQUIPMENT

STEPS	RATIONALE
1. **See Standard Protocol (inside front cover).**	Prevents transmission of microorganisms.
2. **Apply gown**, with opening to the back. Be sure that it covers all outer garments. Pull sleeves down to wrist. Tie securely at neck and waist.	Prevents transmission of infection and protects the NAP when patient has excessive drainage or discharges.
3. **Apply a cap.**	
a. If hair is long, comb back behind ears and secure.	Cap must cover all hair entirely.
b. Secure hair in place with pins.	Long hair should not fall down or cause cap to slip and expose hair.
c. Apply cap over head as you would apply a hair net. Be sure that all hair fits under edges of cap.	Loose hair hanging over sterile field contaminates objects on sterile field.
4. **Apply a mask.**	
a. Find top edge of mask, which usually has a thin metal strip along the edge.	Pliable metal fits snugly against bridge of nose.
b. Hold mask by top two strings or loops, keeping top edge above bridge of nose.	Prevents contact of hands with clean facial portion of mask. Mask covers all of nose.
c. Tie two top strings in a bow at top of back of head over cap (if worn), with strings above ears (see illustration).	Position of ties at top of head provides a tight fit. Strings over ears may cause irritation.
d. Tie two lower ties in a bow snugly around neck, with mask well under chin (see illustration).	Prevents escape of microorganisms through sides of mask as nurse talks and breathes.
e. Gently pinch upper metal band around bridge of nose.	Prevents microorganisms from escaping around nose.
f. *Option:* In some cases you will be required to wear a fitted respirator mask. Type and fit-testing will depend on type of precautions and facility policy.	
5. **Apply protective eyewear.**	
a. Apply protective glasses, goggles, or face shield comfortably over eyes and check that vision is clear.	Positioning can affect clarity of vision.
b. Be sure that eyewear fits snugly around forehead and face.	Ensures that eyes are fully protected.

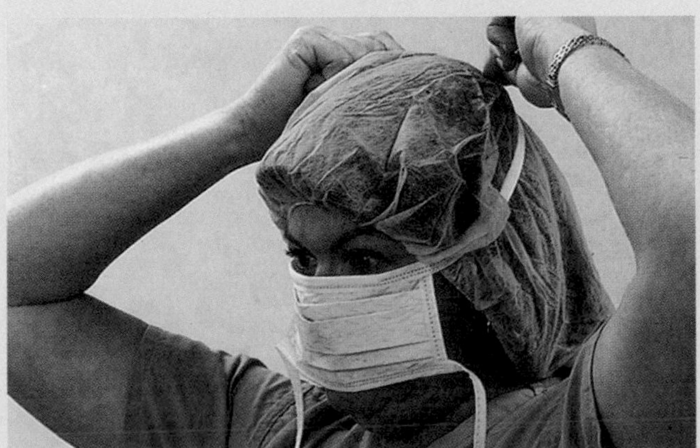

STEP 4c Tie top strings of mask.

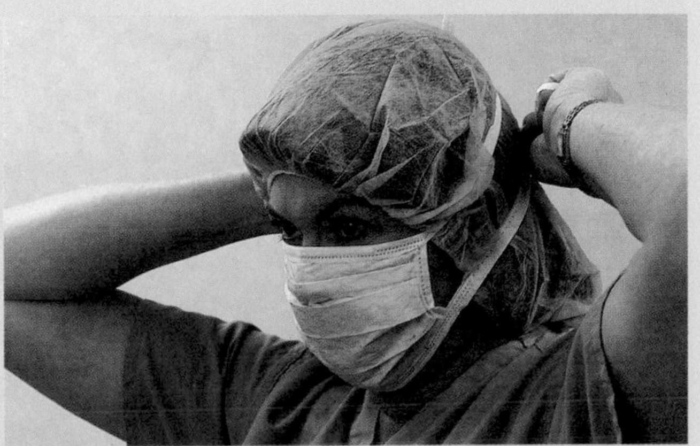

STEP 4d Tie lower strings of mask.

Continued

STEPS	RATIONALE
6. (NOTE: Provide a latex-free environment if the patient or the health care worker has a latex allergy.) Pull up gloves to cover the wrist (see illustration).	Prevents transmission of microorganisms.
7. Removal of PPE:	
a. Remove gloves. Remove one glove by grasping cuff and pulling glove inside out over hand. Hold removed glove in gloved hand. Slide fingers of ungloved hand under remaining glove at the wrist (see illustration). Peel glove off over first glove. Discard gloves in proper container.	Prevents contamination of hair, neck, and facial area.
b. Remove eyewear. Avoid placing hands over soiled lens.	Reduces transmission of microorganisms.
c. Remove gown by unfastening ties and pulling away from neck and shoulders. Touching only the inside of the gown, turn gown inside out, roll or fold into a bundle, and discard.	Front and sleeves of gown are contaminated. Prevents transmission of microorganisms.
d. Untie top strings of mask first, hold strings, untie bottom strings, and pull mask away from face while holding strings. Remove mask from face (see illustrations).	Prevents top part of mask from falling down over nurse's uniform. Contaminated surface of mask could then contaminate uniform.
e. Do not touch outside surface of mask. Discard in plastic-lined receptacle.	Prevents contamination of hands.
f. Grasp outer surface of cap and lift from hair.	Minimizes contact of hands with hair.
g. Discard cap in proper receptacle and perform hand hygiene.	Reduces transmission of microorganisms.
8. See Completion Protocol (inside front cover).	

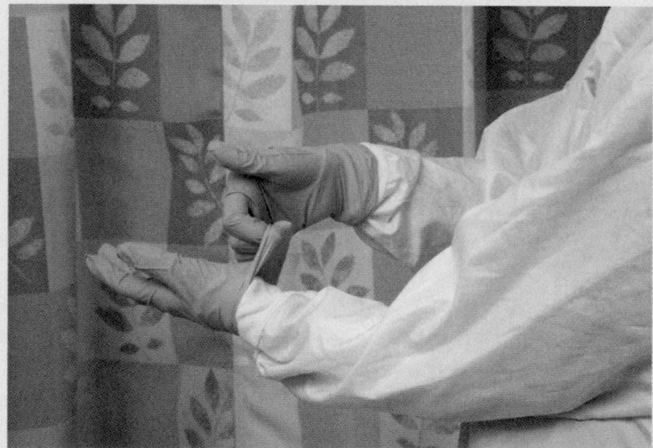

STEP 6 Applying gloves over gown sleeves.

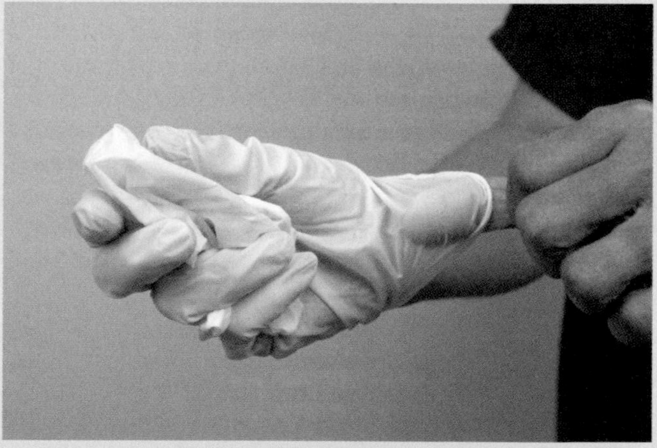

STEP 7a Remove second glove while holding soiled glove.

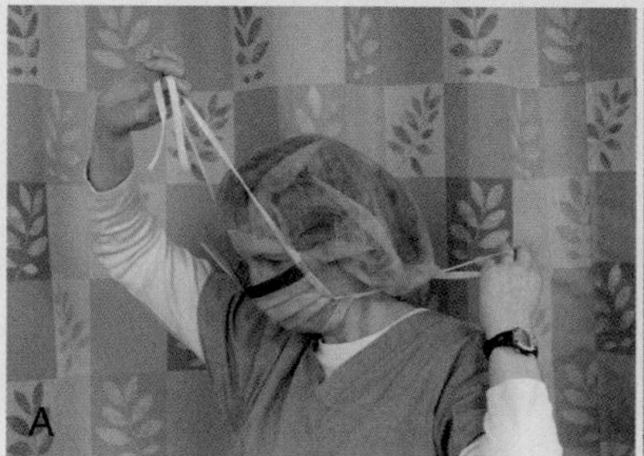

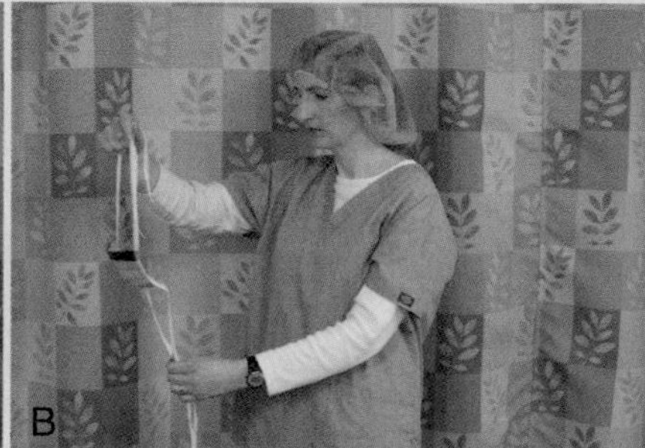

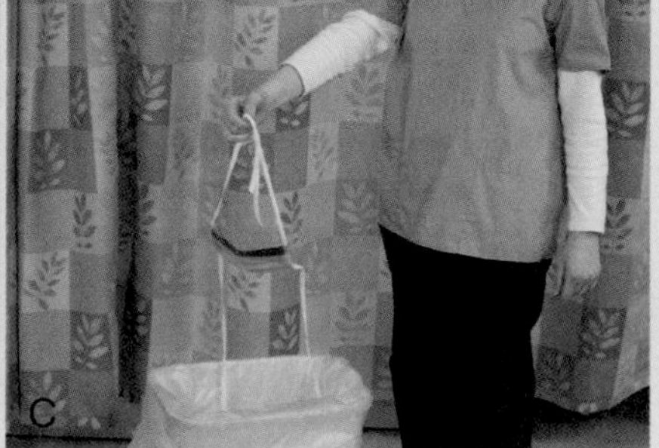

STEP 7d A, Untie top strings of mask. **B,** Remove mask from face. **C,** Drop mask in trash.

EVALUATION

- Inspect glove integrity.

Special Considerations

Home Care

- Instruct a family caregiver on how and when to use PPE.
- Determine ability of family caregiver to observe for signs of infection.

Recording and Reporting

It is unnecessary to document use of PPE.

SKILL 5.3 CARING FOR PATIENTS UNDER ISOLATION PRECAUTIONS

When a patient has a source of infection, health care workers follow specific infection prevention and control practices to reduce the risk of cross-contamination to other patients. Body substances such as feces, urine, mucus, and wound drainage contain potentially infectious organisms. Isolation or barrier precautions include the use of personal protective equipment (PPE) (see Skill 5.2). In 2007 the Hospital Infection Control Practices Advisory Committee of the CDC (2007) published revised guidelines for isolation precautions. The new guidelines contain recommendations for respiratory hygiene/etiquette as part of standard precautions. Standard precautions, or tier one precautions, are part of care for all patients (Table 5-1). The second tier (see Table 5-1) includes precautions for patients with known or suspected infection. Adherence to standard precautions has been associated with decreased skin and mucous membrane exposures and percutaneous injuries (e.g., needlestick injuries) (Brinsko, 2009).

When patients are infected or colonized with specific microorganisms, the CDC recommends transmission-based precautions in addition to standard precautions (CDC, 2007). Health care facilities modify these guidelines according to need and as dictated by state or local regulations. Isolation precautions are based on the assumption that microorganisms are transmitted by several routes: contact, droplet, air, common vehicle, and vector. The guidelines recommend the use of barrier precautions to interrupt the mode of transmission (see Skill 5.2). Isolation or barrier precautions prescribe the specific use of PPE when a patient is infected or colonized with specific organisms.

The three types of transmission-based precautions may be combined for diseases that have multiple routes of transmission. Whether used singularly or in combination, they are to be used in addition to standard precautions. When a patient requires isolation, determine the reason and mode of transmission. Evaluate the tasks to be performed to identify the barrier equipment needed. For example, a patient on airborne precautions for measles has an organism that can be carried by the airborne route. A mask is necessary when entering the room for any reason.

One important aspect of care for a patient in isolation is compliance with hand hygiene and the changing of gloves between exposures to body sites and patient equipment. Inadequate glove changes and hand hygiene between exposures to body sites can lead to contamination of previously uncolonized sites (Haas, 2009). For example, do not allow microorganisms in a patient's respiratory secretions to spread to the hub of a central line catheter on your gloved hands. Change gloves after the patient expectorates, perform hand hygiene, and reapply gloves in such a situation. Noncompliance with glove changing and hand hygiene increases the risk of HAIs.

ASSESSMENT

1. Assess patient's medical history and possible indications for isolation (e.g., purulent productive cough, major draining wound). Review the precautions necessary for the specific isolation category.
2. Review laboratory test results (e.g., wound culture, acid-fast bacillus [AFB] smears, changes in WBC count). *Rationale: Reveals type of organism infecting a patient.*
3. Consider types of care measures to be performed while in patient's room. *Rationale: Allows nurse to organize all equipment needed in room.*
4. Determine from nursing care plan, nursing colleagues, or family members the patient's emotional state and reaction to isolation. Also assess patient's understanding of purpose of isolation. *Rationale: Allows planning for appropriate social support and education.*
5. Assess whether patient has a known latex allergy. If an allergy is present, use latex-free gloves and refer to agency policy and resources available to provide full latex-free care. *Rationale: Protects patient from serious allergic response.*

PLANNING

Expected Outcomes focus on preventing transmission of infection to nurse and other patients and improving patient's knowledge of the purpose of isolation.

1. Patient and/or family verbalize purpose of isolation and treatment plan.
2. Infection does not develop in neighboring patients.

Delegation and Collaboration

Assessment of a patient's status and type of care measures to perform cannot be delegated to nursing assistive personnel

TABLE 5-1 CENTERS FOR DISEASE CONTROL AND PREVENTION ISOLATION GUIDELINES

Standard Precautions (Tier One) for Use with All Patients

- Standard precautions apply to blood, blood products, all body fluids, secretions, excretions (except sweat), nonintact skin, and mucous membranes.
- Perform hand hygiene before direct contact with patients; between patient contacts; after contact with blood, body fluids, secretions, and excretions and with equipment or articles contaminated by them; and immediately after gloves are removed.
- When hands are visibly soiled or contaminated with blood or body fluids, wash them with either a nonantimicrobial soap or an antimicrobial soap and water.
- When hands are not visibly soiled or contaminated with blood or body fluids, use an alcohol-based hand rub to perform hand hygiene.
- Wash hands with nonantimicrobial soap and water if contact with spores (e.g., *Clostridium difficile*) is likely to have occurred.
- Do not wear artificial fingernails or extenders if duties include direct contact with patients at high risk for infection and associated adverse outcomes.
- Wear gloves when touching blood, body fluids, secretions, excretions, nonintact skin, mucous membranes, or contaminated items or surfaces. Remove gloves and perform hand hygiene between patient care encounters and when going from a contaminated to a clean body site.
- Wear PPE when the anticipated patient interaction indicates that contact with blood or body fluids may occur.
- A private room is unnecessary unless the patient's hygiene is unacceptable. Check with the infection prevention and control professional of your agency.
- Discard all contaminated sharp instruments and needles in a puncture-resistant container. Health care facilities must make available needleless devices. Any needles should be disposed of uncapped or a mechanical safety device is activated for recapping.
- Respiratory hygiene/cough etiquette: Have patients cover the nose/mouth when coughing or sneezing; use tissues to contain respiratory secretions and dispose in nearest waste container; perform hand hygiene after contacting respiratory secretions and contaminated objects/materials; contain respiratory secretions with procedure or surgical mask; sit at least 3 feet away from others if coughing.

Transmission-Based Precautions (Tier Two) for Use with Specific Types of Patients

CATEGORY	DISEASE	BARRIER PROTECTION
Airborne precautions	Droplet nuclei smaller than 5 microns, measles, chickenpox (varicella), disseminated varicella zoster, pulmonary or laryngeal tuberculosis	Private room, negative-pressure airflow of at least 6 to 12 exchanges per hour via HEPA filtration, mask or respiratory protection device, n95 respirator
Droplet precautions	Droplets larger than 5 microns; being within 3 feet of the patient; diphtheria (pharyngeal), rubella, streptococcal pharyngitis, pneumonia or scarlet fever in infants and young children, pertussis, mumps, *Mycoplasma* pneumonia, meningococcal pneumonia or sepsis, pneumonic plague	Private room or cohort patients, mask or respirator (refer to agency policy)
Contact precautions	Direct patient or environmental contact, colonization or infection with multidrug-resistant organisms such as VRE and MRSA, *Clostridium difficile,* respiratory syncytial virus, shigella and other enteric pathogens, major wound infections, herpes simplex, scabies, varicella zoster (disseminated)	Private room or cohort patients (see agency policy), gloves, gowns
Protective environment	Allogeneic hematopoietic stem cell transplants	Private room; positive airflow with 12 or more air exchanges per hour; HEPA filtration for incoming air; mask, gloves, gowns

Modified from Centers for Disease Control and Prevention, Hospital Infection Control Practice Advisory Committee: Guidelines for isolation precautions in hospitals, *MMWR Morb Mortal Wkly Rep* 57/RR-16:39, 2007.

(NAP). The skill of caring for patients on isolation precautions can be delegated. Instruct the NAP by:

- Reviewing the reason a patient is on isolation precautions
- Instructing on the type of clinical changes to report
- Warning of high risk factors for infection transmission that pertain to the patient

Equipment

- Clean gloves, mask, eyewear, protective goggles or glasses, face shield, and gown (Gowns may be disposable or reusable, depending on agency policy.)
- Disinfectant swab (e.g., isopropyl alcohol with or without chlorhexidine gluconate)
- Other patient care equipment (as appropriate) (e.g., hygiene items, medication, dressing change items)
- Soiled linen bag and trash receptacle
- Sign for door indicating type of isolation in use and/or for visitors to come to the nurses' station before entering the room

IMPLEMENTATION *for* CARING FOR PATIENTS UNDER ISOLATION PRECAUTIONS

STEPS	RATIONALE
1. See Standard Protocol (inside front cover).	
2. Prepare all equipment to be taken into patient's room. In many cases dedicated equipment, such as stethoscopes, blood pressure equipment, and thermometers should remain in the room until patient is discharged. If patient is infected or colonized with resistant organism (e.g., vancomycin-resistant enterococcus, methicillin-resistant *Staphylococcus aureus*), equipment remains in room and is thoroughly disinfected before removal from room (see agency policy).	The CDC recommends use of dedicated noncritical patient care equipment (CDC, 2007).
3. Enter patient's room and remain by the door. Introduce yourself and explain the care that you are providing and the purpose of isolation precautions before applying PPE.	Allows patient to sense the nurse's caring without exposing nurse to risk of infection transmission.
4. Prepare for entrance into isolation room.	
a. Apply gown, being sure that it covers all outer garments; pull sleeves down to wrist. Tie securely at neck and waist.	Prevents transmission of infection when patient has excessive drainage or discharge. Also reduces contamination of clothing from splashes or splatters.
b. Apply either surgical mask or respirator around mouth and nose (type depends on type of organism and facility policy) if needed. Tie or attach a mask securely to make sure that it fits snugly.	Prevents exposure to airborne microorganisms or microorganisms from splashing of fluids.
c. Apply eyewear or goggles snugly around face and eyes (when needed).	Protects nurse from exposure to microorganisms that may occur during splashing of contaminated fluids.
d. (NOTE: Wear unpowdered latex-free gloves if patient or health care worker has a latex allergy.) When you wear gloves with the gown, bring glove cuffs over edge of gown sleeves.	Gloves are applied last so they can be placed over the cuffs of the gown.
5. Enter patient's room. Arrange supplies and equipment. (If equipment will be removed from room for reuse, place on clean paper towel.)	Minimizes contamination of care items.
6. Assess vital signs (see Chapter 6).	
a. Reusable equipment must be thoroughly disinfected when removed from the room.	Decreases the risk of infection being transmitted to another patient.
b. If stethoscope is to be reused, clean diaphragm or bell and ear tips with 70% alcohol or facility-approved germicide. Set aside on clean surface.	Reduces the chance for spreading infection before reuse and reduces bacterial colonies (CDC, 2007).

Continued

STEPS	RATIONALE
c. Use an individual electronic or disposable thermometer.	Prevents cross-contamination.
7. Administer medications (see Chapters 21 through 23).	
a. Give oral medication in wrapper or cup.	
b. Dispose of wrapper or cup.	
c. Administer injection, being sure to wear gloves.	Reduces risk of exposure to blood.
d. Discard needleless syringe or safety sheathed needle into designated sharps container.	Needleless devices should be used to reduce the risk of needlesticks and sharps injuries to health care workers.
8. Administer hygiene, encouraging patient to discuss questions or concerns about isolation.	
a. Avoid allowing isolation gown to become wet. Carry washbasin outward away from gown; avoid leaning against wet tabletop.	Moisture allows organisms to travel through gown to uniform.
b. Remove linen from bed; avoid contact with isolation gown. Place in leak-proof linen bag.	Linen soiled by patient's body fluids is handled so as to prevent contact with clean gown.
c. Provide clean bed linen and set of towels.	
d. Change gloves and perform hand hygiene if hands become excessively soiled and further care is necessary.	
9. Collect specimens (see Chapter 8).	
a. Place specimen container on clean paper towel in patient's bathroom and follow procedure for collecting specimen of body fluids.	Container will be taken out of patient's room; thus outer surface must not be contaminated.
b. Transfer specimen to container without soiling outside of container. After gloves are removed, place container in plastic biohazard bag, complete and apply biohazard label to outside of bag, and transport to laboratory. Perform hand hygiene and reglove if further procedures are to be performed.	
10. Dispose of linen, trash, and disposable items.	Linen or refuse should be contained completely to prevent exposure of personnel to infective material.
a. Use sturdy moisture-impervious single bags to contain soiled articles. Use double bag if outer bag is torn or contaminated.	Heavy soiling can cause outer side of first bag to become contaminated.
b. Tie bags securely at top in knot.	
11. Remove all reusable pieces of equipment. Clean any contaminated surfaces with disinfectant (see agency policy).	Items must be properly cleaned, disinfected, or sterilized for reuse.
12. Resupply room as needed. Have staff hand new supplies to you.	Limiting trips into and out of room reduces nurse and patient exposure to microorganisms.
13. Leave isolation room. Order for removing PPE depends on what is worn in room. This sequence describes steps to take if all barriers were required to be worn (CDC, 2007).	
a. Remove gloves. (See Skill 5.2, Step 7a)	Prevents nurse from contacting outer surface of contaminated glove.
b. Remove eyewear or goggles.	
c. Untie waist and neck strings of gown. Allow gown to fall from shoulders (see illustration). Remove hands from sleeves without touching outside of gown. Hold gown inside at shoulder seams and fold inside out. Discard disposable gown in trash bag.	Hands do not come in contact with soiled front of gown and therefore have not been soiled.

STEPS	RATIONALE
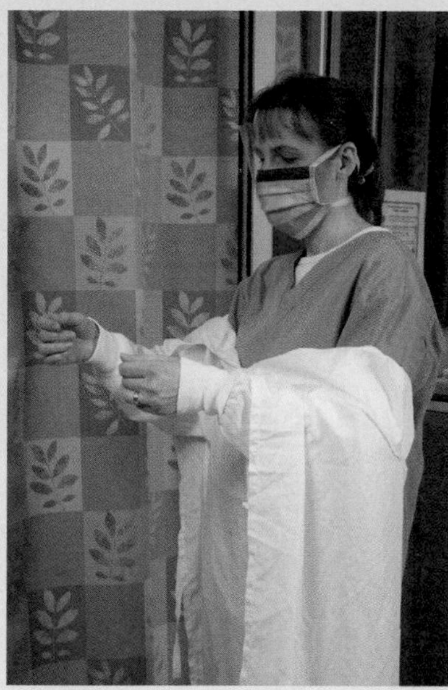 STEP 13c Nurse removes gown.	
d. Remove mask. If mask secures over ears, remove elastic from ears and pull mask away from face. For a tie-on mask, while holding onto strings, untie *top* mask strings. Then hold strings while untying bottom strings. Pull mask away from face and drop into trash container. (Do not touch outer surface of mask.) If body fluids splash onto mask, dispose in biohazard waste container.	Ungloved hands are not contaminated by touching only mask strings.
e. Perform hand hygiene.	
f. Retrieve wristwatch and stethoscope (unless it remains in room) and record vital signs on notepaper or clean paper towel.	Clean hands can contact clean items.
g. Explain to patient when you plan to return to room. Ask if patient requires anything such as personal care items or books or has any requests or needs.	
h. Leave room and close door if necessary. (Close door if patient is on airborne precautions.)	Keeping door open too long equalizes pressure in room and allows organisms to flow out.
14. See Completion Protocol (inside front cover).	

EVALUATION

1. Ask patient and family member to explain purpose of isolation in relation to diagnosed condition.
2. While in room, ask if patient has any health-related questions.

Unexpected Outcomes and Related Interventions

1. Patient avoids social and therapeutic discussions.
   a. Confer with patient, family, and/or significant other and determine best approach to reduce patient's sense of loneliness and depression.
   b. Use therapeutic listening.
2. Infectious organism spreads to other patients.
   a. Confer with provider, who may recommend an infectious disease consultation.
   b. Determine appropriate isolation precautions to take with other affected patients.

Recording and Reporting

- Procedures performed (including education) and patient's response
- Type of isolation in use and the microorganism (if known)
- Patient's response to social isolation

Sample Documentation

1320 Contact isolation in place for *Salmonella* in stool. Patient incontinent of liquid stool. Wife at bedside, asking questions about barrier equipment. Discussed method by which *Salmonella* is transmitted and explained purpose of handwashing and use of gown and gloves. Wife verbalized understanding when she requested gloves and gown to assist in cleanup.

Special Considerations

Pediatric

- Isolation creates sense of separation from family and loss of control. Strange environment confuses child. Preschoolers are unable to understand cause-effect relationship for isolation. Older children may be able to understand cause but still fantasize.
- Children require simple explanations (e.g., "You need to be in this room to help you get better"). All barriers to be used must be shown to child. Involve parents in any explanations. Nurses let children see their faces before applying masks so children do not become frightened (Hockenberry and Wilson, 2007).

Geriatric

- Isolation can be a concern for older adults, especially those who have signs and symptoms of confusion or depression. Many times patients become more confused when confronted by a nurse using barrier precautions or when they are left in a room with the door closed. Assess need for closing door (negative airflow room) along with safety of patient and additional safety measures required.
- Assess older adult for signs of depression: loss of appetite, decrease in verbal communications, or inability to sleep.

Home Care

- If patient returns home with draining wound or productive cough, educate family on potential sources of contamination in the home and techniques for disposing of any biological wastes in accordance with state laws.
- Encourage patients and family to use vigilant hand hygiene and avoid sharing personal care items with other family members.
- Have patients use a 5% (1:100 solution) bleach solution when performing household kitchen and bathroom cleaning of spills containing blood or other body fluids.

PROCEDURAL GUIDELINE 5.1
Special Tuberculosis Precautions

In 1994 the CDC published guidelines for preventing TB transmission in health care facilities. The current CDC guidelines for preventing and controlling TB focus on early detection of infection, protecting close contacts of patients with active TB disease, and applying effective infection control measures in health care settings. Isolation for patients with suspected or confirmed TB includes placing the patient on airborne precautions in a single-patient negative-pressure room.

OSHA and CDC guidelines require health care workers who care for suspected or confirmed TB patients to wear special respirators (e.g., N95 or P100). These respirators are high-efficiency particulate masks that have the ability to filter particles at a 95% or better efficiency. Health care workers who use these respirators must be fit tested, a procedure to determine adequate fit in a reliable way to obtain a face-seal leakage of 10% or less (Roberge, 2008). OSHA also requires employers to provide training concerning transmission of TB, especially in areas where the risk of exposure is high. In addition, the CDC now recommends the use of the QuantiFERON-TB Gold (QFT-G) test (CDC, 2006b), a blood test, in place of the traditional Mantoux TB skin test. The advantages of the QFT-G test are that it does not boost responses measured by subsequent tests and the results are not subject to reader bias.

Delegation and Collaboration

Assessment of a patient's status and type of care to perform cannot be delegated to nursing assistive personnel (NAP). Basic care procedures performed under TB isolation can be delegated. Instruct the NAP by:

- Clarifying precautions used under TB isolation, including fitting of mask
- Instructing on the type of clinical changes to report

Equipment

- TB isolation room with negative airflow
- N95 or P100 respirator
- Clean gloves, gown, protective eyewear (based on patient's clinical condition)
- Basic care items (e.g., medication equipment, hygiene items)

Procedural Steps

1. Assess potential for infectious pulmonary or laryngeal TB (e.g., documentation of positive AFB smear or culture, signs or symptoms of TB).
2. **See Standard Protocol (inside front cover).**
3. Before entering room, apply recommended mask. Be sure that it fits snugly.
4. Explain purpose of AFB isolation to patient, family, and others.
5. Instruct patient to cover mouth with tissue when coughing and to wear disposable surgical mask when leaving the room.
6. Provide hygiene care (see Chapter 10).
7. Leave the room and close the door.
8. **See Completion Protocol (inside front cover).**

PROCEDURAL GUIDELINE 5.1
Special Tuberculosis Precautions—cont'd

9. Place reusable mask in labeled paper bag for storage, being careful not to crush mask. (Check agency policy for number of times it can be reused.)
10. Assess patient's laboratory data for repeated AFB smears that may be negative.
11. Ask patient and/or family to identify method of transmission for TB.
12. Be alert and assess any suspected respiratory symptoms in neighboring patients.

SKILL 5.4 PREPARING A STERILE FIELD

- **Nursing Skills Online: Infection Control, Lesson 3**

Video Clips

Performing sterile aseptic procedures requires a work area in which objects can be handled with minimal risk of contamination. A sterile field provides a sterile surface for placement of sterile equipment. It is an area considered free of microorganisms and may consist of a sterile kit or tray, a work surface draped with a sterile towel or wrapper, or a table covered with a large sterile drape (Church and Bjerke, 2009). Sterile drapes establish a sterile field around a treatment site such as a surgical incision, venipuncture site, or site for introduction of an indwelling urinary catheter. Drapes also provide a work surface for placing sterile supplies and manipulating items with sterile gloves. Drapes are available in cloth, paper, and plastic. They may be wrapped in individual sterile packages or included within sterile kits or trays. These kits or trays contain external and internal sterile (chemical) indicators that indicate that the item has completed a sterilization process. After the kit is opened, the inside surface of the cover can be used as a sterile field. Most drapes are fluid resistant. There are various styles, shapes, and sizes of drapes. For example, bladder catheterization and tracheal suction kits contain sterile items that can be moved with the tray and containers into which sterile solutions can be poured. After you create a sterile field, you are responsible for performing the procedure and making sure that the field is not contaminated.

ASSESSMENT

1. Verify that procedure requires surgical aseptic technique.
2. Assess patient's comfort, oxygen requirements, and elimination needs before procedure. *Rationale: Certain sterile procedures may last a long time. Anticipate patient's needs so patient can relax and avoid any unnecessary movement that might disrupt the procedure.*
3. Instruct patient not to touch the work surface or equipment during the procedure and to remain still.
4. Assess for latex allergies. *Rationale: A focused review may reveal latex allergies even when no known allergies are indicated during the chart review.*
5. Check sterile package integrity for punctures, tears, discoloration, expiration date, and moisture. If using commercially packaged supplies or those prepared by agency, check sterilization indicator. *Rationale: Inspection of packaging ensures that only sterile items are presented to the sterile field (*AORN, 2007*).*
6. Anticipate number and variety of supplies needed for procedure. *Rationale: Ensures that procedure is organized to prevent break in technique.*

PLANNING

Expected Outcomes focus on prevention of localized or systemic infection.

1. Patient remains afebrile 24 to 48 hours after a procedure or during course of repeated procedures.
2. Sterile field is not contaminated.
3. Patient displays no signs of localized infection (e.g., redness, tenderness, edema, drainage) or systemic infection (e.g., fever, change in WBC count) 24 hours after the procedure.

Delegation and Collaboration

The skill of preparing a sterile field cannot be delegated to nursing assistive personnel (NAP), except in the case of surgical technicians trained in surgical aseptic techniques. Instruct the NAP to:

- Assist in positioning patients and obtaining necessary supplies.

Equipment

- Sterile gloves
- Sterile drape or kit that is to be used as a sterile field
- Sterile gown (see agency policy)
- Disposable cap and mask (see agency policy)
- Sterile equipment and solutions specific to the procedure
- Waist-high table or countertop surface
- Protective eyewear

IMPLEMENTATION *for* PREPARING A STERILE FIELD

STEPS	RATIONALE
1. See Standard Protocol (inside front cover).	
2. Complete all priority care tasks before beginning procedure.	Sterile fields should be prepared as close as possible to time of use (AORN, 2007).
3. Ask visitors to step out of room briefly during procedure. Discourage movement by staff assisting with procedure.	Traffic and movement increase potential for contamination through spread of microorganisms by air currents.
4. Apply PPE as needed (consult agency policy) (see Skill 5.2).	
5. Select a clean, flat, dry work surface above waist level.	A sterile object below a person's waist is considered contaminated.
6. Check expiration dates on all kits, packs, and supplies to be sure they are sterile.	
7. Perform hand hygiene.	Reduces transmission of microorganisms.
8. Prepare sterile work surface.	
a. Sterile commercial kit or tray containing sterile items:	
(1) Place sterile kit or package containing sterile items on work surface.	Once created, sterile field is sterile only at table level.
(2) Open outside cover and remove kit from dust cover. Place on work surface.	Inner kit remains sterile.
(3) Grasp outer edge of tip of outermost flap.	Outer surface of package is considered unsterile. There is a 2.5-cm (1-inch) border around any sterile drape or wrap that is considered contaminated.
(4) Open outermost flap away from body, keeping arm outstretched and away from sterile field (see illustration).	Reaching over sterile field contaminates it.
(5) Grasp outer edge of first side flap.	Outer border is considered unsterile.
(6) Open side flap, pulling to side and allowing it to lie flat on table surface. Keep arm to the side and not extended over the sterile surface (see illustration).	Drape or flap should lie flat so it does not rise up accidentally and contaminate inner surface or the sterile items placed on its surface.

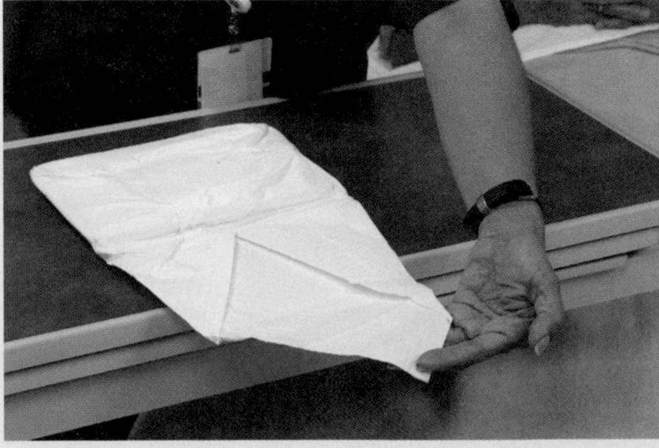

STEP 8a(4) Open outermost flap of sterile kit away from body.

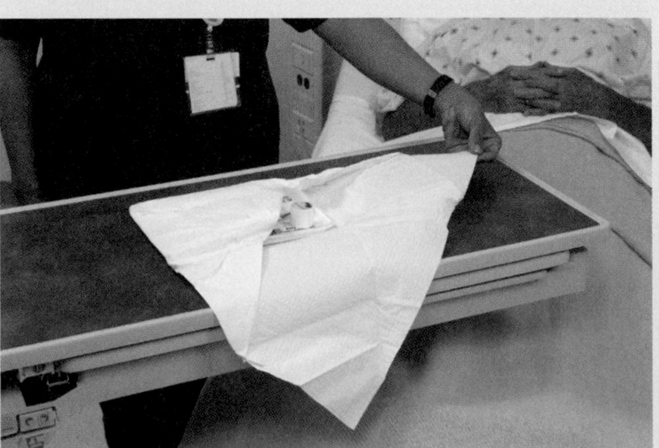

STEP 8a(6) Open first side flap, pulling to side.

STEPS	RATIONALE
(7) Grasp outer edge of second side flap. Repeat Step 8a(6) for opening second side flap (see illustration).	
(8) Grasp outer edge of last and innermost flap.	
(9) Stand away from sterile package and pull flap back, allowing it to fall flat on work surface (see illustration).	Reaching over sterile field contaminates it.
b. Sterile linen-wrapped package	
(1) Place package on work surface above waist level.	Items placed below waist level are considered contaminated.
(2) Remove tape seal and unwrap both layers, following Steps 8a(2) through 8a(9) as with sterile kit.	
(3) Use opened linen wrapper as sterile field.	Inner surface of wrapper is considered sterile.
c. Sterile drape	
(1) Place pack containing sterile drape on work surface and open as described in Steps 8a(2) through 8a(9) for sterile package.	Ensures sterility of packaged drape.
(2) Apply sterile gloves. (NOTE: This is an option, depending on agency policy. You may touch outer 1-inch border of drape without wearing gloves.)	
(3) Grasp folded top edge of drape with fingertips of one hand. Gently lift drape up from its wrapper without touching any object.	If a sterile object touches any nonsterile object, it becomes contaminated.
(4) Allow drape to unfold, keeping it above waist and the work surface and away from the body. (Carefully discard outer wrapper with other hand.)	Object held below person's waist or above chest is contaminated.

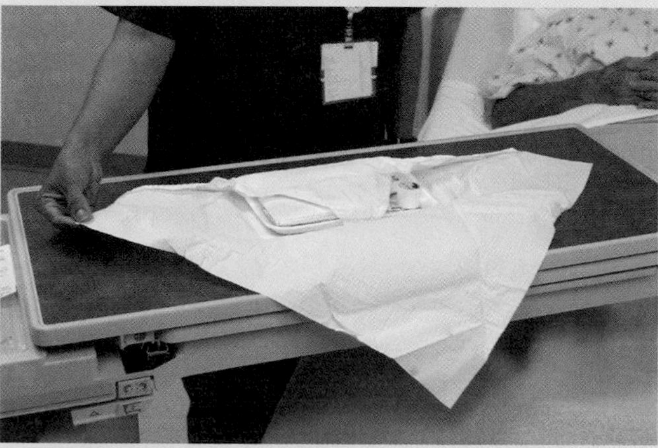

STEP 8a(7) Open second side flap, pulling to side.

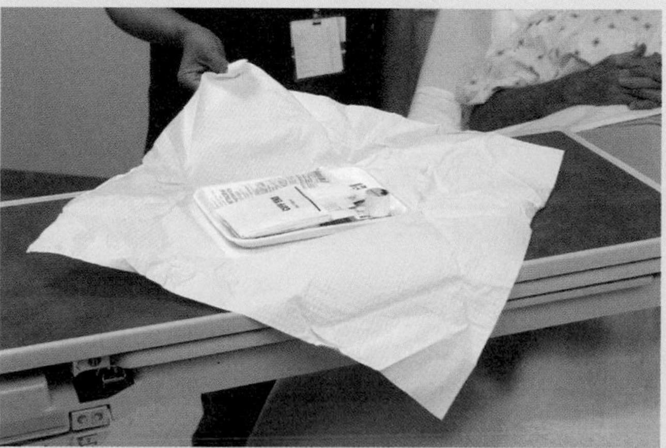

STEP 8a(9) Open last and innermost flap, standing away from sterile field.

Continued

STEPS	RATIONALE
(5) With other hand grasp adjacent corner of drape. Hold drape straight up and away from your body (see illustration).	Drape can now be properly placed with two hands.
(6) Holding drape, first position and lay the bottom half over top half of intended work surface.	Prevents nurse from reaching over sterile field.
(7) Allow top half of drape to be placed over bottom half of work surface (see illustration).	A flat sterile surface is now available for placement of sterile items.
9. Add sterile items to sterile field.	
a. Open sterile item (following package directions) while holding outside wrapper in nondominant hand.	Frees dominant hand for unwrapping outer wrapper.
b. Carefully peel wrapper over nondominant hand.	Item remains sterile. Inner surface of wrapper covers hand, making it sterile.
c. Being sure that wrapper does not fall down on sterile field, place item onto field at an angle. *Do not hold arm over sterile field.*	Secured wrapper edges prevent flipping wrapper and contaminating contents of sterile field (AORN, 2007).

SAFETY ALERT Do not flip or throw objects onto sterile field.

STEPS	RATIONALE
d. Dispose of outer wrapper.	Prevents accidental contamination of sterile field.
10. Pour sterile solutions.	
a. Verify contents and expiration date of solution.	Ensures proper solution and sterility of contents.
b. Be sure that receptacle for solution is located near or on sterile work surface edge. Sterile kits have cups or plastic molded sections into which fluids can be poured.	Prevents reaching over sterile field.
c. Remove sterile seal and cap from bottle in an upward motion.	Prevents contamination of bottle lip. Maintains sterility of inside of cap.
d. With solution bottle held away from sterile field, with the label facing up and bottle lip 1 to 2 inches above inside of sterile receiving container, slowly pour contents of solution container (see illustration). Avoid splashing.	Edge and outside of bottle are considered contaminated. Slow pouring prevents splashing liquids, which causes fluid permeation of the sterile barrier, called *strike-through,* resulting in contamination. Sterility of contents cannot be ensured if cap is replaced.

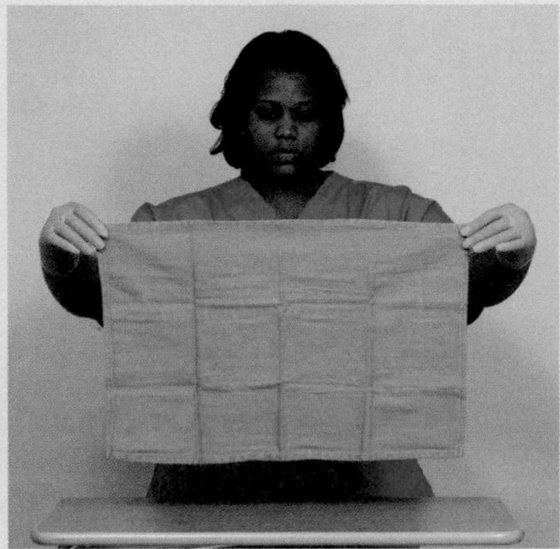

STEP 8c(5) Hold corners of sterile drape up and away from body.

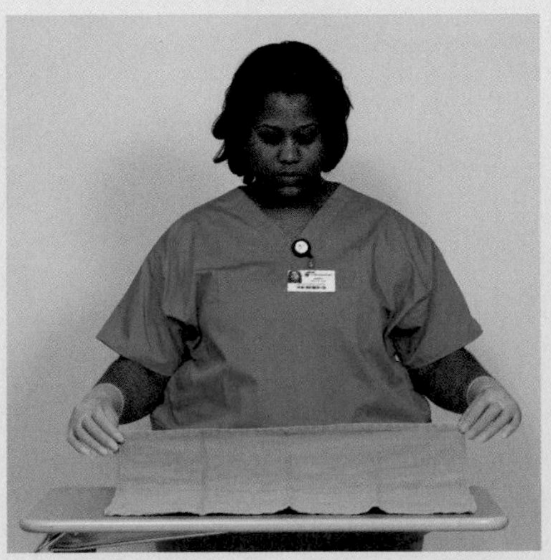

STEP 8c(7) Allow top half of drape to be placed over bottom half of work surface.

STEPS	RATIONALE

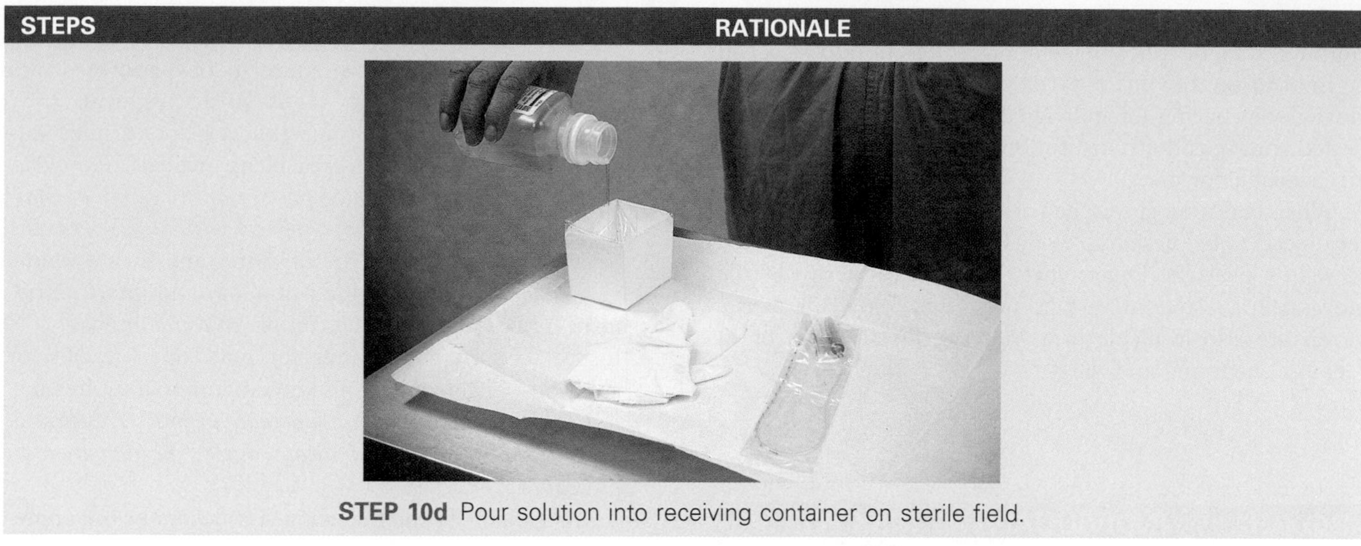

STEP 10d Pour solution into receiving container on sterile field.

EVALUATION

1. Observe for break in sterile technique.
2. Observe patient for fever and signs of localized infection.

Unexpected Outcomes and Related Interventions

1. Patient develops signs of infection.
   a. Notify health care provider of findings.
   b. Continue strict aseptic technique and hand hygiene.
   c. Monitor temperature every 4 hours and as needed.
   d. Encourage intake of fluids
2. Sterile field comes in contact with contaminated object or liquid splatters onto drape, causing strikethrough.
   a. Discontinue field preparation and start over with new equipment.

Recording and Reporting

- No recording or reporting is required for setting up sterile field.
- Record the sterile procedure performed in the nurses' notes.

Special Considerations

Pediatric

- Children may be unable to cooperate during a sterile procedure, depending on their level of developmental maturity.
- Instruct family members about how they may assist so child does not contaminate sterile field (Hockenberry and Wilson, 2007).

Geriatric

- Memory and sensory deficits may impair patient's ability to understand and cooperate with a procedure.

Home Care

- Adaptations may be made for some procedures such as self-catheterization and home tracheostomy care. In some cases patients use medical asepsis rather than surgical technique.
- If possible, teach patient and family to perform sterile procedures well before discharge from acute care so skills can be learned with professional assistance.

SKILL 5.5 STERILE GLOVING

- **Nursing Skills Online: Infection Control, Lesson 4**

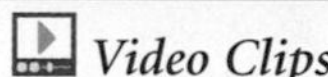 *Video Clips*

Sterile gloves act as a barrier against the transmission of pathogenic microorganisms and are applied before performing any sterile procedure such as a sterile dressing change or urinary catheter insertion. Always remember that sterile gloves do not replace hand hygiene.

You use the open-glove application method for most sterile procedures not requiring a sterile gown. Be careful not to contaminate the gloved hands by touching clean, contaminated, or possibly contaminated items or areas. If a glove becomes contaminated or torn, change it immediately. Once gloved, keep your hands clasped about 12 inches in front of your body, above waist level and below the shoulders, until you are ready to perform a procedure.

It is important to choose not only the right glove size but also the correct material. Many patients and health care workers have known allergies to latex, the natural rubber used in most gloves and other medical products (Church and Bjerke, 2009). Box 5-3 lists individuals who are at risk for latex allergy. Studies have shown that individuals who are highly sensitive to latex develop local and systemic reactions when latex gloves are removed and the latex glove powder particles are suspended in the air, often for hours (Molinari and Harte, 2009). The latex can then be inhaled or settle on clothing, skin, or mucous membranes. Reaction to latex can be mild to severe (Box 5-4). Choose latex-free or synthetic gloves when caring for individuals at high risk or with suspected latex sensitivity. Institutions have latex-free procedure kits available for use.

When choosing gloves, be sure that they are tight enough for objects to be picked up easily but that they do not stretch so tightly over the fingers that they can tear easily. Sterile gloves are available in various sizes (e.g., 6, 6½, 7). Sterile gloves are also available in a "one-size-fits-all" style or in "small," "medium," and "large."

BOX 5-3 INDIVIDUALS AT RISK FOR LATEX ALLERGY

- Spina bifida
- Congenital or urogenital defects
- History of indwelling catheters or repeated catheterization
- History of using condom catheters
- High latex exposure (e.g., health care workers, housekeepers, food handlers, tire manufacturers, workers in industries that use gloves routinely)
- History of multiple childhood surgeries
- History of food allergies

Modified from Mayo Clinic Staff: *Latex allergy,* December 2009, http://www.mayoclinic.com/health/latex-allergy, accessed July 10, 2010.

BOX 5-4 LEVELS OF LATEX REACTIONS

The three types of common latex reactions (in order of increasing severity) are:

1. *Irritant dermatitis:* A nonallergic response characterized by skin redness and itching.
2. *Type IV hypersensitivity:* A cell-mediated allergic reaction to chemicals used in latex processing. Reaction can be delayed as long as 48 hours and can be mild to severe, including redness, itching, and hives. More severe reaction includes localized swelling, red and itchy or runny eyes and nose, difficulty breathing, and coughing may develop.
3. *Type I allergic reaction:* A true latex allergy that can be life threatening. Reactions vary based on type of latex protein and degree of individual sensitivity, including local and systemic. Symptoms include hives, generalized edema, itching, rash, wheezing, bronchospasm, difficulty breathing, laryngeal edema, diarrhea, nausea, hypotension, tachycardia, and respiratory or cardiac arrest.

Modified from Mayo Clinic Staff: *Latex allergy,* December 2009, http://www.mayoclinic.com/health/latex-allergy, accessed July 10, 2010.

ASSESSMENT

1. Consider the type of procedure to be performed and consult institutional policy on use of sterile gloves.
2. Consider patient's risk for infection (e.g., preexisting condition, size or extent of area being treated). *Rationale: Directs nurse to follow added precautions (e.g., use of additional PPE) if necessary.*
3. Select correct size and type of gloves and then examine glove package to determine if it is dry and intact. *Rationale: Torn or wet package is considered contaminated.*
4. Inspect condition of hands for cuts, open lesions, or abrasions. Cover any lesions with an impervious dressing. *Rationale: Lesions harbor microorganisms. Presence of such lesions may contraindicate nurse's participation in procedure.*
5. Assess patient for the following risk factors before applying latex gloves (see Box 5-3):
   a. Previous reaction to the following items within hours of exposure: adhesive tape, dental or face mask, golf club grip, ostomy bag, rubber band, balloon, bandage, elastic underwear, IV tubing, rubber gloves, or condom
   b. Personal history of asthma, contact dermatitis, eczema, urticaria, or rhinitis
   c. History of food allergies, especially avocado, banana, peach, chestnut, raw potato, kiwi, tomato, or papaya
   d. Previous history of adverse reactions during surgery or dental procedures
   e. Previous reaction to latex product
6. If patient is expected to be at risk, check facility procedure for obtaining latex allergy cart. *Rationale: Contains nonlatex patient care items, including gloves.*

PLANNING

Expected Outcomes focus on prevention of localized or systemic infection and latex reaction.

1. Patient remains afebrile with no signs of localized infection 24 to 72 hours after the procedure or during the course of repeated procedures.
2. Patient does not develop signs of latex sensitivity or allergic reaction.

Delegation and Collaboration

The skill of sterile gloving can be delegated to nursing assistive personnel (NAP). However, many procedures that require the use of sterile gloves cannot be delegated (see agency policy).

Equipment

- Package of correct-size sterile gloves: latex or synthetic nonlatex. (NOTE: Hypoallergenic, low-powder, or low-protein latex gloves may still contain enough latex protein to cause an allergic reaction.)

IMPLEMENTATION *for* STERILE GLOVING

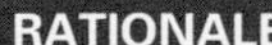

STEPS	RATIONALE
1. See Standard Protocol (inside front cover).	
2. Apply gloves.	
a. Perform hand hygiene.	Reduces transmission of microorganisms.
b. Place glove package near work area.	Ensures availability before procedure.
c. Open sterile gloves by carefully separating and peeling open adhered package sides (see illustration).	Prevents inner glove package from accidentally opening and touching contaminated objects.
d. Grasp inner glove package and lay it on a clean, dry, flat surface at waist level. Open package, keeping gloves on wrappers inside surface (see illustration).	Inner surface of glove package is sterile. Sterile object held below waist level is contaminated.
e. Identify right and left glove. Each glove has a cuff approximately 5 cm (2 inches) wide. Glove dominant hand first.	Proper identification of gloves prevents contamination by improper fit. Gloving of dominant hand first improves dexterity.
f. With thumb and first two fingers of nondominant hand, grasp edge of cuff of glove for dominant hand. Touch only inside surface of glove.	Inner edge of cuff touches skin and is no longer considered sterile.
g. Carefully pull glove over dominant hand, leaving cuff and being sure cuff does not roll up wrist (see illustration). Be careful in working thumb and fingers into correct spaces.	
h. With gloved dominant hand, slip fingers underneath cuff of second glove (see illustration).	Cuff protects gloved fingers; abducting thumb prevents contamination from contact with unsterile surface.

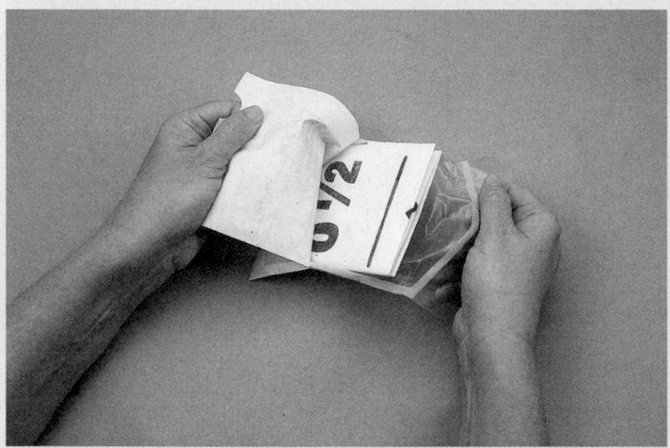

STEP 2c Open outer glove package wrapper.

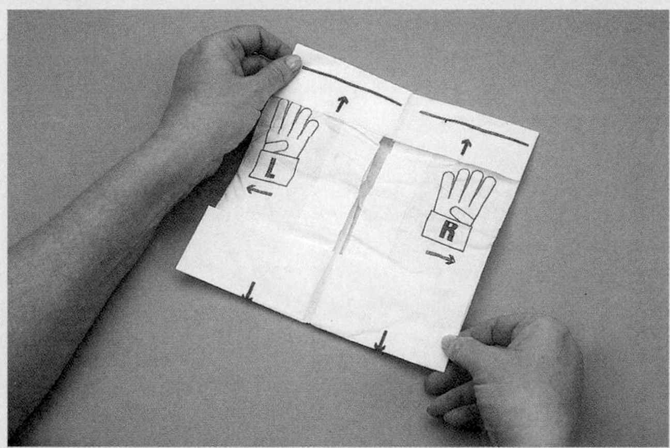

STEP 2d Open inner glove package on work surface.

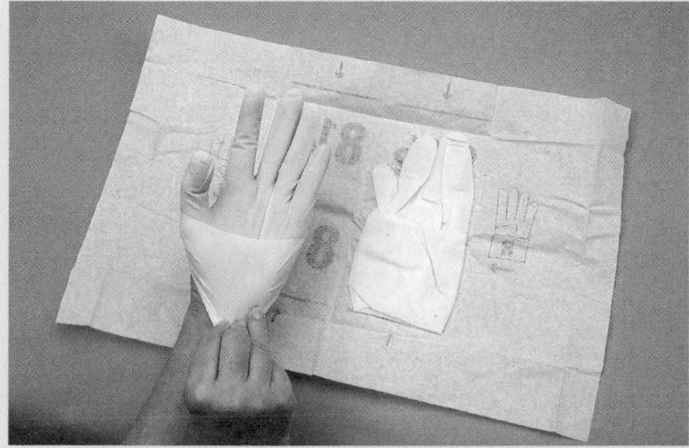

STEP 2g Pick up glove for dominant hand and insert fingers.

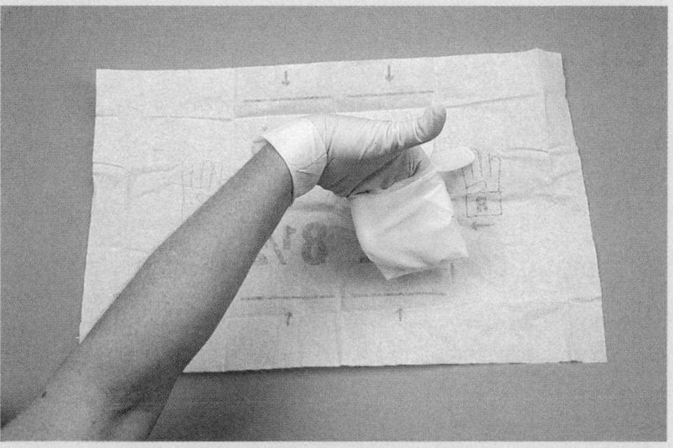

STEP 2h Pick up glove for nondominant hand.

Continued

STEPS	RATIONALE
i. Carefully pull second glove over fingers of nondominant hand (see illustration).	
j. Interlock fingers of gloved hands and hold away from body, above waist level, until beginning procedure (see illustration).	Prevents accidental contamination from hand movement.
3. Proceed with procedure.	
4. Remove gloves.	
a. Grasp outside of one cuff with other gloved hand; avoid touching wrist. Pull glove off, turning it inside out. Discard in proper receptacle.	Outside of glove should not touch skin surface.
b. Take fingers of bare hand and tuck inside remaining glove cuff. Peel glove off inside out. Discard in trash receptacle.	Fingers do not touch contaminated glove surface.
5. See Completion Protocol (inside front cover).	

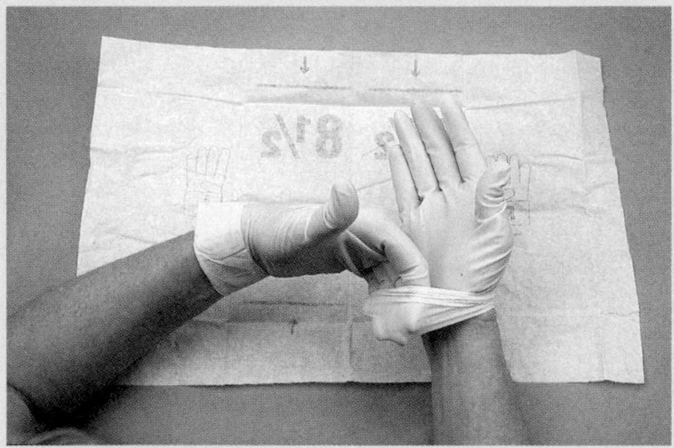

STEP 2i Pull second glove over nondominant hand.

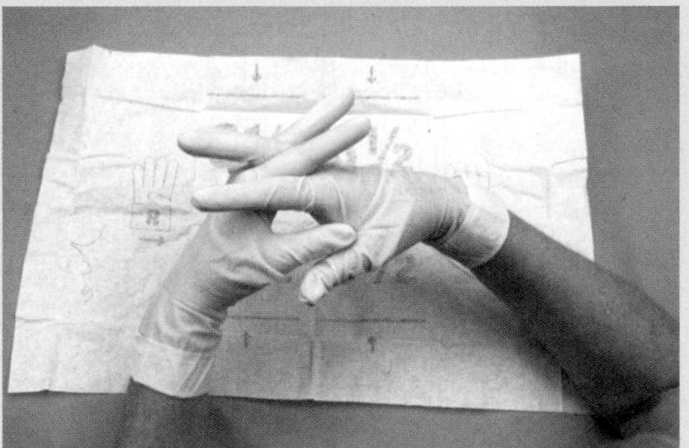

STEP 2j Interlock gloved hands.

EVALUATION

1. Evaluate patient for signs and symptoms of infection (e.g., fever, development of wound drainage) for 48 hours after the procedure.
2. Evaluate patient for signs of latex reaction.

Unexpected Outcomes and Related Interventions

1. Patient develops signs of infection.
   a. Notify physician or health care provider of findings. Wound cultures (see Chapter 8) and antibiotic therapy may be needed.
   b. Apply standard precautions and sterile technique (as appropriate).
   c. Monitor temperature every 4 hours or per orders.
2. Patient develops signs of dermatitis or latex sensitivity.
   a. Notify physician or health care provider of findings.
   b. Remove source of latex. Bring emergency equipment to bedside.
   c. Have dose of epinephrine and Solu-Medrol available, which may be needed for allergic reaction, and be prepared to initiate IV fluids and oxygen.

Recording and Reporting

- No recording or reporting is required for sterile gloving.
- Record the procedure performed in the nurses' notes.

REVIEW QUESTIONS

1. A nurse enters the room of a patient who has been diagnosed with pneumonia. The nurse instructs the patient to cover the mouth when coughing. This will reduce transmission of infection by:
   1. Contact
   2. Small droplet nuclei
   3. Vector
   4. Splashing
2. Put the following steps in order for removal of protective barriers, after leaving an isolation room:
   1. Untie bottom mask strings.
   2. Untie waist and neck strings of gown. Allow gown to fall from shoulders.
   3. Remove gloves.
   4. Remove eyewear or goggles.
   5. Untie top mask strings.
   6. Remove hands from gown sleeves without touching outside of gown; hold gown inside at shoulder seams, fold inside out, and then discard.
   7. Pull mask away from face and drop into container.
3. Identify all of the following that classify as a case of a health care–associated infection:
   1. An infected bedsore on a patient admitted from a nursing home
   2. A urinary tract infection that develops after a Foley catheter placement
   3. A patient tested as human immunodeficiency virus positive
   4. The development of purulent drainage exiting from a central venous catheter insertion site
   5. A *Staphylococcus* infection that develops in an incisional wound
4. When a nurse applies clean gloves when collecting a urine specimen, how does this technique break the chain of infection?
   1. Blocks the portal of entry of a microorganism
   2. Reduces susceptibility of the host
   3. Controls a reservoir source of organism growth
   4. Blocks the portal of exit
5. Which of the following breaks the chain of infection by controlling the reservoir source of microorganism growth?
   1. Changing a soiled dressing
   2. Cleaning a wound site
   3. Avoiding sneezing
   4. Disposing of used needles in a puncture-proof container
6. Place an "S" next to the procedures requiring sterile (aseptic) technique and place an "M" next to those requiring only medical aseptic technique.
   1. Urinary catheterization
   2. Tracheal suctioning
   3. Insertion of rectal suppository
   4. Insertion of a feeding tube
   5. Lumbar puncture
   6. Sitz bath
7. The nurse has applied the first sterile glove on her right hand (dominant) without touching the sterile outer surface. She takes her gloved right hand and picks up the remaining glove at the top of the cuff and slips it over her left hand. Which of the following statements is correct?
   1. The first glove is applied correctly but is contaminated while applying the second glove.
   2. The first glove is applied incorrectly, but the second glove is applied correctly.
   3. The first glove is applied correctly, and the second glove becomes contaminated.
   4. Both gloves have been applied correctly.
8. When opening a sterile pack, which of the following compromises the sterility of the contents?
   1. Keeping the contents of the pack away from the table edge
   2. Holding or moving the object below the waist
   3. Opening the pack just before the procedure
   4. Allowing movement around the sterile field that does not touch near the sterile field
9. Select all of the following persons who are at risk for a latex allergy:
   1. A patient who has had a surgical procedure
   2. A health care worker who works in the operating room
   3. A patient who reports frequent nausea and diarrhea after eating peaches
   4. A patient who develops hives after the taping of his surgical dressing
   5. A health care worker who comes to work with coughing and respiratory congestion
10. In setting up a sterile field, which of the listed actions would require intervention?
    1. The first flap of the sterile package is opened toward the nurse.
    2. The glove for the dominant hand is pulled on first.
    3. The sterile drape is allowed to unfold, keeping it above the waist.
    4. The bottle of solution is poured with the label facing up.

REFERENCES

Association of Operating Room Nurses (AORN): *Standards, recommended practices, and guidelines*, Denver, 2007, The Association.

Brinsko V: Isolation precautions. In Carrico R, editor: *APIC text of infection control and epidemiology*, Washington, DC, 2009, Association for Professionals in Infection Control and Epidemiology.

Centers for Disease Control and Prevention, Healthcare Infection Control Practices Advisory Committee and the HICPAC/SHEA/APIC/IDSA Hand Hygiene Task Force: Guideline for hand hygiene in health-care settings, *MMWR Recomm Rep* 51(RR16):1, 2002.

Centers for Disease Control and Prevention: Controlling tuberculosis in the United States: recommendations from the American Thoracic Society, CDC, and the Infectious Disease Society of America, *MMWR Recomm Rep* 54(RR12):1, 2005a.

Centers for Disease Control and Prevention, US Department of Health & Human Services: *Guidance for the selection and use of personal protective equipment (PPE) in the health care setting*, http://www.cdc.gov/ncidod/dhqp/pdf/ppe/PPEslides6-29-04.ppt, accessed December 2, 2005b.

Centers for Disease Control and Prevention: *Healthcare-associated infections (HAIs)*, http://www.cdc.gov/ncidod/dhqp/healthdis.html, accessed April 17, 2006a.

Centers for Disease Control and Prevention, Division of Tuberculosis Elimination: *Fact sheets: QuantiFERON-TB Gold Test, 2006*, http://www.cdc.gov/nchstp/tb/pubs/tbfactsheets/250103.htm, accessed April 9, 2006b.

Centers for Disease Control and Prevention, Hospital Infection Control Practice Advisory Committee: *Guidelines for isolation precautions in Healthcare Settings 2007*, http://www.cdc.gov/ncidod/dhap/pdf/guidelines/Isolation2007.

Centers for Disease Control and Prevention, Hospital Infection Control Practice Advisory Committee and the HICPAC/SHEA/APIC/IDSA Hand Hygiene Task Force: *Guideline for hand hygiene in health-care settings*, Atlanta, 2008, Centers for Disease Control and Prevention.

Church N, Bjerke N: Surgical services. In Carrico R, editor: *APIC text of infection control and epidemiology*, Washington, DC, 2009, Association for Professionals in Infection Control and Epidemiology.

Fardo R: Geriatrics. In Carrico R, editor: *APIC text of infection control and epidemiology*, Washington, DC, 2009, Association for Professionals in Infection Control and Epidemiology.

Haas J: Hand hygiene. In Carrico R, editor: *APIC text of infection control and epidemiology*, Washington, DC, 2009, Association for Professionals in Infection Control and Epidemiology.

Herud T and others: Association between use of hand hygiene products and rates of healthcare-associated infections in a large university hospital in Norway, *Am J Infect Control* 37(4):311-317, 2009.

Hockenberry MJ, Wilson D: *Wong's nursing care of infants and children*, ed 8, St Louis, 2007, Mosby.

Iwamoto P: Aseptic technique. In Carrico R, editor: *APIC text of infection control and epidemiology*, Washington, DC, 2009, Association for Professionals in Infection Control and Epidemiology.

Molinari J, Harte J: Dental services. In Carrico R, editor: *APIC text of infection control and epidemiology*, Washington, DC, 2009, Association for Professionals in Infection Control and Epidemiology.

Occupational Safety and Health Administration (OSHA): Occupational exposure to bloodborne pathogens; needlesticks and other sharps injuries; final rule, *Fed Reg* 66:5318, 2001.

Roberge R: Evaluation of the rationale for concurrent use of N95 filtering face piece respirators with loose-fitting powered air-purifying respirators during aerosol generating medical procedures, *Am J Infect Control* 36(2):135, 2008.

Rutala W: Disinfection and sterilization. In Carrico R, editor: *APIC text of infection control and epidemiology*, Washington, DC, 2009, Association for Professionals in Infection Control and Epidemiology.

Stricof RL: Endoscopy. In Carrico R, editor: *APIC text of infection control and epidemiology*, Washington, DC, 2009, Association for Professionals in Infection Control and Epidemiology, p. 40.

World Health Organization: *Issues guidelines on hand hygiene in health care*, Geneva, Switzerland, 2009, WHO Press.

CHAPTER

6

Vital Signs

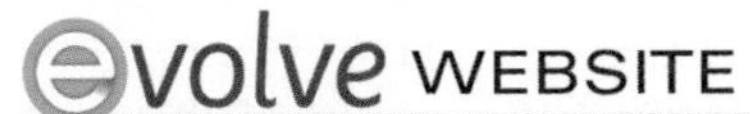

http://evolve.elsevier.com/Perry/nursinginterventions
Video Clips
Nursing Skills Online

Vital signs include temperature, pulse, respirations, and blood pressure (BP). These are indicators of the ability of the body to regulate body temperature, oxygenate body tissues, and maintain blood flow. Pain assessment is considered a fifth vital sign (see Chapter 13). Frequently pain is the symptom that leads patients to seek health care.

PATIENT-CENTERED CARE

Changes in vital signs indicate a patient's response to physical, environmental, and psychological stressors. These changes may reveal sudden alterations in a patient's condition. The nurse uses clinical judgment to determine which vital signs to measure, when to take measurements (Box 6-1), and when measurements can be delegated safely. A change in one vital sign (e.g., pulse) can reflect changes in the other vital signs (temperature, respirations, and blood pressure). The nurse's findings aid in determining whether it is necessary to assess specific body systems more thoroughly. For some patients vital sign assessment may be limited to measuring a single vital sign to monitor a specific aspect of a patient's condition. For example, after administering an antihypertensive medication, you measure the patient's blood pressure to evaluate the effect of the drug. The nurse must measure vital signs correctly, understand and interpret the values, begin interventions as needed, and report findings appropriately. Keeping patients informed of their vital signs promotes understanding of their health status.

SAFETY

Assessing vital signs requires equipment that is clean and in working order. You should carefully clean stethoscopes, thermometers, and blood pressure cuffs before and after use with each patient to avoid contamination by microorganisms. The biomedical department should routinely inspect electronic blood pressure machines for electrical safety. Know how to use each device; if you are unsure, ask for instructions. It is important that each device be used correctly and appropriately to ensure patient safety and to obtain correct, complete patient information.

EVIDENCE-BASED PRACTICE TRENDS

Heinemann M and others: Automated versus manual blood pressure measurement: a randomized crossover trial, *Int J Nurs Pract* 14:296, 2008.

Automatic electronic blood pressure machines are common in many facilities when frequent blood pressure measurements are necessary. Nurses frequently report that blood pressure obtained with electronic machines is not accurate, especially in patients with heart irregularities and during high and low blood pressures. The blood pressure taken with the Dinamapp machine was compared to manual blood pressure obtained using a sphygmomanometer and stethoscope by experienced nurses in medical and surgical adult patients. Systolic and diastolic electronic blood pressure readings were lower than blood pressures obtained manually. The greatest difference was in diastolic readings. Electronic blood pressure devices are more suitable for obtaining blood pressures in normotensive patients than in patients who have unstable blood pressures or require treatment for blood pressure deviations.

TEMPERATURE

The measurement of body temperature is aimed at obtaining an average of the core body tissues. Body tissues and cell processes function best within a relatively narrow temperature range between 36° C and 38° C (96.8° F and 100.4° F). The temperature range of an adult depends on age; physical activity; status of hydration; and state of health, including the presence of infection (Table 6-1). A patient can adjust body temperature by avoiding temperature extremes, adding or removing external clothing or coverings, and ingesting fluids and drugs. Average body temperature varies, depending on the measurement site used. Each site and type of thermometer has unique techniques, contraindications, or limitations and norms (Table 6-2). Several types of thermometers are commonly available to measure body temperature (Box 6-2). You can measure temperature on a Celsius or Fahrenheit scale. Although some electronic thermometers can display both Celsius and Fahrenheit readings, conversion charts are also available to convert from one scale to the other.

BOX 6-1 WHEN TO TAKE VITAL SIGNS

- On admission to a health care facility
- When assessing patient during home health visits
- In a hospital or care facility on a routine schedule according to a physician's or health care provider's order or standards of practice of the institution
- Before and after a surgical procedure or invasive diagnostic procedure
- Before, during, and after a transfusion of any type of blood product
- Before, during, and after the administration of medications or application of therapies that affect cardiovascular, respiratory, and temperature-control functions
- When the patient's general physical condition changes (e.g., loss of consciousness, increased severity of pain)
- Before and after nursing interventions influencing a vital sign (e.g., before and after a patient previously on bed rest ambulates, before and after patient performs range-of-motion exercises)
- When the patient reports specific symptoms of physical distress (e.g., feeling "funny" or "different")

TABLE 6-1 VITAL SIGNS: ACCEPTABLE RANGES

VITAL SIGNS	ACCEPTABLE RANGE
Temperature	36-38° C; 98.6-100.4° F
Oral/tympanic	37.0° C; 98.6° F
Rectal	37.5° C; 99.5° F
Axillary	36.5° C; 97.7° F
Pulse	Adult: 60-100 beats/min, strong and regular
Respirations	Adult: 12-20 breaths/min, deep and regular
Blood pressure*	Systolic: less than 120 mm Hg; diastolic: less than 80 mm Hg; pulse pressure 30-50 mm Hg
Pulse oximetry	Normal SpO_2 greater than 90%

*In some patients blood pressure is measured consecutively lying, sitting, and standing or in both arms. In normal individuals the change from lying to standing causes a decrease in systolic blood pressure of less than 15 mm Hg. Record the position and extremity and compare the measurements for significant differences.

TABLE 6-2 ADVANTAGES AND LIMITATIONS OF SELECTED TEMPERATURE MEASUREMENT SITES

SITE ADVANTAGES	SITE LIMITATIONS
Oral	
Easily accessible—requires no position change Comfortable for patient Provides accurate surface temperature reading Reflects rapid change in core temperature Reliable route to measure temperature for intubated patients	Causes delay in measurement if patient recently ingested hot/cold fluids or foods, smoked, or chewed gum Not used with patients who have had oral surgery, are unable to position in mouth, or have trauma, shaking or chills, or history of epilepsy Not used with infants; small children; or confused, unconscious, or uncooperative patients Risk of body fluid exposure
Tympanic Membrane	
Easily accessible site Minimal patient repositioning required Can be obtained without disturbing, waking, or repositioning patient	More variability of measurement than with other core temperature devices (Lawson and others, 2007) Requires removal of hearing aids before measurement Requires disposable sensor cover with only one size available

TABLE 6-2 ADVANTAGES AND LIMITATIONS OF SELECTED TEMPERATURE MEASUREMENT SITES—cont'd

SITE ADVANTAGES	SITE LIMITATIONS
Used for patients with tachypnea without affecting breathing Provides accurate core reading because eardrum is close to hypothalamus; sensitive to core temperature changes Very rapid measurement (2 to 5 seconds) Unaffected by oral intake of food or fluids or smoking Used in newborns to reduce infant handling and heat loss	Readings distorted by otitis media and cerumen impaction (Lawson and others, 2007) Not used with patients who have had surgery of the ear or tympanic membrane Does not accurately measure core temperature changes during and after exercise Affected by ambient temperature devices such as incubators, radiant warmers, and facial fans Difficult to position correctly in neonates, infants, and children under 3 years old because of anatomy of ear canal Inaccuracies reported caused by incorrect positioning of handheld unit
Rectal Argued to be more reliable when oral temperature is difficult or impossible to obtain	Lags behind core temperature during rapid temperature changes (Henker and Carlson, 2007) Not used for patients with diarrhea or those who have had rectal surgery, rectal disorders, bleeding tendencies, or neutropenia Requires positioning and is a source of patient embarrassment and anxiety Risk of body fluid exposure Requires lubrication Not used for routine vital signs in newborns Readings sometimes influenced by impacted stool
Axilla Safe and inexpensive Used with newborns and unconscious patients	Long measurement time Requires continuous positioning Measurement lags behind core temperature during rapid temperature changes Not recommended for detecting fever in infants and young children Requires exposure of thorax, which results in temperature loss, especially in newborns Affected by exposure to the environment, including time to place thermometer Underestimates core temperature (Lawson and others, 2007)
Skin Inexpensive Provides continuous reading Safe and noninvasive Used for neonates	Measurement lags behind other sites during temperature changes, especially during hyperthermia Adhesion impaired by diaphoresis or sweat Affected by environmental temperature Cannot be used on patients with adhesive allergy
Temporal Artery Easy to access without position change Very rapid measurement No risk of injury to patient or nurse Eliminates need to disrobe or unbundle Comfortable for patient Used in premature infants, newborns, and children Reflects rapid change in core temperature Sensor cover not required	Inaccurate with head covering or hair on forehead Affected by skin moisture such as diaphoresis or sweating

BOX 6-2 TYPES OF THERMOMETERS

Electronic Thermometers

These are rechargeable battery-powered display units with a thin wire cord and a temperature-processing probe covered by a disposable cover.

Within 1 minute after placement the thermometer displays a digital temperature reading.

Separate probes are available for oral and axillary temperature measurement (blue tip) and rectal temperature measurement (red tip) (see illustration *A*).

Tympanic Electronic Thermometers

The probe consists of an otoscope-like speculum with an infrared sensor tip that detects heat radiated from the tympanic membrane of the ear (see illustration *B*).

Within 2 to 5 seconds after placement in the ear canal and depressing the scan button, a digital reading appears on the display unit. A sound signals when the peak temperature has been measured.

Temporal Artery Thermometers

An infrared scanner is swept across the forehead and just behind the ear.

Within 2 to 5 seconds after scanning, a digital reading appears on the display unit.

Chemical Dot Single-Use Or Reusable Thermometers

These are thin strips of plastic with a temperature sensor at one end and chemically impregnated dots formulated to change color at different temperatures (see illustration *C*).

Chemical dots on the thermometer change color to reflect temperature reading, usually within 60 seconds.

They are useful for screening temperatures, especially in infants; during invasive procedures; and in orally intubated critical care patients.

They are not appropriate for monitoring fever in acutely ill patients or monitoring temperature therapies (Fallis and others, 2006).

They may underestimate oral temperature by 0.4° C (32.7° F) or more in 50% of adults.

They are easy to store and disposable, and they can be used for patients requiring isolation.

They can be used at axillary or rectal site if covered by a plastic sheath with a placement time of 3 minutes.

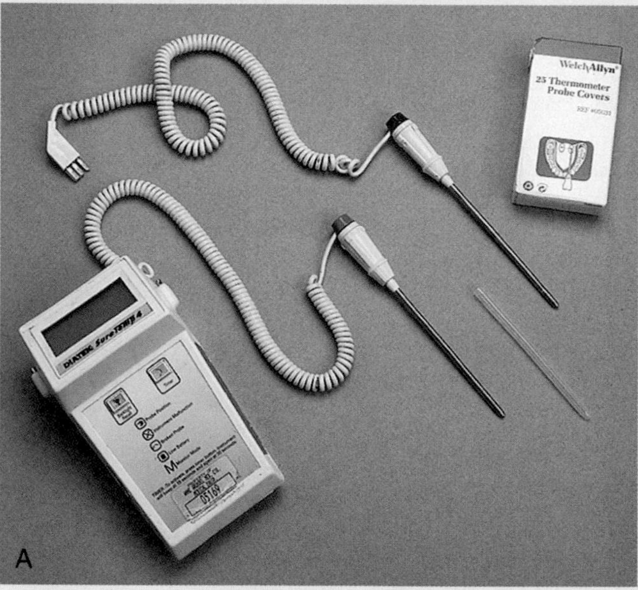

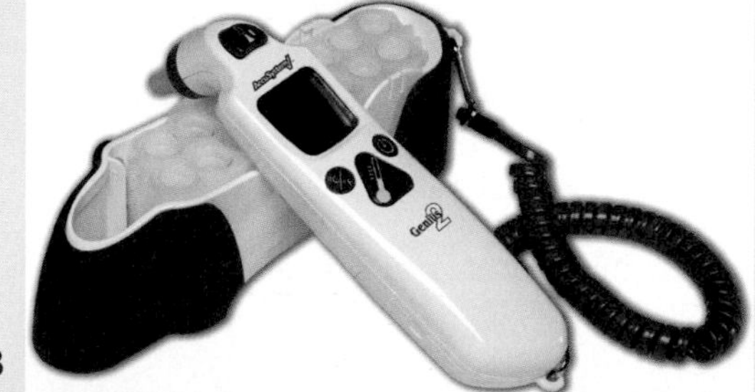

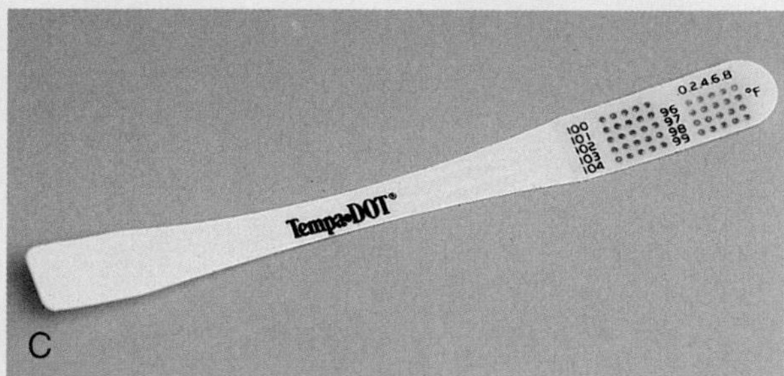

A, Electronic thermometer with disposable plastic sheath. **B,** Electronic tympanic membrane thermometer. (Genius 2 Thermometer used with permission of Covidien. All rights reserved.) **C,** Chemical dot disposable single-use thermometer.

PULSE

The pulse is a palpable bounding of blood flow caused by pressure wave transmission from the left ventricle to the peripheral arteries. Assessing the pulse provides indications of heart function and tissue perfusion (circulation). In adults the radial pulse is the site for routine pulse assessment. The brachial or apical pulse is the site for routine pulse assessment in infants.

Normally the pulse is easily palpable, regular in rhythm, and ranges between 60 and 100 beats per minute in adults. When palpated, a normal pulse does not fade in and out and is not easily obliterated by pressure. Pulse abnormalities include bradycardia (pulse less than 60 beats per minute), tachycardia (pulse greater than 100 beats per minute), and arrhythmia (irregular pulse rate). *Weak, feeble,* and *thready* are descriptive words for a pulse of low volume that is difficult to palpate. *Bounding* is the term used to describe a pulse that

BOX 6-3 LEARNING TO USE A STETHOSCOPE

1. Place earpieces in both ears with tips of earpieces turned toward the face. Lightly blow against the diaphragm (flat side of chestpiece). Now place the earpieces in both ears with the tips turned toward the back of the head, and again blow against the diaphragm. Compare comfort in the ears and amplification of sounds with earpieces in both directions. Earpieces pointing toward the face should fit snugly and comfortably.
2. If the stethoscope has both a diaphragm (flat side) and a bell (bowl shaped with a rubber ring) (see illustration *A*), put earpieces in ears and lightly blow against the diaphragm. The chestpiece can be turned to allow sound to be carried through either side (bell or diaphragm) of the chestpiece. If sound is faint, lightly blow into the bell. Then turn the chestpiece and blow again against both the diaphragm and the bell. The diaphragm is used for higher-pitched heart sounds, bowel sounds, and lung sounds (see illustration *B*). The bell is used for lower-pitched heart sounds and vascular sounds (see illustration *C*).
3. With earpieces in place and using the diaphragm, move the diaphragm lightly over the hair on your arm. The bristling sound mimics a sound heard in the lungs. When listening for significant sounds, hold the diaphragm still and firmly make a tight seal against the skin to eliminate extraneous sounds.
4. Place the diaphragm over the front of your chest directly on your skin and listen to your own breathing, comparing the bell and the diaphragm. Repeat the process while listening to your heartbeat. Ask someone to speak in a conversational tone and note how the speech detracts from hearing clearly. When using a stethoscope, both the patient and the examiner should remain quiet.
5. With the earpieces in your ears, gently tap the tubing. Note that this also generates extraneous sounds. When listening to a patient, maintain a position that allows tubing to extend straight and hang free. Movement may allow tubing to rub or bump objects, creating extraneous sounds. Kinked tubing muffles sounds.

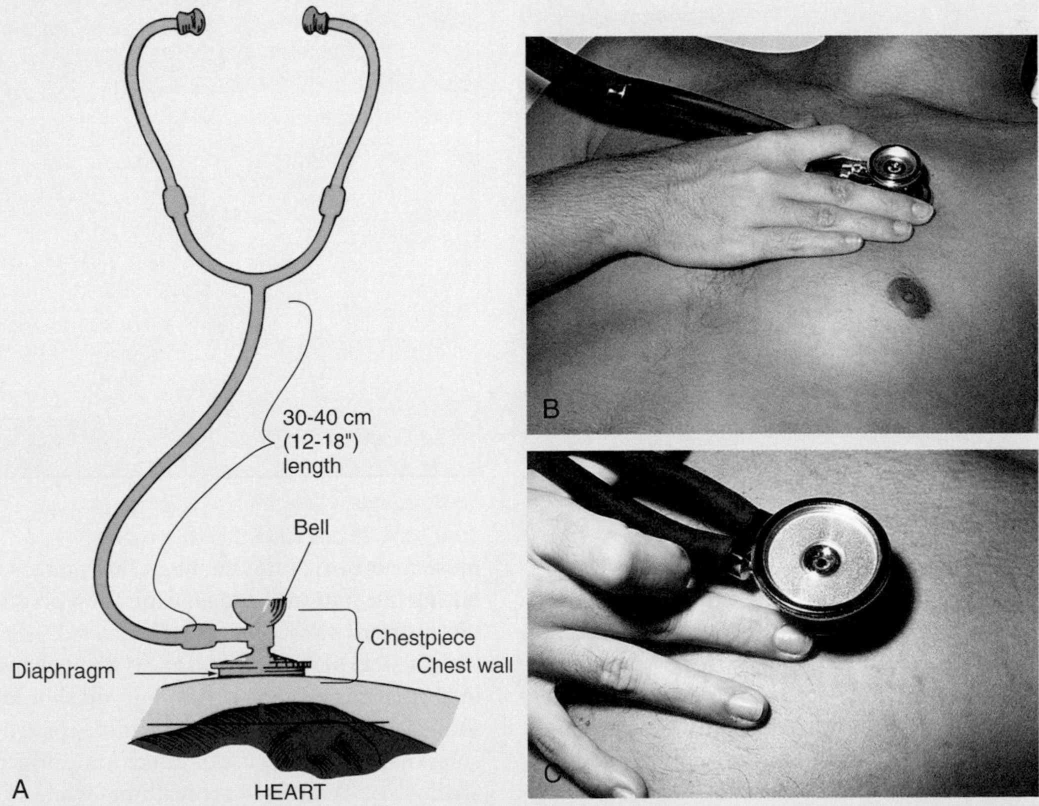

A, Parts of a stethoscope. **B,** The diaphragm is placed firmly and securely when auscultating high-pitched lung and bowel sounds. **C,** The bell must be placed lightly on the skin to hear low-pitched vascular and heart sounds.

is very strong. If you identify abnormalities such as an irregular rhythm or an inability to palpate the radial pulse, you must obtain an apical pulse. The apical pulse is the most accurate noninvasive measure of heart rate; you obtain it by using a stethoscope (Box 6-3). The stethoscope magnifies the sounds as they are transmitted from the chest wall through the tubing to the listener. In adults, you auscultate the apical pulse (heard with a stethoscope) by placing the diaphragm over the point of maximal impulse (PMI) at the fifth intercostal space on the left midclavicular line (Fig. 6-1).

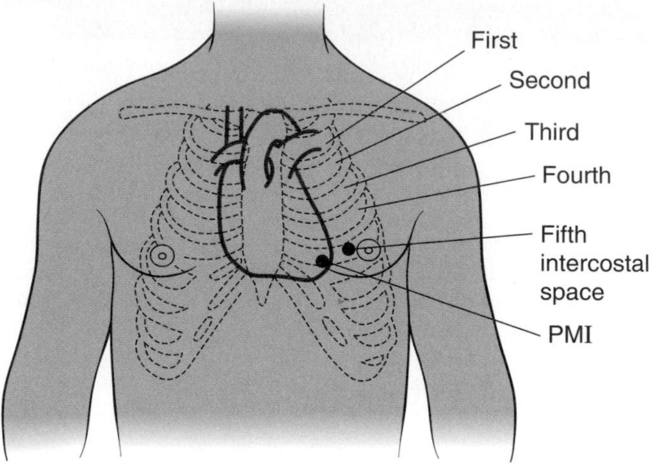

FIG 6-1 Point of maximal impulse (PMI) is at fifth intercostal space.

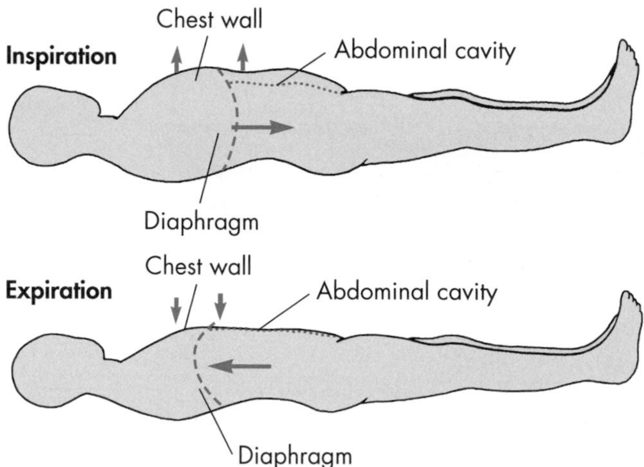

FIG 6-2 Diaphragmatic and chest wall movement during inspiration and expiration.

TABLE 6-3 ALTERATIONS IN BREATHING PATTERN

ALTERATION	DESCRIPTION
Apnea	Respirations cease for several seconds. Persistent cessation results in respiratory arrest.
Biot's respiration	Respirations are abnormally shallow for two to three breaths, followed by irregular period of apnea.
Bradypnea	Rate of breathing is regular but abnormally slow (less than 12 breaths per minute).
Cheyne-Stokes respiration	Respiratory rate and depth are irregular, characterized by alternating periods of apnea and hyperventilation. Respiratory cycle begins with slow, shallow breaths that gradually increase to abnormal rate and depth. The pattern reverses; breathing slows and becomes shallow, climaxing in apnea before respiration resumes.
Hyperpnea	Respirations are increased in depth. Hyperpnea occurs normally during exercise.
Hyperventilation	Rate and depth of respirations increase. Hypocarbia may occur.
Hypoventilation	Respiratory rate is abnormally low, and depth of ventilation may be depressed. Hypercarbia may occur.
Kussmaul's respiration	Respirations are abnormally deep but regular.
Tachypnea	Rate of breathing is regular but abnormally rapid (greater than 20 breaths per minute).

RESPIRATIONS

Assessing respirations involves evaluating the exchange of oxygen and carbon dioxide between the environment, the blood, and the cells. Obtain the respiratory rate by observing the rate, depth, and rhythm of respiratory movements. Rate refers to the number of times the person breathes in and out in 1 minute. Estimate the depth of respirations by observing the movement of the chest during inspiration. Respiration can be described as deep or shallow. Rhythm of respirations is normally regular; however, irregular respiration patterns may occur (Table 6-3).

Determine breathing patterns by observing the patient's chest or the abdomen. Diaphragmatic breathing results from the contraction and relaxation of the diaphragm and is most visible in the abdomen. Healthy men usually demonstrate diaphragmatic breathing (Fig. 6-2), whereas women breathe more with the thorax, most apparent in the upper chest. Labored respirations usually involve the accessory muscles of respiration in the neck. The breathing cycle consists of a period of inspiration followed by a period of expiration. When something such as a foreign body interferes with the movement of air into the lungs, the intercostal spaces retract during inspiration. A longer expiration phase is evident when the outward flow of air is obstructed (e.g., asthma). If a patient is experiencing dyspnea, a subjective experience of inadequate or difficult breathing, you should auscultate lung sounds. Dyspnea is associated with increased effort to inhale and exhale and active use of intercostal and accessory muscles. Orthopnea is difficulty breathing while lying flat and is relieved by sitting or standing. Assess lungs sounds when the patient has excessive secretions, complains of chest pain, or has sustained trauma to the chest (see Chapter 7).

BLOOD PRESSURE

Blood pressure is the force exerted by the blood against the arterial walls. The systolic blood pressure is the peak pressure occurring during cardiac contraction when blood is forced from the ventricles under high pressure into the aorta. The diastolic blood pressure is the pressure present when the ventricles are relaxed and there is minimal pressure exerted

TABLE 6-4 CLASSIFICATION OF BLOOD PRESSURE FOR ADULTS AGE 18 YEARS AND OLDER

CATEGORY	SYSTOLIC* (mm Hg)		DIASTOLIC* (mm Hg)
Normal	Less than 120	and	Less than 80
Prehypertension*	120-139	or	80-89
Stage 1 hypertension	140-159	or	90-99
Stage 2 hypertension	160 or greater	or	100 or greater

Modified from NHBPEP: The seventh report of the NHBPEP on prevention, detection, evaluation, and treatment of high blood pressure, *JAMA* 289:2560, 2003.

*Based on the average of two or more readings taken at each of two or more visits after an initial screening in a patient not taking antihypertensive drugs and not acutely ill. When systolic and diastolic blood pressures fall into different categories, the higher category should be selected to classify the individual's blood pressure status. For example, 160/92 mm Hg should be classified as Stage 2 hypertension.

against the arterial wall. The pulse pressure is the difference between the systolic and diastolic pressure; for a blood pressure of 114/72, the pulse pressure is 42.

Many factors influence blood pressure. A single measurement does not adequately reflect a patient's blood pressure. Blood pressure trends, not individual measurements, guide nursing interventions. The most common alteration in blood pressure is *hypertension,* an often asymptomatic disorder characterized by persistently elevated blood pressure. A diagnosis of prehypertension in nonpregnant adults is confirmed when an average of two or more diastolic readings on at least two subsequent visits is 80 to 89 mm Hg (NHBPEP, 2003) (Table 6-4). Prehypertension places individuals at high risk for the development of hypertension. Early intervention by adoption of healthy lifestyles reduces the risk for or prevents hypertension. Factors that increase the risk for hypertension include obesity, increased sodium intake, smoking, and lack of exercise.

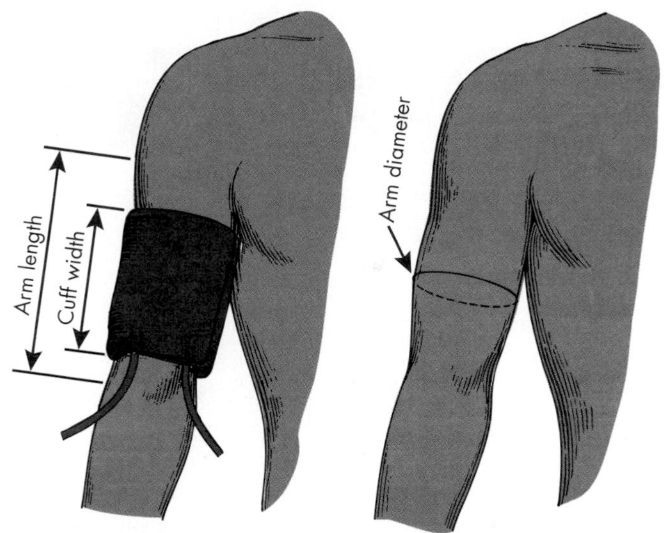

FIG 6-3 Proper cuff size: Length of bladder is 80% of arm circumference; cuff width is at least 40% larger than arm diameter.

Measuring blood pressure using the auscultatory method requires detecting the sounds of the rush of blood (Korotkoff phases) as blood resumes its flow through the artery. The auscultatory method is performed manually with the use of a sphygmomanometer and a stethoscope or electronically with an auscultatory blood pressure machine. The electronic auscultatory blood pressure machine uses a microphone to detect the Korotkoff phases.

A sphygmomanometer includes a pressure manometer, an occlusive cloth or vinyl cuff that encloses an inflatable rubber bladder, and a pressure bulb with a release valve that inflates the bladder. It can be portable or wall mounted. The manometer has a glass-enclosed circular gauge containing a needle that registers millimeter calibrations. The needle of the gauge should point to zero when not in use and move freely when the cuff pressure is released.

The cloth or disposable vinyl compression cuff of the sphygmomanometer contains an inflatable bladder. The cuff is placed around the arm or thigh. Cuffs come in several different sizes, and the blood pressure measurement is not accurate unless you use the correct-size cuff (Fig. 6-3). Many adults require a large cuff. The bladder, enclosed by the cuff, should encircle at least 80% of the arm of an adult; the cuff width should be at least 40% greater than the arm circumference. Quickly inflate the cuff until blood flow ceases and slowly deflate the cuff while the needle begins to fall. Korotkoff phases are auscultated by placing the stethoscope over the artery distal to the blood pressure cuff. In some patients the sounds are clear and distinct, whereas in others only the beginning and ending sounds are audible (Fig. 6-4). You record the blood pressure with the systolic and diastolic numbers written as a fraction. The systolic pressure is the first heart sound. Before the sounds cease, they may become distinctly muffled (second sound). The diastolic pressure is the last sound heard. In adults you identify the systolic and diastolic blood pressure readings and record them by the pressures corresponding to the first of two consecutive sounds heard and the disappearance of sounds (not muffling), respectively. Confirm the last sounds by continuing to listen for 10 to 20 mm Hg below the last sound heard. The nurse promotes accuracy in measurement by being aware of the various factors that influence accurate blood pressure values when a stethoscope and sphygmomanometer are used (Table 6-5).

Electronic blood pressure machines are used when frequent assessment is required such as in critically ill or potentially unstable patients, during or after invasive procedures, or when therapies require frequent monitoring (e.g., trials of

BOX 6-4 ADVANTAGES AND LIMITATIONS OF ASSESSING BLOOD PRESSURE ELECTRONICALLY

Advantages

- Ease of use
- Ability to use a stethoscope not required
- Efficient when frequent repeated measurements are indicated
- Allows blood pressure to be measured frequently, as often as every 15 seconds, with accuracy
- Some devices not sensitive to outside noise

Limitations

- Expensive
- Requires source of electricity and space to position machine
- Sensitive to outside motion interference and cannot be used in patients with seizures, tremors, or shivers
- Not accurate for patients with irregular heart rate or hypotension (blood pressure less than 90 mm Hg systolic) or in situations of reduced blood flow (Bern and others, 2007)
- Accuracy standards for electronic blood pressure manufacturers are voluntary
- Vulnerable to error among older-adult and obese patients (Heinemann and others, 2008)

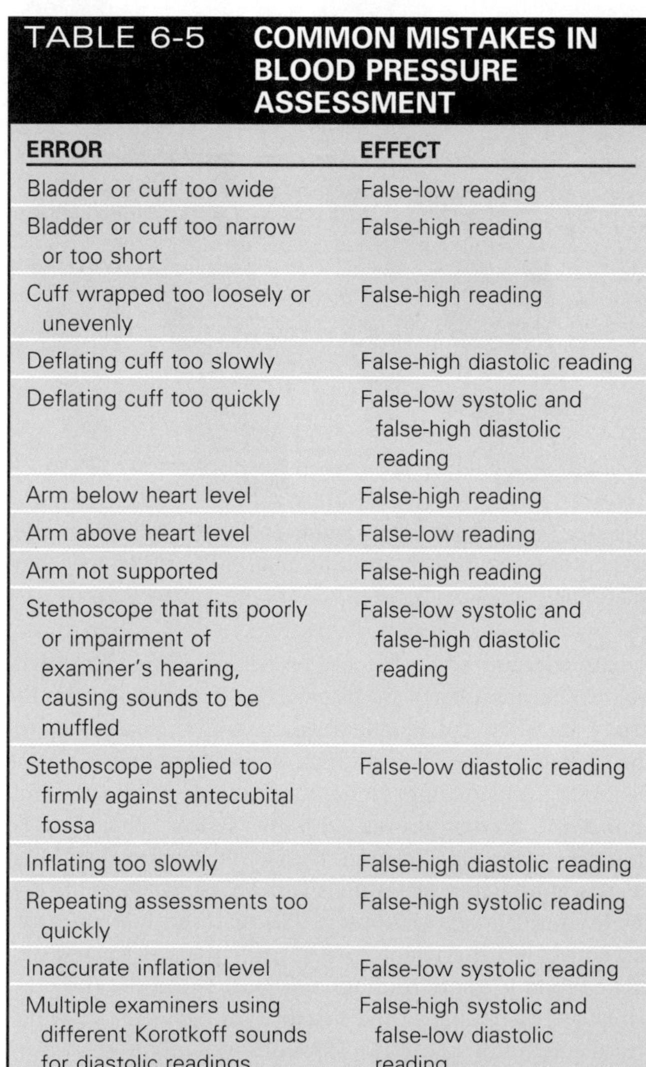

TABLE 6-5 COMMON MISTAKES IN BLOOD PRESSURE ASSESSMENT

ERROR	EFFECT
Bladder or cuff too wide	False-low reading
Bladder or cuff too narrow or too short	False-high reading
Cuff wrapped too loosely or unevenly	False-high reading
Deflating cuff too slowly	False-high diastolic reading
Deflating cuff too quickly	False-low systolic and false-high diastolic reading
Arm below heart level	False-high reading
Arm above heart level	False-low reading
Arm not supported	False-high reading
Stethoscope that fits poorly or impairment of examiner's hearing, causing sounds to be muffled	False-low systolic and false-high diastolic reading
Stethoscope applied too firmly against antecubital fossa	False-low diastolic reading
Inflating too slowly	False-high diastolic reading
Repeating assessments too quickly	False-high systolic reading
Inaccurate inflation level	False-low systolic reading
Multiple examiners using different Korotkoff sounds for diastolic readings	False-high systolic and false-low diastolic reading

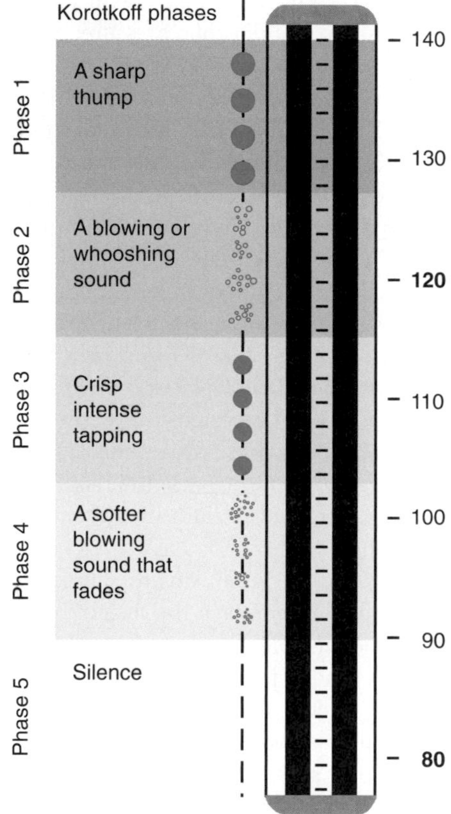

FIG 6-4 Sounds auscultated during blood pressure measurement can be differentiated into five Korotkoff phases. In this example the blood pressure is 140/90 mm Hg.

new drugs). Many different styles of electronic blood pressure machines are available, and you can also find them in public areas such as shopping malls or patient's homes. Although electronic blood pressure machines are fast and free the nurse for other activities, they do have disadvantages (Box 6-4).

SKILL 6.1 MEASURING BODY TEMPERATURE

- **Nursing Skills Online: Vital Signs, Lesson 2**

Video Clips

Assessment of temperature requires making judgments about the site for temperature measurement, type of thermometer, and frequency of measurement. This skill includes temperature measurement with an electronic thermometer using the oral, tympanic, temporal, rectal, or axillary sites.

ASSESSMENT

1. Consider normal daily fluctuations in temperature. *Rationale: Body temperature tends to be lowest in early morning, peak in late afternoon, and gradually decline during the night. When temperatures are taken between 5 and 7 PM, fever is assessed more accurately.*
2. Identify medications or treatments that may influence temperature. *Rationale: Antiinflammatory drugs, steroids, warming or cooling blankets, and fans affect temperature.*
3. Identify factors affecting the patient that influence temperature. *Rationale: Exercise increases metabolism and heat production, resulting in increased temperature.*
4. Identify factors likely to interfere with accuracy of temperature measurement. *Rationale: Smoking, chewing gum, and hot or cold substances cause false temperature readings in oral cavity for up to 15 minutes. Stool decreases accuracy of rectal temperature. Cerumen decreases accuracy of tympanic temperature. Diaphoresis decreases reliability of temporal temperature.*
5. Assess for signs and symptoms that accompany temperature alterations: hyperthermia: decreased skin turgor; tachycardia; hypotension; concentrated urine; heatstroke: hot, dry skin; tachycardia; hypotension; excessive thirst; muscle cramps; visual disturbances; confusion or delirium; hypothermia: pale skin; skin cool or cold to touch; bradycardia and dysrhythmias; uncontrollable shivering; reduced level of consciousness; shallow respirations. *Rationale: Physical signs and symptoms indicate abnormal temperature.*
6. Assess pertinent laboratory values, including complete blood count (CBC). *Rationale: A white blood cell (WBC) count greater than 12,000/mm^3 in a nonpregnant adult suggests the presence of infection, which can lead to hyperthermia; a WBC count less than 5000/mm^3 suggests that the ability of the body to fight infection is compromised, which can lead to ineffective thermoregulation.*
7. Determine previous baseline temperature from patient's record. *Rationale: Allows the nurse to assess for change in condition by comparing future vital sign measurements.*
8. Determine appropriate temperature site and measurement device for patient, considering the advantages and disadvantages of each site (see Table 6-2).

PLANNING

Expected Outcomes focus on identifying abnormalities and restoring homeostasis.

1. Patient's temperature is within acceptable range.
2. Patient identifies the factors that influence body temperature.

Delegation and Collaboration

The skill of temperature measurement may be delegated to nursing assistive personnel (NAP). Instruct the NAP by:

- Communicating the route, device, and frequency for temperature measurement.
- Explaining any precautions needed in positioning the patient for rectal temperature measurement.
- Reviewing patient's usual temperature values and significant changes or abnormalities to report to the nurse.

Equipment

- Thermometer (selected based on site used: see Table 6-2)
- Soft tissue or wipe
- Alcohol swab
- Lubricant (for rectal measurements only)
- Pen, vital sign flow sheet or record, or patient's electronic medical record
- Clean gloves, plastic thermometer sleeve, disposable probe or sensor cover
- Towel

IMPLEMENTATION *for* MEASURING BODY TEMPERATURE

STEP	RATIONALE
1. See Standard Protocol (inside front cover).	
2. Explain route by which you will take temperature and importance of maintaining proper position until reading is complete.	Patients are often curious about such measurements and prematurely remove thermometer to read results.
3. Assess oral temperature (electronic).	
a. *Optional:* Apply gloves when there are respiratory secretions or facial or mouth wound drainage.	Use of oral probe cover, which is removable without physical contact, minimizes need to wear gloves.
b. Remove thermometer pack from charging unit. Attach oral thermometer probe stem (blue tip) to thermometer unit. Grasp top of probe stem, being careful not to apply pressure on the ejection button.	Charging provides battery power. Ejection button releases plastic cover from probe stem.

Continued

STEP	RATIONALE
c. Slide disposable plastic probe cover over thermometer probe stem until cover locks in place (see illustration).	Soft plastic cover will not break in patient's mouth and prevents transmission of microorganisms between patients.
d. Ask patient to open mouth; then gently place thermometer probe under tongue in posterior sublingual pocket lateral to center of lower jaw (see illustration).	Heat from superficial blood vessels in sublingual pocket produces temperature reading. With electronic thermometer, temperatures in right and left posterior sublingual pocket are significantly higher than in area under front of tongue.
e. Ask patient to hold thermometer probe with lips closed.	Maintains proper position of thermometer during recording.
f. Leave thermometer probe in place until audible signal indicates completion and patient's temperature appears on digital display; remove thermometer probe from under patient's tongue.	Makes sure that probe stays in place until signal occurs to ensure accurate reading.
g. Push ejection button on thermometer probe stem to discard plastic probe cover into appropriate receptacle.	Reduces transmission of microorganisms.
h. Return thermometer probe stem to storage position of recording unit.	Returning probe stem automatically causes digital reading to disappear. Storage position protects stem.
4. Assess rectal temperature (electronic).	
a. Draw curtain around bed and/or close room door. Assist patient to side-lying or Sims' position with upper leg flexed. Move aside bed linen to expose only anal area. Keep patient's upper body and lower extremities covered with sheet or blanket.	Maintains patient's privacy, minimizes embarrassment, and promotes comfort.
b. Cleanse anal region when feces and/or secretions are present. Remove soiled gloves and reapply clean gloves.	Maintains standard precautions when exposed to items soiled with body fluids (e.g., feces).
c. Remove thermometer pack from charging unit. Attach rectal thermometer probe stem (red tip) to thermometer unit. Grasp top of probe stem, being careful not to apply pressure on the ejection button.	Charging provides battery power. Ejection button releases plastic cover from probe stem.
d. Slide disposable plastic probe cover over thermometer probe stem until cover locks in place.	Probe cover prevents transmission of microorganisms between patients.
e. Squeeze liberal portion of lubricant onto tissue. Dip probe thermometer probe cover, blunt end, into lubricant, covering 2.5 to 3.5 cm (1 to 1½ inches) for adult.	Lubrication minimizes trauma to rectal mucosa during insertion. Tissue avoids contamination of remaining lubricant in container.
f. With nondominant hand, separate patient's buttocks to expose anus. Ask patient to breathe slowly and relax.	Fully exposes anus for thermometer insertion. Relaxes anal sphincter for easier thermometer insertion.

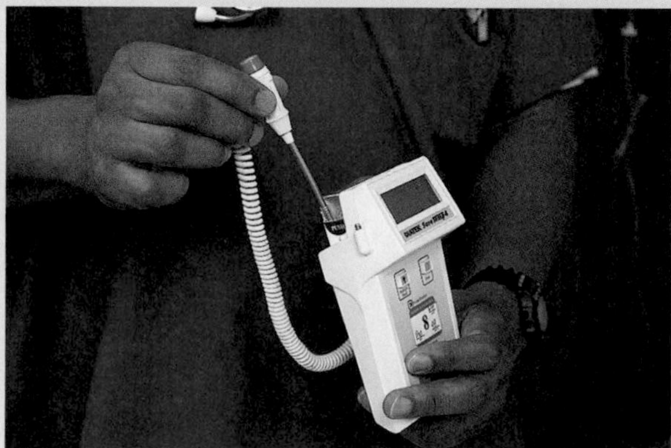

STEP 3c Disposable plastic cover is placed over probe.

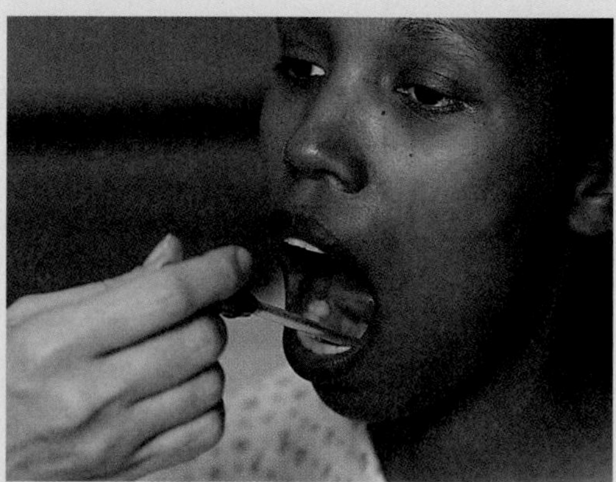

STEP 3d Probe under tongue in posterior sublingual pocket.

STEP	RATIONALE
g. Gently insert thermometer probe into anus in direction of umbilicus 3.5 cm (1½ inches) for adult. If you feel resistance during insertion, withdraw immediately. Do not force thermometer.	Ensures adequate exposure against blood vessels in rectal wall.

SAFETY ALERT If you cannot insert thermometer into rectum adequately, remove it and consider alternative method for obtaining temperature.

STEP	RATIONALE
h. Once positioned, hold thermometer probe in place until audible signal indicates completion and patient's temperature appears on digital display; remove thermometer probe from anus (see illustration).	Probe needs to stay in place until signal occurs to ensure accurate reading.
i. Push ejection button on thermometer stem to discard plastic probe cover into an appropriate receptacle. Wipe probe stem with alcohol swab, paying particular attention to ridges where probe stem connects to probe.	Reduces transmission of microorganisms.
j. Return thermometer stem to storage position of recording unit.	Automatically causes digital reading to disappear. Storage position protects stem.
k. Wipe patient's anal area with tissue or soft wipe to remove lubricant or feces and discard tissue. Assist patient in assuming a comfortable position.	Provides for comfort and hygiene.
5. *Assess axillary temperature (electronic).*	
a. Draw curtain around bed and/or close room door. Assist patient to supine or sitting position. Move clothing or gown away from shoulder and arm.	Maintains patient's privacy, minimizes embarrassment, and promotes comfort. Exposes axilla for correct thermometer probe placement.
b. Remove thermometer pack from charging unit. Attach oral thermometer probe stem (blue tip) to thermometer unit. Grasp top of thermometer probe stem, being careful not to apply pressure on ejection button.	Ejection button releases plastic cover from probe.
c. Slide disposable plastic probe cover over thermometer stem until cover locks in place.	Probe cover prevents transmission of microorganisms between patients.
d. Raise patient's arm away from torso. Inspect for skin lesions and excessive perspiration. Insert thermometer probe into center of axilla (see illustration), lower arm over probe, and place arm across patient's chest.	Maintains proper position of probe against blood vessels in axilla.

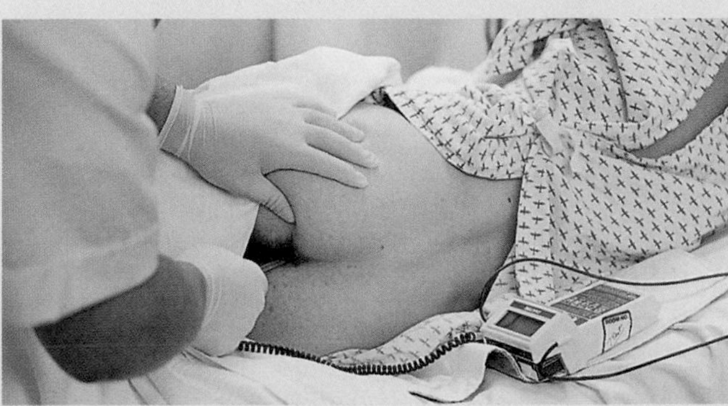

STEP 4h Remove probe smoothly from anus.

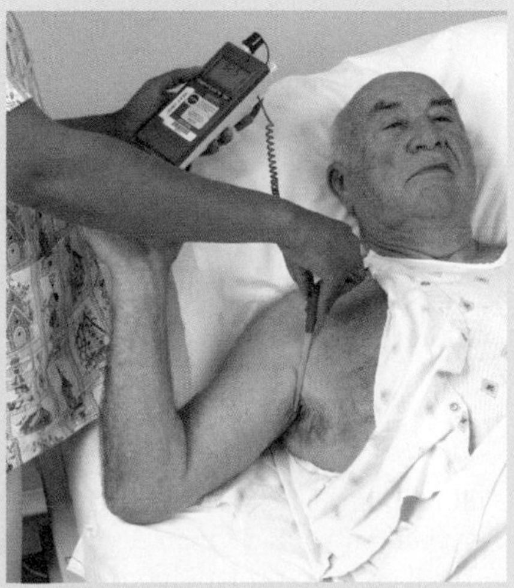

STEP 5d Place thermometer in axilla.

Continued

STEP	RATIONALE

SAFETY ALERT Do not use axilla if skin lesions are present because local temperature may be altered and area may be painful to touch.

STEP	RATIONALE
e. Once positioned, hold thermometer probe in place until audible signal indicates completion and patient's temperature appears on digital display. Remove thermometer probe from axilla.	Thermometer probe needs to stay in place until signal occurs to ensure accurate reading.
f. Push ejection button on thermometer stem to discard plastic probe cover into appropriate receptacle.	Reduces transmission of microorganisms.
g. Return thermometer stem to storage position of recording unit.	Returning thermometer stem to storage position automatically causes digital reading to disappear. Storage position protects stem.
6. ***Assess tympanic temperature.***	
a. Assist patient in assuming comfortable position with head turned toward side, away from you. If patient has been lying on one side, use upper ear. Obtain temperature from patient's right ear if you are right handed. Obtain temperature from patient's left ear if you are left handed.	Ensures comfort and helps expose auditory canal for accurate temperature measurement. Heat trapped in ear facing down causes false-high temperature readings. Using the appropriate hand reduces the angle of approach. The less acute the angle, the better the probe seal.
b. Note if there is obvious earwax in patient's ear canal.	Earwax on the lens cover of the speculum blocks a clear optical pathway. Switch to other ear or select alternative measurement site.
c. Remove thermometer handheld unit from charging base, being careful not to apply pressure to the ejection button.	Base provides battery power. Removal of handheld unit from base prepares it to measure temperature. Ejection button releases plastic probe cover from thermometer tip.
d. Slide disposable speculum cover over otoscope-like tip until it locks into place. Be careful not to touch lens cover.	Soft plastic probe cover prevents transmission of microorganisms between patients. Lens cover must be free of dust, fingerprints, and earwax to ensure clear optical path. Earwax can lower tympanic temperature by 0.3° C (0.5° F).
e. Insert speculum into ear canal, following manufacturer's instructions for tympanic probe positioning (see illustration).	Correct positioning of speculum probe tip with respect to ear canal allows maximum exposure of tympanic membrane.

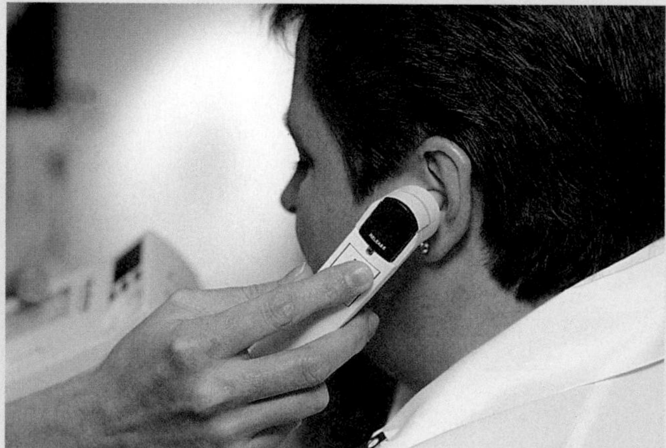

STEP 6e Tympanic membrane thermometer with probe cover placed in patient's ear.

STEP	RATIONALE
(1) Pull ear pinna backward, up and out for an adult. For children younger than 3 years of age, point covered probe toward midpoint between eyebrow and sideburns.	The ear tug straightens the external auditory canal, allowing maximum exposure of the tympanic membrane.

STEP	RATIONALE
(2) Move thermometer in a figure-eight pattern.	Some manufacturers recommend this movement because it allows the sensor to detect maximum tympanic membrane heat radiation.
(3) Fit speculum tip snugly into canal and do not move, pointing speculum tip toward nose.	Gentle pressure seals ear canal from ambient air temperature, which alters readings as much as 2.8° C (5° F). Operator error leads to false-low temperatures.
f. Once positioned, press scan button on handheld unit. Leave speculum in place until audible signal indicates completion and patient's temperature appears on digital display.	Pressing scan button causes detection of infrared energy. Speculum probe tip needs to stay in place until signal-indicating device has detected infrared energy.
g. Carefully remove speculum from auditory canal.	Prevents rubbing of sensitive outer ear lining.
h. Push ejection button on handheld unit to discard speculum cover into appropriate receptacle.	Reduces transmission of microorganisms. Automatically causes digital reading to disappear.
i. If temperature is abnormal or a second reading is necessary, replace speculum cover and wait 2 minutes before repeating the measurement in the same ear or repeat measurement in other ear. Consider trying an alternative temperature site or instrument.	Time allows ear canal to regain usual temperature.
j. Return handheld unit to thermometer base.	Protects sensor tip from damage.
7. *Assess temporal artery temperature:*	
a. Ensure that forehead is dry; wipe with towel if needed.	Moist skin distorts thermometer sensor.
b. Place sensor flush on patient's forehead.	Contact avoids measurement of ambient temperature.
c. Press red scan button with your thumb. Slowly slide thermometer straight across forehead while keeping sensor flush on skin (see illustration).	Continuous scanning for the highest temperature continues until you release the scan button.

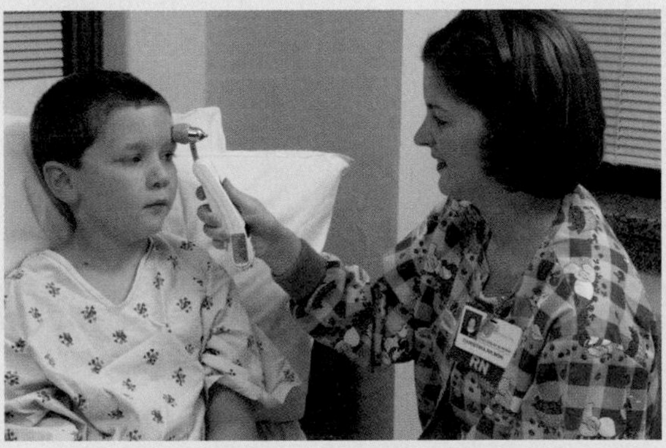

STEP 8c Scanning the forehead.

STEP	RATIONALE
d. Keeping the scan button pressed, lift sensor from forehead and touch sensor to skin on the neck, just behind the earlobe. Peak temperature occurs when clicking sound during scanning stops. Release scan button.	Sensor confirms highest temperature behind earlobe.
e. Clean sensor with alcohol swab.	Prevents transmission of microorganisms.
8. See Completion Protocol (inside front cover).	
9. Return thermometer to charger or thermometer base.	Maintains battery charge of thermometer unit.

EVALUATION

1. Compare temperature measurement with patient's baseline and acceptable range.
2. If patient has fever, take temperature approximately 30 minutes after administering antipyretics and every 4 hours until temperature stabilizes.
3. Ask patient to identify factors that influence temperature.

Unexpected Outcomes and Related Interventions

1. Patient has a temperature 1° C (1.8° F) or more above usual range.

a. Assess possible sites for localized infection and related data suggesting systemic infection, including pain or tenderness; purulent drainage; local area of redness or unusual warmth; loss of appetite; headache; hot, dry skin; flushed face; thirst; general malaise; or chills.
b. Reduce external covering on patient's body to promote heat loss. Do not induce shivering.
c. If fever persists or reaches unacceptable level as defined by health care provider, administer antipyretics and antibiotics as ordered and apply hypothermia blanket.

2. Patient has a temperature 1° C (1.8° F) or more below usual range.
a. Remove any wet clothing or linen, replace with dry garments, and cover patient with warm blankets.
b. Close room doors to eliminate drafts.
c. Encourage warm liquids.
d. Monitor apical pulse rate and rhythm (see Skill 6.2) because hypothermia causes bradycardia and dysrhythmias.

Recording and Reporting

- Record temperature and route in nurses' notes, vital sign flow sheet, or electronic medical record.
- Record temperature after administration of specific therapies in narrative form in nurses' notes.
- Record in nurses' notes any signs or symptoms of temperature alterations.
- Report abnormal findings to nurse in charge or health care provider immediately.

Sample Documentation

1400 Temporal temperature 39.0° C (102.2° F). Reports fatigue. Skin flushed, dry. Acetaminophen (Tylenol) 650 mg PO per order. Patient instructed to increase fluids.

1430 Temporal temperature 38.0° C (100.4° F). Patient napping. Skin pink, dry.

Special Considerations

Pediatric

- Axillary temperature cannot be relied on to detect fevers in infants and young children.
- For children who cry or become restless, take temperature last, after the other vital signs.

Geriatric

- The temperature of older adults is at the lower end of the acceptable temperature range. Temperatures considered within normal range may reflect a fever in an older adult.
- A decrease in sweat gland reactivity in the older adult results in higher threshold for sweating at high temperatures, which can lead to hyperthermia.
- Older adults are at high risk for hypothermia because of diminished sensation to cold, abnormal vasoconstrictor responses, and impaired shivering.

Home Care

- A temperature taken in the home may differ from the temperature assessed in a health care facility because the temperature routes differ.

SKILL 6.2 ASSESSING APICAL PULSE

- **Nursing Skills Online: Vital Signs, Lesson 3**

Video Clips

Assessing the apical pulse is the most accurate noninvasive method of determining heart rate and rhythm. Accurate assessment of the apical pulse requires correct use of a stethoscope (see Box 6-3).

ASSESSMENT

1. Identify medications or treatments that may influence pulse. *Rationale: Antiarrhythmics, cardiotonics, antihypertensives, vasodilators, and vasoconstrictors affect pulse rate and rhythm.*
2. Identify factors affecting the patient that influence pulse. *Rationale: Exercise and anxiety increase heart rate. An elevated temperature increases pulse rate and causes vasodilation, which can affect pulse strength. Certain conditions place patients at risk for pulse alterations: a history of heart disease, cardiac dysrhythmia, onset of sudden chest pain or acute pain from any site, invasive cardiovascular diagnostic tests, surgery, sudden infusion of large volume of intravenous (IV) fluid, internal or external hemorrhage, dehydration, or administration of medications that alter cardiac function.*
3. Identify factors likely to interfere with accuracy of pulse rate. *Rationale: Caffeine and nicotine increase pulse rate. Pulse rate is increased immediately by smoking, which lasts as long as 15 minutes (NHBPEP, 2003).*
4. Assess for signs and symptoms of altered cardiac function such as dyspnea, fatigue, chest pain, orthopnea, syncope, palpitations (person's unpleasant awareness of heartbeat), edema of dependent body parts, cyanosis or pallor of skin (see Chapter 7). *Rationale: Physical signs and symptoms indicate alteration in cardiac function, which affects pulse rate and rhythm.*
5. Assess pertinent laboratory values, including complete blood count (CBC). *Rationale: Low values for hemoglobin are associated with decreased oxygen transport, which can increase pulse rate.*
6. Determine previous baseline pulse rate from patient's record. *Rationale: Allows the nurse to assess for change in condition and effect of cardiac medications.*

PLANNING

Expected Outcomes focus on identifying abnormalities and restoring homeostasis.

1. Patient's pulse rate is regular and within acceptable range for age.
2. A baseline is established for patients with chronic diseases that alter pulse rate such as hypertension or arteriosclerosis.

Delegation and Collaboration

The skill of apical pulse measurement can be delegated to nursing assistive personnel (NAP) if the patient is stable and not at high risk for acute or serious cardiac problems. Instruct the NAP by:

- Communicating the frequency of measurement and factors related to the patient's history such as risk for abnormally slow or irregular pulse.
- Reviewing patient's usual pulse rate and significant changes or abnormalities to report to the nurse.

Equipment

- Wristwatch with second hand or digital display
- Stethoscope
- Pen, vital sign flow sheet or record, or patient's electronic medical record

IMPLEMENTATION *for* ASSESSING APICAL PULSE

STEPS	RATIONALE
1. **See Standard Protocol (inside front cover).**	
2. Assist patient to supine or sitting position. Move bed linen and gown to uncover sternum and left side of chest.	Exposes portion of chest wall for selection of auscultatory site.
3. Locate anatomical landmarks to identify the apical impulse, also called the *point of maximal impulse* (PMI). The heart is located behind and to the left of the sternum with base at top and apex at bottom. Find the angle of Louis just below the suprasternal notch between the sternal body and manubrium; feels like a bony prominence. Slip fingers down each side of the angle to find the second intercostal space (ICS). Carefully move fingers down the left side of the sternum to the fifth ICS and laterally to the left midclavicular line (MCL). A light tap felt within an area 1 to 2.5 cm (½ to 1 inch) of the apical impulse is reflected from the apex of the heart (see Fig. 6-1).	Use of anatomical landmarks allows correct placement of stethoscope over the apex of the heart. This position enhances the ability to hear heart sounds clearly. If unable to palpate the apical impulse, reposition patient on left side. In the presence of serious heart disease, locate the apical impulse to the left of the MCL or at the sixth ICS.
4. Place diaphragm of stethoscope in palm of hand for 5 to 10 seconds.	Warming metal or plastic diaphragm prevents patient from being startled and promotes comfort.
5. Place diaphragm of stethoscope over the apical impulse at the fifth ICS, at the left MCL, and auscultate for normal S_1 and S_2 heart sounds (heard as "lub dub") (see illustration).	Allow stethoscope tubing to extend straight without kinks so it does not distort sound transmission. Normal sounds S_1 and S_2 are high pitched and best heard with the diaphragm.

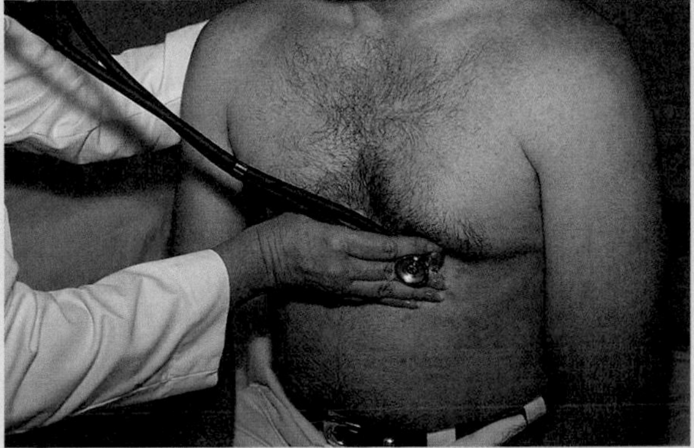

STEP 5 Stethoscope over the apical impulse.

Continued

STEPS	RATIONALE
6. When you hear S_1 and S_2 with regularity, use watch's second hand and begin to count rate: when sweep hand hits number on dial, start counting with zero and then one, two, and so on.	Apical rate is accurate only after you are able to hear sounds clearly. Timing begins with zero. Count of one is first sound auscultated after timing begins.
7. If apical rate is regular, count for 30 seconds and multiply by 2. If heart rate is irregular or patient is receiving cardiovascular medication, count for 1 minute (60 seconds).	Monitor a regular apical rate for 30 seconds. You can assess irregular rate more accurately when measured over a longer interval, usually 60 seconds.
8. Note if heart rate is irregular and describe pattern of irregularity (S_1 and S_2 occurring early or later after previous sequence of sounds; e.g., every third or every fourth beat is skipped).	Irregular heart rate indicates dysrhythmia. Regular occurrence of dysrhythmia within 1 minute indicates inefficient contraction of heart and alteration in cardiac function.
9. See Completion Protocol (inside front cover).	
10. Clean earpieces and diaphragm of stethoscope with alcohol swab routinely after each use.	Stethoscopes are frequently contaminated with microorganisms. Regular disinfection controls nosocomial infections.

EVALUATION

1. Compare apical pulse rate with patient's baseline and acceptable range.
2. Correlate apical pulse rate with data obtained from radial pulse, blood pressure, and related signs and symptoms (palpitations, dizziness).

Unexpected Outcomes and Related Interventions

1. Patient has an apical pulse greater than 100 beats per minute (tachycardia) in an adult or expected normal value.
   a. Identify related data, including pain, fear, anxiety, recent exercise, hypotension, blood loss, fever, or inadequate oxygenation.
   b. Observe for signs and symptoms associated with abnormal cardiac function, including fatigue, chest pain, orthopnea, cyanosis.
2. Patient has an apical pulse less than 60 beats per minute (bradycardia) in an adult or expected normal value.
   a. Observe for factors that alter heart rate such as digoxin (Lanoxin), beta-blockers, and antidysrhythmics; it is sometimes necessary to withhold prescribed medications until the health care provider is able to evaluate the need to adjust the dosage.
   b. Observe for signs and symptoms associated with abnormal cardiac function, including fatigue, chest pain, orthopnea, cyanosis.
3. Patient has an irregular rhythm.
   a. Assess for pulse deficit (see Procedural Guideline 6.1).
   b. Patients with irregular rhythm may require an electrocardiogram or 24-hour heart monitor per health care provider order to detect heart abnormalities.

Recording and Reporting

- Record apical pulse rate in nurses' notes, vital signs flow sheet, or electronic medical record.
- Record apical pulse rate after administration of specific therapies and document in narrative in nurses' notes.
- Report any signs and symptoms of alteration in cardiac function in nurses' notes.
- Report abnormal findings to nurse in charge or health care provider immediately.

Sample Documentation

1200 Apical rate 64, regularly irregular. No pulse deficit noted.

Special Considerations

Pediatric

- Children often have a sinus arrhythmia, which is an irregular heartbeat that speeds up with inspiration and slows down with expiration. Breath holding in a child affects pulse rate.
- Apical or brachial pulse is the best site for assessing infant's or young child's heart rate and rhythm.

Geriatric

- Once elevated, the pulse rate of an older adult takes longer to return to normal resting rate.
- Older adults have a reduced heart rate with exercise because of a decreased responsiveness to catecholamines.

SKILL 6.3 ASSESSING RADIAL PULSE

- **Nursing Skills Online: Vital Signs, Lesson 3**

Video Clips

The radial pulse in an adult is the easiest to access and provides a quick, accurate assessment of peripheral circulation and heart function.

ASSESSMENT

1. Identify medications or treatments that may influence pulse. *Rationale: Antiarrhythmics, cardiotonics, antihypertensives, vasodilators, and vasoconstrictors affect pulse rate.*
2. Identify factors affecting the patient that influence pulse. *Rationale: Exercise and anxiety increase heart rate. An elevated temperature increases pulse rate and causes vasodilation, which can affect pulse strength.*
3. Identify factors likely to interfere with accuracy of pulse rate. *Rationale: Caffeine and nicotine increase pulse rate. Pulse rate is increased immediately by smoking, which lasts as long as 15 minutes (NHBPEP, 2003).*
4. Assess for signs and symptoms of altered cardiac function such as dyspnea, fatigue, chest pain, orthopnea, syncope, or palpitations. *Rationale: Physical signs and symptoms indicate alteration in cardiac function, which affects pulse rate and rhythm.*
5. Determine previous baseline pulse rate from patient's record. *Rationale: Allows the nurse to assess for change in condition and effect of cardiac medications.*

PLANNING

Expected Outcomes focus on identifying abnormalities and restoring homeostasis.

1. Patient's pulse rate is regular and within acceptable range for age.
2. A baseline is established for patients with chronic diseases that alter pulse rate such as hypertension or arteriosclerosis.

Delegation and Collaboration

The skill of pulse measurement can be delegated to nursing assistive personnel (NAP) if the patient is stable and not at high risk for acute or serious cardiac or vascular problems. Instruct the NAP by:

- Communicating the appropriate site for pulse rate, frequency of measurement, and factors related to the patient's history such as risk for abnormally slow or irregular pulse.
- Reviewing patient's usual pulse rates and significant changes or abnormalities to report to the nurse.

Equipment

- Wristwatch with second hand or digital display
- Pen, vital sign flow sheet or record, or patient's electronic medical record

IMPLEMENTATION *for* ASSESSING RADIAL PULSE

STEP	RATIONALE
1. **See Standard Protocol (inside front cover).**	
2. Explain to patient that you will assess pulse or heart rate. Encourage patient to relax and not speak. If patient has been active, wait 5 to 10 minutes before assessing pulse.	Activity and anxiety elevate heart rate. Obtaining pulse rates at rest allows for objective comparison of values.
3. If patient is supine, place patient's forearm straight alongside or across lower chest or upper abdomen with wrist extended straight. If sitting, bend patient's elbow 90 degrees and support lower arm on chair or on your arm.	Relaxed position of lower arm and extension of wrist permit full exposure of artery to palpation.
4. Place tips of first two or middle three fingers of your hand over groove along radial or thumb side of patient's inner wrist (see illustration). Slightly extend the wrist with palm down until you note the strongest pulse.	Fingertips are the most sensitive parts of your hand to palpate arterial pulsation. Your thumb has a pulsation that interferes with accuracy.

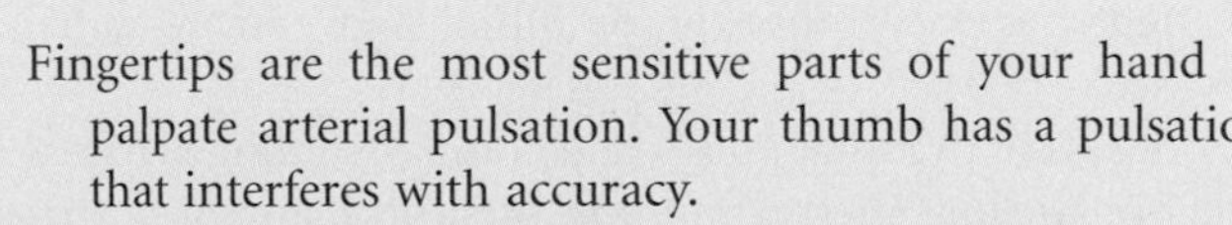

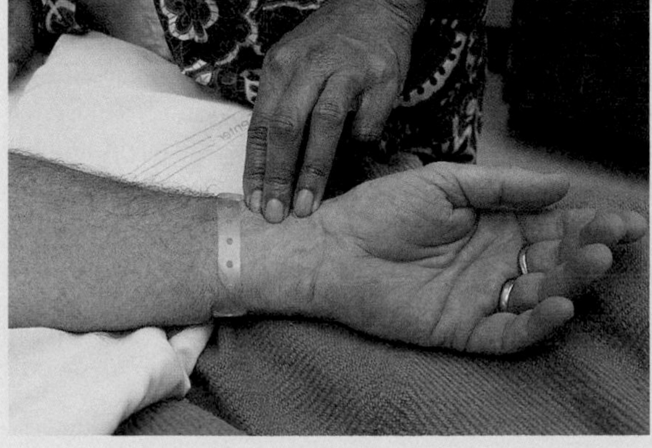

STEP 4 Hand placement for pulse assessment. (From Sorrentino SA, Remmert L, Gorek B: *Mosby's essentials for nursing assistants,* ed 4, St Louis, 2010, Mosby.)

Continued

STEP	RATIONALE
5. Lightly compress against radius, obliterate pulse initially, and then relax pressure so pulse becomes easily palpable.	Pulse is more accurate with moderate pressure. Too much pressure occludes pulse and impairs blood flow.
6. Determine strength of pulse. Note whether thrust of vessel against fingertips is bounding (4+); full, increased (+3); expected (+2); diminished, barely palpable (+1); or absent, nonpalpable (0).	Strength reflects volume of blood ejected against arterial wall with each heart contraction. Accurate description of strength improves communication among nurses and other health care providers.
7. After you feel pulse regularly, look at watch's second hand and begin to count rate: when sweep hand hits number on dial, start counting with zero and then one, two, and so on.	Timing begins with zero. Count of one is first beat palpated after timing begins.
8. If pulse is regular, count rate for 30 seconds and multiply total by 2.	A 30-second count is accurate for rapid, slow, or regular pulse rates.
9. If pulse is irregular, count rate for 60 seconds. Assess frequency and pattern of irregularity.	Inefficient contraction of heart fails to transmit pulse wave, resulting in irregular pulse. Longer time period promotes accurate count.
10. When pulse is irregular, compare radial pulses bilaterally.	A marked inequality indicates compromised arterial flow to one extremity, and you need to take action.

SAFETY ALERT If pulse is irregular, obtain an apical-radial pulse to assess for pulse deficit (see Procedural Guideline 6.1).

11. See Completion Protocol (inside front cover).

EVALUATION

1. Compare pulse rate with patient's baseline and acceptable range.
2. Compare radial pulse equality and note discrepancy. Differences between radial arteries indicate compromised peripheral vascular system.
3. Correlate pulse rate with data obtained from apical pulse, blood pressure, and related signs and symptoms (palpitations, dizziness).

Unexpected Outcomes and Related Interventions

1. Patient has weak, thready, or difficult-to-palpate radial pulse.
   a. Assess both radial pulses and compare findings. Assess for swelling in surrounding tissues or anything that may impede blood flow (e.g., dressing or cast).
   b. Observe for symptoms associated with altered peripheral tissue perfusion, including pallor or cyanosis of tissue distal to pulse and cold extremities.
2. Patient has irregular radial pulse or less than 60 (bradycardia) or greater than 100 (tachycardia) beats per minute.
   a. Auscultate the apical pulse.

Recording and Reporting

- Record pulse rate with assessment site in nurses' notes, vital signs flow sheet, or electronic medical record.
- Record pulse rate after administration of specific therapies and document in narrative in nurses' notes.
- Record any signs and symptoms of alteration in cardiac function in nurses' notes.
- Report abnormal findings to nurse in charge or health care provider immediately.

Sample Documentation

1400 Right radial pulse +2; left radial pulse +1, left hand cool to touch, capillary refill >4 sec, charge nurse notified.

Special Considerations

Pediatric

- Radial artery is difficult to assess in infant. Apical or brachial pulse is best site for assessing pediatric heart rate and rhythm until 2 years of age.

Geriatric

- Once elevated, the pulse rate of an older adult takes longer to return to normal resting rate.
- Older adults have a reduced heart rate with exercise because of a decreased responsiveness to catecholamine.
- Peripheral vascular disease is more common among older adults, making radial pulse assessment difficult.

Home Care

- Patients taking certain prescribed cardiac or antiarrhythmic medications should learn to assess their own pulse rates to detect side effects of medications.

PROCEDURAL GUIDELINE 6.1
Assessing Apical-Radial Pulse Deficit

The difference between pulses assessed from two different sites, or a pulse deficit, provides information about cardiac and vascular integrity. When a pulse deficit exists between the apical and radial pulses, the volume of blood ejected from the heart may be inadequate to meet the circulatory needs of the tissues, and intervention may be required.

Delegation and Collaboration

The skill of assessing an apical-radial pulse deficit cannot be delegated to nursing assistive personnel (NAP). Collaboration between the nurse and a second health care provider is required.

Equipment

- Stethoscope
- Alcohol swab
- Watch that displays seconds

Procedural Steps

1. **See Standard Protocol (inside front cover).**
2. Explain to patient that two people will be assessing heart function at the same time.
3. Nurse auscultates for apical pulse (see Skill 6.2) while second provider obtains radial pulse (see Skill 6.3).
4. Nurse begins pulse count by calling out loud simultaneously when to begin counting pulses.
5. Each nurse completes a 60-second pulse count. Compare apical and radial rates. If pulse count differs by more than 2, a pulse deficit exists, which sometimes indicates alterations in cardiac function.
6. **See Completion Protocol (inside front cover).**
7. Record presence of a pulse deficit in narrative nurses' notes and report findings to health care provider.

SKILL 6.4 ASSESSING RESPIRATIONS

- **Nursing Skills Online: Vital Signs, Lesson 4**

Video Clips

Assessment of respiration includes determining respiratory rate, respiratory depth, and respiratory rhythm.

ASSESSMENT

1. Identify medications or treatments that may influence respiratory rate. *Rationale: Oxygen and bronchodilators affect respiratory rate.*
2. Identify factors affecting the patient that influence respiratory rate, depth, and rhythm. *Rationale: Fever, pain, anxiety, diseases of chest wall or muscles, constrictive chest or abdominal dressings, presence of abdominal incisions, gastric distention, chronic pulmonary disease (emphysema, bronchitis, asthma), traumatic injury to chest wall, presence of a chest tube, respiratory infection (pneumonia, acute bronchitis), pulmonary edema and emboli, head injury with damage to brain stem, and anemia all can affect respiratory assessment.*
3. Assess for signs and symptoms of altered respiratory function:
   - Bluish or cyanotic appearance of nail beds, lips, mucous membranes, and skin
   - Restlessness, irritability, confusion, reduced level of consciousness
   - Pain during inspiration
   - Labored or difficult breathing
   - Orthopnea
   - Use of accessory muscles
   - Adventitious breath sounds (see Chapter 7),
   - Inability to breathe spontaneously
   - Thick, frothy, blood-tinged, or large amounts of sputum produced on coughing

   Rationale: Physical signs and symptoms indicate alterations in respiratory function, which affects respiratory rate, depth, and rhythm.
4. Identify that patient is in comfortable position. *Rationale: Sitting erect promotes full ventilatory movement. Position of discomfort causes patient to breathe more rapidly.*
5. Determine previous baseline respiratory rate from patient's record. *Rationale: Allows the nurse to assess for change in condition and effect of respiratory medications.*

PLANNING

Expected Outcomes focus on identifying abnormalities and restoring homeostasis.

1. Patient's respiratory rate is regular and within acceptable range for age.
2. A baseline is established for patients with chronic diseases such as obstructive lung disease that alters respiratory rate.

Delegation and Collaboration

The skill of assessing respirations can be delegated to nursing assistive personnel (NAP). Instruct the NAP by:

- Communicating the frequency of measurement as determined by the patient's history and factors related to it such as labored breathing or complaints of breathing difficulty.
- Reviewing patient's usual respiratory values and significant changes or abnormalities to report to the nurse.

Equipment

- Wristwatch with second hand or digital display
- Pen, vital sign flow sheet or record, or patient's electronic medical record

IMPLEMENTATION *for* ASSESSING RESPIRATIONS

STEPS	RATIONALE
1. See Standard Protocol (inside front cover).	
2. Be sure that patient's chest is visible. If necessary, move bed linen or gown.	Ensures clear view of chest wall and abdominal movements.
3. Place patient's arm in relaxed position across the abdomen or lower chest or place your hand directly over patient's upper abdomen.	A similar position used during pulse assessment allows you to assess respiratory rate subtly. Patient's arm or your hand rises and falls during respiratory cycle.
4. Observe complete respiratory cycle (one inspiration and one expiration).	The nurse determines an accurate rate only after viewing the entire respiratory cycle.
5. After you observe a cycle, look at watch's second hand and begin to count rate: when sweep hand hits number on dial, begin time frame, counting one with first full respiratory cycle.	Timing begins with count of one. Respirations occur more slowly than pulse; thus timing does not begin with zero.
6. If rhythm is regular, count number of respirations in 30 seconds and multiply by 2. If rhythm is irregular, less than 12, or greater than 20, count for 1 full minute.	Respiratory rate is equivalent to number of respirations per minute. Suspected irregularities require assessment for at least 1 minute (see Table 6-3)
7. Note depth of respirations, subjectively assessed by observing degree of chest wall movement while counting rate. You also objectively assess depth by palpating chest wall excursion or auscultating the posterior thorax (see Chapter 7) after you have counted the rate. Describe depth as shallow, normal, or deep.	Character of ventilatory movement reveals specific disease state that restricts volume of air from moving into and out of the lungs.
8. Note rhythm of ventilatory cycle. Normal breathing is regular and uninterrupted. Do not confuse sighing with abnormal rhythm.	Character of ventilations reveals specific types of alterations. Periodically people unconsciously take single deep breaths or sighs to expand small airways prone to collapse.
9. Observe for evidence of dyspnea (increased effort to inhale and exhale). Ask patient to describe subjective experience of shortness of breath compared with usual breathing pattern.	Patients with chronic lung disease may experience difficulty breathing all the time and can best describe their own discomfort from shortness of breath.
10. See Completion Protocol (inside front cover).	

EVALUATION

1. Compare findings with previous baseline and acceptable range for patient's age.
2. Correlate respiratory rate with data obtained from auscultation, laboratory data, and related respiratory signs and symptoms.

Unexpected Outcomes and Related Interventions

1. Respiratory rate is below 12 (bradypnea) or above 20 (tachypnea). Breathing pattern is irregular. Depth of respirations is increased or decreased; patient complains of feeling short of breath.
   a. Observe for related factors, including obstructed airway, noisy respirations, cyanosis, restlessness, irritability, confusion, productive cough, use of accessory muscles, and abnormal breath sounds (Chapter 7).
   b. Assist patient to supported sitting position (semi- or high-Fowler's) unless contraindicated.
   c. Provide oxygen as ordered (see Chapter 14).
   d. Assess for environmental factors that influence patient's respiratory rate such as secondhand smoke, poor ventilation, or gas fumes.

Recording and Reporting

- Record respiratory rate and character in nurses' notes, vital sign flow sheet, or electronic medical record.
- Record abnormal depth and rhythm in narrative form in nurses' notes.
- Record respiratory rate after administration of specific therapies in narrative form in nurses' notes.
- Record type and amount of oxygen therapy if used by patient during assessment.
- Report abnormal findings to nurse in charge or health care provider immediately.

Sample Documentation

0750 Patient c/o dyspnea. RR 32, shallow and labored. Oxygen at 2 L NC. Bilateral wheezing auscultated. BP 144/56 R arm, R radial pulse 112, strong. Respiratory therapy notified for prn nebulizer treatment. Charge nurse notified.

Special Considerations

Pediatric

- Acceptable average respiratory rate for newborns is 35 to 40 breaths per minute; infant (6 months) is 30 to 50 breaths per minute; toddler (2 years) is 25 to 32 breaths per minute; and child is 20 to 30 breaths per minute.

Geriatric

- A change in lung function with aging results in respiratory rates that are generally higher in older adults, with a normal range of 16 to 25 breaths per minute.

SKILL 6.5 ASSESSING BLOOD PRESSURE

- **Nursing Skills Online: Vital Signs, Lesson 5**

Video Clips

Accurate blood pressure measurement ensures optimum care. This skill describes blood pressure assessment in upper and lower extremities using a sphygmomanometer and stethoscope.

ASSESSMENT

1. Consider normal daily fluctuations in blood pressure. *Rationale: Blood pressure varies throughout the day, with lower blood pressure during sleep, highest blood pressure in the afternoon (Giles, 2006).*
2. Identify patient's medications or treatments that may influence blood pressure. *Rationale: Narcotics, anesthesia, cardiotonics, antihypertensives, vasodilators, vasoconstrictors, blood and IV fluids affect blood pressure.*
3. Identify factors affecting the patient that influence blood pressure. *Rationale: Exercise, stress, anxiety, and hormone stimulation can increase blood pressure.*
4. Identify factors likely to interfere with accuracy of blood pressure measurements. *Rationale: Coffee, smoking, and talking all affect blood pressure.*
5. Assess for signs and symptoms of blood pressure alterations. *Rationale: Physical signs and symptoms sometimes indicate alterations in blood pressure. High blood pressure (hypertension) is often asymptomatic until pressure is very high. Assess for headache (usually occipital), flushing of face, nosebleed, and fatigue in older adults. Low blood pressure (hypotension) is associated with dizziness; confusion; restlessness; pale, dusky, or cyanotic skin and mucous membranes; cool, mottled skin over extremities.*
6. Determine appropriate extremity and blood pressure cuff for patient extremity. *Rationale: Inappropriate site selection results in poor amplification of sounds, causing inaccurate readings (see Table 6-5). Application of pressure from inflated bladder temporarily impairs blood flow and further compromises circulation in an extremity that already has impaired blood flow. Avoid applying cuff to extremity when IV fluids are infusing; an arteriovenous shunt or fistula is present; breast or axillary surgery has been performed on that side; extremity has been traumatized, diseased, or requires a cast or bulky bandage. Use the lower extremities when the brachial arteries are inaccessible.*
7. Determine if patient has a latex allergy. *Rationale: If patient has a latex allergy, verify that blood pressure cuff is latex free.*
8. Determine previous baseline blood pressure from patient's record.

PLANNING

Expected Outcomes focus on identifying abnormalities and restoring homeostasis.

1. Patient's blood pressure is within acceptable range for age, gender, and ethnicity.
2. Patient identifies factors that increase blood pressure.
3. A baseline is established for patients with hypertension and chronic diseases that alter blood pressure.
4. Patient states strategies to reduce personal risk for hypertension.

Delegation and Collaboration

The skill of blood pressure measurement may be delegated to nursing assistive personnel (NAP) unless the patient is considered unstable (i.e., hypotensive). Instruct the NAP by:

- Communicating the frequency of measurement, limb for measurement, and factors related to the patient's history such as risk for orthostatic hypotension.
- Explaining the appropriate size blood pressure cuff and equipment (electronic or manual) to be used.
- Reviewing patient's usual blood pressure values and significant changes or abnormalities to report to the nurse.

Equipment

- Aneroid sphygmomanometer
- Cloth or disposable vinyl pressure cuff of appropriate size for patient's extremity
- Stethoscope
- Alcohol swab
- Pen, vital sign flow sheet or record, or patient's electronic medical record

IMPLEMENTATION *for* ASSESSING BLOOD PRESSURE

STEPS	RATIONALE
1. **See Standard Protocol (inside front cover).**	
2. Explain to patient that you will assess blood pressure. Have patient rest at least 5 minutes before measuring lying or sitting blood pressure and 1 minute when standing. Ask patient not to speak while measuring blood pressure.	Reduces anxiety that falsely elevates readings. Blood pressure readings taken at different times can be compared more objectively when assessed with patient at rest. Exercise causes false elevations in blood pressure. Talking to a patient when assessing the blood pressure increases readings 10% to 40% (NHBPEP, 2003).
3. Be sure that patient has not ingested caffeine or smoked for 30 minutes before blood pressure assessment.	Caffeine or nicotine cause false elevations in blood pressure. Smoking increases blood pressure immediately and lasts up to 15 minutes. Caffeine increases blood pressure up to 3 hours (NHBPEP, 2003).
4. Select appropriate cuff size.	Improper cuff size results in inaccurate readings (see Table 6-5). For example, if the cuff is too small, false-high readings result. If the cuff is too large, false-low readings result.
5. Clean stethoscope earpieces and diaphragm with alcohol swab.	Reduces transmission of microorganisms.
6. Have patient assume sitting position. Be sure that environment is warm, quiet, and relaxing.	Sitting is preferred to lying. Diastolic pressure measured while sitting is approximately 5 mm Hg higher than when measured supine. The patient's perceptions that the physical or interpersonal environment is stressful affect the blood pressure measurement. Talking and background noise result in inaccurate readings.
7. Position patient's forearm, supported at heart level if needed, with palm turned up (see illustration); for thigh, position with knee slightly flexed. If sitting, instruct patient to keep feet flat on floor without legs crossed. If supine, support the patient's arm (e.g., on the mattress or with a pillow so that the cuff is at the level of the right atrium).	If arm is extended and not supported, patient will perform isometric exercise that increases diastolic pressure (Adiyaman and others, 2006). Placement of arm above the level of the heart causes false-low reading 2 mm Hg for each inch above heart level. Leg crossing falsely increases systolic blood pressure by 2 to 8 mm Hg. Even in the supine position a diastolic pressure increases blood pressure up to 3 to 4 mm Hg for each 5-cm change in heart level.

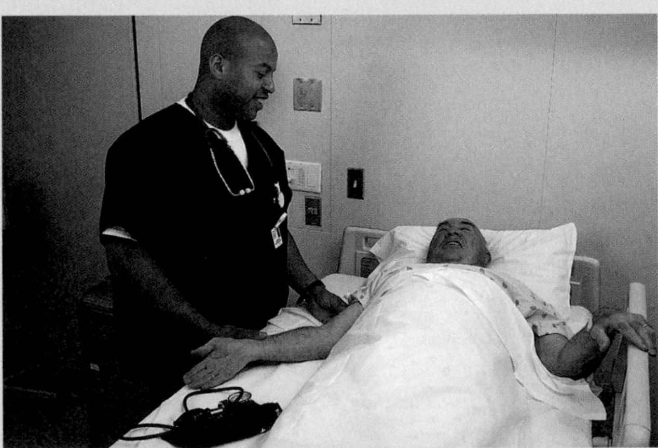

STEP 7 Patient's forearm supported in bed.

STEPS	RATIONALE
8. Expose extremity (arm or leg) fully by removing constricting clothing.	Ensures proper cuff application. Do not place blood pressure cuff over clothing. Tight clothing causes congestion of blood and can falsely elevate blood pressure readings.

STEPS	RATIONALE
9. Palpate brachial artery (arm) or popliteal artery (leg). With cuff fully deflated, apply bladder of cuff above artery by centering arrows marked on cuff over artery. If there are no center arrows on cuff, estimate the center of the bladder and place this center over artery. Position cuff 2.5 cm (1 inch) above site of pulsation (antecubital or popliteal space). With cuff fully deflated, wrap cuff evenly and snugly around extremity (see illustrations).	Inflating bladder directly over artery ensures that proper pressure is applied during inflation. Loose-fitting cuff causes false-high readings.
10. Position manometer gauge vertically at eye level. Make sure that observer is no farther than 1 m (approximately 1 yard) away.	Looking up or down at the scale results in inaccurate readings.
11. Measure blood pressure.	
a. Two-Step Method:	
(1) Relocate brachial pulse. Palpate the artery distal to the cuff with fingertips of nondominant hand while inflating cuff rapidly to a pressure 30 mm Hg above point at which pulse disappears. Slowly deflate cuff and note point when pulse reappears. Deflate cuff fully and wait 30 seconds.	Estimating systolic pressure prevents false-low readings, which result in the presence of an auscultatory gap. Palpation determines maximal inflation point for accurate reading. If unable to palpate artery because of weakened pulse, use an ultrasonic stethoscope (see Chapter 7). Completely deflating cuff prevents venous congestion and false-high readings.
(2) Place stethoscope earpieces in ears and be sure that sounds are clear, not muffled.	Ensures that each earpiece follows angle of ear canal to facilitate hearing.

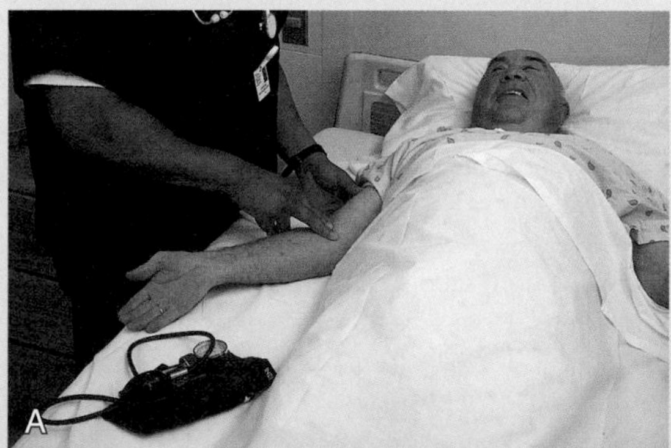

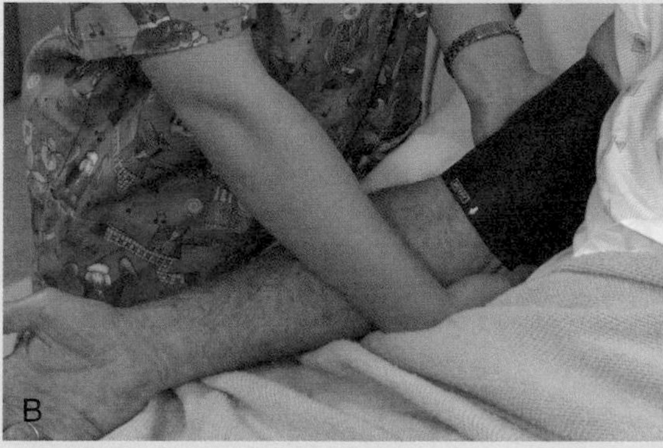

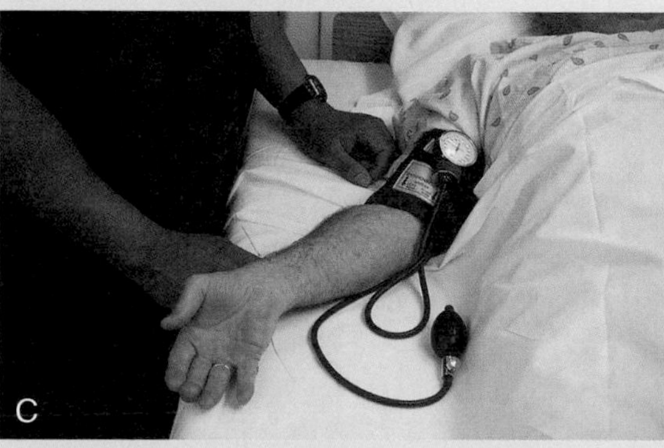

STEP 9 A, Palpating the brachial artery. **B,** Aligning blood pressure cuff arrow with brachial artery. **C,** Blood pressure cuff wrapped around upper arm.

Continued

STEPS	RATIONALE
(3) Relocate brachial artery and place bell or diaphragm of stethoscope over it. Do not allow chestpiece to touch cuff or clothing (see illustration).	Proper stethoscope placement ensures the best sound reception. The bell provides better sound reproduction, whereas the diaphragm is easier to secure with fingers and covers a larger area. Stethoscope improperly positioned causes muffled sounds that often result in false-low systolic and false-high diastolic readings.
(4) Close valve of pressure bulb clockwise until tight.	Tightening valve prevents air leak during inflation.
(5) Quickly inflate cuff to 30 mm Hg above patient's estimated systolic pressure.	Rapid inflation ensures accurate measurement of systolic pressure.
(6) Slowly release pressure bulb valve and allow manometer needle gauge to fall at rate of 2 to 3 mm Hg/sec.	Too-rapid or too-slow a decline in pressure release causes inaccurate readings.
(7) Note point on manometer when the first clear sound is heard. The sound slowly increases in intensity.	First Korotkoff sound reflects systolic blood pressure.
(8) Continue to deflate cuff gradually, noting point at which sound disappears in adults. Note pressure to nearest 2 mm Hg. Listen for 20 to 30 mm Hg after the last sound and then allow remaining air to escape quickly.	Beginning of the fifth Korotkoff sound is an indication of diastolic pressure in adults (NHBPEP, 2003). Fourth Korotkoff sound involves distinct muffling of sounds and is an indication of diastolic pressure in children (NHBPEP, 2003).
b. One-Step Method:	
(1) Place stethoscope earpieces in ears and be sure that sounds are clear, not muffled.	Earpiece should follow the angle of ear canal to facilitate hearing.
(2) Relocate brachial artery and place diaphragm of stethoscope over it. Do not allow chestpiece to touch cuff or clothing.	Proper stethoscope placement ensures optimal sound reception.
(3) Close valve of pressure bulb clockwise until tight.	Tightening valve prevents air leak during inflation.
(4) Quickly inflate cuff to 30 mm Hg above patient's usual systolic pressure.	Inflation above systolic level ensures accurate measurement of systolic pressure.
(5) Slowly release pressure bulb valve and allow manometer needle to fall at rate of 2 to 3 mm Hg/sec. Note point on manometer when you hear the first clear sound. The sound slowly increases in intensity.	Too-rapid or too-slow a decline in pressure release causes inaccurate readings. The first Korotkoff sounds reflect systolic pressure.
(6) Continue to deflate cuff gradually, noting point at which sound disappears in adults. Note pressure to nearest 2 mm Hg. Listen for 20 to 30 mm Hg after the last sound and then allow remaining air to escape quickly.	Beginning of the fifth Korotkoff sound is an indication of diastolic pressure in adults (NHBPEP, 2003). Fourth Korotkoff sound involves distinct muffling of sounds and is an indication of diastolic pressure in children (NHBPEP, 2003).

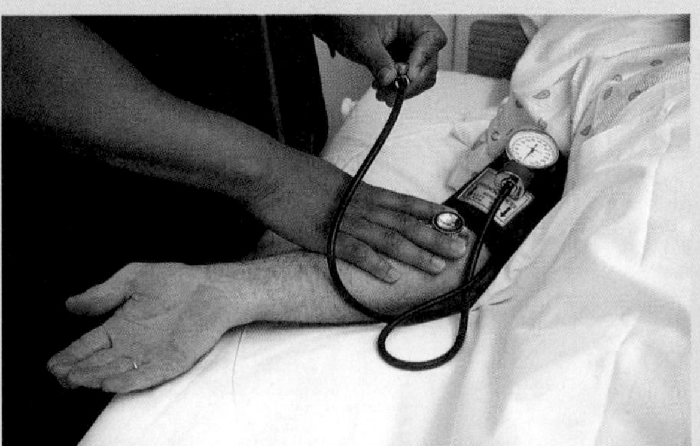

STEP 11a(3) Stethoscope over brachial artery to measure blood pressure.

STEPS	RATIONALE
12. The American Heart Association recommends the average of two sets of blood pressure measurements 2 minutes apart. Use the second set of blood pressure measurements as the patient's baseline.	Two sets of blood pressure measurements help to prevent false positives based on a patient's sympathetic response (alert reaction). Averaging minimizes the effect of anxiety, which often causes a first reading to be higher than subsequent measurements (NHBPEP, 2003).
13. Remove cuff from patient's extremity unless you need to repeat measurement. If this is the first assessment of patient, repeat procedure on the other extremity.	Comparison of blood pressure in both extremities detects circulatory problems. (Normal difference of 5 to 10 mm Hg exists between extremities.)
14. See Completion Protocol (inside front cover). Clean earpieces, bell, and diaphragm of stethoscope with alcohol swab.	Reduces transmission of microorganisms when nurses share stethoscopes.

EVALUATION

1. Compare reading with previous baseline and acceptable value of blood pressure for patient's age.
2. Compare blood pressure in both arms or both legs. If using upper extremities, use the arm with higher pressure for subsequent assessments unless contraindicated.
3. Correlate blood pressure with data obtained from pulse assessment and related cardiovascular signs and symptoms.
4. Ask patient to describe strategies to reduce personal risk factors for hypertension.

Unexpected Outcomes and Related Interventions

1. Unable to obtain blood pressure reading
   a. Determine that no immediate crisis is present by assessing pulse and respiratory rate.
   b. Assess for signs and symptoms of altered cardiac function. If present, notify nurse in charge or health care provider immediately.
   c. Use alternative sites or procedures to obtain blood pressure: auscultate blood pressure in lower extremity, use an ultrasonic stethoscope, or use palpation method to obtain systolic blood pressure.
   d. Repeat any electronic blood pressure measurement with sphygmomanometer. Electronic blood pressure measurements are less accurate in low blood flow conditions.
2. Blood pressure above acceptable range
   a. Repeat blood pressure measurement in other extremity and compare findings.
   b. Verify correct selection of cuff size and placement of cuff. Cuff is placed below the right atrium when blood pressure is measured.
   c. Ask nurse colleague to repeat measurement in 1 to 2 minutes.
   d. Observe for related symptoms, although symptoms sometimes are not apparent until blood pressure is extremely elevated.
3. Blood pressure not sufficient for adequate perfusion and oxygenation of tissues
   a. Compare blood pressure value to baseline. A systolic reading of 90 mm Hg is an acceptable value for some patients.
   b. Position patient in supine position to enhance circulation and restrict activity that may decrease blood pressure further.
   c. Assess for signs and symptoms associated with hypotension, including tachycardia; weak, thready pulse; weakness; dizziness; confusion; cool, pale dusky or cyanotic skin.
   d. Assess for factors that would contribute to a low blood pressure, including hemorrhage, dilation of blood vessels resulting from hypothermia, anesthesia, or medication side effects.

Recording and Reporting

- Record blood pressure and extremity assessed on vital sign flow sheet, nurses' notes, or electronic medical record.
- Record any signs and symptoms of blood pressure alterations in narrative form in nurses' notes.
- Record measurement of blood pressure after administration of specific therapies in narrative form in nurses' notes.
- Report abnormal findings such as elevated blood pressure, low blood pressure, or if patient has a difference of more than 20 mm Hg systolic or diastolic when comparing blood pressure measurements on upper extremities immediately to nurse in charge or health care provider.

Sample Documentation

0400 BP 104/56 R arm, supine, dropping from baseline of 124/72. R radial pulse 112, weak, thready. RR 24, regular. Temporal T 36.8° C (98.2° F). Patient c/o dizziness, nausea. Skin pale. Health care provider notified. Orders received.

Special Considerations

Pediatric

- Blood pressure is not a routine part of assessment in children younger than 3 years.

Geriatric

- Older adults who have lost upper arm mass, especially the frail elderly, require special attention to selection of smaller blood pressure cuff.
- Skin of older adults is more fragile and susceptible to cuff pressure when blood pressure measurements are frequent. More frequent assessment of skin under cuff or rotation of blood pressure sites is recommended.
- Instruct older adults to change position slowly and wait after each change to avoid postural hypotension and prevent injuries.

Home Care

- Assess family's financial ability to afford a sphygmomanometer for performing blood pressure evaluations on a regular basis.
- Consider an electronic blood pressure cuff with large digital display for home if patient or caregiver has hearing or vision difficulties.

PROCEDURAL GUIDELINE 6.2
Assessing Blood Pressure Electronically

- **Nursing Skills Online: Vital Signs, Lesson 5**

Video Clips

Electronic blood pressure machines can be found in health care facilities and public places such as shopping malls. The machines rely on sound waves or vibrations that are interpreted electronically and converted into a blood pressure value. Verify an assessment of an abnormal blood pressure by an electronic machine with a sphygmomanometer and stethoscope.

Delegation and Collaboration

The skill of blood pressure measurement using an electronic blood pressure machine can be delegated to nursing assistive personnel (NAP) unless the patient is considered unstable (i.e., hypotensive). Instruct the NAP by:

- Communicating the frequency of measurement and extremity for measurement.
- Reviewing patient's usual blood pressure and need to report significant changes or abnormalities to the nurse.
- Selecting appropriate-size blood pressure cuff for designated extremity and appropriate cuff for the machine.

Equipment

- Electronic blood pressure machine
- Blood pressure cuff of appropriate size as recommended by manufacturer
- Source of electricity

Procedural Steps

1. **See Standard Protocol (inside front cover).**
2. Determine the appropriateness of using electronic blood pressure measurement. Patients with irregular heart rate, peripheral vascular disease, seizures, tremors, and shivering are not candidates for this device.
3. Determine best site for cuff placement.
4. Assist patient to comfortable position, either lying or sitting. Plug in device and place near patient, ensuring that connector hose between cuff and machine reaches.
5. Locate on/off switch and turn on machine to enable device to self-test computer systems.
6. Select appropriate cuff size for patient extremity and appropriate cuff for machine (Table 6-6). Electronic blood pressure cuff and machine are matched by manufacturer and are not interchangeable.
7. Expose extremity for measurement by removing constricting clothing to ensure proper cuff application. Do not place blood pressure cuff over clothing.
8. Prepare blood pressure cuff by manually squeezing all the air out of the cuff and connecting cuff to connector hose.
9. Wrap flattened cuff snugly around extremity, verifying that only one finger fits between cuff and patient's skin. Make sure that the "artery" arrow marked on the outside of the cuff is correctly placed (see illustration for Skill 6.5, Step 9, *B* on p. 105).
10. Verify that connector hose between cuff and machine is not kinked. Kinking prevents proper inflation and deflation of cuff.
11. Following manufacturer's directions, set the frequency control to automatic or manual, and then press start button. The first blood pressure measurement pumps the cuff to a peak pressure of about 180 mm Hg. After this pressure is reached, the machine begins a deflation sequence that determines the blood pressure. The first

TABLE 6-6 PROPER CUFF SIZE FOR ELECTRONIC MONITOR*

CUFF TYPE	LIMB CIRCUMFERENCE (cm)
Small adult	17-25
Adult	23-33
Large adult	31-40
Thigh	38-50

*It is mandatory that the 12- to 24-foot cord be used for adult monitoring.

PROCEDURAL GUIDELINE 6.2
Assessing Blood Pressure Electronically—cont'd

reading determines the peak pressure inflation for additional measurements.

12. When deflation is complete, digital display provides the most recent values and flash time in minutes that has elapsed since the measurement occurred (see illustration).

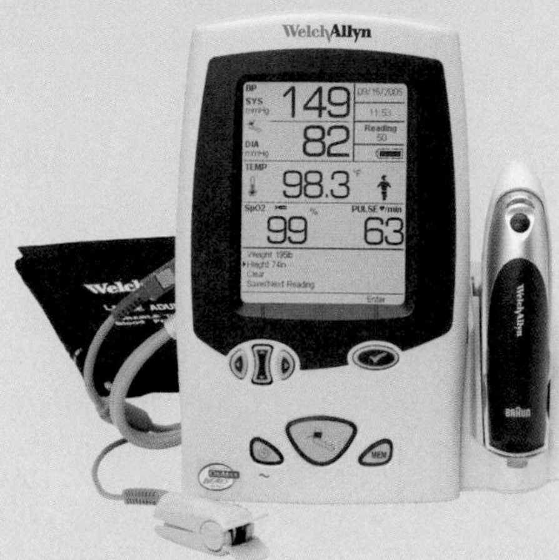

STEP 12 Monitor displays reading. Verify electronic alarm settings. (Image courtesy Welch Allyn.)

> **SAFETY ALERT** If unable to obtain blood pressure with electronic device, verify machine connections (e.g., plugged into working electrical outlet, hose-cuff connections tight, machine on, correct cuff). Repeat electronic blood pressure; if unable to obtain, use auscultatory technique (see Skill 6.5).

13. Set frequency of blood pressure measurements and upper and lower alarm limits for systolic, diastolic, and mean blood pressure readings. Intervals between blood pressure measurements are set from 1 to 90 minutes. The nurse determines frequency and alarm limits based on patient's acceptable range of blood pressure, nursing judgment, facility standards, or health care provider order.
14. Obtain additional readings at any time by pressing the start button. (Sometimes the nurse needs these for unstable patients.) Pressing the cancel button immediately deflates the cuff.
15. If frequent blood pressure measurements are required, leave the cuff in place. Remove cuff every 2 hours to assess underlying skin integrity and, if possible, alternate blood pressure sites. Patients with abnormal bleeding tendencies are at risk for microvascular rupture from repeated inflations. When you are finished using the electronic blood pressure machine, clean blood pressure cuff according to facility policy to reduce transmission of microorganisms.
16. Compare electronic blood pressure readings with auscultatory blood pressure measurements to verify accuracy of electronic blood pressure device.
17. **See Completion Protocol (inside front cover).**
18. Record blood pressure and site assessed on vital sign flow sheet, nurses' notes, or electronic medical record. Record any signs of blood pressure alterations in nurses' notes. Report abnormal findings to nurse in charge or health care provider.

PROCEDURAL GUIDELINE 6.3
Measuring Oxygen Saturation (Pulse Oximetry)

- **Nursing Skills Online: Vital Signs, Lesson 6**

Pulse oximetry is the noninvasive measurement of arterial blood oxygen saturation, the percent to which hemoglobin is filled with oxygen. A pulse oximeter is a probe with a light-emitting diode (LED) connected by cable to an oximeter. Normally SpO_2 is greater than 90%.

The measurement of oxygen saturation is simple, painless, and has few of the risks associated with more invasive measurements of oxygen saturation, such as arterial blood gas sampling. Conditions that decrease arterial blood flow, such as peripheral vascular disease, hypothermia, pharmacological vasoconstrictors, hypotension, or peripheral edema, affect accurate measurement of oxygen saturation in these areas. Factors that affect light transmission, such as outside light sources or patient motion, also affect the accurate measurement of oxygen saturation. Avoid direct sunlight or fluorescent lighting when using an oximeter.

Video Clips

In adults you can apply reusable and disposable oximeter probes to the earlobe, finger, toe, bridge of the nose, or forehead. Pulse oximetry is indicated in patients who have an unstable oxygen status or are at risk for impaired gas exchange.

Delegation and Collaboration

The skill of oxygen saturation measurement can be delegated to an NAP. The nurse instructs the NAP about:

- Specific factors related to patient that can falsely lower oxygen saturation.
- Appropriate sensor site and probe to select.
- Obtaining frequency of oxygen saturation measurements for specific patient.
- Notifying nurse immediately of any SpO_2 reading lower than 90%.

Continued

PROCEDURAL GUIDELINE 6.3
Measuring Oxygen Saturation (Pulse Oximetry)—cont'd

- Refraining from using pulse oximetry as an assessment of heart rate because oximeter will not detect an irregular pulse.

Equipment

- Oximeter
- Oximeter probe appropriate for patient and recommended by oximeter manufacturer
- Acetone or nail polish remover if needed
- Pen, pencil, vital sign flow sheet or record form

Procedural Steps

1. Determine need to measure patient's oxygen saturation. Assess for risk factors for decreased oxygen saturation (e.g., acute or chronic respiratory problems, chest wall injury, recovery from anesthesia).
2. Assess for signs and symptoms of alterations in oxygen saturation (e.g., altered respiratory rate, depth, or rhythm; adventitious breath sounds [see Chapter 7]; cyanotic nail beds, lips, or mucous membranes; restlessness; difficulty breathing).
3. Assess for factors that influence measurement of SpO_2: oxygen therapy, respiratory therapy such as postural drainage and percussion, hemoglobin level, hypotension, temperature, and medications such as bronchodilators.
4. Review patient's medical record for health care provider's order, or consult agency's procedure manual for standard of care for measurement of SpO_2.
5. Determine previous baseline SpO_2 (if available) from patient's record.
6. Determine most appropriate patient-specific site (e.g., finger, earlobe, bridge of nose, forehead) for sensor probe placement by measuring capillary refill. If capillary refill is less than 3 seconds, select alternative site.
   a. Site must have adequate local circulation and be free of moisture.
   b. A finger free of polish or acrylic nail is preferred.
   c. If patient has tremors or is likely to move, use earlobe or forehead.
   d. If patient is obese, clip-on probe may not fit properly; obtain a disposable (tape-on) probe.
7. **See Standard Protocol (inside front cover).**
8. Position patient comfortably. Instruct patient to breathe normally. If finger is the monitoring site, support lower arm.
9. If using the finger, remove fingernail polish from digit with acetone or polish remover.
10. Attach sensor to monitoring site. Instruct patient that clip-on probe will feel like a clothespin on the finger but will not hurt.
11. Once sensor is in place, turn on oximeter by activating power. Observe pulse waveform/intensity display and audible beep. Correlate oximeter pulse rate with patient's radial pulse.
12. Leave sensor in place until oximeter readout reaches constant value and pulse display reaches full strength during each cardiac cycle. Inform patient that oximeter alarm will sound if sensor falls off or if patient moves sensor. Read SpO_2 on digital display (see illustration).
13. If you plan to monitor oxygen saturation continuously, verify SpO_2 alarm limits preset by the manufacturer at a low of 85% and a high of 100%. Determine limits for SpO_2 and pulse rate as indicated by patient's condition. Verify that alarms are on. Assess skin integrity under sensor probe every 2 hours; relocate sensor at least every 4 hours and more frequently if skin integrity is altered or tissue perfusion compromised.
14. If you plan on intermittent or spot-checking SpO_2, remove probe and turn oximeter power off. Store sensor in appropriate location.
15. **See Completion Protocol (inside front cover).**
16. Compare SpO_2 with patient's previous baseline and acceptable SpO_2. Note use of oxygen therapy.

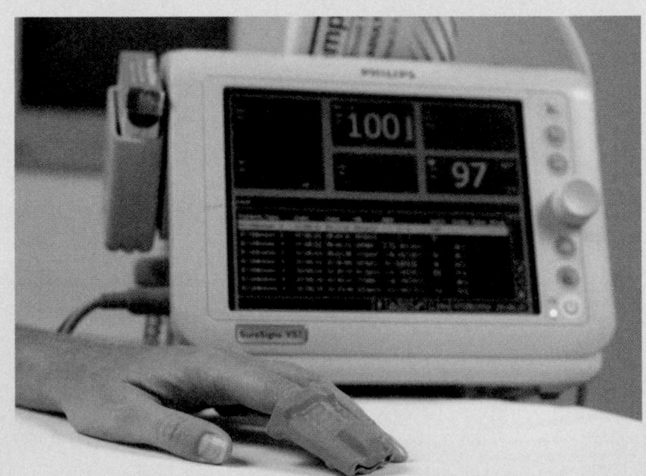

STEP 12 Obtain oximetry reading.

REVIEW QUESTIONS

Case Study for Questions 1 and 2

Mrs. Kilty is a 56-year-old patient who has a history of cerebrovascular accident (stroke). She uses a walker to ambulate, even though her right arm is weaker than the left. She has drooping on the right side of her mouth but is able to eat and swallow safely. She arrives at the urgent care clinic with her daughter complaining of weakness, cough, and general malaise. She appears alert and oriented and is cooperative.

1. When the nurse attempts to place an oral thermometer in her mouth, she is unable to keep it positioned in the right sublingual pocket. What should the nurse do?
   1. Hold the thermometer in place with her gloved hand.
   2. Ask Mrs. Kilty to hold the thermometer herself.
   3. Switch the thermometer to the left sublingual pocket.
   4. Obtain temperature from a different site.
2. When the nurse assesses Mrs. Kilty's blood pressure, she obtains 140/76 on the left arm and 128/72 on the right arm. What action is appropriate at this time? Select all that apply.
   1. Notify Mrs. Kilty's primary health care provider immediately.
   2. Repeat the measurements on both arms after the other vital signs are obtained.
   3. Ask a nurse colleague to obtain the blood pressure.
   4. Ask Mrs. Kilty why she has not taken her blood pressure medications.
   5. Review Mrs. Kilty's medical record for her baseline vital signs.
   6. Conduct a complete assessment of Mrs. Kilty's vascular system.
   7. Obtain blood pressures on the lower extremities.
   8. Obtain a larger blood pressure cuff.

Case Study for Questions 3 and 4

Mr. Ahern is a 66-year-old man who was recently admitted from the emergency department with a fractured hip. He is awaiting surgery, which is scheduled for the morning. As the nurse enters his room, he is moaning. The nursing assistive personnel (NAP) has just obtained his vital signs. The nurse observes that he is restless, perspiring, and complains of pain (7 on a scale of 0 to 10). He has an IV of lactated Ringer's at 100 mL/hr infusing in the left antecubital space.

3. What effect does the nurse anticipate Mr. Ahern's pain will have on his vital signs?
   1. Decrease heart rate
   2. Increase blood pressure
   3. Decrease respiratory rate
   4. Increase temperature
4. Two hours after admission, the NAP reports that Mr. Ahern's vital signs are: BP R arm 112/72, L arm 124/96; HR 98, RR 22, temporal artery temp 36.4. Which action is appropriate?
   1. Report the abnormal L arm pulse pressure to the health care provider.
   2. Direct the NAP to obtain the temperature using an alternative site and repeat the blood pressure in the left arm.
   3. Conduct an assessment of Mr. Ahern's respiratory status and obtain an apical heart rate.
   4. Report the R arm–to–L arm blood pressure difference to the health care provider,
5. Mrs. Malone is admitted with pneumonia. Her vital signs are: BP 112/64 mm Hg, HR 102, RR 26, tympanic temperature 37.9° C (100.2° F). What vital sign requires immediate attention?
   1. Heart rate
   2. Pulse pressure
   3. Respiratory rate
   4. Temperature
6. Mr. Amenta is a 62-year-old retired accountant who arrives at the outpatient clinic complaining of a headache. His BP is 170/88 mm Hg in the right arm and 188/92 mm Hg in the left arm. He reports that he ran out of blood pressure medication last week and has not been able to afford to refill the prescription. What is the nurse's priority nursing action?
   1. Allow the patient to relax for 15 minutes and reevaluate the blood pressure measurements.
   2. Contact the social worker for financial assistance.
   3. Notify the physician.
   4. Retake the blood pressure in the left arm with a different-size cuff.
7. Mr. Meyer is a 69-year-old retired pilot who arrives at the pacemaker clinic for his routine visit. He has had a pacemaker for the past 10 years for a slow heart rate. The NAP reports that, when she obtained his vital signs, his right radial pulse was irregular and his rate was 52. His other vital signs are within normal limits. What action should the nurse take?
   1. Direct the NAP to obtain the left radial pulse rate.
   2. Assess for a pulse deficit with the NAP.
   3. Obtain an apical pulse.
   4. Notify the nurse in charge.
8. During report the nurse obtains information on Mrs. Gardner, a 98-year-old patient who has terminal lung cancer and is admitted for palliative care. The nurse describes her breathing as labored, with periods of apnea alternating with deep breathes. The NAP reports her RR as 12. After the nurse's assessment confirms these findings, she describes this pattern as:
   1. Kussmaul's respirations
   2. Cheyne-Stokes respirations
   3. Agonal respirations
   4. Hypoventilation

9. The NAP obtains a blood pressure of 188/70 when taking frequent vital signs on a postoperative patient. She appropriately notifies the nurse of the value, and the nurse checks the patient. The electronic blood pressure machine reads 112/80, and the patient is awake and alert and offers no complaints. How does the nurse explain the difference in values?
  1. The patient flexed her arm when the machine was inflating during the initial assessment.
  2. The blood pressure cuff is too loose.
  3. The blood pressure cuff is too large.
  4. The patient's blood pressure is very sensitive.

10. Mr. Ryan is admitted to the nurse's unit for observation following a motorcycle accident. He broke his left arm and right leg, both of which are in casts. An IV line is infusing in his right hand. Mr. Ryan complains that his left hand is cool. Which finding would indicate the need for further assessment?
  1. Tympanic temperature of 36.2° C (97.2° F)
  2. Apical pulse rate of 92
  3. Blood pressure R arm 118/84
  4. L radial pulse 1+ strength

REFERENCES

Adiyaman A and others: The position of the arm during blood pressure measurement in sitting position, *Blood Press Monit* 11(6):309, 2006.

Bern L and others: Differences in blood pressure values obtained with automated and manual methods in medical inpatients, *Medsurg Nurs* 16(6):356, 2007.

Fallis WM and others: A multimethod approach to evaluate chemical dot thermometers for oral temperature measurement, *J Nurs Meas* 14(3):151, 2006.

Giles TD: Circadian rhythm of blood pressure and the relation to cardiovascular events, *J Hypertens* 24(Suppl 2):S11, 2006.

Heinemann M and others: Automated versus manual blood pressure measurement: a randomized crossover trial, *Int J Nurs Pract* 14:296, 2008.

Henker R, Carlson KK: Fever: Applying research to bedside practice, *AACN Adv Crit Care* 18(1):76, 2007.

Lawson L and others: Accuracy and precision of noninvasive core temperature measurement in adult intensive care patients, *Am J Crit Care* (16):485, 2007.

National High Blood Pressure Education Program (NHBPEP); National Heart, Lung, and Blood Institute; National Institutes of Health: The seventh report of the NHPBEP on detection, evaluation, and treatment of high blood pressure, *JAMA* 289(19):560, 2003.

CHAPTER

7

Health Assessment

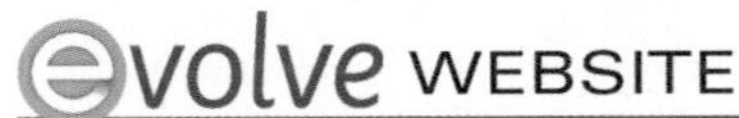

http://evolve.elsevier.com/Perry/nursinginterventions
Video Clips

Nurses perform systematic assessments on a regular basis in nearly every health care setting. In acute care settings a brief assessment at the beginning of each shift identifies any changes in a patient's status for comparison with the previous assessment. This routine assessment takes 10 to 15 minutes and reveals information that adds to the patient's database (Box 7-1). In nursing homes and home care settings nurses complete similar assessments weekly, monthly, or more frequently when a patient's health status changes. Continuity in health care improves when you make ongoing, objective, and comprehensive assessments.

PATIENT-CENTERED CARE

Nurses perform a more comprehensive assessment when a patient is admitted to a health care agency. This assessment involves a detailed review of a patient's condition and includes a nursing history and a behavioral and physical examination. The health history involves an interview with patients to gather subjective data about their current state of health and any presenting conditions. It is important for the interview to be patient centered, in order for the nurse to learn about any problems through the patients' eyes. A patient can be very helpful in describing the most bothersome symptoms so that the nurse can focus the assessment appropriately.

A physical assessment includes a head-to-toe review of each body system that offers objective information about the patient. Use of examination techniques allows you to validate any subjective information the patient shared during the interview. For example, if a patient complains of shortness of breath, checking lung sounds and observing lung excursion will help identify the nature of the problem. The patient's condition and response affect the extent of the examination. After gathering data, you will group significant findings into patterns of data (clusters) that reveal actual or potential nursing diagnoses. Each abnormal finding directs you to gather additional data. Initial assessment and examination provides a baseline for the patient's functional status and serves as a comparison for future assessment findings. In addition, the information is useful in selecting the best nursing measures to manage the patient's health problems.

Nurses are often the first to detect changes in patients' conditions. For this reason the ability to think critically and interpret patient behaviors and physiological changes is essential. The skills of physical assessment are powerful tools for detecting both subtle and obvious changes in a patient's health. The physical assessment is an ideal time to offer patient teaching and encourage promotion of health practices such as breast (Box 7-2) and genital (Box 7-3) self-examination. The American Cancer Society (ACS, 2010a) recommends guidelines for early detection.

ASSESSMENT TECHNIQUES

Inspection, palpation, percussion, auscultation, and olfaction are the five basic assessment techniques. Each skill allows you to collect a broad range of physical data about patients. Nurses need experience to recognize normal variations among patients and ranges of normal for an individual. Remember that cultural diversity is one factor that influences both normal variations and potential alterations that you may find during the assessment. It is very important to take the time needed to carefully assess each body part. Hurrying can cause you to overlook significant signs and form incorrect conclusions about a patient's condition.

Inspection is the visual examination of body parts or areas. An experienced nurse learns to make multiple observations almost simultaneously while becoming very perceptive of any

BOX 7-1 CHECKLIST FOR ROUTINE SHIFT ASSESSMENT

1. **Mental and neurological status**
   a. Level of consciousness (LOC)/responsiveness
   b. Alertness/orientation
   c. Pupils equal, round, and reactive to light and accommodation (PERRLA)
   d. Mood
   e. Behavior
   f. Facial expression
   g. Speech
2. **Vital signs**
   a. Blood pressure
   b. Pulse
   c. Respiration
   d. Temperature
   e. Pain and comfort level
   f. Pulse oximetry
3. **Motor sensory function**
   a. Range of motion of major extremities
   b. Movement
   c. Strength
   d. Presence of numbness or tingling
4. **Integument (skin/mucous membranes)**
   a. Color
   b. Temperature
   c. Turgor
   d. Moisture
   e. Edema
   f. Integrity
5. **Cardiopulmonary system**
   a. Apical rate and rhythm
   b. Lung sounds
   c. Breathing pattern
   d. Peripheral pulses
   e. Capillary refill
6. **Gastrointestinal system**
   a. Bowel sounds
   b. Abdominal palpation
   c. Degree of abdominal distention
   d. Bowel elimination problems (e.g., diarrhea, constipation, flatulence)
7. **Genitourinary system**
   a. Presence of discharge, odor, or pain
   b. Urinary elimination problems (e.g., pain, difficulty with stream)
8. **Wounds**
   a. Cleanliness
   b. Presence of swelling, redness, infection, or drainage
   c. Bandage/dressing, integrity of sutures
9. **Invasive tubes (e.g., intravenous [IV] lines, nasogastric tubes, wound drains, catheters)**
   a. Device and location
   b. IV line: Correct fluid/medication infusing
   c. Patency and position
   d. Presence of redness, swelling, or tenderness at IV site
   e. Drainage rate (wound drain) or infusion rate of IV or NG feeding
   f. Date of last tubing change
10. **Supportive devices**
   a. Oxygen
   b. Bed alarms
   c. Traction

abnormalities. The secret is to always pay attention to the patient. Watch all movements and look carefully at the body part that you are inspecting. It is important to recognize normal physical characteristics of patients of all ages before trying to distinguish abnormal findings.

Inspection requires adequate lighting and full exposure of body parts. Inspect each area for size, shape, color, symmetry, position, and the presence of abnormalities. If possible, inspect each area compared with the same area on the opposite side of the body. When necessary, use additional light such as a penlight to inspect body cavities such as the mouth and throat. *Do not hurry. Pay attention to detail.* Verify and clarify all abnormalities with subjective patient data. In other words, ask the patient for further information about each abnormality or change such as whether the change is recent.

Palpation uses the sense of touch. Through palpation the hands make delicate and sensitive measurements of specific physical signs. Palpation detects resistance, resilience, roughness, texture, temperature, and mobility. You will often use palpation with or after visual inspection. You will also use different parts of the hand to detect specific characteristics. For example, the dorsum (back) of the hand is sensitive to temperature variations. The pads of the fingertips detect subtle changes in texture, shape, size, consistency, and pulsation of body parts. The palm of the hand is especially sensitive to vibration. You measure position, consistency, and turgor by lightly grasping the body part with the fingertips.

Assist the patient to relax and assume a comfortable position because muscle tension during palpation impairs the ability to palpate correctly. Asking the patient to take slow, deep breaths enhances muscle relaxation. Palpate tender areas last because they could cause the patient to become tense and hinder the assessment. Ask the patient to point out areas that are more sensitive and note any nonverbal signs of discomfort. Patients appreciate clean, warm hands; short fingernails; and a gentle approach. Palpation is either light or deep and is controlled by the amount of pressure applied with the fingers or hand. Light palpation precedes deep palpation. Consider the patient's condition, the area being palpated, and the reason for using palpation. For example, when a patient is admitted to the emergency department after an automobile accident, consider the factors surrounding his or her injury and inspect the chest wall carefully before performing any palpation around the area of the ribs.

For light palpation, apply pressure slowly, gently, and deliberately, depressing about 1 cm (½ inch). Check tender areas further, using light intermittent pressure. After light palpation, you may use deeper palpation to examine

BOX 7-2 BREAST SELF-EXAMINATION

Women who are age 20 and over should be told about the benefits and limitations of breast self-examination (BSE) (ACS, 2010a). Emphasize the importance of prompt reporting of any new breast symptoms to a health care professional. Women who choose to do BSE should receive instruction and have their technique reviewed. BSE should be done once a month so that the woman becomes familiar with the usual appearance and feel of her breast. Familiarity makes it easier to notice any changes in the breast from one month to another. Early discovery of a change from "normal" is the main idea behind BSE.

For women who menstruate, the best time to do BSE is the fourth through the seventh day of the menstrual cycle or right after the menstrual cycle ends, when the breasts are least likely to be tender or swollen. Women who no longer menstruate should pick a day such as the first day of the month to remind them to do BSE.

Procedure

1. Stand before a mirror. Inspect both breasts for anything unusual, such as skin redness, discharge from the nipples, puckering, dimpling, or scaling of the skin.

The next two steps are designed to emphasize any change in the shape or contour of the breasts. As you do them, you should be able to feel your chest muscles tighten.

2. Watching closely in the mirror, clasp hands behind your head, and swing elbows forward.
3. Next, press hands firmly on hips and bow slightly toward the mirror as you pull your shoulders and elbows forward.

The next part of the examination may be done in the shower. Fingers glide over soapy skin, making it easy to feel the texture underneath.

4. Raise your left arm. Use three or four fingers of your right hand to explore your left breast firmly, carefully, and thoroughly. Beginning at the outer edge, press the flat part of your fingers in small circles, moving the circles slowly around the breast. Gradually work toward the nipple. Be sure to cover the entire breast. Evidence exists that suggests that using an up-and-down pattern (vertical pattern) is most effective for covering the entire breast and not missing any breast tissue (ACS, 2010b). Pay special attention to the area between the breast and the armpit, including the armpit itself. Feel for any unusual lump or mass under the skin.
5. Gently squeeze the nipple and look for a discharge. Repeat the examination on your right breast.
6. Steps 4 and 5 should be repeated lying down. Lie flat on your back, left arm over your head and a pillow or folded towel under your left shoulder. This position flattens the breast and makes it easier to examine. Use the same circular motion described earlier. Repeat on your right breast.

Call your health care provider if you find a lump or other abnormality.

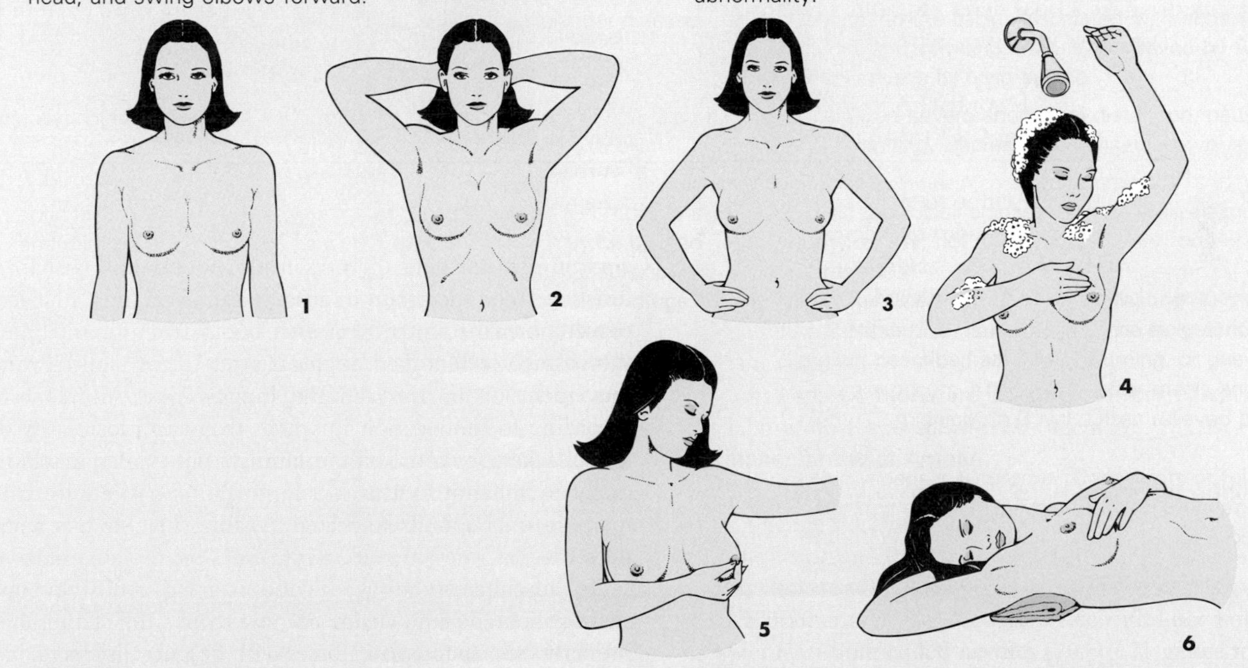

From Seidel HM and others: *Mosby's guide to physical examination*, ed 7, St Louis, 2011, Mosby.

the condition of organs (Fig. 7-1). Depress the area being examined approximately 2 cm (1 inch). Caution is the rule. Bimanual palpation involves one hand placed over the other while applying pressure. The upper hand exerts downward pressure as the other hand feels the subtle characteristics of underlying organs and masses. Seek the assistance of a qualified instructor before attempting deep palpation.

Percussion involves tapping the body with the fingertips to evaluate the size, borders, and consistency of body organs and discover fluid in body cavities. Percussion identifies the location, size, and density of underlying structures. This skill is beyond the scope of this text. Sounds are heard as percussion tones arise from vibrations in body tissues (Jarvis, 2008). The character of sound depends on the density of underlying tissues. The technique requires practice and skill and is typically used by advanced practice nurses.

Auscultation is listening with a stethoscope to sounds produced by the body. To auscultate correctly, listen in a quiet

BOX 7-3 GENITAL SELF-EXAMINATION

All men ages 15 years and older should perform this examination monthly. Perform it after a warm bath or shower when the scrotal sac is relaxed. Call your health care provider if you find a lump or any other abnormality.

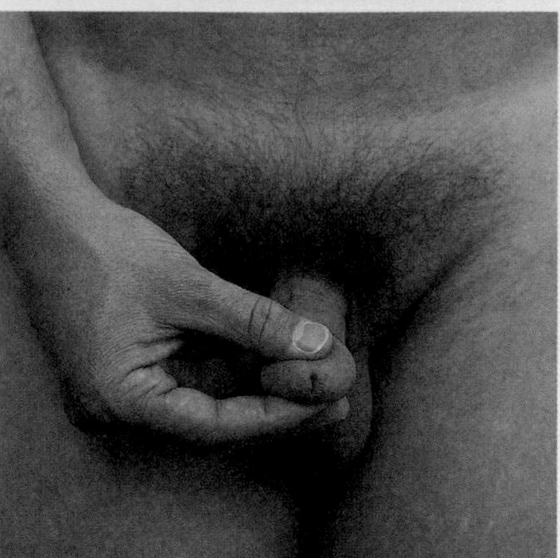

Penile Examination

1. Stand naked in front of a mirror and hold the penis in your hand and examine the head. Pull back the foreskin if uncircumcised.
2. Inspect and palpate the entire head of the penis in a clockwise motion, looking carefully for any bumps, sores, or blisters.
3. Look for any bumpy warts.
4. Look at the opening at the end of the penis for discharge.
5. Look along the entire shaft of the penis for the same signs.
6. Separate pubic hair at the base of the penis and carefully examine the skin underneath.

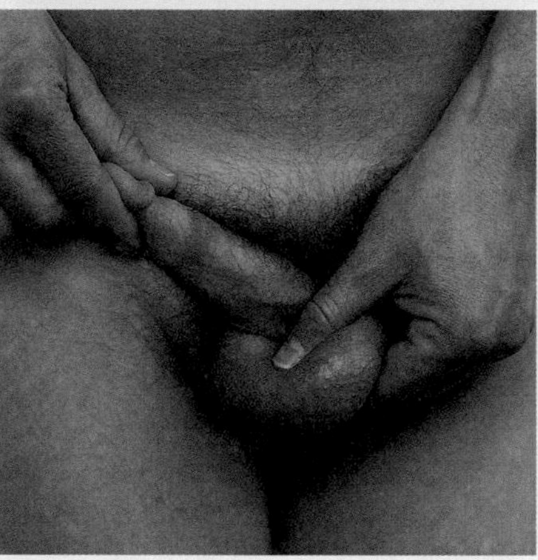

Testicular Examination

1. Look for swelling or lumps in the skin of the scrotum while looking in the mirror.
2. Use both hands, placing the index and middle fingers under the testicles and the thumb on top.
3. Gently roll the testicle, feeling for lumps, thickening, or a change in consistency (hardening).
4. Find the epididymis (a cordlike structure on the top and back of the testicle; it is not a lump).
5. Feel for small, pea-size lumps on the front and side of the testicle. The lumps are usually painless and are abnormal.

From Seidel HM and others: *Mosby's guide to physical examination*, ed 7, 2011, Mosby.

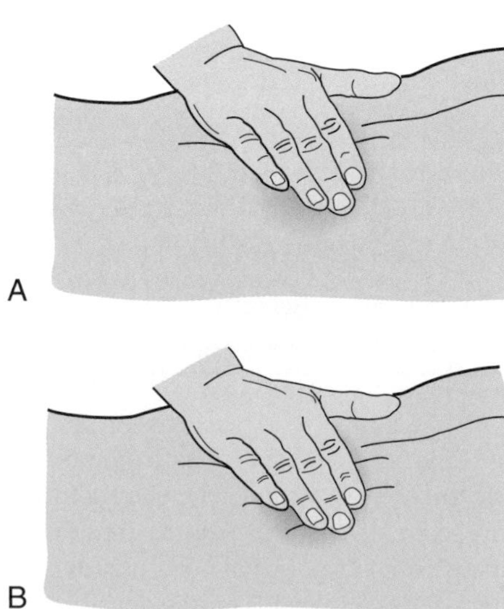

FIG 7-1 A, During light palpation, gentle pressure against underlying skin and tissues can be used to detect areas of irregularity and tenderness. **B,** During deep palpation, depressing tissue can assess condition of underlying organs.

environment for both the presence of sound and its characteristics. To be successful in auscultation, you must first recognize normal sounds from each body structure, including the passage of blood through an artery, heart sounds, and movement of air through the lungs. These sounds vary according to the location in which they can most easily be heard. Likewise, you become familiar with areas that normally do not emit sounds. It is important for you to listen to many normal sounds to recognize abnormal sounds when they arise.

To auscultate, you need good hearing acuity, a good stethoscope, and knowledge of how to use the stethoscope properly (see Chapter 6). Nurses with hearing disorders may purchase stethoscopes with greater sound amplification and may need to ask colleagues to verify some findings through auscultation. It is essential to place the stethoscope directly on the patient's skin because clothing obscures and changes sound. Through auscultation there are four characteristics of sound:

Frequency: Number of sound wave cycles generated per second by a vibrating object. The higher the frequency, the higher the pitch of a sound and vice versa.

Loudness: Amplitude of a sound wave. Auscultated sounds are either loud or soft.

TABLE 7-1 ASSESSMENT OF CHARACTERISTIC ODORS

ODOR	SITE OR SOURCE	POTENTIAL CAUSES
Alcohol	Oral cavity	Ingestion of alcohol
Ammonia	Urine	Urinary tract infection, renal failure
Body odor	Skin, particularly in areas where body parts rub together (e.g., underarms, beneath breasts)	Poor hygiene, excess perspiration (hyperhidrosis), foul-smelling perspiration (bromhidrosis)
	Wound site	Wound abscess; infection
	Vomitus	Abdominal irritation, contaminated food
Feces	Rectal area	Bowel obstruction
	Vomitus/oral cavity (fecal odor)	Fecal incontinence; fistula
Fetid, sweet odor	Tracheostomy or mucus secretions	Infection of bronchial tree (*Pseudomonas* bacteria)
Foul-smelling stools in infant	Stool	Malabsorption syndrome
Halitosis	Oral cavity	Poor dental and oral hygiene, gum disease; sinus infection
Musty odor	Casted body part	Infection inside cast
Stale urine	Skin	Uremic acidosis
Sweet, fruity ketones	Oral cavity	Diabetic acidosis
Sweet, heavy, thick odor	Draining wound	*Pseudomonas* (bacterial) infection

Quality: Sounds of similar frequency and loudness from different sources. Terms such as *blowing* or *gurgling* describe quality of sound.

Duration: Length of time that sound vibrations last. Duration of sound is short, medium, or long. Layers of soft tissue dampen the duration of sounds from deep internal organs.

Olfaction uses the sense of smell to detect abnormalities that go unrecognized by any other means. Some alterations in body function and certain bacteria create characteristic odors (Table 7-1).

SAFETY

The process of assessment begins the moment that you see a patient and continues with each encounter. Always know the patient's health history and the reason for seeking care. Be alert for any changes or problems that may have developed since the last assessment.

Preparation for Assessment

Preparation of the environment, equipment, and patient facilitates a smooth assessment. Provide patients privacy to promote their comfort and the efficiency of the examination. In a health care facility close the door and pull privacy curtains. In the home examine the patient in the bedroom. A comfortable environment includes a warm, comfortable temperature; a loose-fitting gown or pajamas for the patient; adequate direct lighting; control of outside noises; and precautions to prevent interruptions by visitors or health care personnel. If possible, place the bed or examination table at waist level so that you can access the patient easily. The Joint Commission's National Patient Safety Goals for 2009 mandated the need to protect patients from falls and injury; thus returning the bed to a safe height after the assessment is essential (TJC, 2010).

Culture

Respect the cultural differences of patients when completing an examination. It is important to remember that cultural differences influence a patient's behavior. Consider the patient's health beliefs, use of alternative therapies, nutritional habits, relationships with family, and comfort with your physical closeness during the examination and history taking. Be culturally aware and avoid stereotyping on the basis of gender or race. There is a difference between cultural and physical characteristics. Learn to recognize common disorders for ethnic populations within the community. Recognition of cultural diversity helps to respect a patient's uniqueness and provide higher-quality care. Improved patient outcomes can result from recognition and respect for cultural diversity (Giger and Davidhizar, 2008).

Preparing the Patient

Prepare the patient both physically and psychologically for an accurate assessment. A tense, anxious patient may have difficulty understanding, following directions, or cooperating with your instructions. To prepare the patient:

1. Make the patient comfortable by allowing the opportunity to empty the bowel or bladder (a good time to collect needed specimens).
2. Minimize patient's anxiety and fear by conveying an open, receptive, and professional approach. Using simple terms and thoroughly explain what will be done, what the patient should expect to feel, and how the patient can cooperate. Even if the patient appears

unresponsive, it is still important to explain your actions.
3. Provide access to body parts while draping areas that are not being examined.
4. Reduce distractions. Turn down volume or turn off television/radio.
5. Eliminate drafts, control room temperature, and provide warm blankets.
6. Help the patient assume positions during the assessment so body parts are accessible and the patient stays comfortable. A patient's ability to assume positions depends on physical strength and limitations. Some positions are uncomfortable or embarrassing; keep a patient in position no longer than is necessary.
7. Pace assessment according to the patient's physical and emotional tolerance.
8. Use a relaxed tone of voice and facial expressions to put the patient at ease.
9. Encourage the patient to ask questions and report discomfort felt during the examination.
10. Have a third person of the patient's gender in the room during assessment of genitalia. This prevents the patient from accusing you of behaving in an unethical manner.
11. At the conclusion of the assessment, ask the patient if there are any concerns or questions.

PHYSICAL ASSESSMENT OF VARIOUS AGE-GROUPS

Children and Adolescents

1. Routine assessment of children focuses on health promotion and illness prevention, particularly for care of well children with competent parenting and no serious health problems (Hockenberry and Wilson, 2007). Focus on growth and development, sensory screening, dental examination, and behavioral assessment.
2. Children who are chronically ill, disabled, in foster care, or foreign-born adopted may require additional assessments because of their unique health risks.
3. When obtaining histories of infants and children, gather all or part of information from parents or guardians.
4. Parents may think the examiner is testing or judging them. Offer support during examination and do not pass judgment.
5. Call children by their preferred name and address parents as "Mr. and Mrs. Brown" rather than by first names.
6. Open-ended questions often allow parents to share more information and describe more of the child's problems.
7. Older children and adolescents respond best when treated as adults and individuals and often can provide details about their health history and severity of symptoms.
8. The adolescent has a right to confidentiality. After talking with parents about historical information, arrange to be alone with the adolescent to speak privately and perform the examination.

Older Adults

1. Do not assume that aging is always accompanied by illness or disability. Most older adults are able to adapt to change and maintain functional independence (Ebersole and others, 2008).
2. Allow extra time and be calm, relaxed, and unhurried with older adults.
3. Provide adequate space for an examination, particularly if the patient uses a mobility aid.
4. Plan the history and examination, taking into account the older adult's energy level, physical limitations, pace, and adaptability. You may need more than one session to complete the assessment (Touhy and Jett, 2009).
5. Measure performance under the most favorable of conditions. Take advantage of natural opportunities for assessment (e.g., during bathing, grooming, and mealtime) (Touhy and Jett, 2009).
6. Sequence an examination to keep position changes to a minimum. Be efficient throughout the examination to limit patient movement.
7. Be sure that an examination of an older adult includes review of mental status.

EVIDENCE-BASED PRACTICE TRENDS

American Cancer Society: *Cancer facts and figures 2010,* Atlanta, 2010a, ACS.

Katapodi M and others: Underestimation of breast cancer risk: influence on screening behavior, *Oncol Nurs Forum* 36(3):306, 2009.

Excluding skin cancer, breast cancer is the most diagnosed cancer in women. An estimated 207,090 new cases of invasive breast cancer are expected to occur among U.S. women during 2010; about 1970 new cases are expected in men (ACS, 2010a). There has been a 2% decreased incidence in breast cancer between 1999 and 2006. A recent research study sought to describe women's perceived breast cancer risk. Of the 184 participants, 89% perceived that they were not likely to be affected by breast cancer (Katapodi and others, 2009). These inaccurate perceptions do not promote breast cancer screening and have implications for women at high risk. Nursing implications include the use of risk assessment tools to provide education and counseling regarding breast cancer risks and screening.

SKILL GUIDELINES

1. Prioritize the assessment based on a patient's presenting signs and symptoms or health care needs. For example, when a patient develops sudden shortness of breath, first assess the lungs and thorax. If a patient is acutely ill, you may choose to assess only the involved body systems. Use judgment to ensure that an examination is relevant and inclusive.
2. Organize the examination. Compare both sides of the body for symmetry. If patient becomes fatigued, offer

rest periods. Perform painful or intrusive procedures near the end of the examination.

3. Use a head-to-toe approach following the sequence of inspection, palpation, and auscultation (except for abdominal assessment). This sequence facilitates an effective assessment.
4. Encourage the patient's active participation. Patients usually know about their physical condition. Often the patient can let you know when certain findings are normal or when there have been changes.
5. Always identify the patient using at least two patient identifiers other than the room number. For example, use the patient's name and date of birth, comparing with either the armband or medical record (TJC, 2010). In long-term care settings arm bands are not used; however, pictures are available for identification. CAUTION: patients with difficulty hearing or altered level of consciousness (LOC) may answer to name other than their own.
6. Respect the patient's race, gender, age, and cultural beliefs. These important variables often influence assessment findings and examination approaches. Consider a patient's health beliefs, use of alternative therapies, nutritional habits, relationships with family, and comfort with close physical contact (Box 7-4).
7. Follow standard precautions for infection control. During an assessment you may have contact with body fluids and discharge. Always wear gloves when there are lesions, wounds, or breaks in the skin. In some circumstances you will need to wear a gown.
8. Record quick notes to facilitate accurate documentation. Inform the patient that you will be recording this data.

BOX 7-4 CULTURAL CONSIDERATIONS

Cultural behaviors are relevant to the health assessment, and you need to be aware of them before conducting an assessment on a patient. Consider these guidelines but remember that each patient is an individual and may respond differently.

Mexican Americans: Eye behavior is important; always touch a child when examining him or her.

Asians/Pacific Islanders: Excessive eye contact or touch is offensive.

African Americans: Dialect requires careful communication to prevent interpretation errors.

American Indians: Eye contact is considered disrespectful and is avoided.

Data from Giger J, Davidhizar R: *Transcultural nursing: assessment and intervention,* ed 5, St Louis, 2008, Mosby.

9. Use assessment skills during each patient contact, including activities such as bathing, administration of medications, other therapies, or while conversing with a patient.
10. Integrate health promotion and education into physical assessment activities. There are "teachable moments" when you can share findings and educate patients about health promotion.
11. Record a summary of the assessment using appropriate medical terminology and in the sequence that findings are gathered. Use commonly accepted medical abbreviations to keep notes concise. Be thorough and descriptive, especially for abnormal findings.

SKILL 7.1 GENERAL SURVEY

The general survey begins a review of the patient's primary health problems, and it includes assessment of the patient's vital signs, height and weight, general behavior, and appearance. It provides information about characteristics of an illness, a patient's hygiene, skin and body image, emotional state, recent changes in weight, and developmental status. The survey reveals important information about the patient's behavior that can influence how you communicate instructions to the patient and continue the assessment.

ASSESSMENT

1. Note if patient has had any acute distress: difficulty breathing, pain, or anxiety. If such signs are present, defer general survey until later and focus immediately on body system affected. *Rationale: Signs establish priorities regarding what part of the examination to conduct first.*
2. Review graphic sheet for previous vital signs and consider factors or conditions that may alter values (see Chapter 6). *Rationale: Provides baseline data about patient's vital signs.*
3. Determine patient's primary language. If you identify a need for an interpreter, determine the availability of a professional interpreter. It is best to have an interpreter of the same gender who is older and more mature. Have the interpreter translate verbatim if possible. *Rationale: Facilitates patient understanding and promotes accuracy of information provided by patient.*
4. Identify patient's normal height, weight, and body mass index. If a sudden gain or loss in weight has occurred, determine the amount of weight change and period of time in which it occurred. Assess if patient has recently been dieting or is following an exercise program. Use growth charts for children under 18 years of age. *Rationale: Generally a body mass index of 25 to 29.9 for men and women is overweight, whereas 30 and over is obese (Seidel and others, 2011). Fluid retention is one factor that must be ruled out. A person's weight can fluctuate daily because of fluid loss or retention (1 L of water weighs 1 kg [2.2 pounds]).*
5. Review patient's past fluid intake and output (I&O) records. *Rationale: Fluid and electrolyte balance affects health and function in all body systems.*
6. Assess for evidence of latex allergy, which may include contact dermatitis or systemic reactions (see Chapter 5). Ask if patient has risk factors such as food allergies (papaya,

avocado, banana, peach, kiwi, or tomato). *Rationale: Gloves are worn during certain aspects of the assessment. Repeated exposure may result in more serious reactions, including asthma, itching, and anaphylaxis (Ball and Bindler, 2010; Seidel and others, 2011).*

PLANNING

Expected Outcomes focus on accurate assessment data.

1. Patient demonstrates alert, cooperative behaviors without evidence of physical or emotional distress during assessment.
2. Patient provides appropriate subjective data related to physical condition.

Delegation and Collaboration

The general survey cannot be delegated to nursing assistive personnel (NAP). Instruct the NAP to:

- Measure patient's height and weight.
- Obtain vital signs (not the initial set, but subsequent measurements if patient is stable).
- Monitor oral intake and urinary output.
- Report patient's subjective signs and symptoms to the nurse.

Equipment

- Stethoscope
- Sphygmomanometer and cuff
- Thermometer
- Digital watch or wristwatch with second hand
- Tape measure
- Clean gloves (use nonlatex if necessary)
- Tongue blade

IMPLEMENTATION *for* GENERAL SURVEY

STEPS	RATIONALE
1. **See Standard Protocol (inside front cover).**	
2. Throughout the assessment note patient's verbal and nonverbal behaviors. Determine patient's LOC and orientation by observing and talking to patient.	Behaviors may reflect specific physical abnormalities. Dementia and LOC influence ability to cooperate.

> **SAFETY ALERT** Timing of recent medications, especially pain medication and sedatives, may cause patient to be groggy or less responsive.

STEPS	RATIONALE
3. Obtain temperature, pulse, respirations, and blood pressure unless routinely taken within past 3 hours; or repeat if a serious potential change is noted (e.g., change in LOC or difficulty breathing [see Chapter 6]). Inform patient of vital signs.	Vital signs provide important information regarding physiological changes in relation to oxygenation and circulation.
4. Observe the following aspects of appearance: gender, race, and age. Note patient's physical features.	Gender influences type of examination performed and manner in which assessments are made. Different physical characteristics and predisposition to illnesses are related to gender and race.
5. If uncertain whether patient understands a question, rephrase or ask a similar question.	Inappropriate response from a patient may be caused by language barriers, deterioration of mental status, preoccupation with illness, or decreased hearing acuity.
6. If patient's responses are inappropriate, ask short, to-the-point questions regarding information patient should know; for example, "Tell me your name," "What is the name of this place?" "Tell me where you live," "What day is this?" or "What season of the year is this?"	Measures patient's orientation to person, place, and time. You may note this in the documentation as "Oriented × 3." If disoriented in any way, include subjective and/or objective data rather than just documenting "disoriented."
7. If patient is unable to respond to questions of orientation, offer simple commands; for example, "Squeeze my fingers" or "Move your toes."	LOC exists along a continuum that includes full responsiveness, inability to consciously initiate meaningful behaviors, and unresponsiveness to stimuli.
8. Assess affect and mood. Note if verbal expressions match nonverbal behavior and if appropriate to situation.	Reflects patient's mental and emotional status, consciousness, and feelings.

STEPS	RATIONALE
9. Watch patient interact with spouse or partner, older adult child, or caregiver. Be alert for indications of fear, hesitancy to report health status, or willingness to let caregiver control interview. Does partner or caregiver have a history of violence, alcoholism, or drug abuse? Is the person unemployed, ill, or frustrated with caring for patient? Note if patient has any obvious physical injuries.	Suspect abuse in patients who have suffered obvious physical injury or neglect, show signs of malnutrition, or have ecchymoses (bruises) on the extremities or trunk. Health care providers are often the first to identify evidence of abuse because patients may not be able to tell family or friends. Partners or caregivers may have a history of abusive or addictive behaviors.
10. Observe for signs of abuse:	
a. Child: Blood on underclothing, pain in genital area, pain on urination, vaginal or penile discharge, or difficulty sitting or walking. Physical injury inconsistent with parent's or caregiver's account of how injury occurred.	Indicates child sexual abuse (Anbarghalami and others, 2007; Ball and Bindler, 2010). Suggests child physical abuse.
b. Female patient: Injury or trauma inconsistent with reported cause or obvious injuries to face, neck, breasts, abdomen, and genitalia, such as black eyes, broken nose, lip lacerations, broken teeth, burns.	May indicate domestic abuse (Hegarty and others, 2008). These signs also apply to male patient being abused by female partner.
c. Older adult: Injury or trauma inconsistent with reported cause, injuries in unusual locations (such as neck or genitalia), pattern injuries (left when an object with which a person is struck leaves an imprint), parallel injuries (such as bilateral bruises on the upper arms suggesting that the person was held and shaken), burns (shaped like a cigarette, iron, rope), fractures, poor hygiene, and poor nutrition.	Indicates elder abuse/neglect (Touhy and Jett, 2009). Prolonged interval between injury and time patient sought medical treatment also indicates older adult abuse/neglect.

SAFETY ALERT A pattern of findings indicating abuse usually mandates a report to a social service center (refer to state guidelines). Obtain an immediate consultation with health care provider, social worker, and other support staff to facilitate placement in a safer environment.

STEPS	RATIONALE
11. Assess posture, noting alignment of the shoulders and hips when patient stands and/or sits. Observe whether patient has a slumped, erect, or bent posture.	Reveals musculoskeletal problem, mood, presence of pain, or difficulty breathing in certain positions.
a. Assess body movements. Are they purposeful? Are there tremors of the extremities? Are any body parts immobile? Are movements coordinated or uncoordinated?	May indicate neurological or muscular problem or emotional stress (see Skill 7.7).
12. Assess speech. Is it understandable and moderately paced? Is there an association with the person's thoughts?	Alterations reflect neurological impairment, injury or impairment of mouth, improperly fitting dentures, or differences in dialect and language.
13. Observe hygiene and grooming for presence or absence of makeup, type of clothes (hospital or personal), and cleanliness. Hair, teeth, and nails are good places to assess for hygiene status.	Grooming may reflect activity level before examination, resources available to purchase grooming supplies, patient's mood, and self-care practices. May also reflect culture, lifestyle, and personal preferences.
a. Observe the color, distribution, quantity, thickness, texture, and lubrication of hair.	Changes in hair may reflect hormone changes, changes from aging, poor nutrition, or use of certain hair care products.
b. Inspect the condition of nails (hands and feet).	Changes indicate inadequate nutrition or grooming practices, nervous habits, or systemic diseases.
c. Assess the presence or absence of body odor.	Body odor may result from physical exercise, deficient hygiene, or physical or mental abnormalities. Inadequate oral hygiene or unhealthy teeth may cause bad breath.

Continued

STEPS	RATIONALE
14. Inspect exposed skin and ask if patient has noted any changes in the skin, including:	The incidence of melanoma in the United States has been increasing for at least 30 years (ACS, 2010a). It is an aggressive form of skin cancer. The cancer can spread to other parts of the body quickly. Early detection and prompt treatment are critical (Box 7-5).
a. Pruritus, oozing, bleeding	Itching could result from dry skin, oozing could indicate infection, and bleeding may indicate a blood disorder.
b. Change in the appearance of a mole (nevus), bump, or nodule; change in sensation, itchiness, tenderness, or pain	This is a key indicator of a lesion that may be cancerous.
c. Petechiae (pinpoint-size, red or purple spots on the skin caused by small hemorrhages in the skin layers)	Petechiae may indicate serious blood clotting disorder, drug reaction, or liver disease.
15. Inspect skin surfaces. Compare color of symmetrical body parts, including areas unexposed to sun. Look for any patches or areas of skin color variation.	Changes in color can indicate pathological alterations (Table 7-2).

BOX 7-5 THE ABCD RULE OF MALIGNANT MELANOMA

This simple mnemonic helps you remember the characteristics that should alert you to the possibility of malignant melanoma.

- **A**symmetry of lesion
- **B**orders: irregular
- **C**olor blue/black or variegated, pigmentation not uniform, variations/multiple colors (tan, black) with areas of pink, white, gray, blue, or red
- **D**iameter greater than 6 mm

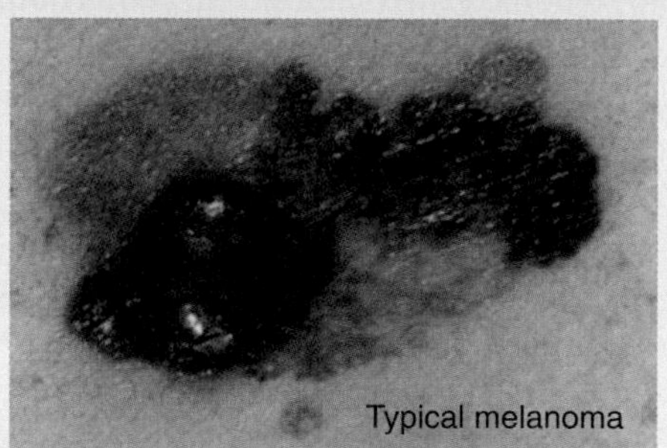
Typical melanoma

Illustration from Zitelli B, Davis H: *Atlas of pediatric physical diagnosis,* ed 5, St Louis, 2007, Mosby.

TABLE 7-2 SKIN COLOR VARIATIONS

COLOR	CONDITION	CAUSE	ASSESSMENT LOCATION
Bluish (cyanosis)	Related to hypoxia (late sign of decreased oxygen).	Heart or lung disease, cold environment	Nail beds, lips, base of tongue, skin (severe cases)
Pallor (decrease in color)	Reduced amount of oxyhemoglobin Reduced visibility of oxyhemoglobin resulting from decreased blood flow	Anemia Shock	Face, conjunctivae, nail beds, palms of hands Skin, nail beds, conjunctivae, lips
Red (erythema)	Increased visibility of oxyhemoglobin caused by dilation or increased blood flow	Fever, direct trauma, blushing, alcohol intake	Face, area of trauma, and areas at risk of pressure such as sacrum, shoulders, elbows, heels
Yellow-orange (jaundice)	Increased deposit of bilirubin in tissues	Liver disease, destruction of red blood cells	Sclerae, mucous membranes, skin
Loss of pigmentation	Vitiligo	Congenital autoimmune condition causing lack of pigment	Patchy areas on skin over face, hands, arms
Tan-brown	Increased amount of melanin	Suntan, pregnancy	Areas exposed to sun: face, arms; areolas, nipples

STEPS	RATIONALE

SAFETY ALERT Be alert for basal cell carcinomas such as an open sore that does not heal, a shiny nodule, a pink or reddish growth, or a scarlike area. These often occur in sun-exposed areas, which frequently occur in sun-damaged skin.

16. Carefully inspect color of face, oral mucosa, lips, conjunctivae, sclera, palms of hands, and nail beds.

Abnormalities are easier to identify in areas of body where melanin production is lowest.

SAFETY ALERT When assessing the skin of a patient with bandages, cast, restraints, or other restrictive devices, note report of pain or tingling and areas of pallor, decreased temperature, decreased movement, and impaired sensation, which may indicate impaired circulation. Immediate release of pressure from the restrictive device may be necessary.

17. Use ungloved fingertips to palpate skin surfaces to feel texture and moisture of intact skin.

Changes in texture may be the first indication of skin rashes in dark-skinned patients. Hydration, body temperature, and environment may affect the skin. Older adults are prone to xerosis, presenting as dry, scaly skin (Touhy and Jett, 2009).

a. Using dorsum (back) of hand, palpate for temperature of skin surfaces. Compare symmetrical body parts. Compare upper and lower body parts. Note distinct temperature differences and localized areas of warmth.

Skin on dorsum of hand is thin, which allows detection of subtle temperature changes. Cool skin temperature often indicates decreased blood flow. A stage I pressure ulcer may cause warmth and erythema (redness) of an area. Environmental temperature and anxiety may also affect skin temperature.

b. Assess skin turgor by grasping fold of skin on the sternum, forearm, or abdomen with the fingertips. Release skin fold and note ease and speed with which skin returns to place (see illustration).

With reduced turgor skin remains suspended or "tented" for a few seconds, then slowly returns to place, indicating decreased elasticity and possible dehydration. With altered turgor, provide measures for prevention of pressure ulcers (see Chapter 25).

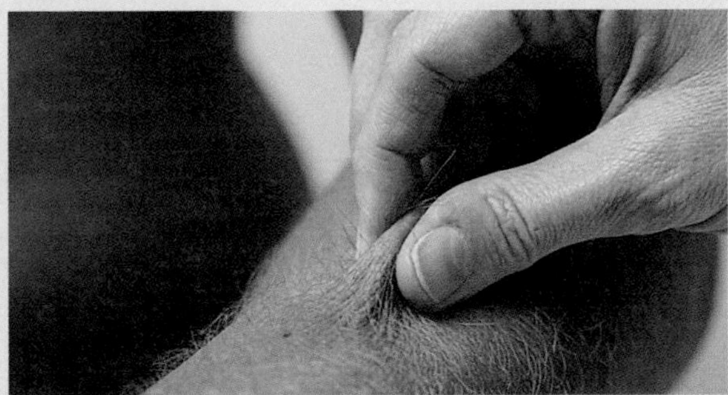

STEP 17b Assessment of skin turgor.

18. Inspect character of any secretions; note color, odor, amount, and consistency (e.g., thin and watery or thick and oily). Remove gloves.

Description of secretions helps to indicate whether infection is present or a wound is healing.

19. Assess condition of skin for pressure areas, paying particular attention to regions at risk for pressure (e.g., sacrum, greater trochanter, heels, occipital area, clavicles). If you see areas of redness, place fingertip over area, apply gentle pressure and then release. Look at skin color.

Normal reactive hyperemia (redness) is a visible effect of localized vasodilation, the normal response of the body to lack of blood flow to underlying tissue. Affected area of skin normally blanches with fingertip pressure. If area does not blanch, suspect tissue injury.

SAFETY ALERT With evidence of normal reactive hyperemia, reposition the patient and develop a turning schedule if patient is dependent (see Chapter 25).

Continued

STEPS	RATIONALE
20. When you detect a lesion, use adequate lighting to inspect color, location, texture, size, shape, and type (Box 7-6). Also note grouping (e.g., clustered or linear) and distribution (e.g., localized or generalized).	Observation of the lesion allows for accurate description and identification.
a. Use gloves if lesion is moist or draining. Gently palpate any lesion to determine mobility, contour (flat, raised, or depressed), and consistency (soft or hard).	Gentle palpation prevents rupture of underlying cysts. Gloves reduce transmission of microorganisms.
b. Note if patient reports tenderness with or without palpation.	Tenderness may indicate inflammation or pressure on body part.
c. Measure size of lesion (height, width, depth) with centimeter ruler.	Provides for baseline to assess changes in lesion over time.
21. See Completion Protocol (inside front cover).	

BOX 7-6 TYPES OF SKIN LESIONS

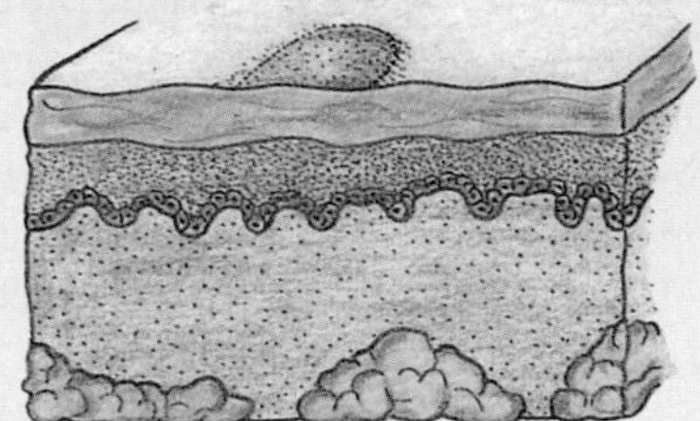

Macule: Flat, nonpalpable change in skin color; smaller than 1 cm (0.4 inch) (e.g., freckle, petechia)

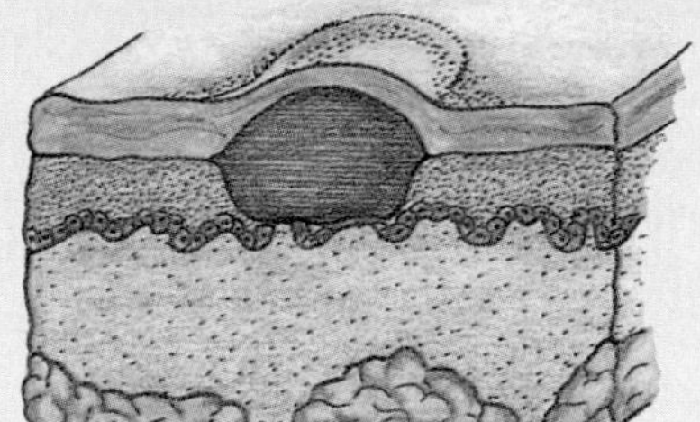

Papule: Palpable, circumscribed, solid elevation in skin; smaller than 0.5 cm (0.2 inch) (e.g., elevated nevus)

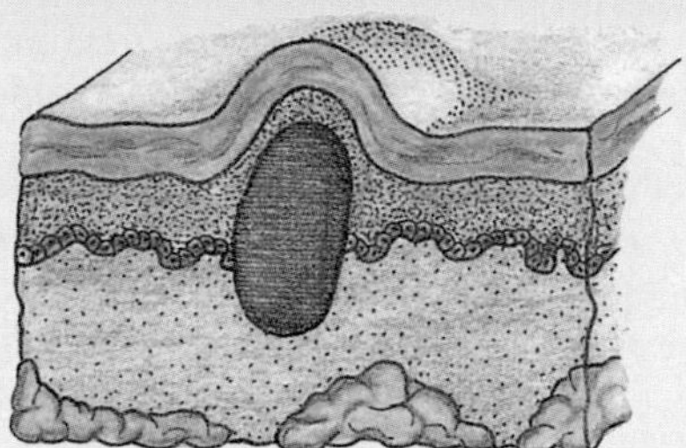

Nodule: Elevated solid mass; deeper and firmer than papule, 0.5 to 2 cm (0.8 inch) (e.g., wart)

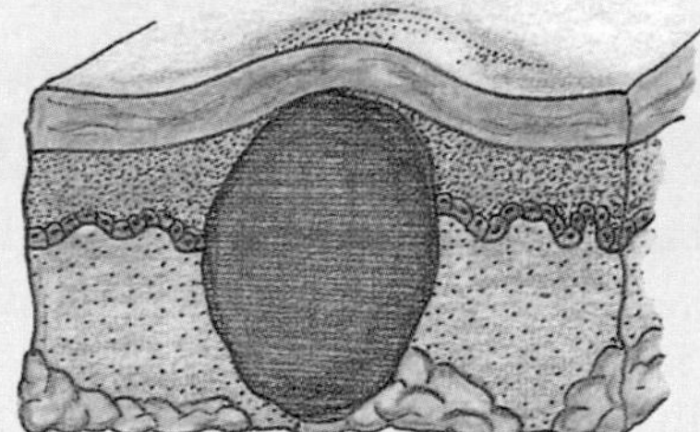

Tumor: Solid mass that may extend deep through subcutaneous tissue; larger than 1 to 2 cm (e.g., epithelioma)

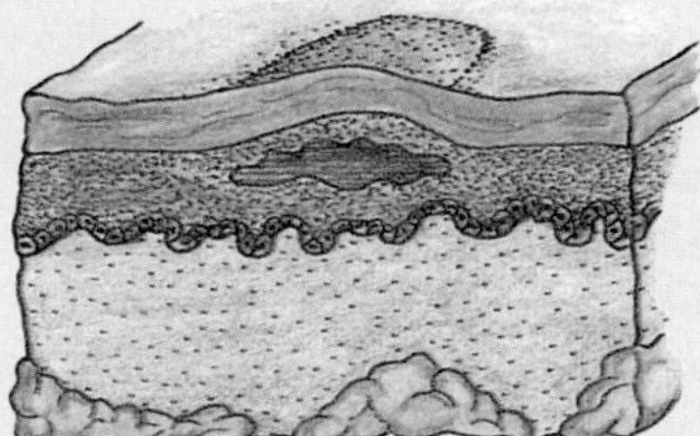

Wheal: Irregularly shaped, elevated area or superficial localized edema; varies in size (e.g., hive, mosquito bite)

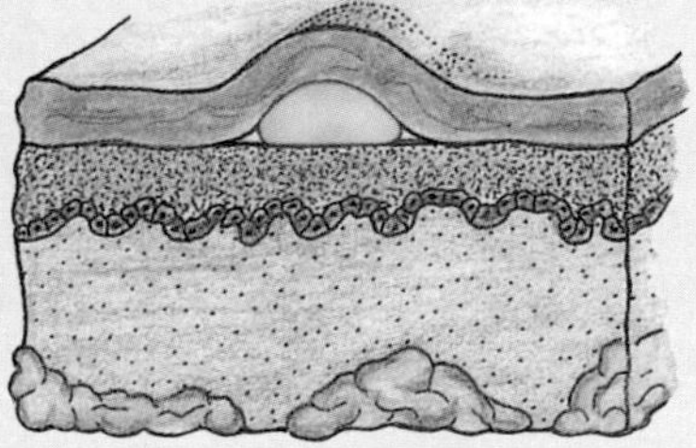

Vesicle: Circumscribed elevation of skin filled with serous fluid; smaller than 0.5 cm (e.g., herpes simplex, chickenpox)

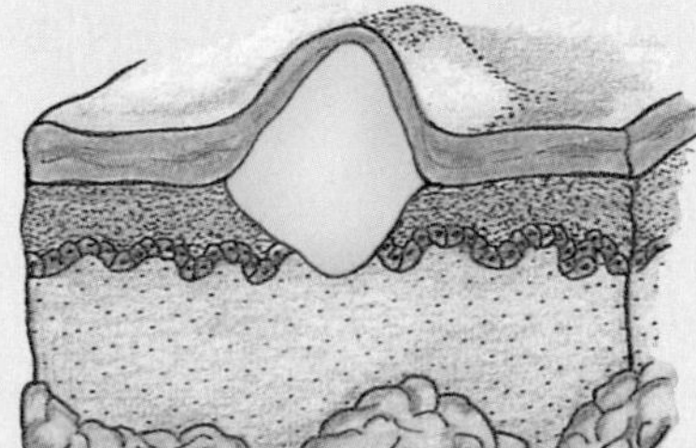

Pustule: Circumscribed elevation of skin similar to vesicle but filled with pus; varies in size (e.g., acne, staphylococcal infection)

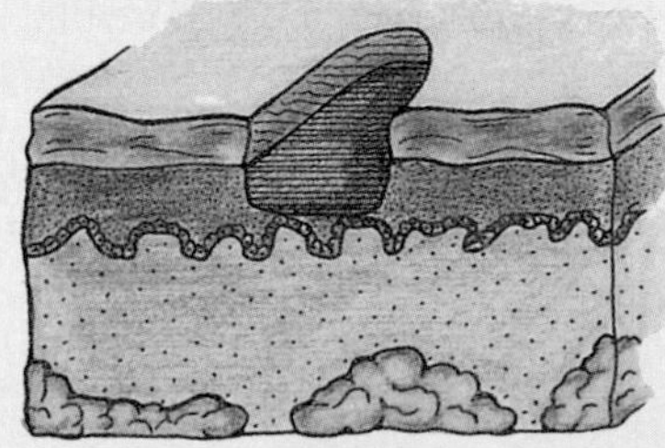

Ulcer: Deep loss of skin surface that may extend to dermis and frequently bleeds and scars; varies in size (e.g., venous stasis ulcer)

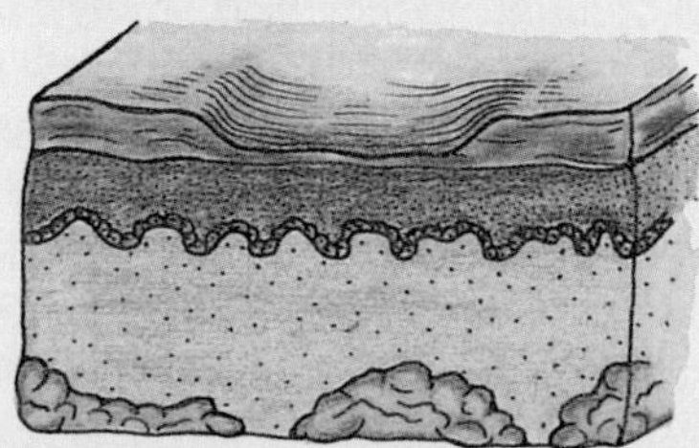

Atrophy: Thinning of skin with loss of normal skin furrow with skin appearing shiny and translucent; varies in size (e.g., arterial insufficiency)

EVALUATION

1. Observe throughout the assessment for evidence of physical or emotional distress, which may alter assessment data.
2. Compare assessment findings with previous observations to identify changes.
3. Ask patient if there is information about physical condition that has not been discussed.

Unexpected Outcomes and Related Interventions

1. Patient demonstrates acute distress (e.g., shortness of breath, acute pain, or severe anxiety).
   a. Respond immediately to identified need (e.g., vital signs, reposition patient with head of bed elevated, apply oxygen, or give medication as appropriate).
   b. Notify health care provider.
2. Patient has abnormal skin condition (e.g., dry texture, reduced turgor, lesions, or erythema).
   a. Identify contributing factors and prevent continued irritation or damage as appropriate.
3. Patient is unwilling or unable to provide adequate information relating to identified concerns.
   a. Seek information from family members if present, and review patient's record for baseline data.

Recording and Reporting

- Record patient's vital signs on vital sign flow sheet.
- Record description of alterations in patient's general appearance.
- Describe patient's behavior using objective terminology. Include patient's self-report of any signs and symptoms.
- Report abnormalities and acute symptoms to nurse in charge or health care provider.

Sample Documentation

0830 Patient reports a "painful bottom." A 2-cm flat, round, erythematous area is noted on sacrum. Area does not blanch following palpation. Skin integrity is intact. Repositioned to left side and will be repositioned every 2 hours.

Special Considerations

Pediatric

- Measure physical growth, including height, weight, length, and head circumference, which are key elements in evaluation of a child's health status (Hockenberry and Wilson, 2007).
- Weigh infants nude. Children may be weighed in light underclothes or gown.
- A child's interactions with parents provide valuable information regarding the child's behavior.

Geriatric

- An older adult's presenting signs and symptoms can be deceiving. An older adult has a diminished physiological reserve that may mask the usual, or "classic," signs and symptoms of a disease. In older adults signs and symptoms are often blunted or atypical (Ebersole and others, 2008).
- Postural hypotension is common in older patients. Check vital signs in lying, sitting, and standing positions, especially when positional dizziness and light-headedness are reported.
- Inspection of the feet is critically important in the presence of impaired circulation, impaired vision, and diabetes. Common foot conditions include ulceration, fungal infection, calluses, bunions, and plantar warts.

Home Care

- In the home the focus may be on patient's ability to perform basic self-care tasks. Be sure that the home assessment builds on all health concerns identified in other settings.
- The home health nurse takes a small portable scale to monitor weight changes.

PROCEDURAL GUIDELINE 7.1 Monitoring Intake and Output

Video Clips

Measuring and recording I&O during a 24-hour period helps complete the assessment database for fluid and electrolyte balance (Table 7-3). You are responsible for recording all intake (liquids taken orally, by enteral feeding, and parenterally) and all output (urine, diarrhea, vomitus, gastric suction, and drainage from surgical tubes). Placing a patient on I&O requires cooperation and assistance from the patient and family. I&O are monitored for patients with a fever or edema, receiving intravenous (IV) or diuretic therapy, or on restricted fluids. It is also important when a patient has electrolyte losses associated with vomiting, diarrhea, gastrointestinal (GI) drainage. or extensive wounds such as burns. You total and evaluate I&O at the end of each shift or at specified times, such as every 24 hours.

Delegation and Collaboration

The skills of assessing I&O totals at the end of each shift; comparing 24-hour totals over several days; and monitoring and recording IV therapy, wound or chest tube drainage, and tube feeding cannot be delegated to nursing assistive personnel (NAP). The nurse emphasizes maintaining standard precautions relating to body fluids, accurately measuring and recording I&O, and using the metric system with standard containers. Instruct the NAP to:

Continued

PROCEDURAL GUIDELINE 7.1
Monitoring Intake and Output—cont'd

- Measure and record oral intake.
- Measure and record urinary output, liquid diarrheal stool, vomitus, and wound drainage device output.
- Report changes in patient's condition such as alterations in intake or changes in color, amount, or odor of output.

Equipment

- Sign to alert personnel of I&O measurement
- Daily I&O record form or computer graphic
- Graduated measuring container
- Bedpan, urinal, bedside commode, or urine "hat" (a receptacle that fits under the toilet seat)
- Clean gloves

Procedural Steps

1. Identify patients with conditions that increase fluid loss (e.g., fever, diarrhea, vomiting, surgical wound drainage, chest tube drainage, gastric suction, major burns, or severe trauma).
2. Identify patients with impaired swallowing or mobility and unconscious patients.
3. Identify patients on medications that influence fluid balance (e.g., diuretics and steroids).
4. Assess signs and symptoms of dehydration and fluid excess (e.g., bradycardia versus tachycardia, hypotension versus hypertension, and reduced skin turgor versus edema).
5. Weigh patients daily using the same scale, at the same time of day, and with comparable clothing.
6. Monitor laboratory results:
   a. Urine specific gravity (normal 1.010 to 1.030)
   b. Hematocrit (normal range is 38% to 47% for females and 40% to 54% for males).
7. Assess patient's and family's knowledge of the purpose and process of I&O measurement.
8. Explain to patient and family the reasons that I&O are important.
9. Measure and record all intake of fluids:
   a. Liquids with meals, gelatin, custards, ice cream, popsicles, sherbets, ice chips (recorded as 50% of measured volume [e.g., 100 mL of ice chips equals 50 mL of water]). Convert household measures to the metric system: 1 ounce equals 30 mL, therefore 12 ounces (soda can) equals 360 mL.
   b. Count liquid medications such as antacids as fluid intake, as are fluids with medications.
   c. Calculate fluid intake from tube feedings (see Chapter 12).

> **SAFETY ALERT** Record intake as soon as you measure it to maintain accuracy.

   d. Calculate fluid intake from parenteral fluids, blood components, and total parenteral nutrition (see Chapter 28).
10. Instruct patient and family to call you or the NAP to empty contents of urinal, urine hat, or commode each time patient uses it. Patient and family also need to monitor incontinence, vomiting, and excessive perspiration and report it to the nurse.
11. Inform patient and family that Foley catheter drainage bag and wound, gastric, or chest tube drainage are closely monitored, measured, and recorded and who is responsible for this. Each patient must have a graduated container clearly marked with name and bed location and used only for the identified patient.
12. Measure drainage at the end of the shift or as indicated, using appropriate containers and noting color and characteristics. If splashing is anticipated, wear mask, eye protection, and/or gown.
   a. Measure urine drainage using a "hat" into which the patient voids or a graduated container.

TABLE 7-3 ADULT AVERAGE DAILY FLUID GAINS AND LOSSES

FLUID INTAKE AND OUTPUT	VOLUME (mL)	FLUID INTAKE AND OUTPUT	VOLUME (mL)
Fluid Intake		**Fluid Output**	
Oral fluids	1100-1400	Kidneys	1200-1500
Solid foods	800-1000	Skin	500-600
Oxidative metabolism	300	Lungs	400
Total gains	2200-2700	Gastrointestinal	100-200
		Total losses	2200-2700

PROCEDURAL GUIDELINE 7.1
Monitoring Intake and Output—cont'd

b. Observe color and characteristics of urine in Foley tubing and drainage bag. Sometimes a measuring device is part of drainage bag. Otherwise measure using a graduated container (see illustration).

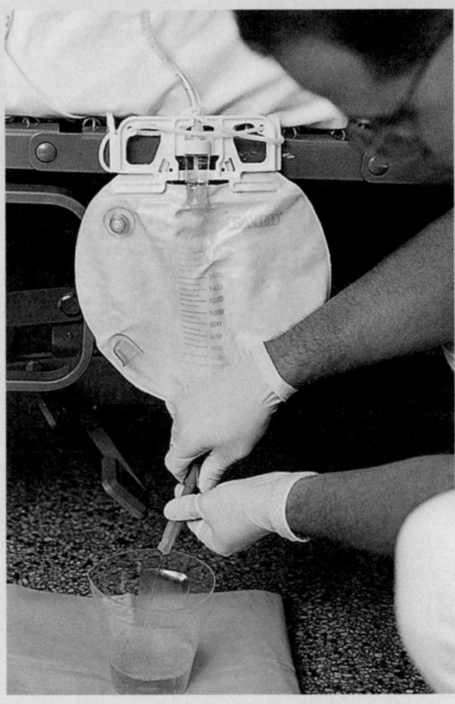

STEP 12b Device for monitoring hourly urine output.

c. Measure chest tube drainage by marking and recording the time on the collection chamber at specified intervals. Empty chest tube drainage *only* when container is nearly full. A closed system is necessary to maintain lung expansion.

d. Measure Jackson-Pratt/Hemovac drainage using a medicine cup (see illustration) (see Chapter 24).

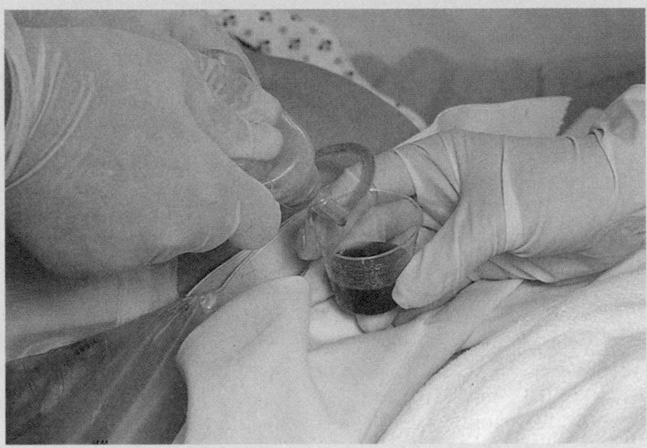

STEP 12d Measuring wound drainage from a Jackson-Pratt drain.

e. Measure gastric drainage or larger drainage pouches by opening clamp and pouring into graduated container with 240-mL capacity.

13. Remove gloves and dispose of them in appropriate receptacle. Perform hand hygiene.
14. Note I&O balance or imbalance and report to health care provider any urine output less than 30 mL/hr or significant changes in daily weight.
15. Document on I&O forms or computer record.

SKILL 7.2 ASSESSING THE HEAD AND NECK

Examination of the head and neck includes assessment of the head, eyes, ears, nose, mouth, and sinuses. Assessment of the head and neck uses inspection, palpation, and auscultation, with inspection and palpation often used simultaneously.

ASSESSMENT

1. Assess for history of headache, dizziness, pain, or stiffness. *Rationale: Headaches and dizziness may be a sign of stress, a symptom of another underlying problem such as high blood pressure, or a result of injury.*
2. Determine if patient has a history of eye disease, diabetes mellitus, or hypertension. *Rationale: Common conditions predispose patients to visual alterations requiring health care provider referral.*
3. Ask if patient has experienced blurred vision, flashing lights, or reduced visual field. *Rationale: These common symptoms indicate visual problems.*
4. Ask if patient has experienced ear pain, itching, discharge, vertigo, tinnitus (ringing in the ears), or change in hearing. *Rationale: These signs and symptoms indicate infection or hearing loss.*
5. Review patient's occupational history. *Rationale: Patient's occupation can create a risk of injury, potential for eye fatigue, or prolonged noise exposure.*
6. Ask if patient has a history of allergies, nasal discharge, epistaxis (nosebleeds), or postnasal drip. *Rationale: History is useful in determining source of nasal and sinus drainage.*
7. Determine if patient smokes or chews tobacco. *Rationale: Tobacco users have greater risk for mouth and throat cancer (ACS, 2010b).*
8. Ask if patient has regular/annual dental examinations. *Rationale: Annual examinations often detect abnormalities early.*

PLANNING

Expected Outcomes focus on identifying alterations in the head and neck.

1. Physical findings are within normal limits.

2. Patient recognizes warning signs and symptoms of eye, ear, sinus, and mouth disease.
3. Patient takes appropriate safety precautions for occupational injury related to the head and neck.

Delegation and Collaboration

The skill of assessing the head and neck cannot be delegated to nursing assistive personnel (NAP). Instruct the NAP to:

- Observe for nasal discharge and nasal bleeding.
- Report any findings found during routine care (e.g., oral care, bathing) to the nurse for further assessment.

Equipment

- Stethoscope
- Clean gloves (use nonlatex if necessary)
- Tongue blade
- Pen light

IMPLEMENTATION *for* ASSESSING THE HEAD AND NECK

STEPS	RATIONALE
1. See Standard Protocol (inside front cover).	
2. Position patient sitting upright if possible.	Provides for a more thorough examination of the head and neck structures.
3. Inspect the head.	
a. Note head position and facial features.	Head tilting to one side may indicate hearing or visual loss.
b. Note patient's facial features for symmetry.	Neurological disorders such as paralysis may affect the symmetry of the face.
4. Assess the eyes.	
a. Inspect position of eyes, color, condition of conjunctivae, and movement.	Asymmetrical positioning may reflect trauma or tumor growth. Differences in color may be congenital; changes in color of conjunctivae may be due to local infection or symptomatic of another abnormality (e.g., pale conjunctiva is associated with anemia).
b. Assess patient's near vision (ability to read newspaper or magazines) and far vision (ability to follow movement or read clock, watch television, or read signs at a distance).	If patient has visual acuity or visual field loss, make adjustments to support self-care measures (e.g., feeding, bathing and hygiene, dressing) and teaching.
c. Inspect pupils for size, shape, and equality (see illustration).	Normal pupils are round, clear, and equal in size and shape.

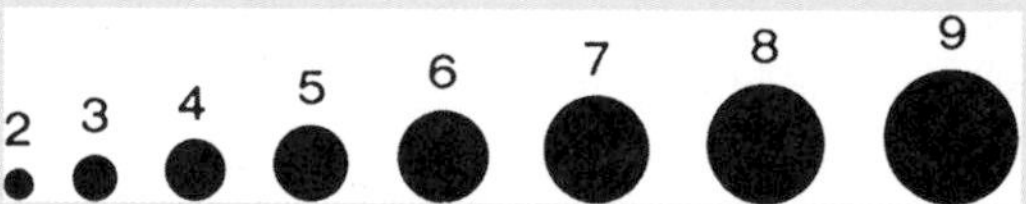

STEP 4c Pupil size in millimeters.

STEPS	RATIONALE
d. Test pupillary reflexes. To test reaction to light, dim room light. As patient looks straight ahead, move penlight from side of patient's face and direct light on pupil. Observe pupillary response of both eyes (consensual response), noting briskness and equality of reflex (see illustrations).	Darkened room normally ensures brisk response of pupils to light. Pupil that is illuminated constricts. Pupil in other eye should constrict equally (consensual light reflex).

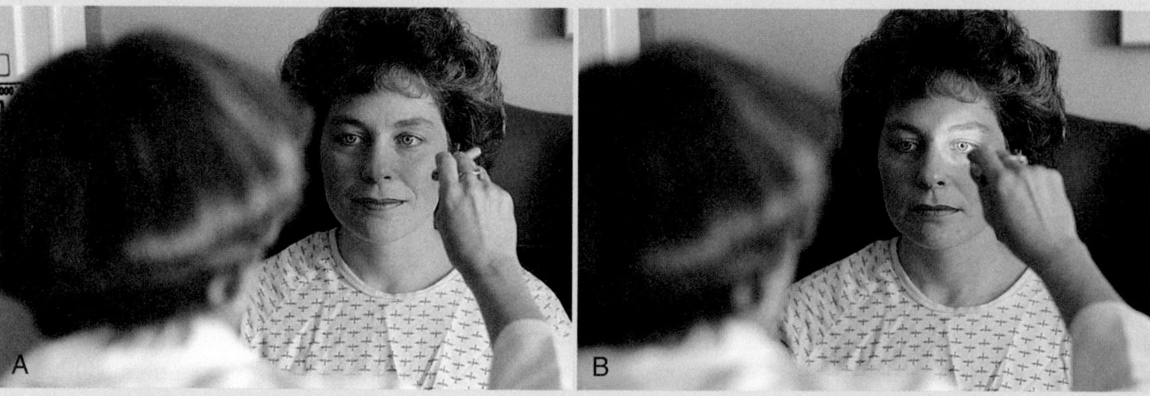

STEP 4d A, Hold penlight to side of patient's face. **B,** Illuminate pupil to cause pupil to constrict.

STEPS	RATIONALE
(1) Test for accommodation by asking the patient to focus on a distant object, which dilates the pupil. Then have the patient shift to a near object about 7 to 8 cm (3 inches) from the nose and observe for pupil constriction and convergence of the eyes. NOTE: Can also ask patient to follow an object (e.g., finger, pen) with eyes from a far to a near point.	Absence of constriction or convergence or an asymmetric response requires further ophthalmologic assessment (Jarvis, 2008).
5. Assess hearing. Note patient's response to questions and presence/use of a hearing aid. If hearing loss is suspected, ask patient to repeat random numbers spoken by the nurse. Use one- or two-syllable words. Repeat, gradually increasing voice intensity until patient correctly repeats the words.	Seidel and others (2011) report that patients normally hear numbers clearly when whispered, responding correctly at least 50% of the time. For patient with obvious hearing impairment, speak clearly and concisely; stand so patient can see face; and speak toward patient's good ear, using a low pitch and without yelling.

> **SAFETY ALERT** If hearing deficit is present, have a qualified nurse inspect patient's ears because impaired hearing may be caused by impacted cerumen, external otitis, or swelling in ear canal because of allergic reaction to material in hearing aid.

STEPS	RATIONALE
6. Inspect the nose externally for shape, skin color, alignment, drainage, and presence of deformity or inflammation. Note color of mucosa and any lesions, discharge, swelling, or presence of bleeding. If drainage appears infectious, consult health care provider about obtaining a specimen.	Character of discharge and inflammation indicates allergy or infection. Perforation and erosion of the septum and puffiness and/or increased vascularity of the mucosa indicate habitual drug use.
7. In patients with a nasogastric (NG), nasointestinal (NI), or nasotracheal tube, inspect the nares for excoriation, inflammation, or discharge. Using a penlight, look up into each nares. Stabilize tube as needed.	Swallowing or coughing reflex causes movement of tubes against nares, and pressure against tissues and mucosa can result in tissue erosion.
8. Inspect the sinuses by palpation over frontal and maxillary areas.	Infection, allergy, or drug use sometimes causes tenderness.
9. Assess the mouth.	
a. Use a tongue blade to depress the tongue and inspect the oral cavity with a penlight. Inspect the oral mucosa, tongue, teeth, and gums for hydration, discoloration, and obvious lesions.	Precancerous lesions can go unnoticed and progress rapidly.
b. Determine if patient wears dentures or retainers and if they are comfortable. You may remove dentures to visualize and palpate gums.	Ill-fitting dentures and retainers chronically irritate mucosa and gums and may pose a risk for mouth cancer.
10. Inspect and palpate the neck. Ask the patient if there is a history of neck pain or difficulty with movement of the neck.	This determines whether all neck structures are present, including neck muscles, lymph nodes of the head and neck, thyroid gland, and trachea. May indicate muscle strain, head injury, local nerve injury, or swollen lymph nodes.
a. Neck muscles: Inspect neck for bilateral symmetry of muscles. Ask patient to flex and hyperextend neck and turn head side to side.	Detects muscle weakness, strain, and range of motion (ROM).
b. Lymph nodes:	

Continued

STEPS	RATIONALE
(1) With patient's chin raised and head tilted slightly, inspect area where lymph nodes are distributed and compare both sides (see illustration).	Lymph nodes may be enlarged from infection or from various diseases such as cancer.

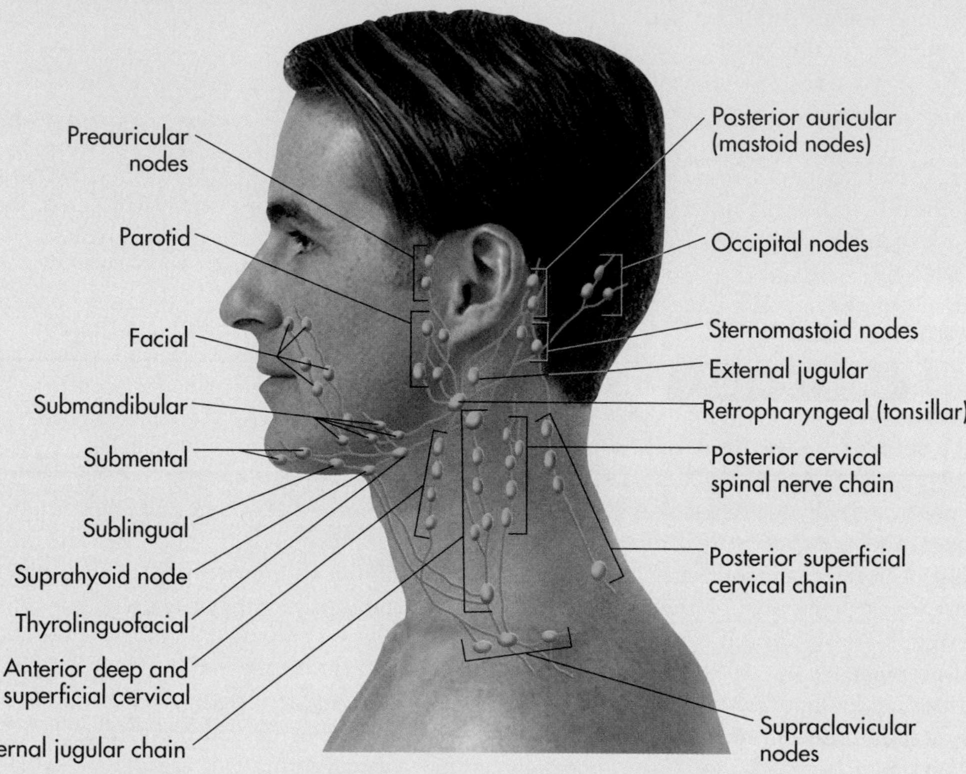

STEP 10b(1) Palpable lymph nodes of head and neck. (From Seidel HM and others: *Mosby's guide to physical examination,* ed 6, St Louis, 2006, Mosby.)

STEPS	RATIONALE
(2) To examine lymph nodes, have patient relax with neck flexed slightly forward. To palpate, face or stand to the side of patient and use pads of middle three fingers of hand. Palpate gently in a rotary motion for superficial lymph nodes (see illustration).	This position relaxes tissues and muscles.

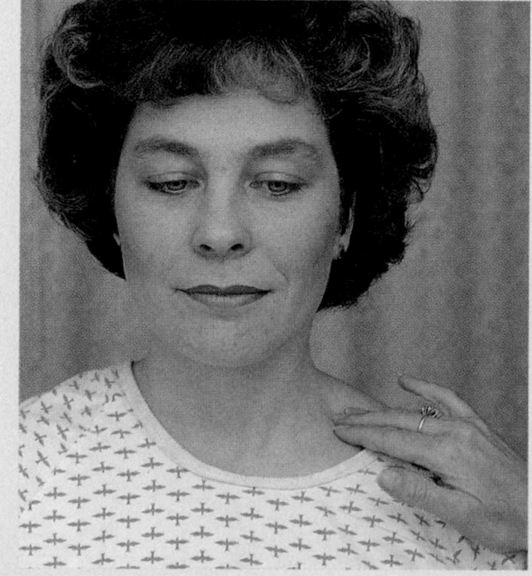

STEP 10b(2) Palpation of cervical lymph nodes.

STEPS	RATIONALE
(3) Note if lymph nodes are large, fixed, inflamed, or tender.	Large, fixed, inflamed, or tender lymph nodes indicate local infection, systemic disease, or neoplasm.

11. See Completion Protocol (inside front cover).

EVALUATION

1. Compare assessment with previous observations to identify changes.
2. Ask patient to describe common symptoms of eye, ear, sinus, or mouth disease.
3. Ask patient to list occupational safety precautions.

Unexpected Outcomes and Related Interventions

1. Patient demonstrates yellow nasal discharge, sneezing, and complaint of sinus pain.
   a. Reposition into semi-Fowler's or other comfortable position to relieve sinus pain.
   b. Monitor temperature for fever.
   c. Notify health care provider if these are new findings.
2. Patient complains of severe headache and dizziness when standing.
   a. Respond immediately by obtaining vital signs, especially blood pressure (lying, sitting, and standing).
   b. Return patient to bed in position of comfort to minimize dizziness and relieve headache.
   c. Identify contributing factors (e.g., stress, pain, or elevated blood pressure).
   d. Notify health care provider.

Recording and Reporting

- Record all findings, including any abnormal findings such as hearing or visual loss, pain and its location, and current infection in nurses' notes or flow sheet.
- Report increased headache, dizziness, or visual changes immediately to charge nurse or health care provider.

Sample Documentation

1200 Copious, green, thick nasal discharge noted from both nares. No odor noted. Patient complains of frontal "headache." Blood pressure 110/70. Head of bed raised to 60 degrees. Health care provider notified.

Special Considerations

Pediatric

- Infants may resist eye examination by closing eyes. Holding the infant in an upright position over caregiver's shoulders may cause eyes to open (Ball and Bindler, 2010).
- Headaches in children are usually caused by loss of sleep, poor nutrition, eye fatigue, and allergies. Children as young as 3 years of age can develop severe migraine headaches, but the symptoms are vague and difficult to diagnose (Hockenberry and Wilson, 2007).

Geriatric

- Older adults commonly have loss of peripheral vision caused by changes in the lens.
- Instruct patients older than age 65 to have regular hearing checks.
- Measurement of visual acuity helps determine level of assistance that patient requires with activities of daily living (ADLs) and ability of patient to safely ambulate and function independently within home.

SKILL 7.3 ASSESSING THE THORAX AND LUNGS

Assessment of respiratory function is one of the most critical assessment skills because alterations can be life threatening. Routine assessment is essential; changes in respirations or breath sounds can occur quickly as a result of a variety of factors, including immobility, infection, and fluid overload. Physical assessment includes auscultation, which assesses the movement of air through the tracheobronchial tree. Recognizing the sounds created by normal airflow allows you to detect sounds caused by obstruction of the airways. Auscultation of the lungs requires familiarity with landmarks of the chest (Fig. 7-2). During the assessment keep a mental image of the location of the lung lobes. To locate the position of each rib anteriorly, locate the angle of Louis by palpating the "speed bump" on the sternum where the second rib connects with the sternum. Count the ribs and intercostal spaces from this point. Auscultation involves listening to breath sounds using a stethoscope. You can hear these sounds best when the person breathes deeply through the mouth.

Adventitious sounds (abnormal sounds) result from air passing through fluid, mucus, or narrowed airways; alveoli suddenly reinflating; or an inflammation between the pleural linings. The four types of adventitious sounds include crackles (rales), rhonchi (gurgles), wheezes, and pleural friction rubs (Table 7-4). Note the location and characteristics of the sounds, diminished breath sounds, or the absence of breath sounds (found with collapsed or surgically removed lobes). Note where in the respiratory cycle the abnormal sounds are heard.

ASSESSMENT

1. Assess history of tobacco or marijuana use, including type of tobacco, duration of use, and amount in pack years. Pack years equal number of years smoking times the number of packs per day (e.g., 4 years × ½ pack per day equals 2 pack years). If patient has quit, determine the length of time since smoking stopped. *Rationale: Smoking is a major cause of lung cancer, heart disease, and chronic lung disease (emphysema and chronic bronchitis) and is responsible for 15% of all lung cancers in the United States (ACS, 2010b).*
2. Ask if patient experiences any of the following: *persistent cough* (productive or nonproductive), sputum production, *blood-streaked sputum*, *chest pain*, shortness of breath,

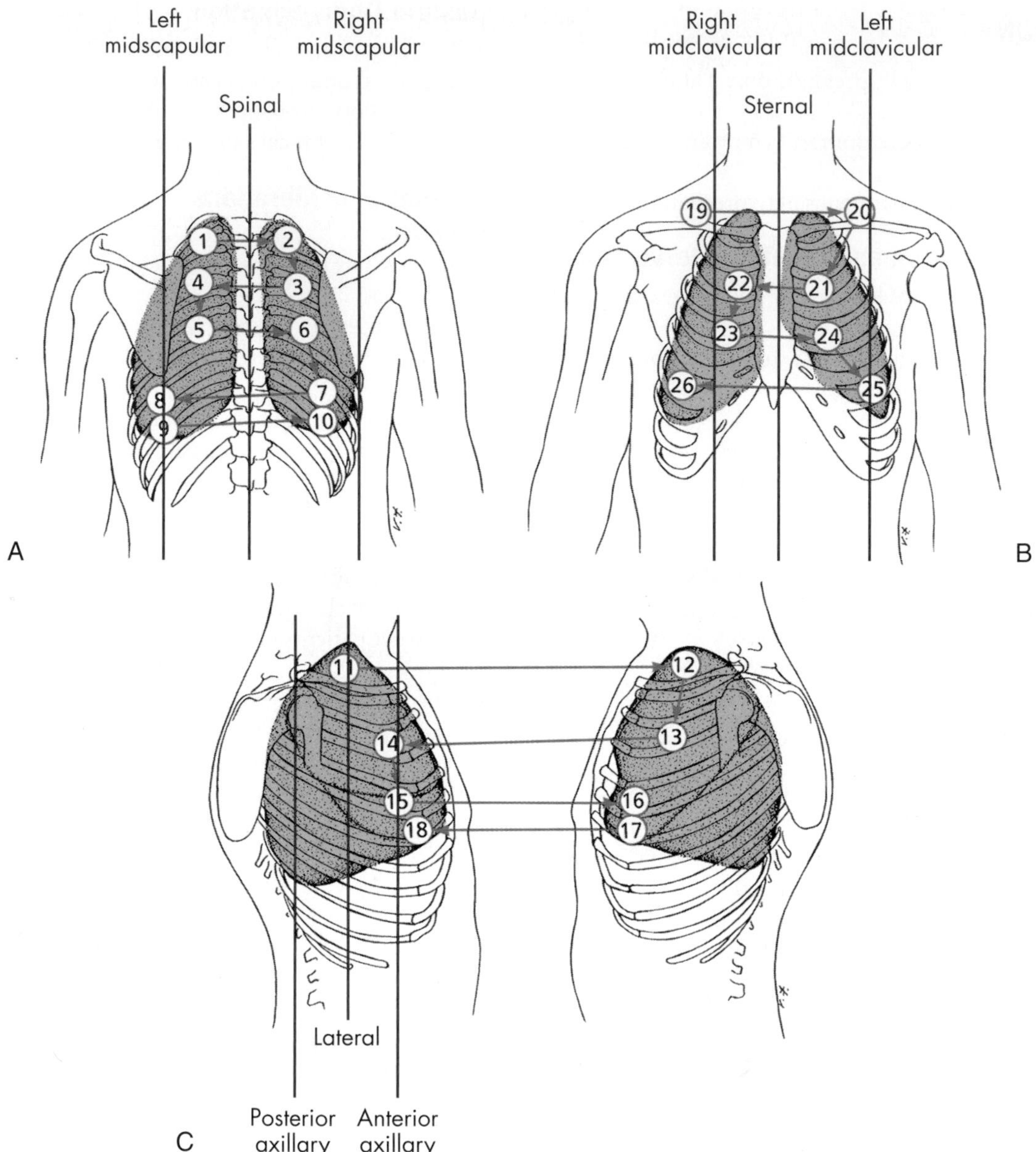

FIG 7-2 Anatomical landmarks and order of progression for examination of the thorax. **A,** Posterior thorax. **B,** Anterior thorax. **C,** Lateral thorax.

orthopnea, dyspnea during exertion, activity intolerance, or *recurrent attacks of pneumonia or bronchitis. Rationale: Symptoms of respiratory alterations help to localize objective physical findings. Warning signs of lung cancer are in italic type.*

3. Assess for history of allergies to pollens, dust, or other airborne irritants and to any foods, drugs, or chemical substances. *Rationale: Allergic response is associated with wheezing on auscultation, dyspnea, cyanosis, and diaphoresis.*
4. Determine if patient works in environment containing pollutants (e.g., asbestos, coal dust, or chemical irritants). Does patient have exposure to secondhand cigarette smoke? *Rationale: Patients with chronic respiratory disease, particularly asthma, have symptoms aggravated by change in temperature and humidity, irritating fumes or smoke, emotional stress, and physical exertion.*
5. Review history for known or suspected human immunodeficiency virus (HIV) infection, substance abuse, low income, residence or employment in nursing home or shelter, homelessness, recent imprisonment, or exposure to family member with tuberculosis (TB). *Rationale: These are known risk factors for exposure to and/or development of TB.*
6. Ask if patient has history of persistent cough, hemoptysis (bloody sputum), unexplained weight loss, fatigue, night sweats, and/or fever. *Rationale: These are signs and symptoms for both TB and HIV infection.*

TABLE 7-4 ADVENTITIOUS SOUNDS

SOUND	SITE AUSCULTATED	CAUSE	CHARACTER
Crackles (formerly called rales)	Most common in dependent lobes: right and left lung bases	Random, sudden reinflation of groups of alveoli; also related to increase in fluid in small airways	Fine, short, interrupted crackling sounds heard during end of inspiration, expiration, or both; may or may not change with coughing; sound like crushing cellophane; medium crackles are lower, more moist sounds heard during middle of inspiration, not cleared with coughing; coarse crackles are loud bubbly sounds heard during inspiration; not cleared with coughing
Rhonchi (sonorous wheeze)	Heard primarily over trachea and bronchi; if loud enough, can be heard over most lung fields	Fluid or mucus in larger airways, causing turbulence; muscular spasm	Loud, low-pitched, continuous sounds heard more during expiration; sometimes cleared by coughing; sound like blowing air through fluid with a straw
Wheezes (sibilant wheeze)	Heard over all lung fields but are more distinct over posterior lung fields	High-velocity airflow through severely narrowed or obstructed bronchus	High-pitched, musical sounds like a squeak heard continuously during inspiration or expiration; usually louder on expiration; do not clear with coughing
Pleural friction rub	Heard over anterior lateral lung field (if patient is sitting upright)	Inflamed pleura, parietal pleura rubbing against visceral pleura	Has grating quality heard best during inspiration, does not clear with coughing; heard loudest over lower lateral anterior surface

Data from Jarvis C: *Physical examination & health assessment,* ed 5, St Louis, 2008, Saunders; Seidel HM and others: *Mosby's guide to physical examination,* ed 6, St Louis, 2006, Mosby.

PLANNING

Expected Outcomes focus on identifying alterations in respiratory function.

1. Physical findings are within normal limits (respirations passive, diaphragmatic or costal, and regular [12 to 20/min in adult] with symmetrical expansion; breath sounds clear to auscultation and equal in all lung fields).
2. Patient is able to describe own risks and factors that predispose to lung disease.

Delegation and Collaboration

The skill of assessing the lungs and thorax cannot be delegated to nursing assistive personnel (NAP). Instruct the NAP to:

- Measure patient's respirations after determining stability.
- Report any respiratory distress, difficulty breathing, and changes in rate or depth of respiration.

Equipment

- Stethoscope
- Clean gloves

IMPLEMENTATION *for* ASSESSING THE THORAX AND LUNGS

STEPS	RATIONALE
1. See Standard Protocol (inside front cover).	
2. Position and prepare patient for examination.	
a. Position patient sitting upright. For bedridden patient, elevate head of bed 45 to 90 degrees. If patient is unable to tolerate sitting, use the supine position or side-lying position.	Promotes full lung expansion during examination. Patients with chronic respiratory disease may need to sit up throughout the examination because of shortness of breath. May require assistance of another caregiver to help position unresponsive patients.
b. Remove gown or drape first from posterior chest, keeping front of chest and legs covered. As examination progresses, remove gown from area being examined.	Avoids unnecessary exposure and provides full visibility of thorax. Allows direct placement of diaphragm or bell of stethoscope on patient's skin, which enhances clarity of sounds.
c. Explain all steps of procedure, encouraging patient to relax and breathe normally through the mouth.	Anxiety alters respiratory function. Breathing through the mouth decreases extraneous sounds from air passing through the nose.
3. *Posterior thorax.*	
a. If possible, stand behind patient. Inspect thorax for shape, deformities; position of the spine; slope of the ribs; retraction of intercostal spaces during inspiration and bulging of intercostal spaces during expiration; and symmetrical expansion during inspiration.	Allows for identification of impairment in chest expansion and any symptoms of respiratory distress. In a child shape of chest is almost circular, with anteroposterior (AP) diameter in 1:1 ratio. In the adult the AP diameter is less than the lateral diameter. Chronic lung disease causes the ribs to become more horizontal and increases the AP diameter, causing a "barrel chest." Patients with breathing problems assume postures that improve ventilation.

SAFETY ALERT When a patient holds the chest wall during breathing, this indicates localized chest pain. Assess the nature of pain, including onset, severity, precipitating factors, quality, region, and radiation.

STEPS	RATIONALE
b. Determine the rate and rhythm of breathing (see Chapter 6). Have patient relaxed.	This is a good time to count respirations, with patient relaxed and unaware of inspection. Awareness could alter respirations.
c. Systematically palpate posterior chest wall, costal spaces, and intercostal spaces, noting any masses, pulsations, unusual movement, or areas of localized tenderness (see Fig. 7-2, *A*, for numbered areas to systematically palpate). If you detect a suspicious mass or swollen area, palpate for size, shape, and typical qualities of lesion. Do not palpate painful areas deeply.	Palpation assesses further characteristics and confirms or supplements findings from assessment. Localized swelling or tenderness may indicate trauma to ribs or underlying cartilage. A fractured rib fragment could be displaced.
d. Standing behind patient, place thumbs along the spinal processes at the tenth rib, with the palms lightly contacting the posterolateral surfaces (see illustration *A*). Keep thumbs about 5 cm (2 inches) apart, with the thumbs pointing toward the spine and the fingers pointing laterally. Press hands toward patient's spine to form small skin fold between thumbs. After exhalation, patient takes deep breath. Note movement of thumbs (see illustration *B*) and symmetry of chest wall movement. Normally symmetrical separation of the thumbs occurs during chest excursion—3 to 5 cm (1½ to 2 inches).	Palpation of chest excursion assesses depth of patient's breathing. This technique is a good measure to evaluate patient's ability to perform deep-breathing exercises (see Chapter 29). Limited movement on one side may indicate that patient is voluntarily splinting during ventilation because of pain. Avoid allowing the hands to slide over the skin, which gives a false measure of excursion.

STEPS	RATIONALE
e. Auscultate breath sounds. Have patient take slow deep breaths with the mouth slightly open. For adult, place diaphragm of stethoscope firmly on chest wall over intercostal spaces (see illustration). Listen to entire inspiration and expiration at each stethoscope position (see Fig. 7-2, *A*). Systematically compare breath sounds over right and left sides. If sounds are faint, ask patient to breathe a little deeper temporarily.	Assesses movement of air through tracheobronchial tree (Table 7-5). Recognition of normal airflow sounds allows detection of sounds caused by mucus or airway obstruction. Characterize sound by length of inspiratory and expiratory phases.

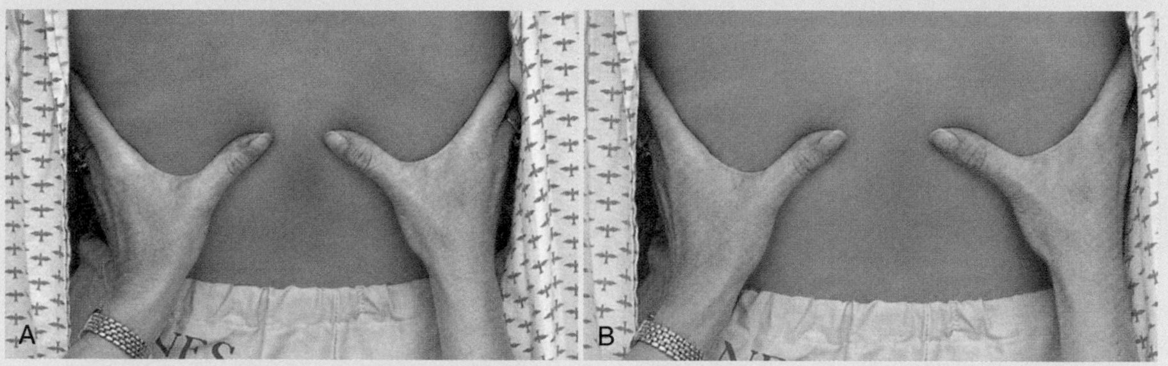

STEP 3d A, Position of hands for palpation of posterior thorax excursion. **B,** As patient inhales, movement of chest excursion separates nurse's thumbs.

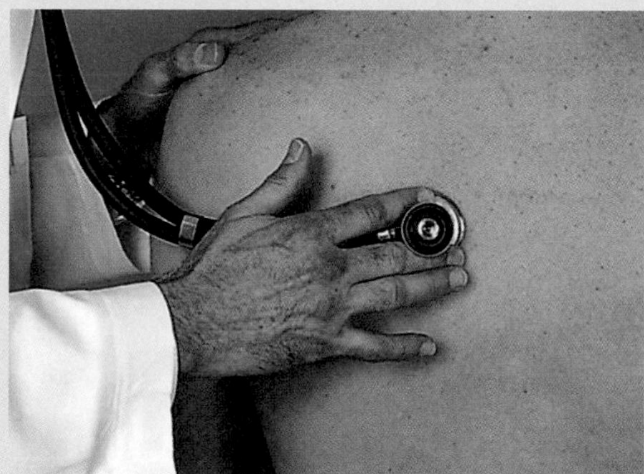

STEP 3e Use of diaphragm of stethoscope to auscultate breath sounds. (From Seidel HM and others: *Mosby's guide to physical examination,* ed 6, St Louis, 2006, Mosby.)

TABLE 7-5 NORMAL BREATH SOUNDS

TYPE	DESCRIPTION	LOCATION	ORIGIN
Bronchial	Loud and high-pitched sounds with hollow quality; expiration lasts longer than inspiration (3:2 ratio).	Best heard over trachea	Created by air moving through trachea close to chest wall
Bronchovesicular	Medium-pitched and blowing sounds of medium intensity; inspiratory phase is equal to expiratory phase.	Best heard posteriorly between scapulae and anteriorly over bronchioles lateral to sternum at first and second intercostal spaces	Created by air moving through large airways
Vesicular	Soft, breezy, low-pitched sounds. Inspiratory phase is 3 times longer than expiratory phase.	Best heard over periphery of lung (except over scapula)	Created by air moving through smaller airways

Continued

STEPS	RATIONALE
f. If you auscultate adventitious sounds, have patient cough. Listen again with stethoscope to determine if sound has cleared with coughing. See Table 7-5 for a description of normal breath sounds.	Coughing may clear adventitious sound. Rhonchi often are eliminated or altered by coughing. Crackles and wheezes are not.
4. *Lateral thorax.*	
a. Instruct patient to raise arms and inspect chest wall for same characteristics as reviewed for posterior chest.	Improves access to lateral thoracic structures.
b. Extend palpation and auscultation of posterior thorax to lateral sides of chest, except for excursion measurement (see Fig. 7-2, *C*).	Locates abnormalities in lateral lung fields.
5. *Anterior thorax.*	
a. Inspect accessory muscles of breathing: sternocleidomastoid, trapezius, and abdominal muscles, noting effort to breathe.	Extent to which accessory muscles are used reveals degree of effort to breathe. Generally these muscles are not used for breathing.
b. Inspect width or spread of angle made by costal margins and tip of sternum. Angle is usually larger than 90 degrees between margins.	Indicates congenital, acquired, or traumatic alterations that may influence patient's chest expansion.
c. Observe patient's breathing pattern, observing symmetry and degree of chest wall and abdominal movement. Respiratory rate and rhythm are more often assessed on the anterior chest wall.	Assesses patient's effort to breathe: symmetrical, passive movement indicates no respiratory distress.
d. Palpate anterior thoracic muscles and ribs for lumps, masses, tenderness, or unusual movement following pattern across and down (see Fig. 7-2, *B*).	Localized swelling or tenderness may indicate trauma to underlying ribs or cartilage.
e. Palpate anterior chest excursion. Place hands over each lateral rib cage, with thumbs approximately 5 cm (2 inches) apart and angled along each costal margin. As patient inhales deeply, thumbs should symmetrically separate approximately 3 to 5 cm (1½ to 2 inches), with each side expanding equally.	Assesses depth of patient's breathing and ability to perform deep-breathing exercises. Certain abnormalities are evident if expansion is not symmetrical.
f. With patient sitting, auscultate anterior thorax. Begin above the clavicles and move across and then down as during palpation.	A systematic pattern of assessment comparing sides helps identify abnormal sounds.
6. See Completion Protocol (inside front cover).	

EVALUATION

1. Compare respiratory findings with assessment characteristics for thorax and lungs to identify changes.
2. Have patient identify factors leading to lung disease.

Unexpected Outcomes and Related Interventions

1. Patient has copious mucus production; audible inspiratory wheezing; or congested cough with thick, tenacious mucus.
   a. Assist patient to cough by splinting chest; teach to inhale slowly through nose, exhale, and cough; encourage expectoration of sputum.
   b. Auscultate breath sounds before and after cough to evaluate cough effectiveness.
   c. Encourage increased oral fluid intake (if permitted).
   d. If unable to clear airway by coughing, suctioning is indicated (see Chapter 14).
   e. Monitor vital signs.
   f. Notify health care provider.
2. Patient demonstrates weakness, fatigue, dyspnea, altered vital signs, or dizziness with exertion.
   a. Provide bed rest and limited activity to conserve oxygen.
   b. Plan interventions alternately with periods of rest.
   c. Monitor for restlessness, anxiety, confusion, and respiratory status.

Recording and Reporting

- Record patient's respiratory rate and character; breath sounds, including type, location, and presence on inspiration, expiration, or both; and changes noted after coughing in nurses' notes or on flow sheet.
- Report any abnormalities immediately to nurse in charge or health care provider.

Sample Documentation

0730 Inspiratory wheezing noted over anterior upper lobes bilaterally; lungs sounds clear and equal bilaterally in all other lung fields. Respirations 26 and regular. Patient complaining of shortness of breath even at rest. Head of bed raised to 90 degrees. Health care provider notified.

Special Considerations

Pediatric

- Infants and young children have thin chest walls, allowing breath sounds from one lung to be heard over entire chest (Ball and Bindler, 2010).
- Children younger than 7 years of age normally exhibit noticeable abdominal or diaphragmatic movement. Older children and adults exhibit more costal or thoracic movement. Use stethoscope bell to auscultate breath sounds in children. Breath sounds are louder in children because of their thin chest walls.
- In children observe for use of accessory muscles, which is a sign of respiratory distress and may involve intercostal, suprasternal, supraclavicular, or sternal muscles. Head bobbing and nasal flaring are signs of significant respiratory distress in infants (Hockenberry and Wilson, 2007).

Geriatric

- Older adults have a costal angle (anteriorly) of slightly less than 90 degrees. The AP diameter may be increased from kyphosis.
- In older adults chest expansion is reduced because of calcification of rib cartilage and partial contraction of inspiratory muscles.
- Adults over 65 years of age should receive influenza and pneumococcal vaccines (Ebersole and others, 2008).

SKILL 7.4 CARDIOVASCULAR ASSESSMENT

A patient who presents with signs or symptoms of heart (cardiac) problems such as chest pain may be suffering a life-threatening condition requiring immediate attention. In this situation you must act quickly and decide on the parts of the examination that are absolutely necessary. When a patient's condition is stable, a more thorough assessment can reveal baseline heart function and any risks for heart disease. Patients tend to seek information about heart disease because it remains a leading cause of death in the United States. The heart, neck vessels, and peripheral circulation are assessed together because the systems work together.

Your assessment can determine the integrity of the circulatory system. Inadequate tissue perfusion results in an inadequate delivery of oxygen and nutrients to cells, a condition called *ischemia*. This is caused by constriction of the vessels or occlusion (blockage) from clot formation. The effects of the ischemia depend on the duration of the problem and the metabolic needs of the tissues. Ischemia results in pain. If lack of oxygen to tissues is unrelieved, tissue necrosis (death) occurs. An embolus is a blood clot that breaks loose and travels through the circulation. If the clot obstructs circulation to the lungs or the brain, it can be life threatening. The nurse assesses the heart after examining the lungs because the patient is already in a suitable position with the chest exposed. Assessment then proceeds to the neck vessels and ends with the peripheral circulation. The skills of inspection, palpation, auscultation, and percussion are used during the examination.

ASSESSMENT

1. Assess patient for history of smoking, alcohol intake, caffeine intake (coffee, tea, soft drinks, energy drinks, and chocolate), use of "recreational" drugs, exercise habits, and dietary patterns and intake. *Rationale: These can contribute to risk factors for cardiovascular disease. In addition, caffeine and alcohol may cause tachycardia.*
2. Determine if patient is taking medications for cardiovascular function (e.g., antiarrhythmics, antihypertensives, antianginals) and if patient knows their purpose, dosage, and side effects. *Rationale: Allows you to assess patient's compliance with and understanding of drug therapies. Medications for cardiovascular function cannot be taken intermittently.*
3. Ask if patient has experienced dyspnea, chest pain or discomfort, palpitations, excess fatigue, cough, leg pain or cramps, edema of the feet, cyanosis, fainting, or orthopnea. Ask if symptoms occur at rest or during exercise. *Rationale: These are the cardinal symptoms of heart disease. Cardiovascular function may be adequate during rest but not during exercise.*
4. If patient reports chest pain, determine onset (sudden or gradual), precipitating factors, quality, region, severity, and if pain radiates. Anginal pain is usually a deep pressure or ache that is substernal and diffuse, radiating to one or both arms, neck, or jaw. *Rationale: Symptoms may reveal acute coronary syndrome or coronary artery disease.*
5. Assess family history for heart disease, diabetes mellitus, high cholesterol and/or lipid levels, hypertension, stroke, or rheumatic heart disease. *Rationale: Family history of these conditions increases risk for heart and vascular disease.*
6. Ask patient about a history of heart trouble (e.g., heart failure, congenital heart disease, coronary artery disease, dysrhythmias, murmurs), heart surgery, or vascular disease (e.g., hypertension, phlebitis, varicose veins). *Rationale: Knowledge reveals patient's level of understanding of condition. A preexisting condition influences which examination techniques to use and the expected findings.*
7. If patient experiences leg pain or cramping in lower extremities, ask if it is relieved or aggravated by walking

or standing for long periods or if it occurs during sleep. *Rationale: Relationship of symptoms to exercise can help determine if problem is vascular or musculoskeletal. Musculoskeletal pain usually is not relieved when exercise ends.*

PLANNING

Expected Outcomes focus on identifying alterations in cardiovascular function.

1. Heart is in normal sinus rhythm with rate from 60 to 100 beats per minute (adolescent through adult), without extra sounds or murmurs.
2. Point of maximal impulse (PMI) is palpable at fifth intercostal space at left midclavicular line in children older than age 7 and in adults (Fig. 7-3). PMI is at the fourth intercostal space at the left midclavicular line in children younger than age 7 (Hockenberry and Wilson, 2007).
3. Patient describes changes in own behavior that may improve cardiovascular function.
4. Patient describes schedule, dosage, purpose, and benefits of medications being taken for cardiovascular function.
5. Blood pressure is within normal limits for patient (see Chapter 6).
6. Carotid pulse is localized, strong, elastic, and equal bilaterally. No change occurs during inspiration or expiration and without carotid bruit. This indicates a patent vessel.
7. Peripheral pulses are equal and strong (2+), extremities are warm and pink with capillary refill less than 2 seconds. There is no dependent edema. Peripheral hair growth is symmetrical and evenly distributed, and the skin is free of lesions.

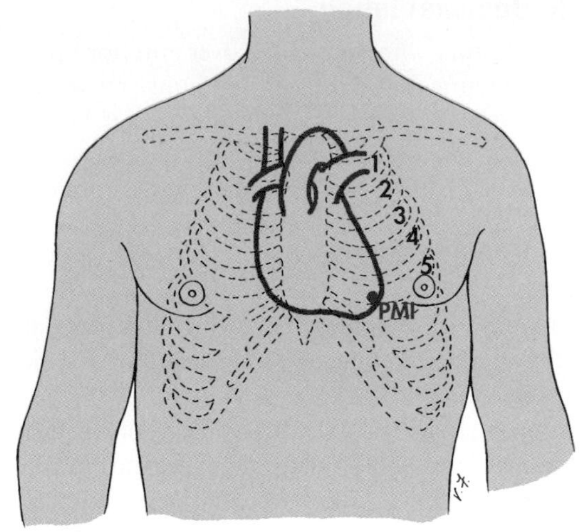

FIG 7-3 Location of point of maximal impulse (PMI) in adult.

Delegation and Collaboration

Comprehensive cardiovascular assessment cannot be delegated to nursing assistive personnel (NAP). Instruct the NAP to:

- Count apical and peripheral pulses if patient is stable.
- Recognize skin temperature and color changes of affected extremities along with changes in peripheral pulses and report any changes to the nurse.

Equipment

- Stethoscope
- Doppler stethoscope (optional)
- Conducting gel (if a Doppler stethoscope is used)

IMPLEMENTATION *for* CARDIOVASCULAR ASSESSMENT

STEPS	RATIONALE
1. **See Standard Protocol (inside front cover).**	
2. Assist patient to be as relaxed and comfortable as possible.	An anxious or uncomfortable patient can have mild tachycardia, which alters findings.
3. Have patient assume semi-Fowler's or supine position.	Provides adequate visibility and access to left thorax and mediastinum. Patient with heart disease often experiences shortness of breath when lying flat.
4. Explain procedure. Avoid facial gestures reflecting concern.	Patient with previously normal cardiac history may become anxious if you show concern.
5. Be sure that room is quiet.	Subtle, low-pitched heart sounds are difficult to hear.
6. *Assess the heart.*	
a. Form a mental image of the exact location of the heart (see illustration). The base of the heart is the upper portion, and the apex is the bottom tip. The surface of the right ventricle composes most of the heart's anterior surface.	Visualization improves ability to assess findings accurately and determine possible source of abnormalities.

STEPS	RATIONALE

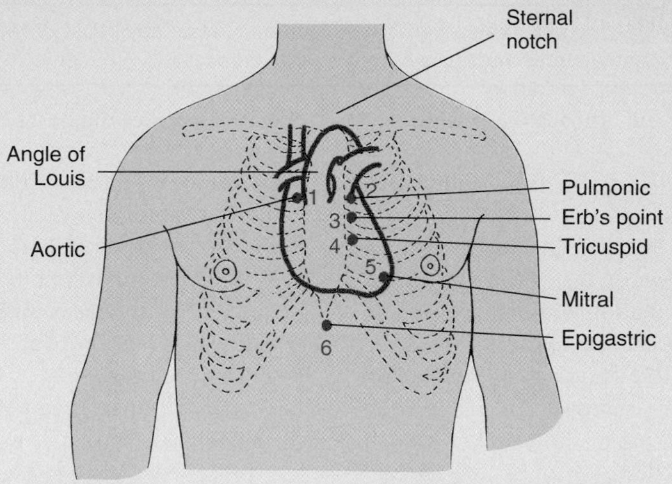

STEP 6a Anatomical sites for assessment of cardiac function.

STEPS	RATIONALE
b. Find the angle of Louis, felt as a ridge in the sternum approximately 5 cm (2 inches) below the suprasternal notch (between the sternal body and manubrium). Slip fingers down each side of angle to feel adjacent ribs. The intercostal spaces are just below each rib.	Provides examiner with landmarks for locating and assessing heart sounds.
c. Find the following anatomical landmarks (see illustration for Step 6a): **(1)** The aortic area is at the second intercostal space, right of the sternum, close to the sternal border *(1)*. **(2)** The pulmonic area is at the second intercostal space, left of the sternum, close to the sternal border *(2)*. **(3)** The second pulmonic area is found by moving down the left side of sternum to the third intercostal space, close to the sternal border *(3)*; also referred to as Erb's point. **(4)** The tricuspid area *(4)* is located at the fourth left intercostal space along the sternum, close to the sternal border. **(5)** The mitral area is found by moving fingers laterally to patient's left to locate the fifth intercostal space at the left midclavicular line *(5)*. **(6)** The epigastric area *(6)* is at the inferior tip of the sternum.	Familiarity with landmarks allows you to describe findings more clearly and ultimately may improve assessment. Listening to the heart sounds from too far away from the sternal border decreases the ability to hear the sounds clearly.
d. Stand to patient's right to inspect and palpate the precordium with patient supine. Note any visible pulsations and more exaggerated lifts. Closely inspect at the area of the apex.	Reveals size and symmetry of the heart. The apical impulse may be visible at the midclavicular line in the fifth intercostal space. The apical impulse (PMI) may become visible only when the patient sits up, bringing the heart closer to the anterior wall. Obesity can easily obscure it. There should be no pulsations or vibrations.
e. Locate the PMI by palpating with fingertips along the fifth intercostal space in the midclavicular line. Note a light, brief pulsation in an area 1 to 2 cm (½ to 1 inch) in diameter at the apex. The PMI is less visible when there is more tissue covering the chest wall.	In the presence of serious heart disease, the PMI is located to the left of the midclavicular line related to the enlarged left ventricle. In chronic lung disease the PMI may be to the right of the midclavicular line as a result of an enlarged right ventricle.

Continued

STEPS	RATIONALE

SAFETY ALERT A stronger-than-expected impulse may be a heave or lift, which may indicate increased cardiac output or left ventricular hypertrophy.

STEPS	RATIONALE
f. If palpating PMI is difficult, turn patient onto left side.	Maneuver moves the heart closer to the chest wall.
g. Inspect the epigastric area and palpate the abdominal aorta. Note a localized strong beat.	Rules out reduced blood flow or diffuse pulse, which may indicate a number of abnormalities.
h. Auscultate heart sounds. Begin by having patient sit up and lean slightly forward; then have patient lie supine; and end the examination with patient in a left lateral recumbent position (see illustrations). In a female patient it may be necessary to lift the left breast to hear heart sounds more effectively.	Different positions help to clarify type of sounds heard. Sitting position is best to hear high-pitched murmurs (if present). Supine is common position to hear all sounds. Left lateral recumbent is best position to hear low-pitched sounds. Listening through breast tissue diminishes sound and impairs assessment.

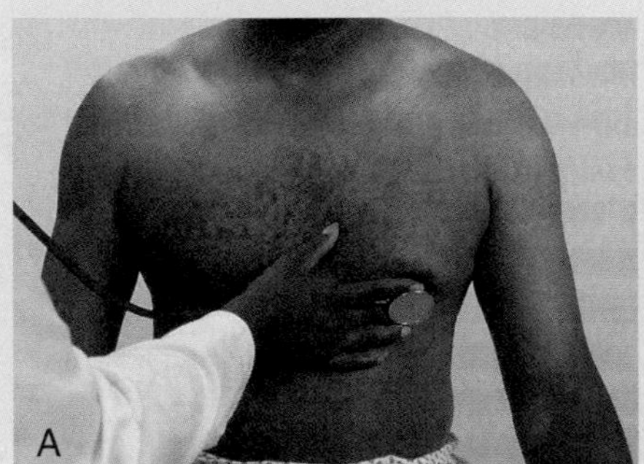
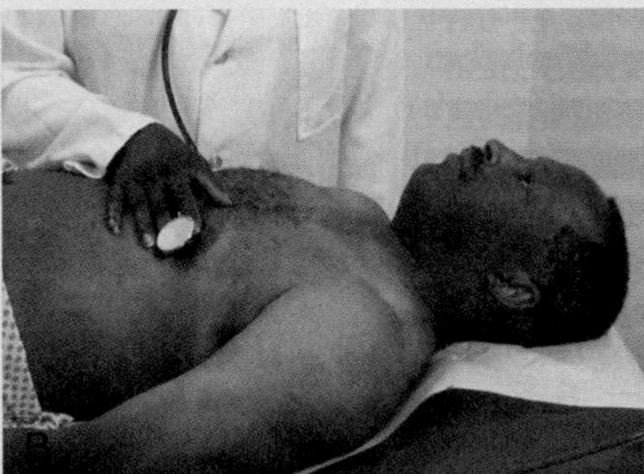
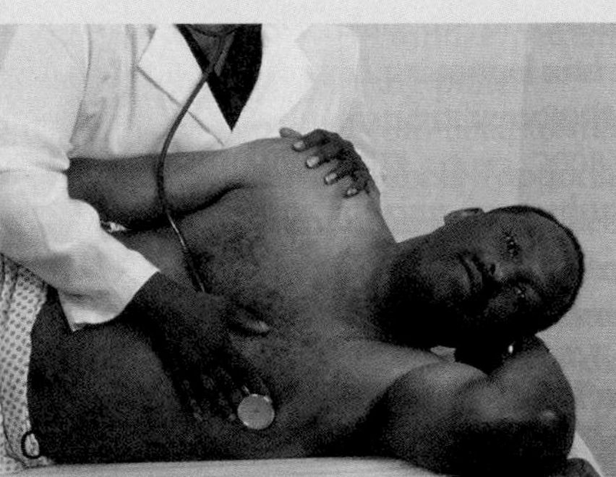

STEP 6h Patient positions for heart auscultation. **A,** Sitting. **B,** Supine. **C,** Left lateral. (From Seidel HM and others: *Mosby's guide to physical examination,* ed 6, St Louis, 2006, Mosby.)

STEPS	RATIONALE
(1) While auscultating sounds, ask patient not to speak but to breathe comfortably. Begin with the diaphragm of the stethoscope; then alternate with the bell. Use very light pressure for the bell. Inch the stethoscope along; avoid jumping from one area to another. Do not try to hear all heart sounds at once.	Auscultation requires the examiner to isolate each heart sound at all auscultation sites, especially in patients with soft heart sounds.
(2) Begin at the apex or PMI; move systematically to the aortic area, pulmonic area, Erb's point, tricuspid area, and mitral area (see illustration for Step 6h). (NOTE: Some examiners use reverse sequence.) S_1 is best heard at the apex and is simultaneous with the carotid pulse. NOTE: a helpful mnemonic for remembering heart sound locations: **A** **P**ig **E**ats **T**oo **M**uch.	At normal slow rates S_1 is high pitched and dull in quality and sounds like "lub." This sound precedes the systolic phase of heart contraction.
(3) Listen for S_2 at each site. This sound is best heard at the aortic area. Heart sounds vary by pitch, loudness, and duration, depending on the auscultatory site.	Normal sounds S_1 and S_2 are high pitched and best heard with a diaphragm. S_2 precedes the diastolic phase and sounds like "dub." For abnormal sounds, note physical location on chest wall and where in the cardiac cycle the sound is heard.

STEPS	RATIONALE
(4) After both sounds are heard clearly as "lub-dub," count each combination of S_1 and S_2 as one heartbeat. Count the number of beats for 1 minute.	Determines apical pulse rate.
(5) Assess heart rhythm by noting the time between S_1 and S_2 (systole) and the time between S_2 and the next S_1 (diastole). Listen to the full cycle at each auscultation area. Note regular intervals between each sequence of beats. There should be a distinct pause between S_1 and S_2.	Failure of heart to beat at regular intervals is a dysrhythmia, which interferes with the ability of the heart to pump effectively.
(6) When the heart rate is irregular, compare apical and radial pulses. Auscultate the apical pulse and then immediately palpate the radial pulse. A colleague can assess the radial pulse while you assess the apical pulse.	Determines if a pulse deficit (radial pulse is slower than apical) exists. Deficit indicates that ineffective contractions of the heart fail to send pulse waves to the periphery.
7. *Assess neck vessels.*	
a. To assess carotid arteries, have patient remain in sitting position.	Allows easier mobility of neck to expose artery for inspection and palpation.
b. Inspect neck on both sides for obvious arterial pulsations. Ask patient to turn head slightly away from artery being examined. Sometimes pulse wave can be seen.	Carotids are the only sites to assess quality of pulse wave. Experience is required to evaluate wave in relation to events of cardiac cycle.
c. Palpate each carotid artery separately with index and middle fingers around medial edge of sternocleidomastoid muscle. Ask patient to raise chin slightly, keeping the head straight (see illustration). Note rate and rhythm, strength, and elasticity of artery. Also note if the pulse changes as patient inspires and expires.	If both arteries were occluded simultaneously, patient could lose consciousness from reduced circulation to brain. Turning head improves access to artery. Change during respiratory cycle may indicate a sinus arrhythmia.

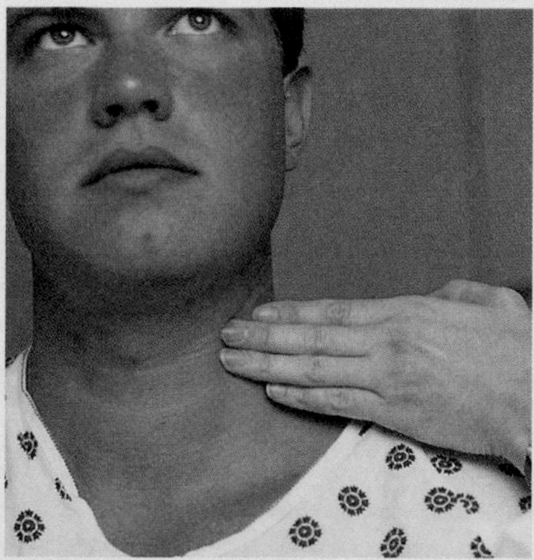

STEP 7c Palpation of internal carotid artery.

SAFETY ALERT Do not vigorously palpate or massage the artery. Stimulation of carotid sinus may cause a reflex drop in heart rate and blood pressure.

Continued

STEPS	RATIONALE
d. Place bell of stethoscope over each carotid artery, auscultating for blowing sound (bruit) (see illustration). Ask patient to hold breath for a few heartbeats so the respiratory sounds will not interfere with auscultation (Jarvis, 2008).	Narrowing of the lumen of the carotid artery by arteriosclerotic plaques causes disturbance in blood flow. Blood passing through narrowed section creates turbulence and emits blowing or swishing sound. Normally you do not hear a bruit.

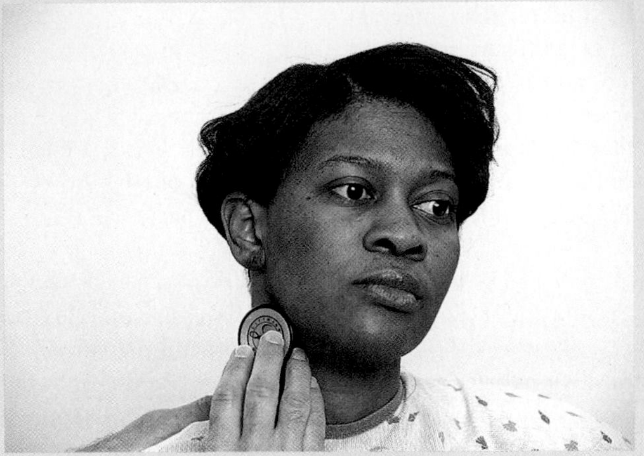

STEP 7d Auscultation for carotid artery bruit. (From Seidel HM and others: *Mosby's guide to physical examination,* ed 5, St Louis, 2003, Mosby.)

STEPS	RATIONALE
8. *Assess peripheral vascular area.*	
a. Inspect lower extremities for changes in color and condition of the skin (Table 7-6). Note skin and nail texture, hair distribution, venous patterns, edema, and scars or ulcers. Compare skin color lying and standing.	Changes may reflect impaired peripheral circulation.
b. Palpate edematous areas, noting mobility, consistency, and tenderness.	Assists in determining extent of edema.

TABLE 7-6 SIGNS OF VENOUS AND ARTERIAL INSUFFICIENCY

ASSESSMENT CRITERION	VENOUS	ARTERIAL
Pain	Aching, increases in evening and with dependent position	Burning, throbbing, cramping, increases with exercise
Paresthesia	None	Numbness, tingling, decreased sensation
Color	Normal or cyanotic	Pale; worsened by elevation of extremity; dusky red when extremity lowered
Capillary refill	Not applicable	>2 seconds
Edema	Often marked	Absent or mild
Pulse	Present	Decreased or absent
Skin changes	Brown pigmentation around ankles	Thin, shiny skin; decreased hair growth; thickened nails
Temperature	Normal to touch	Cool to touch

STEPS	RATIONALE
c. Assess for pitting edema by pressing area firmly for 5 seconds and then releasing. Depth of indentation determines severity (see illustration). Use a tape measure to measure the circumference of the extremity.	Unilateral edema of affected leg is the most common physical finding of deep vein thrombosis (DVT), although many patients with DVT present with no obvious symptoms. Measuring circumference establishes a baseline for comparison.

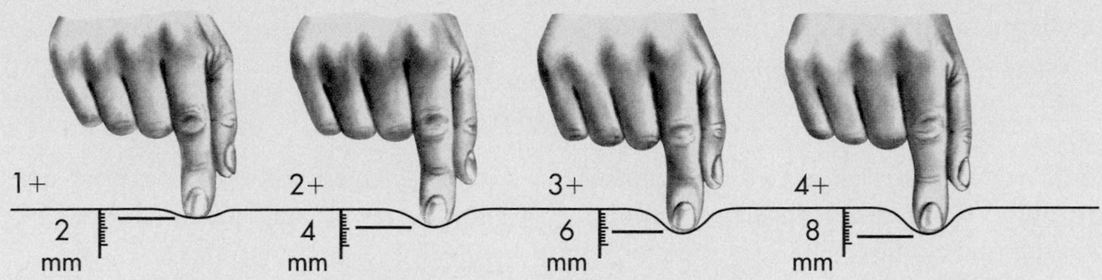

STEP 8c Assessing for pitting edema. (From Seidel HM and others: *Mosby's guide to physical examination,* ed 6, St Louis, 2006, Mosby.)

STEPS	RATIONALE
d. Check capillary refill by grasping patient's fingernail or toenail and noting color of nail bed. Next apply gentle, firm pressure to the nail bed. Release quickly, watching for color change. Circulation is restored and normally returns to pink color in less than 2 seconds.	Capillary refill is measured in seconds; less than 2 seconds is brisk, whereas greater than 4 seconds is sluggish. Cold environmental temperature with vasoconstriction and vascular disease can delay refill. Local pressure from a cast or bandage may also deter refill.
e. Ask if patient experiences pain or tenderness and then gently palpate for heat, firmness, or localized swelling of the calf muscle, which are signs of phlebitis or DVT.	Patients who have been immobilized for several days and those who have bone or joint disease, surgical correction of joint or bone, heart failure, varicose veins, or pain are at risk for impaired tissue perfusion (Farley, 2009).

SAFETY ALERT Homans' sign (pain in calf upon dorsiflexion of foot) is no longer a reliable indicator for the presence or absence of DVT and should not be considered a reliable parameter. If the calf is swollen, red, or tender, notify patient's health care provider for further assessment and evaluation and do not massage the calf muscle.

STEPS	RATIONALE
f. Starting at the most distal part of each extremity, palpate each peripheral artery for equality, comparing side to side; elasticity of vessel wall (depress and release artery, noting ease with which it springs back to shape); and strength of pulse (force of blood against arterial wall) using the following rating scale (Seidel and others, 2011): 0 Absent, no pulse palpable 1+ Diminished, pulse barely palpable, weak and thready, and easy to obliterate 2+ Normal pulse, easy to palpate 3+ Full, easy to palpate, increased 4+ Strong, bounding against fingertips, and cannot be obliterated	Comparison of both arteries allows you to determine any localized obstruction or disturbance in blood flow. Pulses should be symmetrical side to side. If asymmetry is noted, look for other factors related to impaired circulation.

Continued

STEPS	RATIONALE
g. Palpate radial pulse by lightly placing tips of first and second fingers in groove formed along radial side of forearm, lateral to flexor tendon of wrist (see illustration).	Pulse is relatively superficial and should not require deep palpation.
h. Palpate ulnar pulse by placing fingertips along ulnar side of forearm (see illustration).	Palpated when arterial insufficiency to hand is expected or when nurse assesses for radial occlusion, which might affect circulation to hand.
i. Palpate brachial pulse by locating groove between biceps and triceps muscles above elbow at antecubital fossa (see illustration). Place tips of first two fingers in muscle groove.	Artery runs along medial side of extended arm, requiring moderate palpation. If difficult to palpate, hyperextend arm to bring pulse site closer to the surface.
j. Have patient lie supine with feet relaxed and palpate dorsalis pedis pulse. Gently place fingertips between great and first toe; slowly move fingers along groove between extensor tendons of great and first toe until pulse is palpable (see illustration).	Artery lies superficially and does not require deep palpation. Pulse may be congenitally absent.
k. If pulses are difficult to palpate or not palpable, use a Doppler instrument over the pulse site.	Doppler amplifies sounds, allowing you to hear low-velocity blood flow through peripheral arteries.
(1) Apply conducting gel to patient's skin over the pulse site or onto transducer tip of probe.	
(2) Turn Doppler on. Gently apply ultrasound probe to the skin, changing Doppler angle until pulsation is audible. Adjust volume as needed. Wipe off gel from patient and Doppler.	

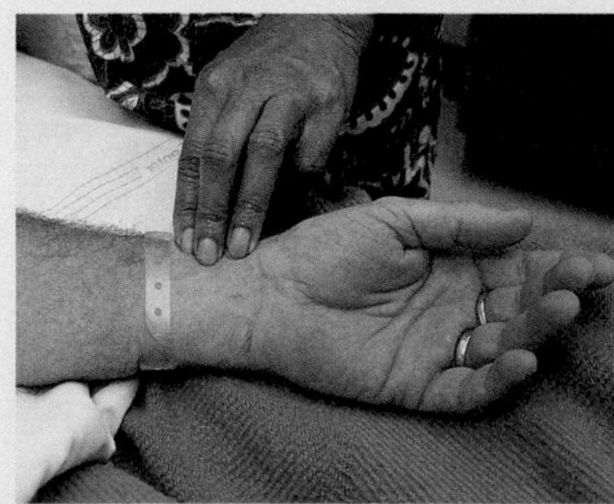

STEP 8g Palpation of radial pulse.

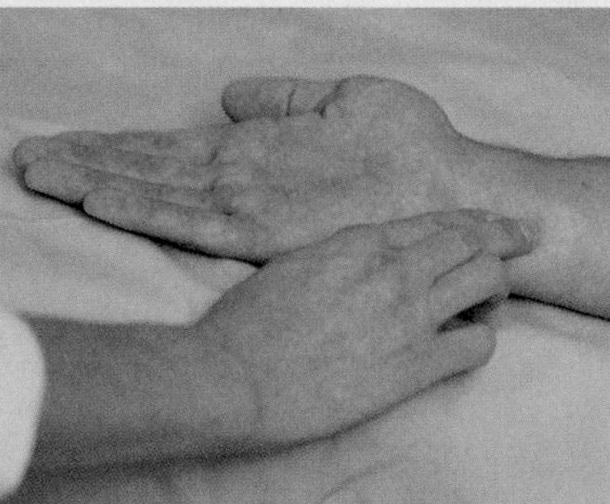

STEP 8h Palpation of ulnar pulse.

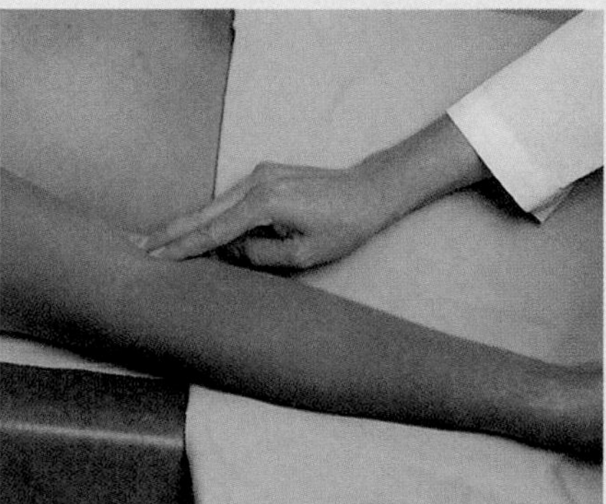

STEP 8i Palpation of brachial pulse.

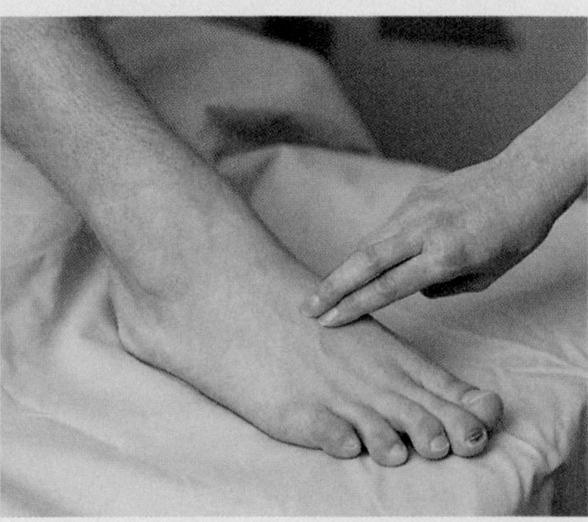

STEP 8j Palpation of pedal pulse.

STEPS	RATIONALE
l. Palpate posterior tibial pulse by having patient relax and slightly extend feet. Place fingertips behind and below medial malleolus (ankle bone) (see illustration).	Artery is easily palpable with foot relaxed.
m. Palpate popliteal pulse by having patient slightly flex knee with foot resting on table or bed. Instruct patient to keep leg muscles relaxed. Palpate deeply into popliteal fossa with fingers of both hands placed just lateral to midline. Patient may also lie prone to achieve exposure of artery (see illustration).	Flexion of knee and muscle relaxation improve accessibility of artery. Popliteal pulse is one of the more difficult pulses to palpate.
n. With patient supine, palpate femoral pulse by placing first two fingers over inguinal area below inguinal ligament, midway between pubic symphysis and anterosuperior iliac spine (see illustration).	Supine position prevents flexion in groin area, which interferes with artery access.
9. See Completion Protocol (inside front cover).	

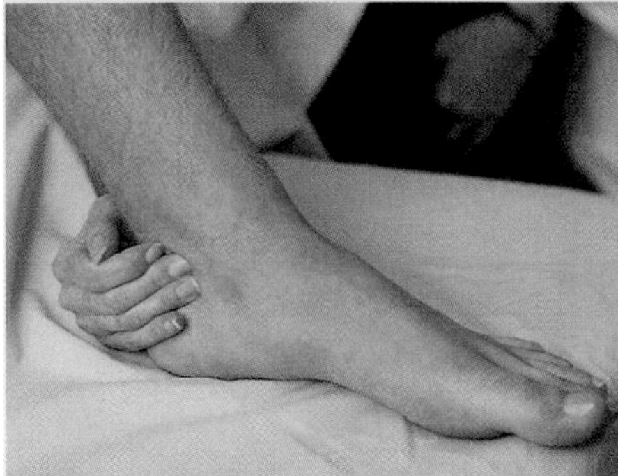

STEP 8l Palpation of posterior tibial pulse.

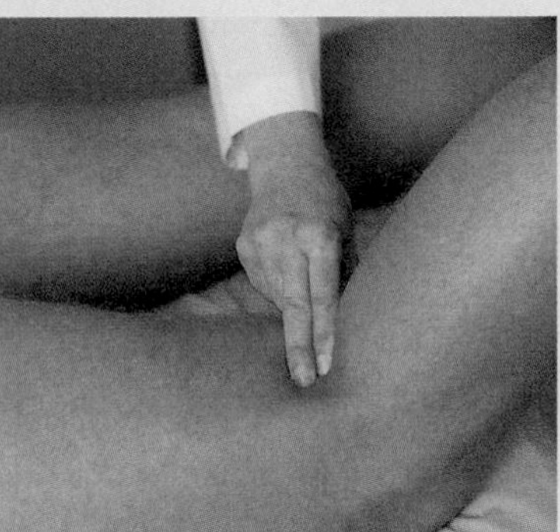

STEP 8m Palpation of popliteal pulse with patient prone.

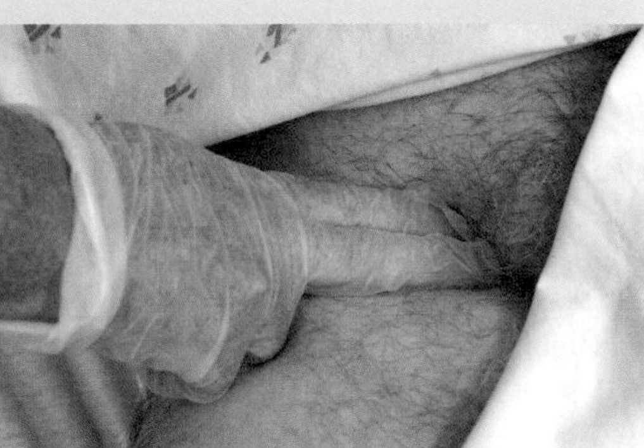

STEP 8n Palpation of femoral pulse.

EVALUATION

1. Compare findings with normal assessment characteristics of heart and vascular system.
2. If heart sounds are not audible or pulses are not palpable, ask another nurse to confirm assessment.
3. Ask patient to describe behaviors that increase risk for heart and vascular disease.

Unexpected Outcomes and Related Interventions

1. Abnormal findings that differ from previous assessments require you to notify health care provider. These include:
   - PMI is found left of the midclavicular line, suggesting cardiomegaly.
   - Extra heart sounds or a murmur is auscultated.

   a. Notify health care provider.
   b. Be prepared to assist with an electrocardiogram (ECG) and obtain vital signs.
2. Heart rate is irregular and/or the rate is less than 60 beats per minute or more than 100 beats per minute.
   a. Check blood pressure. If low, dysrhythmia is contributing to inadequate cardiac output.
   b. Observe for sensations or reports of dizziness or feeling "faint."
   c. Notify health care provider.
   d. Prepare to order ECG.
3. Pulse deficit is noted. There is risk for inadequate cardiac output.
   a. Be prepared to assist with an ECG and obtain vital signs.
   b. Notify health care provider.
4. Previously palpable pedal pulses are diminished or absent.
   a. Notify health care provider.
   b. Elevate extremity.
5. Patient's lower extremities have pale, cool, thin, and shiny skin, with reduced hair growth and thickened nails, indicating chronic arterial insufficiency.
   a. Instruct patient in proper foot care.
   b. Refer to podiatrist for nail trimming.

Recording and Reporting

- Document quality (clear or muffled), intensity (weak or pounding), rate, and rhythm (regular, regularly irregular, or irregularly irregular) of heart sounds and peripheral pulses on nurses' notes or flow sheet.

- Document activity level and subjective data related to fatigue, shortness of breath, and chest pain.
- Document preferred position for rest, medications and/or treatments used, and patient's response.
- Report immediately to health care provider any irregularities in heart function and indications of impaired arterial blood flow.
- Report to charge nurse or health care provider any changes in peripheral circulation, which may indicate circulatory compromise, which can result in permanent nerve damage or tissue death if untreated.

Sample Documentation

0730 Apical pulse rate 104 and irregular. Pulse deficit 6/min. BP 110/70. Denies chest pain or other discomfort. Patient states, "I feel weak, but the pain I had last evening has not come back." Notified health care provider of pulse deficit.

Special Considerations

Pediatric

- Capillary refill in infants is usually less than 1 second.
- It is not uncommon for children to have third heart sounds (S3). Sinus arrhythmia occurs normally in many infants (Hockenberry and Wilson, 2007).
- Children have louder, higher-pitched heart sounds because of their thin chest walls.
- Children cannot increase stroke volume, only heart rate, causing a lack of oxygen to tissues (Ball and Bindler, 2010).

Geriatric

- PMI may be difficult to find in an older adult because AP diameter of the chest deepens.
- Accidental massage of the carotid sinus during palpation of the carotid artery can be a particular problem for older adults, causing a sudden drop in heart rate from vagal nerve stimulation.

SKILL 7.5 ASSESSING THE ABDOMEN

Abdominal assessment is complex because of the multiple organs located within and near the abdominal cavity. This area of the body is associated with many health complaints; and many people are embarrassed by bowel or bladder dysfunction, reproductive problems, or urinary elimination problems. Abdominal pain is one of the most common symptoms patients report when seeking medical care. It can be caused by alterations in organs such as the stomach, pancreas, gallbladder, or intestines; or it may be the result of spinal or muscular injury. An accurate assessment requires matching the patient's history with a careful assessment of the location of physical symptoms (Table 7-7).

To perform an effective abdominal assessment you need to know the location and function of the underlying structures involved, including the lower pelvis, kidneys, rectum, genitalia, liver, gallbladder, stomach, spleen, pancreas, intestines, and reproductive organs (Fig. 7-4). An abdominal assessment is routine after abdominal surgery and for any patient who has undergone invasive diagnostic tests of the GI tract (see Chapter 9). The order of an abdominal assessment differs from that of other assessments. You begin with inspection and follow with auscultation. It is important to auscultate before palpation because assessment maneuvers may alter the frequency and character of bowel sounds.

ASSESSMENT

1. If patient has abdominal or low back pain, assess the character of pain in detail (location, onset, frequency, precipitating factors, aggravating factors, type of pain, severity, course). *Rationale: Knowing pattern of characteristics of pain helps determine its source.*
2. Carefully observe patient's movement and position such as lying still with knees drawn up, moving restlessly to find a comfortable position, lying on one side, or sitting with knees drawn up to chest. *Rationale: Positions assumed by patient may reveal nature and source of pain (e.g., peritonitis, renal stone, pancreatitis). Patients with appendicitis often lie on side or back with knees flexed to reduce pain (Monahan and others, 2007).*
3. Assess patient's normal bowel habits: frequency and character of stools; recent changes in character of stools; measures used to promote elimination such as laxatives, enemas, dietary intake; and eating and drinking habits. *Rationale: These data, compared with information from physical assessment, may help to identify cause and nature of elimination problems.*
4. Determine if patient has had abdominal surgery, trauma, or diagnostic tests of the GI tract. *Rationale: Surgery or trauma to abdomen may result in altered position of underlying organs. Diagnostic tests may change character of stool.*
5. Assess if patient has had recent weight changes or intolerance to diet (nausea, vomiting, or cramping, especially in past 24 hours). *Rationale: Changes may indicate alterations in upper GI tract (e.g., stomach, gallbladder) or lower colon.*
6. Assess for difficulty in swallowing, belching, flatulence, bloody emesis (hematemesis), black or tarry stools (melena), heartburn, diarrhea, or constipation. *Rationale: Indicates GI alterations.*

TABLE 7-7 COMMON CAUSES OF ABDOMINAL PAIN

CONDITION	PHYSICAL ALTERATION	PHYSICAL SIGNS AND SYMPTOMS
Appendicitis	Obstruction of the appendix associated with inflammation, perforation, and peritonitis; patient often lies on back or side with knees flexed to decrease pain	Sharp pain directly over the irritated peritoneum 2-12 hours after onset. Often pain localizes in right lower quadrant between the anterior iliac crest and the umbilicus. Associated with rebound tenderness. Accompanied by anorexia, nausea, and vomiting.
Cholecystitis	Obstruction of the cystic duct causing inflammation or distention of the gallbladder	*Murphy's sign*: Apply gentle pressure below right subcostal arch and below liver margin. Sharp pain and increased respiratory rate occur when patient takes a deep breath (Jarvis, 2008).
Constipation	Disruption in normal bowel pattern, which may occur with opioid use or inadequate fiber and fluid intake	Generalized discomfort accompanied by distention and palpation of a hard mass in left lower quadrant. Nausea and vomiting may begin after several days.
Crohn's disease	Chronic inflammatory lesion of the ileum	Steady colicky pain in right lower quadrant, with cramping, tenderness, flatulence, nausea, fever, and diarrhea. Often associated with bloody stools, weight loss, weakness, and fatigue. A tender mass of thickened intestine may be palpated in right lower quadrant.
Gastroenteritis	Inflammation of the stomach and intestinal tract	Generalized abdominal discomfort accompanied by anorexia, nausea, vomiting, diarrhea, and abdominal cramping.
Pancreatitis	Inflammation of the pancreas associated with alcoholism and gallbladder disease	Steady severe epigastric pain close to the umbilicus radiates to the back. Associated with abdominal rigidity and vomiting. Pain is unrelieved by vomiting and worsens by lying supine.
Paralytic ileus	Obstruction of the small bowel that occurs after abdominal surgery or use of anticholinergic medications	Generalized severe abdominal distention, nausea, and vomiting. Decreased or absent bowel sounds.
Peptic ulcers (gastric and duodenal)	Damage of gastrointestinal (GI) mucosa at any area of the GI tract; may be caused by bacterial infection *(Helicobacter pylori)* or nonsteroidal antiinflammatory drugs; thought to be unrelated to stress; aggravated by smoking and excessive alcohol use	*Gastric ulcer:* Dull epigastric pain, localized midline. Early satiety; not usually relieved by food or antacids. *Duodenal ulcer:* Pain is episodic, lasting 30 minutes to 2 hours. Pain is located midline epigastric region; described as aching, burning, or gnawing. Typically occurs 1 to 3 hours after meals and at night (12 midnight to 3 AM). Often relieved by food/antacid. *Both (dyspepsia syndrome):* Complaints of fullness, epigastric discomfort, vague nausea, abdominal distention, and bloating; anorexia; weight loss (Monahan and others, 2007).

7. Determine if patient takes antiinflammatory medications (e.g., aspirin, steroids, nonsteroidal antiinflammatory drugs), or antibiotics. *Rationale: These medications may cause GI upset or bleeding.*
8. Review patient's history for health care occupation, hemodialysis, intravenous drug use, household or sexual contact with hepatitis B virus (HBV) carrier, sexually active heterosexual person (more than one sex partner in previous 6 months), sexually active homosexual or bisexual man, or international traveler in area of high HBV prevalence. *Rationale: These are risk factors for HBV exposure. Abdominal findings for hepatitis include jaundice, hepatomegaly, anorexia, abdominal discomfort, tea-colored urine, and clay-colored stool (Seidel and others, 2011).*

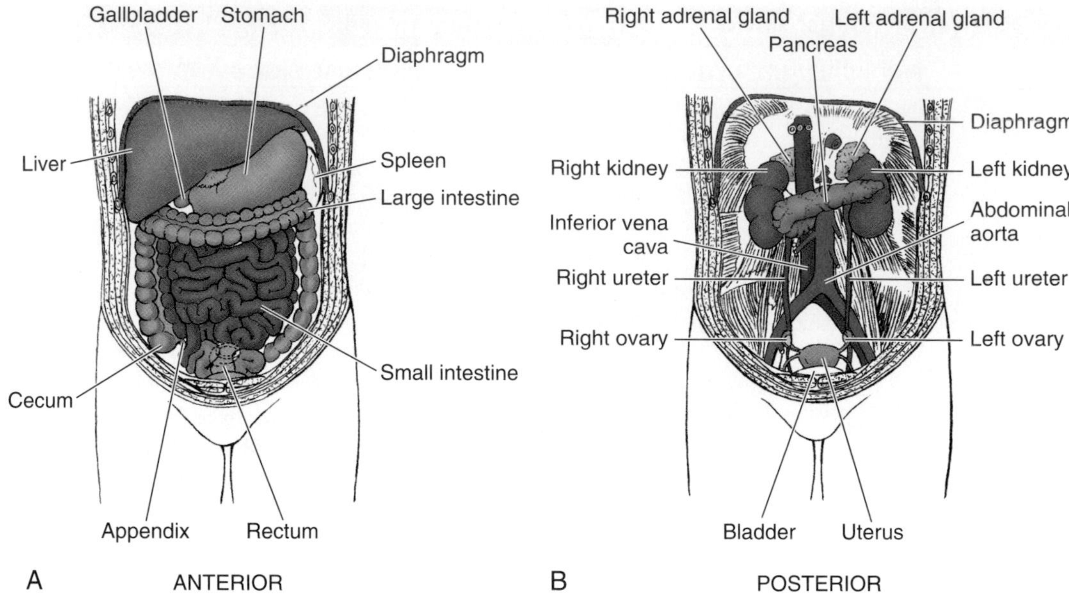

FIG 7-4 Location of organs in the abdomen. **A,** Anterior. **B,** Posterior. (Modified from *Mosby's expert 10 minute physical examinations*, ed 2, St Louis, 2005, Mosby.)

PLANNING

Expected Outcomes focus on identifying alterations in the abdomen.

1. Abdomen is soft and symmetrical with smooth and even contour. No mass, distention, or tenderness is palpable. No forceful visible pulsations are noted.
2. Bowel sounds are active and audible in all four quadrants.
3. Patient denies discomfort or worsening of existing discomfort after examination.
4. Patient is able to list warning signs of colon cancer.

Delegation and Collaboration

The skill of abdominal assessment cannot be delegated to nursing assistive personnel (NAP). Instruct the NAP to:

- Report the development of abdominal pain and changes in the patient's bowel habits or dietary intake to the nurse.

Equipment

- Stethoscope
- Tape measure
- Examination light
- Marking pen
- Drapes

IMPLEMENTATION *for* ASSESSING THE ABDOMEN

STEPS	RATIONALE
1. **See Standard Protocol (inside front cover).**	
2. Prepare patient.	
a. Ask if patient needs to empty bladder or defecate.	Palpation of full bladder can cause discomfort and feeling of urgency and make it difficult for patient to relax.
b. Keep upper chest and legs draped.	Exposes only areas to be examined and maintains patient comfort.
c. Be sure that room is warm.	Provides for patient comfort. Reduces risk of patient tensing muscles.
d. Have patient lie supine or in a dorsal recumbent position with arms down at sides and knees slightly bent. A small pillow may be placed under patient's knees.	Placing the arms under the head or keeping the knees fully extended can cause the abdominal muscles to tighten. Tightening of muscles prevents adequate palpation.
e. Expose area from just above the xiphoid process down to the symphysis pubis.	Exposes areas that you will examine during abdominal assessment.
f. Maintain conversation during assessment except during auscultation. Explain steps calmly and slowly.	When patient is relaxed, it improves accuracy of findings.

STEPS	RATIONALE
g. Ask patient to point to tender areas.	Assess painful areas last. Manipulation of body part can increase patient's pain and anxiety and make remainder of assessment difficult to complete.
3. Identify landmarks that divide abdominal region into quadrants. Boundary begins at tip of xiphoid process to symphysis pubis with line crossing and intersecting the umbilicus, dividing abdomen into four equal sections (Fig. 7-5).	Location of findings by common reference point helps successive examiners to confirm findings and locate abnormalities.
4. Inspect skin of surface of abdomen for color, scars, venous patterns, rashes, lesions, silvery white striae (stretch marks), and artificial openings (stomas). Observe lesions for characteristics described in Skill 7.1.	Scars reveal evidence that patient has past trauma or surgery. Striae indicate stretching of tissue from growth, obesity, pregnancy, ascites, or edema. Venous patterns may reflect liver disease (portal hypertension). Artificial openings indicate bowel or urinary diversion.
5. If you note bruising, ask if patient self-administers injections (e.g., heparin, insulin).	Frequent injections can cause bruising and hardening of underlying tissues.

SAFETY ALERT Bruising may also indicate physical abuse, accidental injury, or bleeding disorders.

STEPS	RATIONALE
6. Inspect contour, symmetry, and surface motion of abdomen. Note any masses, bulging, or distention. (Flat abdomen forms a horizontal plane from xiphoid process to symphysis pubis. Round abdomen protrudes in convex sphere from horizontal plane. Concave abdomen sinks into muscular wall. All are normal.)	Changes in symmetry or contour may reveal underlying masses, fluid collection, or gaseous distention. An everted (pouch extends outward) umbilicus indicates distention. A hernia can also cause the umbilicus to protrude upward.

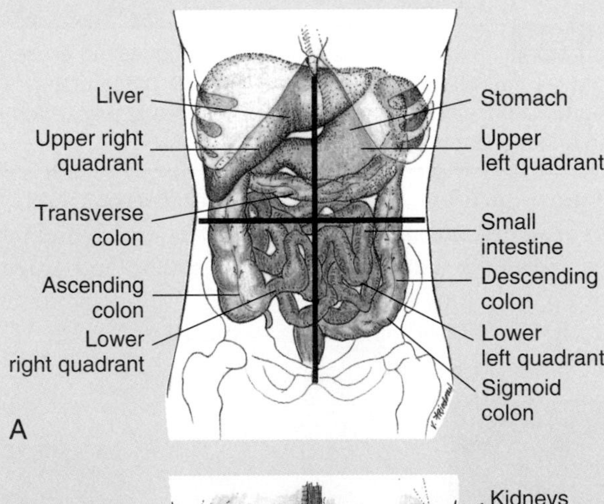

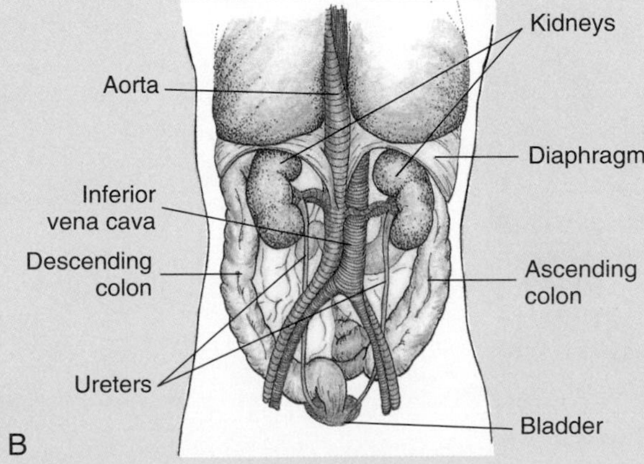

FIG 7-5 A, Anterior view of abdomen divided by quadrants. **B,** Posterior view of abdominal sections.

Continued

STEPS	RATIONALE
7. If abdomen appears distended, note if distention is generalized. Look at flanks on each side.	Distention may be caused by the nine *F's* (*f*at, *f*latus, *f*eces, *f*luids, *f*ibroid, *f*ull bladder, *f*alse pregnancy, *f*atal tumor, and *f*etus) (Seidel and others, 2006). If gas causes distention, flanks do not bulge. If fluid causes distention, flanks bulge. A tumor may cause unilateral bulging or distention. Pregnancy causes symmetrical bulge in lower abdomen.
8. If you suspect distention, measure size of abdominal girth by placing tape measure around abdomen at level of umbilicus. Use marking pen to indicate where tape measure was applied.	Consecutive measurements show any increase or decrease in abdominal distention. Make all subsequent measurements at same level of umbilicus to provide objective means to evaluate changes. Use a water-based pen to make a mark on abdomen for subsequent measurements.
9. If patient has an NG or NI tube connected to suction, turn off momentarily.	Sound of suction obscures bowel sounds.
10. To auscultate bowel sounds, place the diaphragm of the stethoscope lightly over each of the four abdominal quadrants (see illustration). Ask patient not to talk. Listen until you hear repeated gurgling or bubbling sounds in each quadrant (minimum of once in 5 to 20 seconds). Describe sounds as normal, hyperactive, hypoactive, or absent. Listen 5 minutes over each quadrant before deciding that bowel sounds are absent.	Normal bowel sounds occur irregularly every 5 to 15 seconds. Absence of sounds indicates cessation of gastric motility. Hyperactive bowel sounds not related to hunger or a recent meal may indicate diarrhea or early intestinal obstruction. Hypoactive or absent bowel sounds may indicate paralytic ileus or peritonitis. It is common for bowel sounds to be hypoactive after surgery for 24 hours or more, especially after abdominal surgery.
11. Place the bell of the stethoscope over the epigastric region of the abdomen and each quadrant. Auscultate for vascular (whooshing) sounds.	Determines presence of turbulent blood flow (bruit) through thoracic or abdominal aorta, which can indicate an aneurysm.

SAFETY ALERT If aortic bruit is auscultated, suggesting presence of an aneurysm, stop assessment and notify health care provider immediately. Percussion or palpation over abdominal bruit can cause rupture of an already weakened vessel wall in the presence of an abdominal aneurysm.

STEPS	RATIONALE
12. Lightly palpate over each abdominal quadrant, laying the palm of the hand with fingers extended and approximated lightly on the abdomen. Keep the palm and forearm horizontal. The pads of the fingertips depress the skin no more than 1 cm (½ inch) in a gentle dipping motion (see illustration). Palpate painful areas last.	Detects areas of muscle spasm, localized tenderness, degree of tenderness, and presence and character of underlying masses or fluid. Palpation of sensitive area causes guarding (voluntary tightening of underlying abdominal muscles).

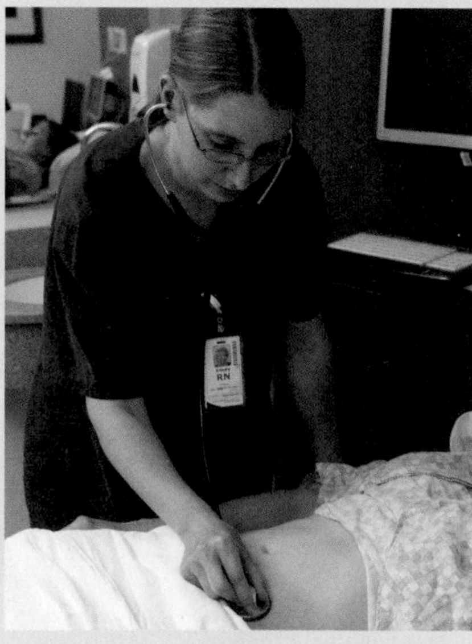

STEP 10 Auscultating bowel sounds.

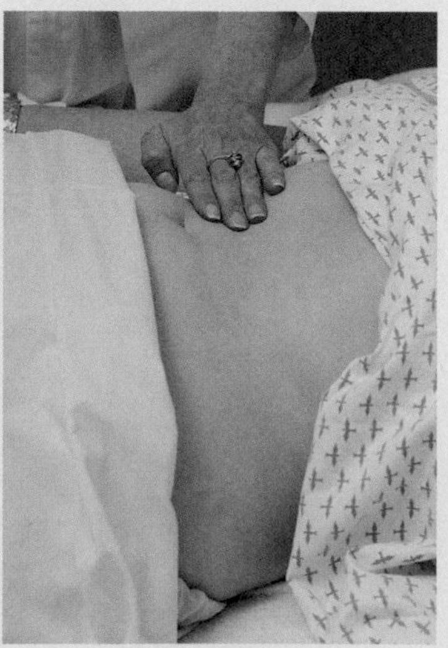

STEP 12 Light palpation of the abdomen.

STEPS	RATIONALE
a. Note muscular resistance, distention, tenderness, and superficial masses or organs while observing patient's face for signs of discomfort.	Patient's verbal and nonverbal cues may indicate discomfort from tenderness. Firm abdomen may indicate active obstruction with fluid or gas building up.
b. Note if abdomen is firm or soft to touch.	Soft abdomen is normal or reveals that obstruction is resolving.
13. Just below umbilicus and above symphysis pubis, palpate for a smooth, rounded mass. While applying light pressure, ask if patient has sensation of need to void.	Detects presence of dome of distended bladder.

SAFETY ALERT Routinely check for distended bladder if patient has been unable to void, patient has been incontinent, or an indwelling Foley catheter is not draining well or patient recently had a Foley catheter removed.

STEPS	RATIONALE
14. If masses are palpated, note size, location, shape, consistency, tenderness, mobility, and texture.	Descriptive characteristics help to reveal type of mass.
15. When tenderness is present, test for rebound tenderness by pressing slowly and deeply into the involved area and then letting go quickly. Note if pain is aggravated.	Results are positive if pain increases. May indicate peritoneal irritation such as appendicitis (Jarvis, 2008).
16. Percussion is an advanced skill used in abdominal assessment and is usually completed before palpation.	Reveals presence of air or fluid in stomach and intestines.
17. See Completion Protocol (inside front cover).	

EVALUATION

1. Observe throughout the assessment for evidence of discomfort.
2. Compare assessment findings with previous assessment to identify changes.

Unexpected Outcomes and Related Interventions

1. Abdomen is asymmetrical, with palpable mass and hypoactive bowel sounds.
   a. Report to health care provider because findings may indicate enlarged liver, spleen, or tumor.
2. Abdomen protrudes symmetrically, with skin taut; patient complains of tightness, and/or bowel sounds are absent. GI motility has ceased. Patient is vomiting.
   a. Keep patient on "nothing by mouth" (NPO) status and encourage ambulation.
   b. Notify health care provider; findings may indicate an obstruction.
   c. Gastric decompression with insertion of NG tube may become necessary.
3. Hyperactive bowel sounds are evident with GI motility. Commonly they result from anxiety, diarrhea, overuse of laxatives, inflammation of the bowel, or reaction of the intestines to certain foods.
   a. Patient may need to be NPO.
   b. Contact health care provider if patient may need antidiarrheal medications.
4. Rebound abdominal tenderness is found.
   a. Avoid palpating area.
   b. Notify health care provider if this is a new finding.
   c. Keep patient on NPO status until health care provider can evaluate.
5. Bladder is palpable over symphysis pubis. Bladder is distended.
   a. Facilitate voiding by placing patient in sitting position or encouraging patient to bear down; run water within hearing distance or have patient place hand in basin of warm water.
   b. Use a bladder scan to determine extent of bladder fullness.
   c. If unable to void, urinary catheterization may be necessary.

Recording and Reporting

- Document quality of bowel sounds, presence of distention, abdominal circumference, and presence of tenderness on nurses' notes or flow sheet.
- Record patient's ability to void and defecate, including description of output.
- Record content of any patient education.
- Report serious abnormalities such as absent bowel sounds or presence of mass or acute pain to nurse in charge and health care provider.

Sample Documentation

0800 Abdomen is distended, no masses palpated. No passage of flatus since surgery, and bowel sounds are hypoactive over all four quadrants. Encouraged to sip on warm fluids and ambulate frequently. Denies nausea, vomiting, or pain at this time.

Special Considerations

Pediatric

- Most common palpable mass in child is feces, usually felt in right lower quadrant (Ball and Bindler, 2010; Hockenberry and Wilson, 2007).
- Have child stand erect and then lie supine during inspection of abdomen. Normal abdomen of infants and young children is cylindrical in erect position and flat in supine position. School-age children may have a rounded abdomen until 13 years of age when standing.
- Infants and children until 7 years of age are abdominal breathers.

Geriatric

- Older adults often lack abdominal tone; underlying organs are more easily palpable.
- A weakened intestinal musculature and decreased peristalsis affect the large intestine.
- Constipation, nausea, flatulence, and heartburn are common.
- Older adults may have increased fat deposits over the abdomen.

SKILL 7.6 ASSESSING THE GENITALIA AND RECTUM

You can perform an external genitalia examination during routine hygiene measures or when preparing to insert or care for a urinary catheter. An examination of female and male external genitalia is part of preventive health screenings. You examine adolescents and young adults because of the growing incidence of sexually transmitted infections (STIs). The average age of menarche among females has declined, and the average age that both males and females become sexually active is 19 (Hockenberry and Wilson, 2007). You can easily combine rectal and anal assessments with this examination because the patient assumes a lithotomy or dorsal recumbent position.

ASSESSMENT

1. Assessment of female patients:
   a. Determine if patient has signs and symptoms of vaginal discharge, painful or swollen perianal tissues, or genital lesions. *Rationale: These signs and symptoms indicate the presence of an STI or other pathological condition.*
   b. Determine if patient has symptoms or history of genitourinary problems, including burning on urination (dysuria), frequency, urgency, nocturia, hematuria, or incontinence. *Rationale: Urinary problems are associated with gynecological disorders, including STIs.*
   c. Ask if the patient has had signs of bleeding outside of normal menstrual cycle or after menopause or has had unusual vaginal discharge. *Rationale: These are warning signs of cervical or endometrial cancer or a vaginal infection.*
   d. Determine if patient has received human papillomavirus (HPV) vaccine. *Rationale: Routine HPV vaccination is recommended for girls ages 11 to 12. Girls as young as age 9 may receive HPV vaccination. There is no scientific evidence to recommend the vaccine for women ages 19 to 26. The HPV vaccination is not currently recommended for women over age 26 or for men (ACS, 2010a).*
   e. Determine if patient has history of HPV (condyloma acuminatum, herpes simplex, or cervical dysplasia); multiple sexual partners; smokes cigarettes; or has had multiple pregnancies. *Rationale: These are risk factors for cervical cancer (ACS, 2010b).*
   f. Determine if patient is over 40 years of age; is obese; has a history of ovarian dysfunction, breast or endometrial cancer, or endometriosis; has a family history of reproductive cancer; has a history of infertility, nulliparity, or use of estrogen (alone) hormone replacement therapy. *Rationale: These are risk factors for ovarian cancer (ACS, 2010a).*
   g. Determine patient's knowledge of risk factors and signs of cervical and other gynecologic cancers. *Rationale: Provides basis for patient education.*
2. Assessment of male patients:
   a. Review normal elimination pattern, including frequency of voiding; history of nocturia; character and volume of urine; daily fluid intake; symptoms of burning, urgency, and frequency; difficulty starting stream; and hematuria. *Rationale: Urinary problems are directly associated with genitourinary problems because of anatomical structures of the male reproductive and urinary systems.*
   b. Ask if patient has noted any penile pain or swelling, genital lesions, or urethral discharge. *Rationale: These are signs and symptoms of STIs.*
   c. Determine if patient has noted any heaviness, painless enlargement, or irregular lumps of testis. *Rationale: These signs and symptoms are early warning signs of testicular cancer.*
   d. Determine if patient reports any enlargement in inguinal area and assess if it is intermittent or constant, associated with straining or lifting, and painful. Assess whether coughing, lifting, or straining at stool causes pain. *Rationale: Signs and symptoms indicate potential inguinal hernia.*
   e. Ask if patient has experienced weak or interrupted urine flow, inability to urinate, difficulty in starting or stopping urine flow, polyuria, nocturia, dysuria, or hematuria. Determine if patient has continuing pain in lower back, pelvis, or upper thighs. *Rationale: These are warning signs of prostate cancer (ACS, 2010b). Symptoms also may indicate infection or prostate enlargement.*

f. Assess patient's knowledge of risk factors and signs of prostate and testicular cancer. *Rationale: provides basis for patient education.*

3. Assessment of all patients:
   a. Determine whether patient has experienced bleeding from rectum, black or tarry stools (melena), rectal pain, or change in bowel habits (constipation or diarrhea). *Rationale: These are warning signs of colorectal cancer (ACS, 2010a).*
   b. Determine whether patient is over 40 years of age or has a personal or family history of colorectal cancer, polyps, or chronic inflammatory bowel disease. *Rationale: These are risk factors for colorectal cancer (ACS, 2010a).*
   c. Determine if patient is obese, physically inactive, smokes cigarettes, or consumes alcohol. *Rationale: These are risk factors for colorectal cancer (ACS, 2010a).*
   d. Assess medication history for use of laxatives or cathartics. *Rationale: Repeated use causes diarrhea and eventual loss of intestinal muscle tone.*
   e. Assess for use of codeine or iron preparations. *Rationale: Codeine causes constipation. Iron turns stool black and tarry.*
   f. Assess patient's knowledge of risks and signs of colorectal cancer. *Rationale: Provides basis for patient education.*

PLANNING

Expected Outcomes focus on accurate genitalia and rectal assessment data.

1. Patient demonstrates alert, cooperative behaviors without evidence of physical or emotional distress during assessment.
2. Patient is able to list warning signs of colorectal cancer; female patient: cervical, endometrial, and ovarian cancer; male patient: testicular and prostate cancer.

Delegation and Collaboration

The skill of assessing the genitalia and rectum cannot be delegated to nursing assistive personnel (NAP). Instruct the NAP to:

- Report changes in patient's urinary or bowel pattern and presence of drainage in perineal area.

Equipment

- Stethoscope
- Examination light
- Clean gloves (use nonlatex if necessary)

IMPLEMENTATION *for* ASSESSING THE GENITALIA AND RECTUM

STEPS	RATIONALE
1. **See Standard Protocol (inside front cover).**	
2. Prepare patient for assessment:	
a. Ask if patient needs to empty bladder or defecate.	Palpation of full bladder causes discomfort and feeling of urgency and makes it difficult for patient to relax.
b. Keep upper chest and legs draped and keep room warm.	Maintains patient's comfort.
c. Position patient: Female should lie in a dorsal recumbent position with arms down at sides and knees slightly bent. Place a small pillow under patient's knees. Male should lie supine with chest, abdomen, and lower legs draped *or* have patient stand during examination.	Placing the arms under the head or keeping knees fully extended causes tightening of abdominal muscles.
3. *Female genitalia examination.*	
a. Expose only perineal area	
b. Inspect surface characteristics of perineum and then retract labia majora; observe for inflammation, edema, lesions, or lacerations. Note if there is any vaginal discharge. Presence of discharge may indicate need for a culture.	Skin of perineum is smooth, clean, and slightly darker than other skin. Mucous membranes are dark pink and moist. Labia majora are symmetrical; may be dry or moist. Normally there is no vaginal discharge.
4. *Male genitalia examination*	
a. Observe genitalia for rashes, excoriations, or lesions.	Normally the skin is clear and without lesions.

Continued

STEPS	RATIONALE
b. Inspect and gently palpate penile surfaces.	
(1) Inspect the corona, prepuce (foreskin), glans, urethral meatus, and shaft. Retract the foreskin in uncircumcised males. Observe for discharge, lesions, edema, and inflammation. Return foreskin to normal position.	Glans should be smooth and pink along all surfaces. Urethral meatus is slitlike and positioned at the tip of the glans. The foreskin should retract easily. The area between the foreskin and glans is a common site for venereal lesions.
c. Inspect and palpate testicular surfaces.	
(1) Inspect size, color, shape, and symmetry; also gently palpate for lesions and edema.	The left testicle normally is lower than the right. Scrotal skin is usually loose, surface is coarse, and skin color is more deeply pigmented than body skin.
d. Palpate the testes.	
(1) Note size, shape, and consistency of tissue.	Testes are normally ovoid and approximately 2 by 4 cm (0.8 to 1.6 inches) in size, feel smooth and rubbery, and are free from nodules. Most common symptom of testicular cancer is an irregular, nontender fixed mass.
(2) Ask if patient experiences tenderness with palpation.	Testes are normally sensitive but not tender.
5. Assess rectum.	
a. Female patient remains in dorsal recumbent position or assumes a side-lying (Sims') position.	This position allows for optimal visualization of the rectum.
b. Male patient stands and bends forward with hips flexed and upper body resting across examination table; examine nonambulatory patient in Sims' position.	
c. View the perianal and sacrococcygeal areas by gently retracting the buttocks using your nondominant hand.	Perianal skin is smooth, more pigmented, and coarser than skin covering the buttocks.
d. Inspect anal tissue for skin characteristics, lesions, external hemorrhoids (dilated veins that appear as reddened skin protrusions), ulcers, inflammation, rashes, and excoriation.	Anal tissues are moist and hairless; the voluntary sphincter holds the anus closed.
6. See Completion Protocol (inside front cover).	

EVALUATION

1. Observe throughout the assessment for evidence of physical or emotional distress, which may alter assessment data.
2. Compare assessment findings with previous assessment characteristics to identify changes.
3. Ask patient to list warning signs of colorectal cancer; female patient: cervical, endometrial, and ovarian cancer; male patient: testicular and prostate cancer.

Unexpected Outcomes and Related Interventions

1. Patient is unable to list warning signs of colorectal cancer; female patient: cervical, endometrial, and ovarian cancer; male patient: testicular and prostate cancer.
   a. Provide additional education.

Recording and Reporting

- Record results of assessment in nurses' notes or flow sheet.
- Record content of any patient teaching.
- Record any abnormalities such as presence of a mass, drainage, or pain to nurse in charge and health care provider.

Sample Documentation

0830 Patient reports "pain in groin when straining to move bowels." No swelling or inflammation noted in inguinal area on palpation. Patient able to lift and cough with no pain. Health care provider notified.

Special Considerations

Pediatric

- Examination of the genitalia may provoke anxiety in children. The best approach is to treat this examination the same as all other parts of the health assessment.
- In male infants, when examining the testes, avoid stimulating the cremasteric reflex, which causes the testes to pull higher into pelvic cavity.

Geriatric

- A weakened intestinal musculature and decreased peristalsis affect the large intestine.
- Promotion of adequate hydration is the key to preventing constipation (Ebersole and others, 2008).

Home Care

- General patient education should focus on the warning signs of colorectal cancer.
- Teach warning signs of STIs, the importance of self-examination for cancer, and the benefit of HPV vaccination in women (age appropriate).

SKILL 7.7 MUSCULOSKELETAL AND NEUROLOGICAL ASSESSMENT

You use the skills of inspection and palpation during the musculoskeletal and neurological assessment. During the general survey (see Skill 7.1) you inspect gait, posture, and body position. A more thorough assessment of major bone, joint, and muscle groups and sensory, motor, and cranial nerve (CN) function is indicated in the presence of abnormalities. The assessment can be performed as you examine other body systems. For example, while assessing head and neck structures, assess neck ROM and examine selected CNs. Integrate assessment into routine activities of care (e.g., while bathing or positioning the patient). Always assess a patient who reports pain, loss of sensation, or impairment of muscle function. Prolonged illness or immobility may result in muscle weakness and atrophy. Neurological assessment is often conducted simultaneously because muscles may be weakened as a result of nerve involvement.

ASSESSMENT

1. Review patient history for use of alcohol/caffeine; cigarette smoking; constant dieting; calcium intake less than 500 mg daily; thin and light body frame; females who have never been pregnant (nulliparous); menopause before age 45; postmenopausal status; family history of osteoporosis; white, Asian, American Indian, or northern European ancestry; sedentary lifestyle; long-term use of certain medications (e.g., corticosteroids, heparin, phenytoin [Dilantin]); and lack of exposure to sunlight. *Rationale: These factors increase the risk for osteoporosis.*
2. Determine if patient has been screened for osteoporosis. *Rationale: Women ages 64 and older or with one or more risk factors need routine screening for osteoporosis (Ebersole and others, 2008).*
3. Ask patient to describe history of alteration in bone, muscle, or joint function (e.g., recent fall, trauma, lifting heavy objects, bone or joint disease with sudden or gradual onset) and location of alteration. *Rationale: Assists in assessing nature of musculoskeletal problem. One in two women and one in four men ages 50 years and older have an osteoporotic-related fracture (Ebersole and others, 2008).*
4. Assess nature and extent of patient's musculoskeletal pain: location, duration, severity, predisposing and aggravating factors, relieving factors, and type of pain. If pain or cramping is reported in the lower extremities, ask if walking relieves or aggravates it. Assess the distance walked and characteristics of pain before, during, and after activity. *Rationale: Pain frequently accompanies alterations in bone, joints, or muscle. Pain has implications for comfort and ability to perform ADLs. Pain caused by certain vascular conditions tends to increase with activity.*
5. Assess for height and weight. Note if there is a decrease in height in a woman older than 50 by subtracting current height from recall of maximum adult height. *Rationale: Body mass index less than 22 is a risk factor. and a loss of height of more than 3 cm (1.2 inches) is one of the first clinical signs of osteoporosis (Ebersole and others, 2008).*
6. Determine if patient uses analgesics, antipsychotics, antidepressants, nervous system stimulants, or recreational drugs. *Rationale: These medications alter LOC or cause behavioral changes.*
7. Determine if patient has recent history of seizures/convulsions: clarify sequence of events (aura, loss of muscle tone, falling, motor activity, loss of consciousness); character of any symptoms; and relationship to time of day, fatigue, or emotional stress. *Rationale: Seizure activity often originates from central nervous system (CNS) alteration. Characteristics of seizure help determine its origin.*
8. Screen patient for headache, tremors, dizziness, numbness, or tingling of body part; visual changes; weakness; pain; or changes in speech. *Rationale: These symptoms commonly result from CNS dysfunction. Identifying patterns may assist in diagnosis.*
9. Discuss with spouse, family member, or friends any recent changes in patient's behavior (e.g., increased irritability, mood swings, memory loss, change in energy level). *Rationale: Behavioral changes may result from intracranial pathology.*

PLANNING

Expected Outcomes focus on identifying deficits in musculoskeletal and neurological function.

1. Patient demonstrates erect posture, strong grasp, and steady gait with arms swinging freely at side.
2. There is bilateral symmetry of extremities in length, circumference, alignment, position, and skin folds.
3. Full active ROM is present in all joints with good muscle tone and absence of contractures, spasticity, or muscular weakness.
4. Patient is alert and oriented to person, place, and time. Behavior and appearance are appropriate for condition/situation.
5. Patient demonstrates normal pupil reaction to light and accommodation (see Skill 7.2); external ocular muscles intact; facial sensation intact; symmetrical facial

expressions; soft palate and uvula midline and rise on phonation; gag reflex intact; speech clear without hoarseness; no difficulty swallowing.

6. Patient distinguishes between sharp and dull sensations and light touch on symmetrical areas of extremities.
7. Gait is coordinated and steady. Romberg test is negative.

Delegation and Collaboration

The skill of assessing musculoskeletal and neurological function cannot be delegated to nursing assistive personnel (NAP). Instruct the NAP to:

- Report patient problems with gait, ROM, and muscle strength.
- Take precautions during ROM exercises to avoid forcing a joint beyond patient's current ROM.
- Be informed of patients at risk for falls (unsteady gait, foot dragging, weakness of lower extremities).
- Assist patients with muscular weakness with transfer and ambulation.

Equipment

- Tape measure
- Cotton balls or cotton-tipped applicators
- Penlight
- Opposite tip of cotton swab or tongue blade broken in half
- Tongue blade
- Tuning fork
- Reflex hammer

IMPLEMENTATION *for* MUSCULOSKELETAL AND NEUROLOGICAL ASSESSMENT

STEPS	RATIONALE
1. See Standard Protocol (inside front cover).	
2. Prepare patient:	
a. Integrate musculoskeletal and neurological assessment during other portions of physical assessment or during care.	As in assessment of the skin, you can conduct an assessment as the patient moves in bed, rises from chair, walks, or goes through movements required during complete physical examination. Integration with care conserves patient's energy and allows observation of patient performing activities more naturally.
b. Plan time for short rest periods during assessment.	Movement of body parts and various maneuvers may fatigue patient. Always plan rest periods with older adults and very ill patients.
3. Assess musculoskeletal system.	
a. Observe ability to use arms and hands for grasping objects (e.g., utensils, pen).	Assesses coordination and muscle strength.
b. Assess muscle strength of upper extremities by applying gradual increase in pressure to muscle group.	Upper and lower extremity on patient's dominant side normally is stronger than that on nondominant side. Pain rather than weakness may cause reduced muscle strength; however, long-term pain can lead to muscle weakening.
c. To assess hand grasp strength, cross your hands and have patient grasp index and middle fingers of both of your hands and squeeze them simultaneously as hard as possible.	It is common for patient's dominant hand to be slightly stronger than nondominant hand. By crossing your hands, patient's right hand grasps your right hand and vice versa. This helps you recall which is patient's right/left hand.
d. Place hand on lower arm or leg and have patient move major joint (e.g., elbow, knee) against resistance (e.g., flex elbow). Have patient maintain resistance until told to stop. Compare symmetrical muscle groups. Note weakness and compare right with left.	Compares strength of symmetrical muscle groups. Rate muscle strength on scale of 0 to 5. Grade as follows: 0 No voluntary contraction 1 Slight contractility, no movement 2 Full ROM, passive 3 Full ROM, active 4 Full ROM against gravity, some resistance 5 Full ROM against gravity, full resistance
e. Observe body alignment for sitting, supine, prone, or standing positions. Muscles and joints should be exposed and free to move to allow for accurate measurement.	Each joint or muscle group may require a different position for measurement.

STEPS	RATIONALE
f. Inspect gait as patient walks. Have patient use their assistive device (cane, walker) if appropriate. Observe for foot dragging, shuffling or limping, balance, presence of obvious deformity in lower extremities, and position of trunk in relation to legs.	Gait is more natural if patient is unaware of your observation. Observations may indicate a neuromusculoskeletal disorder.
g. Perform the Get Up and Go Test: From a sitting position have patient stand without using arms for support; walk several paces, turn, and return to chair; and sit back in chair without using arms for support. Observe gait and ability to sit or stand.	The Get Up and Go Test is an assessment that should be conducted as part of a routine evaluation of older adults. The test detects people at risk for falling.
h. Stand behind patient and observe postural alignment (position of hips relative to shoulders) (see illustration). Look sideways at cervical, thoracic, and lumbar curves.	Abnormal curves of posture include lordosis (swayback, increased lumbar curvature), kyphosis (hunchback, exaggerated posterior curvature of thoracic spine), and scoliosis (lateral spinal curvature). Postural changes may indicate muscular, bone, or joint deformity; pain; or muscular fatigue. Head should be held erect.

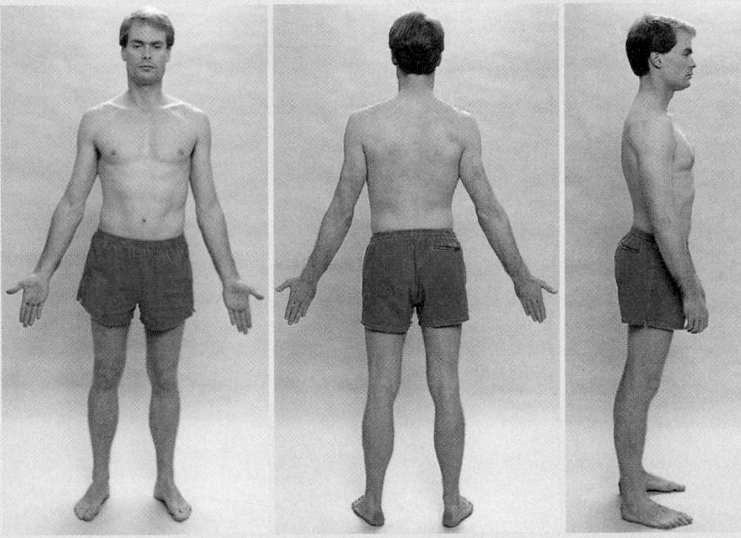

STEP 3h Inspection of overall body posture: *Left,* anterior view; *middle,* posterior view; *right,* right lateral view. (From Seidel HM and others: *Mosby's guide to physical examination,* ed 6, St Louis, 2006, Mosby.)

STEPS	RATIONALE
i. Make a general observation of the extremities. Look at overall size, gross deformity, bony enlargement, alignment, and symmetry.	General review helps to pinpoint areas requiring in-depth assessment.
j. Gently palpate bones, joints, and surrounding tissue in involved areas. Note any heat, tenderness, edema, or resistance to pressure.	Reveals changes resulting from trauma or chronic disease. Do not attempt to move joint when fracture is suspected or when joint apparently is "frozen" by lack of movement over a long period of time.
k. Ask patient to put major joint through its full ROM (Table 7-8). Observe equality of motion in same body parts:	Assessment of patient's normal ROM provides baseline for assessing later changes after surgery or inactivity. Patients with deformities, reduced mobility, joint fixation, or weakness often require passive ROM assessment.
(1) *Active motion:* (Patient needs no support or assistance and is able to move joint independently.) Instruct patient in moving each joint through its normal range. Sometimes it is necessary to demonstrate movements and ask patient to mimic your movements.	Identifies muscle strength and detects limited ROM.

Continued

STEPS	RATIONALE
(2) *Passive motion:* (Joint has full ROM, but patient does not have the strength to move it independently.) Have patient relax and move the same joints passively until the end of the range is felt. Support extremity at joint. Do not force the joint if there is pain or muscle spasm.	Determines ability to perform joint motion in the presence of muscle weakness. Forcing joint causes pain and injury.
l. Palpate joint for swelling, stiffness, tenderness, and heat; note any redness.	Indicates acute or chronic inflammation. ROM causes pain or injury.
m. Assess muscle tone in major muscle groups. Normal tone causes mild, even resistance to movement through entire ROM.	If muscle has increased tone (hypertonicity), any sudden movement of joint is met with considerable resistance. Hypotonic muscle moves without resistance. Muscle feels flabby.

TABLE 7-8 ASSESSING RANGE OF MOTION*

BODY PART	ASSESSMENT PROCEDURE	ROM
Upper Extremities		
Neck	Bend head forward and then backward. Bend neck side to side. Turn head to look over each shoulder.	Flexion; hyperextension; lateral flexion; rotation
Shoulders	Raise both arms to a vertical position level at the sides of the head.	Flexion
	Bring arm across upper chest to touch opposite shoulder.	Adduction
	Place both hands behind the neck, with elbows out to the sides.	External rotation and abduction
	Place both hands behind the small of the back.	Internal rotation
	Have patient make small circles with hands with arms extended at shoulder level.	Circumduction
Elbows	Bend and straighten the elbows.	Flexion and extension
	Place hands at waist with elbows flexed.	Internal rotation
Wrists	Flex and extend wrist (bend and straighten).	Flexion and extension
	Bend wrist to radial then ulnar side.	Radial and ulnar deviation
	Turn palm upward and then downward.	Supination and pronation
Hands	Make a fist with both hands; open hand.	Flexion and extension
	Extend and spread fingers and thumb outward; bring back together.	Adduction and abduction
Lower Extremities		
Hips (with patient supine)	With knees extended, raise one leg upward.	Flexion: expect 90 degrees
	Cross leg over other leg.	Abduction: expect 45 degrees
	Swing legs laterally.	Abduction: expect 30 degrees
	With knee flexed, hold the ankle and rotate the leg inward and outward.	Internal and external rotation: expect 40-45 degrees
Knees (with patient sitting)	Raise the foot, keeping the knee in place.	Extension: expect full extension and up to 15 degrees hyperextension
Ankles	With foot held off the floor, point toes downward, and then bring toes back toward the knee.	Plantar flexion: expect 45 degrees Dorsiflexion: expect 20 degrees
Toes	Turn foot (sole) inward and then sole outward.	Inversion and eversion: expect to reach 5 degrees
	Bend toes down and back.	Flexion and hyperextension: Expect to reach 40 degrees

*This may be done actively by the patient (active ROM [AROM]) or passively by the nurse (passive ROM [PROM]).

STEPS	RATIONALE
4. Neurological assessment.	
a. Assess LOC and orientation by asking patient to identify name, location, day of week, and year; note behavior and appearance. This can be performed during general survey.	A fully conscious patient responds to question spontaneously. As consciousness declines, patient may show irritability, short attention span, or unwillingness to cooperate. As consciousness continues to deteriorate, patient becomes disoriented to name, time, and place. Behavior and appearance reveal information about patient's mental status.
b. Assess CNs.	
(1) For CN III (oculomotor), IV (trochlear), and VI (abducens), assess extraocular movement. Ask patient to follow movement of your finger through the six cardinal positions of gaze; measure pupillary reaction to light reflex and accommodation (see Skill 7.2) using penlight.	These CNs are those most likely affected by increased intracranial pressure (ICP), which causes changes in response or size of pupil; pupils may change shape (more oval) or react sluggishly. ICP impairs movement of external ocular muscles. Accommodation is ability of the eye to adjust vision from near to far.
(2) For CN V (trigeminal), apply light sensation with a cotton ball to symmetrical areas of face.	Sensations should be symmetrical; unilateral decrease or loss of sensation may be caused by CN V lesion.
(3) For CN VII (facial), note facial symmetry. Have patient frown, smile, puff out cheeks, and raise eyebrows.	Expressions should be symmetrical; Bell's palsy causes drooping of upper and lower face; cerebrovascular accident (CVA) causes asymmetry.
(4) For CN IX (glossopharyngeal) and CN X (vagus), have patient speak and swallow. Ask patient to say "ah" while using tongue blade and penlight. Check for midline uvula and symmetrical rise of uvula and soft palate. Use tongue blade and place on posterior tongue to elicit gag reflex.	Damage to CN IX causes impaired swallowing, loss of gag reflex, hoarseness, and nasal voice. When palate fails to rise and uvula pulls toward normal side, this indicates a unilateral paralysis.
c. Assess extremities for sensation. Perform all sensory testing with patient's eyes closed so patient is unable to see when or where a stimulus strikes the skin.	
(1) *Pain*: Ask patient to indicate when sharp or dull sensation is felt as you alternately apply sharp and blunt ends of tongue blade to skin surface. Apply in symmetrical areas of extremities.	Patient should be able to distinguish sharp or dull sensations. Impaired sensations may indicate disorders of the spinal cord or peripheral nerve roots.
(2) *Light touch*: Apply light wisp of cotton to different points along surface of skin in symmetrical areas of extremities.	Patient should be able to distinguish when touched.
(3) *Position*: Grasp finger or toe, holding it by its sides with your thumb and index finger. Alter moving it up and down. Ask patient to state when finger is up or down. Repeat with toes.	Patient should be able to distinguish movements of a few millimeters. Decreased/absent position sense may occur in spinal anesthesia, paralysis, or other neurological disorders.
d. Assess motor and cerebellar function:	
(1) *Gait:* See Step 3f above.	Neurological and musculoskeletal disorders may impair gait and balance.
(2) *Romberg's test:* Have patient stand with feet together, arm at sides, both eyes open and closed (for 20 to 30 seconds). Protect patient's safety by standing at side; observe for swaying.	Romberg's test should be negative; slight swaying is considered normal.
e. Assess deep tendon reflexes (DTRs):	
(1) In patients with back pain or surgery, CVA, or spinal cord compression, it is appropriate to monitor DTRs (Seidel and others, 2011). This requires an advanced level of skill. In most settings this is not part of the routine physical assessment.	Muscle spasticity and hyperactive reflexes may result from disorders such as stroke and paralysis. Diminished DTRs and muscle weakness may suggest electrolyte abnormalities or lower motor neuron disorders such as amyotrophic lateral sclerosis or Guillain-Barré syndrome.
5. See Completion Protocol (inside front cover).	

EVALUATION

1. Compare gait, muscle strength, and ROM with previous physical assessment.
2. Compare neurological status with previous physical assessment.
3. Evaluate level of patient's discomfort after procedure using appropriate pain scale.

Unexpected Outcomes and Related Interventions

1. Joints are prominent, swollen, and tender with nodules or overgrowth of bone in distal joints, indicating signs of arthritis.
   a. Instruct patient in proper ROM.
   b. Determine patient's knowledge regarding antiinflammatory medications and nonpharmacological measures.
2. ROM is reduced in one or more major joints: shoulder, elbow, wrist, fingers, knee, hip.
   a. Assess further for pain during movement, with joint unstable, stiff, painful, or swollen or with obvious deformity.
   b. Notify health care provider.
   c. Reduce mobility in extremity until cause of abnormal joint motion is determined.
3. Patient demonstrates weakness in one or more major muscle groups or has difficulty with gait or ability to walk and sit during Get Up and Go Test, indicating a fall risk.
   a. Provide for patient safety when ambulating.
   b. Place patient on fall precautions.
4. Patient has changes in mental status and pupillary response or other neurological deficits.
   a. Notify health care provider immediately.
   b. Place on fall precautions.
   c. Continue to assess vital signs and patient's LOC closely.

Recording and Reporting

- Record posture, gait, muscle strength, and ROM in nurses' notes or appropriate assessment flow sheet.
- Record LOC, orientation, pupillary response, sensation, and reflex responses in nurses' notes or appropriate assessment flow sheet.
- Report to nurse in charge or health care provider any acute pain or sudden muscle weakness, change in LOC, or change in size or pupillary reaction, which require immediate treatment.

Sample Documentation

1530 Patient out of bed to chair, ambulated without difficulty. Strong, stable gait noted. No complaints of weakness, dizziness, or pain.

Special Considerations

Pediatric

- Examine infants carefully for musculoskeletal anomalies resulting from genetic or fetal insults. An examination includes review of posture, generalized movement, symmetry and skin creases of the extremities, muscle strength, and hip alignment.
- Normally the back of a newborn is rounded or C-shaped from the thoracic and pelvic curves.
- Scoliosis, lateral curvature of the spine, is an important childhood problem, especially in females apparent at puberty. (For closer examination, have child stand erect, wearing only underclothes. Observe from behind, looking for asymmetry of shoulders and hips. Then observe from the back as the child bends forward.) Uneven dress hems or pant leg hems or uneven fit of clothing at the waist may be noted.

Geriatric

- Instruct older adults about fall precautions.
- Older adults tend to assume a stooped, forward-bent posture, with hips and knees somewhat flexed and arms bent at the elbows and the level of the arms raised (Ebersole and others, 2008).
- Instruct older adults and those with osteoporosis in proper body mechanics, ROM exercises, and moderate weight-bearing exercises (e.g., swimming, walking) to minimize trauma.
- Functional assessment is a measurement of older person's ability to perform basic self-care tasks (Ebersole and others, 2008). When patient is unable to perform self-care easily, determine the need for assistive devices (e.g., zippers on clothing instead of buttons, elevation of toilet seat or chairs to minimize bending of knees and hips).

Home Care

- Make modifications in the home for any patient at risk for falls (see Chapter 32).

REVIEW QUESTIONS

1. The nurse's postoperative patient has an intravenous infusion, an abdominal dressing, a Foley catheter to gravity, and a Jackson-Pratt drain in place. What body systems would she assess for this patient? Describe key elements for this patient.
2. The nurse auscultates her postoperative patient's abdomen. After listening for 60 seconds at a site below and to the left of the umbilicus, the nurse is unable to hear bowel sounds. What is the best assessment of this situation?

3. In conducting a general survey of a patient, the nurse knows that the survey should include which of the following? Select all that apply.
   1. Appearance
   2. Obtaining peripheral pulses
   3. Measuring chest excursion
   4. Conducting a detailed history
   5. Behavior
   6. Pupillary response
   7. Posture
4. In teaching a patient about skin lesions, the nurse knows that teaching has been successful when the patient identifies which lesion as abnormal?
   1. A symmetrical lesion
   2. A lesion with regular edges and borders
   3. One that is blue/black or varied in color
   4. One that is less than 7 mm in diameter
5. On respiratory assessment the nurse notes high-pitched, musical sounds on auscultation. The nurse interprets these sounds as:
   1. Normal; vesicular
   2. Rhonchi
   3. Crackles
   4. Wheezes
6. The nurse determines that the patient has an audible S_2 on auscultation during cardiovascular assessment. After documenting this finding, the nurse should:
   1. Reposition the patient for comfort.
   2. Report the finding to the health care provider.
   3. Initiate fluid restriction.
   4. Do nothing as this is a normal finding.
7. Place the following components of the abdominal assessment in the correct order:
   1. Palpation
   2. Inspection
   3. Auscultation
   4. Percussion
8. The patient has an IV infusing in the left arm. The skin looks reddened at the site. Which of the following techniques is most appropriate for the nurse to use to check if there is warmth at the site?
   1. Places palm of hand over site
   2. Grasps skin at site with fingers
   3. Applies dorsum of hand over site
   4. Places pads of fingertips above site
9. Which of the following does the nurse document as an abnormal finding during a muscular-neurological assessment?
   1. Pupils equal, round, and reactive to light and accommodation
   2. Uses hands to sit down in chair during Get Up and Go Test
   3. Negative Romberg's test
   4. Uvula rises symmetrically
10. Calculate the patient's intake in milliliters based on the following fluids: 3 ounces of apple juice, ¼ carton of milk (250 mL per carton), 6 ounces of soda, and an 8-ounce cup of ice.

REFERENCES

American Cancer Society (ACS): *Cancer prevention and early detection facts and figures 2010*, Atlanta, 2010a, ACS.

American Cancer Society (ACS): *Cancer facts and figures 2010*, Atlanta, 2010b, ACS.

Anbarghalami R and others: *When to suspect child abuse, RN* 70(4):34, 2007.

Ball JW, Bindler RC: *Child health nursing: partnering with children and families*, ed 2, Upper Saddle River, NJ, 2010, Pearson Prentice Hall.

Ebersole P and others: *Toward healthy aging: human needs and nursing response*, ed 7, St Louis, 2008, Mosby.

Farley A: Pulmonary embolism: identification, clinical features, and management, *Nursing Standard* 23(28):49, 2009.

Giger J, Davidhizar R: *Transcultural nursing: assessment and intervention*, ed 5, St Louis, 2008, Mosby.

Hegarty K and others: Violence between intimate partners: working with the whole family, *BMJ* 337, 346.

Hockenberry MJ, Wilson D: *Wong's nursing care of infants and children*, ed 8, St Louis, 2007, Mosby.

Jarvis C: *Physical examination & health assessment*, ed 5, St Louis, 2008, Saunders.

Katapodi M and others: Underestimation of breast cancer risk: influence on screening behavior, *Oncol Nurs Forum* 36(3):306, 2009.

Monahan F and others: *Phipps' medical-surgical nursing: health and illness perspectives*, ed 8, St Louis, 2007, Mosby.

Seidel HM and others: *Mosby's guide to physical examination*, ed 7, St Louis, 2011, Mosby.

Seidel HM and others: *Mosby's guide to physical examination*, ed 6, St Louis, 2006, Mosby.

The Joint Commission (TJC): *2010 National Patient Safety Goals*, Oakbrook Terrace, Ill, 2010, The Commission, http://www.jointcommission.org/PatientSafety/NationalPatientSafetyGoals, accessed July 24, 2010.

Touhy T, Jett K: *Ebersole & Hess' Gerontological nursing & healthy aging*, ed 3, St Louis, 2009, Mosby.

CHAPTER

8

Specimen Collection

evolve WEBSITE

http://evolve.elsevier.com/Perry/nursinginterventions

Video Clips

Nursing Skills Online

Laboratory test results aid in the diagnosis of health care problems, provide information about the stage and activity of diseases, and measure patient responses to therapy. Proficiency and judgment in obtaining specimens minimize patient discomfort, ensure patient safety, and ensure accuracy and quality of diagnostic procedures. Nurses are accountable for correctly collecting specimens, monitoring patient outcomes, and ensuring that these tests are collected in a timely manner. When questions arise about laboratory tests, consult the institution's procedure manual or call the laboratory. You can find normal values for laboratory tests in reference books. However, each laboratory also establishes its own values for each test, which are printed on the agency laboratory slips. It is important to know the significance of abnormal findings. Discuss only major deviations with the health care provider immediately.

PATIENT-CENTERED CARE

Confidentiality is an important issue associated with laboratory testing. Agencies must have clearly written and enforced policies regarding disclosure of test results while maintaining confidentiality within the health care system (USDHHS, 2008). Patients often experience embarrassment or discomfort when giving a sample of body excretions or secretions. It is important to handle excretions discreetly and provide the patient with as much privacy as possible.

Given clear instructions, patients are able to obtain their own specimens of urine, stool, and sputum without unnecessary exposure. Choose words that are clearly understood; many patients, especially children, do not understand the terms *void, urine,* or *stool.*

Cultural considerations are important when collecting specimens. Customs may affect the patient's response and willingness to participate in various diagnostic procedures. Southeast Asians consider the blood as a vital life force that should not be wasted. Introduction of a swab or tongue blade into the mouth to collect specimens may be threatening to Southeast Asians who believe that diseases can be introduced through the mouth and that the head is the seat of one's life force. Muslims designate that only the left hand be used for cleaning filth and impurities of the body and the bodily functions such as urination and bowel movement (Stacey, 2009). Whenever possible, use same-gender caregivers when collecting vaginal, rectal, or urinary specimens from patients whose cultural values demand modesty and distinct separation of gender roles. Provide privacy both when giving instructions and collecting the specimen.

SAFETY

When collecting any specimen, know the purpose of the test, how much of the specimen is needed, the appropriate collection, and how the specimen is to be transported to the laboratory (Pagana and Pagana, 2009). A completed laboratory requisition is needed for each specimen to instruct laboratory personnel on the test to be performed and facilitate accurate reporting of the results. Each requisition includes patient

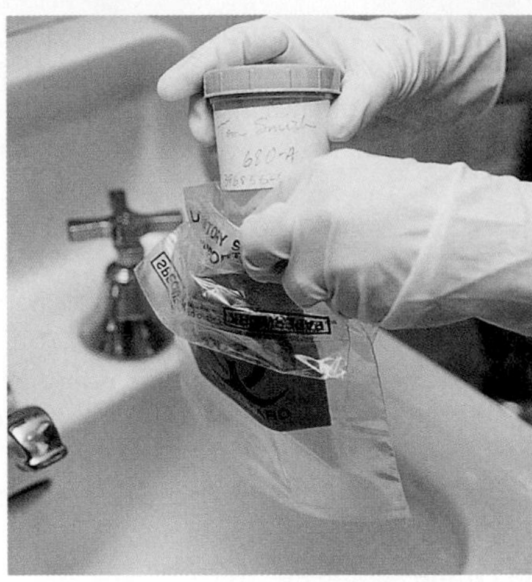

FIG 8-1 Enclose all specimens in a biohazard plastic bag.

identification (name and numbers), the date and time the specimen is obtained, the name of the test, and the source of the specimen/culture for each container (The Joint Commission [TJC], 2010).

Before specimen collection TJC requires the use of at least two identifiers when providing care, treatment, and services. The intent is to reliably identify the individual as the patient for whom the service or treatment is intended and match the service or treatment to that patient (TJC, 2010). After you collect the specimen and in the presence of the patient, you must label the container itself (not the lid) with the same two identifiers (e.g., patient name and hospital identification number), specimen source, collection date and time, series number (if more than one specimen), and anatomical site if appropriate (e.g., wound culture from knee versus abdominal incision).

Everyone who handles body fluids is at risk for exposure to body fluids. The use of hand hygiene and clean gloves is necessary when collecting a specimen. Use a plastic bag marked "biohazard" to enclose the specimen for delivery to the laboratory (Fig. 8-1). Deliver specimens to the laboratory. Specimens left at room temperature are at risk for additional bacterial growth, thereby altering the results of the test.

EVIDENCE-BASED PRACTICE TRENDS

Roark DC, Miguel K: RFID: bar coding's replacement, *Nurs Manage* 37(2):28, 2006.

Identification errors are the most common serious laboratory errors. One of the most important factors in safe and effective collection of laboratory specimens is ensuring that caregivers perform the right test and obtain the right specimen from the right patient. Misidentification of specimens may lead to incorrect diagnoses and unnecessary or inappropriate treatments. New technologies provide simple and accurate identification systems to ensure patient safety and meet the basic requirement of two patient identifiers. Some agencies use bar codes to label specimens. One option is a bar code on the patient's identification bracelet, which is scanned and compared with the labeled specimen. The technology uses a microchip with a radio antenna in an electronic tag on the patient's arm band. Another option uses a bar code implanted under the patient's skin, which transmits a unique code to a special scanner using radio waves. Additional detailed medical information is accessed from an accompanying database.

SKILL 8.1 URINE SPECIMEN COLLECTION—MIDSTREAM, STERILE URINARY CATHETER

- **Nursing Skills Online: Specimen Collection, Lessons 1 and 2; Urinary Catheterization, Lesson 4** *Video Clips*

A urinalysis provides information about kidney or metabolic function, nutrition, and systemic diseases. Urine collection uses a variety of methods, depending on the purpose of the urinalysis and the presence or absence of a urinary catheter. Regardless of the method of collection, guidelines for assessment, planning, and evaluation are similar. Routine urinalysis includes measurement of nine or more elements, including urine pH, protein and glucose levels, ketones, blood, specific gravity, white blood cell (WBC) count, and presence of bacteria and casts (Pagana and Pagana, 2009).

TYPES OF URINE TESTS AND SPECIMENS

A *random urine specimen for routine urinalysis* is collected using a specimen "hat" (Fig. 8-2), which you place under a toilet seat to collect voided urine. You then place approximately 120 mL of urine in a specimen container, properly label it, and send to the laboratory.

A *culture and sensitivity (C&S) of urine* is performed to identify the bacteria causing a urinary tract infection (UTI) (culture) and determine the most effective antibiotic for treatment (sensitivity). Use sterile technique to ensure that any microorganisms present originate in the urine and not from the patient's skin, the hands, or the environment. You collect specimens for C&S either as a clean-voided midstream

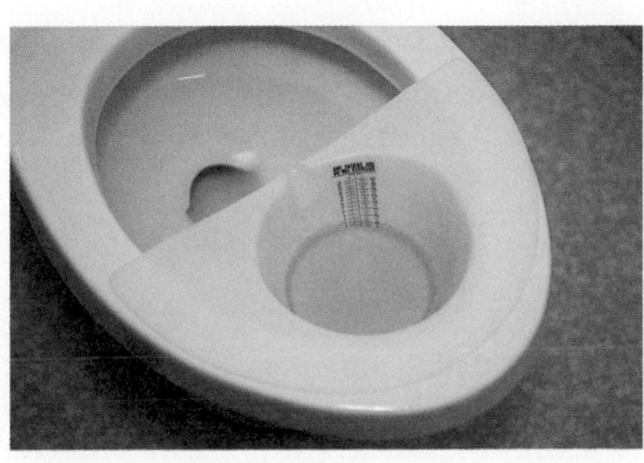

FIG 8-2 Specimen "hat."

specimen or under sterile conditions from a urinary catheter. Urine collected by these methods may also be analyzed for the same components as the routine urinalysis.

A *timed urine specimen for quantitative analysis* requires urine to be collected over 2 to 72 hours. The 24-hour timed collection (see Procedural Guideline 8.1) is most common and allows for measurement and quantitative analysis of elements such as amino acids, creatinine, hormones, glucose, and adrenocorticosteroid excreted.

Chemical properties of urine are tested by immersing a specially prepared strip of paper (Chemstrip) into a clean urine specimen. The test detects the presence of glucose, ketones, protein, or blood *not* normally present in the urine (see Procedural Guideline 8.2). When the screening test for the presence of substances in the urine is positive, additional laboratory tests are used to determine the patient's diagnosis or to measure the effectiveness of treatment.

ASSESSMENT

1. Assess patient's understanding of need for the specimen. *Rationale: This determines the need for health teaching. Patient's understanding of purpose promotes cooperation.*
2. Assess patient's ability to assist with urine specimen collection: able to position self and hold container. *Rationale: This determines the degree of assistance patient requires.*
3. Determine if you need to administer or add fluids, dietary requirements, or medications in conjunction with the test. *Rationale: Certain substances affect excretion and levels of urinary constituents. Specific amounts of fluid may be required for concentration/dilution tests. Drugs such as cortisone preparations, diuretics, and anesthetics increase glucose levels. Anticoagulants increase risk of blood in the urine.*
4. Assess for signs and symptoms of UTI (frequency, urgency, dysuria, hematuria, flank pain, cloudy urine with sediment, foul odor, fever). *Rationale: These are indicators of UTI.*
5. Assess patient's current urinary elimination pattern. *Rationale: Indicates possibility of UTI. Knowledge of frequency of urination facilitates effective planning of specimen collection.*

PLANNING

Expected Outcomes focus on collecting an appropriate uncontaminated specimen with patient knowledgeable of the purpose of the specimen examination.

1. Patient explains procedure for specimen collection.
2. Patient explains purpose of specimen analysis.
3. A specimen free of contaminants is collected.

Delegation and Collaboration

The skill of collecting urine specimens may be delegated to nursing assistive personnel (NAP). Instruct the NAP by:

- Explaining when to collect the specimen.
- Reviewing to observe the amount and appearance of urine and, if the urine is not clear (e.g., contains blood, cloudiness, or excess sediment), to report this information back to the nurse.

Equipment

- Identification labels (with appropriate patient identifiers)
- Completed laboratory requisition, including appropriate patient identification, date, time, name of test, and source of culture
- Small plastic biohazard bag for delivery of specimen to laboratory (or container as specified by agency)

Clean-voided urine specimen

Clean and sterile gloves

Commercial kit for clean-voided urine (Fig. 8-3) containing:

- Sterile cotton balls or antiseptic towelettes
- Antiseptic solution (usually chlorhexidine or povidone-iodine solution)
- Sterile water or normal saline
- Sterile specimen container
- Urine cup

Soap, water, washcloth, and towel

Bedpan (for nonambulatory patient) or specimen hat (for ambulatory patient)

Sterile urine specimen from urinary catheter

Clean gloves

20-mL Luer-Lok safety syringe for routine urinalysis or a 3-mL safety Luer-Lok syringe for culture

Clamp or rubber band

Alcohol, chlorhexidine, or other disinfectant swab

Specimen container (nonsterile for routine urinalysis; sterile for culture)

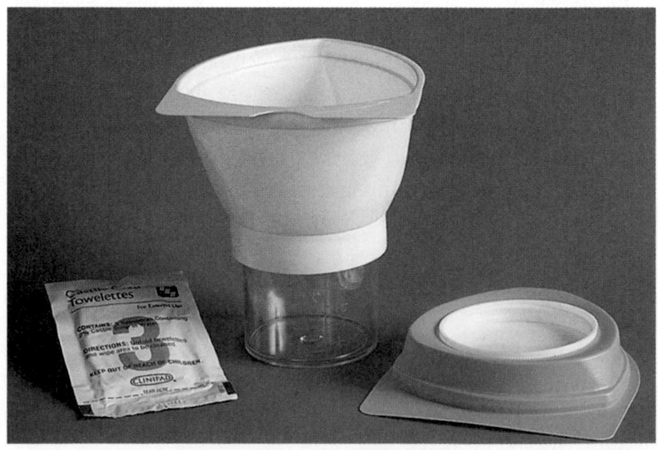

FIG 8-3 Clean-voided urine kit.

IMPLEMENTATION *for* URINE SPECIMEN COLLECTION—MIDSTREAM, STERILE URINARY CATHETER

STEPS	RATIONALE
1. See Standard Protocol (inside front cover).	
2. Identify patient using two identifiers (i.e., name and birth date or name and account number, according to facility policy). Compare identifiers with information in patient's medical record.	Ensures correct patient. Complies with The Joint Commission standards and improves patient safety (TJC, 2010).
3. Explain to patient and/or family member reason specimen is necessary, how patient can assist (when applicable), and how to obtain a specimen that is free of tissue and stool.	Promotes cooperation and patient participation. In some cases patient can collect clean-voided specimen independently. Minimizes contamination of specimen and need for repeat collection.
4. Collect clean-voided urine specimen.	
a. Give patient or family member towel, washcloth, and soap to cleanse perineum or assist with cleansing perineum. If patient is bedridden, you can do this with the patient positioned on the bedpan to facilitate access to the perineum. Remove and dispose of gloves.	Patients usually prefer to wash their own perineal area when possible.
b. Using surgical asepsis, open outer package of commercial specimen kit.	Maintains sterility of specimen container.
c. Apply sterile gloves.	Prevents introduction of microorganisms on nurse's hands into specimen.
d. Pour antiseptic solution over cotton balls (unless kit contains prepared gauze pads in antiseptic towelette).	Cotton ball or gauze pad is used to cleanse perineum.
e. Open specimen container, maintaining sterility of inside of specimen container, and place cap with sterile inside surface up. Do not touch inside of cap or container.	Contaminated specimen is the most frequent reason for inaccurate reporting of urine cultures and sensitivities.
f. Assist or allow patient to independently cleanse perineum and collect specimen. The amount of assistance needed varies with each patient; provide assistance if necessary. Inform patient that the antiseptic solution will feel cold.	Maintains patient's dignity and comfort.
(1) Male:	
(a) Hold penis with one hand; using circular motion and antiseptic towelette, cleanse meatus, moving from center to outside (see illustration). Have uncircumcised male patient retract foreskin for effective cleansing of urinary meatus and keep retracted during voiding. Return foreskin when done.	Reduces number of microorganisms at urethral meatus and moves from areas of least to most contamination. Return of foreskin prevents stricture of penis.

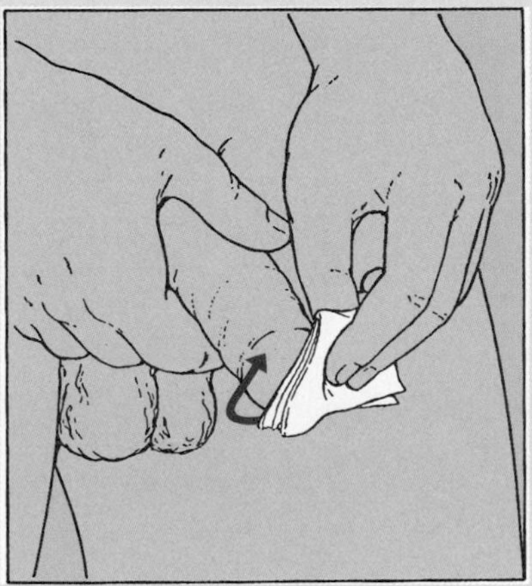

STEP 4f(1)(a) Cleanse penis with a circular motion. (Modified from Grimes D: *Infectious diseases, Mosby's clinical nursing series,* St Louis, 1991, Mosby.)

Continued

STEPS	RATIONALE
(b) If agency procedure indicates, rinse area with sterile water and dry with cotton balls or gauze pad.	Prevents contamination of specimen with antiseptic solution.
(c) Have patient initiate urine stream into toilet or bedpan; then have patient pass urine specimen container into stream and collect 30 to 60 mL of urine (see illustration).	Initial urine flushes microorganisms that normally accumulate at urinary meatus and prevents collection in specimen.
(2) ***Female:***	
(a) Spread labia minora with fingers of nondominant hand.	Provides access to urinary meatus.
(b) With dominant hand, cleanse urethral area with antiseptic swab, cotton ball, or gauze. Move from front (above urethral orifice) to back (toward anus). Use a fresh swab each time; cleanse *three times*; begin with labial fold farthest from you, then labial fold closest, and then down center (see illustration).	Prevents contamination of urinary meatus with fecal material. Move from cleanest to most soiled.
(c) If agency procedure indicates, rinse area with sterile water and dry with cotton.	Prevents contamination of specimen with antiseptic solution.
(d) While continuing to hold labia apart, patient initiates urine stream into the toilet or bedpan; after stream is achieved, patient or nurse passes the specimen container into stream and collects 90 to 120 mL of urine (Pagana and Pagana, 2009) (see illustration).	Initial urine flushes out microorganisms that normally accumulate at the urinary meatus and provides uncontaminated urine from the bladder itself.
g. Remove specimen container before flow of urine stops and before releasing penis or labia. Patient finishes voiding into bedpan or toilet.	Prevents contamination of specimen with skin flora.
h. Replace cap securely on specimen container, touching only outside.	Retains sterility of inside of container and prevents spillage of urine.
i. Cleanse urine from exterior surface of container. Remove and dispose of gloves.	Prevents transfer of microorganisms to others.

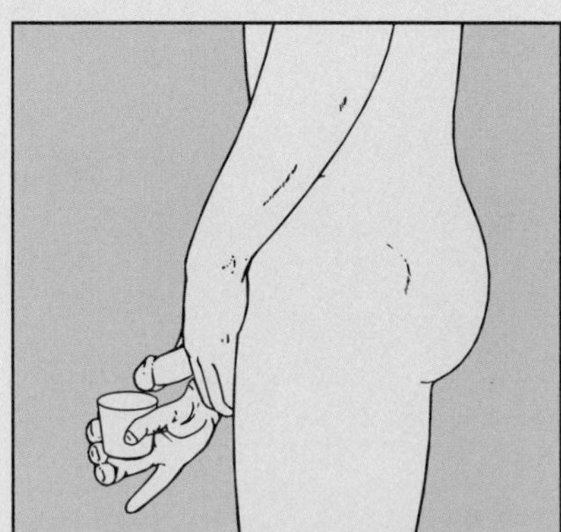

STEP 4f(1)(c) Position of male for collecting midstream urine specimen.

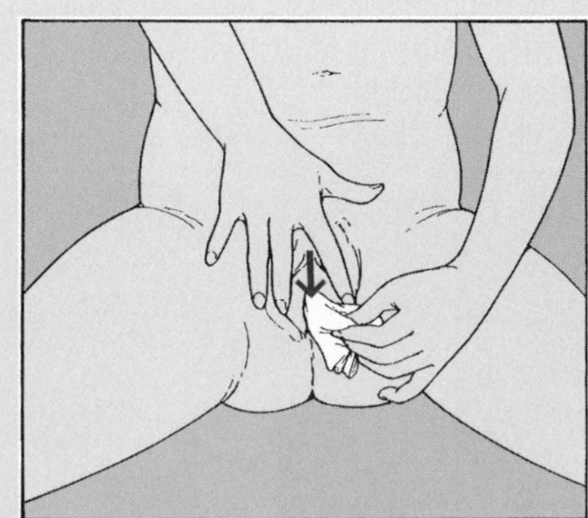

STEP 4f(2)(b) Cleanse from front to back, holding labia apart. (Modified from Grimes D: Infectious diseases, *Mosby's clinical nursing series*, St Louis, 1991, Mosby.)

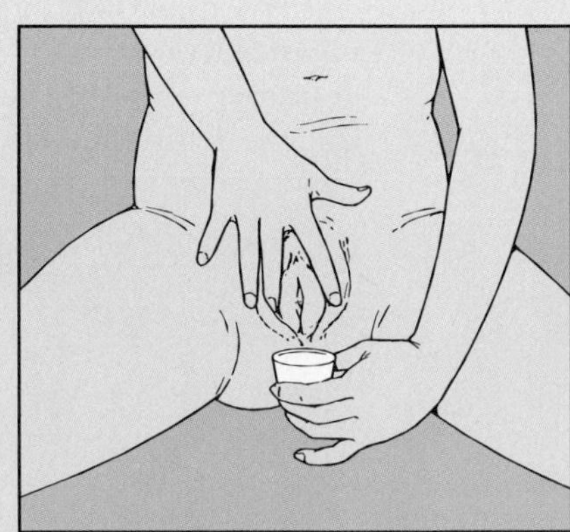

STEP 4f(2)(d) Collection of midstream urine specimen (female).

STEPS	RATIONALE
5. ***Collect urine from an indwelling urinary catheter.***	
a. Explain that you will use a syringe without a needle to remove the urine through the catheter port and patient will not experience discomfort.	Minimizes anxiety when nurse manipulates catheter and aspirates urine with syringe from the catheter port.
b. Explain that you need to clamp the catheter for 10 to 30 minutes before obtaining a urine specimen and that you cannot obtain it from drainage bag.	
c. Clamp drainage tubing with clamp or rubber band for as long as 30 minutes below the site chosen for withdrawal (see illustration).	Permits collection of fresh, sterile urine in catheter tubing. Amount of time depends on amount of urine patient produces.
d. After 30 minutes, position patient so catheter sampling port is easily accessible. Location of the port is where catheter attaches to drainage bag tube (see illustration). Cleanse the port for 15 seconds with a disinfectant swab and allow to dry.	Prevents entry of microorganisms into catheter.
e. Attach a needleless Luer-Lok syringe to the build-in catheter sampling port (see illustration).	

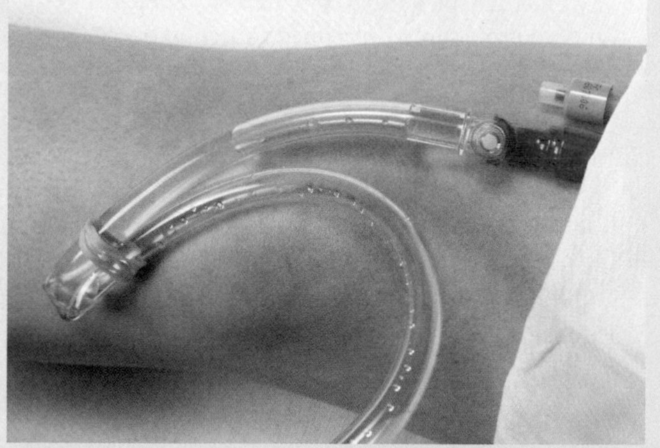

STEP 5c Rubber band used to clamp catheter drainage tube.

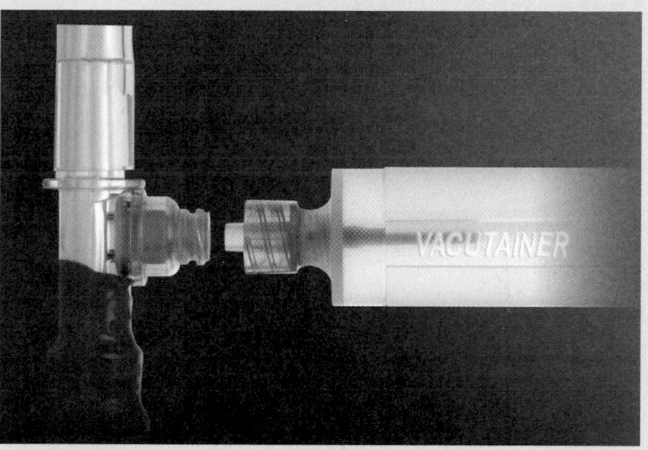

STEP 5d Port with syringe attached. (Courtesy and © Becton, Dickinson and Company.)

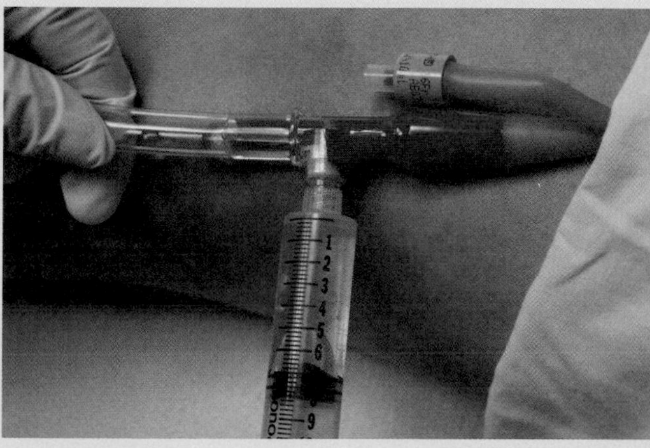

STEP 5e Access urinary catheter port with Luer-Lok syringe or syringe with blunt plastic valve.

Continued

STEPS	RATIONALE
f. Withdraw 3 mL for a culture or 20 mL for routine urinalysis.	Allows collection of urine without contamination. Obtains proper volume for testing.
g. Transfer urine from syringe into clean urine container for routine urinalysis or into a sterile urine container for culture.	Prevents contamination of urine during transfer procedure.
h. Place lid tightly on container.	Prevents contamination of specimen by air and loss by spillage.
i. Unclamp catheter and allow urine to flow into drainage bag. Ensure that urine flows freely.	Allows urine to drain by gravity and prevents stasis of urine in bladder.
6. Securely attach label to container (not the lid). In patient's presence complete label with two identifiers, specimen source, and collection date and time. If patient is female, indicate if patient is menstruating.	Ensures that specimen is identified correctly for proper diagnosis (TJC, 2010).
7. Send specimen and completed requisition to laboratory within 20 minutes. Refrigerate if delay cannot be avoided.	Delay of analysis may alter test results significantly (Pagana and Pagana, 2010).
8. See Completion Protocol (inside front cover).	

EVALUATION

1. Ask patient to identify steps in specimen collection procedure.
2. Ask patient to state purposes of specimen collection.
3. Inspect clean-voided specimen for contamination with toilet tissue or stool.
4. Observe urinary drainage system to be sure that it is intact and patent.

Unexpected Outcomes and Related Interventions

1. Patient is unable to void or urine does not collect in drainage tube.
   a. Offer fluids (if permitted) to enhance urine production.
2. Patient's urine specimen is contaminated with stool and tissue.
   a. Reinforce importance of obtaining specimen free of contaminants.
   b. Collect a new specimen and assist patient with specimen collection; place specimen hat as close to front of commode as possible.
3. Lumen that leads to balloon holding catheter in bladder is punctured.
   a. Notify provider and prepare for insertion of new catheter.
   b. Obtain new specimen.

Recording and Reporting

- Record method used to obtain specimen, date and time collected, type of test ordered, laboratory receiving specimen, characteristics of specimen, and patient's tolerance to procedure of specimen collection.
- Report any abnormal findings to physician or health care provider.

Sample Documentation

1135 Clean-voided specimen of 130 mL dark amber urine obtained and sent to lab. Complains of frequent urge to void, burning sensation with voiding, and voiding small amounts. Dr. Nelson notified.

Special Considerations

Pediatric

- It is not possible to obtain a midstream urine collection on a nontoilet-trained child; consequently, obtain urine for culture by straight catheterization. Consider age-appropriate fears, especially with preschool and school-age children (Hockenberry and Wilson, 2009).

Geriatric

- Older adults may need assistance in positioning to obtain specimen. In confused patients a NAP may be necessary to assist the patient in collecting a specimen.

Home Care

- Instruct a patient collecting a sample at home to keep the specimen on ice until it reaches the laboratory to minimize bacterial growth before applying it to a culture medium in a laboratory setting.

PROCEDURAL GUIDELINE 8.1
Collecting 24-Hour Timed Urine Specimens

To ensure the accuracy of a 24-hour timed urine specimen, the patient and staff must work together to collect all voided urine in a 24-hour period. Obtain an appropriate container with or without preservative from the laboratory. The type of analysis for the 24-hour timed specimen determines the need for any preservative. You may place the specimen container in the patient's bathroom or the "soiled" utility room. Post a sign to remind the patient and staff that a test is in progress. Label the specimen container with all appropriate identification information and the number of the containers sequentially if more than one container is needed. Also note if toxic material is used as a preservative. Documentation and collection of all urine are necessary for an accurate test result.

Delegation and Collaboration

The skill of collecting a timed urine specimen may be delegated to nursing assistive personnel (NAP). Instruct the NAP by:

- Explaining the time to begin specimen collection, how to store collected urine, where to place signs that a timed urine collection is in progress, and to save all urine.
- Reviewing what to observe for and to report blood, mucus, or foul odors present in the specimen or if there is a break in the collection procedure.

Equipment

- Large collection bottle that usually contains a chemical preservative
- Bottle cap
- Bedpan, urinal, or specimen hat
- Graduated measuring cup for intake and output (I&O) measurement
- Large basin to hold collection bottle (surrounded by ice if immediate refrigeration is required)
- Instructional signs that remind patient and staff of timed urine collection
- Clean gloves
- Identification labels and completed laboratory requisition (with appropriate patient identifiers and specimen information)
- Plastic biohazard bag or container (see agency policy).

Procedural Steps

1. **See Standard Protocol (inside front cover).**
2. Identify patient using two identifiers (i.e., name and birth date or name and account number, according to facility policy). Compare identifiers with information in patient's medical record.
3. Explain the reason for specimen collection, how patient can assist, and that urine must be free of feces and toilet tissue.
4. Place signs indicating timed urine specimen collection on patient's door and toileting area. If patient leaves unit for another test or procedure, be sure that personnel in that area collect and save all urine.
5. If possible, have patient drink two to four glasses of water about 30 minutes before timed collection to facilitate ability to void at the appropriate time for the test to begin.
6. Discard the first specimen as test begins. Print time that test began on laboratory requisition. For accurate results the patient must begin the test with an empty bladder. Restart timed period if urine is accidentally lost, discarded, or contaminated.
7. Measure volume of each voiding if I&O is being recorded. Then place all voided urine in labeled specimen bottle with appropriate additive.
8. Unless instructed otherwise, keep specimen bottle in specimen refrigerator or in container of ice in bathroom to prevent decomposition of urine.
9. Encourage patient to drink two glasses of water 1 hour before timed urine collection ends.
10. Encourage patient to empty bladder during last 15 minutes of urine collection period.
11. At end of collection period, label specimen (two identifiers, specimen source, collection date and time, number of bottle) in patient's presence, and attach appropriate requisition (patient identification, date, time, name of test, and specimen source) and send to laboratory.
12. Remove signs and inform patient that specimen collection period is completed.
13. **See Completion Protocol (inside front cover).**

PROCEDURAL GUIDELINE 8.2
Urine Screening for Glucose, Ketones, Protein, Blood, and pH

Test for chemical properties of urine are part of the routine urinalysis completed in the laboratory, as point-of-care at the bed side or in the home. The use of a Multistix reagent test strip may simultaneously assess for up to nine chemical properties, specific gravity, pH, protein, glucose, ketones, blood bilirubin, urobilinogen, leukocytes, and nitrates (Hamill, 2007). The test is easy to perform and causes no pain. This type of screening is used when more detailed laboratory testing is not readily available (e.g., in a physician's office or clinic and in the outpatient, long-term care, or home setting). It may also be done for pregnant women on admission to the hospital in labor. The use of urine

Continued

PROCEDURAL GUIDELINE 8.2
Urine Screening for Glucose, Ketones, Protein, Blood, and pH—cont'd

testing for managing blood glucose is no longer recommended but continues to be useful in detecting the presence of ketones in patients with diabetes (ADA, 2008).

Delegation and Collaboration

The skill of urine screening for chemical properties may be delegated to nursing assistive personnel (NAP). Instruct the NAP by:

- Explaining when to obtain the specimen (e.g., before meals, following a "double-voided" specimen).
- Reviewing the need to report to the nurse the results of the test or any blood, mucus, or odor in the specimen.

Equipment

- Specimen hat, bedpan, urinal, or commode
- Watch with second hand or digital counter
- Clean gloves
- Reagent test strip (check expiration date on container)
- Test strip color chart

Procedural Steps

1. **See Standard Protocol (inside front cover).**
2. Identify patient using two identifiers (i.e., name and birth date or name and account number, according to facility policy). Compare identifiers with information in patient's medical record.
3. Determine if a "double-voided" specimen is needed for glucose testing. If required, ask patient to void, discard, and then drink a glass of water.
4. Assist or ask patient to collect a fresh random urine sample (see Skill 8.1). If patient is catheterized, remove a 5-mL urine specimen from the catheter port.
5. Immerse end of reagent test strip into urine container. Remove the strip immediately and tap it gently against the side of the container to remove excess urine.
6. Hold strip in horizontal position to prevent mixing of chemical reagents.
7. Precisely time the number of seconds specified on container and then compare color of strip with color chart on container.
8. When appropriate, discuss test results with patient.
9. **See Completion Protocol (inside front cover).**

SKILL 8.2 TESTING FOR GASTROINTESTINAL ALTERATIONS—GASTROCCULT TEST, STOOL SPECIMEN, AND HEMOCCULT TEST

- **Nursing Skills Online: Specimen Collection, Lessons 3 and 4**

Video Clips

The collection of gastric secretions involves obtaining a specimen via a nasogastric (NG) or nasointestinal (NI) tube. When a patient has emesis, the nurse tests the material for the presence of blood. Analysis of stool or gastric secretions from the gastrointestinal (GI) tract provides useful information about pathological conditions such as the presence of tumors, infection, and malabsorption problems.

Patients can often assist in providing stool specimens. A meat-free, high-residue diet for 24 hours before testing is desirable to prevent false-positive results. The term *occult blood* refers to blood that is not visible but is present in microscopic amounts. Tests done to detect the presence of occult blood in stool (guaiac test) or emesis and gastric secretions (Gastroccult test) reveal bleeding in the esophagus, stomach, small intestine, or large intestine. The tests verify the presence of blood when the nurse notices red or black coloration of stool or gastric contents or a coffee-grounds appearance of gastric contents in emesis or with NG suction (ACG, 2009).

Hemoccult testing is useful for screening for the presence of occult (invisible) blood in the stool for conditions such as colon cancer, bleeding GI ulcers, and localized gastric or intestinal irritation. Use caution; the stool may appear bloody following a diet that includes red meat, resulting in a false-positive. Hemoccult testing differentiates between blood and other questionable substances in stool. When blood is present, further testing is indicated to determine the source of the bleeding.

ASSESSMENT

1. Assess patient's medical history for GI disorders (e.g., history of bleeding, hemorrhoids, colitis, malabsorption disorders).
2. Determine patient's understanding of need for test and the ability to cooperate with procedure and collect specimen.
3. Assess female patient's menstrual cycle. *Rationale: A woman who is menstruating may have a stool specimen contaminated with blood.*
4. Review medications for drugs that can contribute to GI bleeding. *Rationale: Anticoagulants, steroids, nonsteroidal antiinflammatory drugs (NSAIDs), ascorbic acid (vitamin C), antiinflammatory agents, and alcohol commonly cause bleeding tendency or irritation of GI mucosa.*
5. Check physician's or health care provider's orders for dietary restrictions before testing. *Rationale: Diets rich in red meats, green leafy vegetables, poultry, and fish may produce false-positive guaiac results.*

PLANNING

Expected Outcomes focus on the collection of an appropriate specimen, with patient knowledgeable of the purpose of the specimen test.

1. Patient discusses the purpose of test.
2. Patient maintains a high-residue diet that is free of red meat for specified period.
3. Patient's specimen is appropriate for testing analysis.

Delegation and Collaboration

Assessment of the patient's condition cannot be delegated. The skills of obtaining and testing gastric secretions from an NG or NI tube may not be delegated. The skill of obtaining stool specimens may be delegated to nursing assistive personnel (NAP). Instruct the NAP by:

- Explaining when to obtain stool specimen.
- Reviewing with personnel to report immediately if blood is detected, not to discard stool from a positive test, and to report immediately if blood is observed in patient emesis or NG tube drainage.

Equipment

- Clean gloves
- Soap, water, washcloth, and towel

Gastroccult test

- Facial tissues
- Emesis basin
- Wooden applicator or 3-mL syringe
- 60-mL bulb or catheter tip syringe
- Cardboard Gastroccult slide and developing solution (Fig. 8-4)

Stool specimens

- Plastic container with lid
- Two tongue blades
- Paper towel
- Bedpan, specimen hat, or bedside commode
- "Save stool" signs (24-hour timed specimen)
- Sterile test tube and swab (for culture)
- Identification labels
- Completed laboratory requisition, including appropriate patient identification, date, time, name of test, and source of culture

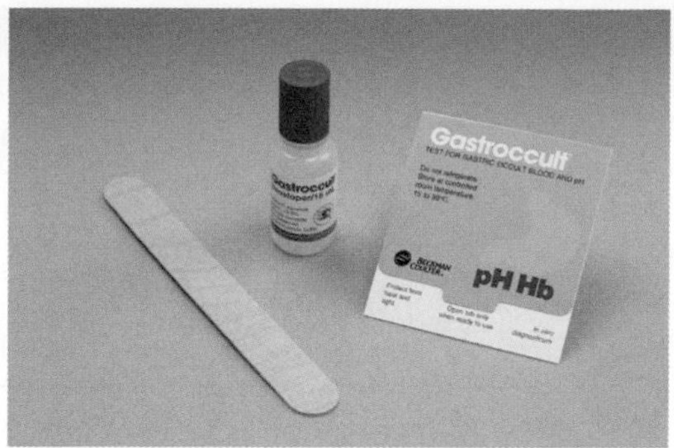

FIG 8-4 Cardboard Gastroccult slide and developing solution.

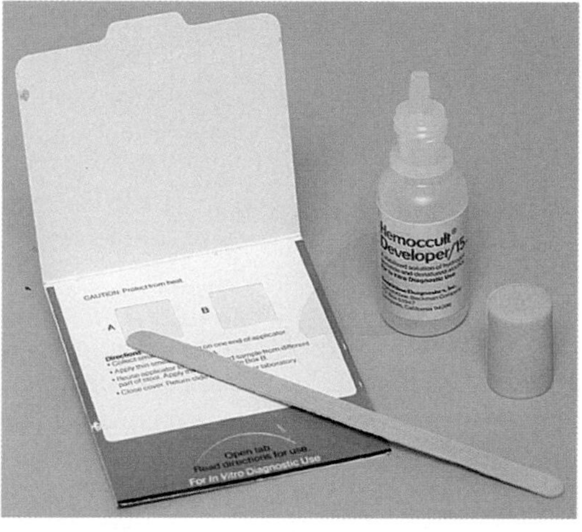

FIG 8-5 Hemoccult slide testing kit for measuring occult blood.

- Small plastic bag for delivery of specimen to laboratory (or container as specified by agency

Hemoccult (guaiac test)

- Paper towel
- Wooden applicator
- Cardboard Hemoccult slide and Hemoccult developing solution (Fig. 8-5)

IMPLEMENTATION *for* TESTING FOR GASTROINTESTINAL ALTERATIONS—GASTROCCULT TEST, STOOL SPECIMEN, AND HEMOCCULT TEST

STEPS	RATIONALE
1. See Standard Protocol (inside front cover).	
2. Identify patient using two identifiers (i.e., name and birth date or name and account number, according to facility policy). Compare identifiers with information in patient's medical record.	Ensures correct patient. Complies with The Joint Commission standards and improves patient safety (TJC, 2010).
3. Arrange for dietary and/or medication restrictions as indicated.	Increases accuracy of test results.

Continued

STEPS	RATIONALE
4. Discuss reason specimen is necessary, how patient can assist in collecting an uncontaminated specimen (for stool specimen), and how you will obtain the gastric specimen.	Promotes patient cooperation.
5. Perform Gastroccult test.	

SAFETY ALERT Gastroccult and Hemoccult slides and developers are *not* interchangeable.

STEPS	RATIONALE
a. To obtain specimen of gastric contents from NG or NI tube, position patient in high-Fowler's position in bed or chair.	Minimizes chance of aspiration of gastric contents. Position relieves pressure on abdominal organs. If patient is nauseated, flat position in bed or one in which patient cannot sit straight may cause abdominal discomfort.
b. Verify enteral tube placement (see Chapter 12).	Ensures aspiration of gastric or intestinal contents.
c. Collect GI contents via NG or NI tube by disconnecting tube from suction or gravity drainage. Draw 30 mL of air (for NG tube) or 10 mL of air (for NI tube) into the bulb or slip-tipped syringe, attach syringe to NG or NI tube, inject air, and then aspirate 5 to 10 mL of fluid.	Only small amount of specimen is needed for pH and occult blood testing.
d. To obtain sample of emesis, use a 3-mL syringe or wooden applicator to gather sample from emesis basin.	
e. Using applicator or syringe, apply 1 drop of gastric sample to Gastroccult blood test slide.	Sample must cover test paper for test reaction to occur.
f. Apply 2 drops of commercial Gastroccult developer solution over sample and 1 drop between positive and negative performance monitors (see illustration).	

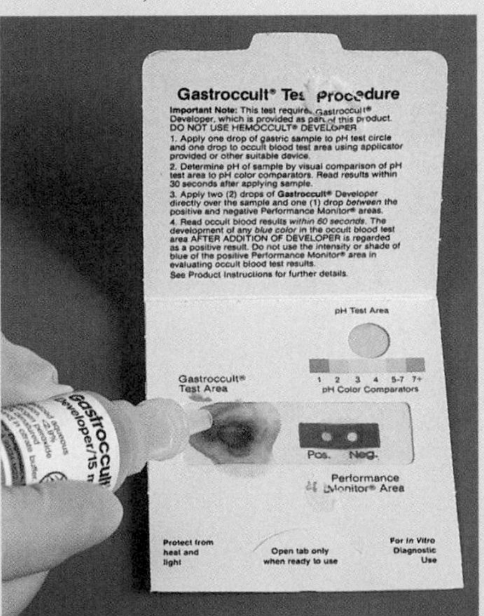

STEP 5f Apply developing solution to Gastroccult test area.

STEPS	RATIONALE
g. Verify that performance monitor turns blue after 30 seconds.	Indicates proper function of the testing paper.
h. After 60 seconds compare color of gastric sample with that of performance monitors.	If sample turns blue, test is positive for occult blood. If sample turns green, test is negative for occult blood.
i. Explain test results to patient.	
j. If needed, reconnect enteral tube to drainage system, suction, or clamp as ordered.	Ensures proper function of enteral tube.

STEPS	RATIONALE
6. Collect stool specimen.	
a. Assist patient as needed into bathroom or to commode or bedpan. Instruct patient to void into toilet or urinal before collecting specimen in container. Provide a clean, dry bedpan or specimen hat in which to defecate.	Feces must not be mixed with urine, water, or toilet tissue. Urine inhibits fecal bacterial growth. Toilet tissue contains bismuth, which interferes with test results.
b. If needed, assist patient in washing after toileting and leave in a comfortable position.	
c. Transport specimen container with stool to bathroom or utility room and gather specimen.	
(1) Culture: Remove swab from sterile test tube, gather bean-size piece of stool, and return swab to tube. If stool is liquid, soak cotton swab in it and return to tube.	Use of sterile swab prevents introduction of bacteria.
(2) Timed stool specimen: Place stool from each collection in waxed cardboard container(s) for specific time ordered and keep in specimen refrigerator.	Tests for dietary products and digestive enzymes such as fat content or bile require analysis of all feces over select time period.
(a) For timed test, place signs that read "Save all stool" (with appropriate date or time) over patient's bed, on bathroom door, and above toilet.	Helps prevent any accidental disposal of stool.
(b) After obtaining the specimen for the laboratory, immediately place lid tightly on container.	Prevents spread of microorganisms by air or contact with other articles.
(3) All other tests, including Hemoccult (guaiac) test: Obtain specimen by using tongue blades and transfer portion of stool to container (2.5 cm [1 inch] of formed stool or 15 mL of liquid stool).	
7. Perform Hemoccult test.	
a. Use tip of wooden applicator to obtain small portion of feces.	
b. Open flap of Hemoccult slide. Apply thin smear of stool on paper in first box.	Guaiac paper inside box is sensitive to fecal blood content.
c. Obtain a second fecal specimen from different portion of stool and apply thinly to second box of slide (see illustration).	Occult blood from upper GI tract is not always dispersed equally through stool. Findings of occult blood are more conclusive when entire specimen is found to contain blood.
d. Close slide cover and turn slide over to reverse side. Open cardboard flap and apply 2 drops of Hemoccult developing solution on each box of guaiac paper (see illustration).	Developing solution penetrates underlying fecal specimen. Blood is indicated by change in color of guaiac paper.

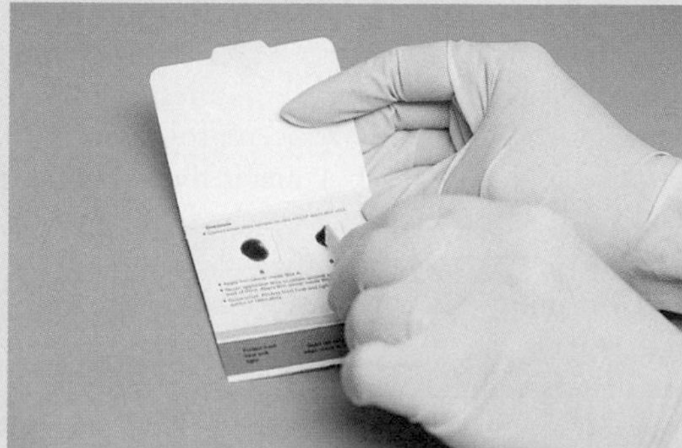

STEP 7c Apply stool to both spots on Hemoccult slide.

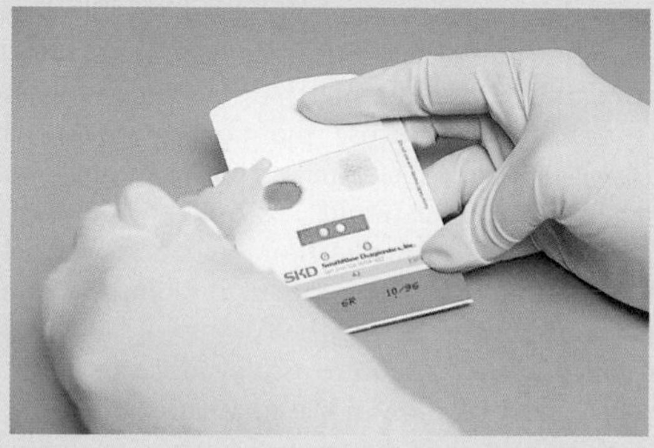

STEP 7d Apply developing solution to Hemoccult slide.

Continued

STEPS	RATIONALE
e. Read results of test after 30 to 60 seconds. Note color changes.	Bluish discoloration indicates occult blood (guaiac positive). No change in color of guaiac paper indicates negative results.
8. For timed specimen, label specimen (two identifiers, specimen source, collection date and time, number of bottle) in patient's presence, attach appropriate requisition (patient identification, date, time, name of test, and specimen source), and send to laboratory.	
9. **See Completion Protocol (inside front cover).**	

EVALUATION

1. Observe quantity, character, and color of stool, emesis, or GI secretions.
2. Compare test findings with normal expected results.
3. Ask patient to explain the purpose of the test.

Unexpected Outcomes and Related Interventions

1. Occult blood test results are positive.
   a. Continue to monitor patient and notify physician or health care provider.

Recording and Reporting

- Record results of test in appropriate records (check agency policy); include characteristics of specimen contents in nurses' notes.
- Report positive results to physician or health care provider.

Sample Documentation

1600 Large, liquid, dark brown stool tested positive for occult blood. Dr. Rains notified. Patient informed that test is to be repeated × 2.

Special Considerations

Pediatric

- Children of school age and older are concrete thinkers, often curious, and ask many questions about tests. Answer honestly and at child's level of understanding. Allow child to watch, if desired, while test is performed (Hockenberry and Wilson, 2009).

Home Care

- Patients are instructed to collect Hemoccult specimens at home and return them to the clinic or physician's office. To collect stool specimen, a piece of plastic wrap can be draped over the toilet. If possible the specimen should not be contaminated with urine. Patient or family caregiver prepares slide with feces, closes cardboard slide, and returns it to the office or clinic.

SKILL 8.3 BLOOD GLUCOSE MONITORING

A blood glucose meter is an effective and efficient method for assessing glucose control in the patient with diabetes mellitus. In the health care setting the monitor used may be different from the type the patient uses at home. The patient needs to know about the general principles for accurate glucose monitoring and reporting results. It is often helpful to request that a family member bring the meter from home to assess the patient's skill. Blood glucose monitoring (BGM) checks glucose levels in a sample of capillary blood, usually obtained from the fingertip. The results are used to direct lifestyle changes such as diet, medication, and physical activity. Regular BGM is an essential component of any diabetes self-management program (AADE, 2006).

Most glucose meters require a skin puncture to obtain a sample of capillary blood. You place the sample on a test strip and the meter calibrates the level of glucose in the sample. Immediate feedback on glucose levels helps patients prevent or recognize and quickly treat abnormal glucose levels according to the health care provider's instructions.

Today's meters are portable, lightweight, and run on batteries. They all provide fast results, usually in a minute or less and some even in 5 seconds (AADE, 2006). Although all meters use a drop of whole blood on a test strip, some read the plasma glucose level or have been programmed to calculate the plasma glucose level. A meter that provides plasma glucose levels has results that are closer to the laboratory results (USFDA, 2009). Many of the meters for home use have memory capability and can store 100 to 450 glucose readings.

Most meters now allow for the use of alternate site or forearm capillary blood testing. Many believe that this is less painful than fingerstick testing. Alternate-site testing is most accurate and correlates best to fingerstick testing when blood glucose levels are not changing rapidly, such as during the period when fasting blood glucose levels are being checked. When blood glucose levels are changing at a rapid level such as after meals or if the patient is experiencing hypoglycemic symptoms, it is best to use the fingertip testing site (AADE, 2006).

Single-use lancets and automatic lancing devices are part of glucose monitoring kits. Current practice in most agencies requires the use of a single-use lancet or a button activating single-use lancing device. Multiple-use lancet devices are intended for use with a disposable lancet with the device retained. Multiple-use lancet devices come with short and long lancet covers to provide different degrees of penetration, and many have adjustable covers or caps (ADA, 2009). A disposable needle needs to be placed in the lancet device for finger and alternate-site testing. It is recommended that the disposable needle be changed after each use and disposed of in an appropriate container such as a home sharps or No. 2 plastic container.

Glucose meters vary in size, shape, weight, ease of use, size of display readout, size of blood sample required, and other features. Medicare and many third-party payers now cover some or all of the cost of supplies for home monitoring if the patient is eligible. Setting goals for blood glucose levels needs to take into consideration the capacity and motivation of the patient to achieve the goals, the age of the patient, other illnesses, and the potential danger that hypoglycemia may occur for the patient (AADE, 2006). In otherwise healthy individuals with diabetes, blood glucose levels often are to remain as close to possible to the normal range (as determined by their physician). The frequency and timing of BGM should be dictated by the particular needs and goals of the patient (AADE, 2006).

This skill describes the technique used to measure blood glucose with a specific style of glucose meter. Specific steps in using meters vary, depending on the make and model of the equipment used. Always follow manufacturer instructions and facility policy and procedure when performing BGM.

ASSESSMENT

1. Assess patient's understanding of the procedure and the purpose and importance of BGM. *Rationale: Provides baseline on which to provide necessary teaching. Adults learn best when the teaching and learning relate to what the patient already knows.*
2. Review all medications that the patient is receiving. *Rationale: Drugs such as corticosteroids, diuretics, and anesthetics increase blood glucose levels. Anticoagulants increase risk for local ecchymosis and/or excessive bleeding from puncture site.*
3. Determine if specific conditions need to be met before or after glucose level is checked (e.g., fasting or postprandial status; medication administration, including insulin). *Rationale: Dietary intake, especially of carbohydrates, alters blood glucose levels. Premeal doses of short- or rapid-acting insulin are based on current blood glucose levels.*
4. Assess area of skin to be used as puncture site. Inspect fingers or forearms for edema, inflammation, or open cuts or sores. Avoid areas of bruising and/or open lesions and the hand on the side of a mastectomy. *Rationale: The puncture site should not be edematous, inflamed, or recently punctured because these factors cause increased interstitial fluid and blood to mix, which increases the risk for infection (Pagana and Pagana, 2010). The sides of the fingertips have fewer nerve endings and good vascularity.*
5. Review the physician's or health care provider's order for timing and frequency of blood glucose measurement. *Rationale: Test schedule is based on the patient's physiological status, risk for glucose imbalance, and any established facility protocols.*

PLANNING

Expected Outcomes focus on minimizing tissue damage at the puncture site, achieving accurate results, and maintaining blood glucose levels within the patient's goal range.

1. Puncture site shows no evidence of excessive or prolonged bleeding or tissue damage.
2. Blood glucose measurements are accurate.
3. Patient can verbalize procedure for self-monitoring of blood glucose and provide feedback on possible causes of results that are out of the target range.

Delegation and Collaboration

Assessment of the patient's condition may not be delegated. When the patient's condition is stable, the skill of obtaining and testing a sample of blood for blood glucose level may be delegated to nursing assistive personnel (NAP). Instruct the NAP by:

- Explaining what sites to use for the puncture and when to obtain glucose levels.
- Reviewing expected values and reminding to report all unexpected glucose levels to the nurse.

Equipment

- Antiseptic swab
- Lancet device, either self-activating or button activated
- Sterile single-use lancet specific to lancet device
- Blood glucose meter (e.g., OneTouch, FreeStyle Freedom)
- Blood glucose test strips appropriate for meter brand used
- Clean gloves

IMPLEMENTATION *for* BLOOD GLUCOSE MONITORING

STEPS	RATIONALE
1. See Standard Protocol (inside front cover).	
2. Identify patient using two identifiers (i.e., name and birth date or name and account number, according to facility policy). Compare identifiers with information in patient's medical record.	Ensures correct patient. Complies with The Joint Commission standards and improves patient safety (TJC, 2010).
3. Instruct patient to thoroughly wash hands and forearm (if applicable) with soap and warm water. Rinse and dry.	Reduces presence of microorganisms. Warmth promotes vasodilation at puncture site. Establishes practice for patient when test is performed at home.
4. Position patient comfortably in chair or in semi-Fowler's position in bed.	Ensures easy accessibility to puncture site.
5. Remove reagent strip from vial and tightly recap.	Protects strips from accidental discoloration caused by exposure to air or light.
6. Check the code on the test strip vial. Use test strips recommended for the glucose meter. Some newer meters do not require entering the code and/or have a disk or drum with 10 or more test strips.	Code on test strip must match code entered into the glucose meter to generate accurate results.
7. Insert the test strip into the meter. Do not bend the strip. The meter turns on automatically.	A bent strip does not measure blood sample accurately.
8. The meter displays a code on the screen. Match the code displayed with the code from the test strip vial. Press the proper button on the meter to confirm matching codes. The meter is ready for use.	Codes must match for meter to operate. Meters have different messages that confirm meter is ready for testing and blood can now be applied.
9. Prepare lancet device. Two types of lancet devices are used to perform skin punctures: single-use and multiple-use.	
a. Single-use lancet (see illustration). Place against skin and press lancet for self-activation lancet or press button on lancet to activate and puncture skin.	Decreases cross-contamination between patients.

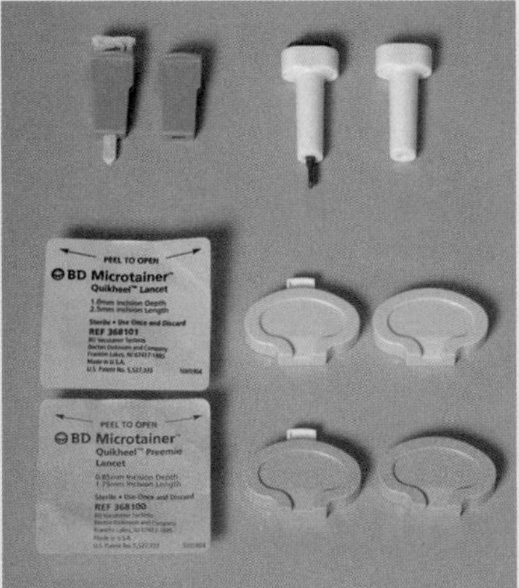

STEP 9a Single-use lancet devices. (Courtesy Zack Bent. From Garrels M, Oatis CS: *Laboratory testing for ambulatory settings: a guide for health care professionals*, Philadelphia, 2006, Saunders.)

STEPS	RATIONALE
b. Prepare a multiple-use lancet device with a new lancet. NOTE: Some meters recommend that this step be completed before preparing the test strip. Remove cap from lancet device. Insert new lancet. Some lancet devices have a disk or cylinder that rotates to a new lancet.	Never reuse a lancet because of risk of infection.

STEPS	RATIONALE
(1) Twist off the protective cover on the tip of the lancet. Replace the cap of the lancet device.	
(2) Cock the lancet device, adjusting for proper puncture depth.	Each patient varies as to depth of insertion needed for lancet to produce blood drop.
10. Obtain blood sample.	
a. Wipe finger or forearm lightly with antiseptic swab. Choose a vascular area for puncture site. In stable adults select lateral side of finger; be sure to avoid central tip of finger, which has a denser nerve supply (Pagana and Pagana, 2010).	Removes resident microorganisms. Too much alcohol can cause blood to hemolyze. Side of finger is less sensitive to pain and has a dense nerve supply. Do not use alternate site when patients are hypoglycemic, prone to hypoglycemia (during peak activity of an injected basal insulin or as long as 2 hours after injecting rapid-acting insulin), after exercise, during illness, or when blood glucose levels are rapidly increasing or decreasing (AADE, 2006).
b. Hold area to be punctured in a dependent position. Do not milk or massage the finger site.	Increases blood flow to area before puncture. Milking may hemolyze the specimen and introduce excess tissue fluid (Pagana and Pagana, 2010).
c. Hold the tip of the lancet device against the area of skin chosen for a test site (see illustration). Press the release button on the device. Some devices allow you to see the blood sample forming. Remove the device.	Placement ensures that lancet enters skin properly.
d. With some devices a blood sample begins to appear (see illustration). Otherwise gently squeeze or massage fingertip until a round drop of blood forms.	Adequate-size blood sample is needed to test glucose.
11. Obtain test results.	
a. Be sure that meter is still on. Bring the test strip in the meter to the drop of blood. The blood will be wicked onto the test strip (see illustration). (Follow specific meter directions to be sure that you obtain a full sample.) Do not scrape or apply blood to wrong side of test strip.	Blood enters strip, and glucose device shows message on screen to signal that enough blood is obtained. Scraping or use of wrong side of test strip prevents proper glucose measurement.
b. The blood glucose test result appears on the screen. Some devices beep when completed.	
12. Turn meter off. Some meters automatically turn off.	Meter is battery powered.
13. See Completion Protocol (inside front cover).	
14. Discuss test results with patient and encourage questions and eventual active participation in personal care if patient is newly diagnosed with diabetes.	Allow assessment of patient understanding for independence and proper use of equipment and supplies.

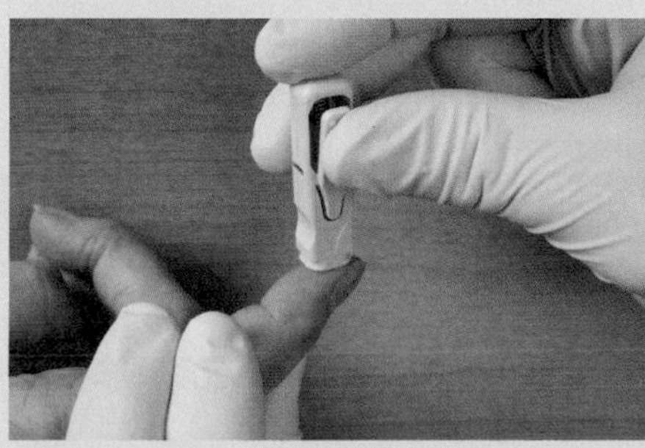

STEP 10c Prick side of finger with lancet.

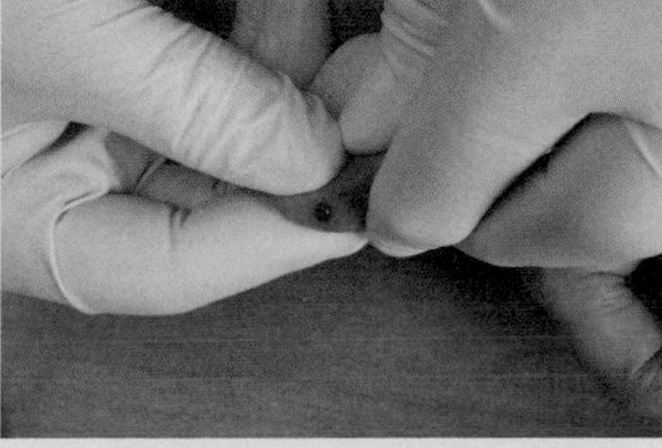

STEP 10d Droplet of blood appears after stick.

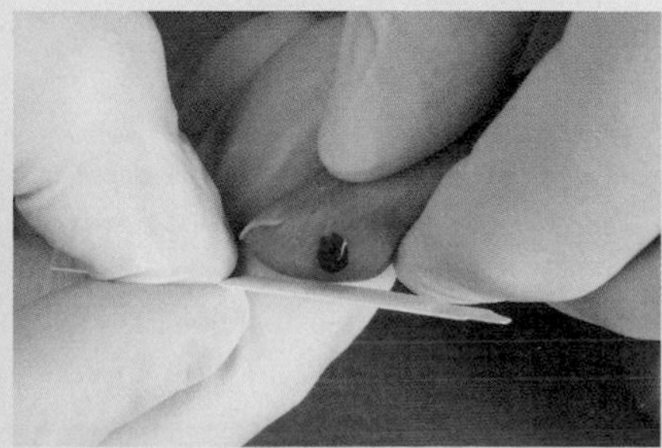

STEP 11a Wick blood onto test strip.

EVALUATION

1. Observe puncture site for evidence of bleeding or bruising.
2. Compare glucose meter reading with target blood glucose levels and prior test results.
3. Ask patient to discuss procedure and test results (have patient demonstrate next test).

Unexpected Outcomes and Related Interventions

1. Puncture site continues to bleed or is bruised.
   a. Apply pressure to site.
   b. Notify health care provider.
2. Glucose meter malfunctions.
   a. Repeat test, following directions.
   b. Follow manufacturer's directions for malfunctions.
3. Blood glucose level above or below target range.
   a. Continue to monitor patient.
   b. Follow agency protocol for laboratory confirmation testing of very high or very low results. Laboratory testing generally is considered more accurate.
   c. Check medical record to see if there is a medication order for deviations in glucose level; if not, notify physician or health care provider.
   d. Administer insulin or carbohydrate source as ordered (depending on glucose level).
   e. Notify health care provider of patient's response.

Recording and Reporting

- Record glucose results on appropriate flow sheet and describe response, including presence or absence of pain or excessive oozing of blood at puncture site.
- Report blood glucose levels out of target range and take appropriate action for hypoglycemia or hyperglycemia (Table 8-1).

Sample Documentation

(For insulin order based on total daily dose [TDD] of 50 units. May be recorded on flow sheet, MAR, and/or in narrative nursing notes.)

0730 Blood glucose 110, finished all food on breakfast tray.

1200 Blood glucose 240. Denies experiencing any signs and symptoms of hyperglycemia. Total of 9 units Humalog administered subcutaneously, 7 units ac plus 2 units per supplemental order.

TABLE 8-1 SIGNS AND SYMPTOMS OF BLOOD GLUCOSE ALTERATIONS

ALTERATION	ASSESSMENT FINDINGS
Hyperglycemia (elevated blood glucose)	Thirst, polyuria, polyphagia, weakness, fatigue, headache, blurred vision, nausea, vomiting, abdominal cramps
Hypoglycemia (low blood glucose)	Sweating, tachycardia, palpitations, nervousness, tremors, weakness, headache, mental confusion, fatigue

Special Considerations

Geriatric

- Older adults who have difficulty seeing the readings on the meter display screen may use a device with a larger display screen and lighted background or an audio blood glucose meter that gives verbal instructions to guide the patient through the procedure and give an audio result.
- Older adults with musculoskeletal alterations may not have the fine-motor coordination necessary to manipulate the device and place blood samples on test strips or insert strips in meter. Some models can be loaded with multiple strips.
- Warming fingertips may facilitate obtaining blood specimen.

Home Care

- Patients should usually assess blood glucose levels before meals, before taking medication, and at bedtime to monitor effectiveness of treatment plan.
- One or more family caregivers should be able to monitor blood glucose levels in the event that the patient is unable to do so independently.
- Some patients with diabetes check blood sugars before driving because they have hypoglycemic unawareness and need to see if their blood sugar is low or getting low before they get behind the wheel of a car.

SKILL 8.4 COLLECTING BLOOD SPECIMENS—VENIPUNCTURE WITH SYRINGE, VENIPUNCTURE WITH VACUTAINER, AND BLOOD CULTURES

Blood tests, one of the most commonly used diagnostic measures, yield valuable information about a patient's nutritional, hematological, metabolic, immune, and biochemical status. These tests allow health care providers to screen patients for early signs of physical illness, monitor changes in acute or chronic diseases, and evaluate responses to therapies.

Because larger veins are sources of blood for both laboratory tests and routes for intravenous (IV) fluid or blood administration, maintaining their integrity is essential. It is important to use the most distal sites first and retain one or more appropriate sites for IV access. Do not draw blood from a site proximal to an IV insertion site.

After obtaining a specimen, place it directly into the appropriate blood tube. A color-coding system for the tops of the collection tubes indicates the types of specimen that can be collected within that tube (see agency procedure). Special blood tubes may contain an additive. For example, a tube with an anticoagulant is used for a test that requires blood to not be clotted or hemolyzed.

Venipuncture is the most common method of obtaining blood specimens. This method involves insertion of a hollow-bore needle into the lumen of a large vein to obtain a specimen using either a needle and syringe or a Vacutainer device that allows the drawing of multiple samples.

Blood cultures aid in the detection of bacteria in the blood. It is important that at least two culture specimens be drawn from two different sites. Because fever and chills may accompany bacteremia, blood cultures may be drawn when symptoms are present (Pagana and Pagana, 2010). If only one culture produces bacteria, the assumption is that the bacteria were skin contaminants rather than the infecting agent. Bacteremia exists when both cultures grow the infectious agent.

ASSESSMENT

1. Determine patient's understanding of purpose of test and ability to cooperate with procedure. *Rationale: Procedure can appear threatening to patient.*
2. Determine if special conditions need to be met for specimen collection (e.g., patient allowed nothing by mouth [NPO], a specific time for collection in relation to time medication is given, need to ice specimen). *Rationale: Some patients have special conditions for accurate measurement of blood elements (e.g., fasting blood sugar, drug peak and trough, ammonia levels).*
3. Assess patient for possible risk factors for venipuncture, which include anticoagulant therapy, low platelet count, or bleeding disorder. Review medication history. *Rationale: Abnormal clotting caused by low platelet count, hemophilia, or medications increases risk for bleeding and hematoma formation.*
4. Assess patient for contraindicated sites for venipuncture: presence of IV infusion, hematoma at potential site, arm on side of mastectomy or axillary surgery, or hemodialysis shunt. *Rationale: Drawing specimens from such sites can result in false test results or may injure patient.*
5. Identify latex allergies, tape sensitivity, or povidone-iodine (Betadine) allergy. *Rationale: Determines the need for avoiding exposure to these items.*
6. When drawing blood cultures, assess for systemic evidence of bacteremia, including fever and chills. *Rationale: Three blood samples should be drawn at least 1 hour apart beginning at the earliest sign of sepsis (Pagana and Pagana, 2010).*
7. Review physician's or health care provider's order for type of blood tests. *Rationale: Order is required. Type of test determines blood tubes to use and amount of specimen.*

PLANNING

Expected Outcomes focus on the collection of an uncontaminated, appropriate blood specimen.

1. Patient explains purpose of blood collections before collection is attempted.
2. Venipuncture site shows no evidence of continued bleeding or hematoma.
3. Patient denies anxiety or discomfort.
4. An adequate sample is collected for testing (see agency report or appropriate laboratory manual).

Delegation and Collaboration

The skill of collecting blood specimens by venipuncture may be delegated to trained nursing assistive personnel (NAP). In some settings phlebotomists are available. Instruct the NAP by:

- Explaining patient's condition (e.g., presence of IV therapy, edema that affects extremity or vein for venipuncture selection).
- Instructing personnel to report patient's discomfort or signs of excessive bleeding to the nurse.

Equipment

All procedures

- Alcohol or antiseptic swab (check agency policy for use of 70% alcohol or other antiseptic solution)
- Clean gloves
- Small pillow or folded towel
- Sterile gauze pads (2 × 2 inch)
- Tourniquet
- Adhesive bandage or adhesive tape
- Appropriate blood tubes
- Identification labels
- Completed laboratory requisition, including appropriate patient identification, date, time, name of test, and source (for culture)
- Small plastic biohazard bag for delivery of specimen to laboratory (or as specified by agency)

Venipuncture with syringe

- Sterile safety needles (20- to 21-gauge for adults; 23- to 25-gauge for children)
- Sterile 10- to 20-mL Luer-Lok safety syringe

Venipuncture with vacutainer

- Vacutainer and safety access device with Luer-Lok adapter
- Sterile double-ended needles (20- to 21-gauge for adults; 23- to 25-gauge for children)
- Appropriate blood tubes (depending on tests being done)

Blood cultures

- Two 20-mL sterile syringes
- Sterile safety needles (20- to 21-gauge for adults; 23- to 25-gauge for children)
- Anaerobic and aerobic culture bottles (check agency policy)

IMPLEMENTATION *for* COLLECTING BLOOD SPECIMENS—VENIPUNCTURE WITH SYRINGE, VENIPUNCTURE WITH VACUTAINER, AND BLOOD CULTURES

STEPS	RATIONALE
1. See Standard Protocol (inside front cover).	
2. Identify patient using two identifiers (i.e., name and birth date or name and account number, according to facility policy). Compare identifiers with information in patient's medical record.	Ensures correct patient. Complies with The Joint Commission standards and improves patient safety (TJC, 2010).
3. Assist patient with lying supine or sitting in semi-Fowler's position or in a chair with arm supported and elbow extended. Place small pillow or towel under upper arm. (Option: lower arm briefly so it fills hand and lower arm with blood.)	Helps to stabilize extremity. Supported position in bed reduces chance of injury to patient if fainting occurs.
4. Apply tourniquet so it can be removed by pulling an end with a single motion.	Tourniquet blocks venous return to heart from extremity, causing veins to dilate for easier visibility.
a. Position the tourniquet 5 to 10 cm (3 to 4 inches) above venipuncture site selected.	
b. Cross the tourniquet over patient's arm (see illustration). May place tourniquet over gown sleeve to protect skin.	Older adult's skin is very fragile.
c. Hold tourniquet between your fingers close to the arm. Tuck a loop between the patient's arm and the tourniquet so you can grasp the free end easily (see illustration).	Pull free end to release tourniquet after the venipuncture.

SAFETY ALERT Palpate distal pulse (e.g., radial) below tourniquet. If pulse is not palpable, the tourniquet is too tight and impeding arterial blood flow. If this happens, remove and wait 60 seconds before reapplying tourniquet more loosely or using other extremity. Keeping the tourniquet in place no longer than 1 minute minimizes effects of hemoconcentration and hemolysis. Prolonged time may alter test results and cause pain and venous stasis (e.g., falsely elevated serum potassium level) (Warekois and Robinson, 2007).

STEPS	RATIONALE
5. Ask patient to *gently* open and close fist several times, finally leaving fist clenched.	
6. Quickly inspect extremity for best venipuncture site, looking for straight, prominent vein without swelling or hematoma. Of the three veins located in the antecubital area, the median cubital vein is preferred (see illustration).	This vein is large, well anchored (does not easily move), closer to the surface of the skin, and less painful to puncture. Straight and intact veins are easiest to puncture. The veins of the lower arm and hand are preferred for administering IV fluids.
7. Palpate selected vein with finger (see illustration). Note if vein is firm and rebounds when palpated or if it feels rigid and cordlike and rolls when palpated. Avoid vigorously slapping vein because this can cause vasospasm.	A healthy vein is elastic and rebounds on palpation. Thrombosed vein is rigid, rolls easily, and is difficult to puncture.

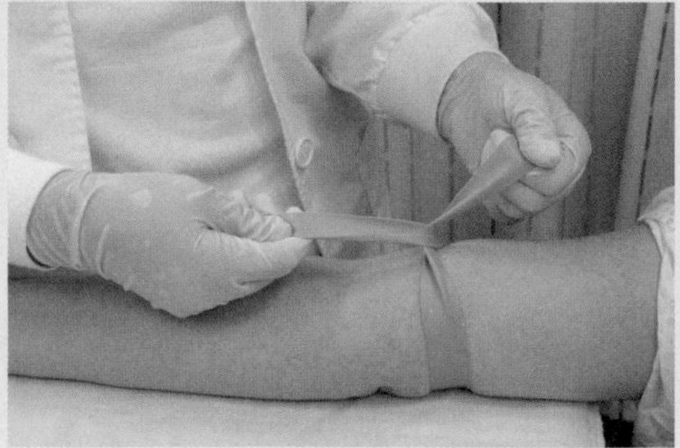

STEP 4b Cross tourniquet over the arm.

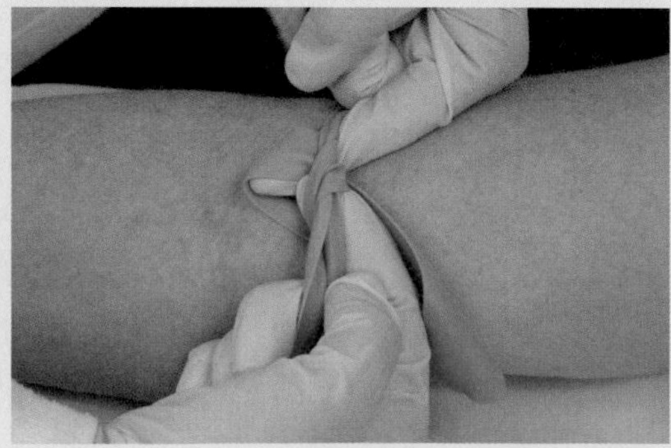

STEP 4c Tuck a loop between patient's arm and tourniquet.

STEPS	RATIONALE
8. Obtain blood specimen.	
a. Syringe method	
(1) Have syringe with appropriate needle attached.	
(2) Cleanse venipuncture site with antiseptic swabs, first swab moving back and forth on horizontal plane, then another swab on a vertical plane, and last in a circular motion from site outward for about 5 cm (2 inches) (see illustration). Allow to dry.	Antimicrobial agent cleans skin surface of resident bacteria so organisms do not enter puncture site. Allowing antiseptic to dry completes its antimicrobial task and reduces "sting" of venipuncture. Alcohol left on skin can cause hemolysis of sample.
(a) If drawing sample for blood alcohol level or blood cultures, use only antiseptic swab rather than alcohol swab.	Ensures accurate test results.
(3) Remove needle cover and inform patient of "stick" lasting only a few seconds.	Prepares patient and prevents sudden movement from the needle.
(4) Place thumb or forefinger of nondominant hand 2.5 cm (1 inch) below site, and gently pull skin taut. Stretch skin steadily until vein is stabilized.	Stabilizes vein and minimizes rolling during needle insertion.
(5) Hold syringe and needle at a 15- to 30-degree angle from patient's arm with bevel up.	Angle and bevel-up position facilitate entry of the needle into the vein.
(6) Slowly insert needle into vein, stopping when a "pop" is felt as needle enters vein (see illustration).	Prevents puncture through the opposite side of the vein.

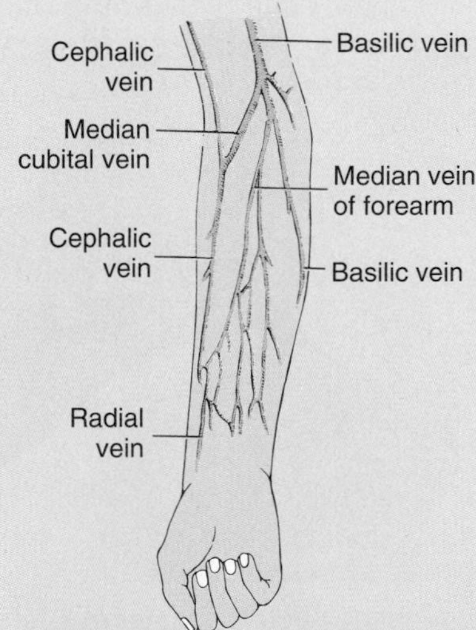

STEP 6 Location of antecubital veins.

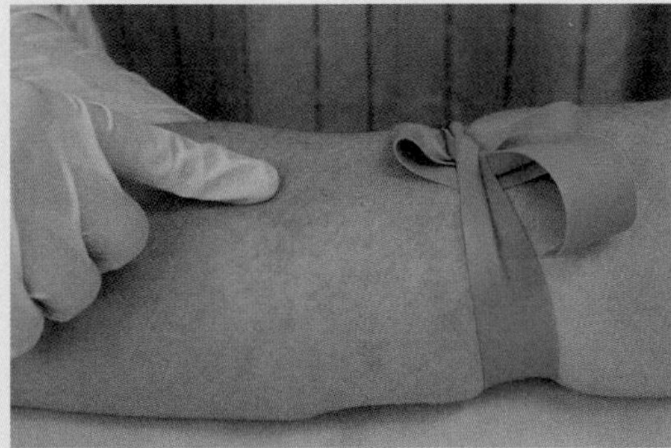

STEP 7 Palpate vein.

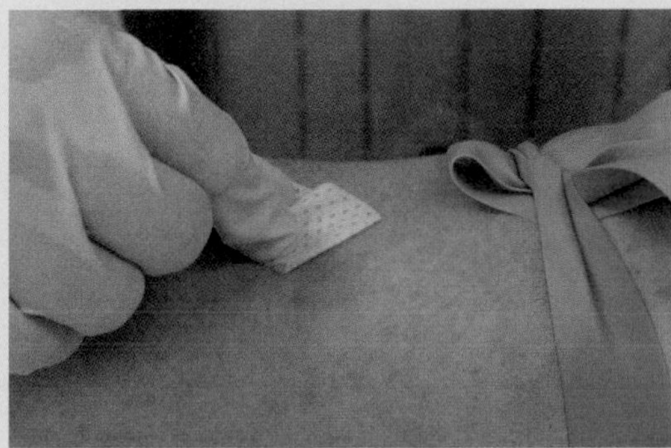

STEP 8a(2) Cleanse venipuncture site with antiseptic solution.

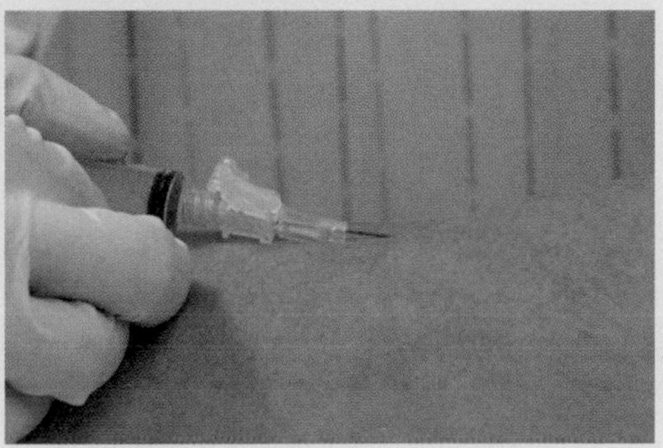

STEP 8a(6) Inserting needle into vein.

Continued

STEPS	RATIONALE
(7) Hold syringe securely and pull back gently on plunger.	Creates a vacuum for withdrawal of blood specimen.
(8) Observe for blood return and withdraw until you obtain the desired amount of blood.	Verifies placement in the vein.
(9) Release tourniquet before removing needle.	Reduces bleeding at site.
(10) Apply 2 × 2–inch gauze pad or alcohol swab over puncture site without pressure (see illustration). Quickly but carefully withdraw needle and apply pressure after removal of needle. If patient is on anticoagulants, hold site for several minutes.	Minimizes discomfort and trauma to vein. Prevents bruising and oozing of blood at venipuncture site.
(11) Activate needle safety cover and immediately discard needle in proper receptacle.	Phlebotomy equipment must include needle safety devices. Reduces risk of needlestick injury (OSHA, 2001).
(12) Attach blood-filled syringe to needle-free blood transfer device. Attach tube and allow vacuum to fill tube to specified level. Remove and fill other tubes as appropriate (see illustration). Gently rotate each tube back and forth 8 to 10 times.	Prevents needlestick injury. Tubes with additives should be inverted as soon as possible. Prevents clotting as additives are mixed with blood.
b. Vacutainer system method	
(1) Attach double-ended needle to Vacutainer tube (see illustration).	
(2) Have proper blood specimen tube resting inside Vacutainer device but do not puncture rubber stopper.	Tubes are color coded to indicate intended use based on size of tube and presence or absence of a chemical additive. Puncture of stopper results in loss of vacuum.

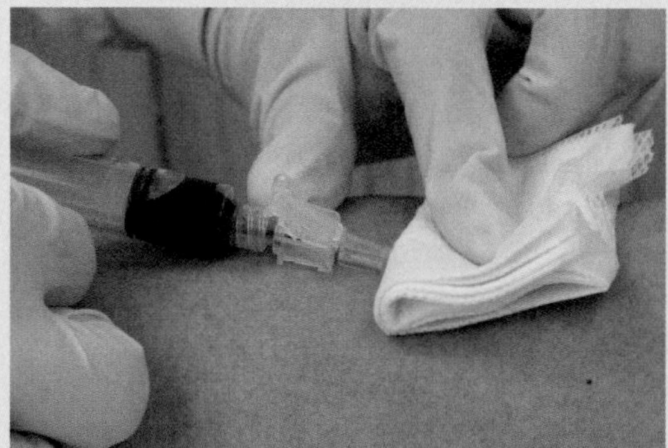

STEP 8a(10) Apply gauze over puncture site.

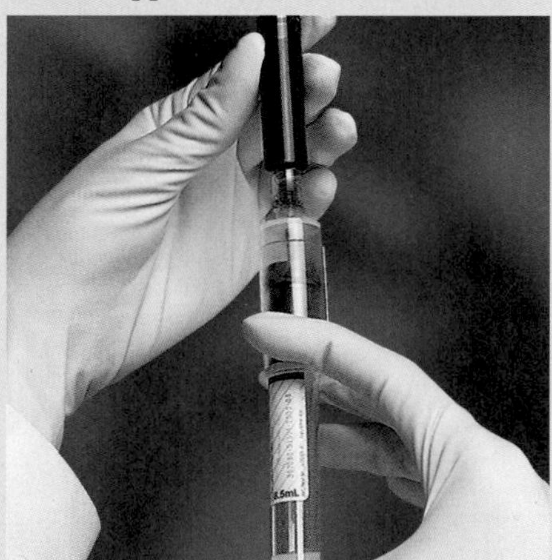

STEP 8a(12) Attach blood-filled syringe to needle-free blood transfer device. (Courtesy and © Becton, Dickinson and Company.)

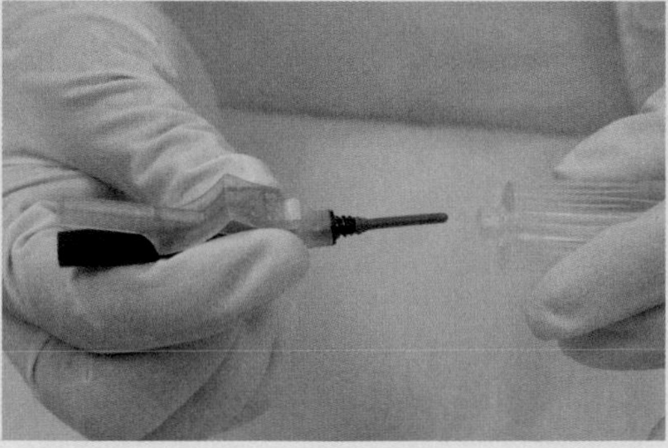

STEP 8b(1) Attach double-ended needle.

STEPS	RATIONALE
(3) Cleanse venipuncture site with alcohol swab (70% isopropyl alcohol) using a circular motion out from site for approximately 5 cm (2 inches). (See Step 8a(2) for antiseptic swab use.) Allow to dry.	Antimicrobial agent cleans skin surface of resident bacteria so organisms do not enter puncture site. Allowing alcohol to dry reduces "sting" of venipuncture. Alcohol left on skin can cause hemolysis of sample.
(4) Remove needle cover and inform patient that he or she will feel "stick" lasting only a few seconds.	Explanation of what to expect reduces anxiety.
(5) Place thumb or forefinger of nondominant hand 2.5 cm (1 inch) *below* site and pull skin taut. Stretch skin down until vein is stabilized.	Position of finger below site prevents accidental needlestick. Stretching helps to stabilize vein and prevents rolling during needle insertion.
(6) Hold Vacutainer needle at 15- to 30-degree angle from arm with bevel of needle up.	Reduces chance of penetrating both sides of vein during insertion and is less traumatic to the vein.
(7) Slowly insert needle into vein (see illustration).	Prevents puncture on opposite side.
(8) Grasp Vacutainer securely and advance specimen tube into needle of holder (do not advance needle in vein).	Pushing needle through stopper breaks vacuum and causes flow of blood into tube. Advancing needle into vein may puncture vein.
(9) Note flow of blood into tube, which should be fairly rapid (see illustration).	Failure of blood to appear indicates that vacuum in tube is lost or needle is not in vein.
(10) After filling specimen tube, grasp Vacutainer firmly and remove tube. Insert additional specimen tubes as needed. Gently rotate each tube back and forth 8 to 10 times.	Prevents needle from advancing or dislodging. Tubes with additives should be inverted as soon as possible. Prevents clotting as additives are mixed with blood.
(11) Release tourniquet before removing needle. Apply gauze and quickly withdraw needle. See Step 8a(10) (see illustration).	Reduces bleeding at site when needle is withdrawn.
c. ***Blood culture***	
(1) Cleanse venipuncture site with antiseptic swab (check agency policy). Allow to dry.	Antimicrobial agent cleans skin surface so organisms do not enter puncture site or contaminate culture. Drying ensures complete antimicrobial action.
(2) Clean bottle tops of culture bottles for 15 seconds with either alcohol or antiseptic swab. Check agency policy regarding cleaning solution.	Ensures that specimen is sterile.
(3) Collect 10 to 15 mL of venous blood using syringe method (Step 8a) from first venipuncture site and repeat procedure in other arm.	Cultures must be obtained from two sites to confirm culture growth.
(4) With each specimen activate needle safety cover, discard needle on syringe, and replace with new sterile needle before injecting blood sample into culture bottles.	Maintains sterile technique and prevents contamination of specimen.
(5) If both aerobic and anaerobic cultures are needed, fill the anaerobic container first (Pagana and Pagana, 2010).	Anaerobic organisms may take longer to grow.

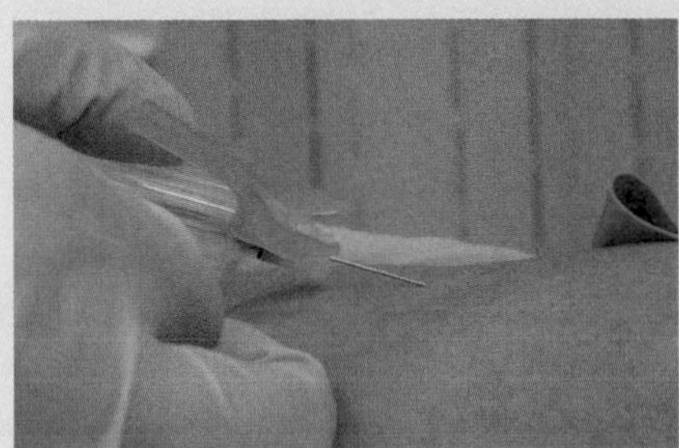
STEP 8b(7) Insert Vacutainer needle into vein.

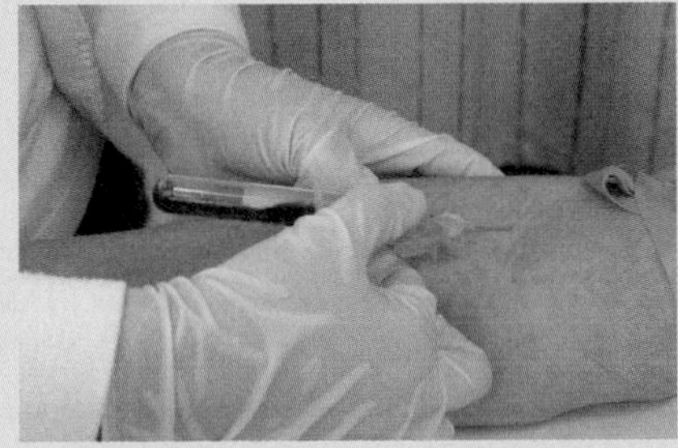
STEP 8b(9) Note rapid flow of blood into tube.

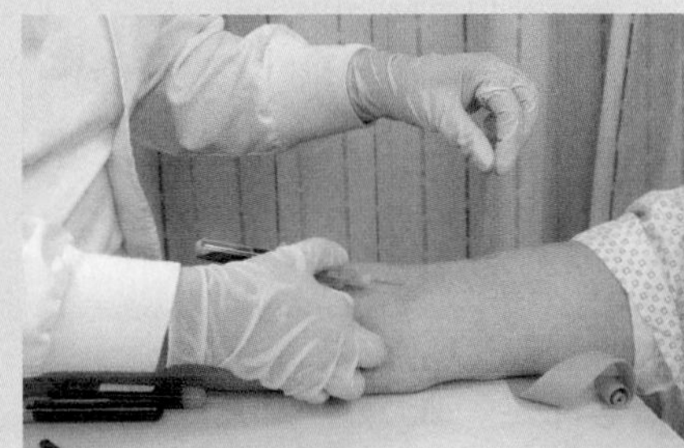
STEP 8b(11) Release tourniquet before removing needle.

Continued

STEPS	RATIONALE
(6) Gently mix blood in each culture bottle.	Mixes medium and blood.
(7) Release tourniquet, apply gauze over puncture site, and withdraw needle; see Step 8a(10).	
9. Observe for any sign of blood on outside of tube; wipe with 70% alcohol.	
10. Double needles have built-in safety cover; activate and then discard in proper receptacle for disposal.	One-handed technique and activation of safe needle devices helps to avoid needlestick injuries and exposure to potentially fatal bloodborne pathogens (OSHA, 2005).
11. In presence of patient, label the specimen with the patient identifiers, date, and time. Label each tube noting the arm from which specimen was drawn. Attach the proper completed requisition to specimen container.	Ensures diagnostic information reported on correct patient.
12. Place all specimens in plastic biohazard bag and send to laboratory. Send cultures immediately to laboratory (or at least within 30 minutes) (Pagana and Pagana, 2009).	Minimize spread of microorganisms.
13. See Completion Protocol (inside front cover).	

EVALUATION

1. Ask patient to explain purposes of tests.
2. Reinspect venipuncture site for hemostasis.
3. Determine if patient is anxious or fearful.
4. Check laboratory report for test results.

Unexpected Outcomes and Related Interventions

1. Hematoma forms at venipuncture site.
   a. Apply pressure using 2 × 2–inch gauze dressing.
   b. Continue to monitor patient for pain and discomfort.
2. Bleeding at site continues.
   a. Apply pressure and have patient help to maintain pressure on site; continue to monitor.
3. Laboratory tests reveal significantly abnormal blood results (see laboratory report or laboratory manual for normal limits).
   a. Report to physician or health care provider.

Recording and Reporting

- Record method used to obtain blood specimen, date and time collected, type of test ordered, site (for blood cultures) and laboratory receiving specimen; describe venipuncture site after specimen collection and patient's response to procedure.
- Report any stat or abnormal results to physician or health care provider.

Sample Documentation

1000 Serum chemistry and CBC specimens drawn from L antecubital fossa, 2 cm hematoma noted. Pressure applied using 2 × 2–inch gauze. Encouraged to elevate arm, continue pressure, and notify nurse if bleeding occurs or hematoma enlarges. Specimens sent to lab.

Special Considerations

Pediatric

- Explain procedure to child using developmentally appropriate language.
- Apply EMLA 60 minutes before procedure; or other local anesthetic cream may be ordered to reduce pain in infants and young children (Hockenberry and Wilson, 2009).
- When performing venipuncture on children, explore a variety of sources for vein access (e.g., scalp, antecubital fossa, saphenous veins, hand veins) to ensure access.
- Vacutainers are not recommended for children under 2 years of age because of possible vein collapse (Hockenberry and Wilson, 2009).

Geriatric

- Older adults have fragile skin and veins that are easily traumatized during venipuncture. Sometimes application of warm compresses may help in obtaining samples.
- A small-bore needle/catheter also may be beneficial.

SKILL 8.5 COLLECTING SPECIMENS FROM THE NOSE AND THROAT

When patients have signs and symptoms of upper respiratory or sinus infection, a nose or throat culture is a simple diagnostic tool to identify the presence and type of microorganisms. You should obtain cultures before antibiotic therapy is started because the antibiotic may interrupt the growth of the organism in the laboratory. If the patient is receiving antibiotics, notify the laboratory and explain what specific antibiotics the patient is receiving (Pagana and Pagana, 2010).

Collection of a specimen from the nose and throat can cause the patient discomfort and gagging because of sensitive mucosal membranes. It is important to collect a throat culture before mealtime or at least 1 hour after eating or drinking to lessen the chance of inducing vomiting and risk for aspiration. Patients should clearly understand how you will collect each specimen to minimize anxiety or discomfort.

ASSESSMENT

1. Assess patient's understanding of purpose of procedure and ability to cooperate. You may need assistance to obtain throat cultures from confused, combative, or unconscious patients. *Rationale: Provides basis to determine need for health teaching, need for assistance, and prevention of injury.*
2. Assess condition of and drainage from nasal mucosa and sinuses. *Rationale: Reveals physical signs that may indicate infection or allergic irritation.*
3. Determine if patient has experienced postnasal drip, sinus headache or tenderness, nasal congestion, or sore throat. *Rationale: Further clarifies nature of problem.*
4. Assess condition of posterior pharynx (see Chapter 7).
5. Assess for systemic indications of infection, including fever, chills, and malaise.

PLANNING

Expected Outcomes focus on obtaining an uncontaminated specimen in the appropriate amount for diagnosis and appropriate treatment.

1. Patient verbalizes understanding of purpose of specimen and how specimen is to be obtained.
2. Culture specimen is obtained without contamination from adjacent skin or tissues.
3. Patient does not experience bleeding of nasal mucosa.

Delegation and Collaboration

The skills of obtaining specimens from the throat and nose may not be delegated.

Equipment

- Two sterile swabs in sterile culture tubes (flexible wire swab with cotton tip may be used for nose cultures)
- Nasal speculum (optional)
- Tongue blades
- Penlight
- Emesis basin or clean container (optional)
- Facial tissues
- Gauze
- Clean gloves
- Identification labels
- Completed laboratory requisition, including appropriate patient identification, date, time, name of test, and source of culture
- Small plastic biohazard bag for delivery of specimen to laboratory (or container as specified by agency)

IMPLEMENTATION *for* COLLECTING SPECIMENS FROM THE NOSE AND THROAT

STEPS	RATIONALE
1. See Standard Protocol (inside front cover).	
2. Identify patient using two identifiers (i.e., name and birth date or name and account number, according to facility policy). Compare identifies with information in patient's medical record.	Ensures correct patient. Complies with The Joint Commission standards and improves patient safety (TJC, 2010).
3. Ask patient to sit erect in bed or on a chair facing you. Acutely ill patient may lie supported at 45-degree angle in semi-Fowler's position. Explain that patient may have tickling sensation or gag during swabbing of throat. Nasal swab may create urge to sneeze. State that procedure takes only a few seconds.	Provides easy access to oral structures.
4. Have swab in tube ready for use. You may want to loosen top so swab can be removed easily.	Most commercial tubes have a top that fits securely over end of swab, which allows nurse to touch outer top without contaminating swab stick.
5. Collect throat culture.	
a. Schedule procedure when patient's stomach is empty. In sitting position have patient tilt head backward. For patients in bed, place pillow behind shoulders.	Obtaining specimen on empty stomach reduces risk of vomiting and aspiration.
b. Ask patient to open mouth and say "ah."	Permits exposure of pharynx, relaxes throat muscles, and minimizes gag reflex.
c. Depress tongue with tongue blade if unable to expose pharynx and note inflamed areas of pharynx or tonsils. Depress anterior third of tongue only and illuminate with penlight as needed.	Area to be swabbed should be clearly visualized.

Continued

STEPS	RATIONALE
d. Insert swab without touching lips, teeth, tongue, or cheeks (see illustration).	Ensures collection of infected drainage.
e. Gently but quickly swab tonsillar area side to side, making contact with inflamed or purulent sites.	Collects microorganisms from the throat tissues without contamination from mouth or tongue.
f. Carefully withdraw swab without touching oral structures.	
6. ***Collect nasal culture.***	
a. Ask patient to blow nose and then check nostrils for patency with penlight. Select nostril with greatest patency.	Clears nasal passage of mucus that contains resident bacteria.
b. In sitting position have patient tilt head backward. Patients in bed should have pillow behind shoulders.	
c. Gently insert nasal speculum in one nostril *(optional)*.	Improves ability to view nasal mucosa and reach back of naris.
d. Carefully pass swab into nostril until it reaches the portion of mucosa that is inflamed or contains exudate. Rotate swab quickly. Note: If you need to obtain a nasopharyngeal culture, use a special swab on a flexible wire that can be flexed downward to reach nasopharynx.	Swab should remain sterile until it reaches area to be cultured. Rotating swab covers all surfaces where exudate is present.
e. Remove swab without touching sides of speculum or nasal canal.	Prevents contamination by resident bacteria.
f. Carefully remove nasal speculum (if used) and place in basin. Offer patient facial tissue.	
7. Insert swab into culture tube. Using gauze to protect your fingers, crush ampule at bottom of tube to release culture medium (see illustration).	Placing tip within culture medium maintains life of bacteria for testing.

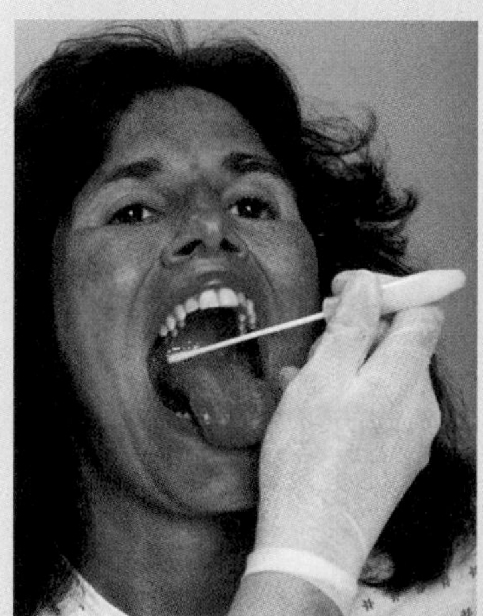

STEP 5d Collection of specimen from posterior pharynx. (From Pagana KD, Pagana TJ: *Mosby's manual of diagnostic and laboratory tests,* ed 4, St Louis, 2010, Mosby.)

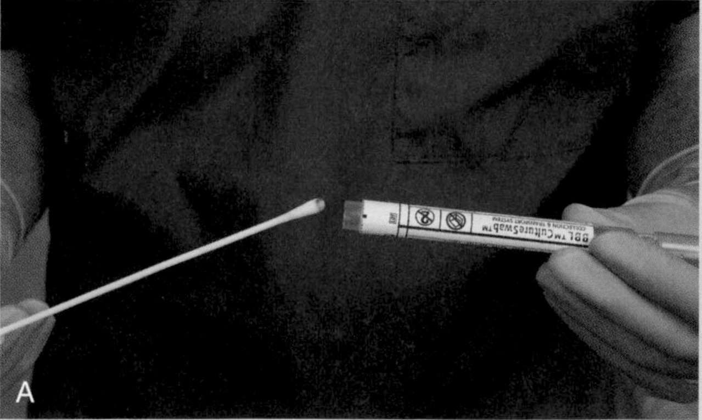

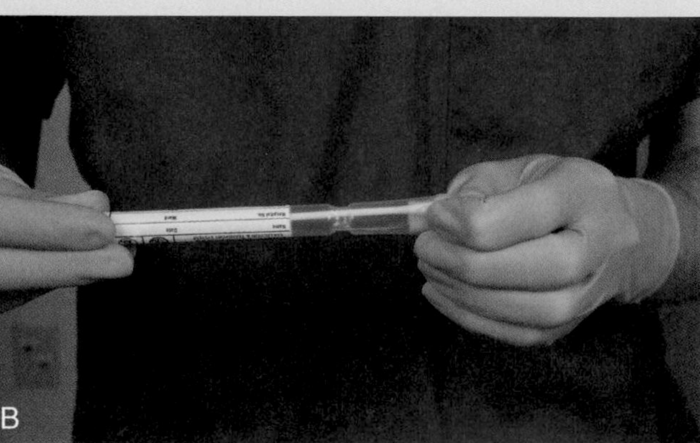

STEP 7 Activating culture tube. **A,** Place swab into tube. **B,** Crush end of tube to release liquid.

STEPS	RATIONALE
8. Push tip of swab into liquid medium.	Preserves specimen for testing.
9. Place top on tube securely.	
10. In presence of patient, complete identification label (two identifiers, specimen source, collection date and time) and attach to tube. Attach properly completed laboratory requisition to tube. Enclose specimen in plastic biohazard bag (according to agency policy) and send immediately to laboratory.	Incorrect identification of specimen could result in diagnostic or therapeutic errors. Specimen not sent to laboratory immediately or refrigerated allows growth of organisms and inaccurate results.
11. See Completion Protocol (inside front cover).	Reduces transmission of microorganisms.

EVALUATION

1. Ask patient to describe purpose of culture.
2. Monitor technique of culture collection process for potential contamination.
3. Inspect specimen for traces of blood and reinspect mucosa if bleeding is apparent.
4. Check laboratory report for test results.

Unexpected Outcomes and Related Interventions

1. Cultures reveal heavy bacterial growth.
   a. Notify physician or health care provider of results.
   b. Administer antibiotics as ordered.
2. Culture was contaminated by bacteria from adjacent skin or tissues.
   a. Notify physician or health care provider and repeat collection of cultures.
3. Patient experiences minor nasal bleeding.
   a. Apply mild pressure and ice pack over bridge of nose.
   b. Notify physician or health care provider of patient's condition.

Recording and Reporting

- Record type of specimen obtained, source, and time and date sent to laboratory; describe appearance of site and presence or absence of signs of local or systemic infection; note any unusual patient response to procedure.
- Report unusual test results to physician or health care provider.

Sample Documentation

0930 C/O sore throat, oral temp 101° F. Pharynx "red hot" with green-colored exudate noted on inspection. Obtained throat culture per order. Tolerated without gagging or discomfort. Specimen sent to lab.

Special Considerations

Pediatric

- Immobilization of child's head and arms is important when obtaining nose or throat culture and should be done in a firm, gentle, kind manner. Ask another nurse or ask and instruct a parent to assist if necessary.
- Showing tongue blade and penlight to child and demonstrating how to say "ah" helps to decrease anxiety.
- Do not attempt throat cultures if you suspect acute epiglottitis because trauma from swab might cause increase in edema and resulting occlusion of airway (Hockenberry and Wilson, 2009).

SKILL 8.6 COLLECTING A SPUTUM SPECIMEN

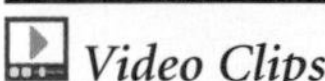
Video Clips

Sputum is mucus secretions produced by the cells of the lungs, bronchi, and trachea. You collect a specimen either by having a patient cough and expectorate into a sterile specimen container or by suctioning into a sterile sputum trap. In a normal health state sputum production is minimal; a disease state can increase the amount and character of sputum. Sputum specimens are collected for three purposes:

1. Cytology to identify cancer cells
2. Culture and sensitivity (C&S) to identify specific pathogens and determine the antibiotics to which they are most sensitive
3. Acid-fast bacillus to support the diagnosis of pulmonary tuberculosis

Nasotracheal suctioning is required to collect a sputum specimen when a patient cannot expectorate sputum. Suctioning can provoke violent coughing, which can induce vomiting and constriction of pharyngeal, laryngeal, and bronchial muscles. Suctioning can also cause direct stimulation of vagal nerve fibers, resulting in cardiac arrhythmias and increased intracranial pressure.

ASSESSMENT

1. Check physician's or health care provider's orders for number and type of specimens needed and time and method of collection.
2. Assess patient's understanding of procedure and its purpose.
3. Assess patient's ability to cough and expectorate sputum. *Rationale: Suction is not necessary when a patient can expectorate mucus.*
4. Determine when patient last ate a meal. *Rationale: It is best to obtain the specimen 1 to 2 hours after or 1 hour before a*

meal to minimize gagging, which can cause vomiting and aspiration.

5. Assess patient's respiratory status, including respiratory rate, depth, and pattern; lung sounds; and lung color. *Rationale: Changes in respiration may indicate the presence of secretions in tracheobronchial tree and potential need for supplementary oxygenation.*
6. Assess patient's anxiety level. Obtain a premedication order (i.e., sedative) if patient is extremely anxious. *Rationale: This procedure may be contraindicated in patients who cannot cooperate or remain still during the procedure (Pagana and Pagana, 2010).*

PLANNING

Expected Outcomes focus on collecting an uncontaminated specimen while maintaining a patent airway, adequate oxygenation, and patient comfort.

1. Patient's respirations are same rate and character before and after procedure.
2. Patient verbalizes understanding of the purpose and process of specimen collection.
3. Patient maintains comfort level and experiences minimal anxiety.
4. Sputum is not contaminated by saliva or oropharyngeal flora.

Delegation and Collaboration

Collection of a sputum specimen by suction may not be delegated. Collection of expectorated sputum specimens may be delegated to nursing assistive personnel (NAP). Instruct the NAP by:

- Instructing to notify nurse if patient expectorates bloody sputum.

Equipment

- Identification labels
- Completed laboratory requisition, including appropriate patient identification, date, time, name of test, and source of culture
- Small plastic biohazard bag for delivery of specimen to laboratory (or container as specified by agency)
- Suction device (wall or portable)
- Sterile suction catheter (size 13, 16, or 18 Fr [not large enough to cause trauma to nasal mucosa]) or suction catheter with sleeve
- Sterile gloves (a single glove if suction catheter has a sleeve)
- Clean gloves
- Sterile specimen container with cover
- Sterile water 100 mL container
- In-line specimen container (sputum trap)
- Oxygen therapy equipment if indicated
- Protective eyewear (if required)
- Facial tissue

IMPLEMENTATION *for* COLLECTING A SPUTUM SPECIMEN

STEPS	RATIONALE
1. **See Standard Protocol (inside front cover).**	
2. Identify patient using two identifiers (i.e., name and birth date or name and account number, according to facility policy). Compare identifiers with information in patient's medical record.	Ensures correct patient. Complies with The Joint Commission standards and improves patient safety (TJC, 2010).
3. Position patient in high- or semi-Fowler's position.	Promotes full lung expansion and facilitates ability to cough.
4. Explain steps of procedure and purpose. Encourage patient not to use mouthwash or toothpaste before procedure. During procedure have patient breathe normally.	Toothpaste and mouthwash may decrease the viability of microorganisms and alter culture results. Prevents hyperventilation.
5. ***Collect sputum specimen by suctioning.***	
a. Apply glove to nondominant hand. Prepare suction machine or device and make sure that it is functioning properly.	Adequate amount of suction is necessary to aspirate sputum.
b. Connect suction tube to adapter on sputum trap. Open sterile water.	
c. Apply sterile glove to dominant hand or use clean glove if suction catheter has sterile plastic sleeve.	Allows handling of suction catheter without introducing microorganisms into the sterile tracheobronchial tree.
d. Connect sterile suction catheter to rubber tubing on sputum trap.	Aspirated sputum goes directly to trap instead of to suction tubing.

STEPS	RATIONALE
e. Lubricate suction catheter tip with sterile water **(with suction off).** Gently insert tip of suction catheter through nasopharynx, endotracheal tube, or tracheostomy without applying suction (see Chapter 14) (see illustration).	Minimizes trauma to airway as catheter is inserted. Lubrication allows for easier insertion.
f. Gently and quickly advance catheter into trachea. Warn patient to expect to cough.	Placement of a catheter into larynx and trachea triggers cough reflex.
g. As patient coughs, apply suction for 5 to 10 seconds, collecting 2 to 10 mL of sputum.	Suctioning longer than 10 seconds can cause hypoxia and mucosal damage.
h. Release suction, remove catheter, and turn off suction. Detach and dispose of catheter into appropriate receptacle.	Releasing suction avoids unnecessary trauma to mucosa as the catheter is withdrawn.
i. Connect rubber tubing on sputum trap to plastic adapter (see illustration).	
6. ***Collect sputum specimen by expectoration.***	
a. Provide sputum cup and instruct patient not to touch inside of container.	Decreases contamination, which can alter results.
b. Instruct patient to take three to four deep slow breaths with full exhalation. Then take full inhalation followed immediately by a forceful cough, expectorating sputum directly into specimen container (see illustration). Repeat until 5 to 10 mL of sputum has been collected.	Sputum must come from tracheobronchial tree, and expectorant must not simply be saliva in mouth.
c. Secure lid on specimen container.	
7. If any sputum is present on outside of container, wipe it off with disinfectant.	Prevents spread of infection to persons handling specimen.
8. Offer patient tissues after suctioning.	
9. In presence of patient, complete label (two identifiers, specimen source, collection date and time) and attach to container. Attach completed laboratory requisition to container. Enclose specimen in a plastic biohazard bag and send immediately to laboratory.	Incorrect patient identification could lead to diagnostic or therapeutic error. Bacteria multiply quickly. Specimen should be analyzed promptly for accurate results.
10. Offer patient mouth care.	
11. **See Completion Protocol (inside front cover).**	

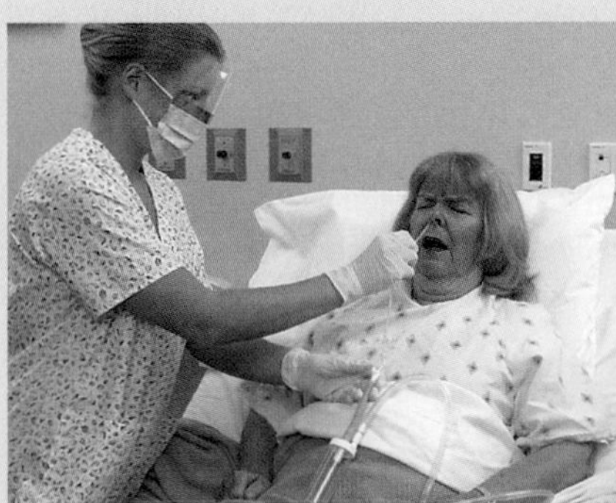

STEP 5e Insert catheter through nasopharynx.

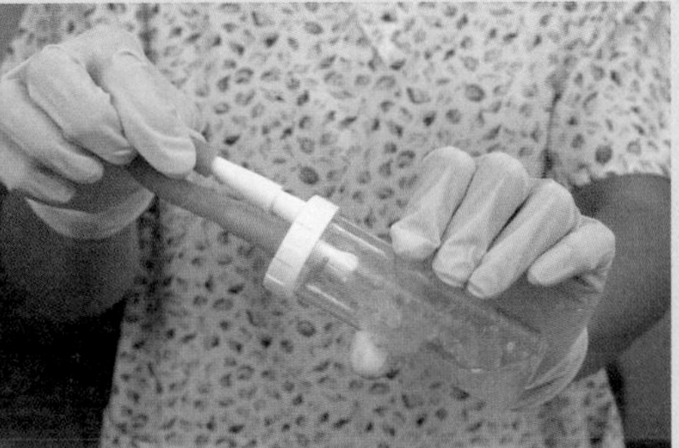

STEP 5i Closing sputum trap.

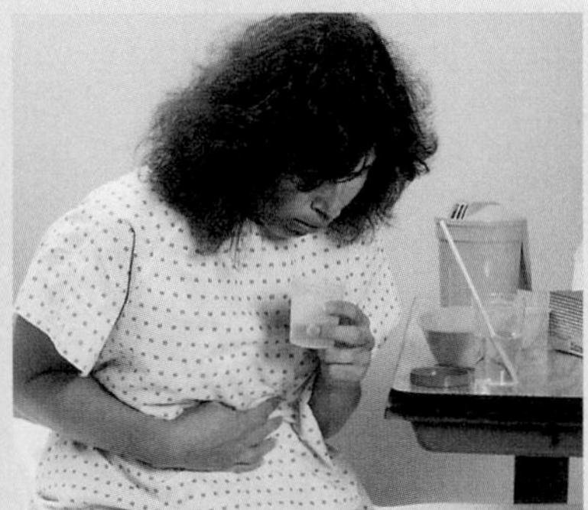

STEP 6b Expectorating sputum. (From Grimes D: Infectious diseases, *Mosby's clinical nursing series*, St Louis, 1991, Mosby.)

EVALUATION

1. Observe respiratory and oxygenation status throughout procedure, especially during suctioning.
2. Note behaviors suggesting anxiety or discomfort.
3. Observe character of sputum, color, consistency, odor, volume, viscosity, and/or presence of blood.
4. Refer to laboratory reports for test results.
5. Evaluate patient's ability to describe/demonstrate sputum collection process.

Unexpected Outcomes and Related Interventions

1. Patient becomes hypoxic with increased respiratory rate and shortness of breath.
   a. Discontinue suctioning immediately.
   b. Administer oxygen (if ordered).
   c. Monitor vital signs and oxygen saturation.
   d. Notify physician or health care provider if distress is unrelieved.
2. Inadequate amount of sputum is collected, or specimen contains saliva.
   a. Repeat collection procedure after patient has rested.
   b. Encourage patient to deep breathe and cough.
3. Patient remains anxious or complains of discomfort from suction catheter.
   a. Discontinue procedure until patient is stable.
   b. Provide oxygen as needed (if ordered).
   c. Notify physician or health care provider of patient's condition.
   d. Continue to monitor patient's vital signs. Consider measuring oxygen saturation.

Recording and Reporting

- Record method used to obtain specimen, date and time collected, type of test ordered, and transport to the laboratory. Describe characteristics of sputum specimen and patient's tolerance of procedure.
- Report any unusual findings such as bloody sputum or patient response such as increased dyspnea.

Sample Documentation

0730 Suctioned 13 mL thick green sputum for culture; immediately transported to lab for C&S. Reports slightly short of breath. Respirations 26. Rales noted bilaterally in all lung fields.

Special Considerations

Home Care

- If patient is to obtain a sputum specimen at home, instruct patient and/or family member regarding proper technique and importance of having sputum (not saliva) specimen sent to laboratory in timely manner.
- Discuss ways to avoid contaminating specimen (e.g., handwashing, using appropriate equipment).

SKILL 8.7 OBTAINING WOUND DRAINAGE SPECIMENS FOR CULTURE

- **Nursing Skills Online: Specimen Collection, Lesson 5**

When caring for a patient with a wound, the nurse assesses the condition of the wound and observes for the development of infection. Localized inflammation, tenderness, warmth at the wound site, and purulent drainage are signs and symptoms of wound infection. Infection is best treated with antibiotics after the causative organism(s) is confirmed from a wound culture.

Always collect a wound culture sample from fresh exudate from the center of a wound after removing old drainage. Resident colonies of bacteria on the skin grow in old wound exudate and may not be the true organisms causing infection.

Use separate techniques to collect specimens for measuring aerobic versus anaerobic microorganism growth. Aerobic organisms grow in superficial wounds exposed to the air. Anaerobic organisms grow deep within body cavities, where oxygen is not normally present.

ASSESSMENT

1. Assess patient's understanding of need for wound culture and ability to cooperate with procedure.
2. Assess patient for fever, chills, malaise, and elevated WBC count. *Rationale: Signs and symptoms indicate systemic infection.*
3. Assess severity of pain at wound site (scale of 0 to 10). *Rationale: If patient requires analgesic before dressing change or a wound culture, ideally medication is given 30 minutes before dressing change to reach peak effect.*
4. Review physician's or health care provider's order for aerobic or anaerobic culture.
5. Wear clean gloves to remove any soiled dressing. Apply sterile gloves to palpate wound. Observe for swelling, separation of wound edges, inflammation, and drainage. Palpate along wound edges and note tenderness or drainage.
6. Determine when dressing change is scheduled. *Rationale: This step may be performed immediately after specimen collection.*

PLANNING

Expected Outcomes focus on obtaining an uncontaminated specimen while maintaining patient comfort.

1. Culture swab is free of contaminants.
2. Patient denies discomfort during procedure.
3. Patient can discuss purpose and procedure for specimen collection.

Delegation and Collaboration

The skill of obtaining wound drainage for culture may not be delegated.

Equipment

- Culture tube with swab and transport medium for aerobic culture
- Anaerobic culture tube with swab (tubes contain carbon dioxide or nitrogen gas)
- 5- to 10-mL safety syringe and 19-gauge needle
- Clean gloves
- Sterile gloves
- Protective eyewear
- Antiseptic swab
- Sterile dressing materials (determined by type of dressing)
- Paper or plastic disposable bag
- Identification labels
- Completed laboratory requisition, including appropriate patient identification, date, time, name of test, and source of culture
- Small plastic biohazard bag for delivery of specimen to laboratory (or container as specified by agency)

IMPLEMENTATION *for* OBTAINING WOUND DRAINAGE SPECIMENS FOR CULTURE

STEPS	RATIONALE
1. See Standard Protocol (inside front cover).	
2. Identify patient using two identifiers (i.e., name and birth date or name and account number, according to facility policy). Compare identifiers with information in patient's medical record.	Ensures correct patient. Complies with The Joint Commission standards and improves patient safety (TJC, 2010).
3. Remove old dressing. Assess drainage. Fold soiled sides of dressing together and dispose in appropriate receptacle.	Provides baseline for condition of wound.
4. Cleanse area around wound edges with antiseptic swab. Wipe from edges outward. Remove old exudate.	Removes skin flora, preventing possible contamination of specimen.
5. Discard swab; remove and dispose of soiled gloves in trash bag.	
6. Open packages containing sterile culture tube and dressing supplies. **Apply sterile gloves.**	Provides sterile field from which nurse can handle supplies.
7. Obtain cultures.	
a. Aerobic culture	
(1) Take swab from culture tube, insert tip into wound in area of drainage, and rotate swab gently. Remove swab from wound and return to culture tube (wrap outside of ampule with gauze to prevent injury to your fingers). Crush ampule of medium and push swab into fluid.	Swab should be coated with fresh secretions from within wound. Medium keeps bacteria alive until analysis is complete.
b. Anaerobic culture	
(1) Take swab from special anaerobic culture tube, swab deeply into draining body cavity, and rotate gently. Remove swab from wound and return to culture tube.	Specimen is taken from deep cavity where oxygen is not present. Carbon dioxide or nitrogen gas keeps organisms alive until analysis is complete. Air injected into tube would cause organisms to die.
Or	
(2) Insert tip of syringe (without needle) into wound and aspirate 5 to 10 mL of exudate. Attach 19-gauge needle, expel all air, and inject drainage into special culture tube.	
8. In presence of patient, complete label (two identifiers, specimen source, collection date and time) and attach to tube. Attach completed laboratory requisition to tube. NOTE: Indicate on specimen requisition if patient is receiving antibiotics. Send specimens to laboratory immediately, no more than 30 minutes after collection (Pagana and Pagana, 2009).	Ensures correct results for correct patient. Bacteria grow rapidly. Cultures should be prepared quickly for accurate results.
9. Clean wound per care provider's orders. Apply new sterile dressing (see Chapter 24). Secure dressing with tape or ties.	Protects wound from further contamination and aids in absorbing drainage and debriding wound.
10. See Completion Protocol (inside front cover).	

EVALUATION

1. Observe character of wound drainage and edges of wound for redness and bleeding.
2. Ask patient to describe any discomfort during procedure.
3. Ask patient to describe purpose of culture.
4. Obtain laboratory report for results of cultures.

Unexpected Outcomes and Related Interventions

1. Wound cultures reveal heavy bacterial growth.
   a. Monitor patient for fever, chills, and increased WBC count.
   b. Inform physician or health care provider of findings.
2. Laboratory report indicates wound culture is contaminated with superficial skin cells.
   a. Monitor patient for fever and pain.
   b. Inform physician or health care provider.
   c. Repeat collection of specimen as ordered.

Recording and Reporting

- Record type of specimen obtained, source, and time and date specimen sent to laboratory; describe appearance of wound and characteristics of drainage; describe patient's tolerance to procedure and response to analgesia.
- Report any evidence of infection to physician or health care provider.

Sample Documentation

1320 Complains of pain from surgical site. Dressing change reveals 4-cm RLQ abdominal wound, separated at top with yellow purulent drainage. Lower half of incision remains well approximated. Aerobic culture obtained from site of drainage, sent to lab as ordered.

Special Considerations

Pediatric

- In some agencies, if you anticipate that the procedure will be painful for the child, perform procedure in area other than child's room, keeping child's room a safe place (Hockenberry and Wilson, 2009).

Home Care

- Risks for wound infections are different in the home setting than in the hospital setting because families are less susceptible to infections from microorganisms in their home environment. Careful handwashing and clean technique are usually adequate for performing dressing changes by patients and their families in the home.
- Inform family regarding signs and symptoms of wound infection and under what circumstances to notify the physician for evaluation of the need for a wound culture.

REVIEW QUESTIONS

Case Study for Questions 1 and 2

Mrs. Juanita Garcia, 82 years of age, was admitted to the medical-surgical unit 3 days ago for uncontrolled diabetes. She lives with her eldest daughter, Lilia Sanchez. Her fasting blood sugar has been decreasing with new medications and moving toward desired level of 110. At 7:00 AM the NAP reports that the patient seems confused, is complaining of frequency and burning with urination. Vital signs: BP 98/80, pulse 86, respiratory rate 20, temperature 38.4° C (101.2° F), fasting blood sugar 165. You recheck the vital signs and fasting blood sugar and her indwelling catheter bag and note that her urine is cloudy, pink tinged and foul smelling; when asked if she knows what this building is called, she is unable to state that she is in a hospital or state her date of birth.

1. The nurse calls the physician and receives an order for a urine culture and sensitivity (C&S). The nurse takes the urine sample from the needleless port of the catheter. Place the following steps in correct order for obtaining a sterile urine specimen: (a) Withdraw 3 to 5 mL of urine and, using sterile technique, instill into a sterile urine container. (b) Perform hand hygiene and apply gloves. (c) Attach completed requisition and immediately send to the laboratory. (d) Wipe needleless port with antiseptic wipe and attach 3-mL Luer-Lok syringe. (e) Attach label to sterile urine container and double bag.
   1. d, b, a, c, e
   2. b, d, c, a, e
   3. d, b, c, e, a
   4. b, d, a, e, c
2. Which of the following indicates that Mrs. Sanchez understands the importance of having a C&S test done on her mother's urine?
   1. "The C&S test is not necessary if her diabetes is under control."
   2. "She always gets the same medication for her urine infections; so she doesn't need a test."
   3. "The C&S test is important so the doctor can order the correct medication for the kind of bacteria in the urine."
   4. "The C&S test is only necessary when she has a catheter."
3. Mrs. Murphy, newly diagnosed with diabetes, performs her blood glucose test before meals and at bedtime. She tells the nurse that her fingers are getting sore and she has trouble getting a droplet of blood large enough for testing. Which of the following interventions would be most appropriate for the nurse?
   1. Instruct her to use the forearm for a blood droplet.
   2. Apply pressure to the puncture site for at least 1 minute before a puncture.
   3. Cleanse site with warm water and allow to dry.
   4. Place the lancet firmly against the site to ensure an appropriate depth of puncture.

4. Which is the preferred vein for venipuncture for phlebotomy?
   1. The antecubital vein, which is less painful
   2. The basilic vein, which is straight
   3. The cephalic vein, which is in the hand and well anchored
   4. The median cubital vein, which is larger and closer to the surface
5. One of the unexpected outcomes of collection of a nasal culture is nasal bleeding. Which of the following interventions would be most appropriate if it occurs?
   1. Provide analgesia as ordered.
   2. Administer antibiotics as ordered.
   3. Perform nasal suctioning of involved naris.
   4. Apply pressure and ice over bridge of nose.
6. The laboratory results for a wound specimen indicated contamination with superficial skin cells. Which of the following actions would the nurse take?
   1. Begin antibiotic therapy.
   2. Monitor patient.
   3. Perform repeat wound specimen collection.
   4. Clean wound with sterile water.
7. Mrs. Henderson started on a 24-hour urine collection at 0800. At 1200 the nurse notes that the hat for collection of urine is on the floor in the bathroom and empty. Questioning indicates that the patient has been voiding in the toilet and flushing. Which is the nurse's most appropriate initial intervention?
   1. Assess Mrs. Henderson's understanding of a 24-hour urine collection.
   2. Continue to collect urine for the remainder of the 24 hours.
   3. Stop the procedure and restart urine collections.
   4. Have patient drink at least one glass of water every hour.
8. This is the third admission for Mr. Burger in 4 months for hyperglycemia. He has insulin-dependent diabetes and has been instructed to perform fingersticks before each meal and at bedtime. Which statement indicates that Mr. Burger understands and does not need further teaching? Select all that apply.
   1. "My sight is poor; so I need to have my son Jeff to help me read the meter."
   2. "My friend Stan said I should do like he does and only poke my finger in the morning to save money."
   3. "I need to be sure that I take my blood sugar before I eat and before bed."
   4. "I take the same amount of insulin every morning but still need to do the fingerstick."
9. The nurse plans to collect a blood specimen. After placing the tourniquet above the elbow, she palpates absence of the radial pulse. Which nursing intervention should be first?
   1. Remove the tourniquet impeding venous blood flow, wait 60 minutes, and then reapply.
   2. Continue performing the phlebotomy; the blood specimen is from the venous system.
   3. Remove the tourniquet to allow arterial blood flow to return, wait 60 seconds, and then reapply the tourniquet.
   4. Palpate for the brachial pulse above the tourniquet.

REFERENCES

American Association of Diabetic Educators (AADE): *The art and science of diabetic self-care management education: a desk reference for health care professionals*, Chicago, 2006, AADE.

American College of Gastroenterology (ACG): *Understanding gastrointestinal bleeding, a consumer's brochure*, Bethesda, Md, 2009, ACG, http://www.acg.gi.org/patients/gibleeding/index.asp, accessed August 2, 2010.

American Diabetes Association (ADA): *2008 Resource guide, diabetes forecast (supplement)*, January 2008, http://www.diabetes.org, accessed July 29, 2010.

American Diabetes Association (ADA): *2009 Resource guide, diabetes forecast (supplement)*, January 2009, http://www.diabetes.org, accessed July 28, 2010.

Hamill T: *Point of care: Multistix 9 and Unistix urinalysis*, San Francisco, March 8, 2007, UCSF Clinical Laboratory; http://pathology.ucsf.edu/labmanual/mftlng-mtzn/dnld/poct-MultistixUristix.pdf, accessed August 31, 2010.

Hockenberry MJ, Wilson D, *Wong's essentials of pediatric nursing*, ed 8, St Louis, 2009, Elsevier.

Occupational Safety and Health Administration (OSHA): *CPL 02-02-069-CPL 2-2.69—enforcement procedures for the occupational exposure to bloodborne pathogens*, November 27, 2001, http://www.osha.gov/pls/oshaweb/owadisp.show_document?p_table=DIRECTIVES&p_id=2570, accessed July 29, 2010.

Occupational Safety and Health Administration (OSHA): Occupational exposure to bloodborne pathogens: final rule, *Fed Reg* 66(12):5318, Update 2005.

Pagana KD, Pagana TJ: *Mosby's manual of diagnostic and laboratory tests*, ed 4, St Louis, 2010, Mosby.

Pagana KD, Pagana TJ: *Mosby's diagnostic and laboratory tests reference*, ed 9, St Louis, 2009, Mosby.

Stacey A: *Personal hygiene (part 2 of 2): the natural way*, June 23, 2009, http://www.islamreligion.com/articles/2178, accessed August 31, 2010.

The Joint Commission (TJC): *2010 National patient safety goals*, Oakbrook Terrace, Ill, 2010, The Commission, http://www.jointcommission.org/PatientSafety/NationalPatientSafetyGoals, accessed July 29, 2010.

US Department of Health and Human Services (USDHHS): Patient safety and quality improvement; final rule, *Federal Register* 73(226):70731-70814, 2008 (codified at 42 C.F.R. Part 3 [73 FR 70732]).

US Food and Drug Administration (USFDA): *Medical device: glucose testing device*, August 31, 2009, http://www.fda.gov/MedicalDevices/ProductsandMedicalProcedures/InVitroDiagnostics/GlucoseTestingDevices/default.htm, accessed July 29, 2010.

Warekois RS, Robinson R: *Phlebotomy: work text and procedures manual*, Philadelphia, 2007, Saunders.

CHAPTER

9

Diagnostic Procedures

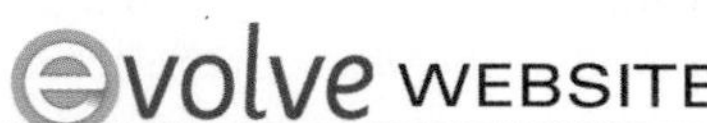

http://evolve.elsevier.com/Perry/nursinginterventions

PATIENT-CENTERED CARE

For patients, diagnostic procedures are often confusing, frightening, and occasionally embarrassing. Some diagnostic procedures are performed at the patient's bedside or in specially equipped rooms. Other testing occurs in an outpatient setting, and the patient has a series of preprocedure medications and activities to complete at home. It is important to educate the patient about the preprocedure activities so they are completed correctly. A delay of the test occurs if preprocedure activities are omitted or not performed correctly.

During diagnostic procedures you are responsible for assessing the patient's knowledge of the procedure; preparing the patient; providing a safe environment throughout the procedure; providing preprocedure assessment, care, teaching, and documentation; and performing postprocedural care.

It is important to know why the patient is having the diagnostic test and what types of outcomes are expected or feared. Anxiety may be related to the preprocedure preparation, the procedure itself, or the potential outcome of the test. For example, a colonoscopy is a routine examination for adults over 50. It is an effective screening mechanism for early-stage colon cancer. However, even though it is a screening procedure, the patient may have some anxiety over the unknown. When there are signs and symptoms such as a change in bowel habits, rectal bleeding, or suspicion of a tumor, the potential diagnosis may cause anxiety.

Often these tests are done for diagnostic purposes to determine the need for surgery. Follow-up diagnostic procedures document the progression of a medical condition or determine the effectiveness of a treatment plan. Approach your patients with concern and provide an opportunity for them to ask questions about the preprocedure preparation and the procedure and to voice concerns about possible outcomes of the test.

SAFETY

If the patient requires moderate sedation for the procedure, maintaining a patent airway following the procedure is a primary safety concern. Patients are usually fully recovered from sedation before being discharged from the diagnostic procedure area. However, patients with renal or liver disease often take longer to metabolize the sedation medications and become drowsy after they return to the hospital unit or discharged home. It is important to ensure that you can awaken the patient and instruct the family to do the same. In the case of an outpatient procedure that requires sedation, the patient must come to the diagnostic center with a designated driver. Instruct the patient not to drive for 24 hours following the procedure. If you are admitting a patient to the diagnostic center, verify that there is a designated driver or that the patient has arranged for transportation before the procedure begins.

Intravenous (IV) sedation is often used for diagnostic or surgical procedures that do not require complete anesthesia in acute care, surgical care, and outpatient care settings. The terminology used for procedural sedation is now classified as "minimal," "moderate," or "deep" sedation/analgesia. In procedures that require sedation, agencies maintain standards for preassessing, preparing, and monitoring patients.

Moderate sedation improves the patient's cooperation with a procedure, allows a rapid return to the preprocedure status, and minimizes the risk of injury. In addition, it often raises the patient's pain threshold and provides amnesia concerning the actual procedural events. Moderate sedation is a drug-induced depression of consciousness during which patients respond purposefully to verbal commands, either alone or accompanied by light tactile stimulation. In addition, no interventions are required to maintain a patent airway, and spontaneous ventilation is adequate (American Society of Anesthesiologists, 2004).

Deep sedation is one risk associated with moderate sedation when the patient's level of consciousness (LOC) decreases past the point where a patent airway cannot be maintained. Because of this risk, the use of IV moderate sedation is closely controlled and normally restricted to physicians and nurses who receive specialized training or credentialing (AANA, 2004). Know the agency policy for recommended and maximum doses of medications monitoring and documentation requirements when using IV sedation.

The most common types of medications used to achieve moderate sedation include benzodiazepines and opiates. Benzodiazepines reduce anxiety and promote muscle relaxation. Midazolam (Versed), in particular, also produces an amnesic effect. Patient risks during IV sedation include hypoventilation, airway compromise, hemodynamic instability, and/or altered LOCs that include an overly depressed LOC or agitation and combativeness. Emergency equipment appropriate for the patient's age and size (see Chapter 30) and staff with skill in airway management, oxygen delivery, and use of resuscitation equipment are essential. During and after the procedure, patients need continuous monitoring of vital signs, airway patency, oxygen saturation, heart rhythm, lung sounds, and LOC. As the patient recovers from sedation, it is imperative that accurate assessments document the level of recovery. Table 9-1 identifies evidence-based objective criteria to monitor a patient's recovery from IV sedation.

Another safety concern is associated with invasive procedures involving injection of radiopaque dye. The physician is responsible for giving an explanation of what is involved with the test, the risks involved, expected benefits, alternative methods of treatment available, and probable outcomes. Some patients are allergic to dye contrast material used in some of the diagnostic procedures to enhance visualization of the internal structures and organs. You must carefully assess a patient for any latex, food, or medication allergies. Ensure that any allergy is noted on the patient's identification according to agency policy. Last, be sure that the physician performing the diagnostic test is aware of the allergy. In some situations when dye is necessary to obtain accurate results and the patient has an allergy to the dye or iodine, the patient is premedicated with an antihistamine such as diphenhydramine (Benadryl), to reduce the chance of an allergic reaction.

TABLE 9-1 ALDRETE SCORING SYSTEM

		SCORE
Activity (moving voluntarily on command)	4 extremities	2
	2 extremities	1
	0 extremities	0
Respiration	Able to deep breathe and cough freely	2
	Dyspnea, shallow or limited breathing	1
	Apneic	0
Circulation	BP ± 20 mm Hg of presedation level	2
	BP ± 20-50 mm Hg of presedation level	1
	BP ± 50 mm Hg of presedation level	0
Consciousness	Fully awake	2
	Arousable on having name called	1
	Not responding	0
Color	Normal	2
	Pale, dusky, blotchy, jaundiced or other change	1
	Cyanotic	0

From Aldrete JA: The post anesthesia recovery score revisited, *J Clin Anesth* 7:89, 1995; and Aldrete JA: Post-anesthetic recovery score, *J Am Coll Surg* 205(5):3, 2007.

EVIDENCE-BASED PRACTICE TRENDS

Ahmed SV and others: Post lumbar puncture headache, *Postgrad Med J* 82(973):713, 2006.

Hon LQ and others: Vascular closure devices: a comparative overview, *Curr Probl Diagn Radiol* 38(1):33, 2009.

Lee LC and others: Prevention and management of post-lumbar puncture headache in pediatric oncology patients, *J Pediatr Oncol Nurs* 24(4):200, 2007.

The use of a vascular closure device (VCD) is now common after procedures involving an arteriotomy. The devices apply manual compression to prevent bleeding at the arterial site. VCDs are available in varieties that mechanically "plug" the arteriotomy or percutaneously apply pressure over the site. Clinical trials on these devices show that VCDs decrease the time needed for hemostasis (cessation of bleeding) and return to ambulation. As a result, the devices increase patient comfort and mobility. However, because each device leaves behind foreign material (e.g., clip, sealant, suture), infection is a concern (Hon and others, 2009).

Postpuncture headaches (PPHDs) after lumbar puncture (LP) can last for several days and are incapacitating. Current literature includes practice guidelines for managing PPHDs and interventions to prevent headaches, including adequate bed rest and hydration (Lee and others, 2007). Another effective intervention includes postprocedure application of an epidural patch for pain management (Ahmed and others, 2006; Lee and others, 2007).

SKILL 9.1 CONTRAST MEDIA STUDIES: ARTERIOGRAM (ANGIOGRAM), CARDIAC CATHETERIZATION, INTRAVENOUS PYELOGRAM

Contrast media studies involve visualization of blood vessel structure of the body by the intravascular injection of a radiopaque medium. An arteriogram (angiogram) permits visualization of the vasculature of an organ and the arterial system of the organ. Arteriography is most frequently performed by an interventional radiologist to diagnose occlusions, stenosis, emboli, thromboses, aneurysms, tumors, congenital malformations, or trauma anywhere in the body.

Cardiac catheterization is a specialized form of angiography in which a catheter is inserted into the left and/or right side of the heart via a peripheral major blood vessel, usually the femoral artery and/or vein. However, the brachial artery/vein can also be used. A contrast medium is injected, and the structures and functions of the heart are assessed. The test studies pressures within the heart and lungs, cardiac volumes, valve function, and patency of coronary arteries. Cardiac catheterizations are performed in specially equipped laboratories (Fig. 9-1). A contrast medium is injected into either the right and/or left side of the heart, and cardiac structure and function are assessed.

Cardiac catheterizations are contraindicated in patients who refuse needed surgery, are allergic to iodine contrast media, are uncooperative or cannot lie still during the entire procedure, or are susceptible to dye-induced renal failure. When a cardiac catheterization is essential for patients with allergies to iodine contrast media, a nonionic media is used, or the patient is pretreated with medications to reduce the allergic reactions. Precautions to help prevent dye-induced renal failure include making sure that the patient is well hydrated; medicating with acetylcysteine (Mucomyst) before, during, and after the procedure; and using nonionic (instead of ionic) contrast media (Murray and others, 2006).

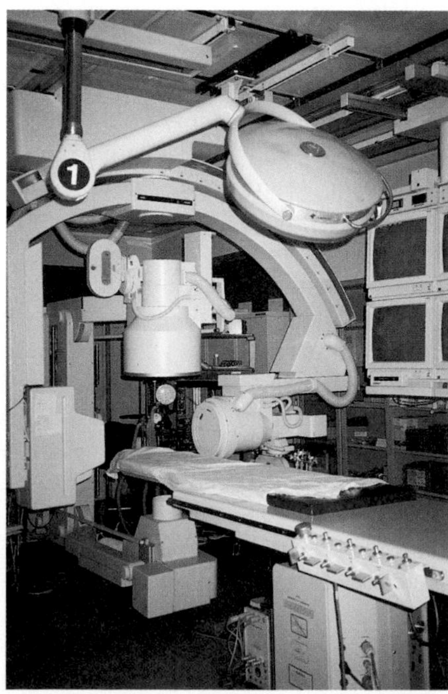

FIG 9-1 Cardiac catheterization procedure room. (From Wong MJ, Wilson D: *Wong's nursing care of infants and children*, ed 8, St Louis, 2007, Mosby.)

Intravenous pyelography (IVP) is an examination of the flow of radiopaque contrast medium through the kidneys, ureters, and bladder to identify obstruction, hematuria, stones, bladder injury, or renal artery occlusion. Dye is injected via a catheter through a peripheral artery, and serial radiographs are taken over the subsequent 30 minutes.

ASSESSMENT

1. Verify that informed consent was obtained. *Rationale: Federal regulations, many state laws, and accreditation agencies require informed consent for procedures.*
2. Determine if patient is taking anticoagulants, aspirin, or any nonsteroidal medication. *Rationale: Medication increases risk of bleeding and needs to be stopped before the procedure.*
3. Assess patient's bleeding and coagulation status (e.g., complete blood count [CBC], platelet count, prothrombin time [PT]). *Rationale: Abnormal clotting factors contraindicate the procedure because of increased risk for bleeding.*
4. Assess patient for allergies to iodine dye, latex, shellfish. If allergies are present, notify the cardiologist or radiologist. *Rationale: Patients with allergies to iodine, shellfish, or other contrast media are at risk for anaphylactic reactions. A hypoallergenic contrast medium is sometimes used.*
5. Examine medical record for contraindications.
   a. All contrast media: Pregnancy unless the benefits to the tests outweigh the risks to the infant. *Rationale: Radioactive iodinated contrast media crosses the blood-placental barrier.*
   b. Angiography: Anticoagulant therapy; bleeding disorders; thrombocytopenia; dehydration; uncontrolled hypertension; renal insufficiency. *Rationale: Anticoagulants and bleeding disorders interfere with the patient's blood clotting abilities. Dehydration and renal insufficiency are contraindications to the use of ionic radiographic contrast media because the patient has an impaired ability to excrete the contrast media via the kidneys.*
   c. Cardiac catheterization contraindications: Severe cardiomyopathy, severe dysrhythmias, uncontrolled congestive heart failure. *Rationale: Introduction of a catheter into the myocardium irritates myocardial tissue and increases the risk for dysrhythmias (Pagana and Pagana, 2007).*
   d. IVP: Dehydration, known renal insufficiency. *Rationale: Dehydration and renal insufficiency impair the ability to excrete the contrast media via the kidneys (Chernecky and Berger, 2008).*

e. Determine whether patient has taken the drug metformin (Glucophage) within the past 48 hours. If so, notify the physician immediately. *Rationale: Metformin taken within 48 hours before receiving iodinated contrast media can lead to renal failure and lactic acidosis. Metformin is contained in the drugs metformin, metformin hydrochloride (Glumetza), and glyburide and metformin (Glucovance) (Ott, 2008).*

6. Obtain vital signs and peripheral pulses. For arterial procedures mark the patient's peripheral pulses before the procedure. For cardiac catheterization, also auscultate heart and lungs and obtain weight. *Rationale: Provides baseline data for postprocedural assessments.*
7. Assess patient's renal function via electrolyte, blood urea nitrogen, and creatinine levels. *Rationale: Elevated urea nitrogen or creatinine levels increase the risk for renal failure.*
8. Assess patient's level of understanding of procedure, including any concerns. *Rationale: Determines extent of preprocedure understanding or level of additional instruction or support needed.*
9. Determine that preprocedure preparation is complete.
   a. For cardiac catheterization: Determine whether the site of catheter insertion needs to be clipped and prepped with antiseptic just before the procedure (check agency policy). Allow antiseptic to dry. *Rationale: Reduces risk of site-related infection.*
   b. For IVP: Verify that patient has taken the orally administered bowel evacuation medication 24 hours before the test or completed an evacuation enema 8 hours before the test (check agency policy). *Rationale: An evacuated lower intestine and bowel improve visualization.*
10. Determine and document time of last ingested fluid or food. *Rationale: Excessive hydration causes dilution of contrast medium, making structure more difficult to visualize. Iodine dye may cause nausea. Patient needs to be NPO for 6 to 8 hours before the procedure.*
11. Remove metal objects and all of patient's jewelry or body piercings. *Rationale: Eliminates objects that interfere with radiography visualization of blood vessels.*
12. Review physician's orders for preprocedure medications, hydration, antihistamines, and IV sedation. *Rationale: Increased hydration is often required for renal insufficiency, antihistamines for possible allergic reaction, or sedation for anxious or confused patients.*
    a. Atropine: *Rationale: Decreases salivary secretions and increases heart rate when bradycardia is present.*
    b. Diphenhydramine: *Rationale: Blocks histamine and decreases allergic response. Often used prophylactically.*
    c. Preprocedure sedative: *Rationale: Decreases anxiety and promotes relaxation.*
    d. IV sedation: Have IV Solu-Medrol, diphenhydramine, and epinephrine available for potential allergic reactions to the dye (check agency policy). *Rationale: These medications are needed immediately in the case of an allergic reaction to the dye.*

PLANNING

Expected Outcomes focus on prevention of respiratory side effects from sedation and cardiovascular complications from catheter placement, puncture site complications, and reactions to contrast medium.

1. Patient assumes the correct position and remains still throughout the entire procedure.
2. Patient has pain less than 4 (on a scale of 0 to 10) that is limited to soreness at catheter insertion site and possible backache.
3. Patient does not experience procedure or postprocedure complications such as:
   a. Flushing, itching, and urticaria, which signify possible allergic reaction to dye.
   b. Diminished or absent peripheral pulses, signifying thrombosis or embolism at puncture site.
   c. Hypotension and tachycardia, signifying hemorrhage or allergic reaction to dye.
   d. Decreased or absent urine output related to renal failure.
4. Patient recovers from IV sedation without respiratory complications or change in LOC.
5. Patient tolerates increased fluid intake and voids sufficiently to excrete radiographic dye.

Delegation and Collaboration

The skill of assisting with angiography and IVP may be delegated to nursing assistive personnel (NAP) if the patient is stable and if no IV sedation is used. Assessment cannot be delegated. Instruct the NAP about the following:

- When to obtain and report vital signs, urinary output, and weight
- What signs and symptoms to report to the nurse
- What to observe and report to the nurse
- Accompanying the patient to the procedure room and assisting specially trained and licensed radiology personnel with the specific angiography procedure

Equipment

- Personal protective equipment: Mask, goggles, sterile gown, and sterile gloves
- Sterile packs containing catheters/equipment for performing procedures
- Equipment for IV access
- Medications such as diazepam (Valium), midazolam, or other sedative for IV sedation as indicated
- Emergency equipment: oxygen, emergency cart, defibrillator, cardiac monitor, sphygmomanometer, pulse oximeter, and sedative reversal agents

IMPLEMENTATION *for* CONTRAST MEDIA STUDIES: ARTERIOGRAM (ANGIOGRAM), CARDIAC CATHETERIZATION, INTRAVENOUS PYELOGRAM

STEPS	RATIONALE
1. See Standard Protocol (inside front cover).	
2. Identify patient using two identifiers (e.g., name and birthday or name and account number, according to facility policy). Compare identifiers on MAR with information on patient's identification bracelet.	Ensures correct patient. Complies with The Joint Commission standards and improves patient safety (TJC, 2010).
3. Have patient empty bowels and bladder before procedure.	Ensures that patient will not need to void during procedure.
4. Prepare equipment for monitoring patient during the procedure, including heart rate and rhythm, oxygen saturation, and blood pressure.	Provides easy access to equipment for monitoring patient status during and after procedure.
5. Provide IV access using large-bore cannula (see Chapter 28). Remove gloves.	Provides access for delivery of IV fluids and/or drugs.
6. Assist patient in assuming a comfortable supine position on x-ray table. Some patients undergoing IVP may be in a supine or in a slight Trendelenburg's position. Immobilize the extremity that will be injected. Pad any bony prominences.	For arterial procedures the patient may need to maintain the position for 1 to 3 hours. Padding of bony prominences reduces the risk for impaired skin integrity.
7. Take "Time Out" to verify the patient's name, type of procedure to be performed, and procedure site with the patient.	"Time Out" verification just before starting an invasive procedure includes the physician and all involved personnel and is a safety precaution to prevent wrong patient, wrong site, and wrong procedure errors (TJC, 2010).
8. Inform patient that, during the injection of the dye, it is common to experience some chest pain and a severe hot flash but it usually lasts only a few seconds.	Dye causes a sensation of warmth, flushing, or a metallic taste shortly after injection (Edmond and others, 2008).
9. Physician cleanses site for catheter insertion (femoral, carotid, or brachial) with antiseptic.	Reduces transmission of infection.
10. Members of the team apply sterile gown and gloves, and the patient is draped with sterile drapes, leaving puncture site exposed.	Maintains surgical asepsis.
11. Physician anesthetizes the skin over the arterial puncture site.	Provides local anesthesia to incision or puncture site.

> **SAFETY ALERT** The physician may end the cardiac catheterization procedure early in the event of severe unrelieved chest pain, neurological symptoms of a cerebrovascular accident, cardiac arrhythmias, or hemodynamic changes (Pagana and Pagana, 2007).

STEPS	RATIONALE
12. For arterial procedures the physician does the following:	
a. Punctures artery; insert guidewire, and threads needle and angiographic (or cardiographic) catheter over the wire.	Permits access to artery and prevents coiling of catheter in the artery.
b. Advances catheter to desired artery or cardiac chamber and injects contrast dye.	Permits radiographic visualization of structures, aneurysms, occlusions, or anomalies.
13. During dye injection specialized machinery takes rapid sequence of x-ray films.	Provides radiographic records of dye through the artery or cardiac chamber and documents any abnormalities.
14. If iodinated dye is administered, observe patient for signs of anaphylaxis, including respiratory distress, palpitations, itching, and diaphoresis.	Allergic reactions can be life threatening.
15. During cardiac catheterization the nurse assists with measuring cardiac volumes and pressures.	Provides data related to cardiac output, central venous pressure, ventricular pressures, and pulmonary artery pressure.

STEPS	RATIONALE
16. Nurse administering IV sedation monitors level of sedation, LOC, and vital signs.	IV sedation should not cause loss of consciousness.
17. The physician withdraws catheter and applies pressure to puncture site until hemostasis occurs (5 to 15 minutes or longer). Commonly a VCD may be used. In patients with severe arteriosclerosis the Angio-Seal VCD is appropriate (Kadner and others, 2008).	Pressure on puncture site promotes clotting and prevents bleeding. VCDs include Angio-Seal, VasoSeal, Duett, and Perclose. Each has a unique method for providing closure of the arterial site. They provide a pretied suture knot that closes the arterial access site after the procedure. This knot provides rapid hemostasis (Kim, 2006).
18. In certain procedures during the cardiac catheterization, a femoral sheath is often left in place and removed in several hours by the nurse caring for the patient.	Postinterventional sheaths provide emergency access to the vasculature in the event that the coronary artery occludes and to allow time for anticoagulants to wear off.

SAFETY ALERT Timing of the removal of the femoral sheath depends on location of the access site, size of the sheath, use of anticoagulants, and agency protocols (Edmond and others, 2008). Manual pressure applied to the groin can stimulate the baroreceptors and cause a vasovagal reaction in which the patient becomes bradycardic and hypotensive. Vasovagal reactions are usually brief and self-limiting. When applying pressure to the groin after sheath removal, be alert for a vasovagal reaction and be prepared to treat it by lowering the head of the bed to the flat position and giving a bolus of IV fluids. Have emergency resuscitation equipment available during sheath removal.

STEPS	RATIONALE
19. Remove and discard gown and gloves.	
20. Postprocedure:	
a. Keep affected extremity immobilized for 6 to 8 hours after removal of catheter. Use orthopedic bedpan for female patient as needed while on bed rest.	Allows time for the body's natural hemostatic mechanisms to form stable initial repair at the insertion site.
b. Emphasize the need to lie flat for 6 to 12 hours (and possibly overnight if the catheters are left in the groin).	Helps prevent disruption of hemostasis at the puncture site.
c. Encourage patient to drink 1 to 2 L of fluid after procedure or administer oral and IV fluids as ordered.	Facilitates elimination of contrast material and prevents renal damage (Pagana and Pagana, 2007).
21. See Completion Protocol (inside front cover).	

EVALUATION

1. Assess patient's body position and comfort during procedure.
2. Postprocedure: Monitor vital signs, oxygen saturation, and urinary output and assess for signs of cardiac complications every 15 minutes for 1 hour, every 30 minutes for 2 hours, or until vital signs are stable.
3. Evaluate patient's level of pain on a pain scale of 0 to 10.
4. Monitor for complications:
   - **a.** Assess vascular site for bleeding and hematoma. Also observe under the patient for blood.
   - **b.** If ordered, monitor postprocedure laboratory values (CBC, electrolytes, creatinine, activated partial thromboplastin time, PT).
   - **c.** Perform neurovascular checks: Palpate peripheral pulses in the affected extremity, use Doppler ultrasonic stethoscope if the pulses are not palpable; observe skin temperature and color and compare to unaffected extremity.
   - **d.** Auscultate heart and lungs and compare findings with preprocedure findings.
   - **e.** Monitor electrocardiogram (ECG) recording as appropriate.
   - **f.** Monitor patient for allergic reactions: (1) assess patient for flushing, itching, and urticaria, and (2) assess patient's respiratory status for sudden, severe shortness of breath.
   - **g.** Monitor patient's LOC and neurological status.
5. If sedation was used, monitor for sedation complications (e.g., excessive sleepiness, inability to arouse patient).
   - **a.** Measure vital signs (see Step 2); compare to baseline and subsequent values.
   - **b.** Measure SpO_2 and compare to baseline.

Unexpected Outcomes and Related Interventions

1. Patient experiences vasovagal response (occurs at time of femoral puncture or after procedure with femoral pressure). Symptoms include feeling faint, dizzy, light-headed,

and possible loss of consciousness for a few seconds. Bradycardic pulse is caused by stimulation of the vagus nerve via baroreceptors.
   a. Support airway, breathing, and circulation.
   b. Lower table or head of bed to the Trendelenburg's position.
   c. Administer IV fluid bolus if ordered.
2. Patient's pedal pulses are nonpalpable bilaterally 2 hours after an angiogram.
   a. Assess pulses with a Doppler scope.
   b. Assess extremity skin temperature, color, and capillary refill time.
   c. Notify physician immediately.
3. Patient develops hematoma or hemorrhage at catheter insertion site.
   a. Maintain direct pressure over insertion site.
   b. Contact physician immediately. Follow specific post-procedure orders related to findings.
   c. Monitor catheter site every 30 minutes for 2 to 3 hours and then as ordered.
4. Oversedation occurs (e.g., decreased oxygen saturation, shallow respirations, decreased blood pressure, tachycardia).
   a. Support patient's airway and breathing.
   b. Immediately notify patient's physician.
   c. Be prepared to administer emergency medications or reversal agents (e.g., naloxone [Narcan] [reversal of opioids] or flumazenil [Romazicon] [reversal of benzodiazepines]).
5. Retroperitoneal bleeding occurs (when femoral access site is used). A hallmark sign of retroperitoneal bleeding is low back pain radiating to both sides of the body.
   a. Prepare patient for emergency surgery.
   b. Monitor vital signs every 5 to 15 minutes.
   c. Monitor distal pulses hourly.

Recording and Reporting

- Record patient's condition: Vital signs, peripheral pulses for equality and symmetry; blood pressure, especially for hypotension; temperature and color of catheterized extremity; condition of IV site; level of comfort and level of patient responsiveness; any drainage from puncture site; dressing appearance; and condition of site.
- Report to physician or charge nurse immediately: Changes in vital signs and/or oxygen saturation, arrhythmias, excessive bleeding or increasing hematoma at puncture site, decreased or absent peripheral pulses, urine output less than 30 mL per hour, and decreased level of patient responsiveness.

Sample Documentation

0800-0900 Returned from angiogram via stretcher awake and alert. Vital signs obtained every 15 minutes, remain stable. Dorsalis pedis and posterior tibial pulses are palpable and equal bilaterally. No bleeding, swelling, or discoloration noted at catheter insertion site in left groin. Left leg extended with soft restraint in place. Complains of mild discomfort at left groin equal to 2 on a 0 to 10 pain scale but denies need for analgesics.

0900-1000 Vital signs obtained every 30 minutes remained stable. Dorsalis pedis and posterior tibial pulses are palpable and equal bilaterally. No bleeding, swelling, or discoloration noted at catheter insertion site in left groin. Left leg extended without soft restraint. Rates pain at 0 on a 0 to 10 pain scale.

Special Considerations

Pediatric

- Infants have the highest risk for complication, and in infants weighing less than 5 kg there is a greater risk of death.
- Infants and children are particularly susceptible to the diuretic effects of radio contrast dyes because of their small body size. In addition, those with congenital cardiac anomalies develop compensatory erythrocytosis and thus experience complications from dehydration very quickly. Emphasize the importance of fluid intake with the child and parent(s) (Hockenberry and Wilson, 2009).

Geriatric

- In the older adult slight alterations in vital signs or behavior are signs of impending problems; therefore close monitoring is very important.
- Physical exposure and room temperature contribute to hypothermia in frail adults. Use heated blankets or forced air heat to maintain core temperature at comfortable, safe levels.
- Renal insufficiency contributes to prolonged sedation.
- The older adult with preexisting dehydration or renal insufficiency in combination with NPO status is at risk for dye-induced renal failure. Carefully monitor intake and output.

Home Care

- Instruct patient to contact the physician (or affiliated emergency department) if any of the following occur after cardiac catheterization:
  - Chest pain or shortness of breath
  - Blood in the urine
  - Bleeding from the catheterization puncture site: Apply gentle pressure with clean gauze or cloth
  - Formation of a knot or lump under the skin that increases in size
  - Worsening of a bruise or its movement down the extremity rather than disappearing
  - Increased pain at puncture site or in the extremity used for the catheterization
  - Extremity with arterial puncture that is pale and cool to touch
  - Appearance of redness, swelling, or warmth of the affected extremity
- Although bathing or showering is allowed the day after the catheterization, the leg used as the access site is often stiff, which increases risk of slipping in the bath or shower.

SKILL 9.2 CARE OF PATIENTS UNDERGOING ASPIRATIONS: BONE MARROW, LUMBAR PUNCTURE, PARACENTESIS, THORACENTESIS

Aspirations are invasive procedures involving removal of body fluids or tissue for diagnostic purposes. The nurse assists the physician during an aspiration procedure. Informed consent is legally required for these procedures (Table 9-2).

Bone marrow aspiration is the removal of a small amount of the liquid organic material in the medullary canals of selected bones. The bones used for aspiration in adults include the sternum and the posterior superior iliac crests. In children the anterior or posterior iliac crests are used, and in infants the proximal tibia is used (Hockenberry and Wilson, 2009; Pagana and Pagana, 2007). A biopsy is the removal of a core of marrow cells for laboratory analysis. Both aspiration and biopsy diagnose and differentiate leukemia, certain malignancies, anemia, and thrombocytopenia. The marrow is examined in a laboratory to reveal the number, size, shape, and development of red blood cells and megakaryocytes (platelet precursors). Bone marrow cultures help differentiate infectious diseases such as tuberculosis or histoplasmosis. This procedure takes about 20 minutes.

A lumbar puncture (LP), called a *spinal puncture* or *tap*, involves the introduction of a needle into the subarachnoid space of the spinal column. The purpose of the test is to measure pressure in the subarachnoid space and obtain cerebrospinal fluid (CSF) for visualization and laboratory examination. An LP is also used to inject anesthetic, diagnostic, or therapeutic agents. CSF is examined in a laboratory to help diagnose spinal cord tumors, central nervous system (CNS) infections, hemorrhage, and degenerative brain disease. The procedure takes about 30 minutes.

TABLE 9-2 SUMMARY OF ASPIRATION PROCEDURES

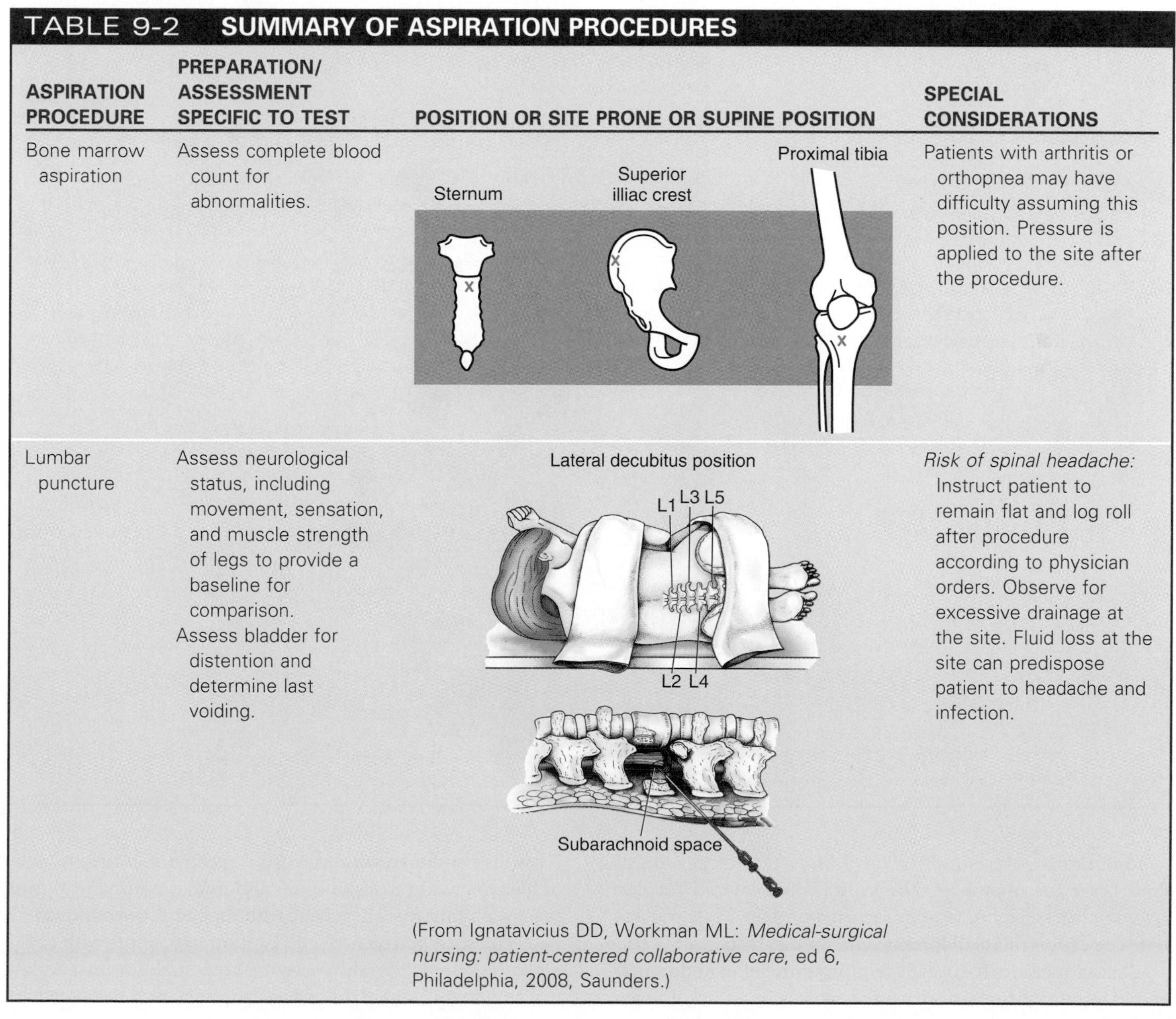

ASPIRATION PROCEDURE	PREPARATION/ ASSESSMENT SPECIFIC TO TEST	POSITION OR SITE PRONE OR SUPINE POSITION	SPECIAL CONSIDERATIONS
Bone marrow aspiration	Assess complete blood count for abnormalities.	Sternum; Superior illiac crest; Proximal tibia	Patients with arthritis or orthopnea may have difficulty assuming this position. Pressure is applied to the site after the procedure.
Lumbar puncture	Assess neurological status, including movement, sensation, and muscle strength of legs to provide a baseline for comparison. Assess bladder for distention and determine last voiding.	Lateral decubitus position (From Ignatavicius DD, Workman ML: *Medical-surgical nursing: patient-centered collaborative care*, ed 6, Philadelphia, 2008, Saunders.)	*Risk of spinal headache:* Instruct patient to remain flat and log roll after procedure according to physician orders. Observe for excessive drainage at the site. Fluid loss at the site can predispose patient to headache and infection.

Continued

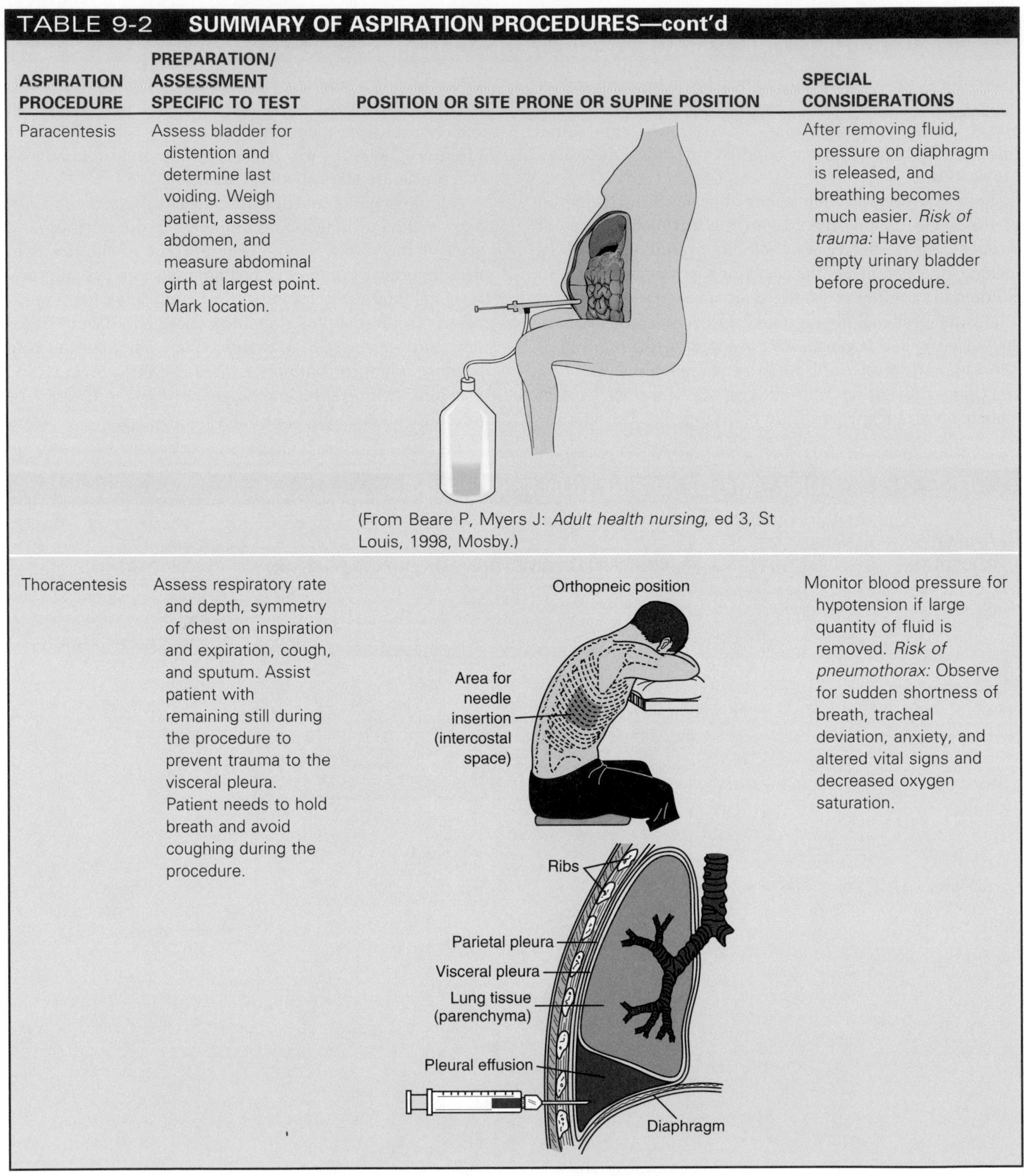

TABLE 9-2 SUMMARY OF ASPIRATION PROCEDURES—cont'd

ASPIRATION PROCEDURE	PREPARATION/ ASSESSMENT SPECIFIC TO TEST	POSITION OR SITE PRONE OR SUPINE POSITION	SPECIAL CONSIDERATIONS
Paracentesis	Assess bladder for distention and determine last voiding. Weigh patient, assess abdomen, and measure abdominal girth at largest point. Mark location.	(From Beare P, Myers J: *Adult health nursing*, ed 3, St Louis, 1998, Mosby.)	After removing fluid, pressure on diaphragm is released, and breathing becomes much easier. *Risk of trauma:* Have patient empty urinary bladder before procedure.
Thoracentesis	Assess respiratory rate and depth, symmetry of chest on inspiration and expiration, cough, and sputum. Assist patient with remaining still during the procedure to prevent trauma to the visceral pleura. Patient needs to hold breath and avoid coughing during the procedure.	Orthopneic position	Monitor blood pressure for hypotension if large quantity of fluid is removed. *Risk of pneumothorax:* Observe for sudden shortness of breath, tracheal deviation, anxiety, and altered vital signs and decreased oxygen saturation.

Abdominal paracentesis involves aspiration of peritoneal fluid from the abdomen. The aspirate is analyzed for cell cytology, bacteria, blood, glucose, and protein to help diagnose the causes of an abdominal effusion. Paracentesis is also a palliative measure to provide temporary relief of abdominal and respiratory discomfort caused by severe ascites. Lavage paracentesis, a process in which a large amount of solution is instilled and then withdrawn, is done to detect the presence of bleeding, as in cases of blunt abdominal trauma or tumor cells when cancer is suspected. Although not contraindicated, paracentesis is performed with caution in patients with coagulopathies, with portal hypertension with abdominal collateral circulation, and in those who are pregnant. The procedure takes about 30 minutes.

Thoracentesis is performed to analyze or remove pleural fluid or instill medications intrapleurally. Specimens are examined for cell cytology, blood, glucose, amylase, lactate dehydrogenase (LD), and cellular composition. Cytologic specimens are examined for malignancy, differentiated between transudative and exudative characteristics, and cultured for pathogens. Therapeutic thoracentesis is used to relieve pain, dyspnea, and signs of pleural pressure. The test takes about 30 minutes.

ASSESSMENT

1. Verify the type of procedure that the physician will perform and procedure site with the patient. *Rationale: Ensures correct patient. Complies with TJC (2010) requirements and improves procedure safety.*
2. Verify that informed consent was obtained. *Rationale: Federal regulations, many state laws, and accreditation agencies require informed consent for procedures.*
3. Review medical record for contraindications:
   a. Bone marrow biopsy: Patient cannot maintain position or lie still during procedure
   b. LP: Increased intracranial pressure (IICP), spinal deformities, and clotting disorders
   c. Paracentesis: Patients with clotting disorders, intestinal obstructions, and pregnancy
   d. Thoracentesis: Patient cannot maintain position during procedure
4. Determine patient's ability to assume position required for procedure and ability to remain still (see Table 9-2). *Rationale: Movement during the procedure can cause complications such as bleeding and injury to nerves or tissue.*
5. Before procedure: Obtain vital signs, oxygen saturation, and weight. For paracentesis obtain an abdominal girth measurement. (Use ink pen to mark location of position of abdominal girth measurement.) For LP obtain baseline assessment of lower extremity movement, sensation, and muscle strength. *Rationale: Provides baseline for comparison with postprocedure vital signs. Patients have decreased abdominal girth and lose weight after parenthesis.*
6. Instruct patient to empty bladder. *Rationale: Reduces risk for bladder trauma during paracentesis. Promotes patient comfort.*
7. Assess patient's coagulation status: Use of anticoagulants, platelet count, and PT. *Rationale: Invasive procedures are contraindicated in patients with coagulation disorders because of risk of bleeding (Pagana and Pagana, 2007).*
8. Determine whether patient is allergic to antiseptic, latex, or anesthetic solutions. *Rationale: Decreases chance of allergic reactions.*
9. Assess patient's level of understanding of procedure, including any concerns. *Rationale: Determines extent of instructions and level of support required.*
10. Obtain baseline pain level. *Rationale: Determines need for preprocedure analgesia. Pain control helps patients maintain proper position and tolerate aspiration procedure.*

PLANNING

Expected Outcomes focus on proper positioning, patient's ability to follow directions, comfort, and absence of complications.

1. Patient assumes the correct position and remains still throughout the entire procedure.
2. There is no bleeding at needle insertion site.
3. The amount of aspirate is sufficient to perform laboratory testing.
4. Patient's level of pain is 4 or less on a pain scale of 0 to 10.
5. Patient's respiratory rate, heart rate, and blood pressure are within normal limits during and after aspiration procedure.

Delegation and Collaboration

The skill of assisting with aspirations may be delegated to nursing assistive personnel (NAP) if the patient is stable (check agency policy). Assessment of the patient's condition cannot be delegated. Instruct the NAP about the following:

- How to properly position the patient during the procedure
- Obtaining baseline and postprocedure vital signs and reporting them to the nurse
- Which signs and symptoms experienced by the patient to immediately report to the nurse

Equipment

Personal protective equipment: Masks, goggles, gowns, gloves for health care personnel

Test tubes, sterile specimen containers, laboratory requisitions, and labels

Analgesia if ordered, given 30 minutes before procedure

Antiseptic solution

Gauze pads (4 × 4 inch), tape, band aid

Aspiration tray: Most institutions provide trays specific to the aspiration procedure. Standard equipment includes antiseptic solution (e.g., chlorhexidine; gauze sponges (4 × 4 inch); sterile towels; local anesthetic solution (e.g., lidocaine 1%); two 3-mL sterile syringes with 16- to 27-gauge needles. Additional equipment for specific aspirations include the following:

- Bone marrow aspiration: Two additional bone marrow needles with inner stylus
- Lumbar puncture: Manometer to measure spinal pressure and at least four test tubes
- Paracentesis: IV fluids as ordered, vacuum bottles, stopcock with extension tubing, sterile collection containers, measuring tape
- Thoracentesis: Vacuum bottles, stopcock with extension tubing

IMPLEMENTATION *for* CARE OF PATIENTS UNDERGOING ASPIRATIONS: BONE MARROW, LUMBAR PUNCTURE, PARACENTESIS, THORACENTESIS

STEPS	RATIONALE
1. **See Standard Protocol (inside front cover).**	
2. Identify patient using two identifiers (i.e., name and birthday or name and account number, according to facility policy). Compare identifiers on MAR with information on patient's identification bracelet.	Ensures correct patient. Complies with The Joint Commission standards and improves patient safety (TJC, 2010).
3. Premedicate patient as ordered.	Reduces pain and any anxiety associated with the procedure.
4. Explain steps of skin preparation, anesthetic injection, needle insertion, and position required. NOTE: For bone marrow biopsy, explain to patient that pain may occur when the bone marrow is aspirated.	Explanation reduces anxiety.
5. Set up sterile tray or open supplies to make accessible for physician.	Reduces risk of contamination of sterile field and promotes prompt completion of procedure.
6. Take "Time Out" to verify the patient's name, type of procedure to be performed, and procedure site with patient.	"Time Out" verification just before starting the procedure includes the physician and all involved personnel and is a safety precaution to prevent wrong patient, wrong site, and wrong procedure errors (TJC, 2010).
7. Assist patient in maintaining correct position (see Table 9-2). Reassure patient while explaining procedure.	Decreases chance of complications during procedure. Explanations increase patient comfort and relaxation.
8. Physician cleanses site with antiseptic solution and drapes site with sterile drape.	
9. Explain to patient that pain can occur when local anesthetic is injected into the tissues. Pressure may also occur when the tissue of fluid is aspirated.	Aspiration is painful but lasts for only a few minutes. Preprocedure analgesia decreases discomfort. If the patient is having a bone marrow aspirate, a deep pressure feeling is frequently experienced as the bone marrow is withdrawn (Pagana and Pagana, 2007).
10. Physician injects local anesthetic and waits for area to become numb.	Discomfort and pressure may still occur when deep tissues are disrupted.
11. Physician inserts needle or trocar into the body cavity involved (see Table 9-2). To aspirate tissue or body fluids for specimen analysis, a syringe is attached to the trocar or needle, and aspirate is placed into a specimen container.	
12. Assess patient's condition during procedure, including respiratory status, vital signs if indicated, and complaints of pain.	Changes indicate complications.

SAFETY ALERT For patients who have a paracentesis or thoracentesis, increased abdominal or thoracic pain is significant. Severe abdominal pain indicates a possible bowel perforation following a paracentesis. Following a thoracentesis abdominal pain results from diaphragmatic, liver, or spleen perforation. Inspiratory chest pain results from perforation of the lung.

STEPS	RATIONALE
13. Note characteristics of aspirate.	
a. **Bone marrow aspirate:** Marrow is red or yellow.	
b. **Lumbar puncture**: Record opening pressure; observe fluid for color, cloudiness, or blood.	Normal CSF is clear and colorless. Cloudy color is the result of protein, which indicates an infection.
c. **Paracentesis**: Fluid is yellow, cloudy, bile-stained green, or blood tinged. Gastric lavage fluid may appear bright red.	Blood-tinged fluid results from a traumatic tap. In a trauma patient a paracentesis tap is used to lavage the peritoneum to identify active bleeding.

STEPS	RATIONALE
d. Thoracentesis: Pleural fluid is clear yellow, puslike, or cloudy.	Transudate and exudates are typically yellow, straw color. Blood-stained fluid indicates a malignancy, pulmonary infarction, or severe inflammation. Puslike fluid indicates an infection (empyema); milky fluid indicates a chylothorax, a leak from the thoracic duct resulting in lymphatic drainage in the pleural cavity (Allibone, 2006).
14. Properly label specimens with patient information and name of test desired. Transport tubes with test requisitions to the laboratory immediately.	Nurse is responsible for labeling tubes with patient's name and tests desired. Test tubes are numbered in sequence of collection (e.g., 1 through 4).
15. Physician removes needle/trocar and applies pressure over insertion site until drainage ceases. Assist with placement of closure device or direct pressure and gauze dressing. Continue to apply pressure for a specific time period if directed.	
16. See Completion Protocol (inside front cover).	

EVALUATION

1. Monitor vital signs, oxygen saturation, and symmetry of chest wall movements according to agency policy; in some situations vital signs are obtained every 15 minutes for 2 hours.

2. Inspect dressing over puncture site for bleeding, swelling, tenderness, and erythema. Inspect area under patient for bleeding. Avoid disrupting a healing clot at the site if a pressure dressing is present.

3. Ask patient to describe level of pain using a scale of 0 to 10.

4. Following paracentesis obtain patient weight and measure abdominal girth.

5. Ask patient to describe postprocedure positioning and activity restrictions.

Unexpected Outcomes and Related Interventions

1. Oversedation occurs (e.g., decreased oxygen saturation, shallow respirations, tachycardia).
   a. Support patient's airway and breathing.
   b. Immediately notify patient's physician.
   c. Be prepared to administer emergency medications or reversal agents (e.g., naloxone [reversal of opioids] or flumazenil [reversal of benzodiazepines]).
2. PPHD after LP is evidenced by headache, blurred vision, and tinnitus.
   a. Medicate for pain as ordered.
   b. Notify physician, who may choose to inject a blood patch into the epidural space.
   c. IV caffeine sodium benzoate has been used with limited success in relieving PPHD.
3. Hematoma develops internally at LP site, evidenced by lower extremity tingling.
   a. Compare to baseline assessment.
   b. Notify physician.
   c. Continue frequent evaluation.
4. LP patient develops excessive loss of CSF, evidenced by large amount of CSF drainage from site and reduced LOC; dilated pupils; and increased blood pressure.
   a. Maintain airway.
   b. Notify physician immediately.
   c. Prepare for transfer to intensive care setting.
5. Paracentesis patient develops leakage of fluid at the aspiration site as evidenced by continuously saturated dressings.
   a. Reinforce dressing. Place collection bag over the site if needed.
   b. Notify physician, who may place a small suture to stop the drainage.
6. Pneumothorax after thoracentesis is evidenced by sudden dyspnea and tachypnea and asymmetrical chest excursion.
   a. Administer oxygen (if ordered).
   b. Monitor vital signs and respiratory status frequently.
   c. Notify physician of findings and obtain further orders.
   d. Anticipate chest x-ray film and possible chest tube insertion.

Recording and Reporting

- Record in patient's chart name of procedure, preprocedure preparation; location of puncture site; amount, consistency, and color of fluid drained or specimen obtained; duration of procedure; patient's tolerance of the procedure (e.g., vital signs, SpO_2) and comfort level; laboratory tests ordered; specimen sent; type of dressing; postprocedure activities (e.g., chest x-ray film); and other

procedure-specific assessments (e.g., extremity assessment, abdominal girth, LOC).
- Immediately report to physician or charge nurse any unexpected drainage or significant changes in vital signs or oxygen saturation status.

Sample Documentation

0930 Voided 300 mL. Abdominal girth measures 42 inches at umbilicus preprocedure. Preprocedure weight 72.7 kg (160 pounds). Assisted with sitting on side of bed. Physician completed abdominal paracentesis with 1100 mL cloudy liquid aspirated. Respirations 18 with moderate depth, pulse 98, and blood pressure 138/86. Rates pain at 6 on scale of 0 to 10. 22-inch gauze dressing applied to puncture site; remains dry and intact.

0940 Morphine sulfate 10 mg given in right vastus lateralis for abdominal pain.

1010 States pain has decreased to 2, which is tolerable. Abdominal girth measures 38 inches at umbilicus. Weight decreased to 71.8 kg (158 pounds).

Special Considerations

Pediatric

- Sedation is recommended for children because of the risk of injury caused by children's movement during LP. Very young children may receive IV moderate sedation or general anesthetic for aspiration procedures. Conscious or unconscious sedation is commonly used. If unconscious sedation is used, an anesthesiologist or nurse anesthetist is needed for the procedure.
- Prepare child of preschool age before the procedure; make a game out of having child recall the next procedural step, using a doll as a model. This can serve as a distraction mechanism (Hockenberry and Wilson, 2009).

Geriatric

- Older adults with arthritis may have difficulty sustaining the position required for the procedure and need help during the procedure.
- During thoracentesis be aware of ineffective breathing patterns in the older adult because of age-related changes such as reduced elastic lung recoil, declining chest expansion, reduced cough efficiency, and weaker thoracic and diaphragmatic muscles.
- Be aware of need to change positions slowly to minimize risks for postural hypotension.

Home Care

- Instruct patient that some patients experience tenderness at the puncture site for several days and the physician may order a mild analgesia.
- Instruct patient to get medical attention immediately if he or she suddenly complains of severe headache or has change in LOC.
- Inform paracentesis patient to notify physician of fever or any swelling, pain, or drainage at puncture site. Instruct men to report scrotal pain, edema, or discoloration to the physician.
- Teach the thoracentesis patient symptoms of complications related to liver and spleen perforation that may not be present for several days after procedure and to notify the physician. Instruct patient to report any new abdominal pain to the physician.

SKILL 9.3 CARE OF PATIENTS UNDERGOING BRONCHOSCOPY

Bronchoscopy is the examination of the tracheobronchial tree through a lighted tube containing mirrors (Fig. 9-2). The tube, or bronchoscope, most commonly used is a flexible fiberoptic bronchoscope that allows both visualization and simultaneous administration of oxygen. The fiberoptic bronchoscope has lumens for visualization and for obtaining sputum, foreign bodies, and biopsy specimens. Laser ablation of endotracheal lesions may be performed through the bronchoscope.

Bronchoscopy is an emergency or elective procedure performed for diagnostic and therapeutic reasons. The main purposes of this procedure are to aspirate excessive sputum or mucous plugs that airway suctioning cannot remove; to visualize the tracheobronchial tree for assessment of abnormalities of the mucosa, abscesses, aspiration pneumonia, strictures, and tumors; to obtain deep-tissue biopsy and sputum specimens; and to remove foreign bodies. Potential complications of bronchoscopy include fever, infection, hypoxemia, bronchospasm and laryngospasm, pneumothorax, aspiration, dysrhythmias and hypotension, hemorrhage (after biopsy), and cardiac arrest. When needed, perform airway suctioning before assisting with the procedure.

The procedure is performed at the bedside or in a specially equipped endoscopy room. Usually a pulmonary specialist or surgeon performs this procedure in about 30 to 45 minutes.

ASSESSMENT

1. Verify that informed consent was obtained. *Rationale: Federal regulations, many state laws, and accreditation agencies require informed consent for procedures.*
2. Assess patient's history and cardiopulmonary status to include response to previous procedures. Report this to the physician. *Rationale: Determines need for oxygen administration during procedure.*

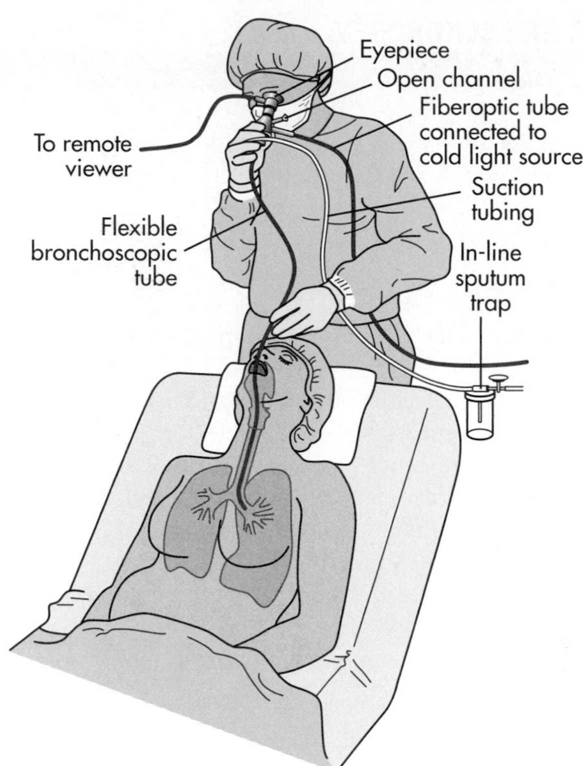

FIG 9-2 Flexible fiberoptic bronchoscopy.

3. Obtain vital signs and oxygen saturation level. *Rationale: Provides baseline data to compare with findings during and after procedure.*
4. Perform respiratory assessment, including lung sounds, chest wall symmetry, pain on inspiration, sputum quantity and color. *Rationale: Provides baseline of respiratory status for comparison during and after procedure.*
5. Review medical record for purpose of procedure: Sputum aspiration, tissue biopsy, sputum culture, removal of foreign object. *Rationale: Anticipates equipment and patient needs.*
6. Determine if patient is allergic to local anesthetic for spraying throat. *Rationale: Allergy produces laryngospasm and laryngeal edema.*
7. Assess need for preprocedure medication (usually atropine and narcotic or sedative). *Rationale: Atropine decreases secretions and inhibits vagally stimulated bradycardia; narcotics or sedatives relieve anxiety and decrease discomfort.*
8. Assess time of last ingested fluid or food. Patients should be NPO 8 hours before bronchoscopy. *Rationale: Excessive hydration causes dilution of contrast medium, making structures more difficult to visualize. NPO decreases chance of aspiration of stomach contents.*
9. Assess patient's knowledge of procedure to determine level of teaching required. *Rationale: Determines level of understanding and level of support needed.*

PLANNING

Expected Outcomes focus on improving patient's knowledge of the procedure, reducing anxiety regarding the procedure and results, and detecting potential complications early.

1. Patient recovers from sedation without respiratory complications or change in LOC.
2. Patient's pain level is 4 or less on a pain scale of 0 to 10.
3. Patient explains what to expect during the procedure before it is begun.
4. Physician is able to observe bronchial structures and obtain desired specimens.
5. Patient's vital signs remain within baseline values.

Delegation and Collaboration

The skill of assisting with bronchoscopy cannot be delegated to nursing assistive personnel (NAP) because this skill requires repeated performance of nursing assessments for patient tolerance of the procedure and for life-threatening complications requiring emergency intervention. The NAP may take baseline and postprocedure vital signs and assist with patient positioning, as long as a nurse is present continuously during the procedure. Instruct the NAP about the following:

- How to assist with patient positioning

Equipment

- Bronchoscopy tray, if available from central supply, which may include: Flexible fiberoptic bronchoscope (see Fig. 9-2; gauze sponges (4 × 4 inch); local anesthetic spray (lidocaine); sterile tracheal suction catheters; diazepam (Valium), midazolam (Versed), or other sedative for IV sedation.
- Oxygen, resuscitative equipment, pulse oximeter, cardiac monitor
- Sterile gloves
- Sterile water-soluble lubricating jelly. (NOTE: Petroleum-based lubricants are not used because of the hazard of aspiration and subsequent pneumonia.)
- Personal protective equipment: Mask, gown, gloves, and goggles for all health care providers or physicians
- Emesis basin
- Tracheal suction equipment

IMPLEMENTATION *for* CARE OF PATIENTS UNDERGOING BRONCHOSCOPY

STEPS	RATIONALE
1. **See Standard Protocol (inside front cover).**	
2. Identify patient using two identifiers (i.e., name and birthday or name and account number, according to facility policy). Compare identifiers on MAR with information on patient's identification bracelet.	Ensures correct patient. Complies with The Joint Commission standards and improves patient safety (TJC, 2010).
3. Remove and safely store patient's dentures and eyeglasses (if applicable).	
4. Assess current IV access or establish new IV access using large-bore cannula (see Chapter 28).	Provides access for IV fluids and/or medications if an emergency occurs.
5. Assist patient in maintaining position desired by physician, usually semi-Fowler's.	Provides maximal visualization of lower airways and adequate lung expansion.
6. Take "Time Out" to verify patient's name, type of procedure to be performed, and procedure site with the patient.	"Time Out" verification just before starting the procedure includes the physician and all involved personnel and is a safety precaution to prevent wrong patient, wrong site, and wrong procedure errors (TJC, 2010).
7. Position tip of suction catheter for easy access in patient's mouth.	Drains oral secretions to reduce risk of aspiration.
8. Physician sprays nasopharynx and oropharynx with topical anesthetic. Lidocaine is commonly used for throat spraying, which is done 10 to 15 minutes before the procedure.	Provides swift local anesthesia to oropharynx.
9. Instruct patient not to swallow local anesthetic; provide an emesis basin.	Swallowed anesthetic is absorbed systemically and causes CNS and cardiovascular reactions.
10. Physician applies goggles, mask, and sterile gloves; introduces bronchoscope into mouth to pharynx and passes through glottis and into trachea and bronchi (see Fig. 9-2). The physician may use more anesthetic spray at glottis to prevent cough reflex. For intubated patients the flexible bronchoscope is introduced through the endotracheal tube.	Bronchoscope must pass through upper airway structures to promote visualization of lower airways. Trachea and bronchi are observed for lesions and obstructions.
11. Physician suctions mucus; bronchial washing performed with cytologic specimens taken with a wire brush or curette. Biopsy specimens may also be obtained.	Cytologic specimens are obtained to diagnose carcinoma.
12. Assist patient by giving explanations, verbal reassurance, and support.	Premedicated and drowsy patients need reminders not to change position and to cooperate.
13. Monitor ECG, pulse, oxygen saturation, and blood pressure for changes every 5 minutes during procedure.	Establishes monitoring for oversedation (see Skill 9.1).
14. Assess patient's respiratory status during procedure: Observe degree of restlessness and respiratory rate; observe capillary refill and color of nail beds; monitor oxygen saturation levels.	Bronchoscope may cause feelings of suffocation; also, because airway is partially occluded, patient may become hypoxic during observations.
15. Note characteristics of suctioned material. A small amount of blood mixed with the aspirate is expected because of tissue trauma.	Information is used to record and report and make further patient observations.
16. Using gloved hand, wipe patient's nose to remove lubricant after bronchoscope is removed.	Promotes hygiene and comfort.
17. Instruct patient not to try to swallow sputum until gag reflex returns. Provide emesis basis for expectoration of sputum.	Helps prevent aspiration pneumonia, which is a risk until gag reflex returns.
18. **See Completion Protocol (inside front cover).**	

EVALUATION

1. Closely monitor patient's vital signs, oxygen saturation, and respiratory status.
   a. Monitor for sudden dyspnea indicating laryngospasm or bronchospasm.
2. Assess level of sedation and LOC.
3. Monitor for return of gag reflex, which usually returns within 2 hours.
4. Observe character and amount of sputum. Physician may order serial sputum collection for 24 hours for cytological examination.
5. Assess patient's level of pain.

Unexpected Outcomes and Related Interventions

1. Laryngospasm and bronchospasm indicated by sudden, severe shortness of breath
   a. Call physician immediately.
   b. Prepare emergency resuscitation equipment.
   c. Anticipate possible cricothyrotomy.
2. Presence of hypoxemia indicated by decreased oxygen saturation, gradual shortness of breath, and decreasing LOC
   a. Maintain airway and oxygenation.
   b. Notify physician immediately.
   c. Monitor oxygen saturation.
3. Vasovagal response during bronchoscope insertion. Vasovagal response is caused by stimulation of the baroreceptors, causing bradycardia. Symptoms include feeling faint, dizzy, and light-headed and being diaphoretic with a slow, steady pulse. Patient may become unconscious for a few seconds.
   a. Lower head of table.
   b. Support airway.
4. Hemorrhage
   a. Call physician immediately.
   b. Emergency resuscitation equipment must be readily available.
   c. Follow specific postprocedure orders related to findings.
5. Oversedation occurs (e.g., decreased oxygen saturation, shallow respirations, tachycardia).
   a. Support patient's airway and breathing.
   b. Immediately notify patient's physician.
   c. Be prepared to administer emergency medications or reversal agent (e.g., naloxone [Narcan; reversal of opioids] or flumazenil [Romazicon; reversal of benzodiazepines]).

Recording and Reporting

- Record name of procedure (include biopsy if performed), duration of procedure, patient's tolerance of procedure and complications, and collection and disposition of specimen. Document return of gag reflex.
- Report excessive bleeding or respiratory difficulty after procedure or changes in vital signs beyond patient's normal limits to physician immediately. Report results of procedure to appropriate health care personnel.

Sample Documentation

0900 To bronchoscopy via stretcher.

1030 Returned from bronchoscopy. Alert and oriented. Vital signs stable. Oxygen saturation 88% on room air. Resting in semi-Fowler's position. Denies dyspnea. Color pale. Respirations 28; rhonchi noted bilaterally at bases, clears some with cough. Occasional cough noted productive of small amount bright red sputum. No gag reflex present.

1130 Vital signs stable and recorded every 15 min × 4. No change in assessment.

1230 Vital signs stable. Gag reflex present. No cough or sputum production since 1130. Taking sips of clear liquids without difficulty.

Special Considerations

Pediatric

- In children the procedure is most frequently performed to remove foreign bodies from larynx or trachea and is done under general anesthesia. Patient is placed in the lateral position after the procedure to prevent aspiration.
- Children are at higher risk of hypoxemia than adults because of their smaller bronchus and because the bronchoscope decreases the available breathing space (Pagana and Pagana, 2007).

Geriatric

- Postprocedure restlessness in the older adult patient often indicates hypoxemia or pain. Thoroughly assess oxygenation status before administration of an opioid analgesic.
- Physical exposure and room temperature contribute to hypothermia in frail older adults, who are unable to communicate that they are cold. Use heated blankets or forced air heat to maintain core temperature at comfortable, safe levels (Negishi and others, 2003).

Home Care

- Instruct patient to notify the physician if the following symptoms develop: fever, chest pain, dyspnea, wheezing, or hemoptysis.
- Throat discomfort is normal after this procedure. Warm saline gargles or throat lozenges are helpful.

SKILL 9.4 CARE OF PATIENTS UNDERGOING GASTROINTESTINAL ENDOSCOPY

Endoscopy is any study that allows direct visualization of an internal organ or structure by means of a long, flexible fiberoptic scope with a light source attached (Fig. 9-3). An esophagoscopy, gastroscopy, gastroduodenojejunoscopy, or duodenoscopy visualizes the upper gastrointestinal (GI) tract; more frequently, these procedures are combined (EGD), which permits visualization of the esophagus, stomach, and duodenum in one examination. Endoscopy enables biopsy of suspicious tissue, polyp removal, and performance of many other procedures such as direct visual guidance for fine-needle aspiration biopsies and dilation and stenting of strictures. For visualization of the hepatobiliary tree and pancreatic ducts, an endoscopic retrograde cholangiopancreatography is performed. For visual examination of the lower GI tract, a proctoscopy, sigmoidoscopy, or colonoscopy is performed. Typically these patients receive IV moderate sedation.

Risks of endoscopic procedures include intestinal perforation, hemorrhage, peritonitis, aspiration, respiratory depression, and myocardial infarction secondary to vasovagal response. Both upper and lower GI endoscopic examinations are performed in a specially equipped endoscopic unit.

ASSESSMENT

1. Verify the type of procedure that the physician will perform and the procedure site with the patient. *Rationale: Ensures correct patient. Complies with TJC (2010) requirements and improves procedure safety.*
2. Verify that informed consent was obtained. *Rationale: Federal regulations, many state laws, and accreditation agencies require informed consent for procedures.*

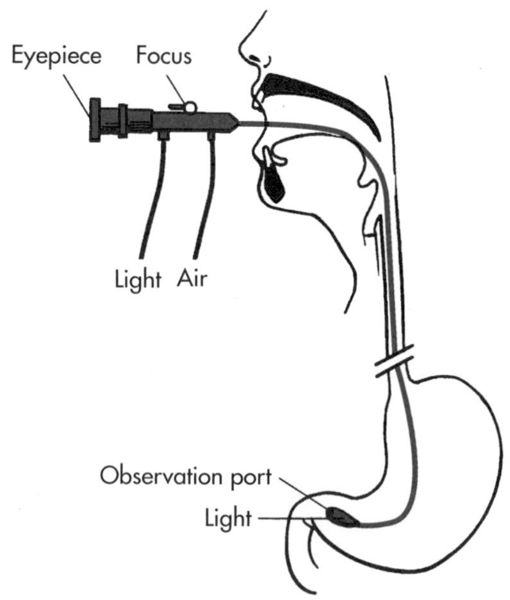

FIG 9-3 Flexible endoscope to visualize stomach.

3. Obtain baseline vital signs and oxygen saturation levels.
4. Determine if signs of GI bleeding are present by observing the character of emesis, stool, and nasogastric tube drainage for frank blood or black material that looks like coffee grounds. *Rationale: Test is contraindicated in patients with severe upper GI bleeding because viewing lens is covered with blood clots, preventing visualization (Pagana and Pagana, 2007).*
5. Determine the purpose of procedure: biopsy, examination, or coagulation of bleeding sites. *Rationale: Anticipates appropriate equipment needs.*
6. Assess patient's knowledge and explain the steps of the procedure. *Rationale: Determines level of teaching required. Answering patient questions helps to relieve anxiety.*
7. Verify that patient has been NPO for at least 8 hours for upper GI. *Rationale: Promotes adequate visualization; helps prevent aspiration if introduction of the endoscope through the oropharynx stimulates the gag reflex and causes vomiting.*
8. For lower GI studies (proctoscopy, sigmoidoscopy, or colonoscopy), verify that the patient has followed a clear liquid diet for 2 days and has completed any ordered bowel cleansing regimen. *Rationale: An empty intestinal tract is necessary to allow the endoscope insertion and good visualization of the interior walls.*
9. Assess patient's ability to understand and follow directions. *Rationale: Procedures require patient to follow directions closely and assume proper position.*
10. Identify designated driver. *Rationale: Patients are not allowed to drive for 24 hours following sedation anesthesia.*

PLANNING

Expected Outcomes focus on preventing complications, promoting patient's ability to follow instructions, and protecting patient's airway.

1. Patient does not aspirate and has no postprocedure bleeding.
2. Patient's level of pain is 4 or less on a pain scale of 0 to 10.
3. Patient is without respiratory complications or change in LOC.
4. Vital signs remain within baseline.

Delegation and Collaboration

The skill of assisting with endoscopy cannot be delegated to nursing assistive personnel (NAP) because this skill requires repeated performance of nursing assessments for patient tolerance of the procedure and life-threatening complications requiring emergency intervention. NAP may take baseline and postprocedure vital signs and assist with patient positioning, as long as a nurse is present continuously during the procedure. Instruct the NAP about the following:

- How to assist with patient positioning

Equipment

- Personal protective equipment: Mask, gown, gloves, goggles for all health care personnel
- Endoscopy tray
- Fiberoptic endoscope and camera (see Fig. 9-3)
- Solutions for biopsy specimens
- Local anesthetic spray
- Tracheal suction equipment (see Chapter 14)
- Blood pressure equipment
- Water-soluble jelly
- Sterile gloves for physician
- Emesis basin
- IV fluid and equipment for IV start (optional)
- Diazepam (Valium), midazolam (Versed), or other sedative for IV sedation (optional)
- Carbon dioxide source (for lower GI procedures)
- Oxygen, resuscitative equipment, and pulse oximeter

IMPLEMENTATION *for* CARE OF PATIENTS UNDERGOING GASTROINTESTINAL ENDOSCOPY

STEPS	RATIONALE
1. See Standard Protocol (inside front cover).	
2. Identify patient using two identifiers (i.e., name and birthday or name and account number, according to facility policy). Compare identifiers on MAR with information on patient's identification bracelet.	Ensures correct patient. Complies with The Joint Commission standards and improves patient safety (TJC, 2010).
3. Administer any preprocedure medication.	Promotes relaxation and reduces anxiety.
4. Remove patient's dentures and dental appliances.	Prevents dislodgement of dental structures during intubation phase.
5. Take "Time Out" to verify patient's name, type of procedure to be performed, and procedure site.	"Time Out" verification just before starting the procedure includes the physician and all involved personnel and is a safety precaution to prevent wrong patient, wrong site, and wrong procedure errors (TJC, 2010).
6. Ensure that IV line is patent and administer IV moderate sedation as ordered.	
7. Assist patient through the procedure:	Helps to minimize patient's anxiety.
a. Anticipate needs and promote comfort.	Patient unable to speak if tube is passed into throat.
b. Tell patient what will happen during each phase.	Reassures patient.
8. Determine patient's level of sedation before initiating procedure.	Properly sedated patient facilitates timely endoscopy and facilitates patient comfort. IV sedation reduces gagging during the procedure.
9. Position patient:	
Upper GI procedures: Assist patient in maintaining left lateral Sims' position.	Sims' position allows easy passage of upper or lower endoscope. Provides for airway clearance if patient gags and vomits gastric contents.
Lower GI procedures: Assist patient in maintaining left lateral decubitus position. Drape patient for privacy and comfort.	Left lateral decubitus position provides access to lower GI tract.
10. Administer atropine if ordered (upper GI studies).	Atropine reduces the quantity of secretions, therefore reducing risk of aspiration for upper GI endoscopic procedures.
11. Position tip of suction cannula for easy access in the patient's mouth (upper GI studies).	Drains oral secretions to reduce risk for aspiration.
12. *Upper GI studies:* Physician slowly passes the endoscope into mouth, esophagus, stomach, or duodenum and advances to desired depth while visualizing the walls.	Provides visualization of structures.
Lower GI studies: A lubricant-coated flexible fiberoptic endoscope is inserted through the anus and slowly advanced through the rectum and colon, visualizing the walls.	

Continued

STEPS	RATIONALE
SAFETY ALERT If patient is bleeding actively, physician may order that the stomach be lavaged and aspirated clear of clots before procedure is attempted.	
13. Physician insufflates air through endoscope into upper GI tract. For colonoscopies carbon dioxide is used. Physician examines, photographs, or performs biopsy of structures. Physician slowly removes the endoscope.	Distends GI structures for better visualization. Carbon dioxide insufflation produces less postprocedure abdominal cramping than air insufflation (Dellon and others, 2009).
14. Place tissue specimens in proper laboratory containers. Provide slides and containers for specimens and fix or seal as needed.	Ensures proper labeling and preparation of specimens for microscopic examination.
15. Assist patient to comfortable position. If sedated, place in a side-lying position.	Promotes rest and relaxation.
16. Suction airway if patient begins to vomit or accumulate saliva. Remove and discard gloves.	Prevents aspiration of gastric contents or oral secretions.
17. Prepare to discharge patient only after return of gag reflex.	Absence of gag reflex increases risk of aspiration. When the gag reflex is absent, the patient needs continuous monitoring.
18. See Completion Protocol (inside front cover).	

EVALUATION

1. Monitor vital signs for signs of bleeding (tachycardia and hypotension) as often as every 15 minutes for 2 hours. Evaluate emesis or aspirate for frank or occult blood.
2. Evaluate level of sedation.
3. Ask patient to describe pain using a 0 to 10 pain scale.
4. Evaluate any emesis or aspirate for frank or occult blood.
5. Asses for return of gag reflex, usually within 2 to 4 hours. Assess breath sounds, labor of respirations, and oxygen saturation.
6. Ask patient to state any postprocedure dietary or activity limitations.

Unexpected Outcomes and Related Interventions

1. For upper GI procedures: Laryngospasm and bronchospasm, as evidenced by sudden, severe shortness of breath
   a. Notify physician immediately. This can be life threatening.
   b. Prepare emergency resuscitation equipment.
   c. Anticipate possible cricothyrotomy.
2. For upper GI procedures: Hypoxemia caused by aspiration, as evidenced by gradually increasing shortness of breath and decreasing LOC
   a. Support airway.
   b. Notify physician immediately.
   c. Monitor oxygen saturation.
3. Hemorrhage, as evidenced by hypotension and tachycardia and decreasing LOC with or without visible signs of hemorrhage
   a. Notify physician immediately. This can be life threatening.
   b. Follow specific postprocedure orders related to findings.
4. Sharp intense pain in chest, stomach, or abdomen and cool, pale skin
   a. Notify physician immediately. These can be signs of GI perforation.
5. Vasovagal response caused by stimulation of the baroreceptors during bronchoscope insertion, as evidenced by feeling faint, dizzy, and light-headed; diaphoresis with a slow, steady pulse; and/or a few seconds of unconsciousness
   a. Lower head of table.
   b. Support airway.

Reporting and Recording

- Record the procedure, duration, patient's tolerance, complications and interventions, and collection and disposition of specimen.
- Report onset of bleeding, abdominal pain, dyspnea, and vital sign changes to physician. Report the duration of procedure, patient's tolerance, and changes in vital signs or condition.

Sample Documentation

0800 NPO since midnight. Transported to endoscopy department via wheelchair for EGD. Vital signs within normal limits. Consent signed. Reports that physician explained procedure and he has no questions at present.

1000 Returned from endoscopy. Reports no discomfort. Vital signs at baseline level. No apparent bleeding. Gag reflex present.

Special Considerations

Pediatric

- Children require deep sedation or general anesthesia (American Academy of Pediatrics, 2006).
- Introduction of the endoscope in infants and small children who have a narrow and collapsible airway can result in respiratory distress.

Geriatric

- Patient is at risk for prolonged sedation because of age-related decreased glomerular filtration rate and decreased hepatic function. Monitor urine output closely.
- Age-related thinning of the gastric mucosa increases the incidence of irritation and ulceration.
- Physical exposure and room temperature contribute to hypothermia in frail older adults. Use heated blankets or forced air heat to maintain core temperature at comfortable, safe levels.
- The older adult is at risk for dehydration, electrolyte imbalance, and exhaustion from test preparation combined with NPO status. If the procedure is done on an ambulatory care basis, it is helpful to have someone stay with the patient.

Home Care

- Instruct ambulatory care patients to notify the physician if the following symptoms develop: fever, chest pain or discomfort, dyspnea, wheezing, or hemoptysis.
- Manage throat discomfort with throat lozenges. Avoid commercial alcohol-based mouthwashes, which further irritate throat discomfort.
- After colonoscopy a warm tub bath minimizes rectal discomfort.
- Inform patient who received sedation not to drive for at least 24 hours after the procedure.

REVIEW QUESTIONS

Case Study for Questions 1 and 2

Mr. Hall, a 67-year-old black man, is a retired executive. He is scheduled for a cardiac catheterization and moderate sedation. The prescription for the procedure faxed from the physician's office lists "new-onset chest pain" as the clinical indication for the procedure. He is currently taking medication to control blood pressure and cholesterol and is on warfarin (Coumadin) for chronic atrial fibrillation. His personal physician instructed him to stop his warfarin two nights before the procedure. Mr. Hall followed the doctor's recommendation and has not had warfarin for 2 days.

1. What laboratory data would the nurse review as part of your preparation of Mr. Hall for his procedure? Select all that apply.
   1. Complete blood count (CBC) and levels of prealbumin and blood gases
   2. CBC and PT
   3. Lipid panel, blood glucose level, and electrolyte levels
   4. Blood urea nitrogen (BUN), creatinine, and urine specific gravity
2. When the nurse reviews Mr. Hall's chart, you see that the consent form for the procedure is unsigned. When you inquire whether the physician explained the procedure and the risks and ask if he has any questions, he replies, "My doctor told me that I needed this to find out why I have chest pain. But I don't know how risky it is." What would the nurse do? Select all that apply.
   1. Ask Mr. Hall to sign the consent form and tell him to ask about the risks when the doctor arrives.
   2. Hold the consent form until physician arrives to speak with Mr. Hall. Proceed with preparation by administering the preprocedure diazepam to Mr. Hall.
   3. Hold the consent form until the physician arrives to discuss the information needed for informed consent.
   4. Administer preprocedure diazepam (Valium) to help patient relax.
   5. Hold the preprocedure diazepam until after informed consent is obtained.
3. The nurse is assessing a patient after a cardiac catheterization. What assessments indicate possible bleeding? Select all that apply.
   1. Catheter site pain and loss of distal pulses
   2. Anxiety, backache, and heart rate increase from 90 to 105
   3. Atrial fibrillation and drowsiness
   4. Fever and bradycardia
4. The nurse has four patients scheduled for an IVP. For which patient is the procedure contraindicated?
   1. The patient with renal failure
   2. The patient with urinary tract infection
   3. The patient with possible kidney stones
   4. The patient with one kidney
5. The nurse's pediatric patient with leukemia is scheduled for a bone marrow aspiration. What nursing intervention is not appropriate?
   1. Apply topical anesthetic to the bone marrow aspiration site 10 minutes before the procedure is scheduled to begin.
   2. Verify that parental informed consent has been obtained.
   3. Use a doll to demonstrate the steps of the procedure for the child.
   4. Check emergency equipment for pediatric sizes.
6. Place the following steps of bronchoscopy preprocedure care in the proper order.
   1. Perform the preprocedure "Time Out."
   2. Administer IV moderate sedation.
   3. Verify that informed consent has been obtained.
   4. Position the patient on the bronchoscopy table.

7. The nurse's patient is unresponsive and febrile, and acute meningitis is suspected. An emergent LP is being done without the normal step of taking a computed tomography scan first to rule out IICP. Appropriate delegation of care to NAP includes:
   1. Instructing the nursing assistant to stay with her during the procedure to help maintain the patient's side-lying position
   2. Assisting the physician during the procedure and notifying you if the patient's vital signs deteriorate
   3. Monitoring patient's airway during the procedure and administering oxygen as needed
   4. Preparing the site and setting up the sterile tray
8. An abdominal paracentesis is performed on a patient, and 1500 mL of fluid is drained. Which of the outcomes indicate a successful procedure?
   1. Increased abdominal girth, decreased respiratory effort, increased respiratory rate
   2. Increased abdominal girth, increased respiratory effort, decreased respiratory rate
   3. Decreased abdominal girth, decreased respiratory effort, decreased respiratory rate
   4. Decreased abdominal girth, increased respiratory effort, increased respiratory rate
9. The nurse is preparing her patient for a colonoscopy. Which of the following are necessary for preprocedure preparation? Select all that apply.
   1. Maintain a side-lying position during the procedure.
   2. Complete the bowel preparation the morning of the procedure.
   3. Have nothing by mouth from midnight the day of the procedure.
   4. Come to the procedure with a designated driver.
10. Following an endoscopy, the patient is nauseated and vomits 200 mL of bright red blood. What are the nurse's correct actions? Select all that apply.
   1. Obtain your patient's vital signs.
   2. Observe and auscultate the abdomen.
   3. Instruct the NAP to obtain the vital signs.
   4. Observe the vomitus.

REFERENCES

Ahmed SV and others: Post lumbar puncture headache, *Postgrad Med J* 82(973):713, 2006.

Allibone C: Assessment and management of patients with pleural effusion, *Nurs Stand* 20(22):55, 2006.

American Academy of Pediatrics: Guidelines and management of pediatric patients during and after sedation for diagnostic and therapeutic procedures: an update, *Pediatrics* 118:2387, 2006.

American Association of Nurse Anesthetists (AANA): *AANA-ASA joint statement regarding propofol administration*, 2004, http://www.aana.com, accessed September 29, 2007.

American Society of Anesthesiologists: *Continuum of depth of sedation: definition of general anesthesia and levels of sedation/analgesia*, 2004, http://www.asahq.org/publicationsAndServices/standards/20.pdf, accessed September 2, 2010.

Chernecky CC, Berger BJ: *Laboratory tests and diagnostic procedures*, ed 5, Philadelphia, 2008, Elsevier.

Dellon ES and others: The use of carbon dioxide for insufflation during GI endoscopy: a systematic review, *Gastrointest Endosc* 69:843, 2009.

Edmond J and others: Introduction to cardiac catheterization. Part one: Diagnostic angiography, *Br J Cardiac Nurs* 3(9):398, 2008.

Hockenberry MJ, Wilson D: *Wong's essentials of pediatric nursing*, ed 8, St Louis, 2009, Mosby.

Hon LQ and others: Vascular closure devices: a comparative overview, *Curr Probl Diagn Radiol* 38(1):33, 2009.

Kadner K and others: Complications associated with the arterial puncture closure device: Angio-Seal, *Vasc Endovasc Surg* 42(3):225, 2008.

Kim MC: Vascular closure devices, *Cardiol Clin* 24:277, 2006.

Lee LC and others: Prevention and management of post-lumbar puncture headache in pediatric oncology patients, *J Pediatr Oncol Nurs* 24(4):200, 2007.

Murray P and others: *Prevention of acute renal failure in the intensive care unit: intensive care in nephrology*, London, 2006, Taylor and Francis.

Negishi C and others: Resistive-heating and forced-air warming are comparably effective, *Anesth Analg* 96(6):1683, 2003.

Ott L: Assessing blood flow with CT angiography, *Nursing* 28(1):26, 2008.

Pagana KD, Pagana TJ: *Mosby's diagnostic and laboratory tests*, ed 8, St Louis, 2007, Mosby.

The Joint Commission (TJC): *2010 National patient safety goals*, Oakbrook Terrace, Ill, 2010, The Commission, http://www.jointcommission.org/PatientSafety/NationalPatientSafetyGoals, accessed September 2009.

CHAPTER

10

Promoting Hygiene

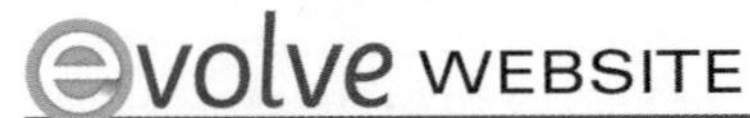

http://evolve.elsevier.com/Perry/nursinginterventions

Video Clips

Providing personal hygiene during an illness or recovery promotes the physical health of the patient's skin and his or her emotional well-being (Biggs, 2009). Personal hygiene provides an opportunity for the nurse and patient to interact about immediate and future emotional, social, and health-related concerns. Personal hygiene maintains skin integrity by promoting adequate circulation and hydration. The functions of intact skin include: (1) defense against infection; (2) awareness of touch, pain, heat, cold, and pressure; and (3) control of body temperature. Bathe the patient and change linens when any body part or linen becomes soiled. Problems such as incontinence, wound drainage, or diaphoresis may require frequent bathing. In addition to cleansing the skin, bathing a patient has several benefits such as stimulating circulation, promoting range of motion (ROM), reducing body odors, and improving self-image.

PATIENT-CENTERED CARE

Because hygiene requires close contact with a patient, ensure as much privacy as possible and convey sensitivity and respect for personal beliefs and cultural customs (Box 10-1). Take time to talk with the patient to identify personal and cultural preferences for the way to perform hygiene. When possible, ask friends or family members to bring in appropriate hygiene soaps, oils, and creams that are not available in the health care setting. Performing hygienic care gives you an opportunity to communicate with the patient and assess the individual's physical and psychological state. The patient may feel embarrassed or even frustrated relying on somebody else to meet his or her intimate needs (Lloyd, 2008). If the patient is anxious, use a calm and gentle manner when talking to him or her. Use a reassuring tone of voice so the patient feels safe and comfortable during bathing. Before performing any aspect of hygiene care, inform the patient of the procedure and acknowledge his or her preferences. Promote independence by encouraging the patient to participate in self-care activities.

SAFETY

Some patients lack the physical energy or functional status to perform self-care and are temporarily dependent on others to enhance the healing and recovery process. Although these patients may want to try to assist with their hygiene, do not leave them unattended because there is a risk for increased falls. If the patient cannot participate, the family or significant other may want to assist when appropriate. Assist the patient and family to understand that a full bath 3 times a week may be adequate for many older patients. Bathing older patients too frequently may contribute to dry skin and cause breaks in the skin. Normally the skin is elastic, well hydrated, firm, and smooth. With age the skin becomes thinner, dry, less vascular, more fragile, and prone to bruising and tears. Bathing is an excellent opportunity to assess the skin for common skin problems or pressure points, which are potential risks for pressure ulcers (Table 10-1). Be aware of other factors such as incontinence, friction, shear, immobility, loss of sensory perception, level of activity, and poor nutrition that contribute to pressure ulcer formation. It is imperative to identify risk factors and immediately begin interventions to reduce or eliminate the negative effects of each factor (see Chapter 25).

Before using showers or baths in health care settings, be sure that the patient has the physical energy and functional status to use the tub or shower. Fully assess the patient's

TABLE 10-1 COMMON SKIN PROBLEMS AND RELATED INTERVENTIONS

PROBLEM	INTERVENTIONS
Dry skin: Flaky, rough texture to skin, which may crack and become infected.	Bathe less frequently; rinse away all soap or use a waterless cleanser rather than soap; increase fluid intake; use moisturizing lotion.
Acne: Inflammatory papulopustular skin eruption, usually involving bacterial breakdown of sebum, typically on face, neck, shoulders, and back.	Wash hair daily. Wash skin twice daily with warm water and soap to remove oils and cosmetics (if used); cosmetics that can accumulate in pores should be used sparingly. If prescribed, topical antibiotics may minimize problems.
Rashes: Skin eruption from overexposure to sun or moisture or from allergic reaction; may be flat, raised, localized, or systemic; may be associated with pruritus (itching).	Wash and rinse thoroughly; apply antiseptic spray or lotion (as ordered) to prevent further itching and aid in healing process; warm or cold soaks relieve inflammation.
Contact dermatitis: Inflammation of skin characterized by abrupt onset with erythema, pruritus, pain, and scaly, oozing lesions; usually results from contact with substance difficult to identify and eliminate.	Wash and rinse thoroughly. Identify and avoid contributing agents; provide linens rinsed and sterilized to minimize irritation.
Abrasion: Scraping or rubbing away of epidermis (like a sheet burn) that results in localized bleeding and later weeping of serous fluid; easily infected.	Wash with mild soap and water; observe dressings for retained moisture, which can increase risk of infection.

BOX 10-1 CULTURAL CONSIDERATIONS FOR PERSONAL HYGIENE

- **For Middle-Eastern and East-Asian** women, avoid uncovering the lower torso and exposing the arms.
- **Orthodox Jews, Amish, Hindus, and Muslims** consider touching unrelated males and females taboo. Therefore males should care for males, and females should care for females. Family members should perform personal care involving the lower torso if gender-appropriate caregivers are not available. Among Hindus and Muslims the right hand is reserved for eating and praying, and the left hand is used only for cleaning gender-private areas.
- **Chinese, Japanese, Koreans, and Hindus** consider the upper body cleaner than the lower parts.
- **Hindus** consider it disrespectful to show any negative nonverbal communication when washing older adults' feet (Galanti, 2008).

activity tolerance and instruct the patient on how to use the emergency call device. In the home setting assess the patient's bath/shower facilities for safety bar, setting on hot water heaters, and the physical layout of the bathroom. Teach family caregivers for a dependent patient how to safely give a bath in the home.

EVIDENCE-BASED PRACTICE TRENDS

Johnson D and others: Patient's bath basins as potential sources of infection: a multicenter sampling study, *Am J Crit Care* 18(1):31, 2009.

Larson E and others: Comparison of traditional and disposable bed baths in critically ill patients, *Am J Crit Care* 13(3):235, 2004.

In 1994 Skewes developed the concept of a disposable bath in a bag. This product continues to be the mainstay in providing hygiene to critically ill and dependent patients. A study by Larson and others (2004) demonstrated that the disposable bath is a desirable form of bathing for patients in critical care and long-term care settings. In another study by Johnson and others (2009) it was found that the traditional soap and water bath using a bath basin can be a conduit for bacterial colonization.

The objectives of the study by Johnson and others (2009) were to identify and quantify bacteria in patients' bath basins and evaluate the bath basins as a possible reservoir for bacterial colonization and a risk factor for subsequent hospital-acquired infection. Results suggest that bath basins may be a reservoir and a way that harmful bacteria are spread. The researchers conclude that there should be increased awareness of bath basins as a possible source of hospital-acquired infections, especially in high-risk patients. According to the researchers, there is a need for further research in this area and further evaluation of alternative bathing methods such as the disposable systems (bag baths).

SKILL 10.1 COMPLETE BATHING

Video Clips

The type of bath, the extent of the bath, and the methods for bathing depend on the patient's ability to participate, the condition of the patient's skin, and in some settings time of day (Box 10-2). Whether to use a basin for bathing or a bag bath often depends on availability of the bag bath (see Procedural Guideline 10.2 and regional differences).

ASSESSMENT

1. Assess degree of assistance needed for bathing. Factors may include vision, ability to sit without support, hand grasp, ROM of extremities, and cognitive ability. *Rationale: Determines patient's ability to perform bathing.*
2. Assess patient's tolerance of activity, level of discomfort with movement, and presence of shortness of breath or chest pain with exertion. *Rationale: Determines type of cleansing bath appropriate for patient.*
3. Assess patient's bathing preferences such as time of day, products used, usual frequency of bathing, and type of bath. *Rationale: Patient participates in plan of care. Promotes patient's comfort and willingness to cooperate.*
4. Ask if patient has noticed any problems related to skin and genitalia. *Rationale: Provides information to direct physical assessment of skin and genitalia during the bath.*

BOX 10-2 TYPES OF BATHS

Complete bed bath: Bath administered to totally dependent patient in bed.

Partial bed bath: Bed bath that consists of bathing only body parts that would cause discomfort if left unbathed such as the hands, face, axilla, and perineal area. Partial bath also includes washing back and providing back rub. Dependent patients in need of partial hygiene or self-sufficient bedridden patients who are unable to reach all body parts receive a partial bed bath.

Sponge bath at the sink: Involves bathing from a bath basin or sink with patient sitting in a chair. Patient is able to perform a portion of the bath independently. Assistance is needed from the nurse for hard-to-reach areas.

Tub bath: Involves immersion in a tub of water that allows more thorough washing and rinsing than a bed bath. Some patients require the nurse's assistance. Some institutions have tubs equipped with lifting devices or panels that swing open to facilitate entry and positioning of dependent patients in the tub.

Shower: Patient sits or stands under a continuous stream of water. The shower provides more thorough cleansing than a bed bath but can be fatiguing.

Bag bath/travel bath: The bag bath contains several soft, nonwoven cotton cloths that are premoistened in a solution of no-rinse surfactant cleanser and emollient. The bag bath is an appealing alternative because of the ease of use, reduced time bathing, and patient comfort (Larson and others, 2004). There are now several commercial body cleansing systems that contain the same ingredients as the bag bath.

5. Before or during bath assess condition of patient's skin. Option: For patients at risk for pressure ulcers use a pressure ulcer assessment tool (see Chapter 25). *Rationale: Provides baseline for comparison over time in determining if bathing improves skin condition. Assessment also influences selection of skin care products.*
6. Carefully assess patients at risk for skin breakdown:
   a. Immobilization or decreased mobility (e.g., patients with paralysis, immobilized extremities, traction; weakened or disabled patients). *Rationale: These patients are more prone to pressure spots in dependent areas.*
   b. Reduced sensation (e.g., paresthesia, circulatory insufficiency, neuropathies).
   c. Nutritional and hydration alterations. *Rationale: Decrease in nutrition and hydration affect the condition of the skin with decreases in skin turgor, thickness, and elasticity.*
   d. Excessive moisture on skin, particularly on skin surfaces that rub against each other (e.g., under breasts, in perineal area. *Rationale: Skin folds trap moisture and cause friction between surfaces, which can lead to breaks in the skin and result in infection.*
   e. Vascular insufficiencies. *Rationale: Result in poor circulation to skin.*
   f. External devices applied to or around skin (e.g., casts, braces, restraints, dressings, catheters, tubes). *Rationale: Improperly placed medical devices or those that move after placement provide pressure or friction that can result in a wound.*
   g. Older-adult patients. *Rationale: Older adults have decreased appetite, which contributes to deficits in caloric intake, nutrients, vitamins, and fluids. This can predispose a patient to breaks in skin integrity.*
   h. Shear or friction (sliding down in bed). *Rationale: Causes damage to underlying tissues.*
   i. Incontinence (bowel or bladder). *Rationale: Accumulation of fluid causes skin maceration.*
7. Identify presence of devices (e.g., catheters, drains, dressings, restraints) and any prescribed limitations of activity or positioning required by patient's illness or treatment plan. *Rationale: Determines patient's safety needs to prevent injury.*
8. Assess room environment for temperature level. *Rationale: Protects patient from discomfort.*

PLANNING

Expected Outcomes focus on promoting comfort, mobility, and self-care abilities.

1. Patient's skin is clean and free of excretions, drainage, and odor.
2. Patient's skin shows decreased redness, cracking, flaking, and scaling.

3. Patient maintains functional ROM of hands and shoulders.
4. Patient demonstrates ability to wash face, hands, and chest independently.
5. Patient expresses comfort and relaxation.

Delegation and Collaboration

Assessment of the patient's skin, pain level, and ROM should not be delegated to nursing assistive personnel (NAP). The skill of bathing may be delegated. Instruct the NAP about the following:

- When a change in type of bath (complete, partial assist, tub, and shower) is planned
- Notifying the nurse of any skin integrity problems so the nurse can inspect areas of breakdown or potential breakdown
- Informing the nurse of concerns regarding changes in comfort level or activity tolerance noticed during bathing

Equipment

- Washcloths and towels
- Bath blanket
- Soap and soap dish
- Toilet tissue or peri-wipes
- Warm water
- Toiletry items (e.g., deodorant, powder, lotion, barrier cream)
- Clean hospital gown or patient's own pajamas
- Laundry bag
- Clean gloves (when body secretions are present)
- Washbasin
- Disposable bed bath if available

IMPLEMENTATION *for* COMPLETE BATHING

STEPS	RATIONALE
1. See Standard Protocol (inside front cover).	
2.  Offer patient bedpan or urinal.	Provides comfort and prevents interruption of bath.
a. If patient is incontinent, check perineum for fecal material. If present, enclose it in a fold of underpad and remove as much as possible with disposable wipes first.	Provides for patient comfort and prevents transmission of infection from fecal material.
b. Cleanse anal area from front to back (see illustration), with special attention to folds of buttocks, using as many washcloths as necessary to cleanse and rinse thoroughly.	Washing from front to back prevents transmission of microorganisms from anus to urethra or genitalia.

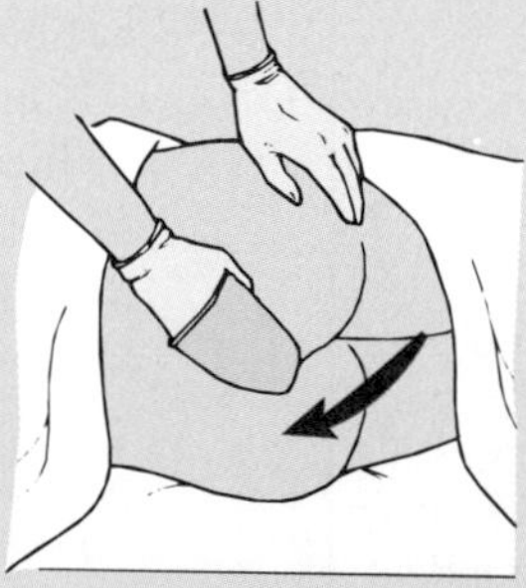

STEP 2b Cleanse buttocks from front to back.

STEPS	RATIONALE
c. Dry area completely.	Prevents skin maceration leading to breakdown.
d. Remove and discard underpad and replace with a clean one.	
e. Remove gloves and perform hand hygiene.	
3. Place bath blanket over patient and remove top sheet without exposing patient. Have patient hold top of bath blanket while removing linen.	Blanket provides warmth and privacy. Covering patient alleviates feeling of being exposed, embarrassed, and without dignity (Rader and others, 2006).
4. Place soiled linen in laundry bag, taking care not to allow it to contact uniform.	Prevents transmission of microorganisms.

STEPS	RATIONALE
5. Remove patient's gown or pajamas. If an extremity is injured or has limited mobility, begin removal from unaffected side first. For patients with an intravenous (IV) line, use a gown with sleeves that have shoulder snaps if possible.	Reduces risk of increased pain or injury.
a. When the gown does not have shoulder snaps, remove it from the arm without the IV line and slide it off the shoulder and arm toward the wrist, keeping the IV line carefully secured (see illustration).	Reduces risk of accidental dislodgement of IV line.
b. Remove bag from IV pole (see illustration).	
c. Slide IV bag and tubing through sleeve (see illustration).	
d. Rehang bag, check flow rate, and regulate if necessary (see illustration).	Manipulation of tubing and container may disrupt flow rate.
e. If IV pump is in use, with the assistance of a registered nurse, turn pump off, clamp tubing, remove tubing from pump, and proceed as before. Insert tubing into pump, unclamp tubing, and turn pump on at correct rate. Observe flow rate and regulate if necessary.	Sterility, patency, and correct rate of infusion must be maintained.

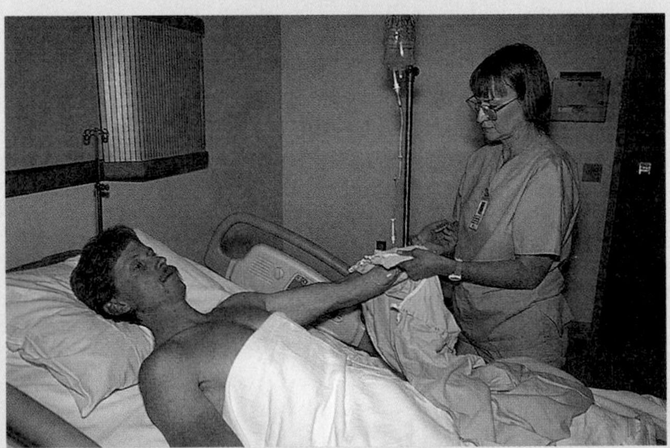

STEP 5a Remove patient's gown.

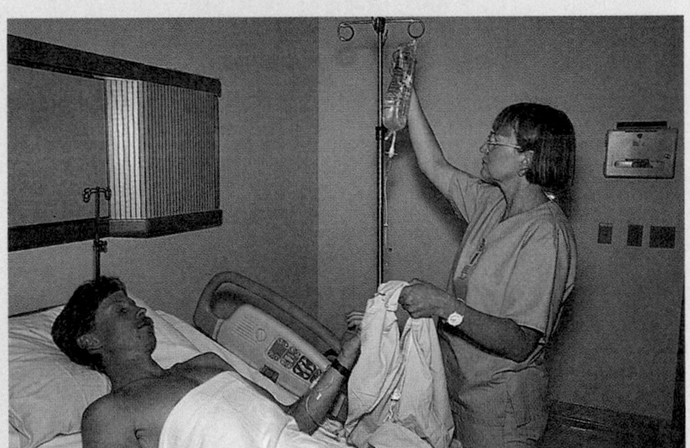

STEP 5b Remove IV bag from pole.

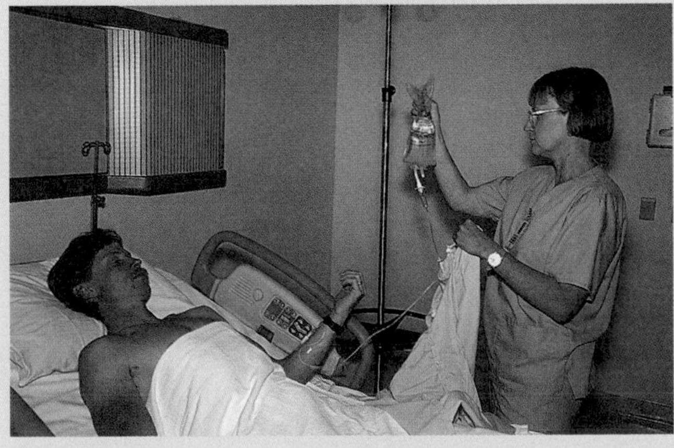

STEP 5c Slide IV tubing and bag through arm of patient's gown.

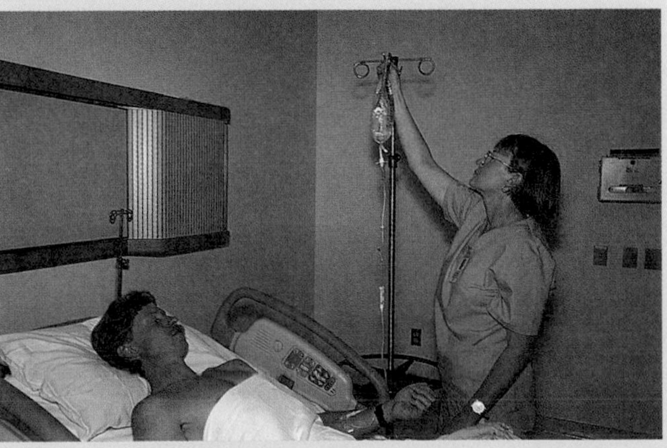

STEP 5d Rehang IV bag.

Continued

STEPS	RATIONALE

SAFETY ALERT For debilitated patients at risk for falls, provide safety by using side rails as appropriate if at any time it is necessary to leave the patient unattended. Check temperature of bath water throughout the bath and change as needed to maintain warmth.

STEPS	RATIONALE
6. Fill washbasin two-thirds full with warm water. Adjust water temperature to be comfortably warm to your wrist and allow the patient to test temperature tolerance. Place washbasin and supplies within easy reach.	Warm water promotes comfort, relaxes muscles, and prevents chilling.
7. Remove pillow. Place one bath towel under patient's head and another over chest.	Removing pillow facilitates bathing ears and neck. Towels absorb moisture.
8. Immerse washcloth in water, wring thoroughly, and form mitt (see illustration).	Mitt retains heat better and prevents loose ends from dripping or annoying patient.
9. Wash face.	
a. Wash patient's eyes with plain warm water using a clean area of cloth for each eye, bathing from inner to outer canthus (see illustration). Dry around eyes gently and thoroughly.	Soap irritates eyes. Bathing inner-to-outer canthus prevents secretions from entering nasolacrimal duct. Using a clean area of the cloth reduces the possibility of infection transmission.
b. Wash, rinse, and dry forehead, cheeks, nose, neck, and ears without using soap. Ask men if they want to be shaved (see Procedural Guideline 10.5).	Soap can be used if patient prefers; however, soap tends to dry face, which is exposed to air more than other body part. If patient has a preferred facial wash, use it.

SAFETY ALERT Patients who are unconscious have lost the normal blink reflex of the eye, which increases their risk for corneal drying, corneal abrasions, and eye infections (Critical Care Extra, 2006). Obtain a physician's order or follow agency policy to instill eyedrops or ointment to help keep a patient's eyes moist. Reassess eyes every 2 to 4 hours for dryness. In the absence of a blink reflex, keep the eyelids closed and covered with an eye patch or shield. Do not tape the eyelid closed because this can injure tissues.

STEPS	RATIONALE
10. Wash trunk and upper extremities.	
a. Expose patient's arm. Place bath towel lengthwise under arm. Bathe with minimal soap and water using long, firm strokes from distal to proximal (fingers to axilla).	Promotes venous blood return to heart.

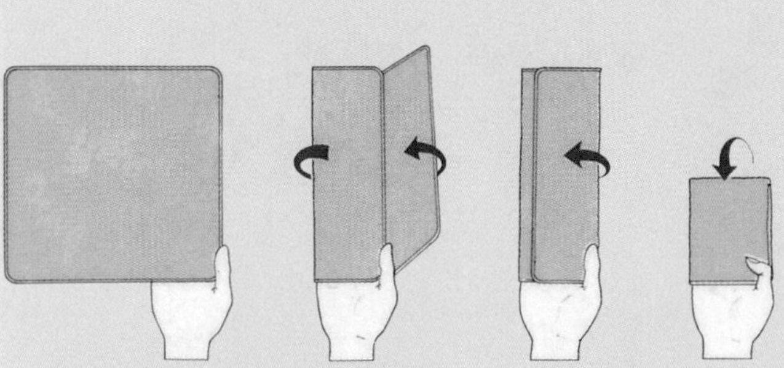

STEP 8 Steps for folding washcloth to form a mitt.

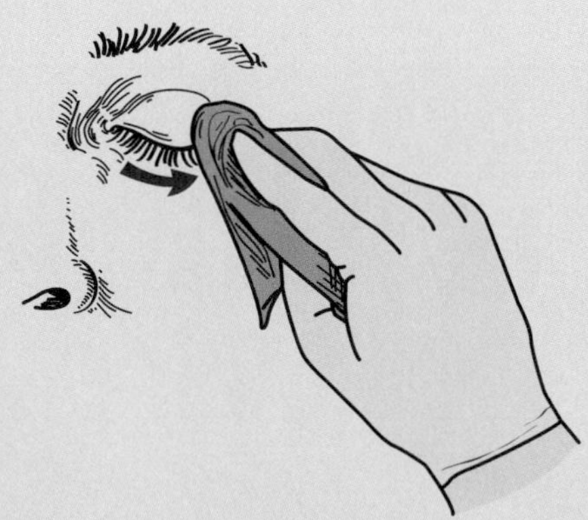

STEP 9a Wash eye from inner to outer canthus.

STEPS	RATIONALE
b. Raise and support arm above head (if possible) to wash, rinse, and dry axilla thoroughly (see illustration).	Raising arm promotes ROM and facilitates thorough cleansing.

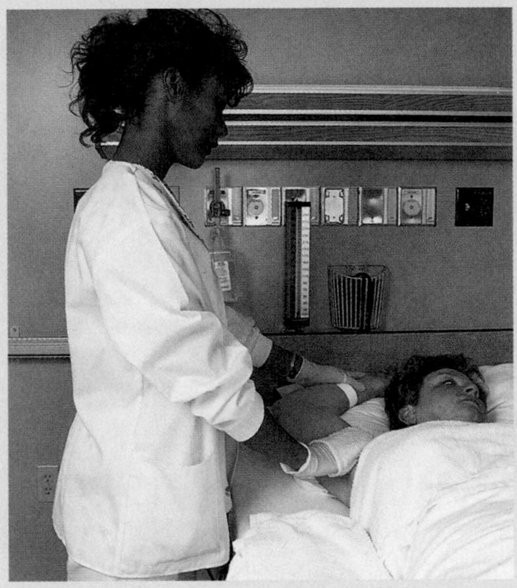

STEP 10b Positioning the arm to wash the axilla.

STEPS	RATIONALE
c. Move to the opposite side of the bed and repeat Steps 10a and 10b. Apply deodorant or powder sparingly to underarms, following patient preference.	Deodorant and powder control body odor.
d. Cover patient's chest with bath towel and fold bath blanket down to umbilicus. Bathe chest using long, firm strokes, lifting breast upward if necessary. Rinse and dry well.	Skin under breasts is vulnerable to excoriation if not kept clean and dry.
11. Wash the abdomen.	
a. Place bath towel over chest and abdomen and fold bath blanket down to just above pubic region. Bathe, rinse, and dry abdomen with special care to umbilicus and skin folds of abdomen and groin.	Keeping skin folds clean and dry helps prevent odor and skin irritation. Moisture and sediment that collect in skin folds predispose skin to maceration.
12. Wash legs.	
a. Expose patient's leg nearest to you, leaving perineum covered.	Provides privacy.
b. Place bath towel under leg, supporting leg at knee and with foot flat on bed.	Keeps linen dry.
c. Place patient's foot in a basin to soak while washing and rinsing. If patient is unable to support leg, assistance is needed, or soaking is omitted.	

SAFETY ALERT Do not soak the feet of patients with diabetes mellitus. This may lead to skin dryness (National Diabetes Education Program, 2003). Dry, scaly skin is susceptible to crack or ulcerate, providing an entry site for bacteria (Pinzur and others, 2005).

Continued

STEPS	RATIONALE
d. Wash leg using short, light strokes. Dry leg thoroughly from ankle to knee and knee to thigh (see illustration). Assess for redness, swelling, tenderness, or pain. Wash between toes. Rinse and dry thoroughly.	Promotes circulation and venous return. Assessing for redness, swelling, tenderness, and pain in the lower extremities is important because these may be early signs of deep vein thrombosis (DVT, i.e., blood clots) (Beck, 2006). Secretions and moisture are often present between toes, predisposing patient to maceration, breakdown, and infection.

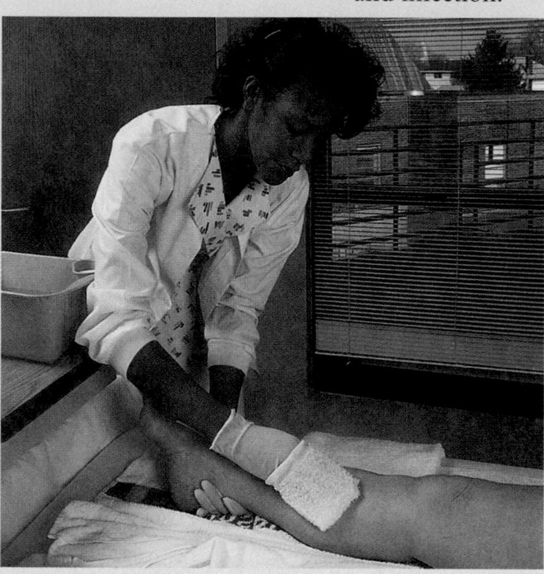

STEP 12d Washing the leg.

> **SAFETY ALERT** Use short, light strokes when washing the legs of a patient at risk of DVT. Long, firm strokes can dislodge a clot, resulting in an embolism. Warmth, redness, swelling, tenderness, and pain in the lower extremities because these might be early signs (Beck, 2006).

STEPS	RATIONALE
e. Raise side rail (if used), move to opposite side, lower side rail, and repeat with other leg and foot. If skin is dry, apply lotion.	Promotes good body mechanics for the nurse. Lotions are effective in moisturizing skin.
f. Cover with bath blanket and raise side rail (if used). Change bath water.	Provides patient warmth and safety.
13. Provide perineal care (see Procedural Guideline 10.1).	
14. Wash back.	
a. Place patient in side-lying position. Place towel lengthwise along patient's side and keep patient covered as much as possible.	Exposes back and buttocks for bathing. Covering promotes warmth and privacy.
b. Wash, rinse, and dry back from neck to buttocks using long, firm strokes. Remove and discard gloves.	Promotes circulation.
15. Cover patient with bath blanket.	
16. Remove gloves, perform hand hygiene, dispose of water, and store basin appropriately.	
17. Apply body lotion to skin as needed and topical moisturizing agents to dry, flaky, or scaling areas. Replace gown.	Dry skin results in reduced pliability and cracking. Moisturizers help prevent skin breakdown.
18. Massage back.	
a. Position patient prone if possible. Side-lying position is used frequently.	

STEPS	RATIONALE
b. Using lotion, begin at sacral area and massage in circular motion, stroking upward from buttocks to shoulders and upper arms and over scapulae with smooth, firm strokes (see illustration). Keep hands on skin and continue massage pattern for 3 to 4 minutes.	Massage stimulates circulation and relaxation.

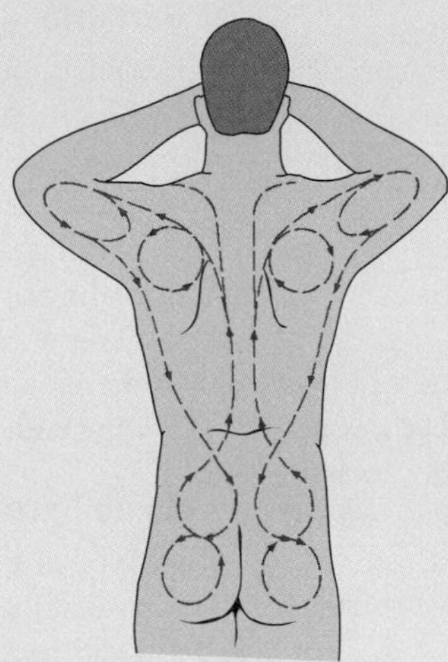

STEP 18b Massage in circular motion upward from buttocks.

STEPS	RATIONALE
c. Knead muscles of upper back and shoulders by grasping tissue between thumb and fingers. Ask the patient if your grasp is uncomfortable. Knead upward along each side of spine and around muscles of neck, avoiding bony prominences.	These muscles are thick and can be massaged vigorously.

> **SAFETY ALERT** Do not massage reddened areas over bony prominences. Evidence suggests that firm massage over these areas may result in decreased blood flow and tissue damage (NPUAP, 2007).

STEPS	RATIONALE
d. End massage with long, stroking movements and tell patient that you are ending massage.	Long strokes promote comfort and relaxation.
e. Observe and report any redness or skin breakdown, paying particular attention to bony prominences.	Assessment is a key intervention to identification of early signs of skin breakdown.
f. Remove excess lotion from back with bath towel.	Excess lotion could promote maceration of skin.
19. Assist patient with grooming, oral hygiene, shaving, hair care, and application of makeup (if desired). (See Procedural Guidelines 10.3 through 10.6.)	Promotes patient's body image.
20. Make patient's bed (see Procedural Guideline 10.7).	
21. See Completion Protocol (inside front cover).	

EVALUATION

1. Observe areas on skin for erythema, exudate, drainage, or breakdown.
2. Measure ROM in hands, arms, and shoulders and compare with baseline.
3. Assess vital signs if patient is experiencing distress or restlessness.
4. Observe for improved ability to assist with self-bathing and hygiene to determine progress.
5. Ask patient to comment on appearance and comfort.

Unexpected Outcomes and Related Interventions

1. Patient's skin on lower extremities is dry, flaky, and itchy.
   a. Limit the frequency of baths to every other day or less.
   b. Use antibacterial soap sparingly. Use a mild soap that is nondrying and rinse thoroughly.
   c. Blot skin dry after bathing and apply lotion to skin.
   d. Administer antipyretics as ordered to control itching.
2. The patient's skin has evidence of rashes, redness, scaling, or cracking.

a. Evaluate the need for a change in frequency of bathing and soap product used.
b. Collaborate with the health care provider regarding application of ointments or creams to provide a protective barrier and help maintain moisture within the skin.
c. For obese patients with fungal growth between skin folds, consider antifungal powders to minimize moisture and treat irritations.

3. The rectum, perineum, or genital region is inflamed, is swollen, or has foul-smelling discharge.
a. Bathe area frequently enough to keep clean and dry.
b. Apply protective barrier or antiinflammatory cream.
c. Report to health care provider.

Recording and Reporting

- Routine documentation may include completion of flow sheet. Record observations made during the bath, which may include type of bath given, patient's ability to assist or cooperate, condition of patient's skin, and any nursing interventions for improving skin integrity.
- Record patient's response to bathing and any concerns voiced by patient regarding self-care needs.

Sample Documentation

0900 Cooperative with turning during bed bath. Stated he felt "very weak." Both legs dry and flaking. Complained of severe itching. Bath oil added to bath water. Emollient lotion applied after bath. States itching is less now.

Special Considerations

Pediatric

- Infants chill easily; keep body covered and work quickly.
- Use only mild soap for bathing infants and children (Hockenberry and Wilson, 2007).
- Families need to be involved in a child's care; children feel more secure in the presence of their family.

Geriatric

- Older adults may chill easily.
- Older adults with urinary incontinence need meticulous skin care to reduce skin irritation from urine and feces.
- Older adults have dry skin and do not need frequent bathing. Reducing the frequency of bathing can prevent scaling or cracking of the skin (Rader and others, 2006).
- Older adults who need assistance with bathing often find the activity to be both physically and emotionally demanding (Rader and others, 2006).

Home Care

- Type of bath chosen depends on assessment of the home, availability of running water, and condition of bathing facilities.
- The two types of bath for the homebound patient are complete and partial.
- Adhesive strips on bottom of tub or shower, hand rails, chairs, or stools in tub or shower help protect patients from falls and injury. Patient also may use portable shower seat.

PROCEDURAL GUIDELINE 10.1
Perineal Care

Perineal care involves thorough cleansing of the patient's external genitalia and surrounding skin. A patient routinely receives perineal care during a complete bath (see Skill 10.1). However, patients who have fecal or urinary incontinence or an indwelling Foley catheter or are recovering from rectal or genital surgery or childbirth need more frequent perineal hygiene. Wear gloves during perineal care because of the risk of contacting infectious organisms present in fecal, urinary, or vaginal secretions. Perineal care may be embarrassing for both the patient and nurse. Always act in a professional and sensitive manner and provide privacy at all times.

Delegation and Collaboration

The skill of perineal care can be delegated to nursing assistive personnel (NAP). Instruct the NAP about:

- Any physical restriction that affects proper positioning of patient
- The proper ways to position male and female patients with an indwelling Foley catheter during perineal care.
- Notifying the nurse of any perineal drainage, excoriation, or rash observed

Equipment

- Washcloths, bath towels, and bath blankets
- Soap and soap dish
- Toilet paper or hygiene wipes and washbasin
- Warm water
- Laundry bag
- Waterproof pad or bedpan
- Clean gloves

PROCEDURAL GUIDELINE 10.1
Perineal Care—cont'd

Procedural Steps

1. **See Standard Protocol (inside front cover).**
2. Provide perineal care:
   a. *For a female:*
      (1) If patient is able to maneuver and handle washcloth, allow cleansing perineum on own.
      (2) Assist patient in assuming dorsal recumbent position. Note restrictions or any limitation in patient's positioning. Be sure to position waterproof pad under buttocks.
      (3) Drape patient with bath blanket placed in the shape of a diamond.
      (4) Fold both outer corners of the bath blanket up around patient's legs onto abdomen and under hip (see illustration). Then you can lift the lower tip of the bath blanket when you are ready to expose the perineum.

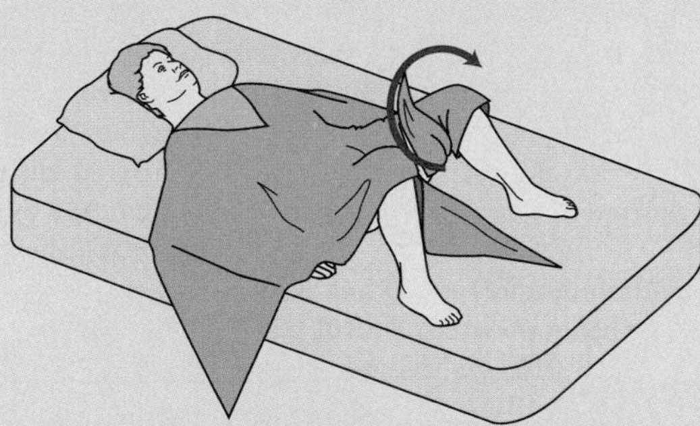

STEP 2a(4) Drape patient for perineal care.

      (5) Wash and dry the patient's upper thighs.
      (6) Wash labia majora. Use nondominant hand to gently retract labia from thigh; with dominant hand, wash carefully in skin folds. Wipe in direction from perineum to rectum (front to back). Repeat on opposite side using separate section of washcloth. Rinse and dry area thoroughly. Discard washcloth.
      (7) Gently separate labia with nondominant hand to expose urethral meatus and vaginal orifice. With dominant hand, use a new washcloth to wash downward from pubic area toward rectum in one smooth stroke (see illustration). Use separate section of cloth for each stroke. Cleanse thoroughly over labia minora, clitoris, and vaginal orifice. Avoid placing tension on indwelling catheter if present and clean around it thoroughly (see Procedural Guideline 19.3 for care of catheter).

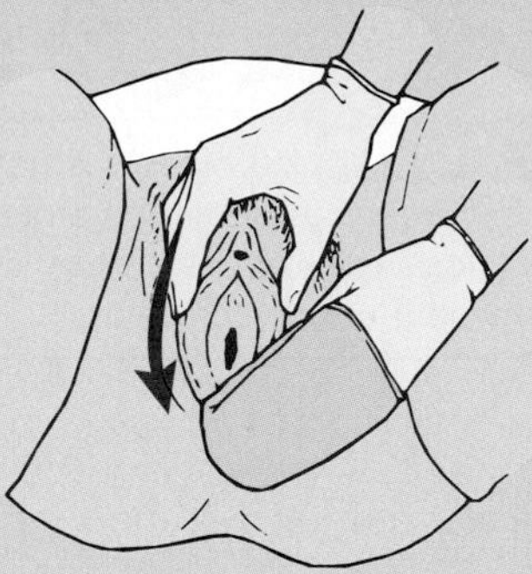

STEP 2a(7) Cleanse from perineum to rectum (front to back).

      (8) Rinse area thoroughly. If patient uses a bedpan, an option is to have patient on the pan and to pour warm water over perineum.
      (9) Ask patient to lower legs and assume comfortable position.
   b. *For a male:*
      (1) If patient is able to maneuver and handle washcloth, allow cleansing perineum on own.
      (2) Assist patient to supine position. Note any mobility restrictions.
      (3) Place bath blanket over patient. Then fold lower half of bath blanket up to expose upper thighs. Wash and dry thighs.
      (4) Cover thighs with bath towels. Raise bath blanket to expose genitalia. Gently raise penis and place bath towel underneath. Gently grasp shaft of penis. If patient is uncircumcised, retract foreskin. If patient has an erection, defer procedure until later.
      (5) Wash tip of penis at urethral meatus first. Using circular motion, cleanse from meatus outward (see illustration). Repeat, using a separate section of the cloth until the penis is clean. Rinse and dry carefully. Discard the washcloth.

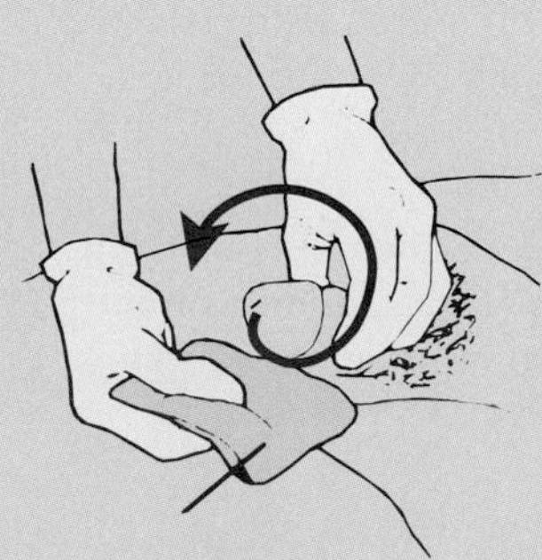

STEP 2b(5) Wash penis in a circular motion.

Continued

PROCEDURAL GUIDELINE 10.1
Perineal Care—cont'd

(6) Return foreskin to its natural position.

SAFETY ALERT If foreskin is not returned to its natural position, tightening of foreskin around shaft of penis can cause local edema; discomfort; and, if not corrected, permanent urethral damage.

(7) Take a new washcloth and gently cleanse the shaft of penis and the scrotum by having patient abduct legs. Pay special attention to underlying surface of penis. Lift scrotum carefully and wash underlying skin folds. Rinse and dry thoroughly.

3. Remove all towels, and then fold bath blanket back over patient's perineum and assist patient to comfortable position.
4. Observe perineal area for any irritation, redness, or drainage that persists after perineal hygiene.
5. **See Completion Protocol (inside front cover).**

PROCEDURAL GUIDELINE 10.2
Use of Disposable Bag Bath

Delegation and Collaboration

Assessment of the patient's skin, pain level, and ROM should not be delegated to nursing assistive personnel (NAP). The skill of bathing may be delegated. Instruct the NAP about the following:

- Notifying the nurse of any skin integrity problems so the nurse can inspect areas of breakdown or potential breakdown
- Notifying the nurse of any skin integrity problem or changes in comfort level or activity tolerance noticed during bathing

Equipment

- Prepackaged, disposable bathing systems are available over the counter (OTC) for use in the home and in health care agencies. Each bath kit contains 8 to 10 disposable cloths premoistened with a cleansing solution that does not require rinsing or towel drying.
- Clean gloves if body fluids present.

Procedural Steps

1. See **Standard Protocol (inside front cover)**.
2. Position patient in a supine position or position of comfort.
3. Assess condition of the skin (see Chapter 7).
4. Warm bath bag or pack in a microwave, following package directions. (The cleansing pack contains 8 to 10 premoistened towels).

SAFETY ALERT Microwaves differ in the power available. Check the temperature of the towels carefully, as inside of towel can retain heat. This could lead to accidental burn of patient's skin.

5. Use a single towel for each body part cleansed. Follow the same order as the total or partial bed bath (see Skill 10.1). No rinsing is needed.
6. Allow the skin to air dry for 30 seconds. It is permissible to lightly cover patient with a bath towel to prevent chilling. No towel drying is needed.

NOTE: If there is excessive soiling (e.g., in the perineal region), an extra bag bath may be necessary; or conventional perineal care using washcloths, water, and towels may be used.

7. **See Completion Protocol (inside front cover)**

PROCEDURAL GUIDELINE 10.3
Oral Care for the Debilitated or Unconscious Patient

Oral hygiene maintains the comfort and integrity of oral cavity mucosa and helps control plaque-associated oral diseases. Inadequate oral hygiene can result in plaque formation, inflammation, pain, and infection (MacNeill and Sorenson, 2009). Poor oral health effects general health, social acceptability, self-esteem, and overall quality of life (Jerreat and others, 2007). Adequate daily oral hygiene includes brushing, flossing, and rinsing. Many factors influence oral hygiene (Box 10-3). Encouraging dependent or chronically ill patients to attend to their own oral hygiene creates a general sense of comfort and improves appetite. Frequency of oral care depends on the condition of the oral cavity and patient's comfort. Oral hygiene may be required as often as every 1 to 2 hours. For unconscious patients, first assess the patient's gag reflex and determine the type of suction apparatus needed to prevent aspiration. Unconscious patients are at risk for oral infections because of the absence of saliva movement and production, which leads to large numbers of gram-negative bacteria in the oral cavity. Critically ill patients with endotracheal tubes and who are on mechanical ventilation are at risk for ventilator-associated pneumonia (VAP) if the saliva is aspirated. Many patients have no gag reflex. Proper hygiene requires keeping the mucosa moist and removing secretions. It appears that mechanical elimination of plaque is a key factor in reducing or eliminating VAP (MacNeill and Sorenson, 2009). Mechanical elimination includes toothbrushing and rinsing of the oral cavity (Munro and Grap, 2004).

Delegation and Collaboration

The skill of oral hygiene (including toothbrushing, flossing, and rinsing) can be delegated to nursing assistive personnel (NAP). However, the nurse is responsible for the assessment of the patient's gag reflex to determine if the patient is at risk for aspiration. Instruct the NAP about the following:

- The patient's level of consciousness, presence or absence of gag reflex, proper positioning, and whether oral suction apparatus is needed for clearing oral secretions
- Reporting any changes in oral mucosa to the nurse
- Reporting excessive coughing or choking during or after oral care

Equipment

- Clean gloves
- Soft-bristled toothbrush or sponge Toothette for edentulous patient
- Fluoridated toothpaste
- Antiinfective or chlorhexidine mouth rinse (order might be required)
- Water-based mouth moisturizer
- Glass of water
- Emesis basin
- Tongue blade
- Face towel, paper towels
- Suction equipment (optional): Suction machine or Yankauer suction
- Water-soluble lubricant
- Oral airway (uncooperative patient or patient who shows bite reflex)

Procedural Steps

1. **See Standard Protocol (inside front cover).**
2. Assess for presence or absence of gag reflex by placing tongue blade on back of tongue.
3. Inspect lips, teeth, gums, buccal mucosa, palate, and tongue using tongue depressor and penlight if necessary (see Chapter 7). Observe for color, texture, moisture, lesions or ulcers, and condition of teeth or dentures.

BOX 10-3 FACTORS INFLUENCING ORAL HYGIENE

- Patient lacks upper-extremity strength or dexterity to perform oral hygiene (e.g., is paralyzed, has limited ROM).
- Patient is unable or unwilling to attend to personal hygiene needs (e.g., is unconscious, depressed, confused).
- Patient has diabetes and is prone to dryness of mouth, gingivitis, periodontal disease, and loss of teeth.
- Patient is prone to dehydration, has a fever, or is NPO (unable to take food or fluids). Thick secretions develop on tongue and gums. Lips become cracked and reddened.
- Radiation therapy causes soreness, mild erythema, swollen mucosa, dysphagia, dryness, taste changes, and possible oral infection.
- Chronic inflammatory disease may be caused by bacteria, viral or fungal infections, or ineffective oral hygiene.
- Chemotherapy causes ulcerations and inflammation of mucosa and possible oral infection. Chemical injury may result from irritating substances such as alcohol, tobacco, acidic foods, or side effects of medications, including chemotherapy, antibiotics, steroids, and antidepressants. Mucositis (inflammation of the mucous membranes in the mouth) is a common complication in patients receiving radiation or chemotherapy.
- Trauma to oral cavity from oral tubes, suctioning, hot foods, broken teeth, or ill-fitting dentures causes swelling, ulcerations, inflammation, and possible bleeding.
- Mouth breathing and use of oxygen may result in dry mucous membranes.

Continued

PROCEDURAL GUIDELINE 10.3
Oral Care for the Debilitated or Unconscious Patient—cont'd

4. Position unconscious patient in side-lying position with bed flat and head turned toward mattress. Place towel under chin. Have emesis basin available.
5. Remove dentures or partial plates if present (see Procedural Guideline 10.4).
6. If patient is uncooperative or having difficulty keeping mouth open, insert an oral airway. Insert it upside down into the mouth, and then turn it sideways as you insert it toward the back of the pharynx and then over the tongue, to keep teeth apart. Insert when patient is relaxed. Do not use force (see illustration).

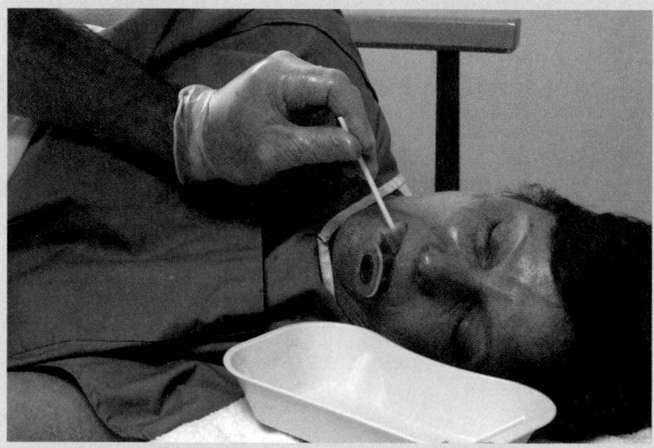

STEP 6 Placement of oral airway; nurse cleans lips with moistened Toothette.

7. Clean mouth using brush moistened in water. Apply toothpaste or use antiinfective solution first to loosen crusts. Hold toothbrush bristles at 45-degree angle to gum line. Brush inner and outer surfaces of upper and lower teeth by brushing from gum to crown. Clean biting surface of teeth by holding top of bristles parallel with teeth and brushing back and forth. Brush sides of teeth moving bristles back and forth (see illustration). A Toothette may be used for patients who have no teeth or have sensitive gums. Moisten brush with chlorhexidine solution to rinse. Use brush or Toothette to clean roof of mouth, gums, and inside cheeks. Gently brush tongue but avoid stimulating gag reflex (if present). Moisten the brush or Toothette to rinse; repeat, rinsing several times.

> **SAFETY ALERT** Suction should be on and ready for use if gag reflex is absent (see Chapter 14).

8. Suction **oral** secretions as they accumulate to reduce risk of aspiration.
9. Apply a thin layer of water-soluble jelly to lips (see illustration).
10. **See Completion Protocol (inside front cover).**

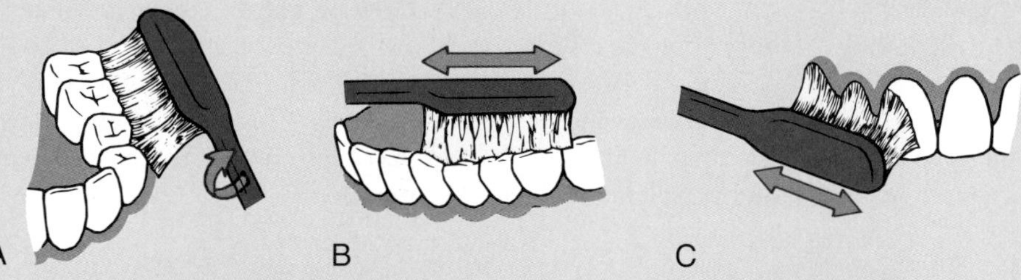

STEP 7 Directions of toothbrush. **A,** A 45-degree angle brushes gum line. **B,** Parallel position brushes biting surfaces. **C,** Lateral position brushes side of teeth.

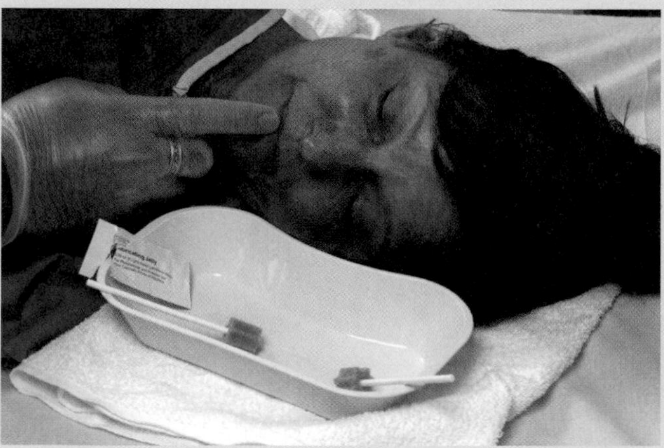

STEP 9 Apply water-soluble moisturizer to lips.

PROCEDURAL GUIDELINE 10.4 Care of Dentures

Video Clips

Clean dentures as regularly as natural teeth to prevent gingival infection and irritation. Loose dentures can cause discomfort and make it difficult for patients to chew food and speak clearly. Loose dentures may result from weight loss. Refer the patient to his or her dentist as needed. Dentures can be easily lost or broken. Store them in an enclosed, labeled cup and soak when not worn (e.g., at night, during surgery or a diagnostic procedure). Reinsert them as soon as possible. The change in appearance when they are not worn may be of major concern to the patient.

Delegation and Collaboration

- The skill of denture care may be delegated to nursing assistive personnel (NAP).

Equipment

- Clean gloves
- Soft-bristled toothbrush or denture toothbrush
- Denture cleaning agent or toothpaste, denture adhesive (optional)
- Glass of water
- Emesis basin or sink
- Washcloth
- 4 × 4–inch gauze
- Denture cup (if dentures are to be stored after cleaning)

Procedural Steps

1. **See Standard Protocol (inside front cover).**
2. Ask patient if dentures fit and if there is any gum or mucous membrane tenderness or irritation.
3. Ask patient about preferences for denture care and products used.
4. Encourage patient to provide denture care independently if able. If patient is unable, it is important for the nurse to provide care.
5. Provide denture care during routine mouth care.
6. Fill emesis basin with tepid water or, if using sink, place washcloth in bottom of sink and fill sink with 1 inch of water.
7. Ask patient to remove dentures. Alternatively, apply gloves, grasp upper plate at front with thumb and index finger wrapped in gauze, and pull downward. Gently lift lower denture from jaw and rotate one side downward to remove from patient's mouth. Hold dentures over emesis basin or sink lined with washcloth and containing 1 inch of water.
8. Apply cleaning agent to brush and brush surfaces of dentures. Hold dentures close to water (see illustration). Hold brush horizontally and use back-and-forth motion to cleanse biting surfaces. Use short strokes from top of denture to biting surfaces to clean outer teeth surfaces. Hold brush vertically and use short strokes to clean inner tooth surfaces. Hold brush horizontally and use back-and-forth motion to clean undersurface of dentures.

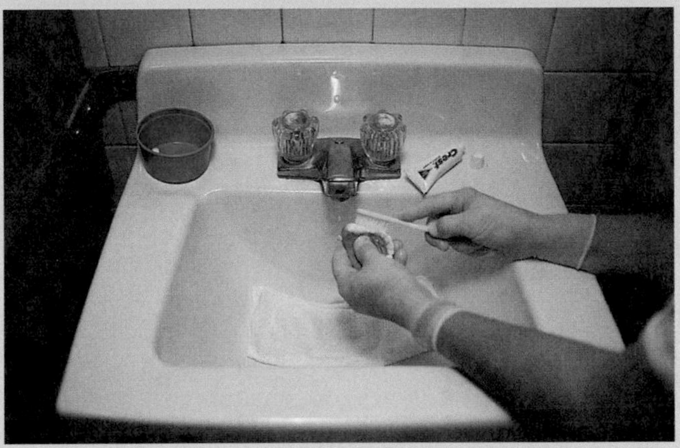

STEP 8 Cleansing dentures in sink.

9. Rinse thoroughly in tepid water.
10. Some patients use an adhesive to seal dentures in place. Apply a thin layer to undersurface of each denture before inserting.
11. If patient needs assistance with insertion of dentures, moisten upper denture and press firmly to seal it in place. Then insert moistened lower denture. Ask if dentures feel comfortable.
12. Some patients prefer to have their dentures stored to give the gums a rest and reduce risk of infection. Keeping dentures moist prevents warping and facilitates easier insertion. Store in tepid water in denture cup. Label the denture cup with patient's name, using either a permanent marker or the patient's identification label and keep in a secure place.
13. **See Completion Protocol (inside front cover).**

PROCEDURAL GUIDELINE 10.5
Hair Care—Shampooing and Shaving

Video Clips

Brushing, combing, and shampooing hair are basic measures for all patients unable to provide self-care. Having the hair groomed makes a person feel more comfortable. Many agencies have a beauty shop where patients can go for professional hair care. Fever, malnutrition, some medications, emotional stress, and depression affect the condition of hair. Diaphoresis leaves hair oily and unmanageable.

Table 10-2 describes common hair and scalp conditions and nursing interventions.

Frequency of shampooing depends on the condition of the hair and the person's personal preferences. Dry hair requires less frequent shampooing than oily hair. Hospitalized patients who have excess perspiration or treatments that leave blood or solutions in the hair may need a shampoo. Positioning with the neck hyperextended over the edge of a sink is contraindicated for patients who have had neck injuries or back pain. Patients may be placed on a stretcher with their head extended over a sink. Bedridden patients use a plastic shampoo trough that drains into a bedside container.

Dependent patients with beards or mustaches need assistance keeping the facial hair clean, especially after eating. Shaving facial hair is a task most men prefer to do for themselves daily. Food particles easily collect in the hair. Because some religions and cultures forbid cutting or shaving any body hair, be sure to obtain consent from these patients (Galanti, 2008).

Delegation and Collaboration

Assessment of the patient's condition may not be delegated. The skills of shampooing and shaving can be delegated to nursing assistive personnel (NAP). Instruct the NAP about the following:

- How to properly position patients with mobility restrictions
- Reporting how the patient tolerated the procedure and reporting any concerns (such as neck pain)
- Any patient at risk for bleeding tendencies and the need to use an electric razor

Equipment

- Hair care:
  - Clean gloves
  - Brush/comb
  - Shampoo board
  - Shampoo and conditioner (optional)
  - Towels (two or more).
  - Dry shampoo cap as an alternative
- Shaving:
  - Disposable or electric razor
  - Shaving cream
  - Basin of very warm water
  - Bath towels

TABLE 10-2 COMMON HAIR AND SCALP CONDITIONS AND RELATED INTERVENTIONS

PROBLEM	INTERVENTIONS
Alopecia (hair loss): Chemotherapeutic agents kill cells that rapidly multiply, including both tumor and normal cells.	Some patients wear scarves. Some prefer hairpieces. Referral may be necessary for professional consultation for long-term interventions.
Dandruff: Scaling of scalp accompanied by itching; if severe, may involve eyebrows.	Shampoo regularly with medicated shampoo.
Pediculosis	
Head lice: Parasites attached to hair strands. Eggs look like oval particles. Bites or pustules may be found behind ears and at hairline. May spread to furniture and other people.	Check the entire scalp. Use a special lice comb to remove lice and nits. The National Pediculosis Association (2005) encourages a nonchemical approach with manual removal. Caution against using products containing Lindane because the ingredient is a neurotoxin and is dangerous. Comb the hair with a nit comb for 2 to 3 days until all lice and nits have been removed. Change bed linens and follow Isolation Precautions for pediculosis according to agency policy.
Body lice: Parasites tend to cling to clothing. Patient itches. Hemorrhagic spots may appear on skin where lice are sucking blood. Lice may lay eggs on clothing and furniture.	Have patient bathe or shower thoroughly. After drying skin, apply medicated lotion for eliminating lice. After about 12 to 24 hours have patient take another bath or shower (follow product directions). Bag infested clothing or linen until laundered. Follow appropriate agency Isolation Precautions.
Crab lice: Found in pubic hair. Are grayish white with red legs. May spread via sexual contact.	For pubic lice, shave hair off affected area, cleanse as for body lice, use medicated product for lice, and notify sexual partner of proper treatment.

PROCEDURAL GUIDELINE 10.5
Hair Care—Shampooing and Shaving—cont'd

Procedural Steps

1. **See Standard Protocol (inside front cover).**
2. Shampoo for patient confined to bed.
   - **a.** Before washing patient's hair, determine that there are no contraindications to procedure such as head and neck injuries, spinal cord injuries, and arthritis. Often a physician's order is required to wash a patient's hair (check agency policy). If exposure to moisture is contraindicated, use a dry shampoo.
   - **b.** Inspect condition of hair and scalp. Note distribution of hair, oiliness, and texture. Inspect scalp for abrasions, lacerations, lesions, inflammation, and infestation. If draining head wounds are suspected, apply clean gloves. If lice are present, wear disposable gown during procedure.
   - **c.** Ask if there are any product preferences or personal items that the patient wants to use.
   - **d.** Explain procedure to patient and family.
   - **e.** Place a towel and waterproof pad under patient's shoulders, neck, and head.
   - **f.** Position patient supine with head and shoulders at top edge of bed. Place plastic trough under head and washbasin at end of trough spout (see illustration). Be sure that spout extends beyond edge of mattress.
   - **g.** Obtain warm water, testing temperature with your wrist. Allow patient to feel water temperature for comfort.
   - **h.** Slowly pour warm water from water pitcher over hair until it is completely wet (see illustration). Protect patient's face with towel or washcloth over eyes as needed. If hair contains matted blood, apply hydrogen peroxide; then rinse hair with saline.
   - **i.** Apply small amount of shampoo and work up lather with both hands. Start at hairline and work toward back of neck. Lift head slightly with one hand to wash back of head. Shampoo sides of head. Massage scalp gently by applying pressure with fingertips.
   - **j.** Rinse thoroughly and repeat if necessary until hair is free of soap. Apply conditioner or creme rinse if requested and rinse thoroughly. Dry hair using a second towel, if needed, or hair dryer (if available).
   - **k.** Assist patient to a comfortable position and complete styling of hair. Braids may be helpful for patients with very long hair.

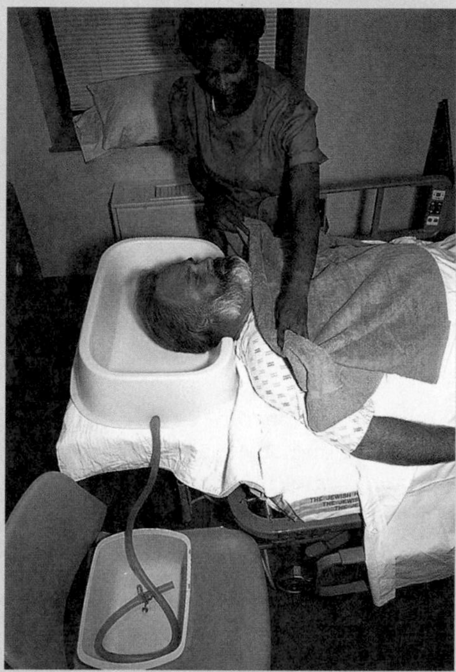

STEP 2f Patient with waterproof pad under shoulders, neck, and head with shampoo board.

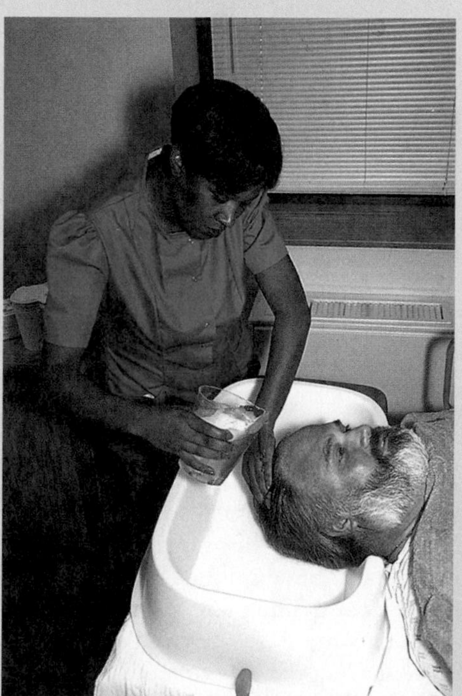

STEP 2h Pour water over hair.

Continued

PROCEDURAL GUIDELINE 10.5
Hair Care—Shampooing and Shaving—cont'd

3. Combing and brushing hair
   a. Part the hair into two sections and then separate it into two more sections (see illustration).

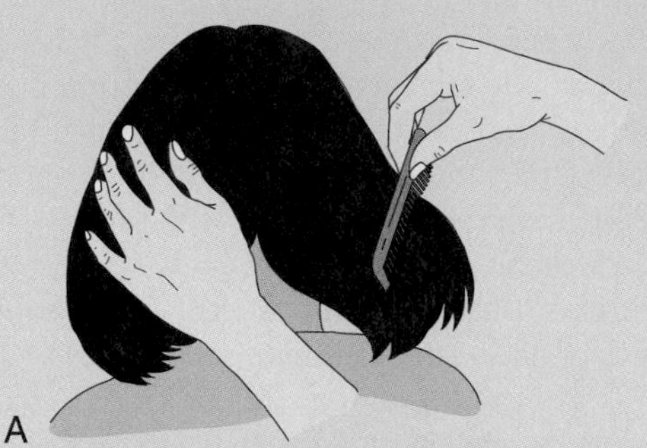

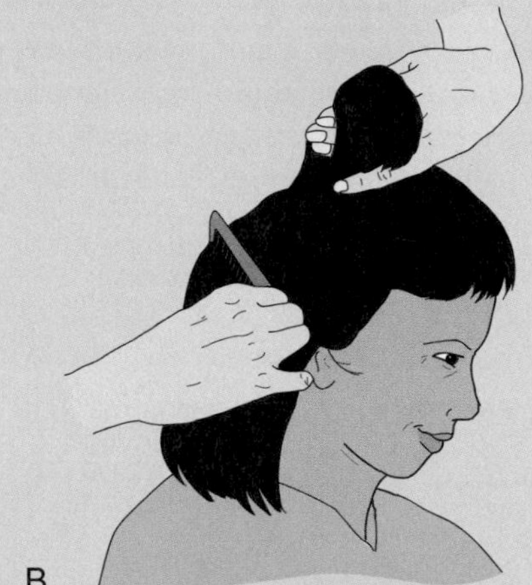

STEP 3a Parting hair: **A,** Part hair down the middle and divide into two main sections. **B,** Part the main section into two smaller sections.

   b. Brush or comb from the scalp toward the hair ends.
   c. Moisten hair lightly with water, conditioner, or an alcohol-free detangle product before combing.
   d. Move fingers through hair to loosen any larger tangles.
   e. Using a wide-tooth comb, start on either side of the head and insert the comb with the teeth upward to the hair near the scalp. Comb through the hair in a circular motion by turning the wrist while lifting up and out. Continue until all hair is combed through and then comb into place to shape and style.
4. Shaving a patient
   a. Before shaving patient with a disposable razor assess for risk of bleeding. Review medical history and laboratory values: platelet count, prothrombin time, and activated partial thromboplastin time.
   b. If patient prefers to shave himself, assess ability to manipulate razor.
   c. Assist patient to sitting position if possible and place towel over chest and shoulders.
   d. Place a warm, moist washcloth over patient's face for several seconds.
   e. Shave using appropriate tools available.
      (1) Apply shaving cream, using product patient prefers. With a disposable razor at a 45-degree angle, shave in direction of hair growth using short strokes. Hold skin taut with nondominant hand (see illustration). Ask patient to tell you if it becomes uncomfortable. Dip razor blade in water; shaving cream accumulates on edge of blade.

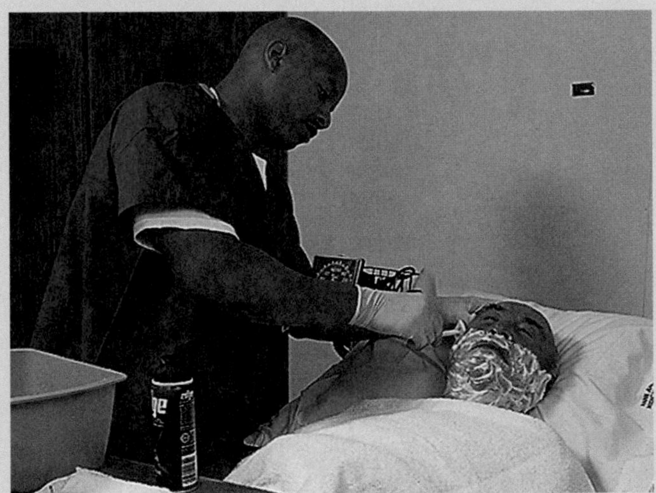

STEP 4e(1) Shaving a patient.

      (2) Apply conditioner for electric razor. Turn electric razor on and shave across side of face using a gentle downward stroke in direction of hair growth.
      (3) If necessary, gently comb mustache or beard. Allow patient to use mirror and direct areas to trim with scissors.
5. Rinse and dry face. Apply aftershave if desired.
6. **See Completion Protocol (inside front cover).**

PROCEDURAL GUIDELINE 10.6
Foot and Nail Care

Care of the nails is important to prevent the occurrence of pain and infection. Neglecting this aspect of care can result in infection, immobility, and increased length of hospital stay (Malkin and Berridge, 2009). Alterations may result from biting nails or trimming them improperly, exposure to harsh chemicals, or wearing poorly fitted shoes (Delmas, 2006). Changes also occur in the shape, color, and texture of nails, which may result from various nutritional, infectious, and circulatory disorders such as diabetes (Table 10-3). Patients with peripheral vascular disease such as diabetes may have inadequate arterial or venous circulation or both. These patients are at high risk for neuropathy, a degeneration of peripheral nerves with loss of sensation. Thus the patients cannot sense pressure or pain from foot lesions. Inspect the feet of patients with altered sensation daily. The inability to feel pain or discomfort can mean that

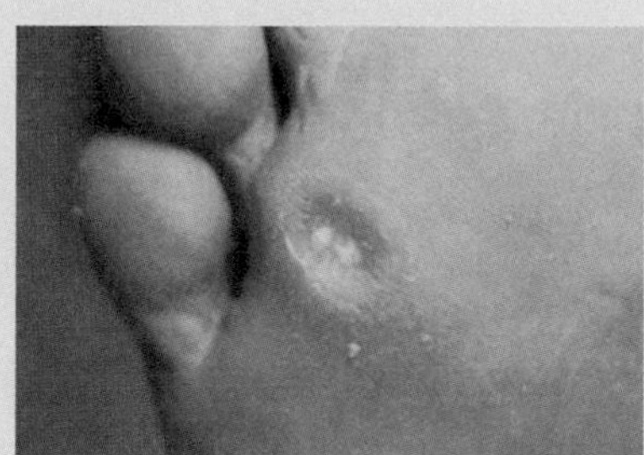

FIG 10-1 Corn. (From Weston WL, Lane AT: *Color textbook of pediatric dermatology,* ed 3, St Louis, 2002, Mosby.)

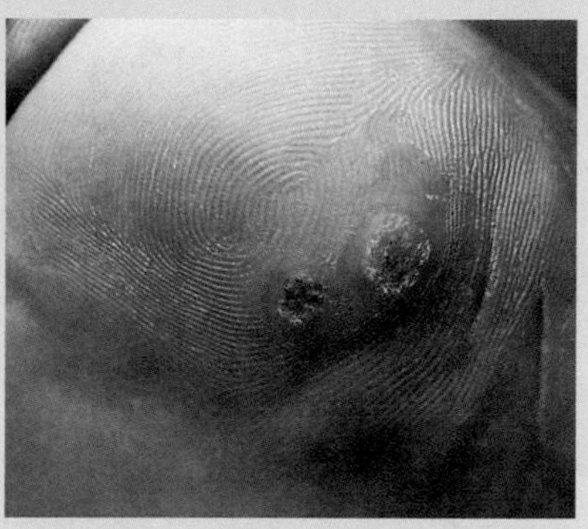

FIG 10-2 Plantar warts. (From Zitelli BJ, Davis HW: *Atlas of pediatric physical diagnosis,* ed 3, St Louis, 1997, Mosby.)

TABLE 10-3 COMMON FOOT AND NAIL PROBLEMS AND RELATED INTERVENTIONS

PROBLEM	PREVENTION	INTERVENTIONS
Callus: Thickened epidermis, usually flat, painless, and on underside of foot; caused by friction or pressure.	Wear proper footwear and always wear clean socks or stockings.	Soak callus in warm water to soften. Creams or lotions can help prevent reformation. Refer patient with diabetes to a podiatrist.
Corns: Caused by friction and pressure from shoes, mainly on toes, over bony prominence; usually cone shaped, round, raised, and tender; may affect gait (Fig. 10-1).	Wear proper footwear; pain is aggravated by tight shoes. Always wear clean socks or stockings.	Surgical removal may be necessary. Use oval corn pads carefully because they increase pressure on toes and reduce circulation.
Plantar warts: Fungating lesions on sole of foot caused by papillomavirus (Fig. 10-2).	Warts are contagious. Avoid going barefoot, especially in public places.	Treatment ordered by physician may include applications of acid, burning, or freezing for removal.
Athlete's foot: Fungal infection of foot; scaling and cracking of skin occur between toes and on soles of feet; may have small blisters containing fluid. Apparently induced by tight footwear (Fig. 10-3).	Feet should be well ventilated. Avoid tight footwear. Dry feet well after bathing; apply powder. Wear clean socks.	Treat with medicated powder or cream. Refer to physician if condition does not improve with medicated products.
Ingrown nails: Toenail or fingernail grows inward into soft tissue around nail; may be painful (Fig. 10-4).	Cut with a nail clipper and file toenails straight across after bathing when they are soft. If nails are thick or vision is poor, have toenails trimmed by a podiatrist.	Treat with frequent warm soaks in antiseptic solution. Surgical removal of portion of nail that has grown into skin may be necessary. Refer patients with diabetes to a podiatrist.
Fungus infection: Thick, discolored nails with yellow streaks.	Keep feet and nails clean and dry. Check feet and nails daily.	Refer to podiatrist.

Continued

PROCEDURAL GUIDELINE 10.6
Foot and Nail Care—cont'd

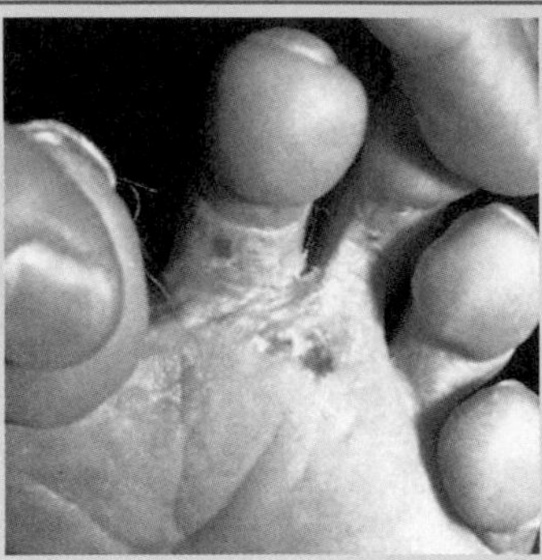

FIG 10-3 Athlete's foot, tinea pedis. (From Greenberger NJ, Hinthorn DR: *History taking and physical examination: essentials and clinical correlates,* St Louis, 1993, Mosby; courtesy Dr Loren Amundson, University of South Dakota, Sioux Falls, SD.)

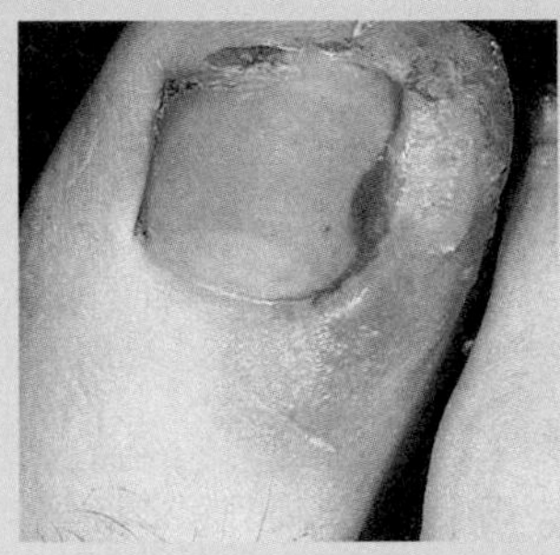

FIG 10-4 Ingrown toenail. (From Habif TP: *Clinical dermatology: a color guide to diagnosis and therapy,* ed 2, St Louis, 1990, Mosby.)

the foot may easily become injured and infected before a problem is detected (National Diabetes Education Program, 2003).

Delegation and Collaboration

The skill of foot and nail care may be delegated to nursing assistive personnel (NAP) *except* for patients with diabetes or patients with peripheral vascular disease or circulatory compromise. Instruct the NAP about the following:

- Reporting any breaks in skin, redness, numbness, swelling, or pain
- Not clipping patient's toenails

Equipment

- Clean gloves
- Basin (appropriate size for soaking)
- Washcloth
- Bath or face towel
- Nail clippers (check agency policy)
- Plastic applicator stick or soft brush, emery board, or nail file
- Soft nail or cuticle brush
- Lotion
- Disposable bath mat

Procedural Steps

1. **See Standard Protocol (inside front cover)**
2. A health care provider's order is usually required for cutting nails, especially when impaired circulation is suspected (e.g., diabetes mellitus, peripheral vascular disease, leg ulcers).
3. Identify patient using two identifiers (i.e., patient's name and birthday or name and account number, according to facility policy).
4. Identify patient risk for foot or nail problems such as reduced visual acuity, history of diabetes, history of stroke.
5. Inspect all surfaces of toes, feet, and nails. Pay particular attention to areas of dryness, inflammation, or cracking. Also inspect areas between toes, heels, and soles of feet.
6. Palpate the dorsalis pedis pulse of both feet simultaneously, comparing the strength of pulses. Note color and warmth of toes and feet. Observe for capillary refill of nails of less than 3 seconds.
7. Assess sensation in the feet by checking for light touch or discrimination between warm and cold.
8. Determine patient's ability to perform self-care.
9. Assess patient's foot and nail care practices for existing foot problems (e.g., home remedies such as cutting corns with razor blade or scissors, applying adhesive tape on foot, or using oval corn pads on toes).
10. Assess type of footwear worn by patients, including type and cleanliness of socks worn, type and fit of shoes, and restrictive garters or knee-high hose.
11. Soak feet and fingers.
    a. Explain that soaking requires 10 to 20 minutes.
    b. Assist ambulatory patient to sit in chair with disposable bath mat under feet. If confined to bed, assist to a semi-Fowler's position with a waterproof pad and bath towel under feet.
    c. Fill washbasin and emesis basin with warm water. Test temperature of water with back of hand.
    d. Place washbasin on bath mat or towel and help patient place one foot in basin. Place emesis basin on over-bed table in front of patient and have him or her immerse the fingers. Place call light within patient's reach. Offer diversional activity.

SAFETY ALERT Patients who have diabetes mellitus or peripheral vascular disease should not soak their feet because of potential of increased dryness of skin and decrease in ability to assess temperature variations related to decreased sensations (ADA, 2007).

12. Foot and nail care
    a. Allow patient's feet and fingers to soak for 10 to 20 minutes. If necessary, rewarm water after 10 minutes.

PROCEDURAL GUIDELINE 10.6
Foot and Nail Care—cont'd

b. Begin care on fingernails. Clean gently under nails with plastic applicator stick or soft brush while immersing fingers (see illustration).

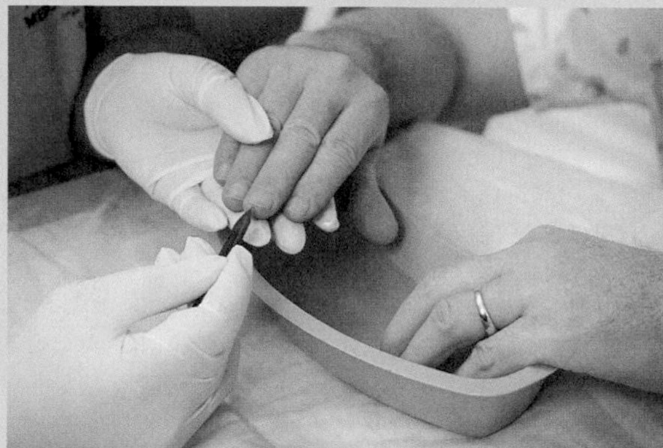

STEP 12b Clean under fingernails.

c. Remove hands from basin and dry thoroughly.
d. File fingernails straight across and even with tops of fingers. Or use nail clippers and clip fingernails straight across and even with tops of fingers (see illustration) and then smooth nail using file.
e. Use soft cuticle brush or nail brush to clean around cuticles.

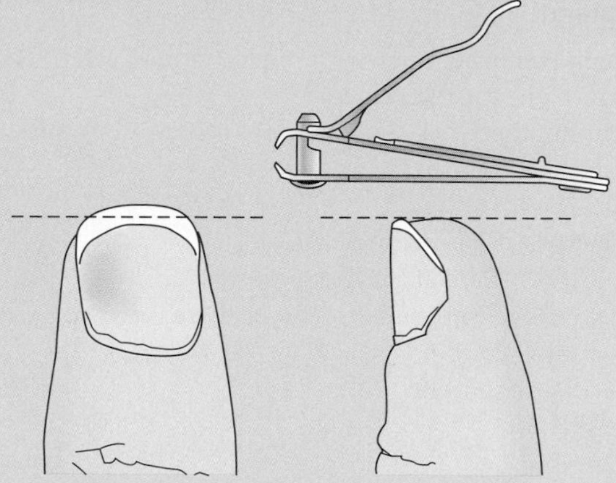

STEP 12d File or clip fingernails straight across.

f. Move over-bed table away from patient.
g. Remove feet from basin and scrub callused areas with washcloth or soft brush.
h. Clean gently under nails with plastic stick applicator or soft brush.
i. Clean and file toenails as in Steps 12d and 12e.

13. Apply lotion to feet and hands to prevent dry skin and susceptibility to cracks, ulcerations, or entry site bacteria (Pinzur and others, 2005).
14. **See Completion Protocol (inside front cover).**

PROCEDURAL GUIDELINE 10.7
Making an Occupied Bed

Because the bed is the piece of equipment most often used by a patient, it should be comfortable, safe, and adaptable to various positions. The typical hospital bed consists of a firm mattress on a metal frame that you can raise or lower horizontally. The frame of the bed is divided into three sections so the operator can raise and lower the head and foot of the bed separately, in addition to inclining the entire bed with the head up or down. Each bed sets on four rollers or casters, which allows you to move the bed easily. See Table 10-4 for common bed positions.

Safety and comfort are primary considerations for bedmaking (Bloomfield and others, 2008; Pegram and others, 2007). Bedmaking may be done with the patient out of the bed (unoccupied) or in the bed (occupied). In some settings bed linen is not changed every day; however, you always need to change any wet or soiled linen promptly.

Occupied bedmaking is limited to patients who cannot tolerate being out of bed. In addition, some patients have activity or positioning restrictions ordered by their health care provider; thus it is important to understand which position the patient can assume while the bed linens are changed. The procedure should be planned carefully and performed in a way that conserves time and the patient's energy. It may be necessary to stop or delay the procedure if the patient's condition is unstable or if his or her reported level of pain makes it inappropriate to continue (Bloomfield and others, 2008). If a patient experiences severe pain with movement, an analgesic administered 30 to 60 minutes before the procedure is helpful in controlling pain and maintaining comfort. Even though the patient is unable to get out of bed, encourage self-help if possible, which helps maintain the patient's strength and mobility. For example, depending on restrictions, the patient can turn, assist in moving up in bed, or hold top sheets while linen is applied.

Delegation and Collaboration

The skill of bedmaking is delegated to nursing assistive personnel (NAP). Instruct the NAP about the following:

- The patient's activity restrictions
- What to do if the patient becomes fatigued or short of breath
- Immediately reporting any unexpected concerns (e.g., excess wound drainage, dislodged IV tubing)

Continued

PROCEDURAL GUIDELINE 10.7
Making an Occupied Bed—cont'd

Equipment

- Linen bag or hamper
- Bath blanket (if available)
- Bottom sheet (in some settings the bottom sheet is a fitted sheet; check agency policy)
- Drawsheet (optional)
- Waterproof pads (optional)
- Top sheet, blanket, spread, pillowcases
- Clean gloves (if linen is soiled or there is risk of exposure to body fluids)
- Antiseptic solution
- Washcloth

Procedural Steps

1. **See Standard Protocol (inside front cover).**
2. Determine if patient has been incontinent or if drainage is present from dressings. If so, put on gloves while making bed. You will need to place waterproof pads on bed.
3. Assess restrictions in mobility/positioning of patient. Explain procedure to patient, noting that you will need to ask the patient to turn over layers of linens.
4. Raise bed to comfortable working height. Loosen all top linens. Remove spread and blanket separately, leaving patient covered with top sheet. If soiled, place in linen bag. If to be reused, fold into square and place over back of chair.
5. Cover patient with bath blanket. Unfold bath blanket over top sheet. Ask patient to hold top edge of bath blanket. If patient is unable to help, tuck top of bath blanket under shoulders. Grasp top sheet under bath blanket at patient's shoulders and bring sheet down to foot of bed. Remove sheet and discard in linen bag.
6. Position patient on the far side of the bed, turned onto side and facing away from you. Encourage use of side rail to aid in turning. Adjust pillow under patient's head. Check that any tubing is not being pulled.
7. Loosen used bottom linens, moving from head to foot. Then fanfold bottom sheet and drawsheet (optional) toward patient—first drawsheet and then bottom sheet. Tuck edges of linen just under buttocks, back, and shoulders (see illustration). Do not fanfold mattress pad (if it is to be reused).

TABLE 10-4 COMMON BED POSITIONS

POSITION	DESCRIPTION	USES
Fowler's	Head of bed raised to angle of 45 degrees or more; semisitting position; foot of bed may also be raised at knee	Used during meals, nasogastric tube insertion, and nasotracheal suction Promotes lung expansion
Semi-Fowler's	Head of bed raised approximately 30 degrees; incline is less than Fowler's position; foot of bed may also be raised at knee	Promotes lung expansion Used when patients receive gastric feedings to reduce regurgitation and risk for aspiration
Trendelenburg's	Entire bed tilted with head of bed down	Used for postural drainage Facilitates venous return in patients with poor peripheral venous perfusion
Reverse Trendelenburg's	Entire bed frame tilted with foot of bed down	Used infrequently Promotes gastric emptying Prevents esophageal reflux
Flat	Entire bed frame horizontally parallel with floor	Used for patients with vertebral injuries and in cervical traction Used for patients who are hypotensive Generally preferred by patients for sleeping

PROCEDURAL GUIDELINE 10.7
Making an Occupied Bed—cont'd

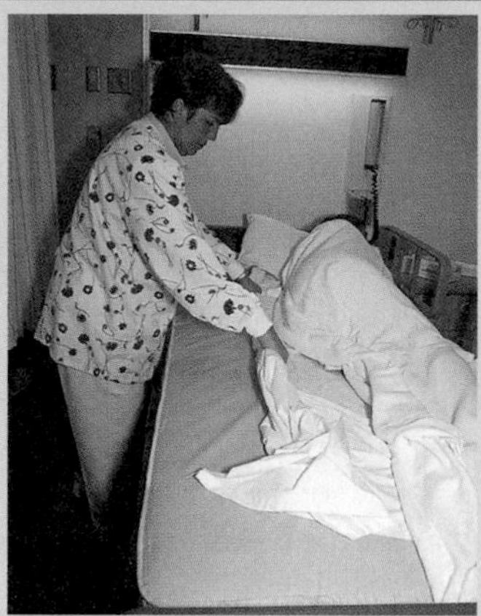

STEP 7 Old linen tucked alongside patient.

8. Clean, disinfect, and dry mattress surface if it is soiled or has moisture.
9. Apply clean linens to exposed half of bed; place clean standard or fitted bottom sheet on bed with seam side down.
   a. Be sure center crease is situated lengthwise along center of bed. Fanfold sheet's top layer toward center of bed alongside the patient (see illustration).

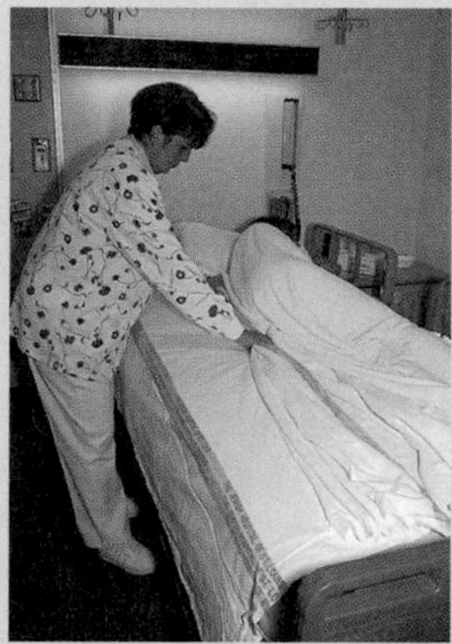

STEP 9a Clean linen applied to bed.

   b. Smooth bottom layer of sheet over mattress and bring edge over closest side of mattress. Pull fitted sheet smoothly over mattress ends. Allow edge of flat unfitted sheet to hang about 10 inches (25 cm) over mattress edge. Lower hem of bottom flat sheet should lie seam down and even with bottom edge of mattress.
10. If flat sheet is used, miter bottom flat sheet at head of bed:
   a. Face head of bed diagonally. Place hand away from head of bed under top corner of mattress, near mattress edge, and lift.
   b. With other hand, tuck top edge of bottom sheet smoothly under mattress so that side edges of sheet above and below mattress meet when brought together.
   c. Face side of bed and pick up top edge of sheet at approximately 18 inches (45 cm) from top end of mattress (see illustration).

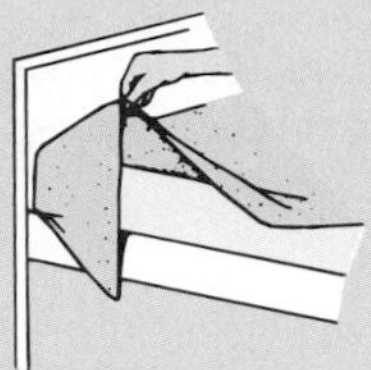

STEP 10c Top edge of sheet picked up.

   d. Lift sheet, and lay it on top of mattress to form a neat triangular fold, with lower base of triangle even with mattress side edge (see illustration).

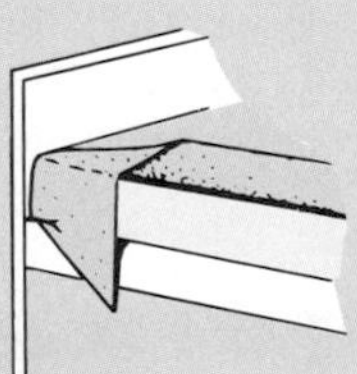

STEP 10d Sheet on top of mattress in a triangular fold.

   e. Tuck lower edge of sheet, which is hanging free below the mattress, under mattress. Tuck with palms down, without pulling triangular fold (see illustration).

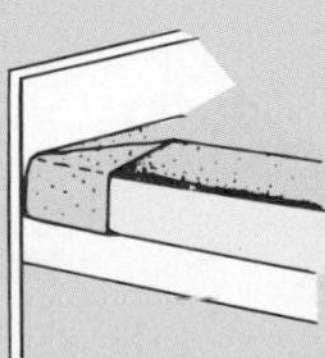

STEP 10e Lower edge of sheet tucked under mattress.

Continued

PROCEDURAL GUIDELINE 10.7
Making an Occupied Bed—cont'd

f. Hold portion of sheet covering side of mattress in place with one hand. With the other hand, pick up top of triangular linen fold and bring it down over side of mattress (see illustrations). Tuck this portion under mattress (see illustration).

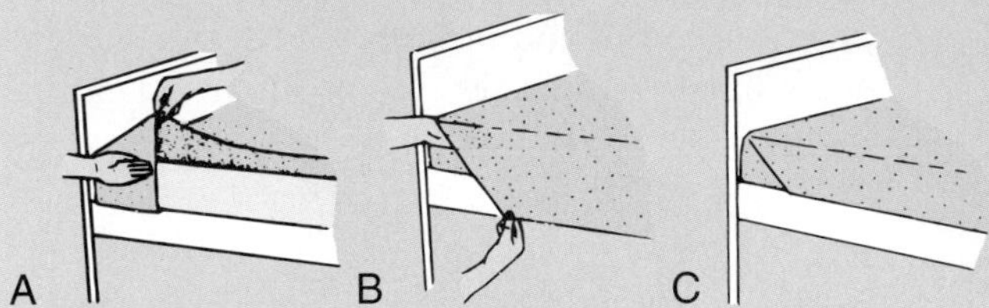

STEP 10f A and **B,** Triangular fold placed over side of mattress. **C,** Linen tucked under mattress.

11. Tuck remaining portion of sheet under mattress, moving toward foot of bed. Keep linen smooth.
12. If needed, place folded drawsheet and/or waterproof pads (absorbent side up) on center of bed with seam side down. Fanfold toward patient. Keep clean and soiled linen separate.
13. Raise side rail. Keeping patient covered, assist patient to roll toward you over layers of linen. Tell patient that he or she will be rolling over layers of linen, and it will feel like a lump. Make sure patient turns slowly. Raise side rail on working side and go to other side of bed.
14. Lower side rail. Assist patient in positioning on other side, over linen folds (see illustration). Loosen edges of soiled linen from under mattress.

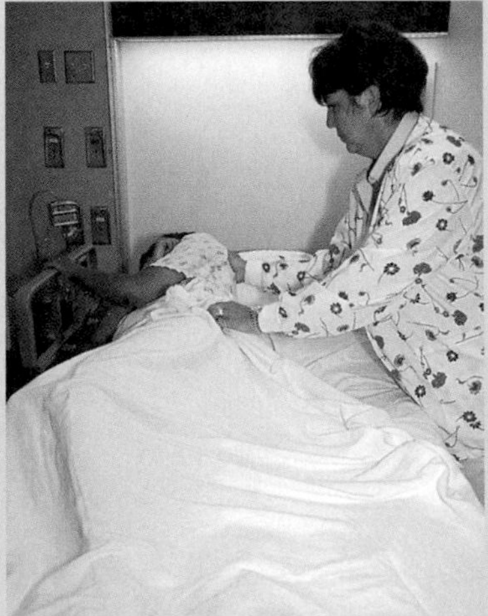

STEP 14 Nurse assists patient with rolling over linen folds.

15. Remove soiled linen by folding into a ball or square, with soiled side turned in. Hold linen away from your body and place in a linen bag.
16. Clean, disinfect, and dry other half of mattress as needed.
17. Gently slide clean linen from beneath patient toward you and smooth it out over mattress. Assist patient to roll back to supine position. Pull fitted sheet over mattress ends. Note: If flat bottom sheet is used, miter the top corner of bottom sheet (see Step 10), Then, facing side of bed, grasp remaining edge of bottom flat sheet. Lean back. Keep back straight and pull while tucking excess linen under mattress from head to foot of bed. Avoid lifting mattress during tucking.
18. Smooth fanfolded drawsheet over bottom sheet. (Tucking is optional.) Smooth out waterproof pads.
19. Place top sheet over patient with centerfold lengthwise down middle of bed. Open sheet out from head to foot and unfold over patient. Be sure that top edge of sheet is even with top edge of mattress.
20. Ask patient to hold clean top sheet (if able). Remove bath blanket and discard in linen bag.
21. Place clean or reused bed blanket on bed over patient. Make sure top edge is parallel with edge of top sheet.
22. Make a cuff by turning edge of top sheet down over top edge of blanket.
23. Make horizontal toe pleat; stand at foot of bed and fanfold in sheet and blanket 5 to 10 cm (2 to 4 inches) across bed. Pull sheet and blanket up from bottom to make fold approximately 15 cm (6 inches) from bottom edge of mattress.
24. Tuck in remaining portion of sheet and blanket under foot of mattress. Tuck top sheet and blanket together. Be sure that toe pleats are not pulled out.
25. Make modified mitered corner with top sheet and blanket.
    a. Pick up side edge of top sheet and blanket and spread about 45 cm (18 inches) from foot of mattress. Lift linen to form a triangular fold, and lay it on bed.
    b. Tuck lower edge of sheet, which is hanging free below mattress, under mattress. Do not pull triangular fold.

PROCEDURAL GUIDELINE 10.7
Making an Occupied Bed—cont'd

c. Pick up triangular fold, and bring it down over mattress while holding linen in place alongside of mattress. Do not tuck in lower edge of triangle (see illustration).

26. Apply clean pillowcase.
27. **See Completion Protocol (inside front cover).**

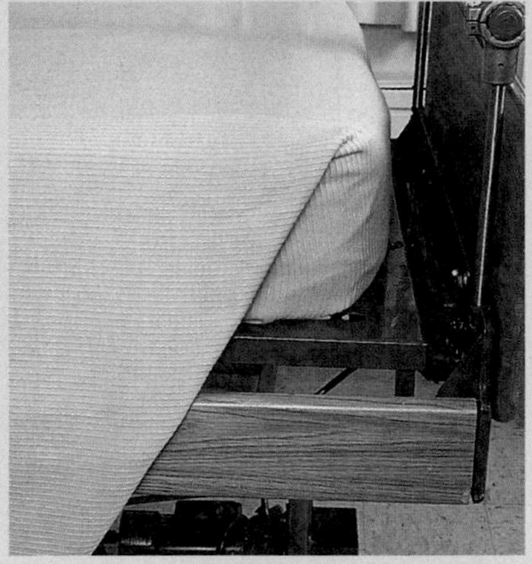

STEP 25c Modified mitered corner.

PROCEDURAL GUIDELINE 10.8
Making an Unoccupied and Surgical Bed

An unoccupied bed is one left open with the top sheets fanfolded down. A postoperative surgical bed is prepared for patients returning from the operating room or procedural area. The bed is left with the top sheets fanfolded lengthwise and not tucked in to facilitate the patient's transfer from a stretcher. A closed bed, which is made with the top sheets pulled up to the head of the bed, is used after a patient is discharged and housekeeping cleans the unit.

Delegation and Collaboration

Bedmaking is delegated to nursing assistive personnel (NAP).

Equipment

- Linen bag or hamper
- Bottom sheet (in some settings the bottom sheet is a fitted sheet; check agency policy)
- Drawsheet (optional)
- Waterproof pads (optional)
- Top sheet, blanket, spread, pillowcases
- Clean gloves (if linen is soiled or there is risk of exposure to body fluids)
- Antiseptic solution
- Washcloth

Procedural Steps

1. **See Standard Protocol (inside front cover).**
2. Assist patient to bedside chair or recliner or encourage ambulation if appropriate.
3. Raise bed to comfortable working position with side rails lowered.
4. Gloves are worn if linen is soiled with body fluids. Remove soiled linen and place in laundry bag, taking care not to contact uniform. Avoid shaking or fanning linen. Cleanse mattress with antiseptic solution if soiled.
5. Apply all bottom linen on one side of bed before moving to opposite side. Make mitered corners at the top corner of the mattress when using a flat sheet (see Procedural Guideline 10.7). Place fitted sheet smoothly over mattress.
6. Optional: Apply waterproof pad or drawsheet, laying center fold along middle of bed lengthwise. Smooth pad or drawsheet over bottom sheet and tuck under mattress.
7. Move to the opposite side of the bed. Repeat Steps 5 and 6.
8. Smooth pad or drawsheet over mattress and tuck excess edge under mattress, keeping palms down.
9. Place top sheet over bed with vertical center fold lengthwise down middle of bed. Open sheet out from head to foot, being sure that top edge of sheet is even with top edge of mattress. Optional: Spread a blanket or spread evenly over bed in same fashion.
10. Standing on one side at foot of bed, lift mattress corner slightly with one hand and with other hand tuck top sheet and blanket or spread under mattress.
11. Make modified mitered corner with top sheet, blanket, and spread. After triangular fold is made, leave tip of triangle untucked (see Procedural Guideline 10.7, Step 25).

Continued

PROCEDURAL GUIDELINE 10.8
Making an Unoccupied and Surgical Bed—cont'd

12. Go to other side of bed. Complete Step 11 to make a modified corner.
13. Make a horizontal toe pleat with all top layers of linen:
    a. Stand at foot of bed and fanfold in sheet 5 to 10 cm (2 to 4 inches) across bed.
    b. Pull sheet up from bottom to make fold approximately 15 cm (6 inches) from bottom edge of mattress.
14. At top of bed make a cuff by turning edge of top sheet down over top edge of blanket and spread.
15. Apply clean pillowcase. Open bed by fanfolding top covers to foot of bed. Leave bed in low position.
16. Surgical bed (variation):
    a. Fold all linen from foot of bed toward center of mattress, even with foot of mattress.
    b. Fold corners toward opposite side of bed, forming a triangle.
    c. Fanfold linen toward you on side of bed away from where patient will be transferred.
17. Leave all side rails down and place bed in high position to match height of stretcher.
18. **See Completion Protocol (inside front cover).**

REVIEW QUESTIONS

Case Study for Questions 1 and 2

Mr. Kline is an 80-year-old patient with a history of heart failure and diabetes. He was admitted to the hospital because of increasing shortness of breath, especially on exertion. He has had diabetes for 30 years, and recently his blood glucose levels have been out of control. He had all of his teeth pulled recently and now wears dentures.

1. Place the following steps for assisting a patient with denture care in the order in which they should be performed.
    a. Rinse dentures thoroughly in tepid water
    b. Perform hand hygiene and don clean gloves; remove upper denture plate by applying gentle downward pressure with 4 × 4–inch gauze.
    c. Hold dentures over emesis basin or sink lined with washcloth and containing 1 inch of water.
    d. Gently lift lower denture from jaw and rotate one side downward to remove from patient's mouth.
    e. Ask patient about preferences for denture care and products used.
    f. Apply cleaning agent to brush and brush surfaces of dentures.
    g. Store dentures in a denture cup with patient's identification label.
    1. b, d, e, a, c, f, g
    2. e, b, d, c, f, a, g
    3. d, b, a, e, f, c, g
    4. g, e, b, d, c, a, f
2. Mr. Kline states that he is feeling uncomfortable and wants a bath. Which type of bath would be most appropriate at this time?
    1. Complete bath
    2. Partial bath
    3. Tub bath
    4. Shower
3. Which of the following actions are appropriate steps when making an unoccupied bed? Select all that apply.
    1. Raise bed to working height.
    2. Wear gloves at all times.
    3. Apply all bottom linen on one side of bed before moving to opposite side.
    4. Remove soiled linen and place on the floor.
    5. Tuck top sheet and spread in at bottom of bed using a modified mitered corner.
    6. Keep top covers at head of bed when procedure is completed.
    7. Make horizontal toe pleat with all top layers of linen.
4. Which of the following is an appropriate guideline when providing perineal care for a patient?
    1. Leave the foreskin in an uncircumcised male retracted after cleansing.
    2. Cleanse from the most contaminated to the least contaminated area for a female patient.
    3. Wash the tip of the penis at the meatus outward in a circular motion.
    4. A patient with a Foley catheter needs minimal perineal care.
5. A patient who has a lowered level of consciousness needs mouth care. When performing mouth care, in what position should the patient be placed?
    1. Supine
    2. Semi-Fowler's
    3. High-Fowler's
    4. Side-lying
6. The nurse begins to prepare a patient for a partial bed bath. The nurse brings a bag bath packet into the room and prepares to bathe the patient. The patient asks, "Why aren't you using soap and water?" The nurse's best response would be:
    1. The bag bath is a bit quicker and causes less discomfort.
    2. The bag bath is easier for me to use.
    3. The bag bath is what our agency uses.
    4. The bag bath poses less risk of infection than using a basin of water.

7. What is the most important reason that the nurse washes the patient's extremities from distal to proximal?
   1. Enhance patient comfort.
   2. Prevent skin irritation.
   3. Promote venous return.
   4. Reduce any noticeable swelling.
8. Which steps should the nurse take to facilitate the shaving of a male patient's facial hair with a disposable razor? Select all that apply.
   1. Use the disposable razor at a 45-degree angle.
   2. Place a cool, moist washcloth over the patient's face.
   3. Shave in the direction of hair growth.
   4. Use long, downward strokes while shaving.
9. The nurse is providing a bed bath to a patient. In which sequence should the nurse bathe the patient (first to last)?
   1. Eyes, face, arms, chest, abdomen, legs, back
   2. Face, eyes, arms, legs, back, chest, abdomen.
   3. Eyes, arms, legs, face, chest, back, abdomen.
   4. Arms, chest, abdomen, legs, back, eyes, face.
10. A patient with diabetes wants to have his nails trimmed. What is the nurse's first step on hearing this request?
   1. Clip the nails to fit the contour of his fingers.
   2. Use manicure scissors to cut the nails straight across.
   3. Use an emery board to shape the nails before being trimmed.
   4. Make sure that there is a physician's order to cut the nails.

REFERENCES

American Diabetes Association (ADA): Position statement on standards of medical care of diabetes, *Diabetes Care* 30:S4, 2007.

Beck DM: Venous thromboembolism (VTE) prophylaxis: implications for medical-surgical nurses, *Medsurg Nurs* 15(5):282, 2006.

Biggs J: Servicing a basic need: bathing and toileting techniques maintain patient well-being, *Rehab Manage* 22(2):18, 2009.

Bloomfield J and others: Recommended procedure for bed making in hospital, *Nurs Stand* 22(23):41, 2008.

Critical Care Extra: Eye care for patients in the ICU, *AJN* 106(1):72AA, 2006.

Delmas L: Best practice in the assessment and management of diabetic foot ulcers, *Rehabil Nurs* 31(6):228, 2006.

Galanti G: *Caring for patients from different cultures*, ed 4, Philadelphia, 2008, University of Pennsylvania Press.

Hockenberry MJ, Wilson D: *Wong's nursing care of infants and children*, ed 8, St Louis, 2007, Mosby.

Jerreat M and others: Denture care of in-patients, *J Research Nurs* 12(2):193, 2007.

Johnson D and others: Patients' bath basins as potential sources of infection: multicenter sampling study, *Am J Crit Care* 18(1):31, 2009.

Larson E and others: Comparison of traditional and disposable bed baths in critically ill patients, *Am J Crit Care* 13(3):235, 2004.

Lloyd DL: Bed bathing patients in hospital, *Nurs Stand* 22(34):35, 2008.

MacNeill BA, Sorenson HM: Oral hygiene for the ventilated patient, *AARC Times* April: 15, 2009.

Malkin B, Berridge P: Guidance on maintaining personal hygiene in nail care, *Nurs Stand* 23(41):35, 2009.

Munro CL, Grap MJ: Oral health and care in the intensive care unit: state of the science, *Am J Crit Care* 13(1):25, 2004.

National Diabetes Education Program: *Take care of your feet for a lifetime*, 2003, http://www.ndep.nih.gov/publications/PublicationDetail.aspx?PubId=67, accessed September 3, 2010.

National Pediculosis Association: *Child care provider's guide to controlling head lice*, 2005, http://www.headlice.org, accessed July 26, 2010.

National Pressure Ulcer Advisory Panel (NPUAP): *Updated staging systems*, 2007, http://www.npuap.org, accessed September 2, 2010.

Pegram A and others: Clinical skills: bed bathing and personal hygiene needs of patients, *Br J Nurs* 16(6):356, 2007.

Pinzur MS and others: Guidelines for diabetic foot care: recommendations endorsed by the diabetes committee of the American orthopaedic foot and ankle society, *Foot Ankle Int* 26(1):113, 2005.

Rader J and others: The bathing of older adults with dementia, *Am J Nurs* 106(4):40, 2006.

Skewes SM: No more bed baths! *RN* 57(1):34, 1994.

CHAPTER 11

Care of the Eye and Ear

evolve WEBSITE

http://evolve.elsevier.com/Perry/nursinginterventions

Meaningful sensory stimuli allow a person to learn about the environment and are necessary for healthy functioning and normal development. Many patients seeking health care have preexisting sensory alterations, whereas others might develop or be at risk for developing alterations after medical treatment. Artificial sensory devices, known as prostheses, replace or restore sensory function to a diseased or lost body part. Eyeglasses and contact lenses help to restore visual loss, and hearing aids improve sound reception. A patient may also depend on a prosthetic device to maintain an attractive appearance. Artificial eyes in particular help patients maintain a normal appearance when an eye is lost as a result of injury or disease.

PATIENT-CENTERED CARE

Any intervention, device, or prosthesis to improve sensory perception must fit and work properly if patients are to function optimally within their environment. It is important to know patients' preferences and have a discussion with them about how to use and care for a device or prosthesis. Breakage or loss of a hearing aid or eye prosthesis often results in costly repair and replacement. When a patient is without visual or hearing aids, it interferes with communication, isolates the patient socially, and increases patient dependence. In addition, especially in the case of an eye prosthesis, the loss of the aid threatens the patient's self-esteem.

When a patient is acutely ill or has mobility limitations, provide more direct care and supervision and communicate the patient's sensory loss to other health professionals. When patients have a hearing deficit, be sure they understand what you communicate. Always face the patient before beginning to speak and make sure there is enough light for the patient to see your lips. Eliminate external noises; speak in a slow, clear, normal tone of voice. Ask patients what communication styles they prefer. Never talk over or exclude a patient from conversation or decisions.

Hospitals, rehabilitation centers, and skilled nursing facilities are poor listening environments. The hard flooring surfaces, medical equipment, televisions, and the constant need to speak with other health care professionals all produce noise. This increased background noise makes hearing even more difficult for the hearing-impaired individual (Wallhagen and others, 2006). When patients have visual impairments, the increased background noise in an unfamiliar environment often makes them more anxious and decreases their abilities to adjust to new surroundings.

Communication is vital to all persons from all cultures. Learn how a change in vision and/or hearing is perceived in terms of the patient's culture. Discuss what a loss in hearing or vision means to a patient. In cultures such as the Navaho Indian and in some Asian and middle-Eastern cultures, limited eye contact is the norm and is a nonverbal form of respect (Galanti, 2008). Changes in the ability to move the eyes, as with a prosthesis, present a social difficulty because the patient is unable to lower the eyes.

The Navajo are comfortable with the soft-spoken word and silence (Galanti, 2008). Hearing impairments may force the patient's family and friends to speak louder. In addition, because of the comfort with silence, you can easily mistake a patient's silence as a measure of comfort and never correctly assess what the patient is able to hear or if he or she heard the information correctly. At times you use touch to get the attention of a patient with decreased hearing; however, in some cultures such as Muslim, it is unacceptable for caregivers of the opposite sex to touch a patient. Remember to learn a patient's preferences before using touch to gain a sensory-impaired patient's attention.

SAFETY

Whenever you care for patients with sensory alterations, safety is a priority. Anticipate how the sensory alteration places the patient at risk for injury. Orient the patient to any new environment or changes within an existing environment to minimize safety hazards. In addition, educate family and friends as to the best way they can help the patient adapt to sensory loss.

Prosthetic devices require regular cleaning to ensure function and prevent injury. Most patients have an established routine for cleaning their prostheses. When patients are unable to care for their eye prostheses and hearing aids, you must understand the correct way to clean, handle, and store them. Careful handling of prostheses is vital to avoid damage to these devices or injury to the patient's eyes or ears.

When patients have visual impairments, they may have difficulty with tasks requiring visual detail (e.g., reading prescriptions or syringes). This increases the risk of improper administration of medications in the home setting. In addition, certain eye conditions such as cataracts and macular degeneration cause the patient difficulty when adjusting to changes in contrast and brightness. Individuals with diabetic retinopathy have changes related to distorted vision, changes in acuity, and loss of depth and contrast cues (Wallhagen, 2010). These changes leave the patient at risk for accidents in the home or health care environments.

EVIDENCE-BASED PRACTICE TRENDS

Cacchione PZ and others: Sensory impairment and associated conditions in LTC elders: a pilot study, *Geriatric Nurs* 28(6):367, 2007.

Maldonado JR: Delirium in the acute care setting: diagnosis and treatment, *Crit Care Clin* 24:657, 2008.

Vision and hearing impairments either as separate problems or in combination have the potential to cause cognitive function decline or contribute to acute confusion, especially in older adults. In determining risk factors associated with acute confusion in the long-term care setting, these studies found that both vision and hearing deficits were significant risk factors. Early identification of sensory loss and prompt interventions to improve vision and/or hearing loss are beneficial in reducing confusion, improving orientation, and increasing patient independence. In some instances hearing loss was related to a buildup of cerumen. Once this buildup was removed, hearing improved, and the residents' cognitive function improved. In addition, these patients were better able to hear, understand, and follow health care instructions relating to self-medication administration, symptom management, and when to return to the health care provider.

SKILL 11.1 EYE IRRIGATION

Eye irrigations effectively flush out exudates, irritating solutions, or foreign bodies from the eye. The procedure typically is used in emergency situations when a foreign object or some other substance has entered the eye. Users of contact lenses or artificial eyes may need eye irrigation to flush out particles of dust or fibers from the eye socket. Patients with artificial eyes are also at risk for socket irritation secondary to the composite material of the artificial eye itself, and irrigation assists in relieving the irritation (Lauren and others, 2009).

When a chemical injury to the eye occurs, the priority is flushing the eye with copious amounts of irrigation fluid. The best type of solution is normal saline or lactated Ringer's. Continue to irrigate the eye because the irrigating solution helps to dilute and flush out the chemical. Once the acute phase is over, an irrigation solution that buffers alkali or acid chemical is then selected (Babineau and Sanchez, 2008; Segal, 2007).

ASSESSMENT

1. Review prescriber's medication order, including solution to be instilled and the affected eye(s) (left, right, or both) to receive irrigation. *Rationale: Ensures safe and correct administration of irrigant.*
2. Assess reason for eye irrigation by obtaining a history of the injury from the patient. *Rationale: Determines amount, type of solution, and immediacy of treatment.*
3. Determine patient's ability to open affected eye. *Rationale: Spasm of the eyelid or pain makes opening the eye difficult. Local anesthetics such as proparacaine or tetracaine cause topical numbness and are used before eye examination procedures.*
4. Conduct an eye examination (Babineau and Sanchez, 2008). Assess eye for redness, excessive tearing, and discharge. Assess pupil response to light and condition of eyelids and lacrimal glands for edema. Assess visual acuity before and after treatment. Ask patient about itching, burning, pain, blurred vision, or photophobia. *Rationale: Provides baseline for condition of eye. You may need to obtain topical anesthetic drops to provide comfort.*
5. Ask patient to rate pain level. Use a scale of 0 to 10. *Rationale: Provides baseline to later evaluate response to irrigation.*
6. Assess patient's ability to cooperate. *Rationale: Extra assistance may be necessary.*

PLANNING

Expected Outcomes focus on patient's physical and psychological comfort and improving vision.

1. Patient demonstrates minimal anxiety during and after irrigation.
2. Patient verbalizes reduced pain/burning/itching and improved visual acuity after eye irrigation.

Delegation and Collaboration

The skill of eye irrigation cannot be delegated to nursing assistive personnel (NAP). Instruct the NAP to:

- Report any patient complaint of discomfort or excess tearing after the irrigation.

Equipment

- Prescribed irrigating solution: volume usually 30 to 180 mL at about 32° to 38° C (90° to 100° F) (For chemical flushing, use normal saline or lactated Ringer's fluid in volume to provide continuous irrigation over 15 minutes.)
- Sterile basin or bag of IV solution
- Curved emesis basin
- Waterproof pad or towel
- 4 × 4–inch gauze pads
- Soft bulb syringe, eyedropper, or intravenous (IV) tubing
- Clean gloves
- Penlight
- Medication administration record (MAR)

IMPLEMENTATION *for* EYE IRRIGATION

STEPS	RATIONALE
1. **See Standard Protocol (inside front cover).**	
2. Check accuracy and completeness of each medication administration record (MAR) with prescriber's written medication or procedure order. Check patient's name, irrigation solution name and concentration, route of administration, and time for administration. Compare MAR with label of eye irrigation solution.	The order sheet is the most reliable source and only legal record of drugs or procedure the patient is to receive. Ensures that patient receives correct medication.
3. Identify patient using two identifiers (e.g., name and birthday or name and account number, according to facility policy). Compare identifiers with information on patient's MAR or medical record.	Ensures correct patient. Complies with The Joint Commission standards and improves patient safety (TJC, 2010).
4. Assist patient to side-lying position on the same side as the affected eye. Turn head toward affected eye. **If both eyes are affected, place patient supine for simultaneous irrigation of both eyes.**	Irrigation solution flows from inner to outer canthus, preventing contamination of unaffected eye and nasolacrimal duct.
5. Remove contact lenses (if possible) before beginning irrigation (Box 11-1).	Prompt removal of lenses is needed to safely and completely irrigate foreign substances from patient's eyes. Contact lens may have absorbed irritant, or it may prevent a thorough irrigation.

SAFETY ALERT In an emergency such as first aid for a chemical burn, do not delay treatment by removing patient's contact lens before irrigation. Do not remove contact unless rapid swelling is occurring. Flush eye from the inner to outer canthus with cool tap water immediately (National Library of Medicine, 2009b). Advise patient to consult prescriber before reusing contact lens.

STEPS	RATIONALE
6. Explain to patient that the eye can be closed periodically and that no object will touch the eye.	Informing patients what to expect decreases anxiety and reassures them.
7. Place towel or waterproof pad under patient's face and place curved emesis basin just below patient's cheek on side of affected eye.	Catches irrigation fluid.
8. With 4 × 4–inch gauze moistened in prescribed solution (or normal saline), gently clean eyelid margins and eyelashes from inner to outer canthus.	Minimizes transfer of debris from lids or lashes into eye during irrigation.
9. Explain next steps to patient and encourage relaxation.	
a. With gloved finger, gently retract upper and lower eyelids to expose conjunctival sacs.	Retraction minimizes blinking and allows irrigation of conjunctiva.
b. To hold lids open, apply gentle pressure to lower bony orbit and bony prominence beneath eyebrow. **Do not apply pressure over eye.**	

STEPS	RATIONALE
10. Hold irrigating syringe, dropper, or IV tubing approximately 2.5 cm (1 inch) from the inner canthus.	Direct contact with irrigation equipment may injure the eye.
11. Ask patient to look toward brow. Gently irrigate with a steady stream toward lower conjunctival sac, moving from inner to outer canthus (see illustration).	Minimizes force of stream on patient's cornea. Flushes irrigant out and away from the other eye and nasolacrimal duct.

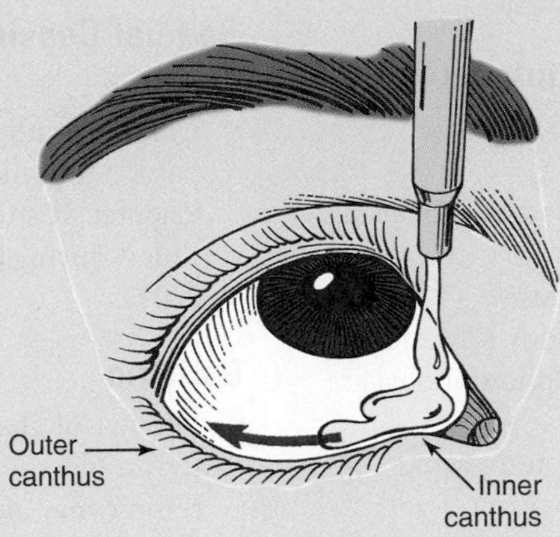

STEP 11 Irrigation of eye from inner to outer canthus.

STEPS	RATIONALE
12. Reinforce the importance of the procedure and encourage patient to lie still by using calm, confident, soft voice.	Reduces anxiety.
13. Allow patient to blink periodically.	Lid closure moves secretions from upper conjunctival sac.
14. Continue irrigation with prescribed solution, volume, or time or until secretions are cleared. (NOTE: An irrigation of 15 minutes or more is needed to flush chemicals.)	Ensures complete removal of irritant. Assessment of eye secretion pH may be necessary if eye was exposed to an acidic or basic solution during injury (National Library of Medicine, 2009b).
15. Blot excess moisture from eyelids and face with gauze or towel.	
16. See Completion Protocol (inside front cover).	

BOX 11-1 REMOVAL OF CONTACT LENSES

Soft Lenses

- Wash hands. Apply powder-free gloves. Place a towel just below patient's face.
- *Option:* Add two to three drops of sterile saline solution to patient's eye.
- If possible, have patient look straight ahead. Retract lower eyelid and expose lower edge of lens.
- Using pad of index finger, slide lens off cornea down onto white of eye.
- Pull upper eyelid down gently with thumb of other hand and compress lens slightly between thumb and index finger.
- Gently pinch lens and lift out without allowing edges to stick together.
- If lens edges stick together, place lens in palm and soak thoroughly with sterile saline.
- Place lens in storage case.
- Follow procedure for cleansing and disinfecting.

Rigid Lenses

- Wash hands. Apply powder-free gloves. Place a towel just below patient's face.
- Be sure lens is positioned directly over cornea. If it is not, have patient close eyelids. Place index and middle fingers of one hand on eyelid just beside the lens and gently but firmly massage lens back over cornea. If lens cannot be repositioned, referral to an ophthalmologist is needed.
- Place index finger on outer corner of patient's eye and draw skin gently back toward ear.
- Ask patient to blink. Do not release pressure on lid until blink is completed.
- If lens fails to pop out, gently retract eyelid beyond edges of lens. Press lower eyelid gently against lower edge of lens to dislodge it.
- Allow both eyelids to close slightly and grasp lens as it rises from the eye. Cup lens in hand.
- If patient is unable to assist, use a specially designed suction cup. Place cup on center of lens and, while applying suction, gently remove lens off patient's cornea.
- Place lens in storage case.
- Follow procedure for cleansing and disinfecting.

EVALUATION

1. Observe for verbal and nonverbal signs of anxiety during irrigation.
2. Assess patient's comfort level after eye irrigation.
3. Ask patient if vision is blurred after irrigation.
4. Inspect eye for presence of discharge and determine if pupils are equal and round and react to light.

Unexpected Outcomes and Related Interventions

1. Anxiety
   a. Reinforce rationale for irrigation.
   b. Allow patient to close eye periodically during irrigation.
   c. Instruct patient to take slow, deep breaths.
2. Patient complains of pain and foreign body sensation in eye after irrigation. Excessive tearing and photophobia are noted.
   a. Advise patient to close the eye and avoid eye movement.
   b. Notify health care provider of findings.

Recording and Reporting

- Record in nurses' notes condition of eye and patient's report of pain and visual symptoms. Record the type and amount of irrigation solution on patient's MAR.
- Report continued symptoms of pain or blurred vision.

Sample Documentation

0800 Patient notes blurred vision and tenderness in left eye. Yellow, crusty drainage noted on eyelids with slight edema and redness of conjunctiva. Eyelids cleaned and eye irrigated with 120 mL warm, sterile, normal saline for 10 minutes. Neosporin ophthalmic ointment applied.

0900 Patient states that eye "feels better." Vision clearer. Pupils equal, round, reactive to light. Normal eye movements noted. Conjunctiva remains red with slight edema, no drainage.

Special Considerations

Pediatric

- Children with foreign bodies or chemicals in the eye often panic. You may need to use a mummy restraint (see Chapter 4) so you can irrigate the eye safely and quickly, thus reducing the risk of injury (Hockenberry and Wilson, 2007).

Geriatric

- Because of changes in fine motor coordination or mobility, an older adult who needs eye irrigations in the home setting may need the assistance of a family member or friend. Therefore the significant other must be present for patient teaching (Ebersole and others, 2008).

Home Care

- If patient suffered injury in the home, instruct in ways to minimize chemical injuries in the future. Have patient wear eye goggles when working with chemicals or in a dusty environment (National Institute for Occupational Safety and Health, 2009).
- Instruct patient and family about how to perform emergency irrigation of the eye.

PROCEDURAL GUIDELINE 11.1
Eye Care for the Comatose Patient

Comatose patients do not have natural protective mechanisms to protect the cornea. Thus patients are at risk for corneal dryness because they are unable to close their eyes. When unprotected, there is an increased risk of corneal dehydration, abrasion, perforation, and infection. Normal protective mechanisms include blinking with lubrication of the eye (Rosenberg and Eisen, 2008). Blinking provides a mechanical barrier to injury and prevents dehydration. Tears maintain a moist environment, lubricate the eyelids, wash away foreign material and cell debris, prevent organisms from adhering to the ocular surface, and transport oxygen to the outer eye surface (Marshall and others, 2008). When patients are in a coma, the nurse is responsible for providing eye care. Left unprotected, damage to the cornea can occur. These damages range from corneal scarring to premature cataract formation or vision changes. Depending on the patient's condition, moisture chambers, lubrication, and corneal surface protection are the best interventions to protect the corneas (Rosenberg and Eisen, 2008).

Delegation and Collaboration

The skill of providing eye care for the comatose patient can be delegated to nursing assistive personnel (NAP). However, it is the nurse's responsibility to assess the patient's eyes and administer the sterile lubricant. Instruct the NAP about the following:

- How to adapt the skill for specific patients (e.g., using skin-sensitive tape to affix eye pads for patients with sensitive skin)
- Immediately reporting any eye drainage or irritation to the nurse for further assessment

Equipment

- Clean gloves
- Water or normal saline solution
- Clean washcloth
- Cotton balls
- Eye pads or patches

PROCEDURAL GUIDELINE 11.1
Eye Care for the Comatose Patient—cont'd

- Paper tape
- Eyedropper bulb syringe
- Sterile lubricant or eye preparations as ordered

NOTE: A moisture chamber (e.g., polyethylene covers or swimming goggles to completely seal off the eye from the environment) is often used; check agency policy.

Procedural Steps

1. **See Standard Protocol (inside front cover)**
2. Observe patient's eyes for drainage, irritation, redness, and lesions.
3. Assess for blink reflex.
4. Perform pupillary examination to determine if pupils are equal and round and react to light (see Chapter 7).
5. Observe patient's eye movements, noting symmetry.
6. Explain procedure to patient and family members.
7. Position patient in supine position.
8. Use clean washcloth or cotton balls moistened with water or saline and gently wipe each eye from inner to outer canthus. Use a separate, clean cotton ball or corner of the washcloth for each eye.
9. Use an eyedropper to instill the prescribed lubricant (e.g., saline, methylcellulose, liquid tears) as ordered.
10. If blink reflex is absent, gently close patient's eyes and apply eye patches, pads, or a moisture chamber. Secure patch, being careful not to tape patient's eyes.
11. **See Completion Protocol (inside front cover).**
12. Remove eye pad or patches every 4 hours or as ordered and observe condition of patient's eye for drainage, irritation, redness, and lesions.
13. Notify health care provider if signs of irritation or infection are present.

PROCEDURAL GUIDELINE 11.2
Caring for an Eye Prosthesis

As a result of tumor, infection, congenital blindness, or severe trauma to the eye, patients may undergo enucleation, the complete surgical removal of the eyeball. During this surgical procedure a spherical implant is placed in the orbit to maintain the natural eye structure and provide support for a cosmetic prosthesis. The muscles and other tissues of the eye are sewn around the implant, holding it in place. Therefore the implant is not visible (Fig. 11-1). Modern implants are made of glass or plastic and are porous so the tissues of the eye grow into the sphere (Center for Ocular Prosthetics, 2009). Like a healthy eye, this integrated implant moves as the companion eye moves.

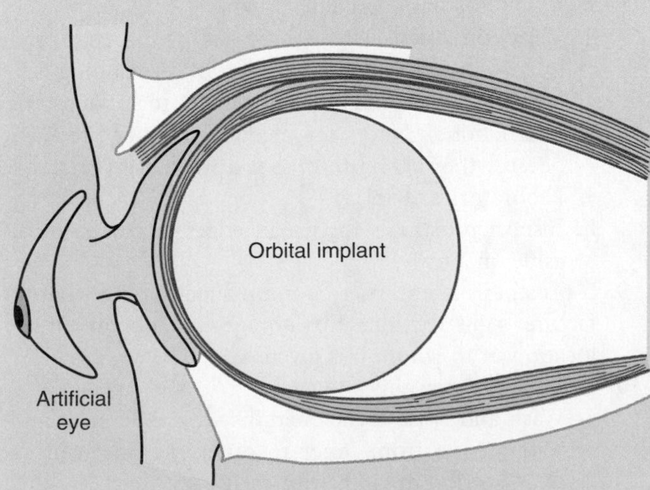

FIG 11-1 Side view of orbital implant, artificial eye removed.

A concave cosmetic prosthesis is placed over the implant, resulting in a nearly normal appearance. Some implants are fitted with a peg that secures and optimally transfers implant movement to the prosthesis. The prosthesis, the artificial eye, is glass or plastic and colored to match the companion eye.

Prostheses are relatively easy to remove and insert and are usually worn day and night. They are cleaned with sterile saline or soap and water at intervals of up to a year based on oculist recommendations and the patient's preference (Kolberg Ocular Prosthetics, 2009). Too much handling of a prosthesis causes socket irritation and increases secretions (Erickson Laboratories, 2009). Patients are instructed to have the artificial eye checked and polished at least twice a year to avoid unnecessary discomfort to the patient as a result of protein deposits or scratches on the surface of the artificial eye. An artificial eye is usually replaced every 5 years (Erickson Laboratories, 2009).

Delegation and Collaboration

The skill of taking care of an artificial eye can be delegated to nursing assistive personnel (NAP). Instruct the NAP about the following:

- Reporting eye pain or discomfort, inflammation, drainage, or odor
- Careful handling of the prosthesis to prevent damage or injury

Equipment

- Bath towels or waterproof pads (2)
- Sterile saline for washing prosthesis

Continued

PROCEDURAL GUIDELINE 11.2
Caring for an Eye Prosthesis—cont'd

- Irrigation bulb or large syringe (without needle)
- Sterile saline: 30 to 180 mL at 32° to 38° C (about 90° to 100° F)
- Emesis basin; 4 × 4–inch gauze pads
- Clean gloves
- Facial tissues (optional)
- Washbasin with warm water and mild soap (optional)
- Suction device (or medicine dropper bulb) (optional)
- Covered plastic storage case (optional).

Procedural Steps

1. **See Standard Protocol (inside front cover).**
2. Ask patient or inspect eyes to determine which is artificial. Some implants allow movement of the prosthesis and can make distinguishing it from the natural eye difficult. An artificial eye pupil does not react to changes in light.
3. Assess patient's frequency and method of cleaning and length of time since last cleaning.
4. Assess patient's ability to remove, clean, and reinsert prosthesis.
5. Before and after removal of prosthesis, assess eyelids and socket for inflammation, tenderness, swelling, drainage, or odor. Pay particular attention to the implant peg if present. Assess patient's pain or other symptoms.

SAFETY ALERT Signs/symptoms such as pain or drainage may indicate infection or injury. Infection can spread easily to neighboring eye, underlying sinuses, or brain tissue. The implant peg is a common site of infection.

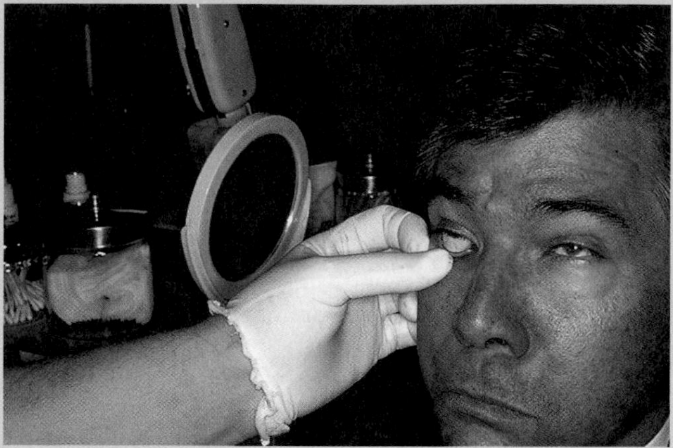

STEP 8c Retraction of lower lid to aid removal of eye prosthesis.

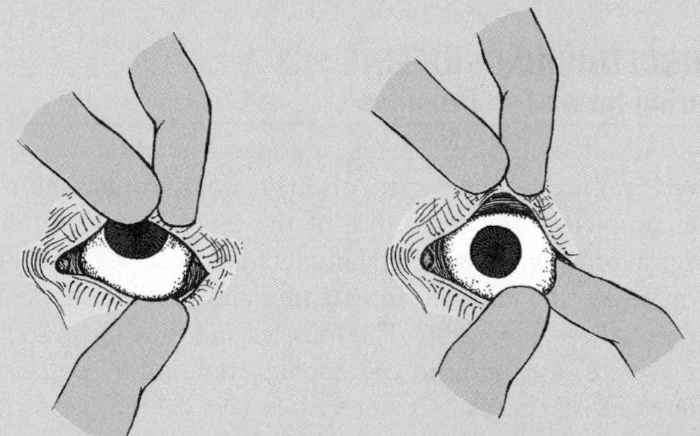

STEP 8d Exertion of pressure below eyelid and removal of eye prosthesis.

6. Discuss procedure with patient.
7. Assemble supplies at bedside. Place one towel over work area.
8. Remove prosthesis.
   a. Position in sitting or supine position with head elevated. Provide privacy.
   b. Place towel just below patient's face.
   c. With thumb or forefinger of dominant hand gently retract lower eyelid against lower orbital ridge (see illustration).
   d. Exert slight pressure below eyelid and slide prosthesis out (see illustration). If prosthesis does not slide out, use moistened suction device to apply direct suction to prosthesis (Kolberg Ocular Prosthetics, 2009).
   e. Note presence and orientation of colored dot at margin of prosthesis.
   f. Place prosthesis in palm of hand.
   g. Clean prosthesis by washing with mild soap and warm water or plain saline solution by rubbing well between thumb and index finger (see manufacturer's instructions). Never use alcohol or other products because they are harmful to the prosthesis (Erickson Laboratories, 2009).
   h. Inspect prosthesis for rough edges or surfaces. Set aside on a towel
9. If prosthesis is not inserted immediately, follow manufacturer's instructions for storage and document its location or to whom it is given.
10. Clean eyelid margins and socket.
    a. Wash and rinse eyelid margins with mild soap and water. Wipe from inner to outer canthus using a clean section of cloth with each wipe.

PROCEDURAL GUIDELINE 11.2
Caring for an Eye Prosthesis—cont'd

b. Retract upper and lower eyelid margins with thumb and index finger.
c. Gently irrigate socket with sterile saline solution. Note presence of discharge or odor.
d. Remove excess moisture with gauze pads by wiping from inner to outer canthus.

11. Insert prosthesis.
    a. Moisten prosthesis in water or sterile saline.
    b. Retract patient's upper eyelid with index finger or thumb of nondominant hand.
    c. With dominant hand, hold prosthesis so iris faces outward and colored dot is oriented properly (see illustration).
    d. Gently slide prosthesis up under upper eyelid and push down lower lid to allow prosthesis to slip into place.
    e. Ask patient if prosthesis fits comfortably and without pain.
12. Inspect eyelids and socket for signs of infection (e.g., excessive, purulent, or foul drainage), excessive tearing or clear discharge, excessive itching, or lashes turned toward prosthesis.
13. Observe patient removing, cleaning, and reinserting prosthesis.

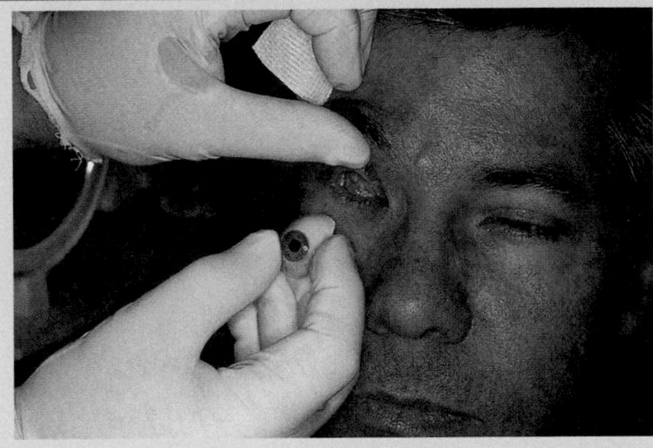

STEP 11c Replacement of eye prosthesis into eye socket.

14. Teach patient and family how to inspect eye socket for redness, drainage, or excessive dryness and when to call oculist.
15. Teach patient and family how to inspect artificial eye for damage, scratches, or areas of roughness. Alert patient to report any odor noted in eye or on prosthesis to the health care provider.
16. **See Completion Protocol (inside front cover).**

SKILL 11.2 EAR IRRIGATION

The common indications for irrigation of the external ear are presence of foreign bodies, local inflammation, and buildup of cerumen in the ear canal. The procedure is not without potential hazards. Usually irrigations are performed with liquid warmed to body temperature to avoid vertigo or nausea in patients. The greatest danger during ear irrigation is rupture of the tympanic membrane caused by forcing irrigant into the canal under pressure. Damage to the external auditory meatus may also occur by scratching the lining of the canal if the patient suddenly moves or if there is inadequate control of the irrigating syringe (Kraszewski, 2008; National Library of Medicine, 2009c). Improperly drying the ear may lead to acute otitis externa (infection of the outer ear).

Ear emergencies can include the presence of foreign bodies, insect bites, or percussion injuries. In addition, the patient can also have damage from inside the ear, which includes blood and drainage. Sometimes the cause of bloody drainage may be the result of a head or neck injury. If you suspect a head or neck injury, (1) do not move the patient, (2) cover the outside of the ear with a sterile dressing (if available), (3) get medical help immediately, and (4) do not irrigate the ear (National Library of Medicine, 2009a). In addition, the ear should not be irrigated if vegetable matter or an insect is present in the canal; the tympanic membrane is ruptured; or the patient has otitis externa, myringotomy tubes, or a mastoid cavity (Hockenberry and Wilson, 2007).

ASSESSMENT

1. Review prescriber's order, including solution to be instilled and affected ear(s) to receive irrigation. *Rationale: Ensures safe and correct administration of irrigation solution.*
2. Review medical record for history of ruptured tympanic membrane, placement of myringotomy tubes, or surgery of auditory canal. *Rationale: These factors contraindicate ear irrigation.*
3. Inspect pinna and external auditory meatus for redness, swelling, drainage, abrasions, and presence of cerumen or foreign objects. Wear clean gloves if drainage is present. *Rationale: Provides baseline information to monitor effects of irrigation.*

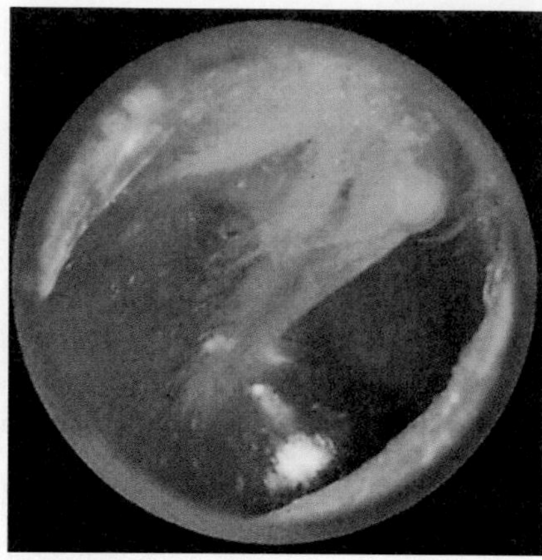

FIG 11-2 Normal tympanic membrane.

a. Attempt to remove foreign object in ear by straightening ear canal. *Rationale: Straightening of canal may cause object to fall out and negate need for irrigation.*

> **SAFETY ALERT** If vegetable matter (e.g., dried bean or pea) is occluding canal, do not perform irrigation because the object may absorb the solution and swell, thus causing further damage (National Library of Medicine, 2009a).

4. Use an otoscope to inspect deeper portions of the auditory canal and tympanic membrane (Fig. 11-2). *Rationale: If the patient's tympanic membrane (eardrum) is not intact, irrigation is contraindicated.*
5. Assess patient's comfort level using a scale of 0 to 10. *Rationale: Provides baseline to evaluate changes in patient's condition. Presence of pain is symptomatic of ear infection or inflammation.*
6. Assess patient's hearing ability in the affected ear. *Rationale: Occlusion of canal by cerumen or foreign object can impair hearing.*
7. Assess patient's knowledge of proper ear care. *Rationale: May indicate need for instruction regarding hygiene.*

PLANNING

Expected Outcomes focus on patient comfort and improved auditory perception.

1. Patient denies increased pain, using a scale of 0 to 10, during instillation.
2. Patient's ear canal is clear of discharge, cerumen, or foreign material after irrigation.
3. Patient demonstrates improved hearing acuity in affected ear after irrigation.
4. Patient describes proper ear care techniques.

Delegation and Collaboration

The skill of irrigating the external ear cannot be delegated to nursing assistive personnel (NAP). Instruct the NAP about the following:

- Reporting any ear drainage or patient's report of ear discomfort

Equipment

- Clean gloves
- Otoscope (optional)
- Irrigation syringe
- Basin for irrigating solution (Use sterile basin if sterile irrigating solution is used.)
- Emesis basin for drainage or irrigating solution exiting the ear
- Towel
- Cotton balls or 4 × 4–inch gauze
- Prescribed irrigating solution warmed to body temperature
- Mineral oil or an over-the-counter ear wax softener
- MAR

IMPLEMENTATION *for* EAR IRRIGATION

STEPS	RATIONALE
1. See Standard Protocol (inside front cover).	
2. If patient is found to have impacted cerumen, instill one to two drops of mineral oil or over-the-counter softener into ear twice a day for 2 to 3 days before irrigation.	Loosens cerumen for easier removal.
3. Check accuracy and completeness of each medication administration record (MAR) with prescriber's written medication or procedure order. Check patient's name, drug name and dosage, route of administration, and time for administration. Compare MAR with label of ear irrigation solution.	The order sheet is the most reliable source and only legal record of drugs or procedure that the patient is to receive. Ensures that patient receives correct medication.
4. Identify patient using two identifiers (e.g., name and birthday or name and account number, according to facility policy). Compare identifiers with information on patient's MAR or medical record.	Ensures correct patient. Complies with The Joint Commission standards and improves patient safety (TJC, 2010).

STEPS	RATIONALE
5. Assist patient to a sitting or lying position with head tilted forward and toward the affected ear. Place towel or waterproof pad under patient's head and shoulder. If possible have patient help hold basin under affected ear.	Position minimizes leakage of fluids around neck and facial area. Solution flows from ear canal to basin.
6. Pour prescribed irrigating solution into basin. Check the temperature of the solution (37° C [98.6° F]) by pouring a small drop on your inner forearm. NOTE: If a sterile solution is prescribed, use a sterile basin.	Warming ear irrigating solutions to body temperature helps to avoid vertigo or nausea (McKenry and others, 2006).

SAFETY ALERT To prevent trauma to the ear or tympanic membrane during irrigation, instruct patient to not make any sudden moves.

STEPS	RATIONALE
7. Gently clean auricle and outer ear canal with moistened gauze or cotton balls. Do not force drainage or cerumen into ear canal.	Prevents infected material from reentering ear canal.
8. Fill irrigating syringe with approximately 50 mL of solution and expel air.	Prevents sudden expulsion of fluid.
9. For adults and children over age 3 years, gently pull pinna up and back. In children 3 years or younger, pinna should be pulled down and back (Hockenberry and Wilson, 2007). Adults can lie supine	Pulling pinna straightens external ear canal and prevents obstruction of canal with device, which can lead to increased pressure on tympanic membrane.
10. Slowly instill irrigating solution by holding tip of syringe 1 cm (½ inch) above opening to ear canal. Leave space between tip and canal; do not occlude canal with syringe. Direct the fluid toward the superior aspect of the ear canal. Allow fluid to drain out during instillation into the basis. Continue until canal is cleansed or solution is used (see illustration).	Prevents occlusion of ear canal with syringe tip. Slow instillation prevents buildup of pressure in ear canal and ensures contact of solution with all canal surfaces.

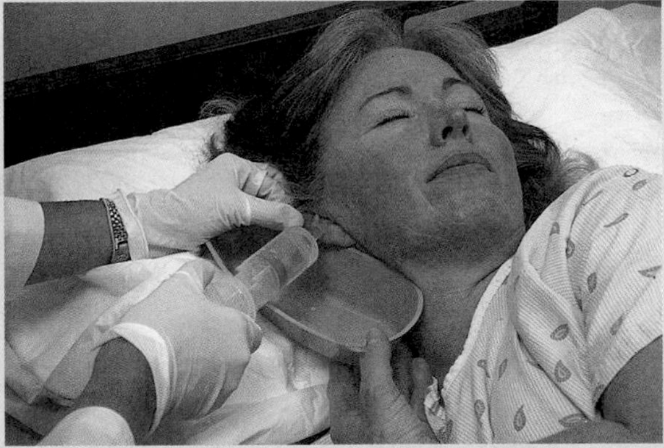

STEP 10 Irrigation of affected ear.

STEPS	RATIONALE
11. Maintain the flow of irrigation in a steady stream until you see pieces of cerumen flow from the canal.	Constant flow of fluid loosens cerumen.
12. Periodically ask if patient is experiencing pain, nausea, or vertigo.	Symptoms indicate irrigating solution is too hot, too cold, or instilled with too much pressure.
13. Drain excessive fluid from ear by having patient tilt head toward affected side.	Excess fluid may promote microorganism growth.
14. Dry outer ear canal gently with a cotton ball. Leave cotton ball in place for 5 to 10 minutes.	Drying prevents buildup of moisture that can lead to otitis externa.
15. **See Completion Protocol (inside front cover).**	

EVALUATION

1. Ask patient if discomfort is noted during instillation of solution.
2. Ask patient about any sensations of dizziness or feeling light-headed.
3. Reinspect condition of external meatus and ear canal.
4. Evaluate hearing acuity in affected ear after irrigation.
5. Ask patient to describe proper ear care techniques.

Unexpected Outcomes and Related Interventions

1. Patient complains of increased ear pain during irrigation.
   a. Discontinue irrigation and notify health care provider.
2. Foreign body remains in the ear canal.
   a. Repeat irrigation.
   b. Refer patient to an otolaryngologist.
3. Patient's ear canal remains occluded. Patient's hearing acuity has not improved in the affected ear.
   a. Repeat irrigation if prescribed.
   b. If condition persists, notify health care provider.

Recording and Reporting

- Record procedure, noting which ear, and record appearance of external ear and patient's hearing acuity after procedure. Record the type and amount of solution, time of administration, and the ear receiving the irrigation on patient's MAR.
- Report adverse effects/patient response to health care provider.

Sample Documentation

1000 Patient reports difficulty hearing in right ear. Cerumen plug noted in canal. Irrigated right ear with 50 mL warm normal saline. Return fluid clear with brown particles. No complaints of pain or discomfort. States that hearing "is fine." Responds appropriately to normal conversation tone. Right ear canal clear. Instructed on ear hygiene.

Special Considerations

Pediatric

- Be certain that child's head is immobilized to prevent puncturing eardrum.
- Ask parent to help calm child during procedure.

Geriatric

- Older adults often require ongoing ear care for cerumen removal. Use of an oil-based softening agent such as slightly warmed mineral oil twice daily for several days before irrigation is helpful (Armstrong, 2009).
- Older adults with higher risk of cerumen impaction include those with large amounts of ear canal hair, those with benign growths that narrow the ear canal, and those who habitually wear hearing aids (Ebersole and others, 2008).

Home Care

- Instruct patient to clean ears with a damp washcloth wrapped around a finger. Do not use a cotton-tipped applicator.
- If patient uses a ceruminolytic agent, instruct that these are softening products and that they will not remove the impaction (McKenry and others, 2006).

SKILL 11.3 CARING FOR A HEARING AID

Hearing is vital for normal communication and orientation to sounds in the environment. Hearing loss affects 36 million American adults according to the National Institute on Deafness and Other Communication Disorders (2010). The institute also notes that only 1 out of 5 people, who actually need a hearing aid, wear one. Those who choose not to wear a hearing aid often dislike the type of sound they hear or they have trouble keeping the hearing aid functional. Sensorineural hearing loss or nerve deafness is more prevalent in the older-adult population. It affects 30% individuals over age 65, 50% of people over age 75, and 50% of nursing home residents (Wallhagen and Pettengill, 2008).

Any hearing loss has social implications, with the person often avoiding social activities. There are also many safety considerations. Not only do people with hearing loss have difficulty hearing car horns and emergency sirens; they also have difficulty understanding patient education and, as a result, may not safely manage their symptoms or therapies (Wallhagen and others, 2006).

For people with hearing loss, a proper hearing aid improves the ability to hear and understand spoken words. Hearing aids amplify sound so it is heard at a more effective level. All aids have four basic components:

1. A microphone, which receives and converts sound into electrical signals
2. An amplifier, which increases the strength of the electrical signal
3. A receiver, which converts the strengthened signal back into sound
4. A power source (batteries)

In addition, programmable hearing aids are now available. They are in analog and digital formats. Digital technology uses a tiny processor to convert the sound before it is amplified (Fransman and Walker, 2007). This allows the signal to be analyzed to remove background nose and automatically adjust the volume. Patients seeking these aids need to be evaluated by a licensed audiologist to determine the type of aid and which frequencies are needed for the individual patient. These aids are adjusted to accommodate the range of the patient's residual hearing. Programmable aids independently amplify high-frequency (soft-spoken consonants) from low-frequency (loudly spoken vowels) sounds; this

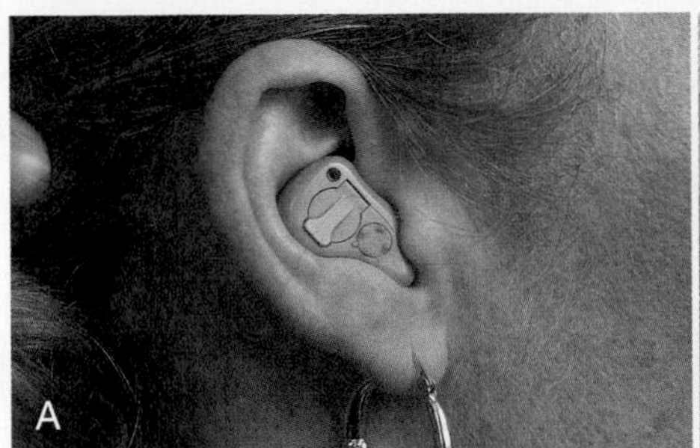
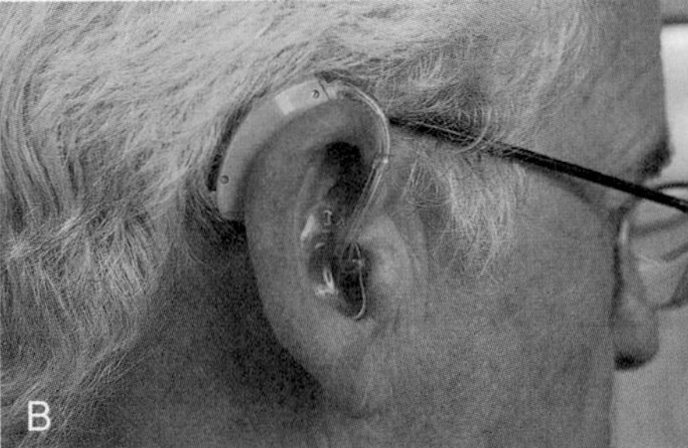
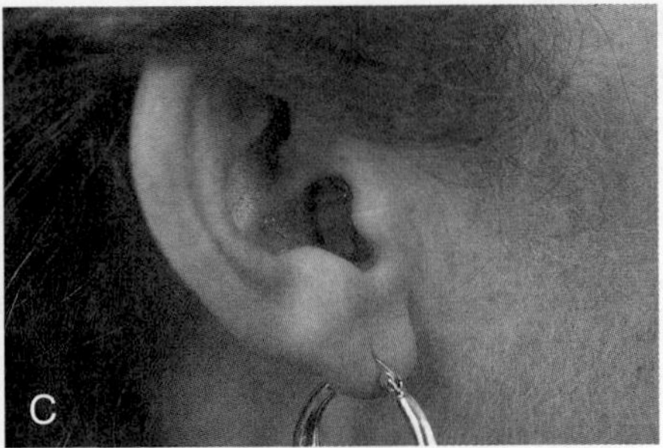

FIG 11-3 **A,** In-the-ear hearing aid. **B,** Behind-the-ear hearing aid. **C,** Completely-in-canal hearing aid.

process occurs rapidly and continuously (Ebersole and others, 2008). Several styles of hearing aids are available to patients today.

1. *In-the-ear (ITE)* hearing aids fit completely in the outer ear and are used for mild-to-severe hearing loss (Fig. 11-3, *A*). The plastic case is large enough to hold internal circuitry and external controls. ITE aids can hold added technical mechanisms such as a telecoil, a small magnetic coil contained in the hearing aid that improves sound transmission during telephone calls. ITE aids can be damaged by earwax and ear drainage, and their small size can cause adjustment problems and feedback. They are not usually worn by children because the casings need to be replaced as the ear grows.
2. *Behind-the-ear (BTE)* hearing aids are worn behind the ear and are connected to a plastic ear mold that fits inside the outer ear. The components are held in a case behind the ear. Sound travels through the ear mold into the ear. People of all ages wear BTE aids for mild-to-profound hearing loss (Fig. 11-3, *B*). Poorly fitting BTE ear molds can cause feedback, a whistling sound caused by the fit of the hearing aid. BTE aids are better protected from earwax.
3. *Canal aids* fit into the ear canal and are available in two sizes. The *in-the-canal* hearing aid is customized to fit the size and shape of the ear canal and is used for mild-to–moderately severe hearing loss. A *completely-in-canal* (CIC) hearing aid is largely concealed in the ear canal and is used for mild-to–moderately severe hearing loss (Fig. 11-3, *C*). Because of their small size, canal aids may be difficult for the user to adjust and remove and may not be able to hold additional devices such as a telecoil. Canal aids can also be damaged by earwax and ear drainage. They are not typically recommended for children.

ASSESSMENT

1. Determine whether patient can hear clearly with use of aid by talking slowly and clearly in normal tone of voice. *Rationale: Inability to hear may indicate faulty function of hearing aid or that aid is no longer effective for patient's auditory loss.*
2. If patient wears an aid, determine if he or she is able to manipulate the hearing aid and batteries. Watch patient insert aid independently. *Rationale: Determines level of assistance required.*
3. Assess patient's knowledge of and routines for cleansing and caring for hearing aid. *Rationale: Determines compliance with and knowledge of self-care.*
4. Assess if hearing aid is working by removing from patient's ear. Close battery case and turn volume slowly to high. Cup hand over hearing aid. If you hear a squealing sound (feedback), it is working. If no sound is heard, replace batteries and test again. *Rationale: May indicate malfunctioning of hearing aid.*
5. Assess patient for any unusual physical or auditory signs/symptoms (pain, itching, redness, discharge, odor, tinnitus, decreased hearing acuity) (see Chapter 7). *Rationale: May indicate injury, infection, or cerumen accumulation.*
6. Inspect ear mold for cracked or rough edges. *Rationale: Poorly fitting hearing aids cause irritation and/or discomfort to external ear canal.*
7. Inspect for accumulation of cerumen around aid and plugging of opening in aid. *Rationale: Cerumen can block sound reception (National Library of Medicine, 2009c).*

PLANNING

Expected Outcomes focus on facilitating communication and promoting comfort and appropriate self-care.

1. Patient hears conversation spoken in normal tone of voice and responds appropriately.
2. Patient responds appropriately to environmental sounds.
3. Patient demonstrates proper care of hearing aid.
4. Patient verbalizes that aid fits comfortably.

Delegation and Collaboration

The skill of caring for a hearing aid can be delegated to nursing assistive personnel (NAP). Instruct the NAP about the following:

- Using patient preferences when cleaning aid
- Communication tips to use for individual patient while aid is being cleaned
- Having care provider report signs and symptoms of hearing loss or presence of ear drainage

Equipment

- Soft towel and washcloth
- Warm soap and water
- Brush or wax loop
- Storage case
- Clean gloves (if drainage is present)
- Spare battery (optional)
- Facial tissue

IMPLEMENTATION *for* CARING FOR A HEARING AID

STEPS	RATIONALE
1. See Standard Protocol (inside front cover).	
2. Removing and cleaning hearing aid	
a. Apply gloves if drainage is present.	Reduces transmission of microorganisms.
b. Have patient turn hearing aid volume off (or assist as needed). Usually you rotate the volume control toward the nose to increase volume and away from the nose to lower volume. Grasp aid securely and gently remove device following natural ear contour. *NOTE: Some ITE and CIC devices do not have a volume control but are turned off by opening the battery door. CIC devices have a clear plastic handle for removal. Grasp handle and gently pull straight out.*	Prevents feedback (whistling) during removal, dropping hearing aid, or injury to ear.
c. Hold aid over towel and wipe exterior with tissue to remove cerumen.	Prevents breakage if dropped. Impaction of cerumen blocks normal sound transmission.
d. Inspect all openings in aid for accumulated cerumen. Carefully remove cerumen with wax loop or brush (supplied with aid) to clean holes in hearing aid.	Cerumen may block sound from receiver. It may also block pressure equalization channel and create feeling of ear pressure.
e. Inspect ear mold for rough edges. Check for any frays in cords.	
f. Open battery door, remove battery, place it in labeled storage container, and allow it to air dry.	Increases battery life and allows moisture to evaporate.
g. Wash ear canal with washcloth moistened in soap and water. Rinse and dry.	Removes cerumen from ear canal. Removes soap residue and water that may harbor microbes or damage hearing aid.
h. If you will be storing the hearing aid, place it in a dry storage case. Most come with a desiccant material for drying. Label case with patient's name and room number. If more than one aid, note right or left.	Protects hearing aid against damage, moisture, and breakage.
3. Inserting hearing aid	
a. 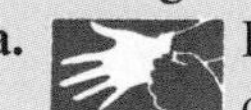 Perform hand hygiene and apply gloves if drainage is present.	Reduces transmission of microorganisms
b. Remove hearing aid from storage case and check battery (see Assessment). Turn hearing aid volume off.	Turning volume off prevents feedback (whistling) during insertion.
c. Identify hearing aid as either right (marked "R" or red color coded) or left (marked "L" or blue color coded).	Proper orientation prevents damage and injury.
d. Allow patient to reinsert aid, if possible. Otherwise, hold hearing aid with thumb and index finger of dominant hand so that canal—long portion with hole(s)—is at the bottom. Insert pointed end of ear mold into ear canal. Follow natural ear contours to guide aid into place.	Proper orientation is important for hearing aid insertion. Ensures correct positioning of aid within ear canal.
e. Adjust or have patient adjust volume gradually to comfortable level for talking to patient in regular voice 3 to 4 feet away. Rotate volume control toward nose to increase volume and away from nose to decrease volume.	

STEPS	RATIONALE

SAFETY ALERT Programmable aids have the volume control located on the remote. For most patients hearing aids work best at lower volume settings.

4. See Completion Protocol (inside front cover).

EVALUATION

1. Ask patient to rate comfort level after removal or insertion.
2. Observe patient during normal conversation and in response to environmental sounds.
3. Observe patient perform hearing aid care (removal, cleaning, and reinsertion).

Unexpected Outcomes and Related Interventions

1. Patient is unable to hear conversations or environmental sounds clearly. Patient's verbal responses are inappropriate.
   a. Remove hearing aid and check battery for power and correct placement.
   b. Inspect ear mold and ear canal for cerumen blockage.
   c. Change volume setting as needed.
   d. If problems persist, contact audiologist or hearing aid specialist.
2. Patient is unable to perform care of hearing aid.
   a. Demonstrate correct aid care and offer return demonstration.
   b. Include family caregiver who will be available to patient.
3. Patient complains of ear discomfort and may complain of whistling sound.
   a. Remove aid and reinsert.
   b. Assess external ear for signs of inflammation.
   c. If problems persist, contact audiologist or hearing aid specialist.

Recording and Reporting

- Record that hearing aid is removed and stored if patient is going for surgery or special procedure. Be sure to document where or with whom aid is stored. Record patient's preferred communication techniques.
- Record and report any signs or symptoms of infection or injury or sudden decrease in hearing acuity to health care provider.
- Report to nursing staff and document on plan-of-care tips that promote communication with patient.

Sample Documentation

1000 Patient responds inappropriately to questions. Unable to hear normal conversation tone. States he hears "an echo." Volume turned down on ITE aid in right ear. Daughter states that patient frequently turns the volume up so he can "hear better." Reviewed proper volume settings and improved listening techniques with patient and daughter.

Special Considerations

Pediatric

- As children grow older, they can become self-conscious of a hearing aid. Changes in hair style may help some children overcome self-consciousness (Hockenberry and Wilson, 2007).
- Store batteries away from children's reach. Batteries are toxic when swallowed.

Geriatric

- The small size of some hearing aids may make it difficult for older adults to handle and manipulate the devices. Patients should contact their hearing aid specialist for assistance. Family members may be able to assist with care of device.
- High-pitched signals associated with consonants *f, p, t, k, ch, sh,* and *st* are more difficult to hear clearly as people age (Ebersole and others, 2008).
- Inappropriate responses to questions or situations, irritation when spoken to, asking to have a statement repeated, inattentiveness, or difficulty following instructions should alert you or family members that the patient may have some hearing loss that needs to be evaluated. People incorrectly may assume that the patient is confused (Ebersole and others, 2008).
- Be alert for patient assessment findings that may indicate some depression. Hearing loss and depression are common, and correction of hearing loss may actually resolve depression in some patients (Wallhagen and others, 2006).

Home Care

- Initial use of hearing aid should be restricted to quiet situations in the home. Patients need to adjust gradually to voices and household sounds (Ebersole and others, 2008).
- Avoid exposure of aid to extreme heat, cold, or moisture. Do not leave in case near stove, heater, or sunny window. Do not use with hair dryer on hot settings or with sunlamp. Do not wear when bathing, during excess sweating, or when shampooing at a hair stylist.
- Do not use hairspray or other hair care products while wearing hearing aids.
- Always keep a set of unused batteries in the home.
- Be sure the person cleans the ears daily. Likewise, a hearing aid should be cleaned daily.

REVIEW QUESTIONS

Case Study for Questions 1 and 2

Mr. Arthur has worn bilateral in-the-ear hearing aids for the last 10 years. He knows how to care for his aids. He notes that, when the aids are working well, he hears his family and co-workers clearly, has minimal distortion in large gatherings, and is able to distinguish emergency sirens and car horns when he is driving.

1. He now complains of diminished hearing in the left ear and senses drainage from the ear. The nurse decides to check the functioning of the hearing aid. Place the following steps in appropriate order for cleaning the hearing aid.
   - a. Wash ear canal.
   - b. Place hearing aid in storage case.
   - c. Apply clean gloves.
   - d. Grasp aid securely and remove from ear following natural ear contour.
   - e. Use brush to clean holes in the aid.
   - f. Have patient turn hearing aid volume off.

   1. f, d, c, a, b, e
   2. c, f, d, e, a, b
   3. c, f, d, a, e, b
   4. f, d, c, e, a, b
2. Mr. Arthur's preschool grandchildren visit frequently and are curious about the hearing aids. What preschool safety concerns should the nurse teach? Select all that apply.
   1. Batteries are toxic if swallowed.
   2. Tell the children to face grandpa when speaking.
   3. Keep batteries and aids out of children's reach.
   4. Show the children how the aid fits in the ear.
3. The nurse should question an order for an ear irrigation if the patient has which of the following conditions?
   1. Foreign body such as a pea
   2. Migraine headaches
   3. Cerumen accumulation
   4. Hearing impairment
4. How should the nurse position a 26-month-old child's ear during irrigation?
   1. Without pulling on the earlobes
   2. While pulling the pinna down and back
   3. While pulling the tragus down and back
   4. While pulling the auricle up and back
5. Which statement best explains nursing actions during an irrigation of the left ear?
   1. Lean the patient's head toward right side.
   2. Hold the irrigation syringe approximately 1 cm (½ inch) above opening to ear canal.
   3. Delegate the procedure to assistive personnel.
   4. Place the patient in supine position with head elevated.
6. A patient is being discharged home and must care for her artificial eye. The nurse knows that further teaching is necessary when the patient states:
   1. "I will clean the eye at least once a week."
   2. "I don't have to use sterile solutions for cleaning the eye."
   3. "The colored dot is there to show me which way to put it in."
   4. "Rubbing alcohol and fingernail polish remover are bad for the eye."
7. After caring for an eye prosthesis, the nurse's priority documentation includes which of the following?
   1. Where the patient stores the eye prosthesis at home
   2. The patient's feelings about wearing the eye prosthesis
   3. Any signs and symptoms of inflammation or infection noted in the eye socket
   4. Which family member was present during the procedure
8. A young man enters the emergency department with a chemical burn from household bleach. His wife ran tap water over the eyes before bringing him to the emergency department. Which sequence represents the nurse's immediate actions in this situation?
   - a. Assess the injured eye.
   - b. Determine the patient's level of pain.
   - c. Prepare to initiate eye irrigation.
   - d. Teach eye safety.
   - e. Wait for the physician because the patient irrigated the eye at home.

   1. a, b, c
   2. a, b, e
   3. a, c, d
   4. b, c, d
   5. b, d, e
9. Routine eye care for a comatose patient facilitates which of the following?
   1. Blinking
   2. Visual acuity
   3. Lubrication
   4. Scleral integrity
10. The nursing assistive personnel (NAP) informs the nurse that, while providing eye care to a comatose patient, she observed yellowish drainage. What is the nurse's immediate reaction?
    1. Instruct her to continue eye care.
    2. Explain that yellow drainage is caused by the environmental eye in contact with eye secretions.
    3. Contact the health care provider.
    4. Completely assess the patient's eyes.

REFERENCES

Armstrong C: Diagnosis and management of cerumen impaction, *Am Fam Physician* 80:1011, 2009.

Babineau MR, Sanchez LD: Ophthalmologic procedures, *Emerg Med Clin North Am* 26:17, 2008.

Center for Ocular Prosthetics: *Custom made artificial plastic eyes*, http://www.artificialeyesplastic.com/new-eye-care.htm, accessed July 2009.

Ebersole P and others: *Toward healthy aging*, ed 7, St Louis, 2008, Mosby.

Erickson Laboratories: *Prosthetic care*, http://www.ericksonlaboratories.com/care.html, accessed July 2009.

Fransman BA, Walker S: Digital hearing aids: a life transformation, *Learn Disabil Res Pract* 10(3):16, 2007.

Galanti GA: *Caring for patients from different cultures*, ed 4, Philadelphia, 2008, University of Pennsylvania Press.

Hockenberry MJ, Wilson D: *Wong's nursing care of infants and children*, ed 8, St Louis, 2007, Mosby.

Kolberg Ocular Prosthetics: *Artificial eye information and patient support page*, 2009, http://www.artificialeye.net, accessed July 2009.

Kraszewski S: Safe and effective ear irrigation, *Nurs Stand* 22(43):45, 2008.

Lauren YC and others: Hand/face/neck localized pattern: sticky resins, *Dermatol Clin* 27:227, 2009.

Marshall AP and others: Eye care in the critically ill: clinical practice guideline, *Aust Crit Care* 21:97, 2008.

McKenry LM and others: *Mosby's pharmacology in nursing*, ed 22, St Louis, 2006, Mosby.

National Institute on Deafness and Other Communication Disorders: *Quick statistics*, 2010, http://www.nidcd.nih.gov/health/statistics/quick.htm, accessed July 2010.

National Institute for Occupational Safety and Health, Centers for Disease Control and Prevention: *Eye Safety*, last updated April 2009, available at http://www.cdc.gov/niosh/topics/eye/, accessed July 2009.

National Library of Medicine: *Medline plus: Ear emergencies*, updated June 2009a, http://www.nlm.nih.gov/medlineplus/ency/article/000052.htm, accessed July 2009.

National Library of Medicine: *Medline Plus: Eye emergencies*, 2009b, http://www.nlm.nih.gov/medlineplus/ency/article/000054.htm, updated January 2009b, accessed July 2009.

National Library of Medicine: *Medline Plus: Wax blockage*, updated June 2009c, http://www.nlm.nih.gov/medlineplus/ency/article/0000979.htm, accessed July 2009.

Rosenberg JB, Eisen LA: Eye care in the intensive care unit: narrative review and meta-analysis, *Crit Care Med* 36(12):3151, 2008.

Segal E: First aid for skin/eye decontamination: are present practices effective? *Chemical Health Safety* 14(4):16, 2007.

The Joint Commission (TJC): *2010 National patient safety goals*, Oakbrook Terrace, Ill, 2010, The Commission, http://jointcommission.org/PatientSafety/NationalPatientSafetyGoals, accessed July 2010.

Wallhagen MI: The stigma of hearing loss, *Gerontologist* 50(1):66, 2010.

Wallhagen MI, Pettengill E: Hearing impairment—significant but underassessed in primary care settings, *J Gerontol Nurs* 34(2):36, 2008.

Wallhagen MI and others: Sensory impairment in older adults. Part 1: Hearing loss, *Am J Nurs* 106(10):40, 2006.

CHAPTER 12

Promoting Nutrition

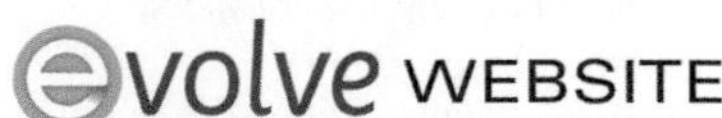

http://evolve.elsevier.com/Perry/nursinginterventions
Video Clips
Nursing Skills Online

Nutrition is a basic component of health. It affects patients' recovery from short-term and chronic illness, surgery, and injury. Your role is to assess patients' risks for nutrition problems, assist patients with oral feeding when needed, and administer enteral nutritional therapies while protecting patients from the risk of aspiration. Routine identification of malnutrition with screening of patients in health care settings is a requirement of The Joint Commission (2009). Nutrition screening involves identifying patient characteristics associated with nutrition problems and risk factors for malnutrition (American Society for Parenteral and Enteral Nutrition [ASPEN], 2007). You learn to conduct an initial nutritional screening with every patient, including a history and physical examination (Table 12-1). Findings determine if there is a need for consultation with a registered dietitian (RD). Box 12-1 provides a list of risk factors for nutritional problems. No single objective measure alone is an effective predictor for nutritional risk. Work closely with RDs to discuss a patient's situation such as resources for buying food and availability of family assistance to devise an appropriate nutritional plan.

PATIENT-CENTERED CARE

Multiple factors affect a patient's nutritional needs. Using a patient-centered approach to care ensures a relevant and appropriate nutritional plan for your patients. In addition to a thorough screening of a patient's physical status, ability to take in nutrients, and nutritional knowledge level (see Skill 12.1), your assessment should include a patient's eating patterns and food choices. Ethnicity, culture, and religious practices all influence what a person eats and the manner in which he or she plans meals and eats socially. Cultural awareness helps you to include patients' preferences in their diet (Box 12-2). Foods are often associated with caring and love, health promotion, maintenance, and restoration. For example, Asians, Hispanics, Eastern Europeans, and Africans believe in the hot and cold theory of health and illness. Foods are classified as cold or hot on the basis of their characteristics, independent of the temperature at which they are served. There is no universal agreement across cultures about which foods are hot or cold.

Mealtime in a health care setting is the ideal time to communicate with patients. During a meal continue your patient assessments and evaluation, encourage decision making, and provide education and counseling. Mealtime is often a social time, but you can use the valuable time to educate patients and family members, especially when planning discharge home. Early identification of potential problems can avoid more serious problems. Your role includes providing information about community resources, referral to an RD, supporting healthy changes, and monitoring dietary progress.

Comfort measures are a part of patient-centered care. Know the types of foods patients avoid or consider adverse. In some cases patients feel nauseated at the simple sight of certain foods. This is common in cancer patients who are taking chemotherapy drugs. If a patient has nausea or pain, offer appropriate antiemetics or analgesics 30 minutes before mealtime. Just before meals, allow patients to toilet and perform hand and oral hygiene. These measures help patients relax at mealtime and promote their appetite.

SAFETY

Difficulty swallowing or dysphagia involves losing control over the ability to chew, move food into a bolus at the back of the mouth, and swallow. Dysphagia is a symptom or

TABLE 12-1 **CLINICAL SIGNS OF NUTRITIONAL STATUS**

BODY AREA	SIGNS OF GOOD NUTRITION	SIGNS OF POOR NUTRITION
General appearance	Alert, responsive	Listless, apathetic, cachectic
Weight	Normal for height, age, body build	Overweight or underweight (special concern for underweight)
Posture	Erect, arms and legs straight	Sagging shoulders, sunken chest, humped back
Muscles	Well-developed, firm, good tone, some fat under skin	Flaccid, poor tone; undeveloped, tender, "wasted" appearance; cannot walk properly
Nervous system control	Good attention span, not irritable or restless, normal reflexes, psychological stability	Inattentive, irritable, confused, burning and tingling of hands and feet (paresthesia), loss of position and vibratory sense, weakness and tenderness of muscles (may affect ability to walk)
Gastrointestinal function	Good appetite and digestion, normal regular elimination, no palpable organs or masses	Anorexia, indigestion, constipation or diarrhea, liver or spleen enlargement
Cardiovascular function	Normal heart rate and rhythm, no murmurs, normal blood pressure for age	Rapid heart rate (above 100 beats per minute), enlarged heart, abnormal rhythm, elevated blood pressure
General vitality	Endurance, energetic, sleeps well, vigorous	Easily fatigued, no energy, falls asleep easily, looks tired, apathetic
Hair	Shiny, lustrous, firm, not easily plucked, healthy scalp	Stringy, dull, brittle, dry, thin and sparse, depigmented; can be easily plucked
Skin (general)	Smooth, slightly moist, good color	Rough, dry, scaly, pale, pigmented, irritated, bruised, petechiae, delayed wound healing, xanthoma (yellowish papules), and presence of pressure ulcers
Face and neck	Skin color is uniform, smooth, healthy looking, not swollen	Greasy, discolored, scaly, swollen, skin dark over cheeks and under eyes, lumpiness or flakiness of skin around nose and mouth
Lips	Smooth, good color, moist, not chapped or swollen	Dry, scaly, swollen, redness and swelling (cheilosis); angular lesions (stomatitis) at corners of the mouth or fissures or scars
Gums	Good pink color, healthy, red, no swelling or bleeding	Spongy, bleed easily, marginal redness, inflamed, gums receding
Tongue	Good pink color or deep reddish in appearance, not swollen or smooth, surface papillae present, no lesions	Swelling, scarlet and raw, magenta color, beefy (glossitis), hyperemic and hypertrophic or atrophic papillae
Teeth	No cavities, no pain, bright, straight, no crowding, well-shaped jaw, clean, no discoloration	Unfilled caries, absent teeth, worn surfaces mottled (fluorosis), malpositioned
Eyes	Bright, clear, shiny, no sores at corner of eyelids, membranes moist and healthy pink color, no prominent blood vessels or mound of tissue or sclera, no fatigue circles beneath	Pale conjunctival membranes, redness of membranes (injection), dryness, redness and fissuring of eyelid corners (angular palpebritis), dryness of eye membrane (conjunctival xerosis), dull appearance of cornea (corneal xerosis)
Neck (glands)	No enlargement	Thyroid enlarged; may indicate iodine deficiency
Nails	Firm, pink	Spoon-shaped (koilonychia), brittle, ridged, blue lunula
Legs and feet	No tenderness, weakness, or swelling; good color	Edema, tender calf, tingling, weakness, muscle wasting
Skeleton	No malformation	Bowlegs, knock-knees, chest deformity at diaphragm, beaded ribs, prominent scapulae

Adapted from Mahan L, Escott-Stump S: *Krause's food nutrition and diet therapy,* ed 12, Philadelphia, 2007, Saunders.

BOX 12-1 RISK FACTORS FOR POTENTIAL NUTRITION PROBLEMS

- Patients on clear- or full-liquid diets for more than 3 days without nutrient supplementation or inappropriate or insufficient nutrient supplementation
- Patients on intravenous feeding (dextrose or saline) or nothing by mouth (NPO) for more than 3 days without supplementation
- Low intake of prescribed diet or tube feeding
- Weight 20% above or 10% below desirable body weight (adjusting for edema)
- Pregnancy weight gain deviating from normal patterns
- Diagnoses that increase nutritional needs or decrease nutrient intake or both: alcoholism, burns, cancer, dementia, diarrhea, hemorrhage, hyperthyroidism, infected or draining wounds, systemic infection, malabsorption, major trauma, postoperative
- Chronic use of drugs, especially alcohol, that affect nutritional intake.
- Alterations in chewing, swallowing, appetite, taste, and smell
- Body temperature consistently above normal for more than 2 days
- Hematocrit: <43% in men, <37% in women; hemoglobin <14 g/dL in men, <12 g/dL in women
- Absolute decrease in lymphocyte count (<1500 cells/mm^3)
- Elevated (>250 mg/dL) or decreased (<130 mg/dL) total plasma cholesterol
- Serum albumin <3 g/dL in patients without renal or liver disease, generalized dermatitis, overhydration
- Older adult living in long-term care facility

Adapted from Grodner M and others: *Foundations and clinical applications of nutrition: a nursing approach*, ed 4, St Louis, 2007, Mosby; Wendland BE and others. Malnutrition in institutionalized seniors: the iatrogenic component, *J Am Geriatr Soc* 51:85, 2003.

complication of a number of conditions, including stroke, serious dementia, cerebral palsy, multiple sclerosis, Parkinson's disease, and oral cancer. Physical impairment of muscles and nerves within the mouth and cognitive conditions that affect concentration and selective attention alter swallowing. Dysphagia leads to disability or decreased functional status, increased length of stay and cost of care, increased likelihood of discharge to institutionalized care, and increased mortality (Ashley and others, 2006). A person with dysphagia is at risk for aspiration, the inhalation of food particles and/or saliva into the lower respiratory tract. When bacteria growing in oral secretions reach the lung, pneumonia develops. As a nurse, assess if your patients are at risk for dysphagia. If so, nursing strategies that include safe feeding techniques and following aspiration precautions can be used (see Skill 12.2).

When educating patients and families, food safety and preparation are important topics. Food safety is a public health issue. Germs enter food from improper cleansing or preparation or poor handwashing practices. Persons most at risk for developing foodborne illnesses are older adults, the very young, and those with lowered resistance to infection. The food safety tips in Box 12-3 help prevent foodborne illnesses such as *Salmonella* and *Escherichia coli.*

BOX 12-2 CULTURAL CONSIDERATIONS TO ENHANCE PATIENT NUTRITION

- The theory of hot and cold foods exists in many cultures. Filipinos, Caribbean Islanders, Mexicans, and Latinos may plan their meals on the basis of these beliefs. Food classification as hot or cold varies slightly from culture to culture. Mexicans believe that hot is warmth, strength, and reassurance; whereas cold is menacing and weak. Classification has nothing to do with spiciness. Hot foods include rice, grains, alcohol, beef, lamb, chili peppers, chocolate, and cheese. Cold foods include beans, citrus fruits, dairy products, most vegetables, honey, raisins, chicken, and goat. Foods can be made hot or cold through methods of preparation.
- Orthodox Judaism requires adherence to kosher food preparation methods and prohibits eating pork, predatory fowl, shellfish (i.e., crab, shrimp), blood, and mixing of milk or dairy products with meat dishes. No cooking is done on the Sabbath (sundown Friday through sundown Saturday). For all Jewish sects no leavened bread is eaten during Passover.
- Muslims prohibit the intake of pork and sometimes practice dietary guidelines similar to kosher, called *halal.*
- The Church of Jesus Christ of Latter-day Saints (Mormons) prohibits the use of alcohol and caffeine.
- Seventh-Day Adventists encourage a vegetarian diet and prohibit intake of pork, shellfish, and alcohol.

BOX 12-3 FOOD SAFETY TIPS

- Wash hands with warm soapy water before touching food.
- Wash all fresh fruits and vegetables thoroughly.
- Do not eat raw meats or drink unpasteurized milk.
- Do not buy or eat food that has passed the expiration date on the package.
- Keep foods properly refrigerated at 4.4° C (40° F) and frozen at −17.8° C (0° F).
- Wash dishes and cutting boards with hot soapy water. Use a dishwasher if available.
- Do not save leftovers for more than 2 days in the refrigerator.
- Wash dishcloths, towels, and sponges regularly or run in a dishwasher cycle. The cleanest option is paper towels.
- Clean the inside of the refrigerator and microwave every month.

EVIDENCE-BASED PRACTICE TRENDS

Lengyel CO and others: Nutrient inadequacies among elderly residents of long-term care facilities, *Can J Diet Pract Res* 69(2):82, 2008.

Determining the dietary intake of elderly long-term care (LTC) residents is important because of their risk for malnutrition. Research shows that the typical diet eaten by elderly residents usually contains insufficient nutrients (Lengyel and others, 2008). Dietary assessment helps nurses and RDs obtain information about patients' nutritional status, dietary adequacy, and risk for progression of medical conditions. Different approaches for assessing these individuals' dietary food intake include self-report through daily diaries and questionnaires and weighing and observing food intake. Self-report is unreliable because of elderly patients' physical and mental limitations. Weighing food requires staff resources. Observing residents' intake has been shown to provide more accurate results of foods consumed than weighing food. With proper training, nurses and RDs can more effectively assess nutritional intake of elderly LTC residents by observing food ingested, beverages poured in dining areas, foods traded among table mates, spillage, and second helpings.

SKILL 12.1 FEEDING DEPENDENT PATIENTS

- **Nursing Skills Online: Safety, Lesson 4**

Video Clips

Patients who require assistance with feeding are unable to feed themselves adequately because of the severity of their illness or the debilitation and fatigue associated with their condition. Some have trouble chewing or swallowing, poor vision, or difficulty holding eating utensils. As a nurse, you are responsible for preparing patients and offering the type of assistance needed to help them successfully eat an adequate amount of food at a comfortable pace. Patients should be involved in selecting food preferences that fit dietary guidelines, choosing where to eat (bed or chair), and selecting the time to eat. It can be difficult to provide meals at times other than when meal trays are delivered in health care institutions. If patients are not hungry at that time, ensuring a good food intake is difficult. Use dietary resources in the agency to provide nutritional snacks between meals. Use common sense when feeding adults and provide a socially meaningful mealtime experience. It is important to encourage independence when possible with the use of adaptive devices or finger foods and with comfortable and safe positioning for swallowing.

Frequently patients receive therapeutic diets, which require a health care provider's order. A therapeutic diet treats many disease states, complementing and at times even replacing drug therapy. Therapeutic diets are available in modified consistencies or texture. For example, patients initially may require a liquid diet for 1 to 2 days after surgery. A mechanical soft diet is used for patients without teeth. When there are no restrictions, the order may be diet as tolerated or regular diet. Table 12-2 summarizes examples of therapeutic diets. For specific information about special diets see the agency dietary manual or contact an RD.

ASSESSMENT

1. Conduct a diet history, including current medications, previous surgeries, food allergies, coexisting medical conditions compromising nutrition, and recent dietary intake. *Rationale: Provides a baseline to determine appropriate therapeutic diet, food options, and educational needs of patient.*
2. Assess if patient passes flatus and is without nausea. Auscultate bowel sounds. *Rationale: Determines status of GI functioning.*
3. On admission and routinely as ordered measure patient's weight and assess pertinent laboratory values (e.g., albumin, prealbumin and transferrin, complete blood count). *Rationale: Provides baseline of nutritional status.*
4. Assess food tolerance, cultural and religious preferences, and food likes and dislikes. *Rationale: Determines type of foods that can potentially improve oral intake and the desire to feed independently.*
5. Review diet orders by health care provider. *Rationale: Ensures that patient receives proper diet. Patients with chronic diseases may need alterations in nutrient content or flavoring.*
6. Place a tongue blade on the back of the patient's tongue to elicit the gag reflex. *Rationale: Patients who do not gag are at risk for aspiration (see Skill 12.2).*
7. Place fingers at level of larynx and ask patient to swallow saliva. *Rationale: Movement of larynx normally occurs during swallowing.*
8. Assess physical motor skills (ability to grasp utensil, hold cup, and move utensil to mouth), level of consciousness or ability to attend to feeding, and visual acuity. *Rationale: Determines appropriate positioning for meals and level of assistance required.*
9. Assess patient's energy level. *Rationale: Patients eat better when well rested.*
10. Assess need for toileting, handwashing, and oral care (including dentures) before feeding. *Rationale: Reduces interruptions and improves patient's appetite during the meal.*

PLANNING

Expected Outcomes focus on increased independence with eating, improved nutritional intake, and safe intake of food.

1. Patient's body weight remains stable or trends toward the desired level.
2. Patient's nutrition-related laboratory values trend toward normal.
3. Patient demonstrates increased ability to self-feed or open items on tray as appropriate.
4. Patient coughs appropriately when eating with no new signs of respiratory compromise.
5. Patient completes meal.

Delegation and Collaboration

The skill of assisting the patient with oral nutrition may be delegated to nursing assistive personnel (NAP). Instruct the NAP by:

- Explaining how to position patient to avoid any swallowing problems.

TABLE 12-2 PROGRESSIVE AND THERAPEUTIC DIETS

DIET	DESCRIPTION
Clear-liquid	Foods that are clear and liquid at room or body temperature (e.g., chicken broth, tea, soda, gelatin, and apple or cranberry juice) and that leave little residue and are easily absorbed; commonly ordered for short-term use (24 to 48 hours) after surgery, before diagnostic tests, and after episodes of vomiting or diarrhea
Full-liquid	Includes foods on clear-liquid diet plus addition of smooth-textured dairy products (e.g., milk and ice cream), strained soups and custard, refined cooked cereals, vegetable juice, and pureed vegetables; commonly ordered before or after surgery for patients who are acutely ill from infection or for patients who cannot chew or tolerate solid foods; must verify that patients are lactose tolerant before providing dairy products
Pureed	Includes food on clear- and full-liquid diets plus easily swallowed foods that do not require chewing (e.g., scrambled eggs; pureed meats, vegetables, and fruits; mashed potatoes); ordered for patients with head and neck abnormalities or who have had oral surgery; can be modified for low sodium, fat, or calorie control
Mechanical or dental-soft	Consists of all previous diets plus addition of lightly seasoned ground or finely diced meats, flaked fish, cottage cheese, cheese, rice, potatoes, pancakes, light breads, cooked vegetables, cooked or canned fruit, bananas, and peanut butter; avoids tough meats, nuts, bacon, and fruits with tough skins or membranes; ordered for patients who have chewing problems or mild gastrointestinal (GI) problems; used as transition diet from liquids to regular
Soft/low-residue	Addition of low-fiber easily digested foods such as pastas, casseroles, moist tender meats, and canned cooked fruits and vegetables; includes foods that are easy to chew and simply cooked; does not permit fatty, rich, and fried foods; is sometimes referred to as low-fiber diet
High-fiber	Addition of fresh uncooked fruits, steamed vegetables, bran, oatmeal and dried fruits; includes sufficient amounts of indigestible carbohydrate to relieve constipation, increase GI motility, and increase stool weight
Regular or diet as tolerated	No restrictions; permits patients' preferences and allows for postoperative diet progression
Sample Therapeutic Diets	
Restricted fluids	Required in severe heart failure and kidney failure
Sodium-restricted	Allows low levels of sodium and may include a 4-g (no added salt), 2-g (moderate), 1-g (strict), or 500-mg (very strict) diet; may be ordered for patients with congestive heart failure, renal failure, cirrhosis, or hypertension
Fat-modified	Low total and saturated fat and low cholesterol; cholesterol intake limited to less than 300 mg daily, and fat intake to 30% to 35%; eliminates or reduces fatty foods for hypercholesterolemia, malabsorptive disorders, and diarrhea
Diabetic	Essential treatment for patients with diabetes mellitus; provides patients with a diet recommended by American Diabetes Association, which allows for patients to select set amount of food from basic food groups

From Grodner M, Lon S, DeYoung S: *Foundations and clinical applications of nutrition*, ed 4, St Louis, 2007, Mosby.

- Reviewing need to observe for coughing, gagging, or difficulty in swallowing and to report information back to the nurse.

Equipment

- Stethoscope and tongue blade for assessment
- Meal tray
- Over-bed table
- Adaptive utensils if appropriate (Fig. 12-1)
- Damp washcloth
- Towel
- Oral hygiene supplies

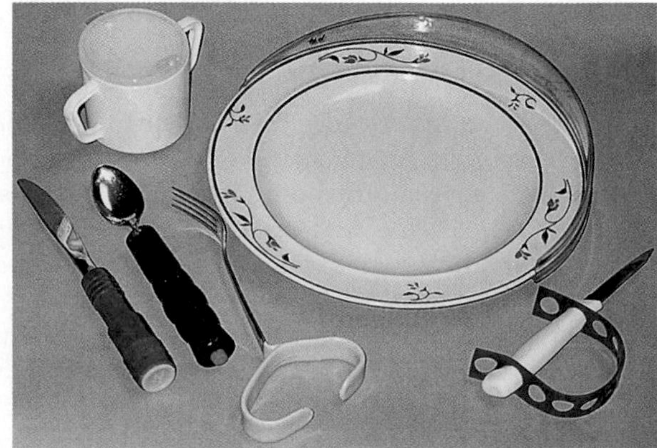

FIG 12-1 Adaptive equipment. Clockwise from upper left: Two-handled cup with lid, plate with plate guard, utensils with splints, and utensils with enlarged handles.

IMPLEMENTATION *for* FEEDING DEPENDENT PATIENTS

STEPS	RATIONALE
1. **See Standard Protocol (inside front cover).**	
2. Prepare patient for meal.	
a. Place patient in high-Fowler's position (see illustration). If unable to sit, turn on side with head elevated.	Upright position helps patient keep food toward front of mouth before swallowing, reducing aspiration.

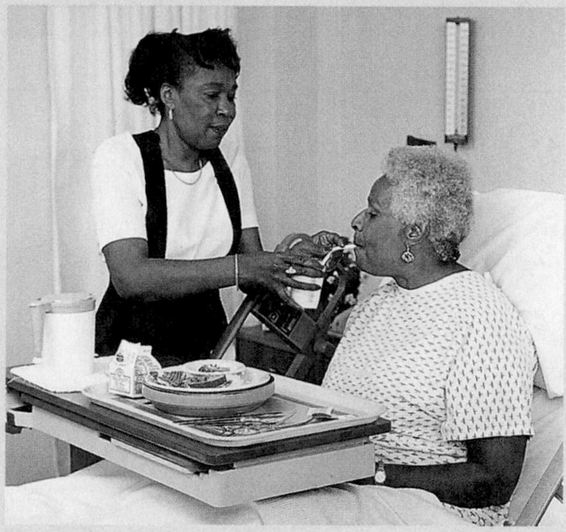

STEP 2a High-Fowler's position.

STEPS	RATIONALE
b. Offer toileting and then handwashing before meal.	Increases level of comfort. Prevents transmission of infection.
c. Offer oral hygiene. If patient has dentures, remove and rinse thoroughly and reinsert.	Moist, clean oral mucosa and teeth improve taste and appetite.
d. Patients with stomatitis (inflammation of mucous membranes) benefit from rinsing with a solution containing hydrogen peroxide, warm saline, and sodium bicarbonate in equal parts. Consult with physician regarding use of an oral analgesic (Munro and others, 2006).	The pain of stomatitis causes some patients to avoid eating.
e. Help patient put on eyeglasses or insert contact lenses if used.	Promotes ability to self-feed and makes meal more visually appealing.
3. Check the environment for distractions. Reduce the noise level if possible. *Option:* If patient enjoys music, play a soothing, low-volume selection.	Pleasant environment enhances mealtime experience.
4. Obtain special assistive devices as needed (see Fig. 12-1) and instruct on use. For example:	Devices facilitate self-feeding by improving ability to grasp, pick up foods with utensils, and drink liquids.
a. Two-handled cup with spout in lid makes it easier to drink and hold and lift a cup. Spills are avoided. Cup has wide base, which prevents tipping over.	
b. Plate with plate guard and nonskid bottom helps a person with limited flexibility of hands or poor motor coordination or who has use of only one hand.	
c. Knife, fork, and spoon with large handles or attached splints help a person with limited hand function or a weak grip.	

Continued

STEPS	RATIONALE
5. Assess tray for completeness and correct diet.	Prevents intake of incomplete or incorrect diet.
6. Assist patient with setting up meal tray if patient is unable to do so. Open packages, cut up food, apply seasonings/condiments, butter bread, and place napkin.	Reduces effort needed to self-feed.
7. If patient is able to eat independently, stop here. Return after 10 to 20 minutes or stay at side for communication and teaching time.	Aim is to make patient as self sufficient as possible for self-feeding.

SAFETY ALERT If patient is at risk for aspiration, stay at his or her side during feeding.

STEPS	RATIONALE
8. Assist patient who cannot eat independently.	
a. Assume a comfortable position.	Being comfortable prevents you from rushing the patient through a meal.
b. If patient is visually impaired, identify food location on plate as if it were a clock (e.g., the chicken is at 12 o'clock) (see illustration).	Visually impaired patient may be able to feed self when given adequate information about food placement on tray.

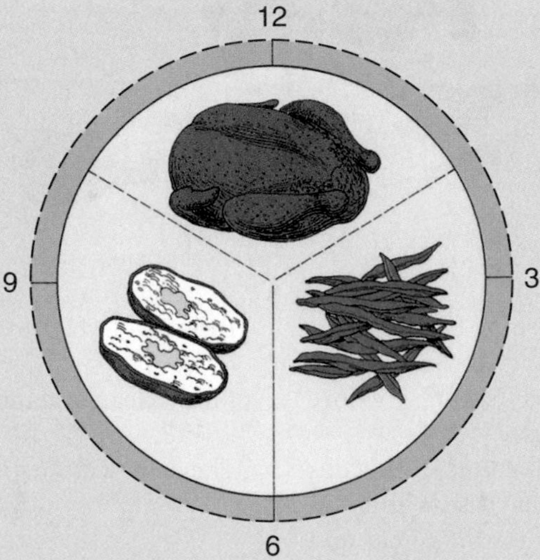

STEP 8b Orient patient to position of food on plate as if it were a clock face.

STEPS	RATIONALE
c. Ask patient in what order he or she would like to eat and cut food into bite-size pieces.	Gives patient more independence and control. Small bites reduce risk of aspiration.
d. Provide fluids as requested. Do not allow patient to drink all fluids at beginning of meal.	Promotes swallowing. Prevents patient from filling up on fluids.
e. Pace feeding to avoid patient fatigue. Interact with patient during mealtime. Verbally encourage self-feeding attempts.	Social interaction may improve appetite.
f. Use meal as an opportunity to educate patient on nutrition topics, discharge plan.	Offers extended time for teaching.
g. Use appropriate feeding techniques for patients with special needs.	
• Older adult: Feed small amounts at a time. Observe biting, chewing, swallowing. Be sure between bites that patient has swallowed food. Offer frequent rest periods (Ebersole and others, 2008).	Decreased saliva production in older adults impairs swallowing. Aspiration results from decreased or absent gag reflex.
• Neurologically impaired: Feed small amounts at a time. Observe ability to chew, manipulate tongue to form bolus of food, and swallow. Ask patient to open mouth and check for pocketed food. Give small amount of thin liquids between bites.	Patients with limited tongue strength and control are unable to move bolus for swallowing. Checking for pocketed food reduces risk of aspiration.

STEPS	RATIONALE
• Patient with cancer: Check for food aversions before and during meal.	Strong, abnormal sense of taste and smell are side effects of chemotherapy.
9. Assist patient with washing hands and mouth care.	
10. Help patient to resting position. If in bed, leave head elevated at least 45 degrees for 30 minutes after meal.	Reduces risk of aspiration.
11. Monitor intake and output (I&O) (see Procedural Guideline 7.1) and complete intake measurement (e.g., observed intake, calorie count).	Physician's orders may require identifying the specific number of calories consumed. The RD usually completes this; however, the nurse is vital in recording percentages of menu items consumed.
12. See Completion Protocol (inside front cover).	

EVALUATION

1. Monitor body weight daily or weekly.
2. Monitor laboratory values as ordered.
3. Observe patient's technique for self-feeding: intake of certain items, part or all of meal.
4. Observe patient for choking, coughing, gagging, or food left in the mouth during eating.
5. Observe amount of food on tray after meal.

Unexpected Outcomes and Related Interventions

1. Patient is unable to eat entire meal or refuses to eat.
   a. Determine if patient has other food preferences, cultural influences, or religious restrictions.
   b. Determine if patient's ability and desire to eat are better at other times of the day.
   c. Determine if patient is in pain, nauseated, has constipation, or is uncomfortable.
   d. If repeated problem, consult with health care provider.
2. Patient chokes on food.
   a. Position on side with head forward and suction food and secretions from mouth and airway.
   b. If choking occurs repeatedly, stop feeding and notify physician.
   c. Make appropriate referrals (e.g., RD or speech therapy) (see Skill 12.2).

Recording and Reporting

- Record the food and fluids actually consumed (including calorie count and I&O), extent of patient self-feeds, patient's ability to swallow and tolerance to diet (including any choking that occurs).
- Report any swallowing difficulties, food dislikes, or refusal to eat to nurse in charge and the RD.

Sample Documentation

0800 Able to feed self 5 bites with encouragement. With assistance, able to consume 60% of meal. Needs much encouragement. Stated, "That is all I can do." No difficulty swallowing or coughing. Discussed food preferences to include in next meal.

Special Considerations

Pediatric

- Food allergies are common in infancy because the immature intestinal tract is more permeable to proteins. They may be prevented by avoiding cow's milk for the first 6 months.
- Human milk is the most desirable complete diet for infants during first 6 months. Infants who are breastfed or bottle fed do not require additional fluids (e.g., water or juice) during the first 4 months. Excessive water intake causes water intoxication, failure to thrive, and hyponatremia. Infants usually do not consume solid foods until 6 months. A common sequence for introducing solid food is one new food every 5 to 7 days (Hockenberry and Wilson, 2007).

Geriatric

- Changes in taste and smell, oral mucus and saliva production, and dentition with aging may affect the patient's food choices, appetite, and ability to chew or swallow.
- Older adults may have difficulty eating because of physical symptoms or lack of teeth or dentures.
- Thirst sensation may diminish in older adults, leading to inadequate fluid intake or dehydration.

Home Care

- Homebound older adults may benefit from Meals on Wheels, which can provide as many as three meals per day, depending on the community services (Meals on Wheels Association of America, 2009).
- Patients who are unable to feed themselves independently may eat better if other family members participate at mealtimes to avoid social isolation.

SKILL 12.2 ASPIRATION PRECAUTIONS

- **Nursing Skills Online: Safety Module, Lesson 4**

Video Clips

Aspiration in adults usually occurs as a result of dysphagia (difficulty swallowing). The condition is associated with muscular, nerve, and obstructive causes (Box 12-4). Dysphagia is a decreased ability to voluntarily pass fluids and/or solids from the mouth to the stomach. Swallowing is complex, requiring the coordination of cranial nerves and the muscles of the tongue, pharynx, larynx, and jaw. Know patients at risk. For example, assess patients with neuromuscular diseases involving the brain, brainstem, cranial nerves, or muscles of swallowing before feeding. Characteristics of dysphagia that are most predictive of aspiration risk include (Nowlin, 2006):

- A wet voice.
- Weak voluntary cough.
- Coughing or choking on food.
- Prolonged swallow.
- A combination of these.
- Additional characteristics of dysphagia: Voice change after swallowing; abnormal lip closure and tongue movement; hoarse voice; slow, weak, imprecise speech; abnormal gag reflex; regurgitation; pharyngeal pooling; and inability to speak consistently

BOX 12-4 CAUSES OF DYSPHAGIA

Muscular Changes
- Aging
- Muscular dystrophy
- Myasthenia gravis
- Polymyositis

Nerve Changes
- Amyotrophic lateral sclerosis (Lou Gehrig's disease)
- Cerebral palsy
- Diabetic neuropathy
- Guillain-Barré syndrome
- Multiple sclerosis
- Parkinson's disease
- Stroke

Obstructive
- Anterior mediastinal masses
- Candidiasis
- Cervical spondylosis
- Esophageal webs
- Head and neck cancer
- Inflammatory masses
- Lower esophageal ring
- Trauma/surgical resection

Other
- Connective tissue disorders
- Gastrointestinal or esophageal resection
- Rheumatological disorders
- Vagotomy

Dysphagia often causes a decrease in food intake, which then leads to malnutrition. In most cases this is caused by difficulty in consuming an adequate volume of solids or liquids. Dietary intake may be affected for long periods of time. The malnutrition that occurs is secondary to insufficient protein, calorie, and micronutrient intake (Ebersole and others, 2008).

In some patients aspiration from dysphagia occurs silently. This means that a patient aspirates without any outward signs of swallowing difficulty. Conditions associated with silent aspiration include local weakness of the pharyngeal muscles, reduced laryngopharyngeal sensation, and impaired ability to cough reflexively (Ramsey and others, 2005). In these cases aspiration is most often identified following chest x-ray film.

There are three techniques for identifying dysphagia. An initial bedside swallow assessment is a brief examination that the nurse can administer with basic clinical swallowing training. Studies of dysphagic patients have shown that penetration into the larynx is more likely when swallowing liquids than semisolid textures (Trapl and others, 2007). Providers often use the 3-ounce water swallow test to screen for aspiration risk (Suiter and Leder, 2008). The test is a good predictor of the ability to tolerate thin liquids. If you suspect dysphagia, a trained swallowing technician (e.g., speech pathologist) conducts a more thorough assessment. The third technique is via video fluoroscopy (x-ray film).

A priority for dysphagic patients is the initiation of safe oral nutrition and hydration (Westergren, 2006). Changes in food consistencies and/or liquid consistencies or even elimination of oral intake and initiation of tube feedings are common diet modifications (Table 12-3). Liquid or pureed foods are sometimes the only consistency tolerated by patients with dysphagia. Liquids often have to be thickened with a commercial thickener to decrease transit time and protect the airway. They pose an increased risk for aspiration. Thickeners added to food or fluids increase the consistency and thus allow the patient more control of the volume of fluid in the mouth. There are four levels of liquid consistencies: thin liquids (low viscosity), nectarlike liquids (medium viscosity), honeylike liquids (honeylike viscosity), and spoon-thick liquids (puddinglike viscosity). After placing a patient on a thickened-liquids diet, carefully monitor and assist as needed at each meal or snack to prevent the patient from choking or aspirating.

ASSESSMENT

1. Perform a nutritional screening (see Skill 12.1). *Rationale: Patients with aspiration from dysphagia may alter their eating patterns or choose foods that do not provide adequate nutrition (White and others, 2008).*
2. Identify patient's risk for aspiration (see Box 12-4). Use a dysphagia screening tool if available. *Rationale: Allows*

TABLE 12-3 NATIONAL DYSPHAGIA DIET STAGES

STAGE	DESCRIPTION	EXAMPLES
NDD 1: Dysphagia pureed	Uniform Pureed Cohesive Puddinglike texture	Smooth hot cereal cooked to a pudding consistency Mashed potatoes Pureed meat Pureed pasta or rice Pureed vegetables Yogurt
NDD 2: Dysphagia mechanically altered	Moist Soft textured Easily forms a bolus	Cooked cereals Dry cereals moistened with milk Canned fruit (except pineapple) Moist ground meat Well-cooked chopped vegetables Cooked noodles in sauce/gravy
NDD 3: Dysphagia advanced	Regular foods (except very hard, sticky, or crunchy foods)	Moist breads (e.g., with butter, jelly) Well-moistened cereals Peeled soft fruits (banana, peach, plum) Tender, thin-sliced meat Baked potato (with no skin) Tender, cooked vegetables
Regular	All foods	No restrictions

Modified from National Dysphagia Diet Task Force (NDDTF): *National dysphagia diet: standardization for optimal care,* Chicago, 2002, American Dietetic Association.
NDD, National Dysphagia Diet.

nurse to identify patients who require precautionary measures during feeding to prevent aspiration.

3. Measure patient's oxygen saturation. *Rationale: Provides baseline to assess for aspiration during meal.*
4. Observe patient during mealtime for signs of dysphagia and allow patient to try to feed self. Note at end of meal if patient tires, has wet voice, or coughs after trying to swallow (White and others, 2008). *Rationale: Detects abnormal eating patterns, increasing risk of aspiration.*
5. Ask patient about any difficulties with chewing or swallowing various textures of food.
6. Take tongue blade and, while asking patient to say "ah," notice movement of tongue. Then gently elicit gag reflex. *Rationale: Tongue movement may reveal weakness on one side of mouth, impairing swallowing.*
7. Assess patient's swallowing reflex before feeding by placing fingers on patient's throat at level of the larynx and asking patient to swallow saliva. *Rationale: Movement of the larynx normally can be palpated.*
8. Place identification on patient's chart or Kardex indicating that dysphagia/aspiration risk is present. *Rationale: Identification reduces risk of patient receiving oral nutrition without supervision.*

PLANNING

Expected Outcomes focus on adequate food and fluid intake to prevent malnutrition and dehydration while avoiding aspiration.

1. Patient exhibits no symptoms of aspiration or new respiratory distress.
2. Patient maintains stable weight.

Delegation and Collaboration

The assessment of patients' risk for aspiration and determination of positioning cannot be delegated to nursing assistive personnel (NAP). However, the NAP may feed patients after receiving instruction in aspiration precautions. Instruct the NAP to:

- Report to the nurse in charge, immediately, any onset of coughing, gagging, a wet voice, or pocketing of food.

Equipment

- Upright chair or bed in high-Fowler's position
- Thickener agent (rice, cereal, yogurt, gelatin, commercial thickener)
- Tongue blade
- Oral hygiene supplies, including antimicrobial mouthwash
- Penlight
- Pulse oximeter
- Suction equipment

IMPLEMENTATION *for* ASPIRATION PRECAUTIONS

STEPS	RATIONALE
1. See Standard Protocol (inside front cover).	
2. Provide thorough oral or denture hygiene (see Chapter 10), including brushing of tongue before meal.	Tongue coating is associated with buildup of bacterial cells in the saliva and aspiration pneumonia, especially in patients without dentures (Abe and others, 2008).
3. Apply pulse oximeter to patient's finger.	Studies have suggested that oxygen desaturation and hypoxia occur with aspiration (White and others, 2008).
4. Position patient upright in a chair or in bed at a 90-degree angle or to highest position allowed by patient's medical condition (Palmer and Metheny, 2008).	Position aims to prevent gastric reflux and reduces occurrence of aspiration. Side-lying position is an option if patient cannot have head elevated.
5. Using penlight and tongue blade, gently inspect mouth for pockets of food.	Pocketing food indicates difficulty swallowing.
6. Have patient assume a chin-tuck position. Begin by having patient try sips of water. Monitor for swallowing and respiratory difficulties continuously. If patient tolerates water, offer a larger volume of water and then different consistencies of foods and liquids.	Chin-tuck or chin-down position helps reduce aspiration. Giving liquids and foods of different textures assesses patient's ability to swallow safely. Gradual increase in types and textures, coupled with monitoring, ensures that patient is able to eat safely (White and others, 2008).
7. Add thickener to liquids, creating the consistency of mashed potatoes.	Thin liquids are easily aspirated (White and others, 2008).
8. Place ½ to 1 teaspoon of food on unaffected side of mouth, allowing utensils to touch the mouth or tongue.	Provides tactile cue to begin eating.
9. Provide verbal coaching while feeding patient. Remind patient to chew and think about swallowing.	Keeps patient focused on swallowing and minimizes distractions (Metheny, 2007).
10. Observe for coughing, choking, gagging, and drooling food; suction airway as necessary.	Indicators of dysphagia and aspiration risk (Nowlin, 2006).
11. During feeding do not rush a patient. Allow time for adequate chewing and swallowing. Alternate solids and liquids (Palmer and Metheny, 2008). Inspect contents of patient's mouth after swallowing for food pocketing.	Enhances swallowing. Checking for pocketed food can prevent aspiration.
12. If needed, demonstrate chewing for patients with dementia (Palmer and Metheny, 2008).	
13. Have patient remain sitting upright for at least 30 to 60 minutes after the meal.	Reduces risk of gastroesophageal reflux, which causes aspiration (Ebersole and others, 2008; Nowlin, 2006).
14. Provide mouth care after meals. Consider using an antimicrobial mouthwash.	Dislodges any food or fluids that may have accumulated inside patient's cheeks. Antimicrobial mouthwash reduces bacterial count in oral cavity (Munro and others, 2006).
15. Advance diet to thicker foods that require more chewing and finally to thin liquids as tolerated.	RD and/or speech pathologist can direct safest advancement of diet.
16. See Completion Protocol (inside front cover).	

EVALUATION

1. Observe patient's ability to swallow foods of various textures and thicknesses.
2. Observe for signs of aspiration, including choking, coughing, wet voice.
3. Monitor I&O, calorie count, weight, and food eaten from tray.
4. Monitor pulse oximetry readings.

Unexpected Outcomes and Related Interventions

1. Patient coughs, gags, develops a wet voice, or complains of food "stuck in throat"; has pocketed food in mouth.
   a. Stop feeding patient.
   b. Be sure that patient is in high-Fowler's position or, if unable, position on side.
   c. Suction airway until clear.
   d. Notify health care provider.

2. Patient avoids certain textures of food.
   a. Change consistency of food in diet.
3. Patient loses weight.
   a. Consult with RD on increasing frequency of meals or providing nutritional supplements.

Recording and Reporting

Record patient's tolerance of liquids and food textures, amount of assistance required, position during meal, absence or presence of any symptoms of dysphagia, fluid intake, and amount of food eaten.

Report any coughing, gagging, choking, or swallowing difficulties to nurse in charge or health care provider.

Sample Documentation

1200 Fed half of pureed diet and 4 oz juice with 1 teaspoon of thickener added. Patient needs much encouragement. Tires easily during feeding. Benefits from coaching to swallow. No coughing or aspiration noted.

Special Considerations

Pediatric

- Infants and children have swallowing problems because of behavioral, developmental, or neurological conditions; respiratory problems; and/or gastroesophageal reflux or structural deficits such as a cleft lip or palate (Prasse and Kikano, 2009).

Geriatric

- Aspiration is a common cause of pneumonia in older adults. No one intervention has been identified to lower an older adult's risk.

SKILL 12.3 INSERTION AND REMOVAL OF A SMALL-BORE FEEDING TUBE

- **Nursing Skills Online: Enteral Nutrition Module, Lessons 1 and 2**

Nasogastric (NG) tubes supply enteral feedings directly into the stomach, whereas nasointestinal (NI) tubes place food directly into the jejunum of the small intestine. Tubes placed into the small bowel are thought to reduce the incidence of pulmonary aspiration of stomach contents because the tube goes beyond the natural sphincters controlling reflux. However, research shows that even NI tubes can migrate back into the stomach.

NG and NI tubes used specifically for feeding are composed of either silicone or polyurethane. They are softer and more flexible and reportedly more comfortable for patients. These tubes are more difficult to insert than large-bore NG tubes used for decompression (see Chapter 19). Some tubes are weighted, and research shows that weighted tubes are superior to nonweighted tubes. Tubes are generally coated with a hydrophilic substance that is activated when exposed to water, making it slippery and easier to insert. A nurse activates the substance immediately before insertion by simply flushing the tube inside and out with water. Wire stylets are included with some tubes but not all. Stylets are thought to improve insertion success but have also been associated with increased risk for nasopulmonary intubation. You can pass a feeding tube without the use of a stylet.

Placement of a feeding tube requires a health care provider's order. Nasal and oral insertion of feeding tubes is commonly performed at a patient's bedside. Confirmation of the correct position of a newly inserted tube is mandatory before any feeding or medication administration (ASPEN, 2009). Nurses use a variety of bedside tests to determine tube placement. However, the gold standard for confirming correct placement of a blindly inserted enteral tube is a chest x-ray film that visualizes the entire course of the tube (ASPEN, 2009). Patients with facial injuries or craniofacial surgery are not candidates for an NG or NI feeding tube. When facial trauma or recent maxillofacial surgery is present, there is a risk for improper placement of the tube such as in the brain. In this type of situation any type of nasally inserted tube should be placed under fluoroscopy by a gastrointestinal (GI) specialist.

There have been multiple reports of adverse events related to enteral nutrition administration across the United States (ASPEN, 2009). These events have included enteral tube misconnections (e.g., connecting an enteral tube to an intravenous [IV] site), access device misplacements (e.g., intubation of the lung instead of GI tract), bronchopulmonary aspiration, and GI intolerance to formulas. Thus the practice of inserting enteral tubes and administering tube feedings requires great care and attention to practice guidelines.

ASSESSMENT

1. Verify health care provider's order for type of tube and enteric feeding schedule. Order should indicate delivery site and device, patient's name and identifying information (see agency policy), formula type, and administration method and rate (see Skill 12.5). *Rationale: Standards for patient-specific enteral nutrition (ASPEN, 2009).*
2. Assess patient's height, weight, hydration status and I&O, electrolyte balance, and caloric needs. *Rationale: Provides baseline information to measure nutritional improvement once enteral feedings are initiated.*
3. Have patient close each nostril alternately and breathe. Examine each naris for patency and skin breakdown. *Rationale: Determines if nasal passage is obstructed or irritated or if septal defect or facial fractures are present.*
4. Review patient's medical history (e.g., for nasal problems, nosebleeds, facial trauma, nasal surgery, deviated septum, anticoagulant therapy, or bleeding tendency). *Rationale:*

History of these problems may require nurse to consult with health care provider to select alternate route (e.g., gastrostomy) for nutritional support.

5. Assess patient's mental status and assess for a gag reflex and ability to swallow. *Rationale: Alert patients are better able to cooperate with procedure. If vomiting should occur, an alert patient can usually expectorate vomitus, which can help to reduce the risk for aspiration.*

> **SAFETY ALERT** Feeding tubes may be inserted in patients with altered or decreased level of consciousness, but risk for inadvertent respiratory placement is increased if there is an impaired gag reflex (Roberts and others, 2007).

6. Auscultate abdomen for bowel sounds. *Rationale: Absence of bowel sounds may indicate decreased or absent peristalsis, contraindicating feedings.*
7. Check medical record orders to determine if the health care provider wants a prokinetic agent (e.g., metoclopramide (Reglan) administered before the placement of tube. *Rationale: Prokinetic agents given* before *tube placement help advance the tube into the intestine (Metheny, 2006).*

PLANNING

Expected Outcomes focus on proper placement of feeding tube into GI tract.

1. Tube is successfully placed in stomach or intestine.
2. Patient has no respiratory distress (e.g., increased respiratory rate, coughing, poor color) or signs of discomfort or nasal trauma during tube insertion.

Delegation and Collaboration

The skill of feeding tube insertion cannot be delegated to nursing assistive personnel (NAP). However, the NAP may assist with patient positioning during tube insertion.

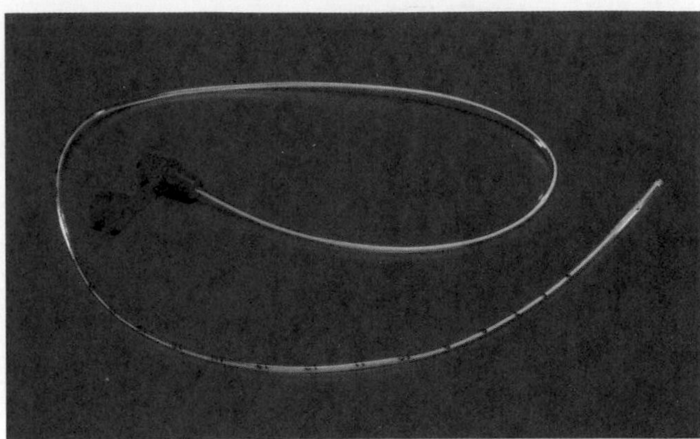

FIG 12-2 Small-bore feeding tube. (Used with permission from Covidien.)

Equipment

Insertion

- NG or nasoenteric feeding tube (8- to 12-Fr) with or without stylet (Fig. 12-2)
- 30-mL catheter-tip Luer-Lok syringe
- Stethoscope
- Hypoallergenic tape, semipermeable (transparent) dressing, or tube fixation device
- Tincture of benzoin or other skin barrier protectant
- pH indicator strip (scale 0.0 to 14.0)
- Cup of water and straw (for patients able to swallow)
- Emesis basin
- Towel
- Facial tissues
- Clean gloves
- Suction equipment in case of aspiration
- Penlight to check placement in nasopharynx
- Tongue blade
- Capnograph (option)

Removal

- Towel
- Facial tissue
- Oral hygiene supplies
- 30-mL Luer-Lok catheter tip syringe

IMPLEMENTATION *for* INSERTION AND REMOVAL OF A SMALL-BORE FEEDING TUBE

STEPS	RATIONALE
1. **See Standard Protocol (inside front cover).**	
Tube Insertion	
2. Identify patient using two identifiers (e.g., name and birthday or name and account number, according to facility policy).	Ensures correct patient. Complies with The Joint Commission standards and improves patient safety (TJC, 2010).
3. Position patient in high-Fowler's position unless contraindicated. If patient is comatose, place in semi-Fowler's position with head propped forward using a pillow. If necessary, have the NAP help with positioning of confused or comatose patients. If patient must lie supine, place in reverse Trendelenburg's position.	Reduces risk for pulmonary aspiration in event patient should vomit (Metheny, 2006). Head propped assists with closure of airway and passage of the tube into the esophagus.

STEPS	RATIONALE
4. Determine length of tube to be inserted and mark location with tape or indelible ink. **a.** Measure distance from tip of nose to earlobe to xiphoid process of sternum (see illustration).	Length approximates distance from nose to stomach in 98% of patients.

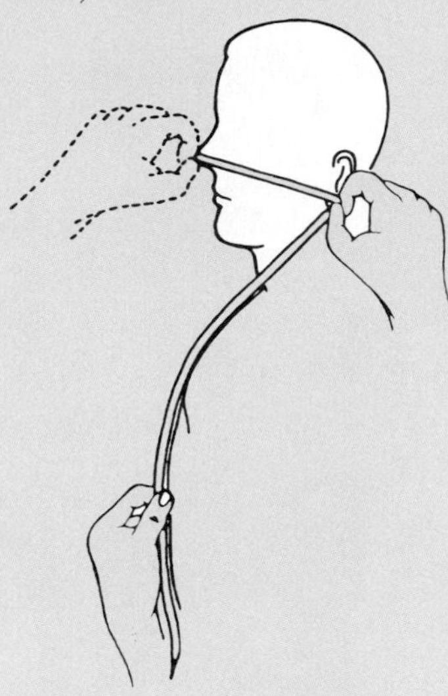

STEP 4a Determine length of tube to be inserted.

STEPS	RATIONALE
5. Prepare NG or nasoenteric tube for intubation. NOTE: Do not use plastic tubes.	
a. Inject 10 mL of water from 30-mL or larger Luer-Lok catheter-tip syringe into the tube.	Activates lubrication of tube for easier passage and ensures that tube is patent. Aids in insertion. Large syringe exerts less pressure, thus minimizing chance of tube rupture (Reising and Neal, 2005),
b. If using stylet, make certain that it is securely positioned against tube tip and that both Luer-Lok connections are snugly fit.	Promotes smooth passage of tube into GI tract. Improperly positioned stylet can induce serious trauma.
6. Cut hypoallergenic tape 10 cm (4 inches) long or prepare membrane dressing or other securing device.	To be used to secure tubing after insertion.
7.	
8. *Option:* Dip tube with surface lubricant into glass of room-temperature water or apply water-soluble lubricant (see manufacturer's directions).	Activates lubricant to facilitate passage of tube into naris and GI tract.
9. Hand the alert patient a cup of water with straw (if able to swallow).	Patient is asked to swallow water to facilitate tube passage.
10. Explain the step and gently insert tube through nostril to back of throat (posterior nasopharynx). This may cause patient to gag. Aim back and down toward ear.	Natural contours facilitate passage of tube into GI tract.
11. Have patient flex head toward chest after tube has passed through nasopharynx. Then encourage patient to swallow by giving small sips of water or ice chips. Advance tube as patient swallows. Rotate tube 180 degrees while inserting.	Closes off glottis and reduces risk for tube entering trachea. Swallowing facilitates passage of tube past oropharynx.
12. Emphasize need to mouth breathe and swallow during the procedure.	Helps facilitate passage of tube and alleviates patient's fears during the procedure.
13. When tip of tube reaches the carina (approximately 25 cm [10 inches] in the adult), stop and listen for air exchange from the distal portion of the tube.	Air may indicate that tube is in the respiratory tract; remove and start over (Baskin, 2006). Never use this step for tube verification.

Continued

STEPS	RATIONALE
14. Advance tube each time patient swallows until desired length has been passed (see illustration).	Reduces discomfort and trauma to patient.

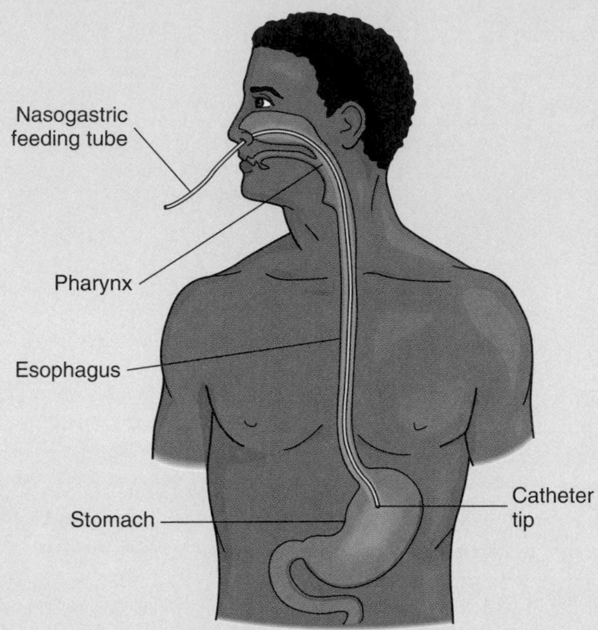

STEP 14 Nasogastric feeding tube inserted through nose and esophagus into stomach.

> **SAFETY ALERT** Do not force tube. If you meet resistance or if patient starts to cough, choke, or become cyanotic, stop advancing the tube, pull it back, and start over.

STEPS	RATIONALE
15. Check for position of tube in back of throat with penlight and tongue blade.	Tube may be coiled, kinked, or entering trachea.
16. Temporarily anchor tube to the nose with a small piece of tape.	Movement of the tube stimulates gagging. Allows for assessment of position before anchoring tube more securely.
17. Check placement of tube by attaching syringe and aspirating small amount of stomach contents (see Skill 12.4). Check pH of contents.	Proper tube position is essential before initiating feeding.

> **SAFETY ALERT** Insufflation of air into tube while auscultating abdomen is not a reliable means to differentiate among gastric, respiratory, and small bowel placement (ASPEN, 2009; Rauen and others, 2008).It may be helpful to use capnography measures to detect the inadvertent entry of the tube into the trachea. However, an x-ray film will still be needed before the tube is used for feedings (ASPEN, 2009).

STEPS	RATIONALE
18. Anchor tube to nose: After you obtain gastric aspirates, attach tube to patient's nose, avoiding pressure on nares. Mark exit site with indelible ink. Select one of the following options for anchoring:	A properly secured tube allows the patient more mobility and prevents trauma to nasal mucosa.
a. Apply tape.	Prevents pulling of tube. Frequent change may be required if tape becomes soiled.
(1) Apply tincture of benzoin or other skin adhesive on tip of patient's nose and allow it to become "tacky."	Helps tape adhere better. Protects skin.
(2) Remove and dispose of gloves and split one end of tape lengthwise 5 cm (2 inches).	

STEPS	RATIONALE
(3) Place the intact end of tape over bridge of patient's nose. Wrap each of the 5-cm (2-inch) strips in opposite directions around tube as it exits nose (see illustration).	Secures tube firmly.
b. Apply membrane dressing or tube fixation device.	Secures tube and minimizes need for frequent dressing change.
(1) Membrane dressing: Apply tincture of benzoin or other skin protector to patient's cheek and portion of tube being secured.	
(2) Place tube against patient's cheek and secure it with membrane dressing, out of patient's line of vision.	Decreases risk for patient's inadvertent extubation.
(3) Tube fixation device: Apply wide end of patch to bridge of nose (see illustration).	
(4) Slip connector around feeding tube as it exits nose (see illustration).	
19. Fasten end of NG tube to patient's gown using a clip (see illustration) or piece of tape. Do not use safety pins to secure tube to patient's gown.	Reduces traction on the naris if tube moves. Safety pins become unfastened and cause injury to patient.

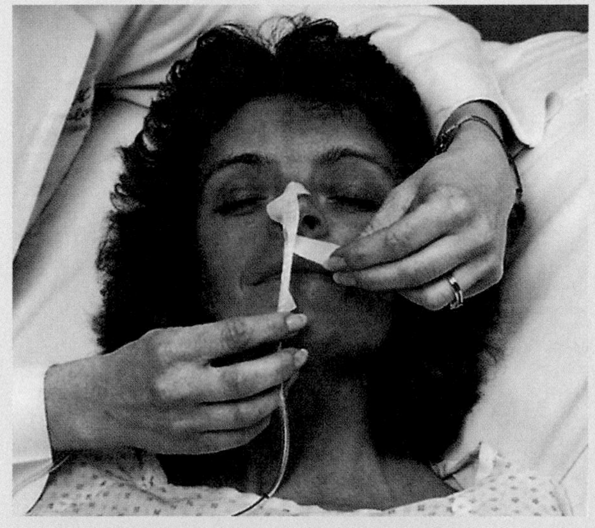

STEP 18a(3) Wrapping tape to anchor nasoenteral tube.

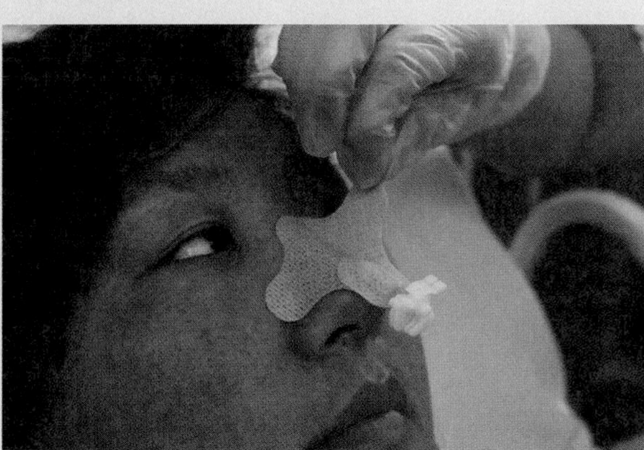

STEP 18b(3) Applying tube fixation patch to bridge of nose.

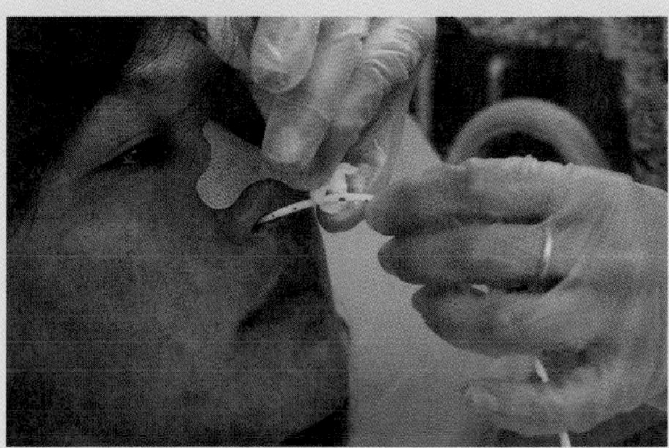

STEP 18b(4) Slip connector around feeding tube.

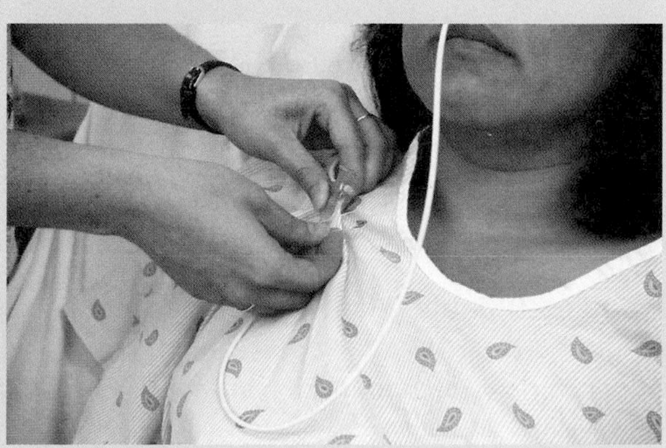

STEP 19 Fasten feeding tube to patient's gown.

Continued

STEPS	RATIONALE
20. Assist patient to a comfortable position.	

> **SAFETY ALERT** Leave stylet in place (if used) until correct position is verified by x-ray film. Never reinsert a partially or fully removed stylet while feeding tube is in place. This can cause perforation of the tube and injure the patient.

STEPS	RATIONALE
21. Obtain x-ray film of chest/abdomen.	X-ray film confirmation is most accurate method to determine that any blindly placed small- or large-bore feeding tube is properly positioned in the GI tract (ASPEN, 2009; Rauen and others, 2008).
22. Administer oral hygiene (see Chapter 10). Cleanse tubing at nostril with washcloth dampened in mild soap and water.	Promotes patient comfort and integrity of oral mucous membranes.
23. See Completion Protocol (inside front cover).	
Tube Removal	
24. See Standard Protocol (inside front cover).	
25. Verify health care provider's order to remove tube. Identify patient using two identifiers (e.g., name and birthday or name and account number, according to facility policy).	Ensures correct procedure performed on correct patient (TJC, 2010).
26. Place towel over patient's chest.	Protects gown from soiling.
27. Remove tape or tube fixation device from patient's nose. Unpin tube from patient's gown.	Allows for free movement of tube during removal.
28. Stand on patient's right side if right handed, left side if left handed. Draw up 30 mL of air into catheter tip syringe, attach syringe to end of feeding tube, flush tube with air.	Allows for easy manipulation of tube. Clears tube of gastric fluids that could irritate esophagus and mouth during removal.
29. Give the patient a facial tissue and ask him or her to take a deep breath and hold it as tube is removed.	Airway is partially occluded during removal of tube.
30. Kink tube securely and pull it out steadily and smoothly onto towel as patient holds breath.	Kinked tube is less likely to expel gastric content. Holding breath reduces risk of aspirating gastric contents.
31. Clean nares and provide mouth care.	Provides patient comfort.
32. See Completion Protocol (inside front cover).	

EVALUATION

1. Observe patient's response to intubation. Have patient speak. Check vital signs. *Option:* You may use capnography in critical care settings to determine if tip of tube is in trachea or lung.
2. Confirm x-ray film results with health care provider.
3. Remove the stylet (if used) after x-ray film verification of correct placement.
4. Routinely check location of external exit site marking on the tube and color and pH of fluid withdrawn from the tube.
5. After tube removal ask patient about level of comfort.

Unexpected Outcomes and Related Interventions

1. The tube was placed into the respiratory tract. This may not be discovered until the x-ray film report. A small-bore tube can enter the airway without causing obvious respiratory symptoms, particularly in a semiconscious or an unconscious patient.
   a. Remove the tube and report the incident to the health care provider.
   b. Obtain order for reinsertion.
2. Stomach contents were aspirated into respiratory tract (immediate response) in the alert patient, evidenced by regurgitation with coughing, dyspnea, cyanosis, or decreases in oxygen saturation during the procedure.
   a. Position patient on side to protect the airway.
   b. Suction patient nasotracheally or orotracheally to remove aspirated substance (see Chapter 14).
   c. Report the event immediately to the health care provider.
3. Stomach contents were aspirated into respiratory tract (delayed response or small-volume aspiration), evidenced by auscultation of crackles or wheezes, dyspnea, or fever.
   a. Report change in patient condition to the health care provider; if there has not been a recent chest x-ray film, suggest ordering one.
   b. Prepare for possible initiation of antibiotics.

Recording and Reporting

- Tube insertion: Record and report type and size of tube placed, location of distal tip of tube, patient's tolerance of procedure, and confirmation of tube position by x-ray film examination.
- Report any type of unexpected outcome and the interventions performed to health care provider.
- Tube removal: Record patient's level of comfort.

Sample Documentation

0800 Small-bore feeding tube inserted nasogastrically into left nares, exit site marked at 52 cm. Patient tolerated insertion well. pH of 3.0 for gastric aspirate. Tube secured with fixation device. Abdominal x-ray obtained, position confirmed by Dr. Madison.

Special Considerations

Pediatric

- Premature infant and neonate: Estimate tube length by measuring from the nose or mouth to the earlobe and then to the xiphoid process (Axelrod and others, 2006).
- In infant observe for vagal stimulation during tube insertion by assessing for decreased heart rate.
- Older child: Estimate tube length by either (1) measuring from the nose to the bottom of the earlobe and then to the lower end of the xiphoid process, or (2) measuring from the nose to the earlobe and then to a point midway between the xiphoid process and the umbilicus (Axelrod and others, 2006).

Geriatric

- Ensure adequate lubrication of tube to decrease discomfort for the older adult because of the potential for decreased oral or nasopharyngeal secretions.

Home Care

- Assess patient's or primary caregiver's ability to maintain tube for a feeding program.
- Assess the environmental safety and sanitation of patient's home environment.
- Teach the family caregiver correct method for resecuring feeding tube and checking tube placement.

SKILL 12.4 VERIFYING FEEDING TUBE PLACEMENT AND IRRIGATION

- **Nursing Skills Online: Enteral Nutrition Module, Lesson 3**

Nurses insert small-bore feeding tubes nasally into the stomach, duodenum, or proximal jejunum for either intermittent or continuous feedings. It is possible for the tip of a feeding tube to move or migrate into a different location (e.g., from the stomach to the intestine or esophagus, from the intestine into the stomach) without any external evidence that the tube has moved. The risk for aspiration of regurgitated gastric contents into the respiratory tract increases when the tip of the tube accidentally dislocates upward into the esophagus.

Following initial x-ray film verification that a tube is positioned correctly (either in the stomach or small intestine), you are responsible for ensuring that the tube has remained in the intended position before administering formula or medications through it. Therefore you must verify tube position every 4 to 6 hours and as needed (Metheny, 2006). Because it is not practical to take x-ray films that often, other methods of determining placement have been used. Characteristics of fluid aspirated from feeding tubes are helpful in assessing tube placement. Color may differentiate gastric from intestinal placement. Because most intestinal aspirates are stained by bile to a distinct yellow color and most gastric aspirates are not, this difference can often distinguish the sites (Rauen and others, 2008). The pH of an aspirate also offers valuable data in assessing placement of a feeding tube (Metheny, 2006). Bedside testing of pH using pH paper covering a range from 0 to 11 is sufficient for this purpose; a properly obtained pH value of 0 to 4 is a good indication of gastric placement (Metheny, 2006).

Adequacy of nutritional support is essential in patient care. For this reason, feeding tubes must remain patent. You routinely irrigate a feeding tube while it is in place and following the administration of medications and feedings. Plain water is the preferred flush solution. However, ASPEN (2009) recommends use of sterile water for flushing before and after medication administration and in immuno-compromised and critically ill patients. All types of feeding tubes require routine irrigation, including gastrostomy and jejunostomy tubes (see Skill 12.5). Question the patency of a tube when you cannot instill air or fluid through the tube.

ASSESSMENT

1. Review policy and procedures for frequency and method of checking tube placement and frequency of irrigation in your facility. *Rationale: Clinicians cannot reliably differentiate between respiratory and gastric placement by auscultation (ASPEN, 2009). Always obtain x-ray film confirmation at the time of placement.*
2. Observe for signs and symptoms of respiratory distress: coughing, choking, or cyanosis. *Rationale: Signs and symptoms indicate accidental migration of feeding tube into the airway. However, their absence does not ensure that respiratory migration has not occurred, especially in a patient with altered level of consciousness and/or altered gag and cough reflexes.*
3. Identify conditions that increase the risk for spontaneous tube migration or dislocation: retching and vomiting, nasotracheal suctioning, or severe bouts of coughing. *Rationale: Feeding tubes migrate by increases in intraabdominal pressure or coughing.*

4. Observe the external portion of the tube for movement of the ink mark away from the mouth or naris (see Skill 12.3). *Rationale: Increased external length of a tube indicates that the distal tip is no longer in the correct position.*
5. Review patient's medication record for a gastric acid inhibitor (e.g., cimetidine [Tagamet], ranitidine [Zantac], famotidine [Pepcid], nizatidine [Axid]) or a proton pump inhibitor (e.g., omeprazole [Prilosec]). *Rationale: H_2 receptor antagonists reduce volume of gastric acid secretion and the acid content of secretions, thus causing the pH value to be higher or more alkaline (Metheny, 2006).*
6. Review patient's record for history of prior tube displacement. *Rationale: Patients are at increased risk for repeated tube displacement.*
7. For irrigation, inspect previous volume color and character of aspirates. *Rationale: Thick secretions and a reduced volume of secretions indicate need to irrigate tube. Excess volume of secretions (more than 200 mL) indicates delayed gastric emptying.*
8. For irrigation, monitor volume of tube-feeding formula administered during a shift and compare with ordered amount. *Rationale: Indicates whether sufficient volume of feeding is infusing.*

PLANNING

Expected Outcomes focus on correct placement and irrigation of feeding tubes.

1. Gastric fluid aspirated from tip insertion tests at a pH of 1.0 to 4.0.
2. Intestinal fluid aspirated from tip insertion tests at a pH of greater than 6.0.

Delegation and Collaboration

The verification of tube placement and irrigation may not be delegated to nursing assistive personnel (NAP). Instruct the NAP to:

- Immediately inform the nurse if patient's respirations change or if shortness of breath, coughing, or choking develops.
- Immediately inform the nurse if the patient vomits or the NAP notices vomitus in patient's mouth during oral hygiene.
- Immediately inform the nurse if displacement of the feeding tube occurs.
- Report when a continuous tube feeding stops infusing.

Equipment

Verifying tube placement

- 60-mL Luer-Lok catheter-tip syringe
- Stethoscope
- Clean gloves
- pH indicator strip (scale of 0.0 to 11.0)
- Small medication cup

Irrigating tube

- 60-mL Luer-Lok or catheter-tip syringe
- Tap water or sterile water (for immunocompromised and critically ill)
- Towel
- Clean gloves

IMPLEMENTATION *for* VERIFYING FEEDING TUBE PLACEMENT AND IRRIGATION

STEPS	RATIONALE
1. See Standard Protocol (inside front cover).	
2. Verify tube placement.	
a. Identify patient using two identifiers (e.g., name and birthday or name and account number, according to facility policy).	Ensures correct patient. Complies with The Joint Commission standards and improves patient safety (TJC, 2010).
b. Verify tube placement at the following times:	
(1) For intermittently tube-fed patients, test placement immediately before each feeding and before medication administration.	Each administration of feeding/medication can lead to aspiration if the tube is displaced.
(2) For continuously tube-fed patients, test placement every 4 to 6 hours and before medication administration.	Determines if tube migration has occurred. Placement confirmed at same time of routine tube irrigation.
(3) Wait to verify placement at least 1 hour after medication administration by tube or mouth.	Premature aspiration of contents removes unabsorbed medication, reducing dose delivered to patient.
c. If an existing tube feeding is infusing, turn off the feeding temporarily. Kink feeding tube while disconnecting it from feeding-bag tubing or while removing plug at end of tube.	Prevents leakage of gastric contents.

STEPS	RATIONALE
d. Draw up 30 mL of air into a 60-mL syringe and attach to end of feeding tube. Release kink and flush tube with 30 mL of air before attempting to aspirate fluid. If there is resistance, reposition the patient from side to side. In some cases more than one bolus of air is necessary.	Burst of air aids in aspirating fluid more easily by forcing ports of tube away from mucosal folds of stomach or intestine (Metheny and others, 2008). It is more difficult to aspirate fluid from the small intestine than from the stomach or from a smaller-bore feeding tube (Metheny and others, 2008).
e. Draw back on syringe slowly and obtain 5 to 10 mL of gastric aspirate (see illustration). Observe appearance of aspirate. Aspirates from continuous tube feeding often have appearance of curdled enteral formula. Aspirates from intermittent tube feeding are not typically bile stained (unless intestinal fluid has refluxed into the stomach).	Drawing back quickly or using a smaller syringe may cause the tube to collapse. Appearance of aspirate helps to assess the position of the tube.
f. Gently mix aspirate in syringe. Expel a few drops into a clean medicine cup. Measure pH by dipping a pH strip into the fluid or applying a few drops of the fluid to the strip. Compare the color of the strip with the color on the chart (see illustration) provided by the manufacturer (Metheny, 2006).	Mixing ensures equal distribution of contents for testing.
(1) Gastric fluid from patient who has fasted for at least 4 hours usually has pH range of 1.0 to 4.0.	Range of 1.0 to 4.0 is a reliable indicator of stomach placement, especially when a gastric acid inhibitor is not being used.
(2) Fluid from tube in small intestine of fasting patient usually has pH greater than 6.0.	Intestinal contents are more alkaline than stomach contents (Metheny, 2006).
(3) Patient with continuous tube feeding may have pH of 5.0 or higher.	Formulas contain solutions that are alkaline.
(4) The pH of pleural fluid from the tracheobronchial tree is generally greater than 6.0.	

SAFETY ALERT Auscultation of an air bolus is no longer considered a reliable or safe method for verification of tube position.

g. If, after repeated attempts, it is not possible to aspirate fluid from a tube that was confirmed by x-ray film to be in desired position, and if (1) there are no risk factors for tube dislocation, (2) tube has remained in original taped position, and (3) patient is not in respiratory distress, assume tube is correctly placed (Roberts and others, 2007). Continue with irrigation.	It is reasonable to assume that tube is correctly placed. When abdominal x-ray films are obtained for clinical reasons, you can take advantage of reports to monitor tube location.

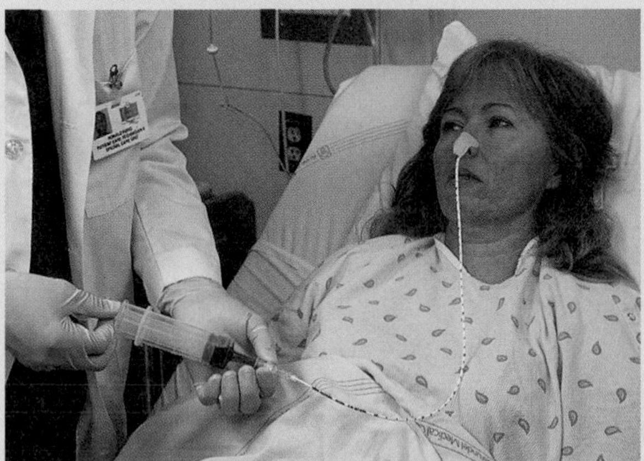

STEP 2e Obtain gastric aspirate.

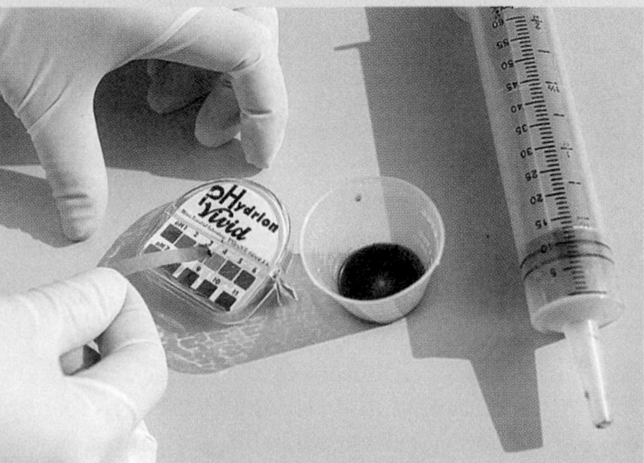

STEP 2f Compare color on test strip with color on pH chart.

Continued

STEPS	RATIONALE
3. *Tube Irrigation*	
a. Elevate patient's head of bed 45 to 90 degrees. Kink tube while it is disconnected from feeding-bag tubing or while plug is removed (see illustration).	Upright position helps to minimize reflux. Prevents leakage of gastric secretions.
b. Draw up 30 mL of water into the syringe. Use sterile water before and after medication administration or in immunocompromised and critically ill patients (ASPEN, 2009). Do not use irrigation fluids from multidose bottles that are used on other patients. Patient should have personal bottle of solution. Change irrigation bottle every 24 hours.	This amount of solution will flush length of tube. Using sterile water prevents contamination of fluids. Not using fluids from multidose bottles ensures sterile solution.
c. Insert tip of syringe into end of feeding tube. Release kink and slowly instill irrigating solution (see illustration).	Infusion of fluid clears tubing.
d. If unable to instill fluid, reposition patient on left side and try again.	Tip of tube may be against stomach wall. Changing patient's position may move tip away from stomach wall.
e. When water has been instilled, remove syringe. Reinstitute tube feeding or administer medication as ordered. Irrigate before, between, and after the final medication (before feedings are reinstituted).	Tubing is clear and patent. Certain formulas may predispose to tube clogging. Irrigation prevents mixing medications in the tube, which may cause clogging. Flushes medications through the tube so medications do not mix with formula.
4. See Completion Protocol (inside front cover).	

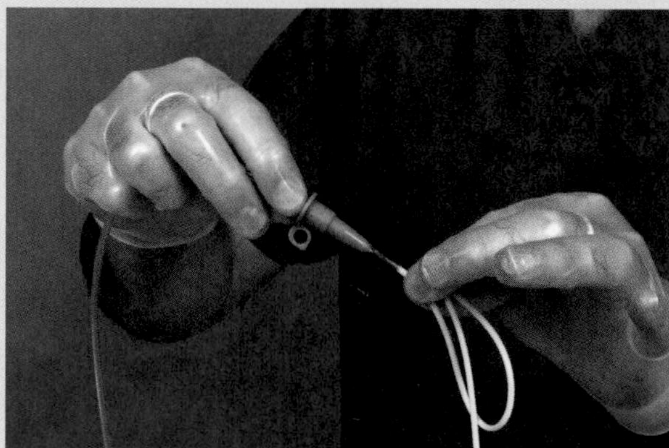

STEP 3a Kink tubing while unplugging feeding tube.

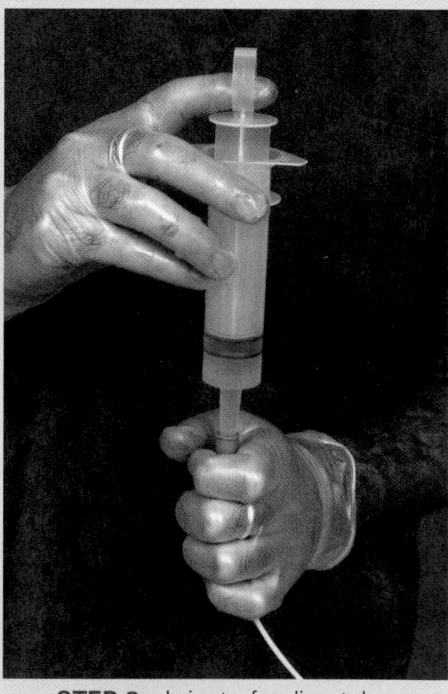

STEP 3c Irrigate feeding tube.

EVALUATION

1. Observe patient for respiratory distress: persistent gagging, paroxysms of coughing, and respiratory patterns (e.g., rate and depth) inconsistent with baseline measures.
2. Verify that color, pH, and appearance of aspirate are consistent with the initial tube placement according to x-ray film results.
3. During irrigation observe ease with which tube feeding instills through tubing.

Unexpected Outcomes and Related Interventions

1. Red or brown coloring (coffee grounds appearance) of fluid aspirated from a feeding tube indicates new blood or old blood, respectively, in the GI tract.

a. If the color is not related to medications recently administered, notify the health care provider.
2. Patient develops severe respiratory distress.
 a. Stop any enteral feeding and notify health care provider.
 b. Prepare to obtain chest x-ray film as ordered.
3. Tube cannot be irrigated and remains obstructed.
 a. Reattempt irrigation; if unsuccessful, notify the health care provider.
 b. Tube may need to be removed, and a new tube placed.
4. Fluid and electrolyte imbalances develop.
 a. Notify the health care provider of abnormal electrolyte levels or imbalanced I&O.

Recording and Reporting

- Record the pH and appearance of aspirate. Report findings if displacement is suspected.
- Record time of irrigation, amount and type of fluid instilled, and patient's tolerance.
- Report if tubing is clogged.

Sample Documentation

1400 Dobhoff feeding tube placement confirmed, aspirant pH 3.0, dark green bile-colored fluid. Tube irrigated easily with 30 mL of sterile water; continuous feeding reconnected and infusing at 60 mL/hr.

Special Considerations

Pediatric

- Decrease the amount of air insufflated before gastric aspiration according to size of patient (e.g., an infant may only need 1 mL of air; a small child 5 mL).
- Flush feeding tubes in neonates and children with the lowest volume of water needed to clear the tube (ASPEN, 2009). Use 1 or 2 mL for small tubes to 5 to 15 mL or more for large ones (Axelrod and others, 2006).
- Sterile water is recommended for irrigation in neonatal and pediatric patients before and after medication administration (ASPEN, 2009).

Home Care

- Instruct patient or primary caregiver not to proceed with feedings or medication administration via the tube if there is any doubt as to proper placement of tube.

SKILL 12.5 ADMINISTERING TUBE FEEDINGS VIA NASOGASTRIC, GASTROSTOMY, AND JEJUNOSTOMY TUBES

- **Nursing Skills Online: Enteral Nutrition Module, Lesson 4**

Video Clips

Enteral nutrition is the administration of nutrients directly into the GI tract by way of a feeding tube. Enteral nutrition is indicated when a patient cannot ingest, chew, or swallow but can digest and absorb nutrients. NG and NI feedings are usually given over short periods of time, usually less than 30 days. Enteral feeding through an NG tube is the most common type of enteral nutrition. The main complication of tube feedings is pulmonary aspiration with possible lung compromise. Other complications include misplaced tubes, infection, diarrhea, tube clogging, and tube displacement. You will collaborate with RDs and health care providers to select an enteral feeding formula based on patients' protein and calorie requirements and digestive ability.

Patients with long-term needs or who have no easy access to the GI tract through the nose or mouth require a more invasive access to the GI tract in the form of gastrostomy and jejunostomy tubes. A gastrostomy tube is surgically placed in the stomach, exits through an incision in the upper left quadrant of the abdomen, and is sutured in place. A more current practice is a percutaneous endoscopic gastrostomy tube, which is inserted during endoscopic viewing of the stomach. A tube is placed in the stomach and exists through the incision, where an external bumper holds it in place (Fig. 12-3). When patients develop a gastric ileus (decreased or absent peristalsis of the stomach but not intestine), delayed gastric emptying, or gastric resection, enteral nutrition is given via a percutaneous endoscopic jejunostomy tube (Baskin, 2006). Jejunostomy tubes are inserted most often by endoscopy through the abdomen and then fed into the jejunum of the large intestine. Always know whether the patient has a gastric or jejunal tube or both. The general indications for enteral feeding include the following:

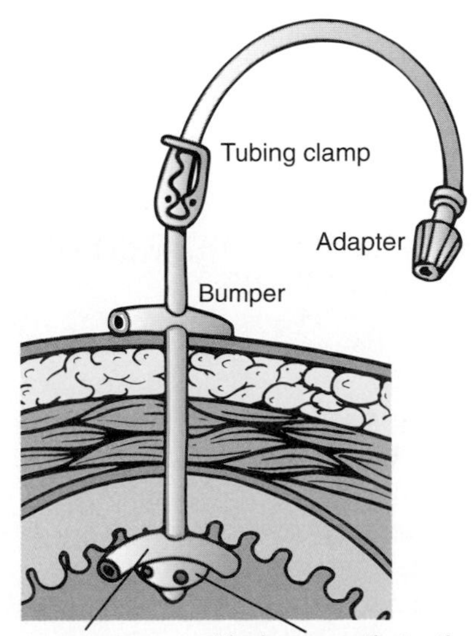

FIG 12-3 Placement of gastrostomy tube into stomach.

1. Patients who can't eat because of surgery, injury, or disease process
2. Nutritional deficit resulting from reduced food ingestion, even when patients are physically able to eat
3. Patients with impaired swallowing or gag reflex

Inadequate delivery of nutrients, potentially leading to malnutrition or electrolyte disturbances, sometimes occurs because of frequent interruptions in feeding (Worthington and Reyen, 2004). Administration of enteral nutrition is often delayed until after bowel sounds can be auscultated in patients, indicating the return of peristalsis. Researchers find it is safe to begin feedings before bowel sounds return, especially in patients with jejunostomy tubes, but this is not without risk. Take care to balance the benefits and risks by assessing for patient tolerance of early enteral feeding (Flesher and others, 2005).

ASSESSMENT

1. Assess patient's need for tube feedings: decreased level of consciousness, a nutritional deficit, head or neck surgery, facial trauma, or impaired swallowing; consult with nutrition support team or health care provider.
2. Assess patient for food allergies. *Rationale: Prevents patient from developing localized or systemic allergic responses to feeding.*
3. Auscultate for bowel sounds before feeding. *Rationale: Absent bowel sounds may indicate decreased ability of GI tract to digest or absorb nutrients. May contraindicate or lead to holding of a feeding.*
4. Obtain baseline weight and review laboratory values (e.g., electrolytes, capillary blood glucose measurement). Assess patient for fluid volume excess or deficit, electrolyte abnormalities, and metabolic abnormalities (e.g., hyperglycemia). *Rationale: Provides baseline to measure patient's response to enteral nutrition.*
5. Review and verify health care provider's order for formula, concentration, route, method of delivery (continuous versus intermittent), and frequency or rate of infusion. *Rationale: Ensures that correct formula will be administered in appropriate volume.*

PLANNING

Expected Outcomes focus on safe administration of tube-feeding formula, patient tolerance of formula, and avoidance of administration complications.

1. Patient experiences slow increase in nutritional status and weight over time.
2. Patient has no sign of respiratory distress.
3. Patient has no fluid or electrolyte imbalance.
4. Patient has no GI distress.

Delegation and Collaboration

The skill of administration of NG, NI, gastrostomy, and jejunostomy tube feeding can be delegated to nursing assistive personnel (NAP). (Refer to agency policy.) However, a registered nurse (RN) or licensed practical nurse (LPN) must first verify tube placement and patency. Instruct the NAP to:

- Position the patient correctly for feeding (see Implementation) and use the reverse Trendelenburg's position when patient cannot tolerate elevated head of bed (ASPEN, 2009).
- Infuse the feeding slowly as ordered.
- Report any difficulty infusing the feeding or any patient discomfort (e.g., abdominal pain or cramping).
- Report any gagging, paroxysms of coughing, or choking.

Equipment

- Disposable feeding bag, tubing, and formula or ready-to-hang system with formula
- 60-mL or larger Luer-Lok or catheter-tip syringe
- Stethoscope
- Infusion pump (required for continuous feedings): Use pump designed for tube feedings.
- pH indicator strip (scale 0.0 to 11.0)
- Cup of tap water or sterile water (immunocompromised and critically ill)
- Clean gloves
- Equipment to obtain blood glucose level by fingerstick, if ordered
- Labels for marking tube connections

IMPLEMENTATION *for* ADMINISTERING TUBE FEEDINGS VIA NASOGASTRIC, GASTROSTOMY, AND JEJUNOSTOMY TUBES

STEPS	RATIONALE
1. See Standard Protocol (inside front cover).	
2. Identify patient using two identifiers (e.g., name and birthday or name and account number, according to facility policy).	Ensures correct patient. Complies with The Joint Commission standards and improves patient safety (TJC, 2010).
3. Prepare feeding container to administer formula.	
a. Check expiration date on formula and integrity of container. Be sure that feeding formula is at room temperature.	Ensures GI tolerance of formula. Prevents leakage of tube feeding. Cold formula causes gastric cramping and discomfort because the liquid is not warmed by mouth and esophagus.

STEPS	RATIONALE
b. Connect tubing of administration set to open system container or prepare ready-to-hang closed system container. Use aseptic technique and avoid handling the feeding system.	The feeding system, including the bag, connections, and tubing, must be free of contamination to prevent bacterial growth (Mathus-Vliegen and others, 2006).
c. For an open system, shake formula container well and fill feeding container bag with formula (see illustration).	Filling the tubing with formula prevents excess air from entering GI tract once infusion begins.
For both closed and open systems, open roller clamp on tubing and fill tubing (prime tubing) with formula. Close roller clamp and cap end of tubing. Hang bag on feeding pump pole. Be sure that formula is at room temperature.	Cold formula causes gastric cramping.

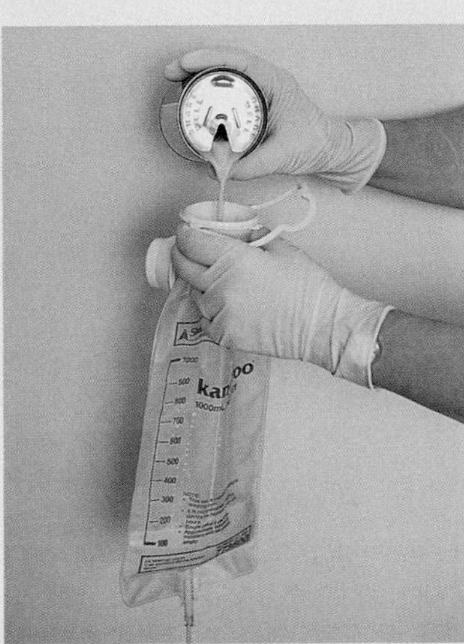

STEP 3c Pour formula into feeding container.

STEPS	RATIONALE
4. Elevate head of bed at least 30 degrees, preferably 45 degrees (unless contraindicated) for all patients receiving enteral nutrition, or sit the patient up in bed or a chair (ASPEN, 2009). For patient who must lie supine, place in reverse Trendelenburg's position (unless contraindicated) (ASPEN, 2009). In critically ill patients elevate head of bed at least 30 degrees.	Elevated head helps to prevent aspiration. Elevating the head-of-bed position to at least 30 degrees and using a small-bowel feeding site can reduce the incidence of aspiration and aspiration-related pneumonia in critically ill tube-fed patients (Metheny and others, 2010).
5. Verify tube placement (see Skill 12.4). Attach syringe and instill 30 mL of air and then aspirate 5 to 10 mL of gastric or intestinal secretions. Observe appearance of aspirate and note pH measure.	Gastric fluid for a patient who has fasted for 4 hours usually has a pH of 1.0 to 4.0. Fluid from the small intestine of fasting patient is usually greater than 6.0. Patient with continuous gastric tube feed may have pH of 5.0 or higher. The pH of pleural fluid is generally greater than 6.0 (Metheny, 2006).
6. Check gastric residual volume (GRV) before each intermittent feeding and every 4 to 6 hours for continuous feedings (Metheny, 2006).	Intestinal residual is very small (≤10 mL); if residual volume is greater than 10 mL, displacement of the tube into the stomach may have occurred.

SAFETY ALERT More fluid can usually be withdrawn from large-bore tubes than from small-bore feeding tubes. Thus high volumes are not always detected when small-bore tubes are in place. Tube ports must rest in fluid for a residual to be aspirated (Metheny and others, 2008).

Continued

STEPS	RATIONALE
a. Draw up 30 mL of air into syringe and connect to feeding tube. Inject the air and pull back slowly; aspirate the total amount of gastric contents (see illustration).	

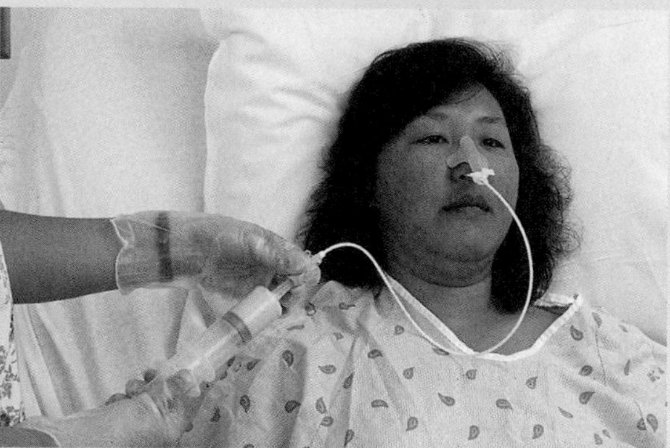

STEP 6a Check for gastric residual volume.

STEPS	RATIONALE
b. Return aspirated contents to stomach unless volume exceeds 200 mL (twice) or 250 mL (once) (check agency policy). In the case of an NI tube, residual should be 10 mL or less.	GRV categories identified as significant were patients having two or more GRVs of at least 200 mL and patients having one or more GRVs of at least 250 mL (Metheny and others, 2008).
7. Flush the tube with 30 mL of water. Remove syringe and replace the cap on tube.	
8. Initiate feeding.	
a. ***Syringe for intermittent feeding***	
(1) Pinch proximal end of feeding tube and remove cap.	Prevents excessive air from entering patient's stomach and leakage of gastric contents.
(2) Remove plunger from syringe and attach barrel of syringe to end of tube.	Barrel receives formula for instillation.
(3) Fill syringe with measured amount of formula. Release tube, raise syringe to no more than 45 cm (18 inches) above insertion site, and allow it to empty slowly by gravity. Repeat until you have given prescribed amount of formula.	Height of syringe allows for safe, slow gravity flow. Total delivery of syringe feeding takes several minutes, depending on volume. Rapid infusion causes abdominal discomfort and increases the risk of aspiration.
b. ***Feeding bag for intermittent feeding***	
(1) Pinch proximal end of feeding tube and remove cap.	Prevents excessive air from entering patient's stomach and leakage of gastric contents.
(2) Attach end of administration set tubing to end of feeding tube. Label administration set as "Tube feeding only." (NOTE: Some manufacturers now provide feeding tubes labeled "for feeding only.")	An enteral misconnection is an inadvertent connection between enteral tubing and nonenteral tubing such as an intravascular catheter, a peritoneal dialysis catheter, or medical gas tubing (ASPEN, 2009). Labeling prevents a misconnection.
(3) Set rate by adjusting roller clamp on tubing or placing on a feeding pump. Allow bag to empty gradually over 30 to 60 minutes until completed (see illustration). Turn off roller clamp. Label bag with tube-feeding type, strength, and amount. Include date, time, and initials.	Gradual emptying of tube feeding by gravity from feeding bag reduces risk for abdominal discomfort, vomiting, or diarrhea induced by bolus or too-rapid infusion of tube feedings.

STEPS	RATIONALE

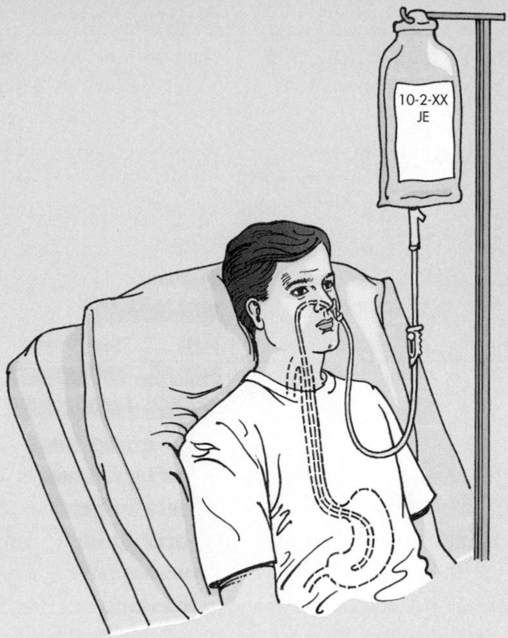

STEP 8b(3) Administer intermittent feeding.

STEPS	RATIONALE
(4) Change bag and tubing every 24 hours.	Decreases risk for bacterial colonization.
c. ***Continuous-drip method***	Continuous-feeding method is designed to deliver prescribed hourly rate of feeding. This method reduces risk for abdominal discomfort.
(1) Connect distal end of administration set tubing to proximal end of feeding tube as in Steps 8b(1) and 8b(2).	
(2) Connect tubing through tube feeding pump, open roller clamp on tubing, set rate on pump, and turn on. Continue to monitor during infusion.	Delivers continuous feeding at a steady rate and pressure. Feeding pump alarms when increased resistance is detected.

SAFETY ALERT Maximum hang time for formula is 8 hours in an open system, 24 to 48 hours in closed, ready-to-hang system (if it remains closed). Refer to manufacturer's guidelines (ASPEN, 2009).

SAFETY ALERT Use pumps designated for tube feeding (not pumps for IV fluids).

STEPS	RATIONALE
9. Advance rate of concentration of tube feeding gradually (Table 12-4).	Helps to prevent diarrhea and gastric intolerance to formula.
10. At the end of a feeding, flush feeding tube with 30 mL of water. Repeat every 4 to 6 hours (check agency policy) (see Skill 12.4).	Provides patient with source of water to help maintain fluid and electrolyte balance. Clears tubing of formula.
11. When patient is receiving intermittent tube feeding, cap or clamp the proximal end of the feeding tube.	Prevents air from entering stomach between feedings.
12. Rinse bag and tubing with warm water whenever feedings are interrupted. Use a new open administration set every 24 hours. Administration sets for closed-system formulas should be changed per manufacturer guidelines (ASPEN, 2009).	Prevents bacterial contamination of feeding solution.
13. See Completion Protocol (inside front cover).	

TABLE 12-4 ADVANCING THE RATE OF TUBE FEEDING

INTERMITTENT	CONTINUOUS
Start formula at full strength for isotonic formulas (300 to 400 mOsm) (ASPEN, 2009) or at ordered concentration.	Start formula at full strength for isotonic formulas (300 to 400 mOsm) (ASPEN, 2009). Usually hypertonic formulas are also started at full strength but at a slower rate.
Infuse formula over at least 20 to 30 minutes via syringe or feeding container.	Begin infusion rate at designated rate.
Begin feedings with no more than 150 to 250 mL at one time. Increase by 50 mL per feeding per day to achieve needed volume and calories In six to eight feedings. (Note: Concentrated formulas at full strength may be infused at slower rate until tolerance is achieved.)	Advance rate slowly (e.g., 10 to 20 mL/hr/day) to target rate if tolerated (tolerance indicated by low gastric residuals and absence of nausea and diarrhea).

EVALUATION

1. Measure residual volume per policy, usually every 4 to 6 hours.
2. Monitor fingerstick blood glucose level as ordered, especially in patients at risk (e.g., diabetes, renal failure).
3. Monitor I&O at least every 8 hours and calculate daily totals every 24 hours (Worthington and Reyen, 2004).
4. Weigh patient daily until maximum tube feeding rate is reached and maintained for 24 hours and then weigh patient 3 times per week.
5. Monitor laboratory values.
6. Observe patient's respiratory status.
7. Evaluate patient's level of comfort (cramping).
8. Auscultate bowel sounds.

Unexpected Outcomes and Related Interventions

1. The feeding tube becomes clogged. Frequent aspiration of gastric contents and frequent administration of medications without adequate flushing increase clogging of feeding tubes (Reising and Neal, 2005).
   a. Attempt to flush the tube with water.
   b. Special products are available for unclogging feeding tubes; do not use soda and juice.
   c. Hold feeding and notify health care provider.
   d. Maintain patient in semi-Fowler's position.
2. Gastric residual volume exceeds 250 mL once or 200 mL twice (see agency policy).
   a. Hold feeding and notify health care provider.
3. Patient aspirates formula.
   a. See Skill 12.2, Unexpected Outcomes and Related Interventions.
4. Patient develops large amount of diarrhea (more than three loose stools in 24 hours).
   a. Notify health care provider. Meet with RD to determine if need to change formula to provide fiber.
   b. Consider other causes (e.g., bacterial contamination of the feeding).
   c. Provide skin care.
   d. Determine if patient is receiving medications (e.g., containing sorbitol) that induce diarrhea.
5. Patient develops nausea and vomiting, which may indicate gastric ileus.
   a. Withhold tube feeding and notify health care provider.
   b. Be sure that tubing is patent; aspirate for gastric residual.
6. Gastric residual fluid has foul odor or unusual appearance.
   a. Do not return residual volume material of unusual odor or appearance without first consulting health care provider.

Recording and Reporting

- Record amount and type of feeding, gastric residual volume (GRV), infusion rate (continuous feeding), patient's response to tube feeding, patency of tube, and condition of skin at tube site.
- Record volume of formula and any additional water on I&O form.
- Report type of feeding, infusion rate (continuous feeding) status of feeding tube, patient's tolerance, and adverse outcomes.

Sample Documentation

1500 Nasogastric Dobhoff feeding tube in place, position confirmed with pH of 4.0. GRV 80 mL, returned to stomach. Continuous feeding of full-strength Isosource HN infusing at 55 mL/hr. Tube irrigates without difficulty. No nasal irritation noted.

Special Considerations

Pediatric

- In acutely ill children receiving continuous feedings, check the GRV every 4 hours and hold if the volume exceeds or is equal to the hourly rate. If feedings are bolus, check the GRV before the next feeding and hold if the GRV is more than half of the previous feeding volume (ASPEN, 2009).
- Intermittent feeding is preferred in infants because of possible perforation of the stomach, nasal airway obstruction, ulceration, and irritation to mucous membranes with

continuous feedings. It usually takes 20 to 30 minutes to give an intermittent feeding to a small child, about as long as it takes to bottle feed the child. Hold the infant and offer a pacifier during the feeding to simulate a more natural bottle-feeding experience (Axelrod and others, 2006).

- Temporary small-bore NG tubes are often placed in infants just before each feeding and removed afterward.
- For a neonate an excessive GRV is more than 20% of the ordered amount. For an older child an excessive GRV is greater than 50% of the ordered amount.

Geriatric

- Some older adults are more susceptible to hyperglycemia related to glucose intolerance from diabetes or other factors.
- Some older adults have decreased gastric emptying so formula remains in the stomach longer than for younger patients. GRV checks are of special importance in patients with impaired cognition to decrease the risk for aspiration during gastric feeding.

Home Care

- Instruct family caregiver and/or patient on:
    - How to administer feedings and monitor for symptoms of discomfort, diarrhea, and aspiration.
    - How to monitor I&O using household measuring devices.
    - How to provide skin care around tube insertion sites (see Procedural Guideline 12.1).

PROCEDURAL GUIDELINE 12.1
Site Care of Enteral Feeding Tubes

The exit site for feeding tubes, including the nose and abdominal surface, can easily become irritated from rubbing of a tube against the skin. Patients develop small ulcers of the nasal mucosa when feeding tubes have been in place a prolonged period and when adequate site care has not been provided. Even though gastrostomy and jejunostomy tubes often have small dressings in place around the tube insertion site, irritation and erosion of the skin can lead to infection. Routine assessment and provision of site care make patients more comfortable and reduce the incidence of skin complications.

Delegation Considerations

Care of an enteral feeding tube site cannot be delegated to nursing assistive personnel (NAP). Instruct the NAP to:

- Inform the nurse of any patient complaints of discomfort at the insertion site.
- Inform the nurse of any drainage on the insertion site dressing.

Equipment

- Normal saline, dated and initialed container at patient's bedside
- 4 × 4–inch gauze dressings
- Tube fixation device; hypoallergenic tape, or transparent dressing (for NG tube)
- Prepared drain-gauze dressing (for gastrostomy and jejunostomy tubes)
- Tape, tincture of benzoin, skin barrier protectant
- Clean gloves.

Procedural Steps

1. Inspect the condition of the skin at the tube exit site, looking for inflammation, bleeding, excoriation, drainage, and tenderness. In the case of gastrostomy and jejunostomy tubes, if a dressing is in place defer inspection until dressing is removed. *Rationale: Provides baseline for condition of exit site.*
2. For an NG tube note the position of the ink mark at exit site indicating tube location. *Rationale: Provides reference point to prevent accidental pulling or advancement of tube.*
3. Determine whether gastrostomy or jejunostomy exit site is to be left open to air or covered with a dressing. Check health care provider's order or verify agency policy.
4. **See Standard Protocol (inside front cover).**
5. *Care of NG tube site*
    a. Use your nondominant hand to anchor the NG tube as you remove the old tape, fixation device, or transparent dressing that anchors the tube.
    b. With tape or fixation device removed, inspect once again the condition of the skin and naris.
    c. Take a 4 × 4–gauze dressing moistened in normal saline and gently cleanse around the exit site. Remove any tape residue.
    d. Replace the old fixation device with new tape, transparent dressing, or commercial fixation device (see Steps 18a and 18b, Skill 12.3).
6. ***Care of gastrostomy and jejunostomy site***
    a. Remove old dressing (if present) and discard in appropriate container.
    b. Assess exit site for evidence of excoriation, drainage, infection, or bleeding.
    c. Cleanse skin around site with warm water and mild soap using 4 × 4–inch gauzes (Vukson, 2008).
    d. Rotate external bumper 90 degrees (see Fig. 12-3).
    e. Dry site completely. Apply thin layer of protective skin barrier to exit site if indicated (e.g., site excoriated).

Continued

PROCEDURAL GUIDELINE 12.1
Site Care of Enteral Feeding Tubes—cont'd

f. If dressing is ordered, place drain-gauze dressing over external bar. NOTE: Do not place dressing under external bar; this can cause gastric tissue erosion or internal abdominal wall pressure.
g. Secure dressing with tape.
h. Place date, time, and initials on new dressing.

7. **See Completion Protocol (inside front cover).**
8. Document in nurse' notes appearance of exit site, drainage noted, and dressing application.
9. Report to health care provider any exit site complications.
10. Routinely evaluate condition of exit site every shift.

REVIEW QUESTIONS

Case Study for Questions 1 and 2

After 4 days of hospitalization a patient has developed serious sepsis and has not tolerated oral feedings. An NG small-bore feeding tube was inserted 12 hours ago. The patient is receiving a continuous infusion of tube-feeding formula. The patient weighed 165 pounds before feedings were initiated.

1. When the nurse checks the position of the tube, which of the following pH values should be expected?
   1. 7.0
   2. 4.0
   3. 5.0
   4. 3.0
2. The nurse prepares to irrigate the feeding tube to prevent clogging. The use of sterile water for irrigation is indicated in which situation? Select all that apply.
   1. When the pH of gastric aspirate is <4
   2. During routine irrigation every 4 hours
   3. After administering a medication through the tube
   4. When the patient receiving a tube feeding is immunocompromised
3. A nurse is assigned to a patient with the diagnosis of stroke, which is affecting the left side of his body. The patient is right handed. During breakfast that morning as the patient is feeding himself, the nurse notices a number of clinical signs. Which of the following suggest that the patient is at risk for aspiration? Select all that apply.
   1. Wet voice
   2. Difficulty smiling
   3. Coughing on food
   4. Aversion to food
   5. Change in taste
4. When feeding a patient who is known to have dysphagia, which of the following interventions prevents gastric reflux?
   1. Monitoring pulse oximetry readings
   2. Providing patient oral hygiene before feeding
   3. Positioning patient upright in a chair
   4. Adding thickener to thin liquids
5. A nurse observes a student nurse performing an irrigation of a feeding tube. The patient is receiving a continuous tube feeding. Which of the following observations by the nurse suggests the student is correctly following the irrigation protocol?
   1. Four hours after the last irrigation the student draws up 30 mL of air into an irrigating syringe, instills it into the feeding tube, withdraws fluid to verify placement, kinks tubing, draws up 30 mL of water into irrigating syringe, inserts syringe tip into end of feeding tube, and irrigates tube.
   2. Eight hours after the last irrigation the student draws up 30 mL of air into an irrigating syringe, instills it into the feeding tube, withdraws fluid to verify placement, kinks tubing, draws up 30 mL of water into irrigating syringe, inserts syringe tip into end of feeding tube, and irrigates tube.
   3. Four hours after the last irrigation the student draws up 30 mL of air into an irrigating syringe, instills it into the feeding tube, draws up 30 mL of water into irrigating syringe, inserts syringe into end of feeding tube, and irrigates tube.
   4. Eight hours after the last irrigation the student draws up 30 mL of air into an irrigating syringe, instills it into the feeding tube, draws up 30 mL of water into irrigating syringe, inserts syringe into end of feeding tube, and irrigates tube.
6. A patient on a medical oncology unit has been receiving continuous tube feedings for the last 2 days. During a morning assessment the nurse gathers information about the patient's tolerance and response to NG feedings. Which of the following are unexpected outcomes of the feedings? Select all that apply.
   1. The patient shows signs of aspiration.
   2. The patient develops symptoms of constipation.
   3. The patient's tube yields a gastric residual volume of 300 mL.
   4. The patient's tube cannot be irrigated.
   5. The patient has a small ulcer on the inner naris.
7. When a nurse educates patients and families about their nutritional needs, food safety is an important topic. Which of the following precautions ensure that it is safe to eat prepared foods? Select all that apply.
   1. Wash hands with warm soapy water before touching food.
   2. Encourage intake of unpasteurized milk.
   3. Keep foods properly refrigerated at 4.4° C (40° F).
   4. Do not save leftovers for more than a week in the refrigerator.

8. A patient who is 2 days postoperative and has normal GI function but is unable to chew because of facial surgery would benefit most from:
   1. Clear-liquid diet
   2. High-fiber diet
   3. Mechanical diet
   4. Pureed diet
9. The nurse caring for a patient in the nursing home notices that the patient routinely has a bowel movement every 3 to 4 days and sometimes the stool is reportedly hard in consistency. The patient is alert and able to tolerate solid foods. The patient wears dentures. The best diet selection for this patient would be:
   1. Pureed diet
   2. High-fiber diet
   3. Fat-modified diet
   4. Low-residue diet
10. A patient on the neurosurgery unit is recovering from a traumatic injury resulting in an unstable vertebral fracture. He is ordered to remain supine and is on an air fluidized bed to prevent pressure ulcers. Which of the following positions does the nurse have the patient assume before a tube feeding?
    1. Head of bed elevated 90 degrees
    2. Reverse Trendelenburg's position
    3. Side-lying position
    4. Trendelenburg's position

REFERENCES

Abe S and others: Tongue-coating as risk indicator for aspiration pneumonia in edentate elderly, *Arch Gerontol Geriatr* 47(2):267, 2008.

American Society for Parenteral and Enteral Nutrition (ASPEN): *The science and practice of nutrition support: a case-based core curriculum*, Dubuque, Iowa, 2007, Kendall Hunt.

American Society for Parenteral and Enteral Nutrition (ASPEN): ASPEN Enteral Nutrition Practice Recommendations, *JPEN J Parenter Enteral Nutr* 22:122, 2009.

Ashley J and others: Speech, language, and swallowing disorders in the older adult, *Clin Geriatr Med* 22:291, 2006.

Axelrod D and others: Pediatric enteral nutrition, *JPEN J Parenter Enteral Nutr* 29(Suppl):S21, 2006.

Baskin WN: Acute complications associated with bedside placement of feeding tubes, *Nutr Clin Pract* 21:40, 2006.

Ebersole P and others: *Toward healthy aging*, ed 7, St Louis, 2008, Mosby.

Flesher ME and others: Assessing the metabolic and clinical consequences of early enteral feeding in the malnourished patient, *JPEN J Parenter Enteral Nutr* 29:108, 2005.

Hockenberry MJ, Wilson D: *Wong's nursing care of infants and children*, ed 8, St Louis, 2007, Mosby.

Lengyel CO and others: Nutrient inadequacies among elderly residents of long-term care facilities, *Can J Diet Pract Res* 69(2):82, 2008.

Mathus-Vliegen EMH and others: Analysis of bacterial contamination in an enteral feeding system, *JPEN J Parenter Enteral Nutr* 29:519, 2006.

Meals on Wheels Association of America: *FAQ*, http://www.mowaa.org/index.asp, accessed June 2009.

Metheny N: Preventing aspiration in older adults with dysphagia, *Medsurg Nurs* 16(4):271, 2007.

Metheny NA: Preventing respiratory complications of tube-feeding: evidence-based practice, *Am J Crit Care* 15:360, 2006.

Metheny NA and others: Gastric residual volume and aspiration in critically ill patients receiving gastric feedings, *Am J Crit Care* 17(6):512, 2008.

Metheny NA and others: Effectiveness of an aspiration risk-reduction protocol, *Nurs Res* 59(1):18, 2010.

Munro C and others: Oral health measurements in nursing research: state of the science, *Biol Res Nurs* 8(1):35, 2006.

Nowlin A: The dysphagia dilemma: How you can help, *RN* 69(6):44, 2006.

Palmer JL, Metheny NA. Preventing aspiration when a patient eats or during hand-feeding of the patient. *AJN* 108(2):40, 2008.

Prasse JE, Kikano GE: An overview of pediatric dysphagia, *Clin Pediatr* 48(3):247, 2009.

Ramsey D and others: Silent aspiration: what do we know? *Dysphagia* 20(3):218, 2005.

Rauen C and others: Seven evidence-based practice habits: putting some sacred cows out to pasture, *Crit Care Nurs* 28(2):98, 2008.

Reising DL, Neal RS: Enteral tube flushing, *Am J Nurs* 105(3):58, 2005.

Roberts S and others: Devices and techniques for bedside enteral feeding tube placement, *Nutr Clin Pract* 22:412, 2007.

Suiter DM, Leder SB: Clinical utility of the 3-ounce water swallow test. *Dysphagia* 23(3):244, 2008.

The Joint Commission (TJC): *Comprehensive accreditation manual for hospitals: the official handbook*, Oakbrook Terrace, Ill, 2009, JCAHO; http://www.jointcommission, accessed June 2009.

The Joint Commission (TJC): *2010 National Patient Safety Goals*, Oakbrook Terrace, Ill, 2010, The Commission, available at http://jointcommission.org/PatientSafety/NationalPatientSafetyGoals/.

Trapl M and others: Dysphagia bedside screening for acute-stroke patients: the Gugging Swallowing Screen, *Stroke* 38(111):2948, 2007.

Vukson K: G-tubes and skin care, Oh My! *Gastroenterol Nurs* 31(4):305, 2008.

Westergren A: Detection of eating difficulties after stroke: a systematic review, *Int Nurs Rev* 53(2):143, 2006.

White G and others: Dysphagia: causes, assessment, treatment, and management, *Geriatrics* 63(5):15, 2008.

Worthington PH, Reyen L: Selecting candidates and delivery methods for enteral nutrition. In Worthington PH, editor: *Practical aspects of nutrition support*, Philadelphia, 2004, Elsevier.

CHAPTER

13

Pain Management

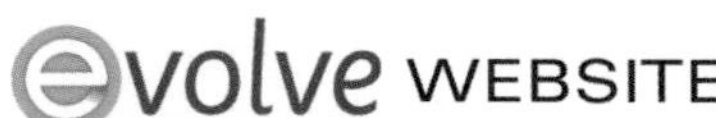

http://evolve.elsevier.com/Perry/nursinginterventions

Video Clips

Pain is the most common reason a person seeks health care. Patients experience various forms of stress, undergo painful procedures, and experience painful illnesses. In addition, the experience of staying in a health care environment and the symptoms of diseases disrupt a patient's comfort level. Assisting patients with achieving comfort is a challenge. Your responsibilities as a nurse include creating a comfortable environment and applying principles of pain management.

Adequate pain management is a priority for health care agencies. Patients expect good pain control. Accrediting organizations such as The Joint Commission (TJC) have set standards for timely and effective pain management (TJC, 2009). The Agency for Healthcare Research and Quality (AHRQ), the American Pain Society (APS), and the World Health Organization (WHO) also have written guidelines for pain management. The pain management skills in this text are for use alone or in combination, depending on patient needs.

PATIENT-CENTERED CARE

Because pain is unique to each individual, it is important to recognize all factors influencing a patient's pain and then integrate these factors into an individualized approach for pain management. Effective pain management begins with a complete patient assessment, which includes a person's coping style, physical status, past experience with pain, culture and ethnicity, and emotional health. A factual, timely, and accurate pain assessment requires you to work closely with patients and their families and to explore the pain experience through the eyes of the patient. Remain objective, listen, and thoroughly explore any symptoms that the patient expresses. Effective therapeutic communication is the key to gathering the information needed to accurately diagnosis the patient's pain and then intervene appropriately.

Cultural diversity is a factor that influences a person's pain experience and your approach to pain assessment and management. Im and colleagues (2009) studied Caucasian, Hispanic, African American, and Asian patients' cancer pain experience by conducting online interviews. All patients talked about "communication breakdowns" with their health care provider. This is important for you to consider when caring for any patient because a caring, nonjudgmental approach is needed to win a patient's trust and to then learn how the pain affects the patient. The researchers also learned that Caucasian patients focus on how to control pain and treatment selection, whereas the ethnic minorities try to control pain by minimizing and acting as though pain is normal (Im and others, 2009). Learning about how a patient hopes to manage pain can help you select pain strategies. For example, a Caucasian patient might accept use of a patient-controlled analgesic (PCA) device more readily than a patient from a minority group. Always assess the meaning of pain to patients, how they express pain, and the various approaches they use for pain relief.

SAFETY

Patient safety during pain management begins with trying the least invasive therapy first along with previously used successful pain remedies. For example, a home health nurse might learn that simply by repositioning a patient, controlling room noise, and giving a patient a cup of herbal tea helps him or her relax and fall asleep even while experiencing chronic back pain. Do not undertreat pain. Acute, uncontrolled pain can threaten a person's well being. For example, if a patient is getting insufficient pain relief from pain medicine given as needed (prn), consult with the health care provider for an around-the-clock (ATC) medication schedule instead. Finally, safety in pain management requires you to

BOX 13-1 PAIN ASSESSMENT IN A NONVERBAL PATIENT

Recommended Assessment Approaches
- Attempt a self-report of pain using simple yes/no response or vocalizations.
- Explain why self-report cannot be used.
- Search for the potential cause of pain by using physical examination techniques (e.g., palpation).
- Assume that pain is present after ruling out other problems (infection, constipation) that cause it.
- Identify pathological conditions or procedures that may cause pain.
- Observe patient behaviors (e.g., facial expressions, vocalizations, body movements such as guarding, changes in mental status or interactions) that indicate pain. These vary based on patient's developmental level.
- Ask family members, parents, and caregivers for a surrogate report.

Using a Behavioral Pain Assessment Tool
- Use reliable and valid tools to ensure that appropriate criteria are used in assessment (e.g., the NOPPAIN for older adults).
- Select an appropriate scale for each patient (such as a visual analog scale versus a FACES scale); no one scale is required for all specific groups of patients.
- Vital signs are not sensitive indicators for the presence of pain.

Adapted from Herr K and others: Pain assessment in the nonverbal patient: position statement with clinical practice recommendations, *Pain Manag Nurs* 7(2):44, 2006; Horgas AL and others: Assessing pain in persons with dementia: relationships among the noncommunicative patient's pain assessment instrument, self-report, and behavioral observations, *Pain Manag Nurs* 8(2):77, 2007.
NOPPAIN, Non-Communicative Patient's Pain Assessment Instrument.

know the action and side effects of analgesic medications available for pain relief so you can competently monitor patients and respond when adverse responses develop.

EVIDENCE-BASED PRACTICE TRENDS

Herr K and others: Pain assessment in the nonverbal patient: position statement with clinical practice recommendations, *Pain Manag Nurs* 7(2):44, 2006.

Horgas AL and others: Assessing pain in persons with dementia: relationships among the noncommunicative patient's pain assessment instrument, self-report, and behavioral observations, *Pain Manag Nurs* 8(2):77, 2007.

Pain assessment is complicated when a patient has an alteration in reasoning, recognition, communication, and ability to verbally report pain. Thus it is important for nurses to use appropriate techniques for pain assessment (Box 13-1). A task force of the American Society for Pain Management Nursing (ASPMN, 2006) has developed clinical practice guidelines for pain assessment and associated treatment principles. To add to this evidence, Horgas and colleagues (2007) have tested and further refined a new pain assessment tool, the Non-Communicative Patient's Pain Assessment Instrument (NOPPAIN) that offers promise for assessing pain in nonverbal older adults. The NOPPAIN is concise and easy to use. The evidence suggests that no single assessment strategy is sufficient and that nurses must use a comprehensive pain assessment approach for vulnerable nonverbal patients.

SKILL 13.1 NONPHARMACOLOGICAL PAIN MANAGEMENT

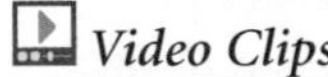 *Video Clips*

Effective pain management does not mean the elimination of pain. Using a combination of nonpharmacological and pharmacological interventions allows your patients to achieve a level of pain relief, which in turn helps them function within their limitations. Always work with a patient to ensure that the level of pain control is acceptable. In addition, collaboration with other health care providers is essential for the best possible pain relief.

A variety of nonpharmacological interventions are available to lessen a patient's pain in any health care setting. Use these interventions in combination with pharmacological measures, not in place of medications, unless the pain is minor. Nonpharmacological techniques diminish the physical effects of pain, alter a patient's perception of pain, and provide a patient with a greater sense of control (Box 13-2). Many of these techniques trigger a relaxation response by stimulating the parasympathetic nervous system (PNS). Because pain often causes muscle tension and anxiety, PNS stimulation relieves these responses. Nonpharmacological interventions are appropriate for patients who find such interventions appealing, express anxiety or fear, may benefit from avoiding or reducing drug therapy, and have incomplete pain relief with pharmacological interventions alone (Whitehead-Pleaux and others, 2006).

ASSESSMENT

1. Assess patients' risk for pain (e.g., those undergoing invasive procedure, anxious patients, those unable to communicate). *Rationale: Allows you to anticipate need for pain control.*
2. Ask patients if they are in pain. Older adults and patients from various cultures may not admit to having pain. Try using other terms such as hurt or discomfort. *Rationale:*

BOX 13-2 NONPHARMACOLOGICAL MEASURES FOR PAIN*

Relaxation and Power of the Mind
- Self-comfort
- Progressive muscle relaxation
- Autogenics training
- Breathing exercises
- Music relaxation
- Visual imagery
- Yoga

Put Your Body to Work
- Exercise
- Pacing
- Conserving energy
- Body mechanics

Spirituality and Reflection
- Engaging in religious practices
- Humor
- Setting aside time to focus on what *is*
- Sharing your stress with others
- Journaling
- Praying

What to Do When Pain Flares
- Cold and hot therapies
- Ball therapy
- Contrast baths
- Hand and foot massage
- Herbals†

*Should be used with analgesic medication.
†Herbals could interact with prescribed analgesics; check with health care provider.

There is no objective test to measure pain. Accept a patient's report of pain (APS, 2008). In patients of differing cultures, watch for nonverbal indicators of pain such as grimacing or clenching teeth and ask significant others if they believe that patient is in pain. Many see pain as a sign of advancing age (Hadjistaviapoulos and others, 2007).

3. Assess characteristics of a patient's pain. Follow agency policy regarding frequency. Use the PQRSTU of pain assessment:
   P: *Precipitating/palliative factors (e.g., "What makes your pain better or worse?"):* Consider patient's experience with over-the-counter (OTC) drugs (including herbals and topicals) that have helped to reduce pain in the past. *Rationale: Identifies possible sources of pain and what the patient uses to reduce the discomfort.*
   Q: *Quality:* Use open-ended questions such as, "Tell me what your pain feels like." *Rationale: Assists in determining underlying pain mechanism (e.g., somatic versus neuropathic pain).*
   R: *Region/radiation:* (e.g., "Show me where your pain is").
   S: *Severity:* Use a valid pain rating scale (Figs. 13-1, 13-2, and 13-3) appropriate to patient's age, developmental level, and comprehension. Have patients rate pain before any intervention. Also assess pain when patient is moving, not just lying in bed or a chair. *Rationale: An appropriate pain rating scale is reliable, easy to use and understand, and reflects changes in pain severity (Ware and others, 2006).*
   T: *Timing:* Ask patient if pain is constant, intermittent, continuous, or a combination. Does pain increase during specific times of day or during certain activities? *Rationale: Stimuli, such as temperature extremes, changes in barometric pressure, and light, often affect a patient's response to pain.*
   U: How is pain affecting *U* (patient) regarding activities of daily living (ADLs), work, relationships, and enjoyment of life? *Rationale: Provides important baseline to later gauge effectiveness of interventions.*

4. Examine site of patient's pain or discomfort. Inspect (discoloration or swelling) and palpate (change in temperature, area of altered sensation, areas that trigger pain, painful area, and range of motion [ROM] of involved joints) the area. Percussion and auscultation help to identify abnormalities (e.g., underlying mass or lung crackles) and determine cause of pain. When assessing abdomen, always auscultate first and then inspect and palpate. *Rationale: Reveals the nature of the pain and directs you toward appropriate interventions.*

5. Assess patient's response to previous pain medications, especially ability to function (e.g., sleeping, eating, and other ADLs). Determine if any analgesic side effects are likely based on medication and patient's previous responses (e.g., itching or nausea). *Rationale: Determines if therapies have been successful or not in the past.*

6. Assess factors that influence perception of pain (e.g., past pain history and ability to cope, depression, fatigue, loneliness, anxiety, helplessness, fear). *Rationale: These factors significantly reduce patients' ability to cope with pain.*

7. Assess patients' culturally determined beliefs about pain and how they express pain. *Rationale: Culture influences the meaning pain holds for a patient and how a patient reacts to discomfort.*

8. Assess physical, behavioral, and emotional signs and symptoms of pain. *Rationale: Signs and symptoms may reveal source and nature of pain. Nonverbal responses to pain are especially useful in assessing pain in patients who are cognitively impaired or nonverbal.*
   a. Moaning, crying, whimpering, vocalizations
   b. Decreased activity
   c. Facial expressions (e.g., grimace, clenched teeth)
   d. Change in usual behavior
   e. Abnormal gait (e.g., shuffling) and posture (e.g., bent, leaning).
   f. Irritability
   g. Guarding of body part
   h. Diaphoresis
   i. Increased blood glucose level reflecting stress of unrelieved pain
   j. Decreased gastrointestinal (GI) motility, nausea, and vomiting
   k. Insomnia, anorexia, and fatigue
   l. Depression, hopelessness, anger, fear, social withdrawal
   m. Concomitant symptoms: Symptoms that often occur with pain (e.g., headache, nausea, constipation)

9. In cognitively impaired patients, obtain a proxy pain intensity rating from the primary caregiver (e.g., family member, friend). *Rationale: Proxy ratings (ratings by*

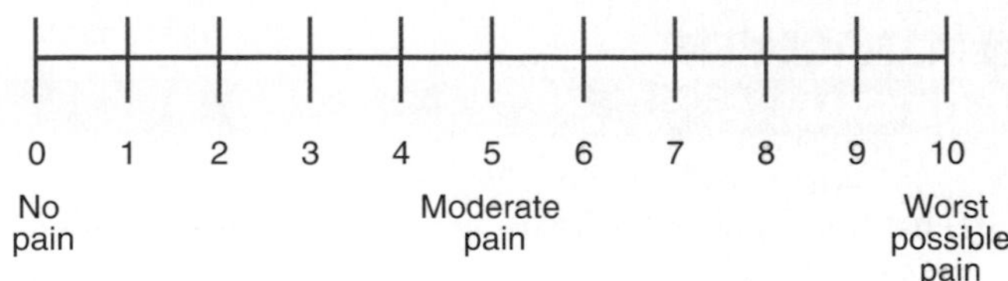

FIG 13-1 0-10 Numeric Pain Rating Scale. (From McCaffery M, Pasero C: *Pain: clinical manual*, ed 2, St Louis, 1999, Mosby.)

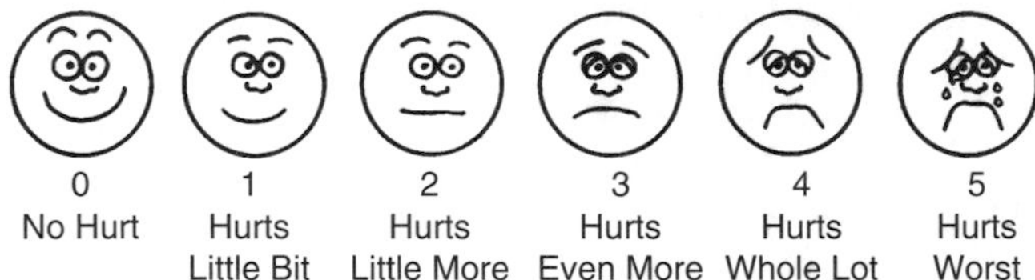

FIG 13-2 Wong-Baker FACES Pain Rating Scale. (From Wong DL and others: *Wong's essentials of pediatric nursing*, ed 7, St Louis, 2005, Mosby.)

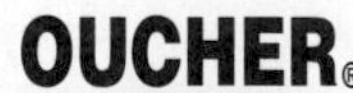

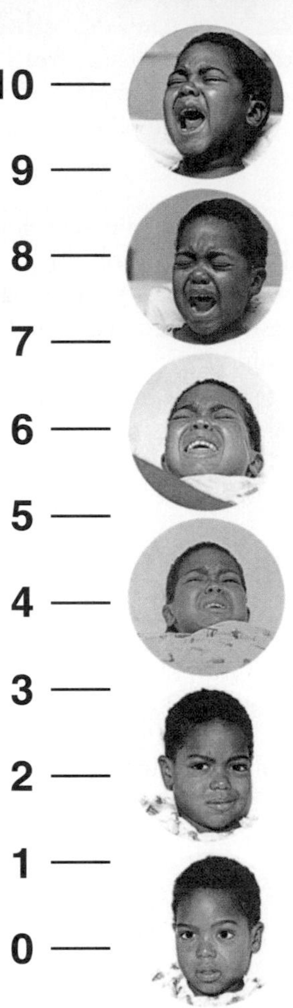

African-American

FIG 13-3 The Oucher Pain Scale. Hispanic and Caucasian versions are also available. (African-American version developed and copyrighted in 1990 by Mary J. Denyes, PhD, RN [Wayne State University], and Antonia M Villarruel, PhD, RN [University of Michigan]. Cornelia P. Porter, PhD, RN, and Charlotta Marshall, RN, MSN, contributed to the development of the scale).

someone who knows patient) may closely approximate patient's pain intensity.

10. Assess for presence of noise, temperature, or bright lights that may aggravate patient's pain perception or tolerance. *Rationale: Environmental factors may intensify perception of discomfort.*
11. Consider health care provider's orders regarding activity or positioning restrictions. *Rationale: Affects choices used in positioning and massage.*
12. Assess activities patient participates in at home that serve as distraction: patient's music preferences (vocal, instrumental, both), style of music (classical, jazz, other), and favorite artist; interactive activities (e.g., puzzles, board games); crochet or knitting; listening to relaxation tapes. *Rationale: Assists in selection of individualized music for relaxation. In older adults with dementia, music can be effective in reducing agitation (Park and Pringle Specht, 2009). Offering activities from home in the health care setting increases likelihood that patient will participate.*

PLANNING

Expected Outcomes focus on attaining comfort and pain relief and improving patient's ability to participate in routine activities.

1. Patient verbalizes full or partial relief from pain.
2. Patient expresses nonverbal behaviors suggesting relief of pain such as a relaxed face and absence of squinting.
3. Patient's function improves in sleep, appetite, physical activity (e.g., initiates walking) and personal relationships (e.g., interacts socially).

Delegation and Collaboration

Assessment of the patient's pain cannot be delegated to nursing assistive personnel (NAP). The skill of nonpharmacological pain management strategies may be delegated to NAP. Instruct the NAP to:

- Eliminate environmental conditions that enhance pain.
- Provide patient with appropriate rest periods.
- Adapt interventions based on any positioning or ambulation restrictions (e.g., administer massage in side-lying versus prone position).

Equipment

- Pain rating scale
- *Distraction:* Patient's preference (e.g., reading material, video game, puzzles)
- *Relaxation:* Patient's music preference for relaxation, using player, CD, or radio
- *Massage:* Lotion or oil (consider aroma therapy lotion), sheet, bath towel

IMPLEMENTATION *for* NONPHARMACOLOGICAL PAIN MANAGEMENT

STEPS	RATIONALE
1. See Standard Protocol (inside front cover).	
2. Prepare patient's environment. • Temperature suited to patient • Lighting • Sound • Eliminate unnecessary interruptions and coordinate care activities; allow for rest.	Temperature and sound extremes can enhance patient's perception of pain. Bright or very dim lighting can aggravate pain sensation. Fatigue increases pain perception.
3. Teach patient how to use pain rating scale (Box 13-3). Explain range of intensity scores and how they relate to measure of pain.	Accurate reporting by patient or family (surrogate) improves pain assessment and treatment.
4. Set pain-intensity goal with patient (when able).	Pain is unique to each individual. Patient sets individual goal for tolerable pain severity.
5. Give pain-relieving medications as ordered (see Skill 13.2) at least 30 minutes before a nonpharmacological intervention.	When analgesics reach their peak effect, other pain relief measures may be more effective.
6. Remove or reduce painful stimuli.	Reduction of the stimulation of pain and pressure receptors maximizes response to other pain relief measures.
a. Assist patient into comfortable position within normal body alignment. Reposition underlying tubes or equipment.	
b. Use pillows prn for alignment and support and to position off of pressure areas (see illustration).	Repositioning reduces strain on muscles and pressure areas, resulting in less stimulation of pain receptors.

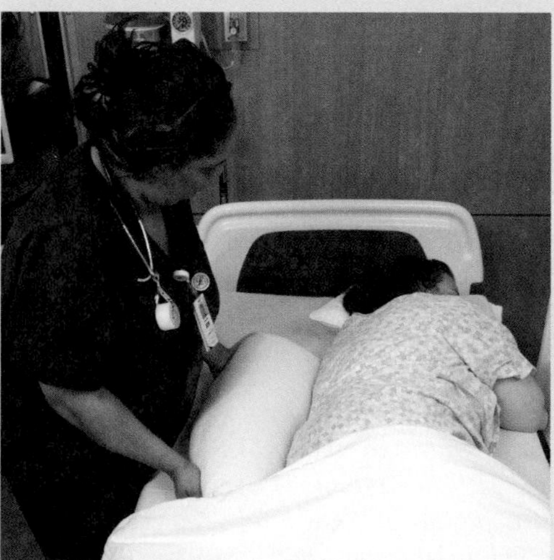

STEP 6b Positioning patient in side-lying lateral position for comfort.

BOX 13-3 TEACHING PATIENT AND FAMILY HOW TO USE A PAIN RATING SCALE

- Show and briefly explain available pain rating scales and ask which one the patient prefers. Offer vertical and horizontal scales as options.
- Explain the purpose of the scale: "This scale allows us to know the level of your pain and how it changes over time as we provide you comfort measures."
- Explain the parts of the scale (e.g., 0 means no pain, whereas 10 means the worst pain you can imagine).
- Discuss pain as a broad concept that is not restricted to a severe or intolerable sensation. Discomfort, hurt, and ache are also pain sensations.
- Verify that patient understands the concept of pain. Ask patient to give an example of pain experienced in the past.
- Ask patient to practice using the pain rating scale with present pain or select one of patient's examples. Also ask to rate worst and average pain in past 24 hours.
- Set mutual goals for comfort and function/recovery.

STEPS	RATIONALE
c. Smooth wrinkles in bed linens.	Reduces irritation to skin.
d. Loosen any constrictive bandage or device (e.g., blood pressure cuff, elastic bandages, band of elastic hose, intravenous (IV) dressing, and identification band).	Bandage or device encircling extremity may apply pressure and restrict circulation.
7. Reduce or eliminate emotional factors that increase the pain experience.	Fear or anxiety may cause muscle tension and vasoconstriction, which intensify the pain experience.
a. Offer information that reduces anxiety, (e.g., explaining the cause of pain if known).	
b. Offer patient opportunity to pray (if appropriate).	
c. Accept patient, and acknowledge patient's report of pain.	
d. Spend time to allow patient to talk about pain; answer questions and listen attentively. Ask, "What makes your pain feel better (or worse)?"	Conveys a sense of caring and interest in patient's welfare.
e. Answer call lights promptly.	Patients in pain expect caregivers to respond quickly when pain worsens.
8. Teach patient how to splint over the site of pain (e.g., using hand or pillow).	Splinting reduces pain by minimizing muscle movement.
a. Explain purpose of splinting.	Improves patient's ability to deep breathe, cough, and move.
b. Place pillow or a blanket over site of discomfort and then assist patient to place hands firmly over area (see illustration).	Splinting immobilizes painful area.

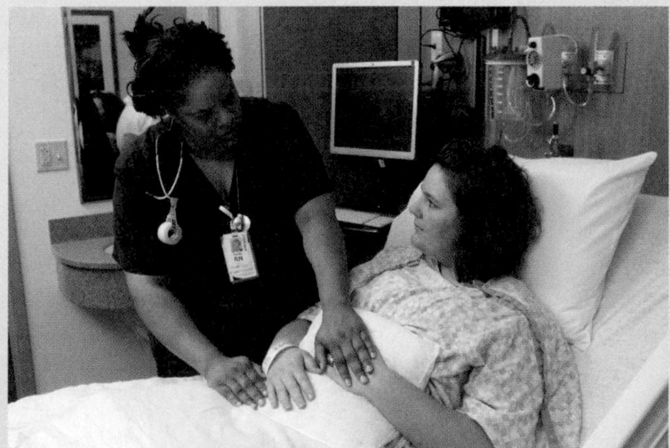

STEP 8b Patient splinting painful area.

STEPS	RATIONALE
c. Have patient hold area firmly while coughing, deep breathing, and turning.	Splinting decreases movement and subsequent pain during activity.
9. ***Massage***	
a. Place patient in comfortable position such as prone or side-lying. Have patients with breathing difficulties lie on side with head of bed elevated.	Enhances relaxation and exposes area to be massaged.
b. Turn on soft, pleasing music of patient's preference.	Promotes relaxation.
c. Drape patient to expose only the area that you will massage.	Maintains patient's privacy and warmth.
d. Be sure that patient is not allergic to lotion and then warm lotion in hands or basin of warm water. (NOTE: If you choose to massage head and scalp, defer use of lotion until completed.)	Warm lotion is soothing, and warmth helps to produce local muscle relaxation. Aroma therapy lotion used in hand massage has been shown to reduce pain and depression in terminal cancer hospice patients (Chang, 2008).
e. Choose stroke technique based on desired effect or body part.	Ensures fuller relaxation of body part.

Continued

STEPS	RATIONALE
SAFETY ALERT Patients who are heavily medicated or unable to communicate verbally need very gentle massage because they cannot inform the nurse if massage becomes uncomfortable.	
(1) Effleurage (see illustration): Massaging upward and outward from vertebral column, and back again	Gliding stroke, used without manipulating deep muscles, smoothes and extends muscles, increases nutrient absorption, and improves lymphatic and venous circulation.
(2) Pétrissage (see illustration)	Kneading tense muscle groups promotes relaxation and stimulates local circulation.
(3) Friction	Strong circular strokes bring blood to surface of skin, thereby increasing local circulation and loosening tight muscle groups.
f. Encourage patient to breathe slowly and deeply and relax during massage.	Potentiates effects of massage.
g. Standing behind patient, touch scalp and temples.	Avoids startling the patient.
h. Supporting patient's head, use friction to rub muscles at base of head.	Strong circular strokes stimulate local circulation and relaxation.
i. Massage hands and arms for 5 minutes as appropriate:	Releases tension in hands and arms. A brief hand massage has been show to reduce levels of stress in palliative care patients (Osaka and others, 2009).
(1) Support hand and apply friction to palm using both thumbs.	
(2) Support base of finger and work each finger in corkscrew-like motion.	
(3) Complete hand massage using effleurage strokes from fingertips to wrist.	
(4) Knead muscles of forearm and upper arm between thumb and forefinger.	Encourages relaxation; enhances circulation and venous return.
j. After determining that patient has no neck injury or condition that contraindicates neck manipulation, massage neck as appropriate.	Massage may be contraindicated after spinal cord injuries or surgery to head and neck because of risk of further injury.
(1) Place patient prone unless contraindicated.	Provides access to neck muscles.
(2) Knead each neck muscle gently between thumb and forefinger.	Reduces tension that often localizes in neck muscles.
k. Massage back as appropriate.	
(1) Keep patient in prone position unless contraindicated; side-lying is an option.	

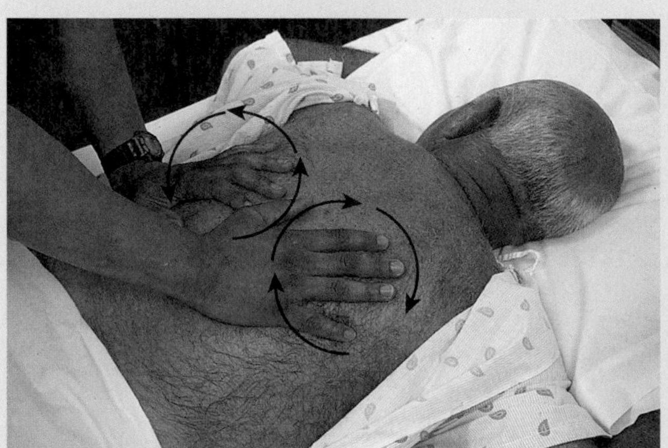

STEP 9e(1) Effleurage.

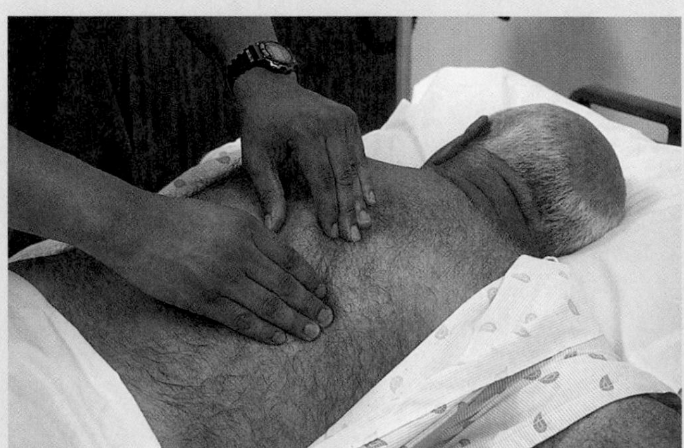

STEP 9e(2) Pétrissage.

STEPS	RATIONALE
(2) Do not allow hands to leave patient's skin.	Continuous contact with skin is soothing and stimulates circulation to tissues. Breaking contact with skin can startle patient.
(3) Apply hands first to sacral area; massage in circular motion. Stroke upward from buttocks to shoulders. Massage over scapulas with smooth, firm stroke. Continue in one smooth stroke to upper arms and laterally along sides of back down to iliac crest (see illustration). Continue massage pattern for 3 minutes.	General firm pressure applied to all muscle groups promotes relaxation.

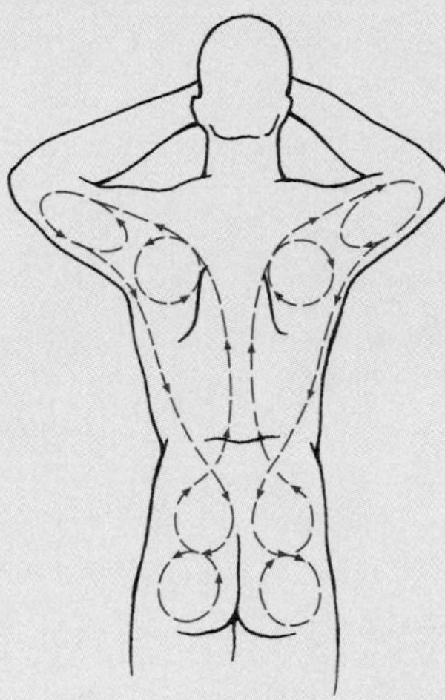

STEP 9k(3) Circular massage of the back.

STEPS	RATIONALE
(4) Use effleurage along muscles of spine in upward and outward motion.	Massage follows distribution of major muscle groups.
(5) Use pétrissage on muscles of each shoulder toward front of patient.	Area often tightens because of tension.
(6) Use palms in upward and outward circular motion from lower buttocks to neck.	Brings blood to surface of skin.
(7) Knead muscles of upper back and shoulder between thumb and forefinger.	These muscles are thick and can be massaged vigorously.
(8) Use both hands to knead muscles up one side of back and then the other side.	
(9) End massage with long, stroking effleurage movements.	Most soothing of massage movements.
l. Massage feet as appropriate.	
(1) Place patient supine; determine if patient is ticklish.	If patient is ticklish, massage may become a source of discomfort.
(2) Hold foot firmly. Support ankle with one hand or support sides of foot with each hand while performing massage.	Maintains joint stability during massage.
(3) Make circular motions with thumb and fingers around bones of ankle and top of foot.	Relaxes muscles.
(4) Trace space between tendons with firm finger pressure, moving from toe to ankle.	
(5) Massage sides and top of each toe. Use top of fist to make circular motions on bottom of foot.	
(6) Knead sides of foot between index finger and thumb.	

Continued

STEPS	RATIONALE
(7) End massage with firm, sweeping motions over top and bottom of foot.	Light strokes may tickle and be uncomfortable.
(8) If using lotion, wipe feet dry to prevent slipping when standing.	Reduces risk of fall.
m. Tell patient that you are ending massage. Ask patient to inhale deeply and exhale. Caution patient to move slowly after resting a few minutes.	Returns patient to a more awake and alert state. When deeply relaxed, patient may experience dizziness on arising too rapidly from postural hypotension.
n. Wipe excess oil or lotion from patient's back with towel.	Excess lotion or oil can irritate skin and cause breakdown.
10. ***Distraction***	Redirection of attention alters emotional or cognitive aspects of pain. The reticular activating system in the brain inhibits painful stimuli if a person receives sufficient or excessive sensory input.
a. Direct patient's attention away from pain.	
b. Use a distraction technique preferred by patient.	
(1) *Music:* Provide a music intervention session for approximately 30 minutes in a location where the patient spends majority of time. Set volume or loudness at a comfortable level. Emphasize listening to rhythm and adjust volume as pain increase or decreases. Offer earphones if desired.	Music produces an altered state of consciousness through sound, silence, space, and time.
(2) Prayer	This coping resource helps minimize physical and psychological symptoms of distress.
(3) Describing pictures or discussing pleasant memories	Reminiscing is an effective distraction, allowing patient to focus on pleasant experiences that were pain free.
11. See Completion Protocol (inside front cover).	

EVALUATION

1. Following an intervention, ask patient to use a pain rating scale (0 to 10) to rate comfort level. (NOTE: The Joint Commission [2009] requires reassessment of pain based on criteria set by agency [e.g., 60 to 90 minutes after intervention].)
2. Observe patient's facial expression, body language, position, mobility, and relaxation.
3. Ask patient to describe ability to rest, sleep, eat, and participate in usual activities.

Unexpected Outcomes and Related Interventions

1. Patient's pain intensity is greater than desired, patient describes worsening of pain, or patient displays nonverbal behavior reflecting pain.
   a. Perform a complete pain reassessment.
   b. Implement alternative nonpharmacological pain relief measures.
   c. Ask family members what might be helpful.
   d. Consult with health care provider about analgesic necessity.
2. Patient is not able to concentrate on pain relief techniques.
   a. Administer analgesics before nonpharmacological measure.
   b. Ensure that environment is conducive to technique.

Recording and Reporting

- Record findings of assessment, interventions, and patient's response to interventions in nurses' notes.
- Refer to agency policy regarding frequency of pain assessment.
- Report inadequate pain relief (not reaching goal), a reduction in patient function, and/or adverse effects from pain interventions (pharmacological and nonpharmacological). Box 13-4 lists suggestions for how to communicate with health care providers about pain.

BOX 13-4 NURSE-PHYSICIAN PAIN COMMUNICATION (SBAR FORMAT)

Situation: Give your name, state patient by name, describe the general nature of the call (e.g., patient's pain intensity increased following analgesic and use of positioning); report the most recent analgesic given, dose, and patient response.

Background: Summarize patient's medical diagnosis and condition pertinent to pain event (e.g., recently removed surgical dressing, up ambulating first time). Describe use of nonpharmacological measures and their effects.

Assessment: Report character of patient's pain, including current pain rating and effect of pain on patient behavior and activities.

Recommendation: Suggest a solution on the basis of a clinical practice guideline or your expertise.

Sample Documentation

0700 Patient rates pain in left shoulder at 6 (scale 0 to 10). Pain is intermittent and nonradiating. Grimaces during turning, holds shoulder when shifting position. Tylenol No. 3, 2 tablets PO given. Repositioned to R side. Back massage provided, with soft jazz music played per request.

0730 Rates shoulder pain at 4. Repositions self more easily.

Special Considerations

Pediatric

- Validity and reliability of pain rating scales generally increase with age. You can use some rating scales with a child as young as 3 years of age (Wilson and Helgadotter, 2006).
- Some children may not report pain because they may have misconceptions about the cause of their pain or fear the consequences (e.g., receiving an injection).
- Infants and children experience pain but may respond differently than adults. For example, they may cry and thrash about, have a shortened attention span, suck or rock, or be quiet and withdrawn. Others may become active when they are in pain. Variations in activity levels are related to the child's personality and development (Hockenberry and Wilson, 2007).
- Parents are helpful in providing pain relief through their presence and conversation and by holding and cuddling small children (Whitehead-Pleaux and others, 2006).
- Adapt distraction strategies to the developmental level of a child (e.g., using a pacifier for an infant, reading or playing a recording of a favorite story for a preschooler, playing music on a CD for a teenager). Play therapists are usually available in children's hospitals.

Geriatric

- Pain is not a natural part of aging. The presence of pain requires aggressive assessment, diagnosis, and management (Ebersole and others, 2008).
- Barriers to pain management in older adults include patient's fear of medication side effects, fear of being a "bad patient" if reporting or complaining about pain, and personal beliefs and experiences (Ebersole and others, 2008).
- Use terms other than pain such as hurt or pressure when assessing older adults because they may reserve the word pain for severe discomfort.
- Most forms of touch such as massage are pleasurable to older adults. Use with caution in patients with bone metastases or osteoporotic bones (Meiner and Lueckenotte, 2006).
- Reminiscence (e.g., sharing stories from the past) is an effective form of distraction in older adults.

Home Care

- Consider patient's home living conditions such as the type of bed and environmental stimuli. A supportive bed and quiet environment enhance sleep and promote pain management.
- Assess the pain management attitudes of family caregivers. Without family caregivers' participation, a patient may not achieve successful pain management.

PROCEDURAL GUIDELINE 13.1 Relaxation and Guided Imagery

Relaxation and guided imagery are mind-body therapies (MBTs) used by almost 17% of adults in the United States (Bertisch and others, 2009). MBT therapies are frequently used for anxiety/depression and musculoskeletal conditions. Approximately 50% of patients who use MBTs do so along with conventional medical treatment (Bertisch and others, 2009).

The ability to relax physically promotes mental relaxation. Relaxation techniques such as guided imagery and progressive relaxation exercises provide patients with self-control when pain occurs. Patients who use relaxation techniques sometimes achieve physiological and behavioral changes (e.g., decreased pulse, blood pressure, and muscle tension). For effective relaxation, the patient needs to participate and cooperate. Teach relaxation only when the patient is not in acute discomfort or severe pain and thus is able to concentrate. Explain the techniques in detail. It often takes several coaching sessions before patients effectively reduce pain. A patient can practice relaxation training at any time and usually with no side effects. Relaxation techniques are especially useful for arthritic pain, jaw relaxation, and relief of certain types of postoperative pain (Kwekkeboom and Gretarsdottir, 2006).

Guided imagery involves using focused concentration to effectively reduce pain perception and minimize reaction to pain. In guided imagery a patient draws on personal memories, dreams, and visions to create an image in the mind; concentrates on that image; and gradually becomes less aware of pain. The goal of imagery is to have the patient use one or several of the senses to create a desired image. This image creates a positive psycho-physiological response. You may use imagery with progressive relaxation or massage or as a distraction. For competence in guided imagery, certification is available nationally through the Academy for Guided Imagery.

Delegation and Collaboration

The assessment of the appropriateness of relaxation and guided imagery for patients cannot be delegated. The exercises of relaxation and guided imagery can be delegated to nursing assistive personnel (NAP). Instruct the NAP by:

Continued

PROCEDURAL GUIDELINE 13.1
Relaxation and Guided Imagery—cont'd

- Identifying and explaining which techniques work best for the patient.
- Making clear the expected patient response.
- Instructing to report a worsening of patient's pain.

Equipment

- Relaxation audiotape, tape player, or disk and DVD player

Procedural Steps

1. Assess character of patient's pain, including severity, to establish baseline (see Skill 13.1).
2. Assess facial expressions, verbal indications of discomfort or distress (e.g., grimacing, frowning, tone of voice), and body position and movement (e.g., restlessness, muscle tension) to establish baseline.
3. Assess character of patient's respirations to establish baseline.
4. Assess underlying probable cause of pain to determine if relaxation approaches are appropriate to use.
5. Site of pain may indicate specific types of pain relief measures.
6. Review health care provider orders (if required by agency).
7. Assess the type of image that patient would prefer to use in guided imagery to avoid using an image that could prove frightening.
8. Review any restrictions on patient's mobility or positioning.
9. Assess patient's willingness to receive nonpharmacological relief measure.
10. Assess patient's language level and identify descriptive terms that you will use when guiding patient through relaxation.
11. Administer an analgesic 30 minutes before implementing relaxation techniques so patient can gain a level of comfort needed to practice noninvasive approaches.
12. **See Standard Protocol (inside front cover).**
13. Explain purpose of each technique and what will be expected of patient during activity.
14. Plan time to perform technique when patient is able to concentrate and prepare patient's environment by controlling lighting and distractions from visitors or staff, keeping a comfortable room temperature for patient, closing curtains around patient's bed, or closing door.
15. *Progressive Relaxation*
    a. Have patient assume a comfortable sitting position (if tolerated) or one of patient's preference.
    b. Instruct patient to take several slow, deep diaphragmatic breaths. Avoid hyperventilation.
    c. Have patient close eyes, if desired.
    d. Have patient establish a regular breathing pattern; coach him or her to locate any area of muscle tension and alternate tightening and relaxing all muscle groups for 6 to 7 seconds, beginning at feet and working upward toward head.
        (1) Instruct patient to tighten muscles during inhalation and relax muscles during exhalation.
        (2) As each muscle group relaxes, ask patient to enjoy relaxed feeling and allow mind to drift and think how nice it is to be relaxed. Have patient breathe deeply.
        (3) Calmly explain during exercise that patient may feel sensations of tingling, heaviness, floating, or warmth as relaxation occurs.
        (4) Have patient continue slow deep breaths throughout exercise.
        (5) When finished, have patient inhale deeply, exhale, and then initially move about slowly after resting a few minutes.
16. *Deep Breathing*
    a. Instruct patient to sit comfortably with feet uncrossed. If patient is unable to sit, move to a supine position with small pillow under head.
    b. Place one of patient's hands on the chest and the other hand on the abdomen.
    c. Coach patient to inhale deeply through the nose, allowing the abdomen to rise and the hand to move outward.
    d. With the abdomen partially expanded, tell patient to continue to breathe and allow chest to expand, moving the upper hand outward.
    e. Pause for a few seconds. Then have patient exhale slowly through pursed lips to ensure slow, controlled, release of air. Repeat for 4 to 6 minutes.
17. *Guided Imagery*
    a. Direct patient through exercise.
        (1) Instruct patient to imagine that inhaled air is a ball of healing energy.
        (2) Have patient imagine that the inhaled air travels to his or her area of pain.
        (3) Alternatively select an image that patient would like to think about.
        (4) Have patient begin with slow deep breathing.
        (5) Suggest that patient think about going to a pleasant place (e.g., beach, field of flowers, top of mountain) to direct mental image toward a restful place.
        (6) Direct patient to experience all sensory aspects of the restful place (e.g., for beach: warm breeze, warm sand between toes, sound of surf hitting beach, water birds in background, smell of salt air).
        (7) Direct patient to continue deep, slow, rhythmic breathing to achieve relaxation.

PROCEDURAL GUIDELINE 13.1
Relaxation and Guided Imagery—cont'd

(8) Direct patient to count to three, inhale, and open eyes.
(9) End the experience. "Experience comfort and relaxation. When you open your eyes, you will feel alert and renewed. Breathe deeply. Be aware of where you are now; stretch gently; and, when you are ready, open your eyes." Suggest that patient move about slowly initially.

18. **See Completion Protocol (inside front cover).**
19. Observe character of patient's respirations, body position, facial expression, tone of voice, mood, mannerisms, and verbalization of discomfort.
20. Ask patient to rate pain on a pain scale 0 to 10.
21. Observe and ask patient to demonstrate relaxation technique at a time of low stress.

SKILL 13.2 PHARMACOLOGICAL PAIN MANAGEMENT

Analgesics are the most common and effective method of pain relief. However, undertreatment continues to be a problem because health care providers access incorrect drug information, have concerns about addiction, and have anxiety over errors in using opioids. Nursing judgment is critical in the safe use and management of analgesics to ensure the best approach for pain management.

There are three types of analgesics: (1) nonopioids, including acetaminophen (Tylenol) and nonsteroidal antiinflammatory drugs (NSAIDs); (2) opioids (traditionally called narcotics); and (3) adjuvants or coanalgesics (e.g., anticonvulsants, antidepressants, and muscle relaxants) that enhance analgesics or have analgesic properties. Common nonopioids include acetaminophen (Tylenol), aspirin (Ecotrin), and ibuprofen (Advil). Acetaminophen is used for mild pain and has no antiinflammatory or antiplatelet effects. It works peripherally on nerves and centrally on the brain. Its major side effect is liver toxicity. It is often combined with opioids (e.g., Percocet [oxycodone], hydrocodone [Vicodin]) for moderate pain relief because it reduces the dose of opioid needed for pain control. Nonselective NSAIDs such as aspirin and ibuprofen provide relief for mild-to-moderate acute intermittent pain such as headache or muscle strain. Treatment of mild-to-moderate postoperative pain usually begins with an NSAID unless contraindicated. NSAIDs do not depress the central nervous system (CNS), nor do they interfere with bowel or bladder function.

Opioid or opioid-like analgesics are generally prescribed for moderate-to-severe pain. The term *opioid* is preferred to *narcotic* because the word narcotic generally infers illegal use of substances. Common opioid analgesics include codeine, morphine, hydromorphone (Dilaudid), fentanyl, oxycodone, propoxyphene (Darvon), and other natural and synthetic medications. Meperidine (Demerol) is no longer a drug of choice because of its potential for causing seizures.

Opioid analgesics work on higher centers of the brain and spinal cord by binding with opiate receptors to modify pain perception. Opioids may cause some respiratory depression. It is important to note that sedation *always* occurs before respiratory depression. Patients receiving opioids can also experience side effects such as nausea, vomiting, constipation, and altered mental processes.

Except for constipation, these side effects usually stop once the patient has been receiving opioids around the clock (ATC) for 4 to 7 days. One way to maximize pain relief while minimizing drug toxicity is to give analgesics on a regular ATC basis rather than on an as-needed basis. ATC administration ensures a more constant blood level of analgesic. Patients receiving ATC opioids report lower pain intensity scores than patients receiving prn opioids.

Adjuvants or coanalgesics such as sedatives, anticonvulsants, steroids, antidepressants, antianxiety agents, and muscle relaxants have analgesic properties to enhance pain control. For example, corticosteroids relieve pain associated with inflammation and bone metastasis. Adjuvants also relieve symptoms associated with pain, including nausea, anxiety, and depression. Although adjuvants enhance pain control, they have *no* direct analgesic effect. Adjuvants are given alone or with analgesics, especially for treatment of chronic pain. Many adjuvants are more effective than opioids in relieving neuropathic pain. The drugs can cause drowsiness and impaired coordination. Do not automatically attribute these side effects to opioids. Always assess a patient carefully to determine the source of side effects.

The proper use of analgesics requires careful assessment and critical thinking in the application of pharmacological principles. Remember that each patient's response to an analgesic is highly individualized.

ASSESSMENT

1. Perform complete pain assessment (see Skill 13.1). *Rationale: Provides baseline for pain condition and assists in selection of type of analgesic to administer.*
2. Check physician or health care provider's orders against medication administration record (MAR) for name of medication(s), dosage, route, frequency of medication (prn or ATC). If the patient has a range order, one in which the dose varies over a prescribed range depending on patient's status, be sure that order follows agency policy (TJC, 2010). *Rationale: Ensures that right drug is administered to patient. Range orders offer flexibility to treat pain in a timely way while allowing for differences in patient response to analgesia.*

3. Consider the type of pain and the form of analgesic most suitable for patient's condition when conferring with health care provider (e.g., nonopioid analgesics or opioid combination drugs for mild-to-moderate pain; fentanyl patches, morphine, or hydromorphone for long-term management of severe pain; opioid and nonopioid analgesic for severe pain; sustained-release oral formulations ATC for chronic pain). *Rationale: Ensures that appropriate analgesic is selected for that specific patient's pain relief.*
4. Check last time medication was administered and dose, route, frequency, and degree of relief experienced. *Rationale: Determines if next dose can be administered and whether dose adjustment is necessary.*
5. Determine if patient has allergies to medications. *Rationale: Avoids possible allergic reaction to the analgesia.*
6. Assess patient's risk for using NSAIDs (e.g., history of GI bleeding or renal insufficiency) or opioids (e.g., history of obstructive or central sleep apnea). *Rationale: Presence of risk factors contraindicates NSAID use.*
7. Consider the duration of action of ordered analgesics. IV medications act quickly and can relieve severe acute pain within 1 hour; oral medications may take up to 2 hours for relief. Injectable medications generally act within 15 to 30 minutes. Immediate-release oral medications may take 1 hour to be effective, whereas some extended-release preparations may take as long as 2 hours to be effective. Oral analgesics usually have a longer duration of action than injectables. *Rationale: Allows for planning pain relief measures with patient activities, anticipating peak and duration of analgesic, and evaluating effectiveness of analgesic.*
8. Know the comparative potencies of analgesics in oral and injectable form. Refer to an equianalgesic chart. *Rationale: If nurses on succeeding shifts choose different routes for the same doses, the patient will not receive the same level of pain control.*

PLANNING

Expected Outcomes focus on elimination or reduction of pain and return to optimal functioning with minimal side effects.

1. Patient sets mutually agreeable pain intensity goal with health care providers.
2. Patient achieves comfort with a self-report of pain intensity at or below pain intensity goal.
3. Patient achieves comfort with reduction in pain behaviors (e.g., guarding, moaning, restlessness).
4. Patient is able to function adequately and perform ADLs (e.g., walking, working, eating, sleeping, interacting).
5. Patient does not experience intolerable or unmanageable adverse effects from the analgesic.

Delegation and Collaboration

The skill of analgesic administration cannot be delegated to nursing assistive personnel (NAP). Instruct the NAP by:

- Explaining the behaviors and physical changes associated with pain and to report their occurrence immediately.
- Reviewing comfort measures to use to support pain relief.

Equipment

- Prescribed medication
- Pain scale (0 to 10 range)
- Necessary administration device (see Chapters 22 and 23)
- Controlled substance record (for opioids only)

IMPLEMENTATION *for* PHARMACOLOGICAL PAIN MANAGEMENT

STEPS	RATIONALE
1. **See Standard Protocol (inside front cover).**	
2. Prepare selected analgesic, following "six rights" for administration of medications (see Chapter 21).	Ensures safe and appropriate medication administration.
3. Identify patient using two identifiers (e.g., name and birthday or name and account number, according to facility policy). Compare identifiers with information on patient's MAR or medical record.	Ensures that right patient receives analgesia. Complies with The Joint Commission standards and improves patient safety (TJC, 2010).
4. At the bedside compare the MAR or computer printout with the name of the medication on the medication label. Administer analgesic or adjuvant (see Chapters 22 and 23) following these guidelines:	Timely administration improves pain management. Final check of medication ensures that right patient receives right medication.

SAFETY ALERT If a patient is unable to swallow or has a gastrostomy or jejunostomy tube in place, remember that, with the exception of methadone, the extended-release opioid formulations may not be crushed for administration. Some capsules may be opened, and contents mixed in applesauce or other soft food; but they may not be crushed.

STEPS	RATIONALE
a. As soon as pain occurs	Pain is easier to prevent than to treat.
b. Before pain increases in severity	Higher levels of pain may not respond to ordered analgesic.

STEPS	RATIONALE
c. Before pain-producing procedures or activities	Reduces or blocks pain transmission in the CNS, allowing procedure to be completed with less discomfort.
d. Routinely, ATC	Maintains analgesic within therapeutic range ATC, reducing pain intensity and minimizing side effects. The ATC schedule avoids the low plasma concentrations that permit breakthrough pain.
5. Provide nonpharmacological comfort measures in addition to analgesics (see Skill 13.1 and Procedure Guideline 13.1).	Increases effectiveness of pharmacologic agents; treats nonphysiological aspects of pain.
6. Administer nursing care measures during times of peak effects of analgesics. Consider duration of action of analgesics when planning activities.	Effects vary depending on the type of medication used; allows for anticipation of next dose; permits evaluation of analgesic effects; maximizes effectiveness of nursing measures to prevent complications.
7. Monitor for adverse effects.	Anticipation of adverse effects leads to more timely intervention.

SAFETY ALERT Patients receiving ATC opioids should also receive stimulant laxatives. Opioids decrease intestinal propulsion (peristalsis) but not intestinal motility (churning); thus stool softeners alone are ineffective. Recommend stimulant laxatives.

8. See Completion Protocol (inside front cover).

EVALUATION

1. Ask patient to rate pain intensity using appropriate pain scale both at rest and with activity.
2. Evaluate PQRSTU aspects of pain, use nonverbal assessment if patient unable to respond (see Skill 13.1).
3. Observe patient's position; mobility; relaxation; and ability to rest, sleep, eat, and participate in usual activities.
4. Observe for adverse side effects of medications.

Unexpected Outcomes and Related Interventions

1. Patient reports that pain intensity is greater than desired and/or shows nonverbal behaviors reflecting pain.
   a. Evaluate the dose of medication administered.
   b. Try an alternative nonpharmacological intervention.
   c. Consult with health care provider if alternative analgesic or adjuvant can be given.
   d. Discomfort that is unrelieved or worse may indicate need for additional diagnostic, medical, or surgical intervention or a change in the pain management plan.
2. Patient develops respiratory depression.
   a. Give no additional dose of analgesic.
   b. Administer naloxone (Narcan) (0.4 mg diluted with 9 mL of saline) IV push at a rate of 0.5 mL every 2 minutes until the respiratory rate is greater than 8 breaths per minute with good depth.
   c. Continue to monitor vital signs, including pulse oximetry.

Recording and Reporting

- Record patient's pain rating (before and 30 minutes after medication), behavioral response to analgesic, and additional comfort measures given in nurses' notes. Incorporate pain relief techniques in nursing care plan.
- Record medication, dose, route, and time given in MAR.
- Report unsuccessful or untoward patient response to analgesics to health care provider.

Sample Documentation

0800 Morphine 5 mg IV push over 3 minutes for c/o low back pain, pain rated 7 on 0 to 10 scale that increases when sitting. Positioned on L side with legs supported. Back massage given. States pain decreased to a rating of 4 within 5 minutes of IV push med.

0830 States, "I feel better now; the pain is still there but less than before." Rates pain 4 (scale 0 to 10).

Special Considerations

Pediatric

- Children (except infants under 3 to 6 months of age) metabolize drugs more rapidly than adults; younger children may require higher doses of opioids to achieve the same analgesic effect (Hockenberry and Wilson, 2007).
- Children should not have to endure pain such as from intramuscular (IM) injections to achieve pain relief. Use the least traumatic route of administration.
- You can enhance the effectiveness of an analgesic by offering a supportive attitude toward a child. Reinforce the cause and effect of the analgesic; then you can condition the child to expect pain relief (provided the regimen is effective) (Hockenberry and Wilson, 2007).

Geriatric

- Generally opioids are not used enough with older adults. Start with a short-acting, low-dose analgesic and increase

dose slowly; but increase to the desired effect or to intolerable side effects. Use ATC whenever possible (Ebersole and others, 2008).
- Do not use meperidine at any age, and do not use propoxyphene hydrochloride in older adults (Willens, 2006) because of the risk of cardiovascular, CNS, renal, and/or liver toxicity.
- Avoid adjuvants with potent anticholinergic effects. Neuroleptics may have the least sedating, cardiotoxic, and hypotensive effects. Avoid tranquilizers that produce sedation and have a long half-life (Ebersole and others, 2008).
- Cognitive impairment or dementia affects some older adults' ability to report pain severity on a pain scale. Be alert for subtle behaviors that indicate pain (see Box 13-1).
- Avoid IM analgesic administration in older adults because IM injections hurt and because analgesic uptake from the muscle into the cardiovascular system is unpredictable.
- Avoid administering a combination of opioids.
- Because of renal and liver decline, maximum daily dosages of NSAIDs and acetaminophen may need to be lower.
- If an older adult is cognitively impaired and had a procedure that usually causes pain, consult with the health care provider about ordering an appropriate analgesic ATC instead of prn.

Home Care

- Family caregivers need to know how to observe and recognize pain in the person they care for and to accept and acknowledge patient's report of pain.
- Explain to family caregivers the importance of following ATC analgesic administration to maximize effect.
- Family caregivers who manage a patient's pain while at home need to have access to health care providers on a 24-hour basis.

SKILL 13.3 PATIENT-CONTROLLED ANALGESIA

Video Clips

Patient-controlled analgesia (PCA) is an interactive method of pain management that permits patient control over pain through self-administration of analgesics (ASPMN, 2006). It is a safe method of analgesic administration for acute and chronic pain, including conditions such as postoperative, traumatic, labor and delivery, sickle cell crisis, myocardial infarction, cancer, and end-of-life pain. A patient depresses the button on a PCA device to deliver a regulated dose of analgesic. Thus patients using PCA must be able to understand how, why, and when to self-administer medication and be able to physically depress the device (APS, 2008). Routes for PCA administration traditionally included subcutaneous and IV but now also include epidural, oral, and transdermal (Kastanias and others, 2006; Pasero and others, 2007). The transdermal route has been shown to be simpler, easier to use, and more satisfactory for nurses than IV PCA (Lindley and others, 2009).

More controversial is nurse-controlled analgesia, whereby the nurse caring for the patient depresses the button after first assessing the patient. This is called PCA by proxy. In addition, family-controlled analgesia (FCA) is used in children with cognitive or physical disabilities (ASPMN, 2006). In FCA one person is chosen as the patient's primary pain manager. In 2004 The Joint Commission issued a "sentinel event alert" on *unauthorized* PCA administration. Nurses must advise patients, family, and other visitors that PCA is for patient use only (TJC, 2004). PCA is not recommended in situations in which oral analgesics could easily manage pain (APS, 2008).

A PCA device may be electronic or nonelectronic and consists of an infusion device, a prefilled drug reservoir, and tubing that delivers the medication from the infuser through the patient-control module to tubing connected to the patient's IV line. PCA devices are individually programmed to automatically deliver a specific physician-prescribed continuous infusion (basal rate) of medication, a bolus dose (patient initiated), or both. The PCA prevents overdosing by having a preprogrammed delay time or "lockout" (usually 6 to 16 minutes) between patient-initiated doses. In addition, a prescriber may limit the total amount of opioid that the patient may receive in 1 to 4 hours. Use basal (continuous) infusions cautiously because studies have not shown superior analgesic benefit.

PCA has several advantages. It allows more constant serum levels of the opioid and thus avoids the peaks and troughs of a large bolus. Patients receive better pain relief and fewer side effects from opioids because blood levels are maintained at a level of minimum effective analgesia concentration for the individual. When used after surgery, fewer complications arise because earlier and easier ambulation occurs as a result of effective pain relief. Increased patient control and independence are other advantages. Because a PCA provides medication on demand as soon as the patient feels the need, the total amount of opioid use can be reduced. PCA allows the patient to manage pain with minimal nursing intervention. Since patients must be awake to push the device button to receive a dose, overdosing is less likely.

Concerns involving PCA use are patient related, pump failure, and operator errors. Patients may not understand how PCA therapy works, mistake the PCA button for a nurse call button, or have family members operate the demand button (ASPMN, 2006). The pump may fail to deliver drug on demand, have a faulty alarm, have a low battery, or lack free-flow protection. Operators may incorrectly program the dose, concentration, or rate. They also may fail to clamp or unclamp tubing, improperly load the syringe or cartridge, fail to monitor for side effects/overdose, or not respond to alarms. PCA requires careful, ongoing monitoring. Never try to operate a PCA without fully understanding the particular model in use.

ASSESSMENT

1. Check health care provider or physician's orders against medication administration record (MAR) for name of

medication, dosage, route, frequency of medication (continuous, demand, or both), and lockout settings. *This is the first check for accuracy.* Verify that patient is not allergic to prescribed medication. *Rationale: Ensures that right drug is administered to patient.*

> **SAFETY ALERT** Nausea is not an allergic reaction and can be treated. Itching alone is not an allergic reaction but is a common side effect of opioids. Itching is treatable and should not preclude use of PCA.

2. Assess patient's cognitive ability and physical ability to press device button. *Rationale: Determines appropriateness of patient to be able to use PCA for pain management.*
3. Assess nonverbal pain responses of cognitively impaired or non–English-speaking patients. *Rationale: Because patient cannot verbalize pain intensity, nonverbal responses help to determine the presence of pain and response to medication.*
4. Assess character of patient's pain, including behavioral and emotional signs and symptoms (see Skill 13.1). *Rationale: Establishes baseline to determine patient's response to analgesia.*
5. Assess environment for factors that heighten pain (e.g., noise, temperature of room). *Rationale: Elimination of irritating stimuli may be effective in further reducing pain perception.*
6. If patient has had surgery, apply clean gloves and inspect incision. Palpate gently around the area for tenderness. Use sterile gloves if placing hand on incision. *Rationale: Reveals nature of pain and provides a baseline to determine response to analgesia.*
7. Assess existing IV infusion line (peripheral or central) for patency and condition of venipuncture site for infiltration or inflammation. *Rationale: IV line must be patent with fluid infusing for medication to reach venous circulation safely and effectively. Never attach a PCA to an IV line with blood running or to IV lines with cardiovascular drugs infusing. If necessary, start another IV site.*
8. Assess if patient has history of sleep apnea. *Rationale: Opioid analgesia contributes significantly to risk of respiratory depression and airway obstruction in sleep apnea (Blake and others, 2009).*

PLANNING

Expected Outcomes focus on proper use of the PCA device and adequate pain control without oversedation and with no or manageable adverse effects.

1. Patient reports pain relief.
2. Patient exhibits relaxed facial expression and body position.
3. Patient correctly operates PCA device.
4. Patient remains alert and oriented.
5. Patient increasingly participates in self-care activities.

Delegation and Collaboration

The skill of PCA administration cannot be delegated to nursing assistive personnel (NAP). Instruct the NAP by:

- Explaining the signs of sedation and unrelieved pain to report to the nurse when they occur.
- Instructing personnel to report any new symptom or change in patient status to the nurse.
- Cautioning personnel to never administer a PCA dose for the patient (ASPMN, 2006).

Equipment

- PCA system and tubing
- Identification label and time tape (may already be attached and completed by pharmacy)
- Needleless connector
- Alcohol swab
- Adhesive tape
- Clean gloves (when applicable)
- Have opioid reversal agent (e.g., naloxone [Narcan]) closely available
- Equipment for vital signs and pulse oximetry

IMPLEMENTATION *for* PATIENT-CONTROLLED ANALGESIA

STEPS	RATIONALE
1. **See Standard Protocol (inside front cover).**	
2. Check the prepared analgesic, following "six rights" for administration of medications (see Chapter 21). NOTE: Pharmacy prepares cartridge.	Ensures safe and appropriate medication administration. *This is the second check for accuracy.*
3. Identify patient using two identifiers (e.g., name and birthday or name and account number, according to facility policy). Compare identifiers with information on patient's MAR or medical record.	Ensures correct patient. Complies with The Joint Commission standards and improves patient safety (TJC, 2010).
4. At the bedside compare the MAR or computer printout with the name of medication on the drug cartridge. Have a second registered nurse (RN) confirm prescriber's order and the correct setup of the PCA. The second RN should check the prescriber's order and the device independently and not just simply look at the first RN's setup.	*This is the third check for accuracy* and ensures that right patient receives right medication. Prevents medication error.

Continued

STEPS	RATIONALE
5. Before initiating analgesia, explain purpose of PCA and demonstrate function of PCA to patient and family, as follows:	Thorough explanation allows patient participation in care and independence in pain control. Preoperative education about PCA improves postoperative pain relief (ASPMN, 2006).
a. Explain type of medication in PCA device.	
b. Explain that device safely administers self-initiated small but frequent amounts of medication prn to provide comfort and minimize side effects from analgesia. Tell patient that self-dosing before repositioning, walking, or coughing and deep breathing will help in performing activities more easily.	Helps patient to understand the value of controlling pain. Small, frequent dosing with PCA produces constant serum drug levels with minimal fluctuation rather than peaks and troughs associated with prn analgesics (Lehne, 2007).
c. Explain that device is programmed to deliver ordered type and dose of pain medication, lockout interval, and 1- or 4-hour maximum dosage limit.	Confirms with patient the safety of a PCA device.
d. Demonstrate to patient how to push medication demand button on PCA unit. Explain that pressing the PCA button delivers a small dose of medication into the IV line, thus eliminating the need to wait for a nurse to draw up medication for a shot.	Gives patient control of pain.
e. Explain how the lockout time prevents overdose.	Relieves patient's fear of possible overdose.
f. Instruct patient to notify the nurse for possible side effects (be specific as to possible effects), problems in attaining pain relief, changes in severity or location of pain, alarm sounding, or questions that arise.	Ensures nurse's more timely response to developing problems.
6. Check infuser and patient-control module for accurate labeling or evidence of leaking.	Avoids medication error and injury to patient.
7. Program computerized PCA pump as ordered to deliver prescribed medication dose and lockout interval.	Ensures safe, therapeutic drug administration.
8. Position patient to ensure that venipuncture or central line site is accessible.	Ensures unimpeded flow of infusion.
9. Insert drug cartridge into infusion device (see illustration) and prime tubing.	Locks system and prevents air from infusing into IV tubing. Wearing gloves reduces potential contact with blood when working with IV line.
10. Attach needleless adapter to tubing adapter of PCA module.	Connects device with IV line.
11. Wipe injection port of main IV line with alcohol.	Alcohol is a topical antiseptic that minimizes entry of microorganisms during needle insertion.
12. Insert needleless adapter into injection port nearest patient.	Establishes route for medication to enter main IV line.
13. Secure connection with tape and anchor PCA tubing. Label PCA tubing and remove gloves.	Prevents dislodging of needleless adapter from port. Facilitates patient's ability to ambulate. Label prevents error from connecting tubing from different device to PCA (TJC, 2006).
14. Administer loading dose of analgesia as prescribed.	The nurse may manually give a one-time dose or program dose into PCA pump to establish a level of analgesia.
15. If patient is having pain, demonstrate use of PCA system (see illustration); if not, have patient repeat instructions given earlier.	Repeating instructions reinforces learning. Return demonstration reveals patient's understanding and ability to manipulate device.
16. To discontinue PCA:	
a. Obtain necessary PCA information from pump for documentation, including amount infused and amount to discard.	Ensures correct documentation of Schedule II drugs.

STEPS	RATIONALE
b.  Turn pump off.	
c. Disconnect PCA tubing from IV maintenance line but maintain IV access.	Ensures continued IV therapy.
d. Dispose of empty cartridge according to institutional policy.	Control and dispensation of opioids are regulated by the Controlled Substances Act.

SAFETY ALERT If PCA is discontinued before device is completely empty, record drug waste on PCA medication record per institutional policy. Note date, time, amount of drug wasted, and reason for waste. Waste must be witnessed and the record signed by two RNs to comply with documentation of Schedule II drugs.

17. See Completion Protocol (inside front cover).

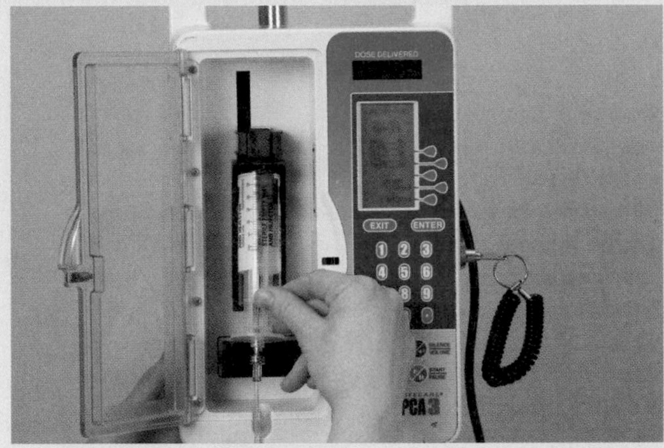

STEP 9 Nurse inserting drug cartridge into patient-controlled analgesia device.

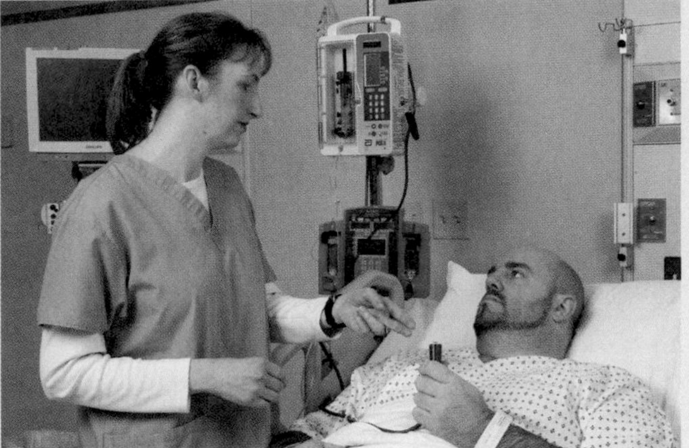

STEP 15 Patient learns how to press patient-controlled analgesia device button.

EVALUATION

1. Use pain rating scale to determine if pain intensity has decreased.
2. Monitor patient's level of sedation, vital signs, and pulse oximetry every 2 hours for the first 12 hours (APS, 2008).
3. Observe patient for signs of adverse reactions, especially excessive sedation (Box 13-5).
4. Have patient demonstrate dose delivery.
5. Evaluate number of attempts (number of times patient pushed the button) and delivery of demand doses (number of times drug actually given) and basal dose, if ordered, according to agency policy (usually every 4 to 8 hours). This maintains compliance with Controlled Substances Act.
6. Observe patient initiate self-care activities.

Unexpected Outcomes and Related Interventions

1. Patient verbalizes continued or worsening discomfort or displays nonverbal behaviors indicating pain.
   a. Perform complete pain reassessment.
   b. Evaluate number of attempts and deliveries initiated by patient.

BOX 13-5 MODIFIED RAMSAY SEDATION SCALE

LEVEL	STATUS
Minimal sedation (anxiolysis)	1. Anxious and agitated or restless or both
	2. Cooperative, oriented, and tranquil
Moderate sedation/ analgesia	3. Responds to commands spoken in normal voice
Deep sedation/ analgesia	4. Brisk response to a light forehead tap or loud auditory stimulus
	5. Sluggish response to light forehead tap or loud auditory stimulus
	6. No response to light forehead tap or loud auditory stimulus

From Sessler C and others: Evaluating and monitoring analgesia and sedation in the critical care unit, *Crit Care* 12(suppl 3):S2, 2008.

c. Evaluate for possible complications other than pain.
d. Inspect IV site for possible catheter occlusion or infiltration and check tubing for possible kinking.
e. Check that maintenance IV fluid is running continuously.
f. Evaluate pump for operational problems.
g. Check to see if patient manipulates PCA button correctly.
h. Use nonpharmacological comfort measures as appropriate.
i. Consult with physician or health care provider, who may need to adjust the dosage. Blood levels of analgesics need to remain stable to be effective. A continuous rate of administration may be needed to provide coverage during hours of sleep, the PCA dose may need to be increased, or an adjuvant may need to be added.

> **SAFETY ALERT** Do not increase demand or basal dose and decrease the interval time (e.g., from 10 to 5 minutes) simultaneously because this increases the risk for oversedation, respiratory depression, and other adverse effects.

2. Patient is sedated and not easily arousable.
   a. Stop PCA and elevate head of bed 30 degrees unless contraindicated.
   b. Instruct patient to take deep breaths.
   c. Notify health care provider.
   d. Apply ordered oxygen at 2 L/min via nasal cannula.
   e. Measure vital signs, including pulse oximetry.
   f. Evaluate amount of opioid delivered within past 4 to 8 hours.
   g. Ask family members if they depressed PCA button without patient knowledge.
   h. Review MAR for other possible sedating drugs.
   i. Prepare to administer opioid-reversing agent.
   j. Continue monitoring patient.
3. Patient is unable to manipulate PCA device.
   a. Consult with prescriber about alternative medication route and possible basal dose.
   b. Assess patient support system for family member who can responsibly manipulate PCA device (check agency policy) (ASPMN, 2006).

Recording and Reporting

- Record drug, concentration, dose (basal and/or demand), time started, lockout time, and amount of solution infused and remaining on appropriate medication form. Many institutions have a separate flow sheet for PCA documentation.
- Record assessment of patient's response to analgesic on PCA medication form, narrative notes, and/or patient assessment flow sheet (see agency policy).This includes vital signs, sedation status, pain rating, and status of vascular access device.
- Calculate infused dose by adding demand and continuous dose together. Follow agency policy.

Sample Documentation

1700 IV PCA with hydrocodone 0.5 mg/mL infusing at 5 mL/hr basal rate into L forearm. IV site without redness or swelling; dressing clean, dry, and occlusive. Dozing at intervals, arouses easily. Resp. 16/min, regular in rate, rhythm, and depth. C/O burning at abdominal incision 4 on 0-10 scale when turning. Reports no pain when lying still.

Special Considerations

Pediatric

- PCA is effective in children who can understand the concept. When selecting a child for PCA use, consider the developmental and cognitive level and motor skills. PCA is usually safe and effective for children beginning at 5 to 6 years of age (Hockenberry and Wilson, 2007).

Geriatric

- Older adults appear more sensitive to analgesic properties and side effects of opioids. Older adults' reduced renal and liver function slows opioid metabolism and excretion. This causes a faster peak effect and a longer duration of action of the opioid. Health care provider or physician's order should start with a low dose and titrate upward slowly.
- If an older adult becomes confused while using a PCA device, lower the dose, lengthen the lockout, or add a nonopioid analgesic to reduce the opioid dose. Nurse-activated ATC dosing is another option (ASPMN, 2006).

Home Care

- PCA should not be used in patients physically or cognitively unable to activate device. However, it is used commonly in patients under hospice care.
- Home care nurses should be available to patient and family members through regular telephone contact and scheduled nursing visits.
- Provide instruction regarding appropriate dosage adjustment and potential errors.
- Notify health care provider or physician if, after dosage adjustments, pain intensity remains unacceptable.

SKILL 13.4 EPIDURAL ANALGESIA

The administration of analgesics into the epidural space is a popular technique for managing acute pain during labor; following surgery; and for chronic pain, especially for patients with cancer. Studies have shown that patient-controlled epidural analgesia (PCEA) offers superior postoperative pain control after a variety of surgeries when compared with IV PCA (Cata and others, 2008; Ferguson and others, 2009; Popping and others, 2008). Use of PCEA is safe and efficient,

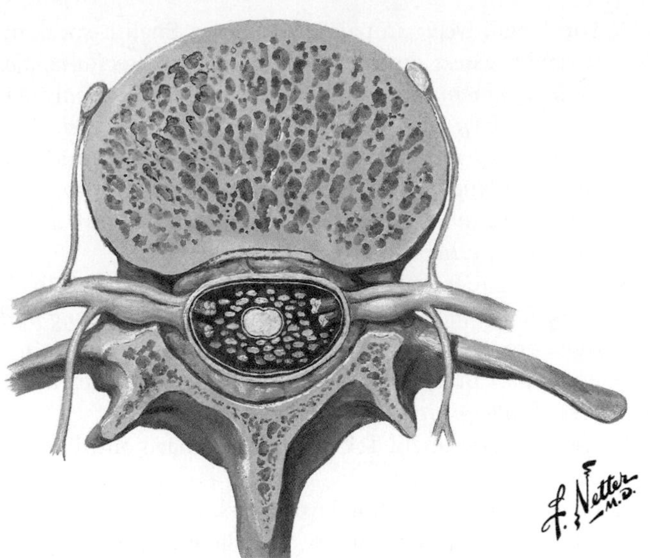
FIG 13-4 Anatomical drawing of epidural space.

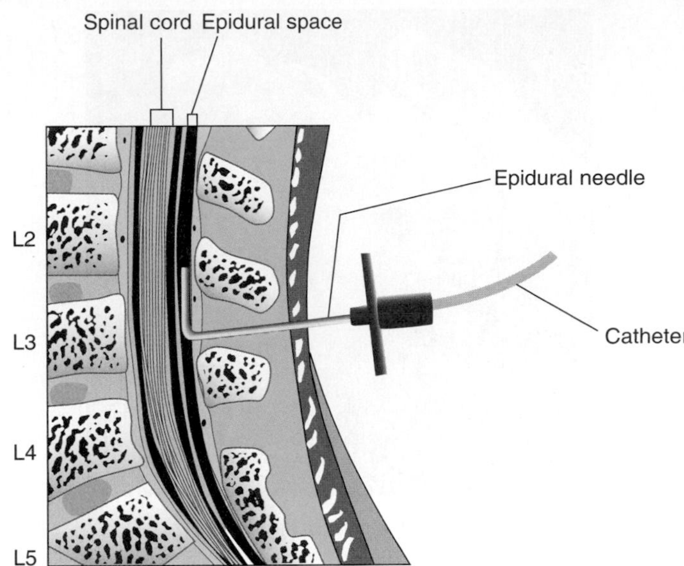

FIG 13-5 Placement of epidural catheter.

and complications of analgesic techniques are rare (Popping and others, 2008). Epidural opioids have reduced the total amount of opioids required to control pain, thus producing fewer side effects (Cata and others, 2008).

The epidural space is a potential space that contains a network of vessels, nerves, and fat located between the vertebral column and the dura mater, the outermost meninges covering the spinal cord (Fig. 13-4). Analgesics delivered into this space distribute (1) by diffusion through the dura mater into the cerebrospinal fluid (CSF), where they act directly on receptors in the dorsal horn of the spinal cord; (2) via blood vessels in the epidural space and deliver systemically; and/or (3) by absorption by fat in the epidural space, creating a depot where the drug is slowly released systemically. The analgesic acts by binding to opiate receptors in the dorsal horn of the spinal cord, thus blocking pain impulse transmission to the cerebral cortex.

Opioids and local anesthetics, separately or in combination, are used in epidural analgesia (Chang and others, 2006). Opioids are delivered close to their site of action (CNS) and thus require much smaller doses to achieve pain relief. Common opioids given epidurally include morphine, hydromorphone, fentanyl, and sufentanil. These opioids differ by their lipophilic "fat-loving" and hydrophilic "water-loving" properties that affect absorption rate and duration of action. Fentanyl and sufentanil are fat loving, causing them to have a quicker onset and shorter duration of action (2 hours). Morphine and hydromorphone are water loving, resulting in longer onset and duration of action (as long as 24 hours with a single bolus dose).

A physician places an epidural catheter with the patient placed in the lateral side-lying or sitting position with shoulders and hips in alignment and hips and head flexed. An anesthesia provider places a catheter in the epidural space below the second lumbar vertebra, where the spinal cord ends (Fig. 13-5). However, epidurals may also be placed at the thoracic level of the spinal cord. Catheters intended for temporary or short-term use are not sutured in place and exit from the insertion site on the back. A catheter intended for permanent or long-term use is "tunneled" subcutaneously and exits on the side of the body (Fig. 13-6) or on the abdomen. Tunneling reduces infection and catheter dislodgement. A sterile occlusive dressing covers the catheter exit site and is secured to the patient. An x-ray film is the only way to confirm an epidural catheter placement.

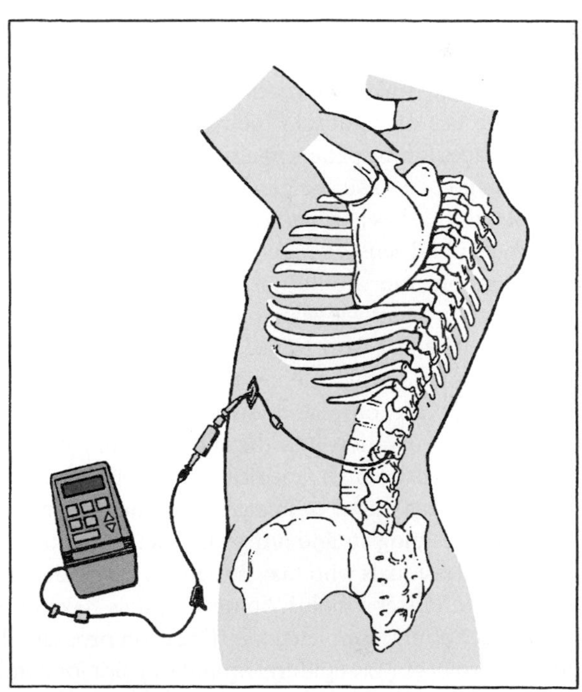
FIG 13-6 External epidural catheter attached to ambulatory infusion pump. (Courtesy SIMS Deltec, Inc., St Paul, Minn.)

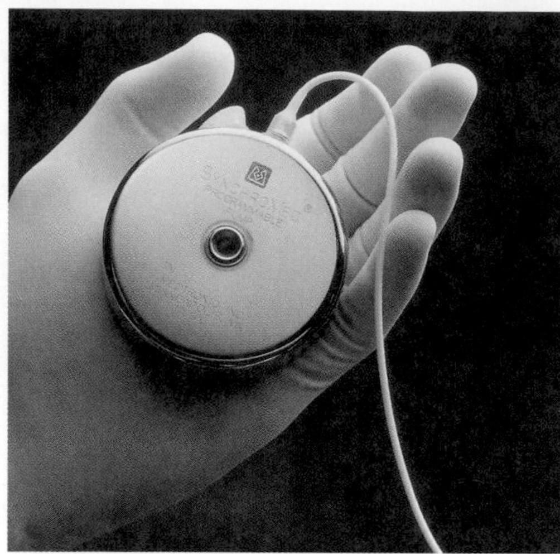

FIG 13-7 Synchromed implantable pump. (Courtesy Medtronic, Inc., Columbia Heights, Minn.)

A clinician administers epidural medication intermittently via bolus injection. Epidural medication is also administered by demand injection with a patient using PCEA or continuously via an implanted infusion pump (Fig. 13-7). An infusion pump injects opioids intermittently and continuously. Although the use of epidural opioids for pain control has many advantages for the patient, it also requires astute nursing observation and care. The analgesic affects spinal cord transmission below the level of catheter insertion. Monitor the patient's motor and sensory function, including any onset of urinary retention. You should not administer other supplemental opioids or sedatives when patients are on an epidural. The combined effect can cause respiratory depression. Because of its anatomical location, the epidural catheter can migrate through the dura and disrupt spinal nerves and vessels. Catheter migration into the subarachnoid space can produce dangerously high medication levels. You must monitor the patient's level of analgesia frequently. In many hospitals anesthesiologists and nurse anesthetists are the only health care professionals who may initiate an epidural opioid infusion or administer a bolus. Some hospitals have nurses who have successfully completed a certification program that enables them to begin the epidural opioid infusion or administer a bolus after the catheter has been placed (check agency policy).

ASSESSMENT

1. Assess level of patient's comfort and character of patient's pain (see Skill 13.1). *Rationale: Establishes baseline pain level.*
2. Assess presenting medical/surgical condition and appropriateness for epidural analgesia, (e.g., major abdominal or thoracic surgery, trauma, advanced cancer, women in labor, and patients predisposed to cardiopulmonary complications because of preexisting medical condition or surgery). *Rationale: Certain conditions may make epidural analgesia the treatment of choice.*
3. For cognitively impaired or non–English-speaking patients, assess nonverbal pain responses. *Rationale: Because patient cannot verbalize pain intensity, nonverbal responses help the nurse establish baseline pain level.*
4. Check to see if patient receives anticoagulants. *Rationale: Anticoagulation may contraindicate placement of epidural catheter because of the inability to apply pressure at the epidural insertion site and risk of bleeding.*
5. Assess if patient takes herbal medicines and, if so, which ones. *Rationale: Herbals may interfere with clotting and could predispose to bleeding at the epidural insertion site.*
6. Assess patient's history of drug allergies. *Rationale: Avoids possible allergic reaction to the analgesia.*
7. Assess environment for factors that may contribute to pain.
8. Assess patient's sedation level by assessing level of wakefulness or alertness, ability to follow commands, and drowsiness (see Box 13-5). *Rationale: Establishes a baseline before first dose. Sedation always precedes respiratory depression from opioids (Chang and others, 2006).*
9. Assess rate, pattern, and depth of respirations and blood pressure. *Rationale: Establishes baseline. Vasodilation can occur; and hypotension, including orthostatic hypotension, is common. Respiratory depression may also occur.*
10. Assess initial motor and sensory function (see Chapter 7). Test sensation in lower extremities. Have patients flex both feet and knees and raise each leg off the bed. Give special attention to patients with preexisting sensory or motor abnormalities. *Rationale: Establishes a baseline. Excess analgesia causes adverse neurological effects. Preexisting conditions may mask sensory/motor changes from analgesia.*
11. Check to see if epidural catheter is secured to patient's skin from the back, side, or front. *Rationale: Prevents accidental catheter dislodgement.*
12. Assess around catheter insertion site for redness, warmth, tenderness, swelling, and drainage. Apply sterile gloves if it is necessary to remove occlusive dressing. *Rationale: Establishes baseline. Local inflammation and superficial skin infection at insertion site can develop. Purulent drainage is a sign of infection. Clear drainage may indicate CSF leaking from punctured dura. Bloody drainage may indicate that catheter entered blood vessel.*
13. Check health care provider or physician's orders against MAR for name of medication, dosage, route, infusion method (bolus, continuous, or demand), and lockout settings. Verify that patient is not allergic to prescribed medication. *Rationale: Ensures that right drug is administered to patient. This is the first check for accuracy.*
14. If continuous infusion, check patency of IV tubing and check infusion pump for proper calibration and operation. Keep IV line patent until 24 hours after epidural analgesia has ended. *Rationale: Ensures that patient will obtain prescribed analgesic dose. Kinked tubing interrupts analgesic infusion. Patent IV line allows for IV access in case you need to give medications to counteract adverse reactions.*

PLANNING

Expected Outcomes focus on elimination or reduction of pain and prevention of complications of epidural analgesia.

1. Patient verbalizes pain relief within 30 to 60 minutes of initiation of epidural infusion.
2. Patient has no headache during epidural analgesia or as long as 72 hours after discontinuation.
3. Patient experiences no redness, warmth, exudate, tenderness, or swelling at catheter insertion site during time epidural catheter is in place. The patient is afebrile.
4. Patient's respirations are regular, of adequate depth, and equal to or greater than 8 breaths per minute.
5. Patient remains normotensive, and heart rate remains at or above patient's baseline.
6. Patient is easily awakened; alert; and oriented to person, place, and time.
7. Patient voids without difficulty; averages 30 to 60 mL per hour.
8. Patient has no or minimal pruritus and no paresthesias of lower extremities.
9. Epidural system remains intact and functioning.

Delegation and Collaboration

The skill of epidural analgesia administration cannot be delegated to nursing assistive personnel (NAP). Instruct the NAP to:

- Pay attention to the insertion site when repositioning or ambulating patients to prevent catheter disruption.
- Report any catheter disconnection immediately.
- Report immediately to the nurse any change in patient status or comfort level.

Equipment

- Clean gloves
- Prediluted preservative-free opioid as prescribed by health care provider or physician and prepared for use in IV infusion pump (usually prepared by pharmacy)
- Infusion pump and compatible tubing. (Do not use Y ports for continuous infusions; some infusion pumps have color-coded tubing for intraspinal use.)
- 20-gauge needless adapter
- Filter needle; per agency policy
- Antiinfective swab (e.g., povidone iodine or chlorhexidine)
- Syringe
- Tape
- Label (for injection port)
- Equipment for vital signs

IMPLEMENTATION *for* EPIDURAL ANALGESIA

STEPS	RATIONALE
1. **See Standard Protocol (inside front cover).**	
2. Prepare analgesic, following "six rights" for administration of medications (see Chapter 21). NOTE: Pharmacy prepares medication for pump. In the case of a bolus injection, draw up prediluted, preservative-free opioid solution through filter needle into syringe.	Ensures safe and appropriate medication administration. *This is the second check for accuracy.*
3. Identify patient using two identifiers (i.e., name and birthday or name and account number, according to facility policy). Compare identifiers with information on patient's medication administration record (MAR) or medical record.	Ensures correct patient. Complies with The Joint Commission standards and improves patient safety (TJC, 2010).
4. Explain purpose and function of epidural analgesia and expectations of patient during procedure (e.g., having patient call for assistance to get out of bed). Demonstrate to patient how to use pump on demand.	Proper explanation of therapy enhances patient cooperation.
5. Attach "epidural line" label to the epidural infusion tubing. Be sure that there are *no* Y *ports* for continuous or demand infusions.	Labeling helps to ensure that medication analgesic is administered into correct line and the epidural space. Labeling of high-risk catheters prevents connection with an inappropriate tube or catheter (TJC, 2009). Using tubing without Y ports prevents accidental injection or infusion of other medication.
6. At the bedside compare the MAR or computer printout with the name of medication on the drug container.	*This is the third check for accuracy* and ensures that the right patient receives right medication.

Continued

STEPS	RATIONALE
7. Administer epidural analgesic.	
a. ***Administer dose on demand.*** Refer to Skill 13.3 for preparation of patient and method of delivery.	Gives patient control over administration of analgesic.
b. ***Administer continuous infusion.***	
(1) Attach container of diluted preservative-free medication to infusion pump tubing and prime the tubing (see Chapter 23).	Tubing filled with solution and free of air bubbles avoids an air embolus.
(2) Insert tubing into infusion pump (see Chapter 23) and attach distal end of tubing to epidural catheter.	Pump propels fluid through tubing.
(3) Check infusion pump for proper calibration and operation. Many agencies have two nurses check settings.	Ensures that patient is receiving proper dosing.
(4) Tape all connections. Give ordered bolus or start infusion (see Chapter 23).	Taping maintains a secure closed system to prevent infection. A filter on tubing may be needed (check agency policy).
c. ***Administer bolus dose of analgesic.***	
(1) Take prepared syringe and change filter needle to regular 20-gauge needless adapter.	Prevents infusion of microscopic glass particles and allows medication to be injected.
(2) Clean injection cap of epidural catheter with antiinfective swab. **(Do not use alcohol.)**	Cleaning agent prevents introduction of microorganisms into CNS. Alcohol causes pain and is toxic to neural tissue.
(3) Dry the injection cap with sterile gauze.	Reduces possible injection of povidone-iodine.
(4) Insert needleless adapter of syringe into injection cap. Aspirate.	Aspiration performed to determine position of catheter. Should aspirate less than 1 mL of clear fluid.

SAFETY ALERT If you aspirate more than 1 mL of clear fluid or bloody return, catheter may have migrated into subarachnoid space or a blood vessel. Do not inject drug. Notify anesthesiologist or nurse anesthetist immediately.

STEPS	RATIONALE
(5) Inject opioid at a rate of 1 mL over 30 seconds.	Slow injection prevents patient discomfort by lowering the pressure exerted by fluid as it enters the epidural space.
(6) Remove syringe from injection cap. There is no need to flush with saline.	The catheter is in a space, not a blood vessel.
8. Explain that nurses will monitor patient's response to epidural analgesic routinely. Also instruct patient on signs or problems to report to nurse.	Builds trust to encourage patient to be a partner in care.
9. **See Completion Protocol (inside front cover).**	
10. Before removal of epidural catheter, check for presence of therapeutic coagulation. Check agency policy.	Removal of catheter while a patient is anti-coagulated increases the risk for spinal hematoma because of anticoagulation and inability to compress blood vessels.

EVALUATION

1. Evaluate patient's comfort level; use pain rating scale.
2. Evaluate sedation level; respiratory rate, rhythm, depth, and pattern; and pulse oximetry every 2 hours for 12 to 14 hours after a bolus of opioid is given to an opioid-naïve patient (one who has not received opioids on an ATC basis for more than 5 to 7 days). Closely monitor a patient who is not opioid naïve (see agency policy), is receiving a larger dose of opioid than usual, or has other risk factors (e.g., sleep apnea) (Pasero and others, 2007).

SAFETY ALERT Be prepared to deliver an ampule of naloxone 0.4 mg diluted in 9 mL of saline at 1 to 2 mL/min (for adults) if respirations fall below 8 breaths per minute and are shallow. Goal is to increase respirations, not reverse analgesia. Rapid reversal can cause serious side effects.

3. Monitor blood pressure and pulse. Assist patient when changing positions to avoid postural hypotension.
4. Evaluate catheter insertion site every 2 to 4 hours for redness, warmth, tenderness, swelling, or drainage (note

character of drainage [e.g., purulent, clear, or bloody]). Monitor body temperature.

5. Inspect site for disruption or displacement of catheter.
6. Evaluate for presence of headache and observe for nonverbal signs of headache.
7. Monitor intake and output. Evaluate for bladder distention (see Chapter 7). Observe for frequency or urgency. Consider consulting with health care provider or physician to order intermittent catheterization.
8. Observe for pruritus, especially of face, head, neck, and torso. Inform the patient that this is a side effect but is not an allergic response. Itching is most common side effect.
9. Evaluate for motor weakness or numbness and tingling of lower extremities (paresthesias). Have patient flex both feet and knees and then raise each leg off the bed. Ask patient if numbness or tingling is felt in lower extremities.
10. Assess patient for pharmacological side effects: nausea, vomiting, presence of tinnitus, or mouth numbness. Nausea may worsen by movement.

Unexpected Outcomes and Related Interventions

1. Patient states that pain is still present or has increased.
   a. Check all tubing, connections, medication doses, and pump settings.
   b. Confer with prescriber regarding adequacy of medication dose.
2. Patient is sedated or not easily arousable.
   a. Stop epidural infusion and elevate patient's head of bed 30 degrees (unless contraindicated).
   b. Prepare to give opioid-reversing agent per prescriber order.
   c. Monitor vital signs and sedation level continuously until patient is easily arousable.
3. Patient experiences periods of apnea; or respirations are fewer than 8 breaths per minute, shallow, or irregular.
   a. Instruct patient to take deep breaths.
   b. Stop or reduce rate of epidural infusion and notify physician.
   c. Prepare to give opioid-reversing agent (e.g., naloxone) per physician order.
   d. Monitor every 30 minutes until respirations are 8 or more and of adequate depth; continue for 2 hours, observing for return of respiratory depression. Naloxone has a shorter half-life than immediate-release opioids.
4. Patient reports sudden headache. Clear drainage is present on epidural dressing, or more than 1 mL of fluid can be aspirated from catheter.
   a. Stop infusion or bolus doses.
   b. Notify prescriber.
5. Blood is present on epidural dressing or can be aspirated from catheter.
   a. Stop infusion.
   b. Notify prescriber.
6. Redness, warmth, tenderness, swelling, or exudate is noted at catheter insertion site. Patient is febrile.
   a. Notify prescriber.
7. Patient experiences minimal urinary output, urinary frequency or urgency, bladder distention, pruritus, or nausea and vomiting.
   a. Consult with prescriber about reducing opioid dose and discuss treatment for side effects.

Recording and Reporting

- Record drug, dose, method (bolus, demand, or continuous), and time given (if injection) or time begun and ended (if continuous or demand infusion) on appropriate medication record. Specify concentration and diluent.
- With continuous or demand infusion, obtain and record pump readout hourly for first 24 hours after infusion begins and then every 4 hours. Review pump settings and usage with staff on next shift.
- Record regular periodic assessments of patient's status in nurses' notes or on appropriate flow sheet, including vital signs, intake and output, sedation level, pain severity score, neurological status, appearance of epidural site, presence or absence of adverse reactions to medication, and presence or absence of complications resulting from placement and maintenance of epidural catheter.
- Report any adverse reactions or complications to physician or health care provider.

Sample Documentation

0800 Fentanyl 2000 mcg in 500 mL 0.9 NS infusing at 15 mL/hr into epidural catheter via infusion pump. Respiratory rate 10 with moderate depth and regular pattern. States abdominal surgical pain is 5 compared with previous 7 at 0700.

1000 Respiratory rate 6 with shallow depth and periods of apnea, O_2 saturation 90%, HR 70, BP 110/70. Arouses with verbal stimulation. Anesthesia notified. Epidural infusion stopped, and Narcan 0.2 mg IV push given in titrated doses per Dr. Arnold's order.

1005 Respiratory rate 8, shallow depth, regular pattern, O_2 saturation 94%, HR 78, BP 118/72. Alert, awake, oriented ×3.

1020 Respiratory rate 12, moderate depth, regular pattern. HR 82, BP 124/78. Rates abdominal surgical incision pain 4 on 0 to 10 scale.

Special Considerations

Pediatric

- Apply EMLA cream to the epidural site a minimum of 60 minutes before catheter insertion to minimize discomfort from procedure.
- Epidural analgesia may be used in all pediatric age-groups; dose of analgesic is by milligram or microgram per kilogram.
- Epidural analgesia is used in infants and children for acute pain conditions (Hockenberry and Wilson, 2007).

- Infants and children require continuous cardiac, respiratory, and oxygen saturation monitoring.

Geriatric

- Because older adults often receive medications for hypertension, evaluating for hypotension during epidural analgesia is essential.

Home Care

- Patients who need home therapy are discharged with a tunneled catheter. Before considering catheter placement and care in the home, assess patient's fine motor skills, cognitive ability, stage of disease and prognosis, and degree of family caregiver involvement (Pasero and others, 2007).
- Teach patient and caregiver the proper dosage and technique for administrating medication. Assess patient's or family caregiver's technique for catheter care and administering medication. Reinforce instructions.
- Explain pain assessment using the pain scale. Observe family member assess patient's pain.
- Explain available drug and dosage for breakthrough pain. Inform patient how to contact clinician for increase in dosage if highest level prescribed is ineffective.
- Teach patient and caregiver aseptic technique for medication administration and for all catheter care procedures, including dressing changes. Instruct patient to change dressing every week (policy varies among home health agencies). Teach signs and symptoms of infection and signs and symptoms to report to nurse or health care provider or physician.
- Provide patient and family list of all supplies needed for procedures and where to purchase.
- Teach patient and caregiver about signs and symptoms of adverse reactions to medications and interventions used to treat side effects.
- *Pruritus:* Advise patient to wear clean, lightweight cotton clothing; keep room cool; use cool moist compresses; lubricate skin; and apply cornstarch.

SKILL 13.5 LOCAL ANESTHETIC INFUSION PUMP FOR ANALGESIA

During surgery for joint replacement, some surgeons inset a one-way catheter into the surgical site and attach it to an infusion pump (Fig. 13-8). The pump delivers a local anesthetic (e.g., bupivacaine [Marcaine], lidocaine, ropivacaine [Naropin], or mepivacaine [Carbocaine]) directly into the wound bed to provide pain relief to the surgical site. Patients may still require oral analgesics, but the total dosage is often reduced. The pump has a demand (4 to 6 mL per bolus) and a continuous rate (2 to 4 mL/hr) feature. Continuous-flow reservoirs hold 100 mL, whereas the patient-controlled units have a 60-mL reservoir. The device is for one-time use only and left in for about 48 hours. Rarely is the pump removed during hospitalization. Patients learn how to remove the catheter at home. Nursing care involves assessment of catheter connections, evaluation of local anesthetic side effects, and patient teaching.

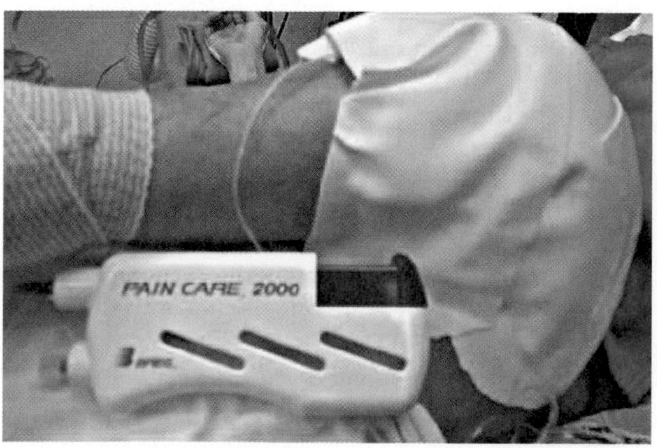

FIG 13-8 Local anesthetic infusion pump. (Courtesy Breg, Inc., Vista, Calif.)

ASSESSMENT

1. Apply clean gloves and assess surgical dressing and site of catheter insertion. Dressing should be dry and intact. *Rationale: Determines if catheter is placed properly.*
2. Assess catheter connections. If connections become detached, do NOT reattach; instead notify surgeon. *Rationale: Reattachment could lead to infection. Also, misconnection could lead to infusion of inappropriate agent into joint site.*
3. Perform complete pain assessment as for Skill 13.1, including type of activities influenced by pain (e.g., sleeping, eating, moving affected extremity). *Rationale: Provides baseline to determine efficacy of analgesia.*
4. Review surgeon's operative report for position of catheter. *Rationale: Confirms catheter location.*
5. Read label on device. *Rationale: Informs you about type of anesthetic, concentration, volume, flow rate, date and time prepared, and name of person who prepared it.*
6. Assess for blood backing up in tubing. If present, stop infusion and notify health care provider or physician. *Rationale: Indicates possible displacement of catheter into blood vessel.*
7. Determine the level of extremity activity patient can perform per health care provider or physician's order. *Rationale: Excessive activity may displace catheter.*
8. Assess for signs of local anesthetic toxicity: hypotension, dizziness, tremor, severe itching, swelling of the skin or throat, irregular heartbeat, palpitations, confusion, ringing in the ears, muscle twitching, numbness around the mouth, metallic taste, seizures. *Rationale: Early identification of toxicity prevents or lessens the possibility of complications.*

9. Assess patient's knowledge of infusion pump. *Rationale: Determines level of teaching and support required by the patient.*

PLANNING

Expected Outcomes focus on pain relief and improvement in patient's ability to resume activity.

1. Patient verbalizes full or partial pain relief from pain.
2. Patient achieves reduction of nonverbal pain behaviors such as grimacing, clenching teeth, or rocking.
3. Patient is free of adverse drug reactions.
4. Patient moves about in bed, sleeps and eats better, is more active, and communicates easily with family and friends.
5. Catheter is removed correctly without injury to patient.

Delegation and Collaboration

The skill of managing local infusion pump analgesia cannot be delegated to nursing assistive personnel (NAP). Instruct the NAP to:

- Pay close attention to the insertion site when providing care to avoid dislocation.
- Report to the nurse any catheter disconnection immediately.
- Notify the nurse immediately of a change in patient's status or level of comfort.

Equipment

- Pump in place from surgery

Home catheter removal

- Clean gloves
- Sterile 4 × 4–inch gauze pads
- Tape
- Plastic bag

IMPLEMENTATION *for* LOCAL ANESTHETIC INFUSION PUMP FOR ANALGESIA

STEPS	RATIONALE
1. **See Standard Protocol (inside front cover).**	
2. When repositioning or ambulating patient, use caution to avoid catheter dislodgement.	
3. Teach patient or family caregiver how to remove catheter (may also be done by home health nurse).	Prevents exposure to body fluids.
a. Instruct patient or family member to perform hand hygiene and apply clean gloves.	Reduces transmission of infection.
b. Have patient assume a relaxed position in bed or chair.	Relaxes joint muscles, reducing traction from muscle tension, and provides distraction.
c. Gently remove surgical dressing.	Provides access to infusion catheter.
d. Explain to patient what he or she will feel when removing the catheter.	Helping patient to anticipate nature of discomfort can relieve anxiety.
e. Place 4 × 4–inch gauze pad over site. Grasp catheter firmly and pull outward from skin with steady motion. If resistance occurs, stop pulling. If tubing continues to stretch and demonstrates resistance, stop pulling, cover area with sterile dressing, and notify surgeon.	Approach minimizes tissue trauma.
f. Look for mark on end of catheter tip.	Indicates complete removal of catheter.
g. After removing the catheter, place a new sterile gauze dressing over the area and apply pressure for at least 2 minutes.	Prevents hematoma formation.
h. Place catheter in plastic bag using standard precautions.	Patient is to bring catheter to physician's office on first visit.
4. Remind patient of follow-up appointment with surgeon.	Improves likelihood of patient adherence.
5. **See Completion Protocol (inside front cover).**	

EVALUATION

1. Ask patient to rate pain intensity using appropriate pain scale both at rest and with activity.
2. Observe patient's position; mobility; relaxation; and ability to rest, sleep, eat, and participate in usual activities.
3. Observe for signs of adverse drug reaction.
4. Inspect condition of surgical dressing.
5. During home visit inspect catheter exit site.

Unexpected Outcomes and Related Interventions

1. Dressing is moist and intact.
   a. Stop infusion and notify physician or health care provider. Catheter may not be placed properly or has been displaced.

2. Patient verbalizes pain intensity greater than previously determined goal or demonstrates nonverbal behaviors indicative of pain. Catheter may be displaced or clogged, or surgical site may be developing complications.
   a. Check reservoir for presence of medication.
   b. Check patency of tubing.
   c. Notify physician or health care provider.
3. Patient reports symptoms of local anesthetic adverse reaction.
   a. Stop pump and call surgeon immediately.

Recording and Reporting

- Record drug, concentration, date inserted, and type of demand feature (continuous or demand) in medication record.
- Record location of catheter, patient's pain rating, response to anesthetic, and additional comfort measures given in nurses' notes.
- Record additional analgesics necessary to control pain.
- Record any adverse reactions to local anesthetic.
- Report damp dressing, displaced catheter to surgeon.

Sample Documentation

1000 Returns from OR after right total knee replacement. Dressing dry and intact. Local anesthetic pump in place, catheter connections intact, receiving continuous 0.125% Marcaine infusion at 3 mL/hr. Patient currently rates knee pain at 3 (scale 0 to 10).

Special Considerations

Pediatric

- Local infusion pumps have been used for children undergoing certain types of orthopedic surgery. Explain to parents importance of not dislodging catheter.

Geriatric

- No special considerations are necessary unless patient is mentally compromised. Continuous dosing may be administered, but demand doses require a mentally competent adult.

Home Care

- If device is on demand (not continuous), instruct patient to depress button every 6 hours.
- Instruct patient to notify home health nurse or surgeon if pain meets or exceeds pain intensity goal.
- Have patient notify physician or health care provider if excessive fluid or bleeding on the dressing occurs.
- Provide written instructions regarding the possible adverse reactions to bupivacaine (Marcaine) that patient should report to surgeon immediately.
- Provide written and verbal instruction as to how and when to discontinue device when at home. Place catheter in a plastic bag and have patient bring it to first follow-up surgeon visit.
- Provide instructions regarding extremity movement.

REVIEW QUESTIONS

Case Study for Questions 1 and 2

Mrs. Salem has had chronic arthritis for over 5 years. When her pain reaches a level affecting her ability to perform ADLs such as cooking and grooming, she takes an NSAID for pain relief. Her joint pain usually involves a deep ache, and it limits her ROM. She does not always get complete relief from taking an analgesic, but it "lessens my pain so I can get around." She tries to avoid taking analgesics as much as she can because she knows the side effects of NSAIDs.

1. What factors make Mrs. Salem a good candidate for nonpharmacological pain therapy?
2. What advice would the nurse give Mrs. Salem to improve the likelihood of the NSAIDs providing pain relief?
3. A patient had a knee replacement performed 48 hours ago and has a local analgesia infusion pump with catheter in place. The nurse notes that the gauze dressing over the infusion catheter is damp and clear in color. What does this indicate?
   1. The patient is developing an infection at the surgical site.
   2. The infusion catheter has become dislodged and is leaking medication.
   3. Nothing; the patient is postop at 48 hours, and clear drainage is normal.
   4. The gauze dressing has become soiled from excess perspiration.
4. A nurse caring for a patient with Alzheimer's suspects that the patient is in pain. Unfortunately the patient's advanced stage of dementia prevents him from being able to verbally describe if something hurts. Which of the following will improve the nurse's ability to assess if the patient is in pain? Select all that apply.
   1. Assume that the patient is having pain and rule out any other problems such as constipation.
   2. Ask a family member to explain the location of the patient's pain.
   3. Observe the patient's facial expressions, body movements, and vocal noises.
   4. Conduct a physical examination, using gentle palpation to find the source of pain.
   5. Consult the last nurse's pain assessment and assume that the pain is unchanged.
5. A nurse is completing a massage for a patient and tells him to inhale deeply, exhale, and then move slowly as he sits up in bed. Why does the nurse end the massage in this manner?
   1. To prevent muscle cramping
   2. To prevent intravascular clotting
   3. To prevent a Valsalva maneuver
   4. To prevent postural hypotension

6. Review each of the clinical cases below and identify the patient most at risk for respiratory depression from opioid use.
   1. Respirations 20, deep; sedation level 1 at baseline. Respirations 14, shallow; sedation level 2 after analgesia.
   2. Respirations 18, deep; sedation level 2 at baseline. Respirations 12, deep; sedation level 4 after analgesia.
   3. Respirations 18, deep; sedation level 1 at baseline. Respirations 10, shallow; sedation level 4 after analgesia.
   4. Respirations 16, shallow; sedation level 2 at baseline. Respirations 12, shallow; sedation level 2 after analgesia.
7. A nurse would suspect bupivacaine (Marcaine) toxicity in a patient connected to a local infusion pump when observing which of the following symptoms:
   1. Hypotension, dizziness, and severe itching
   2. Reduced sensation in lower extremities, urinary urgency, and distended bladder
   3. Reduced respiratory rate and depth with increase in sedation level
   4. Orthostatic hypotension and tingling in extremities
8. The nurse enters the room of a patient who underwent major abdominal surgery in the morning. The patient's epidural catheter is intact, the dressing is dry, and the infusion pump is running at the ordered rate. The nurse finds the patient breathing shallowly at 8 breaths per minute and difficult to arouse. Which of the following steps should she take? Select all that apply.
   1. Try to arouse patient and have him take deep breaths.
   2. Check the infusion tubing to be sure that it is connected to the epidural catheter.
   3. Discuss with physician need for possible basal dose of analgesic.
   4. Prepare to administer naloxone per physician order.
   5. Stop or reduce rate of epidural infusion and notify physician.
9. Following the acronym PQRSTU allows the nurse to complete a comprehensive pain assessment. Fill in the blanks to describe each of the assessment parameters:
   P = ____________________
   Q = ____________________
   R = ____________________
   S = ____________________
   T = ____________________
   U = ____________________
10. The nurse is caring for a 71-year-old patient who had a recent stroke and suffers from expressive aphasia, the inability to express oneself verbally. He is found lying flat in bed with head slightly elevated. He acts irritable when the nurse awakens him. As he rolls onto his right side, he places his left hand over his abdomen. The nurse assesses the vital signs and finds HR 88 and regular, BP 134/88, and respirations 12 and deep. The patient's skin is slightly diaphoretic. The nurse suspects that he is in pain because of which factors? Select all that apply.
    1. Flat position with head raised.
    2. Irritability
    3. Respiratory rate
    4. Diaphoresis
    5. Placement of hand over abdomen

REFERENCES

American Pain Society (APS): *Analgesic use in the treatment of acute pain and cancer pain*, ed 6, Glenview, Ill, 2008, APS.

American Society for Pain Management Nursing (ASPMN): Patient-controlled analgesia: authorized agent-controlled analgesia: a position statement, *Pain Manag Nurs* 7(4):134, 2006.

Bertisch SM and others: Alternative mind-body therapies used by adults with medical conditions, *J Psychosom Res* 66(6):511, 2009. Epub Mar 3, 2009.

Blake DW and others: Postoperative analgesia and respiratory events in patients with symptoms of obstructive sleep apnea, *Anaesth Intensive Care* 37(5):720, 2009.

Cata J and others: Patient-controlled epidural analgesia (PCEA) for postoperative pain control after lumbar spine surgery, *J Neurosurg Anesthesiol* 20(4):256, 2008.

Chang K and others: Determination of patient-controlled epidural analgesic requirements, *Clin J Pain* 22(9):751, 2006.

Chang SY: Effects of aroma hand massage on pain, state anxiety and depression in hospice patients with terminal cancer, *Taehan Kanho Hakhoe Chi* 38(4):493, 2008.

Ebersole P and others: *Toward healthy aging*, ed 7, St Louis, 2008, Mosby.

Ferguson SE and others: A prospective randomized trial comparing patient-controlled epidural analgesia to patient-controlled intravenous analgesia on postoperative pain control and recovery after major open gynecologic cancer surgery, *Gynecol Oncol* 114(1):111, 2009.

Hadjistaviapoulos T and others: An interdisciplinary expert consensus statement on assessment of pain in older persons, *Clin J Pain* 23(suppl 1):S1, 2007.

Hockenberry MJ, Wilson D: *Wong's nursing care of infants and children*, ed 8, St Louis, 2007, Mosby.

Horgas AL and others: Assessing pain in persons with dementia: relationships among the noncommunicative patient's pain assessment instrument, self-report, and behavioral observations. *Pain Manag Nurs* 8(2):77, 2007.

Im EO and others: A national online forum on ethnic differences in cancer pain experience, *Nurs Res* 58(2):86, 2009.

Kastanias P and others: Patient-controlled oral analgesia: a low-tech solution in a high-tech world, *Pain Manag Nurs* 7(3):126, 2006.

Kwekkeboom KL, Gretarsdottir E: Systematic review of relaxation interventions for pain, *J Nurs Scholarsh* 38(3):269, 2006.

Lehne RA: *Pharmacology for nursing care*, ed 6, St Louis 2007, Saunders.

Lindley P and others: Comparison of postoperative pain management using two patient-controlled analgesia methods: nursing perspective, *J Adv Nurs* 65(7):1370, 2009.

Meiner SE, Lueckenotte AG: *Gerontologic nursing*, ed 3, St Louis, 2006, Mosby.

Osaka I and others: Endocrinological evaluations of brief hand massages in palliative care, *J Altern Complement Med* 15(9):981, 2009.

Park H, Pringle Specht JK: Effect of individualized music on agitation in individuals with dementia who live at home, *J Gerontol Nurs* 35(8):47, 2009.

Pasero C and others: Registered nurse management and monitoring of analgesia by catheter techniques: position statement, *Pain Manag Nurs* 8(2):48, 2007.

Popping DM and others: Effectiveness and safety of postoperative pain management: a survey of 18,925 consecutive patients between 1998 and 2006 (2nd revision): a database analysis of prospectively raised data, *Br J Anaesth* 101(6):832, 2008.

The Joint Commission (TJC) on Accreditation of Healthcare Organizations: Sentinel event alert: patient controlled analgesia by proxy, December 20, 2004; http://www.jointcommission.org/SentinelEvents/SentinelEventAlert/sea_33.htm.

The Joint Commission (TJC): Tubing misconnections, a persistent and potentially deadly occurrence, *Sentinel Event Alert*, issue 36, April 3, 2006, TJC.

The Joint Commission (TJC): Accreditation program: critical access hospital, 2009 National patient safety goals, http://www.jointcommission.org/PatientSafety/NationalPatientSafetyGoals/09_cah_npsgs.htm, accessed August 10, 2009.

The Joint Commission (TJC): *2010 National Patient Safety Goals*, Oakbrook Terrace, Ill, 2010, The Commission, http://www.jointcommission.org/PatientSafety/NationalPatientSafetyGoals/, accessed February 14, 2010.

Ware L and others: Evaluation of the revised FACES pain scale, verbal descriptor scale, numeric rating scale, and Iowa pain thermometer in older minority adults, *Pain Manag Nurs* 7(3):11, 2006.

Whitehead-Pleaux AM and others: The effects of music therapy on pediatric patients' pain and anxiety during donor site dressing changes, *J Music Ther* 43(2):136, 2006.

Willens J: Consumer group urges food and drug administration to ban drug Darvon, *Pain Manag Nurs* 7(2):43, 2006.

Wilson M, Helgadotter H: Patterns of pain and analgesic use in 3- to 7-year-old children after tonsillectomy, *Pain Manag Nurs* 7(4):159, 2006.

CHAPTER

14

Promoting Oxygenation

evolve WEBSITE

http://evolve.elsevier.com/Perry/nursinginterventions

Video Clips

Nursing Skills Online

The physiological need for air is one of Maslow's hierarchy of human needs. Respirations are effective when the body obtains sufficient oxygen at the cellular level and removes cellular waste and carbon dioxide via the bloodstream and lungs. When this system is interrupted such as by lung tissue damage, obstruction of airways by inflammation and excess mucus, or impairment of the mechanics of ventilation, intervention is required to achieve adequate oxygenation.

PATIENT-CENTERED CARE

When a person needs respiratory support, an artificial airway may be necessary. However, when an artificial airway is present, the patient is unable to speak. Many patients become stressed when they are unable to communicate with their health care providers and family members. Use positive verbal and nonverbal communication with direct eye contact and questions that only require yes or no responses. Alphabet charts, pen and paper, slates, or magnetic pen boards are examples of common communication tools (Coyer and others, 2007).

Encourage family members to be present for these patients because of feelings of loneliness, helplessness, and isolation. To alleviate these emotions use the following interventions: orient the patient to the day and time; place family photos and personal items within sight; and use music therapy, relaxation techniques, and prayer (Coyer and others, 2007; Wang and others, 2008).

SAFETY

Patients with impaired oxygenation require supplementary oxygen delivery (see Skill 14.1). When oxygen levels are low, patients are at risk for confusion and falls. Orienting the patient and instituting fall precautions are a must when this occurs. In addition, there are other safety risks when oxygen is in use in any health care setting or in the home (see Table 14-2).

Artificial airways require airway suctioning, which poses risks. The most serious relate to hypoxemia, which often result in cardiac dysrhythmias; laryngeal spasm; and bradycardia, which is associated with stimulation of the vagus nerve. In addition, risks related to insertion of the suction catheter include nasal trauma and bleeding (Pederson, 2009).

In most cases you will suction the oropharynx and trachea. Differences between oropharyngeal and tracheal airway suctioning are the depth of suctioning, sterile versus clean procedure, and the potential for complications. Oropharyngeal suctioning removes secretions from the back of the throat. When the secretions are only in the nose and mouth, only the oropharynx requires suctioning.

Tracheal airway suctioning removes secretions from the lower airway. In a health care setting, sterile procedures are usually necessary when suctioning extends into the lower airways. Suctioning removes respiratory secretions and maintains optimum ventilation and oxygenation in patients who are unable to remove these secretions. The frequency for suctioning depends on the patient assessment; some patients require suctioning every hour or two, and others require it only once or twice a day.

EVIDENCE-BASED PRACTICE TRENDS

Celik S, Kanan N: A current conflict: use of isotonic sodium chloride solution on endotracheal suctioning in critically ill patients, *Dimens Crit Care Nurs* 25(1):11, 2006.

Couchman B and others: Nursing care of the mechanically ventilated patient: what does the evidence say? Part One, *Intens Crit Care Nurs* 23:4, 2007.

Rauen CA and others: Seven evidence-based practice habits: putting some sacred cows out to pasture, *Crit Care Nurse* 28(2):98, 2008.

The routine use of normal saline instillation (NSI) into an airway prior to endotracheal (ET) and tracheostomy suctioning is no longer standard. Review of literature indicates that suctioning with or without isotonic normal saline (INS) produces similar amounts of secretions, significant decreases in oxygen saturation, and increases in heart rate for 4 to 5 minutes following the procedure. In addition, the level of a patient's dyspnea after suctioning with or without INS was not significantly different. NSI in conjunction with ET suction leads to the spread of microorganisms into the lower respiratory tract (Celik and Kanan, 2006; Couchman and others, 2007); Rauen and others, 2008). Normal saline is not effective in thinning secretions or improving removal of secretions (Rauen and others, 2008). Clinical studies comparing the results of suctioning using NSI with standard suctioning do not show any clinical or significant results (Celik and Kanan, 2006).

SKILL 14.1 OXYGEN ADMINISTRATION

- **Nursing Skills Online: Airway Management, Lesson 1**

Video Clips

Oxygen therapy supplies supplemental oxygen to prevent or relieve hypoxia. Hypoxia results from hypoxemia, which is a deficiency of oxygen in the arterial blood. Hypoxia occurs when there is insufficient oxygen to meet the metabolic needs of tissues and cells. Normal PaO_2 for an adult is 80 to 100 mm Hg. Supplemental oxygen is indicated when the partial pressure of oxygen (PaO_2) is less than 60 mm Hg or oxygen saturation (SpO_2) is less than 90% (Biddle, 2008). Supplemental oxygen is needed for temporary relief of hypoxia or long term, when it is required for a chronic condition (Eastwood and others, 2007).

Room air has an oxygen concentration, or fraction of inspired oxygen (FIO_2) of 21%. Supplemental oxygen delivery is based on the FIO_2 required to maintain adequate oxygenation (Table 14-1), whether hospital or home use, and the portability desired.

ASSESSMENT

1. Perform respiratory assessment (see Chapter 7). Assess for impaired gas exchange (hypoxia or hypercapnia), during both rest and activity, including the following:
   a. Observe for behavioral changes (e.g., apprehension, anxiety, decreased ability to concentrate, decreased level of consciousness, fatigue, and dizziness). *Rationale: Decreased levels of oxygen (hypoxia) or increased levels of carbon dioxide (hypercapnia) affect a person's cognitive abilities, interpersonal interactions, and mood (Biddle, 2008).*
   b. Obtain vital signs, including rate, rhythm, and depth of respirations and SpO_2 via pulse oximetry. *Rationale: Provides baseline of oxygenation status and enables early detection of hypoxia. In the presence of hypoxemia, the percent of hemoglobin saturated with oxygen declines, and the patient's pulse oximetry level declines.*
   c. Observe skin and mucosa for changes in color: pallor, cyanosis, or flushing. *Rationale: Pallor may occur when patient's oxygen levels decline. Cyanosis is a late sign of hypoxia. Flushing may be noted when hypercapnia is present.*
2. When available check arterial blood gas (ABG) or pulse oximetry results. *Rationale: ABG objectively quantifies changes in oxygen and carbon dioxide that affect acid-base balance.*
3. Observe for patent airway. *Rationale: Secretions obstruct airway and decrease the amount of oxygen that is available for gas exchange.*

PLANNING

Expected Outcomes focus on optimum oxygenation, safe application of oxygen therapy, and an understanding of and compliance with the oxygen prescription.

1. Patient's oxygen saturation (SpO_2) and/or ABGs return to or remain within normal limits or baseline levels.
2. Patient verbalizes improved comfort; subjective experiences of anxiety, fatigue, and breathlessness return to normal.
3. Patient's pulse, respirations, and color return to normal.
4. Patient is able to state the indications for supplemental oxygen by discharge.
5. Patient follows safety guidelines for supplemental oxygen therapy by discharge.
6. Patient uses supplemental oxygen as prescribed by discharge.

Delegation and Collaboration

- Assessment of the patient's condition and setup of oxygen therapy and liter flow cannot be delegated to

TABLE 14-1 OXYGEN DELIVERY SYSTEMS

DELIVERY SYSTEM	FIO_2* DELIVERED	ADVANTAGES	DISADVANTAGES
Nasal cannula	1-6 L/min: 24%-44%	Safe and simple Easily tolerated Effective for low concentrations Does not impede eating or talking Inexpensive, disposable	Unable to use with nasal obstruction Drying to mucous membranes Can dislodge easily May cause skin irritation or breakdown around ears or nares Patient's breathing pattern affects exact FIO_2
Oxymizer	1-15 L/min: 24%-60% (see Skill 14.1, Step 6d)	Higher concentrations without mask Releases O_2 only on inhalation Conserves O_2, increased portability Does not require humidification; however, may be used at flow rates of 6 L and up Two types available with nasal reservoir and pendant reservoir	Nasal reservoir type may interfere with drinking from cup Potential reservoir membrane failure
Simple mask	5-10 L/min: 30%-60%	Usually well tolerated.	Contraindicated for patients who retain CO_2 May induce feelings of claustrophobia Therapy interrupted with eating and drinking
Venturi mask	4-12 L/min: 24%-80%	Delivers exact preset FIO_2 despite patient's breathing pattern Does not dry mucous membranes Can be used to deliver humidity	Hot and confining; mask may irritate skin FIO_2 may be lowered if mask does not fit snugly Interferes with eating and talking
Partial rebreathing mask	6-12 L/min: 40%-70%	Delivers increased FIO_2 Easily humidifies O_2 Does not dry mucous membranes	Hot and confining; may irritate skin; tight seal necessary Interferes with eating and talking Bag may twist or kink; should not totally deflate
Nonrebreathing mask	6-15 L/min: 60%-80%	Delivers highest possible FIO_2 without intubation Does not dry mucous membranes	Requires tight seal; difficult to maintain and uncomfortable May irritate skin Bag should not totally deflate

*FIO_2, Fraction of inspired oxygen concentration. From Beattie, 2006; Biddle, 2008; Eastwood and others, 2007; Higginson and Jones, 2009.

nursing assistive personnel (NAP). However, the skill of nasal cannula or mask placement may be delegated. Instruct the NAP about the following:

- How to adapt the oxygen delivery device for a specific patient
- To immediately report to the nurse changes in vital signs or pulse oximetry, changes in patient's anxiety or behavior, or changes in skin color

Equipment

- Delivery device ordered by health care provider
- Oxygen tubing (consider extension tubing)
- Humidifier if indicated
- Sterile water for humidifier
- Oxygen source
- Oxygen flowmeter
- "Oxygen in use" sign

IMPLEMENTATION *for* OXYGEN ADMINISTRATION

STEPS	RATIONALE
1. **See Standard Protocol (inside front cover).**	
2. Identify patient using two identifiers (e.g., name and birthday or name and account number, according to facility policy). Compare identifiers with information on patient's medication administration record (MAR) or medical record.	Ensures correct patient. Complies with The Joint Commission standards and improves patient safety (TJC, 2010).
3. Attach delivery device (e.g., cannula, mask) to oxygen tubing. Consider using extension tubing for patients who are not confined to bed.	Extension tubing increases patient's ability to move about and assists in avoiding complications of bed rest.

> **SAFETY ALERT** Increase in extension tubing length may pose a fall risk for the older adult.

STEPS	RATIONALE
4. Attach tubing to appropriate flowmeter and humidified oxygen source (see illustration).	Humidity prevents nasal drying. Flowmeters with smaller calibrations may be safer for patients requiring low-dose oxygen when larger doses may be harmful, as in patients with chronic obstructive pulmonary disease (COPD) (McGloin, 2008).
5. Adjust oxygen flow rate to prescribed dosage. The oxygen flow rate is correct when the ball is at the middle of the mark. Verify that water is bubbling when using a humidifier.	Oxygen is a medication; correct dosage is required and must be prescribed by health care provider.
6. Observe for proper fit, function, and FiO_2 of delivery device.	
a. *Nasal cannula:* Place tips of cannula into patient's nares and adjust headband or plastic slide until cannula fits snugly and comfortably (see illustration).	Effective mechanism of oxygen delivery up to 6 L/min. Useful for low oxygen concentration for patients with chronic lung disease (Higginson and Jones, 2009).
b. *Venturi mask*: Oxygen delivered by turning barrel to preset intervals (see illustrations). Be sure setting matches prescribed dosage.	Delivers exact preset FiO_2 despite patient's breathing pattern.
c. *Partial rebreathing mask:* Mask seals tightly around mouth. Reservoir fills on exhalation and almost collapses on inhalation (see illustration).	Easily humidifies oxygen and does not dry mucous membranes. Useful for short-term therapy of 24 hours or less. Patient may not be able to tolerate the fit of the mask (Beattie, 2006).

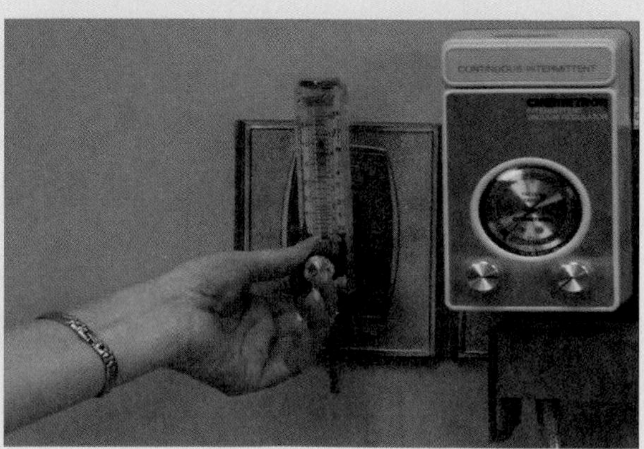
STEP 4 Flowmeter attached to oxygen source.

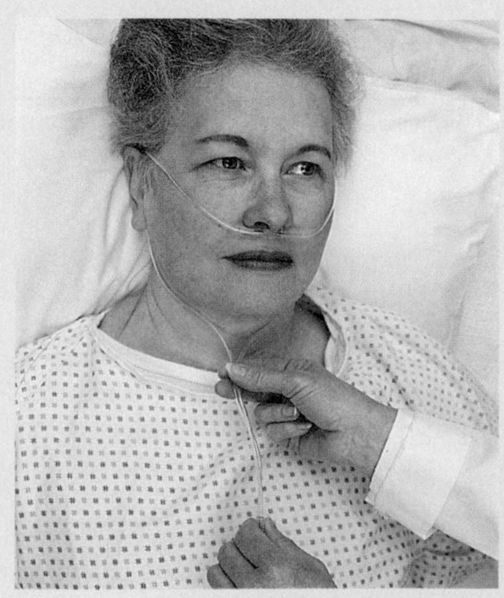
STEP 6a Nasal cannula adjusted for proper fit.

STEPS	RATIONALE
d. *Reservoir nasal cannula (Oxymizer):* Fit as for nasal cannula. Reservoir is located under nose or as a pendant.	Delivers higher flow of oxygen than cannula without changing to a mask, which is claustrophobic for some patients. Delivers a 2:1 ratio (e.g., 6-L nasal cannula is approximately equivalent to 3.5-L reservoir device or Oxymizer).

SAFETY ALERT Observe the reservoir bag to ensure that patient's inspiratory demands are being met. The bag should not collapse completely on inspiration.

STEPS	RATIONALE
e. *Nonrebreathing mask:* Contains one-way valves with a reservoir. Can be combined with a nasal cannula to provide higher FIO_2. A tight seal around the mouth is necessary to prevent room air from entering and decreasing the FIO_2. If a tight seal is required, a nasal cannula cannot be added.	Device of choice for short-term high FIO_2 delivery. Valve prevents exhaled air from entering the reservoir. Patient may not be able to tolerate mask (Beattie, 2006). A leak-free nonrebreathing mask with competent valves and enough flow (10 to 15 L/min) should deliver FIO_2 of 60% to 80% (Beattie, 2006).

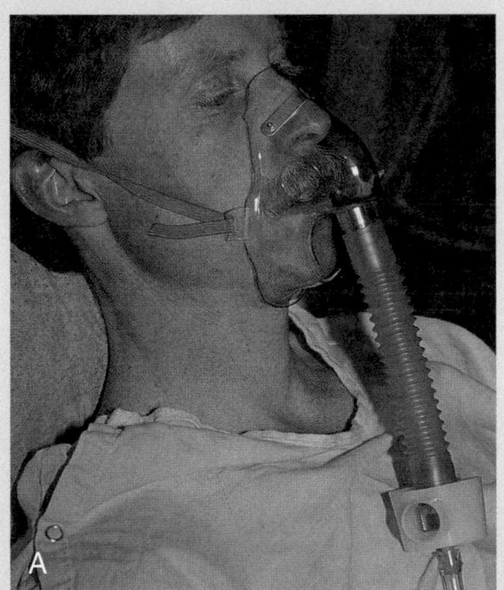

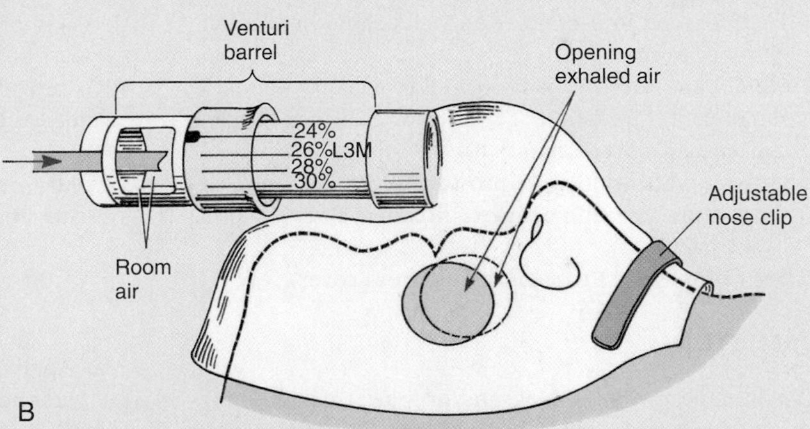

STEP 6b **A,** Venturi mask. **B,** Oxygen is delivered by turning barrel to preset intervals.

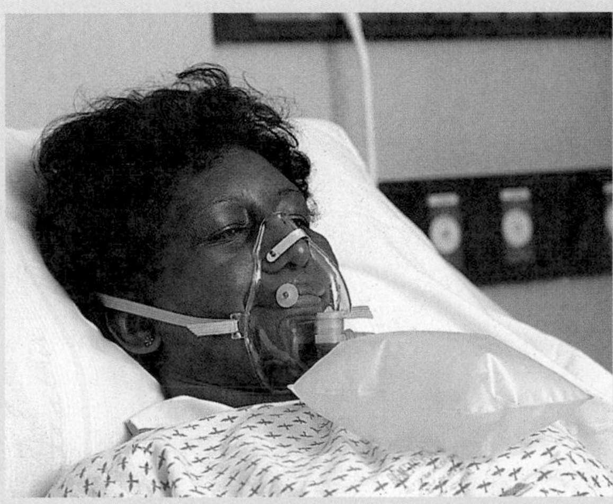

STEP 6c Partial rebreathing mask.

Continued

STEPS	RATIONALE
f. *Simple face mask:* Place securely over patient's nose and mouth (see illustration).	A simple face mask can deliver concentrations of 30% to 60% using flow rates of 5 to 10 L/min. It is a little easier to tolerate than other masks (Beattie, 2006).

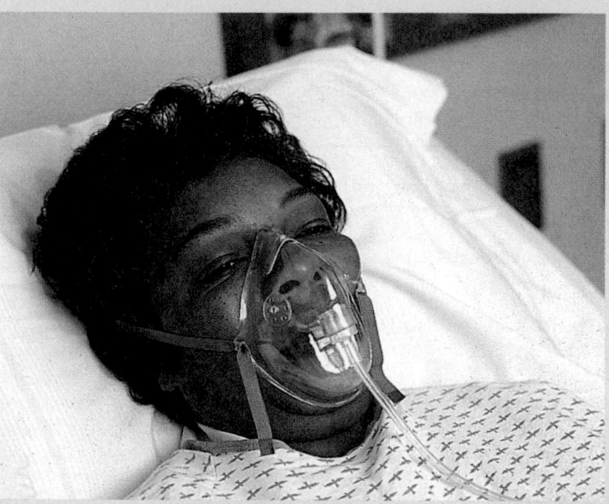
STEP 6f Simple face mask.

STEPS	RATIONALE
7. Post "Oxygen in use" signs on wall behind bed and at entrance to room.	Alerts visitors and care providers that oxygen is in use.
8. Obtain an order for ABGs or pulse oximetry 10 to 15 minutes after initiation of therapy or change in oxygen concentration (see Chapter 6).	ABGs provide objective data regarding blood oxygenation and acid-base status.
9. Consult with health care provider regarding the need for continuous pulse oximetry if patient's oxygen level is not stable.	Oximetry provides objective data regarding blood oxygenation and is used for trending.
10. **See Completion Protocol (inside front cover).**	

EVALUATION

1. Obtain repeat ABG values and/or pulse oximetry for objective measurement of improvement. Whenever possible obtain values both at rest and with activity.
2. Observe patient for decreased anxiety, improved level of consciousness and cognitive abilities, decreased fatigue, and absence of dizziness.
3. Monitor vital signs and pulse oximetry, if ordered; review ABG results. Expect a decreased pulse with regular rhythm, decreased respiratory rate, and improved color.
4. Observe use of accessory muscles.
5. Ask patient to verbalize indications for supplemental oxygen.
6. Observe if patient follows safety guidelines in present setting and ask patient to verbalize safety guidelines for home use.
7. Observe patient or caregiver demonstrate use of supplemental oxygen (Higginson and Jones, 2009).

Unexpected Outcomes and Related Interventions

1. Patient experiences skin and nasal irritation from cannula or mask, drying of nasal mucosa, sinus pain, or epistaxis.
   a. Apply a water-soluble lubricant to areas of irritation around nares.
   b. Recommend use of an isotonic saline nasal spray.
   c. Determine if a reservoir cannula is appropriate (decreased liter flow without reducing FIO_2, oxygen delivery on inspiration only); if so, obtain order.
   d. Consider humidification.
2. Patient has continued hypoxia: increased and/or irregular heart rate, SpO_2 declines.
   a. Monitor ABGs and/or pulse oximetry (see Chapter 6) and perform respiratory assessment.
   b. Notify health care provider.
   c. Identify methods to decrease oxygen demand (e.g., total bed rest, positioning).
3. Patient develops carbon dioxide retention with confusion, headache, decreased level of consciousness, flushing, somnolence, carbon dioxide narcosis, or respiratory arrest.
   a. Monitor ABGs and/or pulse oximetry.
   b. Notify health care provider of symptoms.
   c. Attempt to maintain PaO_2 at 55 mm Hg for patients with COPD. Hypoxia must be treated, but PaO_2 levels that exceed 60 to 70 mm Hg may worsen hypoventilation in patients with obstructive airway diseases (Eastwood and others, 2007).

Recording and Reporting

- Record the respiratory assessment findings: method of oxygen delivery and flow rate.
- Record and report patient's response and any adverse reactions.

Sample Documentation

0800 Alert and oriented. Respirations 20, regular rate, rhythm and depth noted and nonlabored. Lungs clear to auscultation. Mucous membranes pink. O_2 4 L/min nasal cannula. SpO_2 90%. Cough productive of yellow sputum. Fluids encouraged as tolerated.

1000 Reddened area noted behind right ear. Foam ear protector added to nasal cannula tubing.

Special Considerations

Pediatric

- Oxygen hoods are transparent enclosures that surround the head of the neonate or small infant and deliver continuous humidified oxygen. Larger "tents" are available for larger children.

Geriatric

- Decrease in PaO_2 that occurs with aging is about 0.3% per year. After age 75 healthy nonsmokers do not show a noticeable decline. The decrease in oxygen is related to the loss of elasticity in the lungs and the increase in physiological dead space.
- The drive to breathe in patients who have chronically increased CO_2 levels is based on their oxygen levels. Providing oxygen flow rates greater than 2 L/min may increase oxygen levels to a degree that would decrease spontaneous respirations.

Home Care

- Teach patient and family about the hazards of home oxygen and how to safely administer oxygen based on which system is selected for home use (see Chapter 32; Table 14-2).
- Stress the dangers of changing the oxygen flow rate from the prescribed flow.
- Teach patient and family signs and symptoms of hypoxia.

TABLE 14-2 OXYGEN SAFETY GUIDELINES

GUIDELINE	EXPLANATION
"Oxygen in use" sign is on patient's door.	Notifies all personnel of oxygen in patient's room.
Make sure that oxygen is set at prescribed rate.	Oxygen is a medication, and you should not adjust it without a health care provider's order.
Smoking is not permitted. Avoid electrical equipment that may result in sparks.	Oxygen supports combustion. Delivery systems and cylinders must be kept 10 feet from open flames and at least 5 feet from electrical equipment.
Store oxygen cylinders upright. Secure with chain or holder.	Prevents tipping and falling while stationary or when patient is being transported.
Check oxygen available in portable cylinders before transporting or ambulating patients.	Gauge on cylinder should register in green range, indicating that oxygen is available. Have backup supply available if level is low.

SKILL 14.2 AIRWAY MANAGEMENT: NONINVASIVE INTERVENTIONS

The airways must remain open and free of obstruction to decrease resistance of airflow to and from the lung. Positioning enhances airway patency in all patients. A high-Fowler's or semi-Fowler's position promotes chest expansion with the least amount of effort. A patient with COPD who is short of breath may gain relief by sitting with the back against a chair and rolling the head and shoulders forward or leaning over a bedside table while in bed.

Deep-breathing and coughing techniques help patients effectively clear their airways while maintaining their oxygen levels. Teach controlled coughing techniques described in this skill to assist patients to cough effectively and efficiently. There are devices to assist with secretion clearance such as vests that inflate with large volumes of air and vibrate the chest wall and handheld devices that assist in providing positive expiratory pressure to prevent airway collapse in exhalation (Garvey, 2005). Usefulness of these therapies depends on the individual patient situation and preference of both the patient and care provider.

Pharmacological management is essential for patients with respiratory disease. Medications such as bronchodilators effectively relax smooth muscles and open airways in certain disease processes such as asthma. Glucocorticoids relieve inflammation and also assist in opening air passages. Mucolytics and adequate hydration decrease the thickness of pulmonary secretions so they are easily expectorated.

Patients with obstructive sleep apnea (OSA) are often unable to maintain a patent airway. In OSA nasopharyngeal abnormalities that cause narrowing of the upper airway produce repetitive airway obstruction during sleep, with the potential for periods of apnea, carbon dioxide retention, and hypoxemia. Continuous positive airway pressure (CPAP) or bi-level positive airway pressure (BiPAP) delivers pressurized oxygen by mask to reduce carbon dioxide levels. The mask delivers pressure during the inspiratory and expiratory phases of the respiratory cycle to maintain airway patency. The use of this device is individualized and requires assessment of each patient's ability of use the equipment as instructed (Barnes, 2007).

ASSESSMENT

1. Assess patient's work of breathing, sense of breathlessness, and ability to clear copious or tenacious secretions by coughing. *Rationale: Indicates risk for impaired airway clearance. Secretions can plug the airway, decreasing the amount of oxygen available for gas exchange in the lung.*
2. Auscultate lung sounds for adventitious sounds (see Chapter 7). *Rationale: Decreased lung sounds can indicate plugging of the airway from mucus rather than an improvement in condition. Adventitious sounds indicate obstructed air flow; these sounds result from bronchospasm, laryngospasm, or mucus.*
3. Observe for shortness of breath, use of accessory muscles of respiration, pallor, or cyanosis. *Rationale: Indicators of respiratory distress from decreased oxygenation levels.*
4. Monitor patient's vital signs and SpO_2 with oximetry or collect ABGs. *Rationale: Establishes baseline for determining response to therapy.*
5. Ask about interrupted sleep, snoring respirations. Ask patient about history of sleep apnea. *Rationale: Indications for use of CPAP or BiPAP. Refer patient for evaluation.*

PLANNING

Expected Outcomes focus on patient's airway patency, comfort, and ability for self-care.

- Patient maintains a position that promotes maximum lung expansion and comfort.
- Patient's airways are clear of retained secretions.
- Patient's periods of sleep apnea are reduced to fewer than two episodes in 6 hours.
- Patient's ABGs and pulse oximetry readings improve or remain normal.

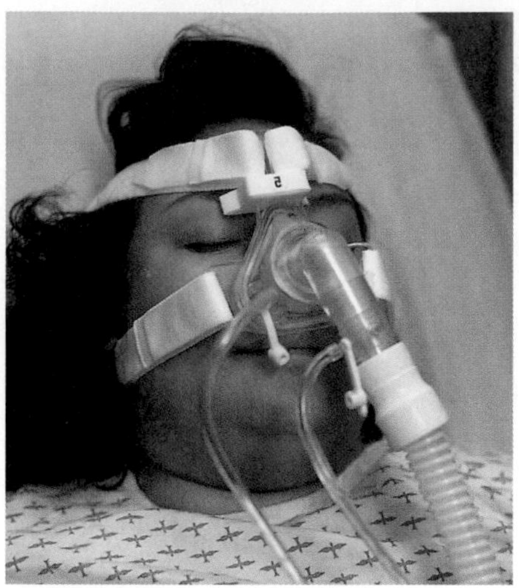

FIG 14-1 CPAP mask/BiPAP mask.

- Patient and family demonstrate correct use of CPAP/BiPAP and express comfort using equipment by discharge.

Delegation and Collaboration

Assessment of patient's condition cannot be delegated. The skills of positioning, therapeutic coughing, and CPAP/BiPAP mask application can be delegated to nursing assistive personnel (NAP). Instruct the NAP to:

- Immediately report to the nurse the patient's difficulty breathing or any change in vital signs, pulse oximetry, skin color, or behavior.

Equipment

- CPAP or BiPAP mask (Fig. 14-1) (NOTE: Several types of masks are available because of the difficulties in achieving a comfortable fit.)
- Mask straps (face or nasal)
- Valve (CPAP or BiPAP)
- Oxygen source
- Generator (CPAP or BiPAP)
- Appropriate signs

IMPLEMENTATION *for* AIRWAY MANAGEMENT: NONINVASIVE INTERVENTIONS

STEPS	RATIONALE
1. **See Standard Protocol (inside front cover).**	
2. Explain to patient that you are aware of the discomfort he or she is experiencing (e.g., breathlessness, pain) and that correct positioning is necessary.	
a. *Sitting:* Assist to semi-Fowler's or high Fowler's, sitting on side of bed or in chair with elbows resting on knees. Patients with COPD may benefit from leaning over table with arms propped up (see illustrations).	Promotes optimum lung expansion and maximizes use of accessory muscles. Decreases patient's work of breathing.

STEPS	RATIONALE

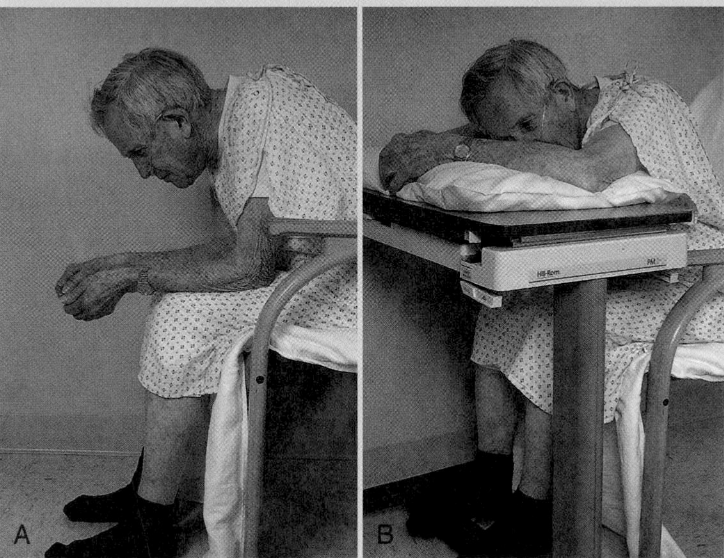

STEP 2a A, Positioning optimizes chest expansion and reduces the work of breathing. **B,** Leaning position allows lungs to expand.

STEPS	RATIONALE
b. *Leaning:* Have patient lean forward over the back of a chair or against the wall.	Leaning forward allows the lungs to expand with less transdiaphragmatic pressure.
c. *Supine:* Most patients are more comfortable supported by two pillows or with the head of the bed up at least 30 degrees.	Decreases orthopnea. Obese patients may experience increased abdominal interference of full lung expansion when lying flat.
d. *Turning*: Turn at least every 2 hours. Turn to drain areas of lungs with retained secretions by gravity if tolerated by patient. If unilateral reexpansion is needed (e.g., after general surgery), have patient lie with side requiring expansion up: "good side down, affected lung up."	Encourages drainage of secretions and promotes lung expansion on the affected side. Promotes gas exchange by increasing blood flow to area of greater surface area available for gas exchange.
3. Controlled coughing	
a. Place patient in upright position, high-Fowler's, leaning forward, or with knees bent and a small pillow or hand to support the abdomen.	Facilitates inhalation and lung expansion during coughing maneuver. May augment expiratory pressure.
b. Instruct patient to take two slow, deep breaths, inhaling through the nose and exhaling through the mouth.	Control of respiratory rate facilitates coughing and minimizes risk of paroxysms of coughing.
c. Instruct patient to inhale deeply a third time, hold this breath, and count to three; then to cough deeply for two or three consecutive coughs without inhaling between coughs. Instruct patient to push air forcefully out of the lungs.	Ensures full, effective cough. Explain to patient that controlled coughing clears secretions that may obstruct the airway by allowing air behind the mucus to move during the cough.
d. Have patients with difficulty coughing use a "huff" cough by taking a medium breath and then making a sound like "ha" to push the air out fast with their mouth slightly open. Repeat three or four times and then instruct patient to cough.	Assists patients to generate more pressure to force secretions through airways.
e. Repeat coughing to ensure airway is clear. Do not continue past patient's tolerance.	
4. CPAP/BiPAP administration	
a. Position patient comfortably with head elevated.	Allows for maximum lung expansion.

Continued

STEPS	RATIONALE
b. Position face mask or nasal mask tightly and adjust head strap until seal is maintained and patient is able to tolerate it (see Fig. 14-1).	Patient may experience claustrophobic sensations and feel discomfort from continuous pressure.
c. Instruct patient to breathe normally.	Reduces hyperventilation and fatigue. Promotes optimum lung expansion.
d. Apply at ordered setting for prescribed length of time.	Like oxygen, administer CPAP/BiPAP at prescribed level.
5. See Completion Protocol (inside front cover).	

EVALUATION

1. Observe patient's body alignment and position whenever in visual contact with patient.
2. Auscultate lung fields for adventitious lung sounds.
3. Observe patient's respiratory status during sleep to determine response to CPAP.
4. Observe vital signs and pulse oximetry. Review ABGs when available.
5. Observe patient's and caregiver's use of CPAP/BiPAP mask and compliance with therapy.
6. Ask patient to explain purpose and benefits of positioning and CPAP/BiPAP (Barnes, 2007).

Unexpected Outcomes and Related Interventions

1. Patient is unable to maintain a patent airway.
   a. Evaluate positioning. Consider suctioning and use of artificial airway (see Skill 14.4).
   b. Monitor ABGs/pulse oximetry.
2. Patient experiences worsening dyspnea with bronchospasm and hypoxemia.
   a. Notify health care provider.
   b. Monitor ABGs/pulse oximetry.
   c. Medicate as ordered.
   d. Evaluate for methods to decrease oxygen demand (bed rest, positioning).
3. Patient is unable to tolerate CPAP/BiPAP.
   a. *Carbon dioxide retention:* Notify health care provider.
   b. *Mask fit:* Check fit of device. Consider alternative (alternate type of mask, nasal pillows) if difficulties continue. If skin breakdown occurs across bridge of nose, apply porous tape until skin becomes adjusted to the pressure. If generalized breakdown occurs, consider a reaction to the mask material (e.g., latex) (Barnes, 2007).
   c. *Pressure:* Feelings of suffocation, shortness of breath, and discomfort related to pressure from CPAP/BiPAP. Determine if another pressure setting will give similar results with more comfort or if BiPAP is required (Barnes, 2007).

Recording and Reporting

- Record activity level, including assistance needed with positioning, coughing effectiveness, and respiratory assessment.
- For CPAP/BiPAP, record patient compliance and tolerance, mask fit and skin assessment beneath mask, effectiveness of therapy, witnessed periods of apnea, and status of daytime hypersomnolence.

Sample Documentation

2400 Observed sleeping. Respirations 18; regular in rate, rhythm, and depth without snoring. Skin is pink, warm, and dry and intact. No jerking movements noted. CPAP continues per face mask with good seal at 7.5 cm H_2O.

Special Considerations

Home Care

- Frequent follow-up may be necessary to enhance CPAP/BiPAP compliance and address unexpected outcomes promptly.

PROCEDURAL GUIDELINE 14.1
Peak Expiratory Flow Rate

For patients who have measurable changes in the air flow through their airways such as patients with asthma or reactive airway disease, peak expiratory flow rate (PEFR) measurements are useful. The PEFR is the maximum flow that a patient forces out during one quick, forced expiration and is measured in liters. Use these measurements as an objective indicator of the patient's current status or the effectiveness of treatment. Decreased PEFR may indicate the need for further interventions such as increased doses of bronchodilators or antiinflammatory medications. Normal values vary according to a person's age, sex, and size. Use a "traffic light" pattern to help the patient know what to do when the peak flow number changes. For example, if the patient's peak flow value is in the green zone, no action is necessary. However if the value is in the yellow (caution) zone, the health care provider might instruct the patient to

PROCEDURAL GUIDELINE 14.1
Peak Expiratory Flow Rate—cont'd

use a different type of inhaler. For helpful information, refer the patient to the NIH government website (http://www.nhlbi.nih.gov).

Delegation and Collaboration

Initial assessment of the patient's condition cannot be delegated. The skills of follow-up PEFR measurements in a stable patient can be delegated to nursing assistive personnel (NAP). Instruct the NAP to:

- Immediately report to the nurse patient's difficulty breathing.

Equipment

- Peak flowmeter
- Patient diary/action plan, if appropriate

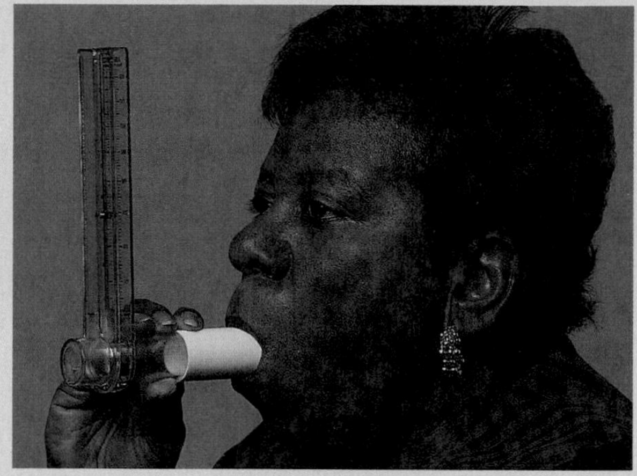

STEP 6 Peak expiratory flowmeter.

Procedural Steps

1. **See Standard Protocol (inside front cover).**
2. Assist patient to high-Fowler's position, which promotes optimum lung expansion.
3. Assess patient's baseline knowledge of when and how to use PEFR and correct response to results.
4. Slide mouthpiece into base of the numbered scale.
5. Instruct patient to take a deep breath.
6. Have patient place meter mouthpiece in mouth and close lips, making a firm seal (see illustration).
7. Have patient blow out as hard and fast as possible through mouth only.
8. Monitor PEFR results and assess if patient is in expected range.
9. Instruct patient as to his or her individualized acceptable range.
10. If patient is to record PEFR at home, have him or her demonstrate PEFR technique independently and assess ability to record PEFR accurately on chart using "traffic light" pattern. Observe a return demonstration by patient or family to determine if patient is using correct technique with PEFR.
11. Determine patient's PEFR and compare with his or her personal best.
12. Record PEFR measurement before and after therapy and patient's ability and effort to perform PEFR.
13. **See Completion Protocol (inside front cover).**

SKILL 14.3 CHEST PHYSIOTHERAPY

Chest physiotherapy (CPT) is used to mobilize pulmonary secretions. CPT includes postural drainage, chest percussion, and vibration, followed by productive coughing or suctioning. CPT is for patients who produce more than 30 mL of sputum per day or have evidence of atelectasis by chest x-ray film.

Chest percussion involves striking the chest wall over the area being drained. Position the hand so your fingers and thumb touch, cupping the hand (Fig. 14-2). Percussion on the surface of the chest wall sends waves of varying amplitude and frequency through the chest, changing the consistency and location of the sputum. Perform chest percussion by alternating hand motion against the chest wall over a single layer of clothing, not over buttons, snaps, or zippers (Fig. 14-3). Use only a single layer of clothing to prevent slapping the patient's skin.

Use caution and do not percuss on the scapular area or trauma will occur to the skin and underlying musculoskeletal structures. Percussion is contraindicated in patients with bleeding disorders, osteoporosis, or fractured ribs.

Vibration is a fine, shaking pressure applied to the chest wall only during exhalation. This technique increases the velocity and turbulence of exhaled air, facilitating secretion removal. Vibration increases the exhalation of trapped air, shakes mucus loose, and induces a cough. It is used with patients with cystic fibrosis or conditions causing thick secretions.

Postural drainage is the use of positioning techniques that drain secretions from specific segments of the lungs and bronchi into the trachea. Each position drains a specific corresponding section of the tracheobronchial tree, either from the upper, middle, or lower lung field, into the trachea. The procedure for postural drainage includes most lung segments (Table 14-3). Use patient history and clinical assessment findings to determine which lung segments require postural drainage. For example, some patients with left lower lobe

TABLE 14-3 POSITIONS AND PROCEDURES FOR DRAINAGE, PERCUSSION, VIBRATION, AND SHAKING

AREA AND PROCEDURE	ANATOMICAL AREA	POSITION OF PATIENT
Left and Right Upper Lobe Anterior Apical Bronchi Position patient in chair, or high-Fowler's, leaning back. Percuss and vibrate with heel of hands at shoulders and fingers over collarbones (clavicles) in front; do both sides at same time. Note body posture and arm position of nurse. Nurse's back is kept straight, and elbows and knees are slightly flexed. Direction of mucus flow through upper lobe anterior apical bronchi.	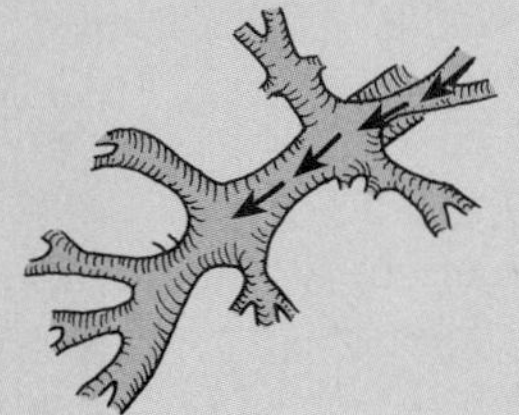	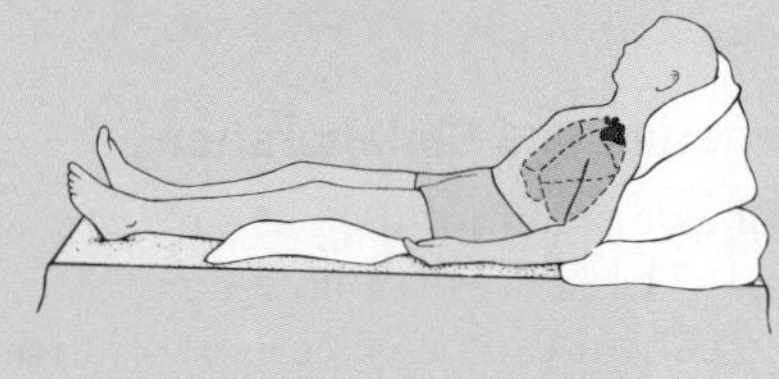 Anterior apical segments Position hands for chest physiotherapy over left and right upper lobe anterior apical bronchi.
Left and Right Upper Lobe Posterior Apical Bronchi Position patient in chair, leaning forward on pillow or table. Percuss and vibrate with hands on either side of upper spine. Do both sides at same time. Direction of mucus flow through upper lobe posterior apical bronchi.	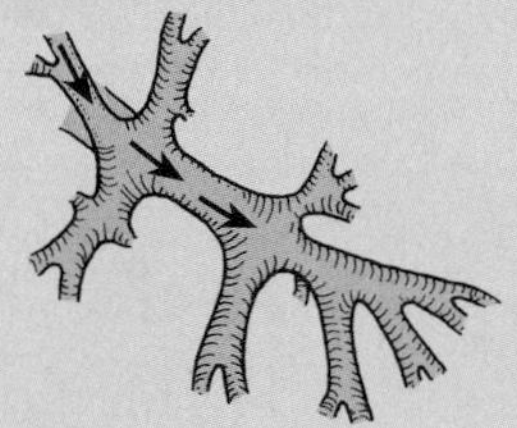	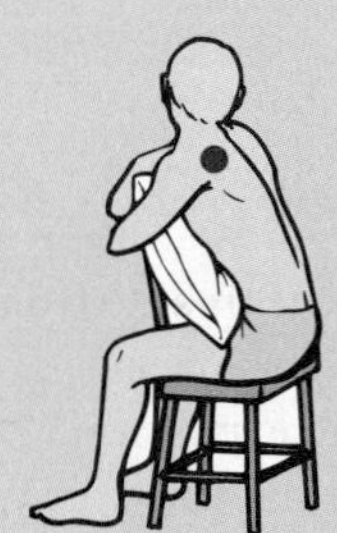 Posterior apical segments Position hands for chest physiotherapy over left and right upper lobe posterior apical bronchi.
Right and Left Anterior Upper Lobe Bronchi Position patient flat on back with small pillow under knees. Percuss and vibrate just below clavicle on either side of sternum. Direction of mucus flow through anterior upper bronchi.	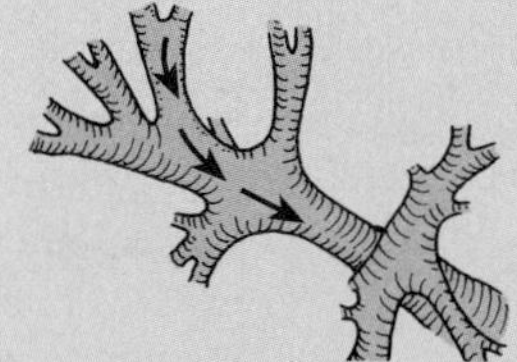	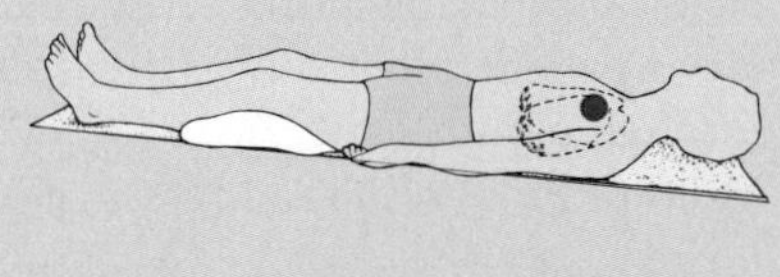 Left and right anterior upper lobe segments Position hands for chest physiotherapy over right and left anterior upper lobe bronchi.
Left Upper Lobe Lingular Bronchus Position patient on right side with arm overhead in Trendelenburg's position, with foot of bed raised 30 cm (12 inches), as tolerated.* Place pillow behind back, and roll patient one-quarter turn onto pillow. Percuss and vibrate lateral to left nipple below axilla. Direction of mucus flow through left upper lobe lingular bronchus.	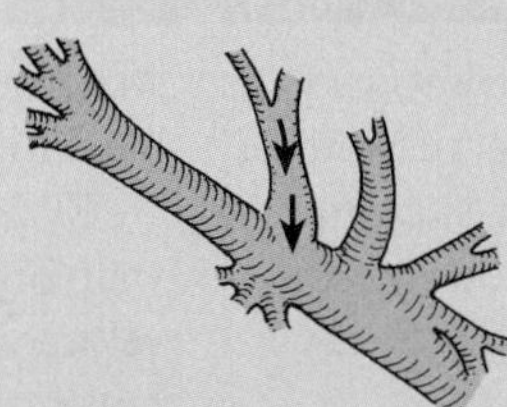	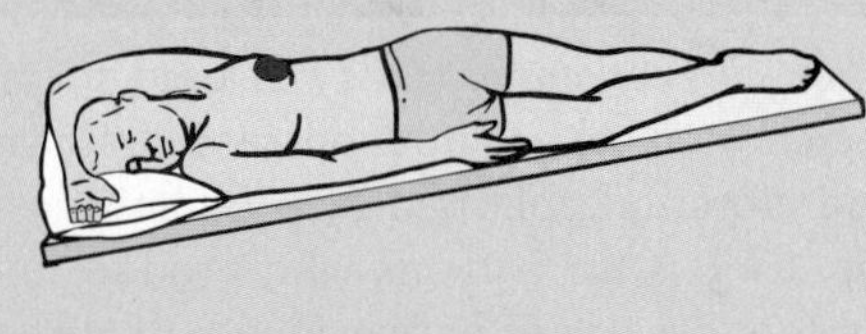 Left upper lobe lingular segment Position hands for chest physiotherapy over left upper lobe lingular bronchus.
Right Middle Lobe Bronchus Position patient on left side or abdomen. Place pillow behind back, and roll patient one-quarter turn onto pillow. Percuss and vibrate to right nipple below axilla. Direction of mucus flow through right middle lobe bronchus.	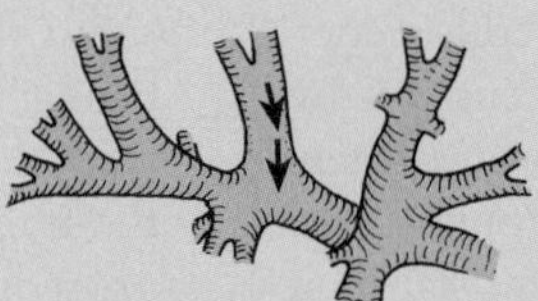	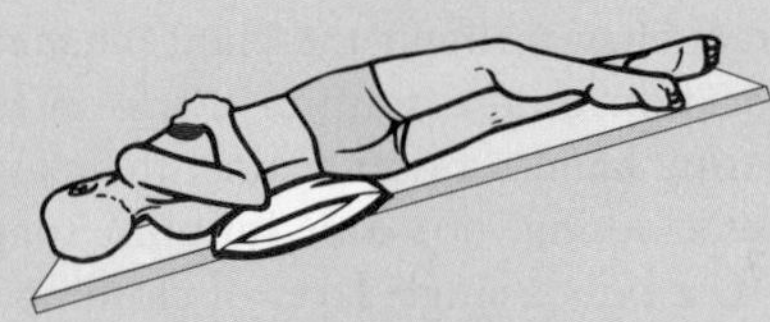 Right middle lobe segment Position hands for chest physiotherapy over right middle lobe bronchus.

TABLE 14-3 POSITIONS AND PROCEDURES FOR DRAINAGE, PERCUSSION, VIBRATION, AND SHAKING—cont'd

AREA AND PROCEDURE	ANATOMICAL AREA	POSITION OF PATIENT
Left and Right Anterior Lower Lobe Bronchi Position patient on back, with foot of bed elevated to 45 to 50 cm (18 to 20 inches). Have knees bent on pillow. Percuss and vibrate over lower anterior ribs on both sides. Direction of mucus flow through anterior lower lobe bronchi.	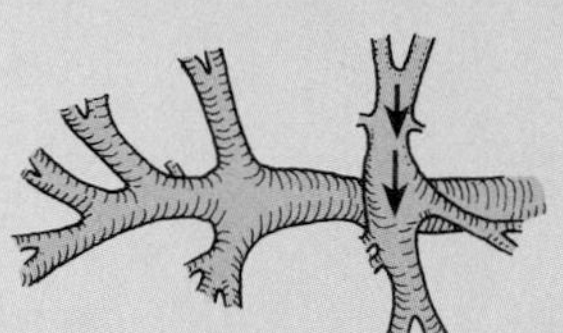	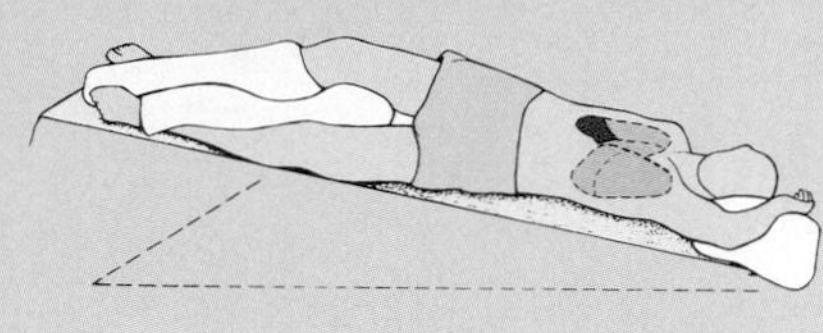 Left and right anterior lower lobe segments Position hands for chest physiotherapy over left and right anterior lower lobe bronchi.
Right Lower Lobe Lateral Bronchus Position patient on abdomen in Trendelenburg's position with foot of bed raised 45 to 50 cm (18 to 20 inches), as tolerated. Percuss and vibrate on left and right sides of chest below shoulder blades (scapulas) posterior to midaxillary line. Direction of mucus flow through right lower lobe lateral bronchus.	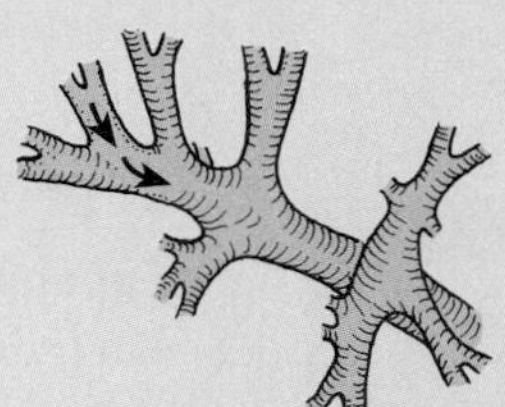	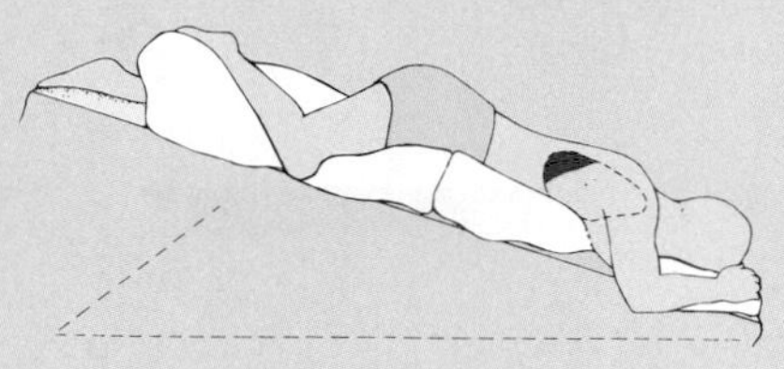 Right lower lateral lobe segment Position hands for chest physiotherapy over right lower lobe lateral bronchus.
Left Lower Lobe Lateral Bronchus Position patient on right side in Trendelenburg's position with foot of bed raised 45 to 50 cm (18 to 20 inches), as tolerated. Percuss and vibrate on left side of chest below scapulas posterior to midaxillary line. Direction of mucus flow through left lower lobe lateral bronchus.	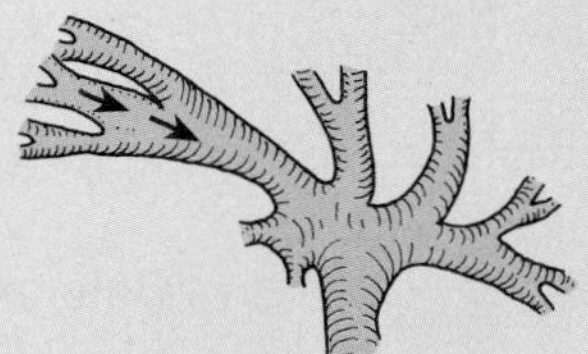	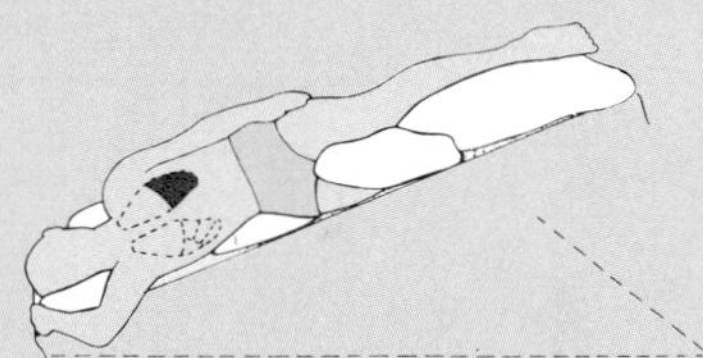 Left lower lobe lateral segment Position hands for chest physiotherapy over left lower lobe lateral bronchus.
Right and Left Lower Lobe Superior Bronchi Position patient flat on stomach with pillow under stomach. Percuss and vibrate below scapulas on either side of spine. Direction of mucus flow through lower lobe superior bronchi.	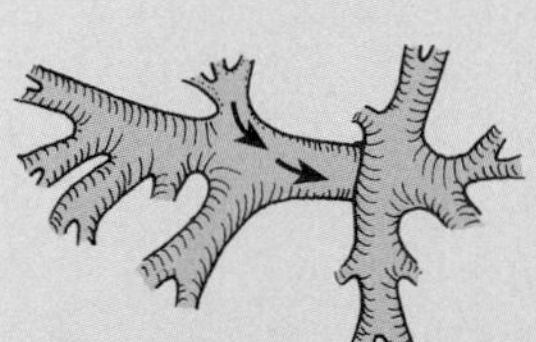	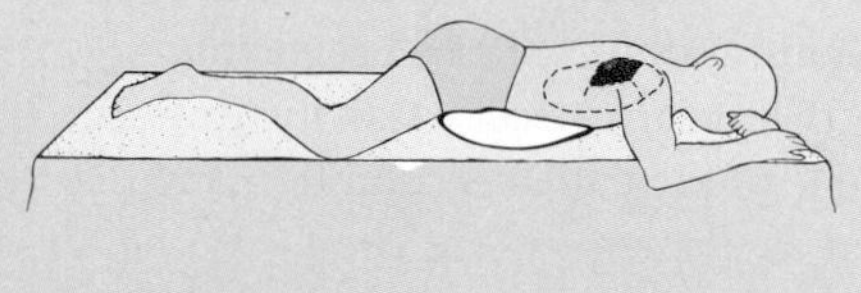 Right and left lower lobe superior segments Position hands for chest physiotherapy over right and left lower lobe superior bronchi.
Right and Left Posterior Basal Bronchi Position patient on stomach in Trendelenburg's position with foot of bed raised 45 to 50 cm (18 to 20 inches), as tolerated. Percuss and vibrate over low posterior ribs on either side of spine. Direction of mucus flow through posterior basal bronchi.	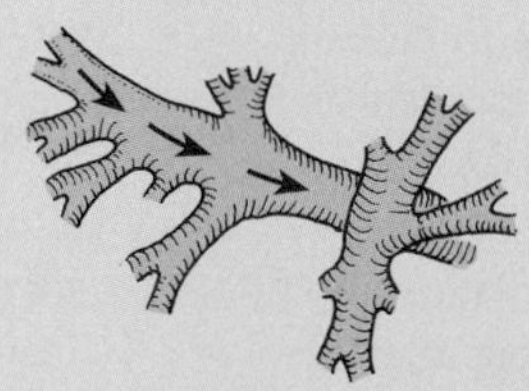	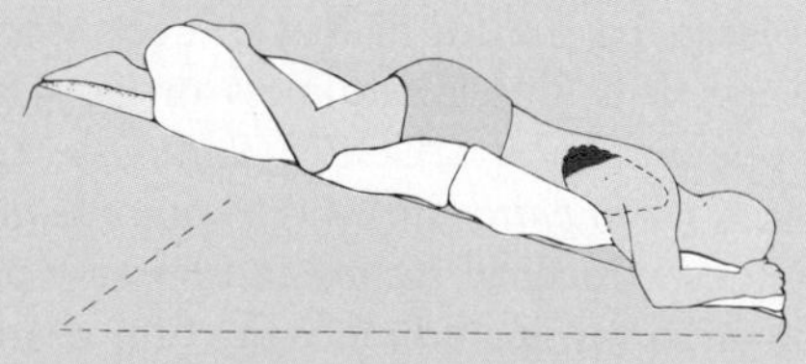 Right and left posterior segments Position hands for chest physiotherapy over right and left posterior lower lobe bronchi.

*In adult settings Trendelenburg's position is not used as frequently. Verify use with agency policy and heath care provider's order.

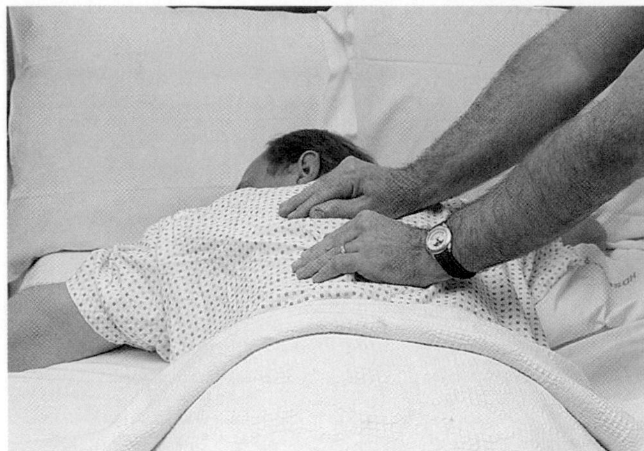

FIG 14-2 Hand position for chest wall percussion during physiotherapy.

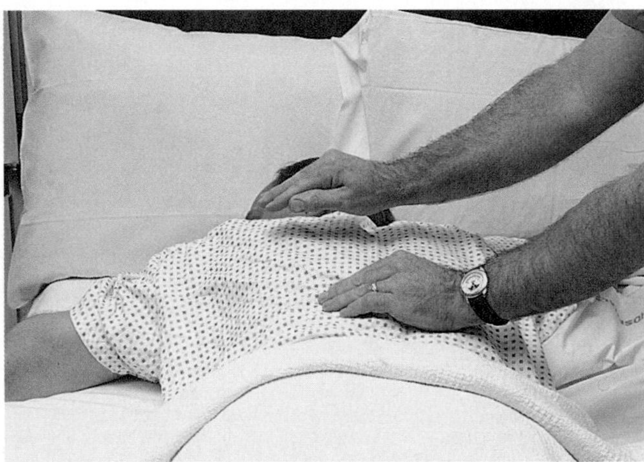

FIG 14-3 Chest wall percussion, alternating hand motion against the patient's chest wall.

bronchiectasis or pneumonia require postural drainage of the affected region, whereas a child with cystic fibrosis requires postural drainage of all segments.

Clinicians select areas for drainage based on (1) knowledge of the patient's condition and disease process, (2) physical assessment of the chest, (3) chest x-ray film results, and (4) the extent of the pathological condition and lobe involvement based on the physical examination and chest x-ray film findings.

ASSESSMENT

1. Assess patient for history of decreased level of consciousness and muscle weakness or disease processes such as pneumonia and COPD. *Rationale: Conditions that pose risk for impaired airway clearance require CPT.*
2. Review medical record and observe patient for signs and symptoms, including: x-ray film changes consistent with atelectasis, lobar collapse pneumonia, or bronchiectasis; ineffective coughing; or thick, sticky, tenacious, and discolored secretions that are difficult to cough up. *Rationale: Indicates need to perform postural drainage. X-ray film data and signs and symptoms indicate accumulation of pulmonary secretions and ineffective airway clearance.*
3. Auscultate all lung fields for decreased breath sounds and adventitious lung sounds. *Rationale: Findings identify bronchial segments needing drainage. Areas of lung congestion and postures for drainage vary, depending on disease process, patient condition, and clinical problems.*
4. Obtain vital signs and pulse oximetry. *Rationale: Provides baseline to evaluate patient's response to therapy.*
5. Determine patient's understanding of and ability to perform home postural drainage. *Rationale: Identifies potential areas for instruction. Home care CPT is indicated in patients with chronic inability to clear lung secretions adequately such as those with cystic fibrosis, chronic bronchitis, asthma, or bronchiectasis.*

PLANNING

Expected Outcomes focus on airway clearance and clear lung sounds.

- Lung sounds improve or become clear.
- Sputum is more easily coughed and expectorated or suctioned out.
- Secretions appear more normal in color and consistency.
- Dyspnea decreases.
- Health care provider confirms chest x-ray shows improvements.
- Patient is able to relax and breathes more deeply.

Delegation and Collaboration

The skill of CPT can be delegated to nursing assistive personnel (NAP) in special situations. It is the nurse's responsibility to assess the patient, review laboratory and x-ray film results, and determine that the patient is stable and able to tolerate the procedure. Instruct the NAP about the following:

- To immediately report to the nurse change in patient's comfort level, tolerance of the procedure, and/or changes in breathing pattern
- Specific patient precautions related to disease, mobility status, positioning restrictions, or treatment

Equipment

- Stethoscope
- Pulse oximeter
- Trendelenburg's hospital bed or tilt table, more common in pediatric agencies
- Water in pitcher and glass
- Chair (for draining upper lobes)
- One to four pillows
- Tissues and paper bag
- Clear graduated screw-top container
- Clean gloves (if there is a risk of exposure to patient's respiratory secretions)
- Suction equipment (if patient is unable to cough and clear own secretions)

IMPLEMENTATION *for* CHEST PHYSIOTHERAPY

STEPS	RATIONALE
1. See Standard Protocol (inside front cover).	
2. Identify patient using two identifiers (e.g., name and birthday or name and account number, according to facility policy).	Ensures correct patient. Complies with The Joint Commission standards and improves patient safety (TJC, 2010).
3. Prepare patient for procedure. **a.** Explain positioning, sensations, how long it will take, and any discomforts or side effects.	Helps promote cooperation. Well-prepared patient is usually more relaxed and comfortable, which is essential for effective drainage.
b. Encourage high–fluid intake program unless contraindicated by other diseases and if health care provider approves. Fluid thins secretions and makes them easier to cough up. Patients need close monitoring and encouragement when first starting high fluid–intake program.	
c. Coordinate therapy at appropriate times (e.g., 20 minutes after bronchodilator therapy). Plan treatments so they do not overlap with meals or tube feeding. Avoid postural drainage 1 to 2 hours before a meal or 1 to 2 hours after meals or bolus tube feedings. Stop all continuous gastric tube feedings for 30 to 45 minutes before postural drainage. Check for residual feeding in patient's stomach; if greater than 100 mL, hold treatment.	Scheduling after bronchodilator enhances movement of secretions out of airways. Scheduling of CPT should avoid conflict with other interventions and/or diagnostic testing. Performing postural drainage when patient's stomach is empty helps avoid gastric reflux or vomiting and aspiration of stomach contents.
d. Have patient remove any tight or restrictive clothing.	
4. Identify selected lung segments for draining based on assessment findings.	Individualized treatment helps relieve specific areas of congestion identified during patient assessment.
5. Position patient to drain the first lung segment (see Table 14-3). Assist patient to assume position as needed. Place pillows for support and comfort. Drape patient appropriately.	Proper patient positioning promotes drainage of pulmonary secretions.
6. For each selected segment perform chest percussion, vibration, and shaking.	Provides mechanical forces to help move airway secretions.
7. After each 10 to 15 minutes of drainage, have patient sit up and cough, using controlled coughing (see Skill 14.2). If patient cannot cough, suctioning is necessary (see Skill 14.4). Any secretions moved to the central airways are removed by cough or suctioning before placing patient into next drainage position.	Coughing is most effective when patient is sitting up and leaning forward.

SAFETY ALERT Sometimes patients experience transient dyspnea and fatigue because of airway irritation and bronchospasm from the secretions. These patients often benefit from an oscillating or vibrating device such as an Acapella device.

STEPS	RATIONALE
8. Have patient rest briefly if necessary.	Short rest periods between postures help prevent fatigue and increase tolerance for the therapy.
9. Repeat Steps 6 through 8 until all congested areas selected are drained. Make sure that each treatment does not exceed 30 to 60 minutes.	Postural drainage is used only in the involved areas and is based on individual assessment.
10. Offer or assist patient with oral hygiene. Have patient take sips of water.	Promotes comfort and reduces bad breath. Keeping mouth moist aids in expectoration of secretions.
11. See Completion Protocol (inside front cover).	

EVALUATION

1. Auscultate lung fields.
2. Inspect character and amount of sputum.
3. Review diagnostic reports, including sputum collections/cultures, chest x-ray films, and ABG levels, with health care provider.
4. Obtain vital signs, pulse oximetry.

Unexpected Outcomes and Related Interventions

1. Patient experiences severe dyspnea, bronchospasm, hypoxemia, hypercarbia, and/or is unable to tolerate treatment.
   a. Discontinue, modify, or shorten treatments.
   b. Administer bronchodilator or nebulizer therapy 20 minutes before CPT.
   c. Suction and ventilate with bag-valve-mask as needed and closely monitor ABG levels, O_2 saturation, and vital signs.
2. There is no improvement in respiratory condition, assessment, or chest x-ray film results.
   a. Initially increase treatments and encourage and teach coughing exercises.
   b. Notify health care provider because patient may need sputum culture, change in antibiotics, mucolytics, or a bronchoscopy to remove thick mucus plugs.
   c. Increase hydration.
3. Hemoptysis occurs; or patient develops acute hypotension, severe chest pain, vomiting, aspiration, and/or dysrhythmias.
   a. Stop therapy, place patient in high-Fowler's position, and obtain vital signs.
   b. Notify health care provider.
   c. Obtain vital signs and remain with patient, call for help, and keep patient calm.
   d. If patient vomits or aspirates, suction airway and place patient on his or her side.

Recording and Reporting

- Record pretherapy and posttherapy assessment of chest findings; frequency and duration of treatment; postures used and bronchial segments drained; cough effectiveness; need for suctioning; color, amount, and consistency of sputum; hemoptysis or other unexpected outcomes; and patient's tolerance and reactions.
- Record if patient and family receive instruction in home care, chart instructions given, understanding of therapy, demonstration of skill, patient acceptance of home care, barriers to learning and implementation, and referrals for home care or rehabilitation.

Sample Documentation

1340 Patient complaining of shortness of breath. Noted respirations elevated at 20 but regular in rate, rhythm, and depth. Crackles noted in right lower lobe. Patient asked to cough and deep breathe. Minimal sputum noted with weak cough. CPT completed in lower lobes. Noted moderate amount yellow sputum when patient asked to cough. Patient relates, "Breathing better." Lung sounds are now clear.

Special Considerations

Pediatric

- In the child with cystic fibrosis, CPT is usually performed at least twice daily, on rising in the morning and in the evening (Hockenberry and Wilson, 2009). Many cystic fibrosis patients use the chest vest when at home so they are independent.

Geriatric

- Take extra care and assessment when using postural drainage in older adults. Change positions more slowly and closely assess for any changes in oxygen saturation or vital signs with position changes.
- Older adults with chronic cardiac and pulmonary conditions do not always tolerate a supine or side-lying position for CPT. In these positions patients experience decline in forced vital capacity and subsequent decline in oxygen saturation.

Home Care Considerations

- Refer patient to pulmonary nurse specialist, pulmonary rehabilitation team, or home care personnel.
- Obtain foam wedge or multiple pillows for correct positioning.

SKILL 14.4 AIRWAY MANAGEMENT: SUCTIONING

- **Nursing Skills Online: Airway Management, Lessons 3-5**

Video Clips

For some patients noninvasive techniques and medications are insufficient to maintain a patent airway. In these cases suctioning is appropriate. Use patient assessment findings, the presence of an artificial airway, and the thickness and volume of the airway secretions to determine the best method of suctioning. Suction the oral cavity by oropharyngeal suctioning, using a rigid plastic catheter (called a *Yankauer*) with one large and several small eyelets to remove mucus (Fig. 14-4). The catheter supplies continuous suction once you connect it to a suction source. Teach patients how to use this catheter to clear secretions from their oral cavity.

Suctioning of the lower airway is needed when patients cannot cough forcefully enough to clear secretions. When lower airway suctioning is required, sterile technique is usually used. Endotracheal tubes (ETs) (Fig. 14-5) and tracheostomy tubes (Fig. 14-6) allow direct access to the lower airways for suctioning. Physicians or certified personnel insert these artificial airways to create a route for mechanical ventilation, relieve mechanical airway obstruction, or protect the airway from aspiration because of impaired cough or gag reflexes.

ASSESSMENT

1. Auscultate for coarse breath sounds, noisy breathing, or adventitious breath sounds. *Rationale: Provides baseline to determine effects of suctioning.*
2. Observe for increased or decreased pulse, increased or decreased respirations, increased or decreased blood pressure, prolonged expiratory breath sounds, and decreased lung expansion. Secretions in the airway, decreased oxygen saturations or level of consciousness, anxiety, lethargy, unilateral breath sounds, and cyanosis may also indicate a need for suctioning. *Rationale: Physical signs and symptoms result from airway obstruction and decreased oxygen to tissues. Never perform suctioning as a "routine" without assessment (Pedersen and others, 2009).*
3. Observe and assess nasal and oral cavity for nasal or oral secretions, drooling, gastric secretions, or vomitus in mouth. *Rationale: Removal of oral secretions prevents aspiration pneumonia, especially in mechanically ventilated patients.*
4. Identify patients with an increased risk for ineffective airway clearance (e.g., patients with a decreased level of consciousness or other neuromuscular or neurological impairment, those with decreased swallowing ability or dysphagia, and those with ineffective cough). *Rationale: Changes in neurological status and neuromuscular impairment increase the likelihood that the patient may need to be suctioned.*
5. Identify contraindications to nasotracheal suctioning: facial trauma or surgery, bleeding disorder, nasal bleeding, epiglottitis or croup, laryngospasm, and irritable airway (AARC, 2004). *Rationale: Passage of catheter can cause additional trauma, increased bleeding, or severe bronchospasm.*
6. Determine patient's understanding of procedure. *Rationale: Procedure can be distressing.*

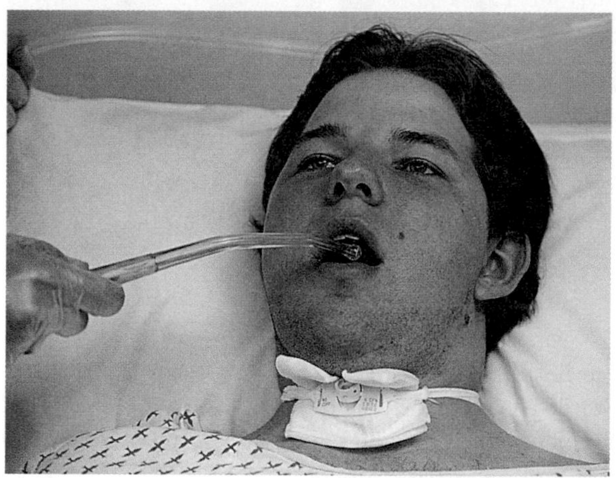

FIG 14-4 Oropharyngeal suctioning with Yankauer catheter.

PLANNING

Expected Outcomes focus on airway patency, avoidance of infection, and patient's comfort and understanding.

1. Patient's airways are cleared of secretions.
2. Adventitious breath sounds are decreased or cleared.
3. Patient reports easier breathing.
4. SpO_2 improves or remains the same.

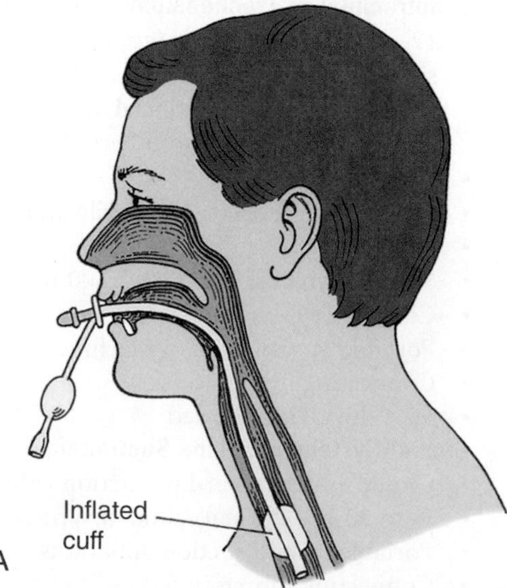

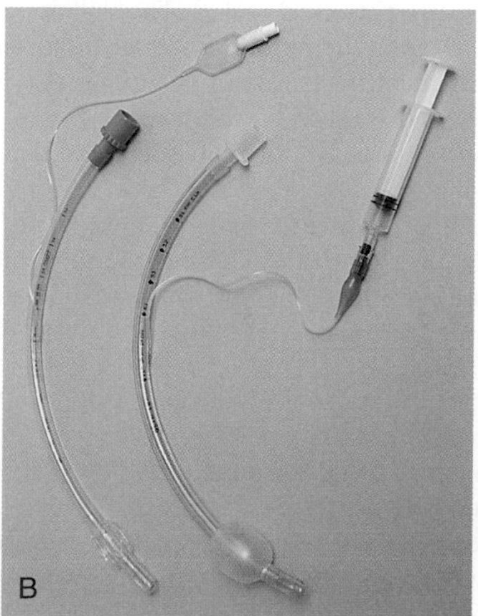

FIG 14-5 A, Endotracheal tube with inflated cuff. **B,** Endotracheal tubes with uninflated and inflated cuffs with syringe for inflation.

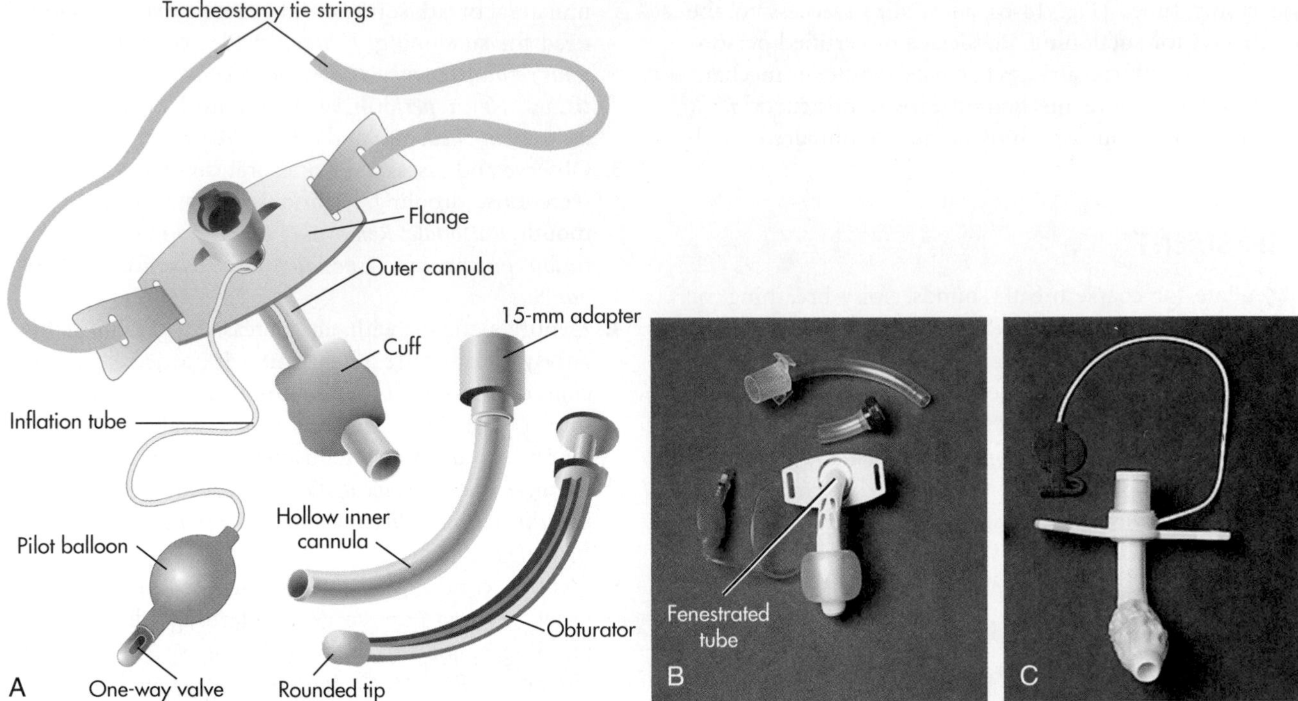

FIG 14-6 A, Parts of a tracheostomy tube. **B,** Fenestrated tracheostomy tube with cuff, inner cannula, decannulation plug, and pilot balloon. **C,** Tracheostomy tube with foam cuff and obturator. (From Lewis SL and others, *Medical-surgical nursing: assessment and management of clinical problems,* ed 7, St Louis, 2007, Mosby.)

5. Patient performs correct oropharyngeal suctioning technique.
6. Indication of aspiration is absent.

Delegation and Collaboration

The skill of deep tracheal suctioning in acutely ill patients cannot be delegated. Oropharyngeal suctioning can be delegated to nursing assistive personnel (NAP). The skill of performing tracheostomy tube suctioning in stable chronically ill patients with permanent tracheostomy tubes may also be delegated. Instruct the NAP about the following:

- To avoid mouth sutures and to apply suction to sensitive tissues
- How to vary the procedure for patients on ventilators
- To immediately report to the nurse changes in vital signs or pulse oximetry, bloody sputum, difficulty breathing, or discomfort during or after the procedure

Equipment

Oropharyngeal (Nonsterile) and Nasotracheal (Sterile) Suctioning

- Sterile suction catheter (12 to 16 Fr) (smallest diameter that will effectively remove secretions) for nasotracheal suctioning
- Clean, nonsterile suction catheter or Yankauer suction tip catheter for oropharyngeal suctioning
- Sterile gloves or one sterile and one clean
- Sterile basin (e.g., sterile disposable cup)
- Sterile water or normal saline (about 100 mL)
- Clean towel or paper drape
- Portable or wall suction
- Connecting tubing (6 feet)
- Face shield if indicated

Endotracheal or Tracheostomy Suctioning

- 12- to 16-Fr catheter (approximate, adult: size of the suction catheter should be no more than half of the internal diameter of the artificial airway to minimize decrease in PaO_2) (Pedersen and others, 2009)
- Bedside table
- Two sterile gloves or one sterile and one clean glove
- Sterile basin
- Sterile normal saline (about 100 mL)
- Clean towel or sterile drape
- Portable or wall suction machine
- Connecting tubing (6 feet)
- Face shield, if indicated

Closed-System or In-Line Suctioning

- Closed-system or in-line suction catheter
- 5- to 10-mL normal saline in syringe or vials
- Portable or wall suction apparatus
- Connecting tubing (6 feet)
- Two clean gloves

IMPLEMENTATION *for* AIRWAY MANAGEMENT: SUCTIONING

STEPS	RATIONALE
1. See Standard Protocol (inside front cover).	
2. Position patient in semi-Fowler's or high-Fowler's position.	Aligns the airway and aids in maximal lung expansion.
3. Preparation for all types of suctioning	
a. Open suction kit or catheter using aseptic technique. If sterile drape is available, place it across patient's chest. Do not allow suction catheter to touch any nonsterile surfaces.	Prepares catheter and prevents transmission of microorganisms.
b. Fill basin or cup with approximately 100 mL of sterile water or normal saline.	Sterile water or saline lubricates the suction catheter and helps check the patency of the tube.
c. If performing nasotracheal suctioning, open packet of lubricant.	
d. Connect one end of connecting tubing to suction machine or port. Check that suction is functioning properly by suctioning a small amount of water or saline from basin.	Always check for proper functioning of equipment before starting procedure.
e. Set regulator to appropriate negative pressure: suggested wall suction: 100 to 150 mm Hg for adults, 40 to 60 mm Hg for infants, and 60 to 100 mm Hg for children (Hockenberry and Wilson, 2009).	Elevated pressure settings increase risk of trauma to mucosa. The best practice is to use the lowest suction pressure. Follow facility guidelines and clinical judgment (Pedersen and others, 2009).
4. *Oropharyngeal suctioning*	
a. Apply mask or face shield if applicable. Attach suction catheter to connecting tubing. Remove oxygen mask if present, but keep near patient's face.	Suction may cause splashing of body fluids. The Centers for Disease Control and Prevention (CDC) guidelines suggest using masks or shields whenever there is the risk of airborne body fluids. Reduces chance of hypoxia.
b. With suction not applied, insert catheter into patient's mouth along gum line to pharynx. Then apply suction and move catheter around mouth until secretions are cleared.	If catheter does not have a suction control to apply intermittent suction, take care not to allow suction tip to damage oral mucosal surfaces with continuous suction.
c. Encourage patient to cough and repeat suctioning if needed. Replace oxygen mask if used.	Coughing moves secretions from lower and upper airways into mouth.
d. Suction water or saline from basin through catheter until catheter is cleared of secretions.	Clearing secretions before they dry reduces probability of transmission of microorganisms and clears catheter.
e. Place catheter in a clean, dry area for reuse with suction turned off. If patient is capable of self-suction, place it within reach.	Facilitates prompt removal of airway secretions when suctioning is needed in the future.
5. *Nasotracheal suctioning*	
a. Apply mask or face shield as appropriate. Apply sterile gloves or clean glove to nondominant hand and sterile glove to dominant hand. Attach nonsterile suction tubing to sterile catheter, keeping hand holding catheter sterile.	Suction may cause splashing of body fluids. CDC guidelines suggest using masks or shields whenever there is the risk of airborne body fluids. Gloving reduces transmission of microorganisms and allows you to maintain sterility of suction catheter.
b. Secure catheter to suction tubing aseptically. Coat distal 6 to 8 cm (2 to 3 inches) of catheter with water-soluble lubricant from suction kit.	Eases passage of catheter and reduces mucosal surface trauma.
c. If indicated, increase supplemental oxygen therapy as ordered by health care provider. Have patient deep breathe with oxygen delivery device in place. If patient is unable to take deep breaths, hyperoxygenate him or her with ventilation bag with mask attached.	Hyperoxygenation before suctioning can minimize postsuctioning hypoxemia (Pedersen and others, 2009).

SAFETY ALERT If mucus is visible at tracheostomy or ET opening, suction to remove secretions *before* hyperoxygenation. This prevents secretions from being pushed back into the trachea.

Continued

STEPS	RATIONALE
d. Remove oxygen delivery device, if present, with nondominant hand. Insert catheter into nares during inspiration without applying suction. Do not force catheter through nares. Have patient extend neck slightly (if not contraindicated) and breathe in. Do not force through nares.	Forcing the catheter causes trauma to the airway tissues. Extending patient's neck may facilitate passage of the catheter.

SAFETY ALERT Keep oxygen delivery device readily available in case patient exhibits symptoms of hypoxemia.

STEPS	RATIONALE
e. As patient takes deep breath, advance catheter to just above entrance into trachea, without applying suction. Quickly insert catheter (approximately 15 to 20 cm [6 to 8 inches] in adults, 8 to 14 cm [3 to 5½ inches] in infants and young children) into trachea until resistance is met or patient coughs; then pull back 1 to 2 cm (½ inch).	Ensures proper placement of catheter in airway to remove secretions. Pulling back on catheter before initiating suction prevents invagination of the tracheal membrane (Pedersen and others, 2009).
f. Apply suction no longer than 15 seconds by placing and releasing nondominant thumb over vent of catheter and slowly withdrawing catheter while rotating it back and forth between dominant thumb and forefinger (Pedersen and others, 2009). Encourage patient to cough. Replace oxygen device if applicable. Do not perform more than two passes with the catheter during *any suctioning session.*	Suctioning longer than 15 seconds can worsen existing hypoxemia. Observe patient for any signs of distress during suctioning. Stop suctioning and apply oxygen. Close observation is necessary after the procedure to assess for cardiovascular, respiratory, and neurological adverse effects (Celik and Kanan, 2006; Pedersen and others, 2009).
g. Rinse catheter and connecting tubing by suctioning water or normal saline from the basin until tubing is clear.	
h. Assess need to repeat suction procedure. Observe for alterations in cardiopulmonary status. Allow adequate time (1 to 2 minutes) between suction passes.	
6. ***ET or tracheostomy tube suctioning***	
a. Apply mask or face shield as appropriate. Apply sterile gloves or clean glove to nondominant hand and sterile glove to dominant hand. Attach nonsterile suction tubing to sterile catheter, keeping hand holding catheter sterile (see illustration).	Suction may cause splashing of body fluids. CDC recommends wearing mask or shield when there is risk of airborne body fluids. Reduces transmission of microorganisms and allows you to maintain sterility of suction catheter.

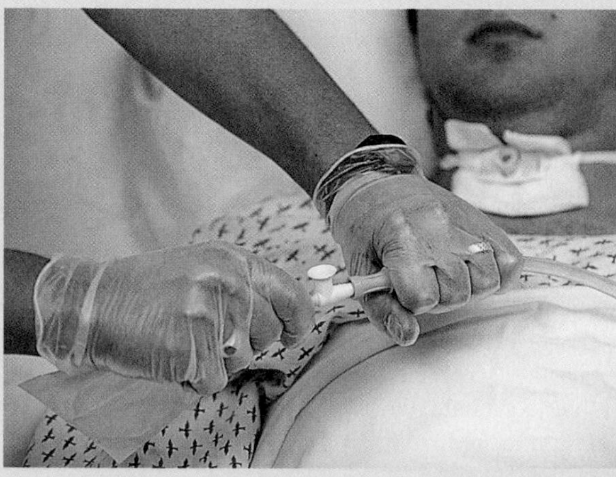

STEP 6a Attaching catheter to suction.

STEPS	RATIONALE
b. Check that equipment is functioning properly by suctioning small amounts of saline from basin.	Lubricates catheter and tubing.
c. Hyperoxygenate patient before suctioning, using manual resuscitation bag and increasing F_{IO_2} for several minutes; or, if mechanically ventilated, use the ventilator to provide additional breaths without increasing tidal volume. Up to 2 minutes may be necessary to provide for time for the increased oxygen to reach the mechanically ventilated patient.	Hyperoxygenation before suctioning decreases suctioning-induced hypoxemia (Pedersen and others, 2009). Most sources recommend hyperoxygenating with 100% F_{IO_2}; yet no clear guidelines are established for patients with COPD, who may not tolerate increased levels of oxygenation. Use hyperinflation with caution in the patient who has or is at risk for increased intracranial pressure or who is hemodynamically unstable.
d. Advise the patient that you are beginning to suction and that the patient may feel like his or her breath is being taken away.	Prepares patient for discomfort and reduces anxiety.
e. Open swivel adapter on tracheostomy or ET tube or, if necessary, remove oxygen or humidity delivery device with nondominant hand.	Exposes artificial airway.
f. Without applying suction and using dominant thumb and forefinger, gently but quickly insert catheter into artificial airway (time catheter insertion with patient's inspiration) until resistance is met or patient coughs; then pull back 1 cm (½ inch) (Pedersen and others, 2009).	Application of suction pressure while introducing catheter into trachea increases risk of damage to tracheal mucosa. Pulling back on catheter 2 cm before initiating suction prevents invagination of the tracheal membrane (Pedersen and others, 2009).
g. Apply suction by placing and releasing nondominant thumb over vent of catheter (see illustration). Slowly withdraw catheter while rotating it back and forth between dominant thumb and forefinger. If catheter "grabs" mucosa, remove thumb to release suction. The maximum time that catheter may remain in airway is 15 seconds (Pedersen and others, 2009). Encourage patient to cough.	No more than two passes with the suction catheter are recommended during any one suctioning session to decrease the risk of hypoxia. Continuous suctioning on withdrawal rather than intermittent suctioning is recommended to reduce the risk of injuring the mucosa (Pedersen and others, 2009).

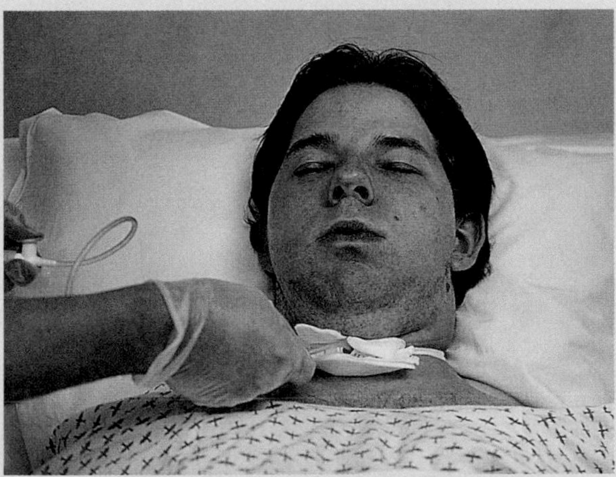

STEP 6g Suctioning tracheostomy.

STEPS	RATIONALE
h. Close swivel adapter or replace oxygen delivery device. Encourage patient to deep breathe. Some patients respond well to several manual breaths from the mechanical ventilator or resuscitation bag.	Reoxygenates and reexpands alveoli. Suctioning can cause hypoxemia and atelectasis. Monitor patient for signs of postsuctioning distress.
i. Rinse catheter and connecting tube with sterile water or normal saline until clear. Use continuous suction.	Removes catheter secretions. Secretions left in tubing decrease suction efficiency and provide environment for growth of microorganisms.

Continued

STEPS	RATIONALE
j. Evaluate patient's cardiopulmonary, neurological, and hemodynamic status. Repeat Steps 6e through 6i one time if you determine that secretion clearance was inadequate. Allow adequate time (up to 2 minutes) between suction passes to reestablish baseline oxygenation.	The effects of hypoxia from suctioning can cause dysrhythmias, hemodynamic instability, and increased intracranial pressure, among other complications. A maximum of two suction passes is recommended to minimize effects of hypoxemia (Celik and Kanan, 2006; Couchman and others, 2007).
k. Perform nasopharyngeal and oropharyngeal suctioning to clear upper airway of secretions. After suctioning upper airway, the catheter is contaminated, and you should not reinsert it into the lower airway.	Removes upper airway secretions. Upper airway is considered "clean," whereas lower airway is considered "sterile." Therefore you can use the same catheter suction from sterile to clean areas but not from clean to sterile areas.
l. Disconnect catheter from connecting tubing. Roll catheter around fingers of dominant hand. Pull glove off inside out so catheter remains in glove. Pull off other glove in same way. Discard into appropriate receptacle. Perform hand hygiene. Turn off suction device.	Reduces transmission of microorganisms. Do not touch clean equipment with contaminated gloves.
m. Place new, unopened suction kit at bedside.	
7. ***ET or tracheostomy tube suctioning with a closed-system (in-line) catheter (see illustration)***	

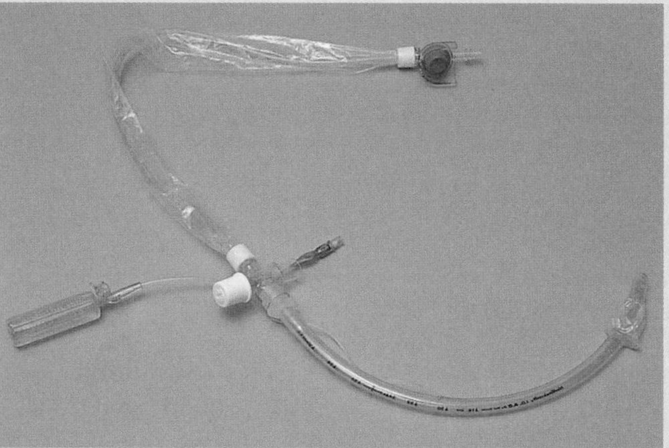

STEP 7 Closed-system suction catheter attached to an endotracheal tube.

STEPS	RATIONALE
a. Apply face shield.	
b. Attach suction.	
(1) In many institutions the catheter is attached to the mechanical ventilator circuit by personnel from respiratory therapy. If not already in place, open suction catheter package using aseptic technique. Attach closed-system suction catheter to ventilator circuit by removing swivel adapter and placing closed-system catheter apparatus on ET or tracheostomy tube. Connect Y on mechanical ventilator circuit to closed-system catheter with flex tubing.	Catheter becomes part of the circuit and is often changed by respiratory therapist with each circuit change, when contaminated, or per agency policy.
(2) Connect one end of connecting tube to suction machine. Connect other end to end of closed-system or in-line suction catheter if not already done. Turn suction device on and set vacuum regulator to appropriate negative pressure (80 to 120 mm Hg for adults) (Pedersen and others, 2009).	Prepares suction apparatus. Excessive negative pressure damages tracheal mucosa and can induce greater hypoxia.

STEPS	RATIONALE
c. Hyperinflate (1 to 2 lung inflations with an increased volume) and/or hyperoxygenate (increase F_IO_2) patient using resuscitation bag or manual breathing mechanism on mechanical ventilator according to institution protocol and clinical status (100% oxygen usually recommended).	Decreases atelectasis caused by negative pressure and increases oxygen available to tissues during suctioning. Both hyperinflation and hyperoxygenation are recommended before and after suctioning (Pedersen and others, 2009).
d. Unlock suction control mechanism if required by manufacturer. Open saline port and attach saline syringe or vial.	
e. Pick up suction catheter enclosed in plastic sleeve with dominant hand.	Plastic sheath provides catheter sterility and secretion containment.
f. Wait until patient inhales to insert catheter, while repeatedly pushing catheter and sliding (or pulling) plastic back between thumb and forefinger until you feel resistance or if patient coughs (see illustration). Pull back 1 cm (½ inch) before applying suction to avoid tissue damage to the carina (Couchman and others, 2007). (NOTE: Some catheters contain depth markings that are useful in positioning catheter.)	Mechanical ventilator breaths, oxygen, and positive end-expiratory pressure are not interrupted during suctioning. Catheter slides within plastic sheath. Coughing occurs or resistance is felt when catheter touches carina.

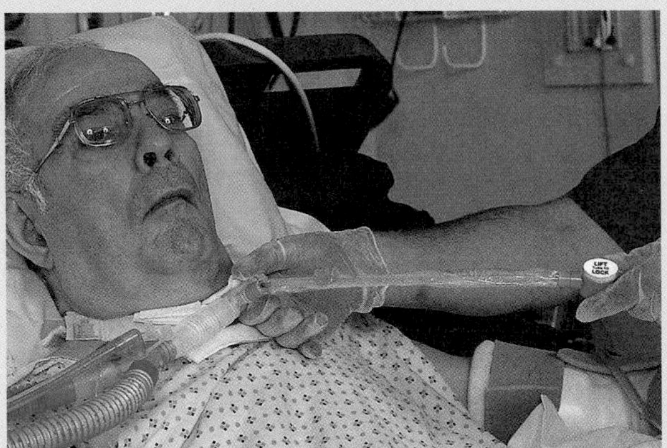

STEP 7f Suctioning tracheostomy with closed-system suction.

STEPS	RATIONALE
g. Encourage patient to cough and apply suction while withdrawing.	Removes secretions from airway.
h. Evaluate cardiopulmonary status, including pulse oximetry, to determine need for subsequent suctioning or complications. If cardiac monitoring is available, observe rhythm during suctioning. Repeat Steps 7c through 7g one or two more times to clear secretions. Allow adequate time (at least 1 full minute) between suction passes for ventilation and reoxygenation.	Repeated passes clear airway of secretions to promote ventilation and oxygenation. Suctioning can cause complications such as irregular heartbeats, hypoxia, and bronchospasm.
i. When airway is clear, withdraw catheter completely into sheath. Be sure that black line on catheter is visible in sheath. Squeeze vial or push syringe while applying suction to rinse inner lumen of catheter. Use at least 5 to 10 mL of normal saline to clear catheter of retained secretions. Lock suction mechanism, if applicable, and turn off suction.	Black line is reference point to determine correct position of catheter when not in use. Inability to see black line suggests that catheter is in airway and may be impeding airflow. Rinsing interior of catheter prevents bacterial growth.
j. Patient may require suctioning of oral cavity (see Step 4).	Separate suction catheter is necessary for oral cavity.
k. Place new, unopened suction kit on suction machine or at head of bed.	Provides immediate access to suction catheter when needed.
8. See Completion Protocol (inside front cover).	

EVALUATION

1. Auscultate lungs and compare patient's respiratory assessments before and after suctioning.
2. Ask patient if breathing is easier and if congestion is decreased.
3. Observe the amount, color, and consistency of suctioned content.
4. Observe patient's respirations and color; measure pulse oximetry (SpO_2).
5. Observe patient's oropharyngeal suctioning technique.

Unexpected Outcomes and Related Interventions

1. Patient becomes cyanotic or restless or develops tachycardia, bradycardia, or other abnormal heart rhythm.
   a. Discontinue attempt at suctioning until stabilized unless patient's condition is deteriorating because of secretions in airway.
   b. Provide supplemental oxygen.
   c. Monitor vital signs and pulse oximetry.
2. Bloody secretions are returned, which may indicate trauma.
   a. Evaluate technique and frequency of suctioning.
   b. If bleeding continues, notify health care provider of potential hemorrhage and monitor vital signs.
3. Thick secretions are present and difficult to suction.
   a. Monitor patient's hydration status. Dehydration contributes to thick secretions.
   b. Increase fluids if not contraindicated.

Recording and Reporting

- Record respiratory assessments before and after suctioning; size of catheter used; route; amount, consistency, and color of secretions obtained; frequency of suctioning.
- Report patient's intolerance to procedure or worsening of oxygenation status.

Sample Documentation

1200 Occasional productive cough. Requires hourly suctioning per ET tube. Moderate amount (5 mL or less) of thick yellow sputum. Patient able to use Yankauer catheter to suction mouth with good technique. Lungs clear after cough and suctioning. SpO_2 92% to 94%. Respirations regular in rate, rhythm, and depth after suctioning, 14 per minute.

Special Considerations

Pediatric

- Diameter of suction catheter should be no more than one half the internal diameter of the child's tracheostomy or other artificial airway (Hockenberry and Wilson, 2009).
- Unless secretions are thick, lower range of vacuum pressure is recommended (Hockenberry and Wilson, 2009).
- Closed suction systems are used only on older children. Use care so the weight of the closed system does not displace the child's ET tube.

Geriatric

- Older adults with ischemic cardiac or obstructive pulmonary disease may benefit from maintenance of oxygen supply during suctioning to reduce the risk of irregular heartbeats.
- Because of increased tissue fragility, older adults may have bloody secretions on suctioning. Monitor the suction return for clearing and avoid unnecessary suctioning.

Home Care

- In the home patients should follow best practices for infection control while weighing the necessity of cost-effectiveness in a chronic situation. For example, clean suctioning techniques may be acceptable, and the patient may clean secretion collection container and disinfect it every 24 hours.

SKILL 14.5 AIRWAY MANAGEMENT: ENDOTRACHEAL TUBE AND TRACHEOSTOMY CARE

- **Nursing Skills Online: Airway Management, Lessons 7 and 8** *Video Clips*

ET tubes are short-term artificial airways used to administer mechanical ventilation, relieve upper airway obstruction, protect against aspiration, or clear secretions (see Fig. 14-5, *A*). The tubes generally are removed within 14 days. If the patient requires continued assistance from an artificial airway, a tracheostomy is considered for long-term use (see Fig. 14-6).

An artificial airway places the patient at high risk for infection. However, correct care of the artificial airway helps to prevent infection. Ventilator-associated pneumonia (VAP) occurs in 10% to 65% of ventilated patients, causes 90% of health care–acquired infections in mechanically ventilated patients, and causes an increase in hospital length of stay and mortality (O'Keefe-McCarthy and others, 2008). VAP typically develops 48 hours after insertion of an artificial airway. Best practice guidelines for preventing VAP include:

1. Elevating the head of bed 30 to 45 degrees to prevent aspiration (O'Keefe-McCarthy and others, 2008).
2. Changing patient position every 2 hours to decrease risk for atelectasis and pulmonary infections (Coyer and others, 2007).
3. Providing oral care with chlorhexidine, which decreases colonization of bacteria, particularly in cardiothoracic surgery patients (AACN, 2007; Stokowski, 2009). Use a toothbrush every 8 hours to remove dental plaque organisms. Toothettes are not adequate to clean the dental plaque but they may be used between brushing for comfort.

4. Maintaining ET cuff pressures at 20 cm of H_2O to decrease movement of secretions to the lower airways.
5. Monitoring patient for aspiration when enteral feedings are infusing (Abbott and others, 2006; O'Keefe-McCarthy and others, 2008; Tolentino-DelosReyes and others, 2007).
6. Increasing patient mobility to promote pulmonary function and decrease pooling of secretions. Intervention such as repositioning, sitting, or standing at the bedside or ambulation decrease the risk of VAP (Stokowski, 2009).

ASSESSMENT

1. Observe condition of tube and inspect mouth and surrounding skin. ET tube: soiled or loose tape; pressure sores on nares, lip, or corner of mouth; unstable tube; excessive secretions. Tracheostomy tube: soiled or loose ties or dressing; unstable tube; excessive secretions. *Rationale: A patient with an artificial airway is at risk for impaired skin integrity and infection because of difficulty controlling secretions and pressure points of the artificial airway.*
2. Identify factors that increase risk of complications from ET tubes: type and size of tube, movement of tube up and down trachea, amount of inflation of tube cuff, and duration of placement. *Rationale: Tube moving up and down trachea predisposes patient to tracheal trauma or dislodgement. Cuff underinflation may allow aspiration, whereas overinflation may cause ischemia or necrosis of tracheal tissue. Use of tubes for longer periods of time increases the risk of lower airway complications such as pneumonia.*
3. Auscultate lungs. *Rationale: Provides baseline confirming bilateral lung inflation.*
4. Determine proper ET tube depth as noted by the number of centimeters at lip or gum line. This line is marked and recorded in patient's chart at time of intubation. *Rationale: Ensures that tube is at proper depth to adequately ventilate lungs.*
5. Assess patient's knowledge and comfort with procedure. *Rationale: Facilitates patient's learning, and participation in care and may help to decrease anxiety.*
6. If applicable, assess patient's understanding of and ability to perform own tracheostomy care. *Rationale: Increases patient's feeling of autonomy and decreases feelings of lack of control over condition/secretions.*

PLANNING

Expected Outcomes focus on the preventing infection and breakdown of skin and mucosa around the artificial airway.

1. Patient's artificial airway/tube is in correct position and properly secured.
2. Patient remains afebrile without signs and symptoms of infection.
3. Patient's oral mucous membrane/stoma remains free of breakdown or accumulation of secretions.
4. Patient's artificial airway is intact without persistent dried secretions.
5. Patient cooperates with care.
6. Patient is able to demonstrate correct technique of tracheostomy care when appropriate.

Delegation and Collaboration

The skill of ET care cannot be delegated. The skill of tracheostomy care can be delegated to nursing assistive personnel (NAP) when a permanent or long-term tracheostomy is in place in chronically ill patients. Instruct the NAP about the following:

- How to adapt the skill for a specific patient
- What to observe and report back to the nurse
- Emergency procedures for acutely ill patients in case the tracheostomy tube inadvertently becomes dislodged

Equipment

Endotracheal Tube Care

- Towel
- ET and oropharyngeal suction equipment
- 1 to 1½-inch adhesive or waterproof tape (not paper tape) or commercial ET tube stabilizer (follow manufacturer's instructions for securing)
- Two pairs of clean gloves
- Adhesive remover swab
- Mouth care supplies (e.g., pediatric-size toothbrush, sponge toothette for edentulous patients, toothpaste, and nonalcohol-based mouthwash)
- Face cleanser (e.g., wet washcloth, towel, soap, shaving supplies)
- Clean 2 × 2–inch gauze
- Tincture of benzoin or liquid adhesive
- Face shield (if indicated)

Tracheostomy Care

- Bedside table
- Towel
- Tracheostomy suction supplies
- Sterile tracheostomy care kit if available or:
- Three sterile 4 × 4–inch gauze pads
- Sterile cotton-tipped applicators
- Sterile tracheostomy dressing
- Sterile basin
- Small sterile brush (or disposable cannula)
- Tracheostomy ties (e.g., twill tape, manufactured tracheostomy ties, Velcro tracheostomy ties)
- Normal saline
- Scissors
- Pair of sterile and clean gloves
- Face shield

IMPLEMENTATION *for* AIRWAY MANAGEMENT: ENDOTRACHEAL TUBE AND TRACHEOSTOMY CARE

STEPS	RATIONALE
1. See Standard Protocol (inside front cover).	
2. ET tube care	
a. Suction ET tube (see Skill 14.4).	Removes secretions. Diminishes patient's need to cough during procedure.

> **SAFETY ALERT** Keep an oral airway or bite block immediately accessible in the event that patient bites down and obstructs the ET tube.

STEPS	RATIONALE
b. Connect oral Yankauer suction catheter to suction source.	Prepares for oropharyngeal suctioning.
c. Prepare method to secure ET tube.	
(1) *Tape method:* Cut piece of tape long enough to go completely around patient's head from nares to nares plus 15 cm (6 inches): total length for adult, about 30 to 60 cm (1 to 2 feet). Lay the tape adhesive side up on bedside table. Cut and lay an 8 to 15 cm (3 to 6 inches) strip of tape in center of long strip, adhesive sides together.	Adhesive tape must be placed around head from cheek to cheek below ears. Placing adhesive sides together in center of strip prevents the tape from adhering to hair. Cotton tape ties may also be used.
(2) *Commercially available ET tube holder:* Open package and set device aside with the head guard in place and Velcro strips open.	
d. Have an assistant apply a pair of gloves and hold ET tube firmly so tube does not move throughout procedure. Note the number marking once again on the ET tube at the lip line.	Reduces transmission of microorganisms. Maintains proper tube position and prevents accidental extubation.
e. Remove old tape or commercial tube holder.	Provides access to skin under tape for assessment and hygiene. Reduces transmission of microorganisms.
(1) *Tape:* Carefully remove tape from ET tube and patient's face. If tape is difficult to remove, moisten with water or adhesive tape remover. Discard in receptacle.	Adhesive can cause damage to skin and prevent adhesion of new tape.
(2) *Commercial tube holder:* Remove Velcro strips from ET tube and remove tube holder.	Devices are latex free, fast, and convenient.
f. Remove oral airway or bite block if present and place in towel. (Do not remove oral airway if patient is actively biting ET tube. This may result in occlusion of the airway.)	Provides access to and complete observation of patient's oral cavity.
g. Keep ET cuff inflated. As assistant continues to hold tube, clean mouth, gums, and teeth opposite ET tube with nonalcohol-based mouthwash solution (e.g., chlorhexidine) and 4 × 4–inch gauze or soft toothbrush. Suction fluid from oral cavity with Yankauer catheter or use toothbrush made to be connected to suction. Use sponge-tipped applicators to apply moisture to gums and buccal mucosa.	Inflated cuff on the ET tube reduces risks for aspiration and accidental extubation. Alcohol-based mouthwashes dry oral mucosa (Lewis and others, 2007).
h. *Oral ET tube only:* Note "cm" ET tube marking at lips. With help of assistant, move ET tube to opposite side or center of mouth. Do not change tube depth.	Prevents pressure-sore formation at sides of patient's mouth. Ensures correct position of tube (Vollman, 2006).
i. Repeat oral cleaning as in Step 2g on opposite side of mouth.	Removes secretions from oropharynx; removes plaque from teeth.
j. Clean face and neck with soapy washcloth; rinse and dry. Shave male patient after ET tube secured.	Moisture and beard growth prevent adhesive tape adherence.
k. Secure ET tube (assistant continues holding tube).	
(1) Tape method	Positions tape to secure ET tube in proper position.

STEPS	RATIONALE
(a) Pour small amount of tincture of benzoin on clean 2 × 2–inch gauze or swab and dot on skin above upper lip (oral ET tube) or across nose (nasal ET tube) and cheeks to ear. Allow to dry completely.	Protects and makes it easier for tape to adhere to skin.
(b) Slip the prepared tape under patient's head and neck, adhesive side up. Take care not to twist tape or catch hair. Do not allow tape to stick to itself. It helps to stick end of tape gently to tongue blade, which serves as a guide while sliding under neck. Center the strip of tape so that double-faced tape extends around back of neck from ear to ear.	
(c) On one side of face secure tape from ear to nares (nasal ET tube) or edge of mouth (oral ET tube). Tear remaining tape in half lengthwise, forming two pieces that are ½ to ¾ inch wide. Secure bottom half of tape across upper lip (oral ET tube) or across top of nose (nasal ET tube) (see illustration *A*). Wrap top half of tape around tube and up from bottom. Tape should encircle tube at least two times for security (see illustration *B*).	Secures tape to face. Using top tape to wrap prevents downward drag on ET tube.
(d) On other side of face, gently pull tape firmly to pick up slack and secure to remaining side of face (see illustration). Assistant can release hold when tube is secure. You may want assistant to help reinsert oral airway.	Secures tape to face and tube. ET tube should be at same depth at the lips. Check earlier assessment for verification of tube depth in centimeters.

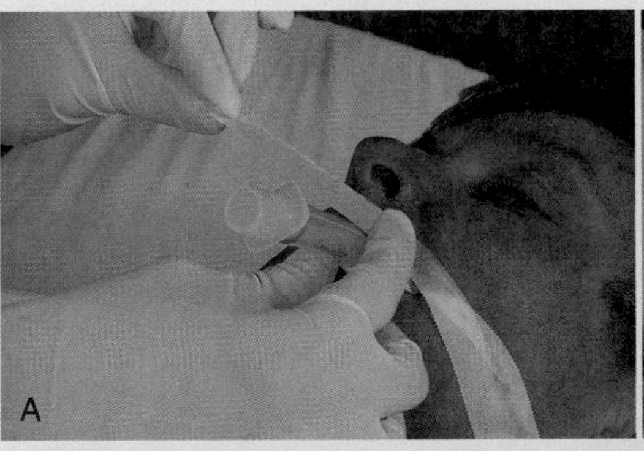

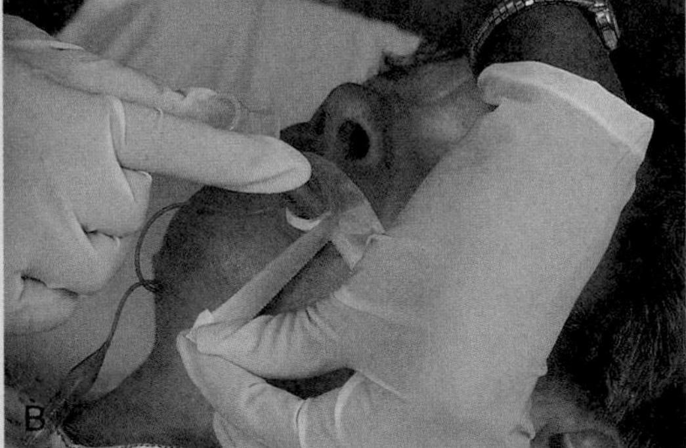

STEP 2k(1)(c) A, Securing bottom half of tape across patient's upper lip. **B,** Securing top half of tape around tube.

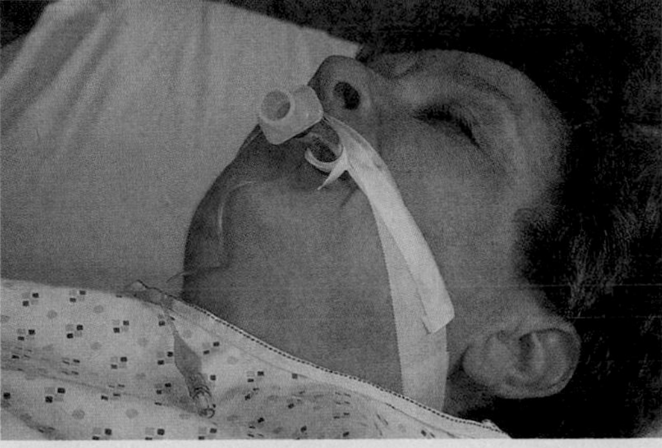

STEP 2k(1)(d) Tape securing endotracheal tube.

Continued

STEPS	RATIONALE
(2) Commercial tube holder	
(a) Thread ET tube through opening designed to secure it. Be sure that the pilot balloon is accessible. Place strips of ET tube holder under patient's head at the occiput.	Commercial holders have a slit in the front of the holder designed to secure the ET tube.
(b) Verify that ET tube is at the established depth, using the lip line marker as a guide. Attach Velcro strips at the base of the patient's head. Leave 1-cm (½-inch) slack in strips. Verify that tube is secure.	Ensures that ET tube remains at correct depth as determined during assessment.
l. Clean oral airway in warm water and rinse well. Shake excess water from oral airway.	Promotes hygiene. Reduces transmission of microorganisms.
m. Reinsert oral airway without pushing tongue into oropharynx by initially inserting upside down until the tip is beyond the end of the tongue and then rotating 180 degrees into place (see Skill 30.1).	Prevents patient from biting ET tube and allows access for oropharyngeal suctioning by sliding catheter along outer edge.
3. *Tracheostomy care*	
a. Suction tracheostomy (see Skill 14.4). Remove soiled tracheostomy dressing, discard in glove with coiled catheter, remove gloves, and perform hand hygiene.	Removes secretions so as not to occlude outer cannula while inner cannula is removed.
b. Have patient deep breathe or use AMBU bag to deliver supplemental oxygen. Prepare equipment on bedside table.	Replenishes oxygen lost in suctioning of tracheostomy.
(1) Open sterile tracheostomy kit. Open three 4 × 4–inch gauze packages using aseptic technique and pour normal saline on the gauze in two packages. Leave gauze in third package dry.	Preparation and organization of equipment allows you to complete procedure efficiently and reconnect patient to oxygen source in a timely manner.
(2) Open two packages of cotton-tipped swabs and pour normal saline on the tip of swabs, keeping packages sterile. Do not recap bottles.	
(3) Open sterile tracheostomy dressing package.	
(4) Unwrap sterile basin and pour about 2 cm (¾ inch) with normal saline. Open small sterile brush package and place aseptically into sterile basin.	
(5) Prepare length of twill tape long enough to circle around patient's neck twice (about 60 to 75 cm or 24 to 30 inches for an adult). Cut ends on diagonal.	Diagonal cut ends allow for easy threading through the tracheostomy device.
(6) If using commercial tracheostomy tube holder, open package.	
c. Apply sterile gloves. Keep dominant hand sterile throughout procedure.	Reduces transmission of microorganisms.
d. Remove oxygen source.	
e. If a nondisposable inner cannula is used (see Fig. 14-6):	

STEPS	RATIONALE
(1) While touching only the outer aspect of the tube, remove the inner cannula with nondominant hand. Drop inner cannula into basin with normal saline.	Normal saline loosens crusted secretions from inner cannula.
(2) Place tracheostomy collar or T tube and ventilator oxygen source over or near tracheostomy opening. NOTE: T tube and ventilator oxygen devices cannot be attached to most outer cannulas when inner cannula is removed. You may insert a new inner cannula quickly so the oxygen source can be maintained. Clean the old inner cannula in normal saline and store it in a sterile container for use the next time the tracheostomy is cleaned (two cannulas would be on hand at all times).	Maintains supply of oxygen to patient to prevent desaturation. Allows quick reconnection to oxygen source.
(3) To prevent oxygen desaturation in affected patients, quickly pick up inner cannula and use small brush to remove secretions inside and outside cannula (see illustration).	Brush removes thick or dried secretions.
(4) Hold inner cannula over basin and rinse with normal saline, using nondominant hand to pour.	Removes secretions from inner cannula.
(5) Replace inner cannula and secure "locking" mechanism (see illustration). Reapply ventilator or oxygen sources once inner cannula is in place.	
f. If a disposable inner cannula is used:	
(1) Remove new cannula from manufacturer's packaging.	
(2) While touching only the outer aspect of the tracheostomy tube, withdraw old inner cannula and replace with new cannula. Lock into position.	Maintains sterility of the inner aspect of the new cannula.
(3) Dispose of contaminated cannula in appropriate receptacle.	

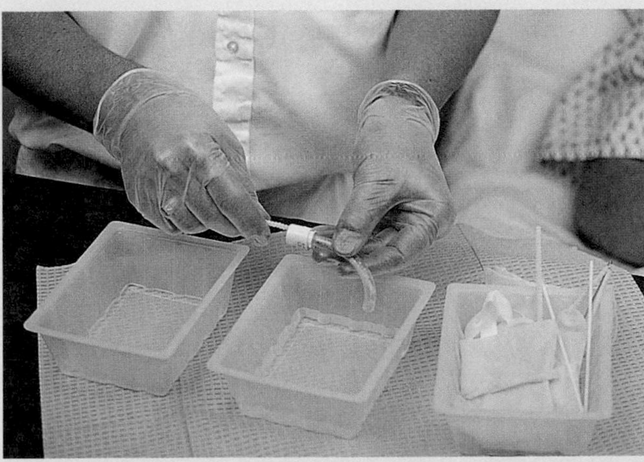
STEP 3e(3) Cleaning tracheostomy inner cannula.

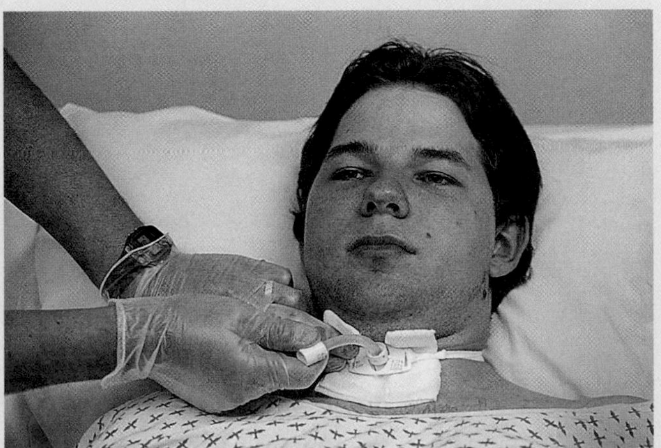
STEP 3e(5) Reinserting inner cannula.

Continued

STEPS	RATIONALE
g. Using normal saline–saturated cotton-tipped swabs and 4 × 4–inch gauze, clean exposed outer cannula surfaces and stoma under faceplate, extending 5 to 10 cm (2 to 4 inches) in all directions from stoma (see illustration). Clean in circular motion from stoma site outward, using dominant hand to handle sterile supplies.	.
h. Using dry 4 × 4–inch gauze, pat skin and exposed outer cannula surfaces lightly.	Dry surfaces decrease growth of microorganisms and skin excoriation.
i. Secure tracheostomy.	
(1) Instruct assistant, if available, to apply clean gloves and hold tracheostomy tube securely in place.	Promotes hygiene, reduces transmission of microorganisms, and secures tracheostomy tube.

SAFETY ALERT Assistant must not release hold on tracheostomy tube until new ties are firmly attached to reduce risk of injury, discomfort, or accidental extubation. If no assistant is present, do not remove old ties until you secure the new ones. (Follow manufacturer's guidelines for Velcro ties.)

STEPS	RATIONALE
(2) Insert one end of prepared tie through faceplate eyelet (see illustration) and pull ends of tie even.	
(3) Slide both ends of tie behind head and around neck to other eyelet and insert one tie through second eyelet. Cut old ties and remove.	
(4) Pull new ties snugly.	Prevents tube displacement.
(5) Tie ends securely in double square knot, allowing space for only one finger in tie.	One-finger slack prevents ties from being too tight. Knot should be to the side of the neck. Foam and Velcro tracheostomy holders are also commonly used.
(6) Insert fresh tracheostomy dressing under clean ties and faceplate (see illustration).	Absorbs drainage. Dressing prevents pressure on clavicle heads.
j. Position patient comfortably and assess respiratory status.	Promotes relaxation. Some patients may require post-tracheostomy care suctioning.

SAFETY ALERT For accidental extubation, call for assistance and manually ventilate patient with resuscitation bag if necessary. Keep tracheostomy obturator at bedside with a fresh tracheostomy to facilitate reinsertion of the outer cannula if dislodged. Keep an additional tracheostomy tube of the same size and shape on hand for emergency replacement.

4. See Completion Protocol (inside front cover).

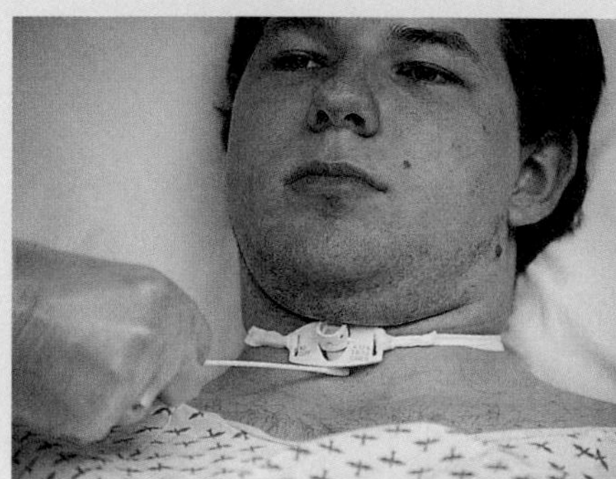
STEP 3g Cleaning around stoma.

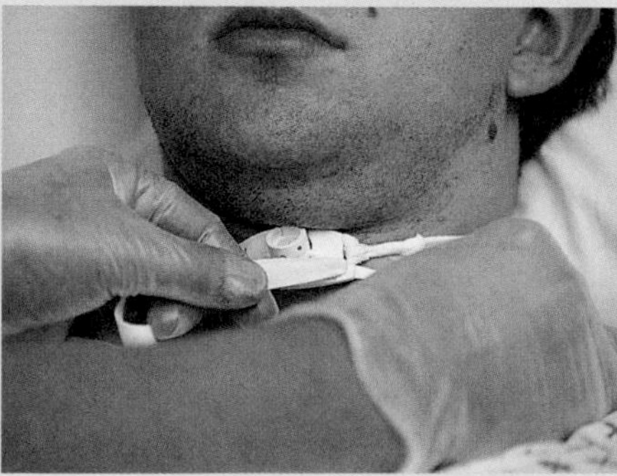
STEP 3i(2) Replacing tracheostomy ties.

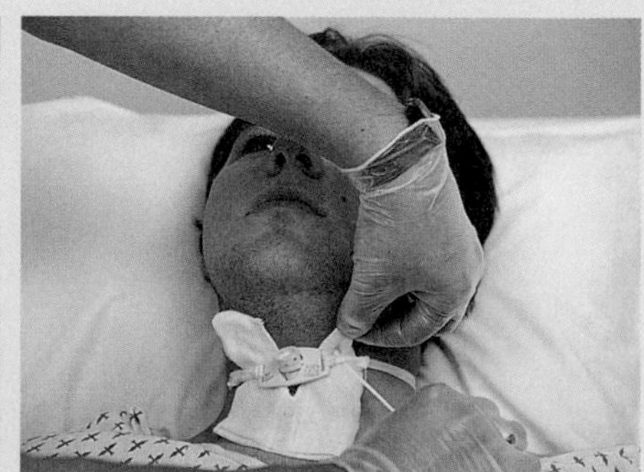
STEP 3i(6) Applying tracheostomy dressing.

EVALUATION

1. Auscultate lungs and observe that airway is in proper position with tape/ties secure and comfortable for patient. ET tube should be at the same depth as before care (as per physician order), with the same centimeter marking at lips and equal bilateral breath sounds.
2. Observe stoma for signs of infection.
3. Compare oral mucosa and airway assessments before and after artificial airway care. Observe for signs of tissue breakdown or persistent dried secretions.
4. Observe patient's actions to determine compliance with the procedure.
5. Have patient indicate when tracheostomy care is required and independently demonstrate the technique for tracheostomy tube care.

Unexpected Outcomes and Related Interventions

1. Tube is not secure. Artificial airway moves in or out or is coughed out by patient.
   a. Adjust or apply new ties.
2. Breath sounds not equal bilaterally with an ET tube in place.
   a. Evaluate ET tube for proper depth. If incorrect, arrange for ET tube to be repositioned as allowed by institution.
   b. Obtain order for chest x-ray study to verify placement if applicable.
   c. Assess patient's respiratory status and observe for the presence of mucus plugs.
3. Breakdown, pressure areas, or stomatitis (tracheostomy tube) develop around tube.
   a. Increase frequency of tube care.
   b. Make sure that skin areas are clean and dry.
4. Accidental extubation
   a. Call for assistance, monitor vital signs, and keep head of bed elevated.
   b. Maintain patent airway by replacing old tracheostomy tube with new tube for established tracheostomy. Use obturator to insert new tube and then remove obturator.
   c. For a new tracheostomy, cover the site with gauze and ventilate via bag-valve-mask. Do not attempt to recannulate because of potential for damage to stoma or trachea.

Recording and Reporting

- Record respiratory assessments before and after tube care, depth of ET tube or type and size of tracheostomy tube, frequency and extent of care, patient tolerance, and any complications related to presence of the tube.
- Report signs of infection or displacement of ET or tracheostomy tube immediately.

Sample Documentation

0800 Routine ET tube care done. Size 7.5-cm tube remains with 22-cm marking at lips. No irritation or skin breakdown noted. Mouth care given. Respirations regular in rate, rhythm, and depth at 16 breaths per minute. Clear breath sounds bilaterally.

Special Considerations

Pediatric

- Monitor children with new tracheostomy for complications such as hemorrhage, edema, accidental decannulation, and airway obstruction (Hockenberry and Wilson, 2009).
- Because of infants' delicate skin, you do not always use skin preparation before securing ET tube. ET tube holders are best to use in this population.

Geriatric

- Older adult skin may be more fragile and prone to breakdown from secretions or pressure or tearing when removing tape.
- Additional communication difficulties may occur for older adults who have visual or auditory deficits. Ensure that glasses and hearing aids are available and working properly.

Home Care

- Caregivers in the home must know how to clean established tracheostomy tubes and the signs and symptoms of respiratory and stoma infections.

SKILL 14.6 MANAGING CLOSED CHEST DRAINAGE SYSTEMS

- **Nursing Skills Online: Chest Tubes, Lessons 1 to 3**

Trauma, disease, or surgery can interrupt the closed negative-pressure system of the lungs, causing lung collapse. Air (pneumothorax) or blood or fluid (hemothorax) may leak into the pleural cavity. A chest tube is inserted, and a closed chest drainage system is attached to promote drainage of air and fluid from the pleural space so the lung can reexpand. A one-way valve prevents the air or fluid from flowing back into the pleural cavity. This type of tube is also called a thoracostomy tube or thoracic catheter. Suction may be added to assist gravity in draining fluid (Sullivan, 2008).

The placement of the chest tube depends on the type of drainage that is necessary. Because air rises, apical and anterior chest tube placement promotes removal of air. Chest tubes are placed low and posterior or lateral to drain fluid (Fig. 14-7). Mediastinal chest tubes are placed just below the sternum (Fig. 14-8) and drain blood or fluid, preventing

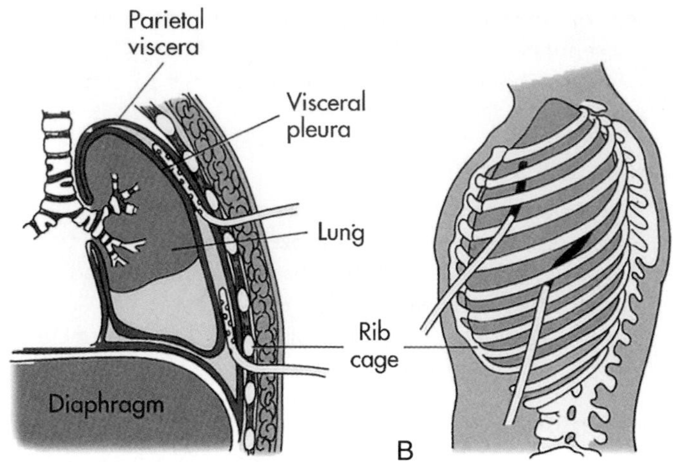

FIG 14-7 Diagram of sites for chest tube placement. **A,** Anatomic drawing showing upper tube placement (for air) and lower tube placement (for blood and fluid). **B,** View of tubes exiting through intracostal sites.

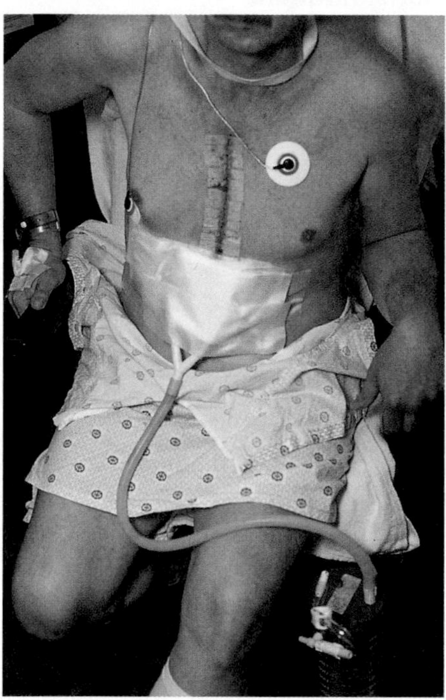

FIG 14-8 Mediastinal chest tube following open heart surgery.

its accumulation around the heart (e.g., after open-heart surgery).

Although single-bottle systems are available, single-unit water-seal or waterless systems are most often used. The water-seal system contains two or three compartments or chambers (Fig. 14-9). Fluid drains into the first chamber. The second chamber contains the water seal, which allows air to escape because of the force of expiration but not to reenter on inspiration. If suction is needed, a third chamber is used. The suction pressure should not exceed 20 cm of H_2O because lung tissue damage may occur (Sullivan, 2008).

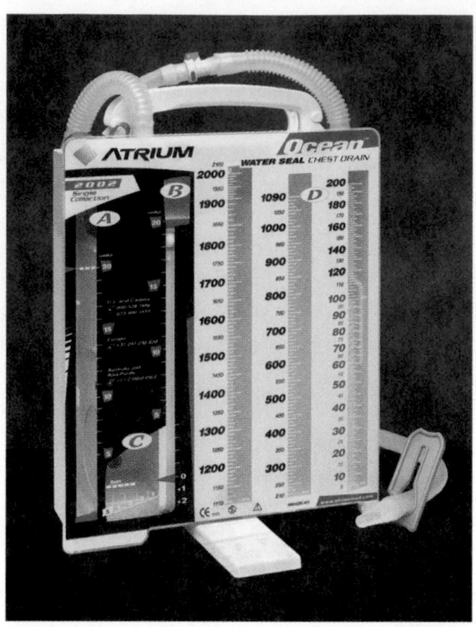

FIG 14-9 Disposable water-seal chest drainage system with suction. (Courtesy Atrium Medical.)

The waterless system follows the same principles, except that sterile water is not required for suction. The suction control chamber is replaced by a one-way valve located near the top of the system. The drainage chamber takes up most of the space in the drainage unit. The suction control chamber contains a suction control float ball that is set by a suction control dial after the suction is connected and turned on.

ASSESSMENT

1. Perform a complete respiratory assessment (see Chapters 6 and 7), baseline vital signs, and oximetry. *Rationale: Baseline vital signs are essential for any invasive procedure (Moore, 2007). Chest tube insertion often causes respiratory distress.*
2. Assess patient's comfort level on a scale of 0 to 10. *Rationale: Determines need for and level of pain management.*
3. Assess if patient is able to breathe deeply and comfortably. *Rationale: Detects early signs and symptoms of complications. Promotes reexpansion of the lung.*
4. Review patient's hemoglobin and hematocrit levels. *Rationale: Parameters reflect if blood loss is occurring, which may affect oxygenation.*

PLANNING

Expected Outcomes focus on removal of air and fluid from the pleural space and reexpansion of the lung with maximum patient comfort.

1. Patient's respirations are nonlabored.
2. Patient's breath sounds are present in all lobes.
3. Patient's lung expansion is symmetrical.

4. Patient's vital signs, oxygenation saturation, hemoglobin level, and hematocrit improve or are within normal ranges by discharge.
5. Patient performs breathing exercises correctly.
6. Patient reports improved comfort on a scale of 0 to 10.
7. Chest drainage system remains intact and functioning properly.

Delegation and Collaboration

The skill of chest tube management cannot be delegated to nursing assistive personnel (NAP).

Equipment

- Local anesthetic, if not an emergent procedure
- Prescribed drainage system
- Water-seal system versus waterless system: sterile water or normal saline per manufacturer's directions
- Suction, if used
- Chest tube tray (all items are sterile), typically: knife handle, chest tube clamp, small sponge forceps, needle holder, knife blade, suture, sterile drape, two clamps, 4 × 4–inch sponges, suture scissors
- Dressings: Petroleum gauze, large dressing of choice, additional 4 × 4–inch dressings, tape
- Two rubber-tipped hemostats (shodded) for each chest tube
- 1-inch waterproof adhesive tape for taping connections
- Face mask/face shield
- Sterile gloves

IMPLEMENTATION *for* MANAGING CLOSED CHEST DRAINAGE SYSTEMS

STEPS	RATIONALE
1. See **Standard Protocol (inside front cover).**	
2. Identify patient using two identifiers (e.g., name and birthday or name and account number, according to facility policy). Compare identifiers with information on patient's medication administration record (MAR) or medical record.	Ensures correct patient. Complies with The Joint Commission standards and improves patient safety (TJC, 2010).
3. Check agency policy to determine if informed consent is needed.	Invasive medical procedures typically require informed consent.
4. Set up water-seal system.	
a. Obtain a chest drainage system. Remove wrappers and prepare to set up as a two- or three-chamber system.	Maintains sterility of system for use under sterile operating room conditions.
b. While maintaining sterility of the drainage tubing, stand system upright and add sterile water or normal saline to appropriate compartments.	Reduces possibility of contamination (Sullivan, 2008).
(1) For a two-chamber system (without suction), add sterile solution to water-seal chamber (second chamber), bringing fluid to the required level as indicated.	Water-seal chamber acts as a one-way valve so air cannot enter pleural space.
(2) For a three-chamber system (with suction); add sterile solution to the water-seal chamber (second chamber). Add amount of sterile solution prescribed by physician to the suction control (third chamber), usually 20 cm of H_2O pressure. Connect tubing from suction control chamber to suction source. Tailor length of drainage tube to patient.	Depth of rod below fluid level dictates highest amount of negative pressure that can be present within system. For example, 20 cm of water is approximately 20 cm of water pressure (Sullivan, 2008). Any additional negative pressure applied to system is vented into the atmosphere through suction control vent. This safety device prevents damage to pleural tissues from an unexpected surge of negative pressure from suction source. Excessively long drainage tube may result in occlusions.
NOTE: **Suction control chamber vent must not be occluded when using suction.**	Provides safety factor of releasing excess negative pressure into the air through suction control vent.
5. Set up waterless system.	
a. Remove sterile wrappers and prepare to set up.	Maintains sterility of system for use under sterile operating room conditions.
b. For a two-chamber system (without suction), nothing is added or needs to be done to system.	Waterless two-chamber system is ready for connecting to patient's chest tube after opening wrappers.
c. For a three-chamber system with suction, connect tubing from suction control chamber to suction source.	Suction source provides additional negative pressure to system.

Continued

STEPS	RATIONALE
d. Instill 15 mL of sterile water or normal saline into diagnostic indicator injection port located on top of system.	Allows for observation of a rise and fall in water in diagnostic air leak window. This is not necessary for mediastinal drainage because there is no tidaling. In an emergency, system *does not* require water for setup.
6. Tape all tubing connections in a double-spiral fashion using 2.5 cm (1-inch) adhesive tape. Then check the system for patency by: **a.** Clamping the drainage tubing that will connect to the patient's chest tube. **b.** Connecting tubing from float ball chamber to suction source. **c.** Turning on suction to prescribed level.	Prevents atmospheric air from leaking into system and patient's intrapleural space. Provides chance to ensure airtight system before connecting it to patient. Allows correction or replacement of system if it is defective before connecting it to patient.
7. Turn off suction source and unclamp drainage tubing before connecting patient to system. Make a second check to be sure drainage tubing is not excessively long. Suction source is turned on again after patient is connected (Step 10).	Having patient connected to suction when it is initiated could damage pleural tissues from sudden increase in negative pressure. Tubing that is coiled or looped may become clotted, impeding drainage while draining a hemothorax, and may potentially cause a tension pneumothorax (Sullivan, 2008).
8. Position patient for tube insertion so the side in which you will place the chest tube is accessible to the physician.	
9. Assist physician with chest tube insertion by providing needed equipment and local analgesic and offering patient support and instruction. Physician will insert and clamp tube, suture it in place, and apply occlusive dressing.	
10. Help physician attach drainage tube to chest tube; remove clamp. Turn on suction to prescribed level.	Connects drainage system and suction (if ordered) to chest tube.
11. Tape tube connection between chest tube and drainage tube. One method: One long strip of tape on each side with an overlapping tape wrapped spirally enables connections to be observed and remain secure.	Secures chest tube to drainage system and reduces risk of air leaks that cause breaks in airtight system.
12. Check system for proper functioning; physician will order a chest x-ray.	Verifies intrapleural placement of tube.
13. After tube placement, position patient:	
a. Use semi-Fowler's to high-Fowler's position to evacuate air (pneumothorax).	Permits optimum drainage of fluid and/or air. Air rises to highest point in the chest (Sullivan, 2008).
b. Using high-Fowler's position to drain fluid (hemothorax).	Permits optimum drainage of fluid.
14. Check patency of air vents in system.	
a. Water-seal vent must have no occlusion.	Permits displaced air to pass into atmosphere.
b. Suction control chamber vent must not be occluded when using suction.	Provides safety factor of releasing excess negative pressure into atmosphere.
c. Waterless systems have relief valves without caps.	
15. Position tubing on mattress next to patient. Secure with clamp provided so it does not obstruct tubing.	Excess tubing hanging over the edge of mattress may form a dependent loop where drainage could pool, causing a blockage (Sullivan, 2008).
16. Adjust tubing to hang in a straight line from top of mattress to drainage chamber.	Promotes drainage.
17. Place two rubber-tipped hemostats (for each chest tube) in an easily accessible position such as taped to the top of patient's headboard. These should remain with patient if ambulating.	Chest tubes are double clamped under specific circumstances: (1) to assess for an air leak (see Table 14-4), (2) to empty or quickly change disposable systems, or (3) to assess if patient ready to have tube removed.
18. Care for patient with chest tubes	

STEPS	RATIONALE
a. Assess vital signs; oxygen saturation; skin color; breath sounds; and rate, depth, and ease of respirations every 15 minutes for first 2 hours, then at least every shift (see agency policy).	Provides data to compare with baseline and information about procedure-related complications.
b. Monitor color, consistency, and amount of drainage every 15 minutes for the first 2 hours. Indicate level of drainage fluid, date, and time on chamber's write-on surface.	Provides baseline for continuous assessment of type and quantity of drainage. Ensures early detection of complications.
(1) From a mediastinal tube, less than 100 mL/hr immediately after surgery is expected and no more than 500 mL in first 24 hours.	Sudden gush of drainage may result from coughing or changing patient's position, releasing pooled/collected blood rather than indicating active bleeding.
(2) From a posterior chest tube between 100 and 300 mL is expected during first 3 hours after insertion, with a total of 500 to 1000 mL expected in the first 24 hours. Drainage is grossly bloody during the first several hours after surgery and then changes to serous.	Acute bleeding indicates hemorrhage.
(3) From an anterior chest tube that is inserted for a pneumothorax, there should be little or no output.	
c. Observe chest dressing for drainage.	Drainage around tube may indicate blockage.
d. Palpate around tube for swelling and crepitus (subcutaneous emphysema) as evidenced by crackling.	Indicates presence of air trapping in subcutaneous tissues. Small amounts are commonly absorbed. Large amounts are potentially dangerous.
e. Check tubing to ensure that it is free of kinks and dependent loops.	Promotes drainage.
f. Observe for fluctuation of drainage in the tubing and water-seal chamber during inspiration and expiration. Observe for clots or debris in tubing.	If fluctuation or tidaling stops, it means that either the lung is fully expanded or the system is obstructed (Sullivan, 2008).
g. Keep drainage system upright and below level of the patient's chest.	Promotes gravity drainage and prevents backflow of fluid and air into the pleural space (Sullivan, 2008).
h. Check for air leaks by monitoring the bubbling in water-seal chamber: Intermittent bubbling is normal during expiration when air is being evacuated from the pleural cavity, but continuous bubbling during both inspiration and expiration indicates a leak in the system.	Absence of bubbling may indicate that the lung has fully expanded if patient had pneumothorax (Sullivan, 2008). Bubbling occurs at first because there is air in tubing and system. This should stop after a few minutes unless other sources of air are entering system. If bubbling continues, check connections and locate source of air leak as described in Table 14-4.

SAFETY ALERT Stripping the chest tube is controversial and generally not recommended since it greatly increases negative pressure within the tube, causing lung injury. Gentle milking of a chest tube by squeezing and releasing one hand at a time is sometimes performed on tubes with high volumes of bloody drainage. Research is inconclusive in this area, and the nurse should refer to hospital policy (Sullivan, 2008).

STEPS	RATIONALE
19. Assist in chest tube removal.	
a. Administer prescribed medication for pain relief about 30 minutes before procedure.	Reduces discomfort and relaxes patient by allowing time for medication to take effect (Sullivan, 2008).
b. Assist patient with sitting on edge of bed or lying on side without chest tubes.	Physician prescribes patient's position to facilitate tube removal.
c. Physician prepares an occlusive dressing of petroleum gauze on a pressure dressing and sets it aside on a sterile field.	Essential to prepare in advance for quick application to wound during tube withdrawal.
d. Physician asks patient to take a deep breath and hold it or exhale completely and hold it.	Prevents air from being sucked into chest as tube is removed.

Continued

STEPS	RATIONALE
e. Physician holds prepared dressing at point of tube insertion and quickly pulls out chest tube.	Prevents entry of air through chest wound.
f. Physician quickly and firmly secures it in position with elastic bandage (Elastoplast) or wide tape. Physician sometimes uses skin clips or draws purse-string sutures together before applying dressing.	Keeps wound aseptic. Prevents entry of air into chest. Wound closure occurs spontaneously. Clips or sutures aid in skin closure (Sullivan, 2008).
20. See Completion Protocol (inside front cover).	

TABLE 14-4 PROBLEM SOLVING WITH CHEST TUBES

ASSESSMENT	INTERVENTION
1. Air leak can occur at insertion site, connection between tube and drainage device, or within drainage device itself. Continuous bubbling is noted in water-seal chamber that is attached to suction. If a water-seal unit is not attached to suction, a total absence of bubbling and drainage would indicate a leak.	Locate leak by clamping tube at different intervals. Leaks are corrected when constant bubbling stops.
2. Assess for location of leak by clamping chest tube with two rubber-shod or toothless clamps close to the chest wall. If bubbling stops, air leak is inside patient's thorax or at chest insertion site (Sullivan, 2008).	**SAFETY ALERT** Unclamp tube, reinforce chest dressing, and notify physician immediately. *Rationale: Leaving chest tube clamped can cause collapse of lung, mediastinal shift, and eventual collapse of other lung from buildup of air pressure within the pleural cavity.*
3. If bubbling continues with clamps near the chest wall, gradually move one clamp at a time down drainage tubing away from patient and toward suction control chamber. When bubbling stops, leak is in section of tubing or connection between clamps.	Replace tubing, or secure connection and release clamps.
4. If bubbling still continues, this indicates that leak is in the drainage system.	Change the drainage system.
5. Assess for tension pneumothorax: • Severe respiratory distress • Low oxygen saturation • Chest pain • Absence of breath sounds on affected side • Tracheal shift toward unaffected side • Hypotension and signs of shock • Tachycardia	Make sure that chest tubes are patent: remove clamps, eliminate kinks, or eliminate occlusion. Notify physician immediately and prepare for another chest tube insertion. You may use a flutter (Heimlich) valve or large-gauge needle for short-term emergency release of pressure in the intrapleural space. Have emergency equipment, oxygen, and code cart available because condition is life threatening.
6. Water-seal tube is no longer submerged in sterile fluid because of evaporation.	Add sterile water to water-seal chamber until distal tip is 2 cm (1 inch) under surface level.

EVALUATION

1. Assess patient for decreased respiratory distress and chest pain.
2. Auscultate patient's lungs and observe chest expansion.
3. Monitor vital signs, hematocrit, hemoglobin level, and oxygen saturation.
4. Evaluate patient's ability to use deep-breathing exercises while maintaining comfort.
5. Reassess patient level of comfort (on a scale of 0 to 10), comparing level with comfort before chest tube insertion.
6. Monitor continued functioning of system as indicated by reduction in the amount of drainage, resolution of the air leak, and complete reexpansion of the lung (tidaling or bubbling noted) (Sullivan, 2008).

Unexpected Outcomes and Related Interventions

1. Air leak is unrelated to patient's respiration.
   a. See Table 14-4 for determining the source of an air leak and problem solving.
2. Chest tubes become obstructed by a clot or kinked tube.
   a. Observe patient for mediastinal shift or respiratory distress, which may constitute a medical emergency.
   b. Determine source of obstruction, as noted by lack of flow through tube or clot detected in system. If kinked, reposition patient and straighten tubing and adjust to prevent continued problems.
   c. If clot is identified, notify physician.
3. Chest tube becomes dislodged.
   a. Immediately apply pressure over chest tube site with anything that is within immediate reach (e.g., several

layers of patient's hospital gown, bed sheet, towel, gauze dressings).
   b. Have assistant obtain a sterile petroleum dressing. Apply as patient exhales. Secure dressing with a tight seal.
   c. Notify physician and remain with patient.
4. Substantial increase in bright-red drainage is observed.
   a. Observe for tachycardia and hypotension.
   b. Report to physician because this may indicate that patient is actively bleeding.

Recording and Reporting

- Record respiratory assessment; amount of suction, if used; amount of drainage since the previous assessment; type of drainage in chest tubing; and presence or absence of an air leak, including amount if present.
- Record integrity of dressing and presence of drainage on dressing.
- Record patient comfort and tolerance.

Sample Documentation

0800 Resting comfortably, denies complaint. Respirations regular in rate, rhythm, and depth at 16 breaths/min. Lungs generally clear with breath sounds heard over right and left upper lung fields. Left posterior lung sounds diminished. Left posterior chest tube and dressing intact with tidaling present in water-seal chamber. No air leak noted. 50 mL serous drainage collected in past 8 hours. Taking deep breaths as instructed without complaints of discomfort.

REVIEW QUESTIONS

Case Study for Questions 1 to 3

Mr. G is a 48-year-old fireman who is married with three young children and has a 25-year history of smoking. He had a recent diagnosis of lung cancer and consequently a right thoracotomy (removal of right lung). He has a right chest tube and is receiving oxygen via a nasal cannula with the oxygen regulator set at 2 L/min. The chest tube with a three-chamber system is set on suction at 20 cm. Bubbling is noted during expiration.

1. The nurse performs a respiratory assessment on this patient, who is short of breath. Which of the following are appropriate when assessing respiratory status? Select all that apply.
   1. Inspect the patient for rate, rhythm, and depth of breathing.
   2. Auscultate anterior lung sounds while he is flat on his side.
   3. Obtain vital signs and a pulse oximeter reading to assess oxygenation.
   4. Evaluate the chest tube for working order.
2. The nurse caring for this patient recognizes the need for supplemental oxygen therapy. It is determined that Mr. G needs an FIO_2 of 80%. Which oxygen delivery devices can deliver oxygen at this FIO_2 level? Select all that apply.
   1. Nasal cannula at 6 L/min
   2. Venturi mask at 12 L/min
   3. Nonrebreathing mask at 6 L/min
   4. Partial rebreathing mask at 6 L/min
3. The nurse notices that this patient's chest tube is bubbling continuously. Which of the following steps is/are appropriate for the nurse to complete? Select all that apply.
   1. Check to ensure that all connections are secure.
   2. Determine that no kinks are affecting the tubing from the chest tube to the drainage system.
   3. Disconnect the chest tube from the drainage tube to assess for adequate suction.
   4. Assess for location of leak by clamping chest tube with two rubber-shod or toothless clamps close to the chest wall.
4. An RN is mentoring a new graduate RN who is suctioning a patient through an ET tube. Which of the following steps indicate acceptable technique?
   1. Hyperoxygenates patient with 21% oxygen before suctioning
   2. Uses a clean catheter for suctioning
   3. Inserts catheter with nurse's thumb covering the suction control port
   4. Dips catheter in saline before suctioning
5. Suctioning the patient may cause which of the following complications? Select all that apply.
   1. Hypoxia
   2. Dysrhythmias
   3. Increased intracranial pressure
   4. Thick secretions
6. Which activities could a nurse delegate to assistive personnel? Select all that apply.
   1. Suctioning an ET tube
   2. Tracheostomy care for a chronically ill patient on humidified oxygen
   3. Application of functioning nasal cannula
   4. Tracheostomy care on an acutely ill mechanically ventilated patient
7. The nurse is assessing a patient with an artificial airway. Which of the following would indicate that the patient might need to be suctioned? Select all that apply.
   1. Wheezes auscultated on inspiration
   2. Decreased breath sounds in the bases
   3. Weak cough
   4. Thick secretions

8. Current best practice indicates that the following interventions are advantageous in preventing VAP. Select all that apply.
   1. Elevating the head of the bed at 30 to 45 degrees to prevent aspiration
   2. Changing patient position every 2 hours to decrease risk for atelectasis and pulmonary infections
   3. Providing oral care with a toothette daily to remove dental plaque organisms
   4. Limiting patient mobility to promote rest and conserve oxygen
9. Patients are unable to speak when they have an ET tube. What are some of the recommended ways to communicate with these patients? Select all that apply.
   1. Talk to patients as if they have a hearing loss by speaking very loudly.
   2. Leave a pen and paper within reach of patient so he or she can write comments to health care providers and family members.
   3. Provide an alphabet board for family and friends to communicate with patient.
   4. Ask family members to explain the plan of care to patient.
10. Patients with chest tubes to remove blood drainage from the chest cavity have many care priorities. Which of the two pairs of priorities are the most important?
   1. Monitoring chest tube drainage and maintaining chest tube patency
   2. Monitoring chest tube drainage and promoting activity
   3. Promoting airway clearance and maintaining chest tube patency
   4. Promoting airway clearance and promoting activity

REFERENCES

Abbott C and others: Adoption of a ventilator-associated pneumonia clinical practice guideline, *Worldviews on Evidence-Based Nursing* 3(4):139, 2006.

American Association of Critical Care Nurses: Practice alert, oral care in the critically ill, 2007, http://www.aacn.org/WD/Practice/Docs/Oral_Care_in_the_Critically_Ill.pdf, accessed August 9, 2009.

American Association of Respiratory Care: AARC clinical practice guideline, nasotracheal suction—2004 revision and update, *Respir Care* 49:1080, 2004, http://www.rcjournal.com/cpgs/pdf/09.04.1080.pdf, accessed August 9, 2009.

Barnes D: Non-invasive ventilation in COPD 2: starting and monitoring NIV, *Nurs Times* 103(40):26, 2007.

Beattie S: Back to the basics with O_2 therapy, *RN* 69(9):37, 2006.

Biddle C: Oxygen: The two-faced elixir of life, *AANA J* 76(1):61, 2008.

Celik S, Kanan N: A current conflict: use of isotonic sodium chloride solution on endotracheal suctioning in critically ill patients, *Dimens Crit Care Nurs* 25(1):11, 2006.

Couchman B and others: Nursing care of the mechanically ventilated patient: what does the evidence say? Part One, *Intens Crit Care Nurs* 23:4, 2007.

Coyer F and others: Nursing care of the mechanically ventilated patient: what does the evidence say? Part Two, *Intens Crit Care Nurs* 23:71, 2007.

Eastwood G and others: Low-flow oxygen therapy: selecting the right device, *Aust Nurs J* 15(4):27, 2007.

Garvey C: *Secretion clearance devices: coverage policies/cost*, 2005, American Thoracic Society Website Practice Tips.

Higginson R, Jones B: Respiratory assessment in critically ill patients: airway and breathing, *Br J Nurs* 18(8):456, 2009.

Hockenberry MJ, Wilson D: *Wong's essentials of pediatric nursing*, ed 8, St Louis, 2009, Mosby.

Lewis SL and others: *Medical surgical nursing, assessment and management of clinical problems*, ed 6, St Louis, 2007, Mosby.

McGloin S: Administration of oxygen therapy, *Nurs Stand* 22(21):46, 2008.

Moore T: Respiratory assessment in adults, *Nurs Stand* 21(49):48, 2007.

National Institute of Health: http://www.nhlbi.nih.gov, 2009, accessed August 9, 2009.

O'Keefe-McCarthy S and others: Ventilator-associated pneumonia bundled strategies: an evidence-based practice, *Worldviews on Evidence-Based Nursing* 4:193, 2008.

Pederson C and others: Endotracheal suctioning of the adult intubated patient—what is the evidence? *Intens Crit Care Nurs* 25:21, 2009.

Rauen CA and others: Seven evidence-based practice habits: putting some sacred cows out to pasture, *Crit Care Nurse* 28(2):98, 2008.

Stokowski LA: An update on preventing ventilator-associated pneumonia, http://cme.medscape.com/viewarticle/591015, 2009, accessed August 9, 2009.

Sullivan B: Nursing management of patients with chest drain, *Br J Nurs* 17(6):388, 2008.

The Joint Commission (TJC): *2010 National Patient Safety Goals*, Oakbrook Terrace, Ill, 2010, The Commission, http://jointcommission.org/PatientSafety/NationalPatientSafetyGoals/.

Tolentino-DelosReyes AF and others: Evidence-based practice: use of ventilator bundle to prevent ventilator-associated pneumonia, *Am J Crit Care* 16(1):20, 2007.

Vollman K: Ask the experts, *Crit Care Nurse* 26(4):53, 2006.

Wang K and others: Qualitative analysis of patients' intensive care experience during mechanical ventilation, *J Clin Nurs* 18:183, 2008.

CHAPTER

15

Safe Patient Handling, Transfer, and Positioning

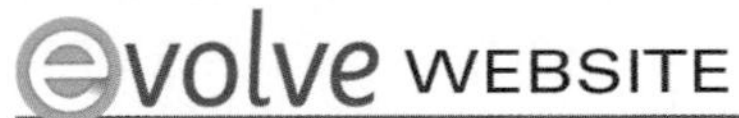

http://evolve.elsevier.com/Perry/nursinginterventions
Video Clips
Nursing Skills Online

Health care providers are required to provide employees with safety information and training to use when transferring, positioning, and lifting patients. The Occupational Safety and Health Administration (OSHA) has identified guidelines on back safety and the prevention of musculoskeletal injuries (OSHA, 2009; United States Department of Labor, 2003). Before lifting, assess the weight you will be lifting and what assistance, if any, is needed (Nelson and others, 2009; United States Department of Labor, 2003). If you need help, assess if a second person is adequate or if you need mechanical assistance. Once you determine the amount of assistance needed, use the following steps for proper body mechanics:

- Before lifting tighten stomach muscles and tuck pelvis to provide balance and protect the back.
- Bend at the knees to help maintain your center of gravity. Let the strong muscles of the legs do the lifting.
- Keep the weight (patient) to be lifted as close to the body as possible; this action places the weight in the same plane as the lifter and close to the center of gravity for balance.
- Maintain the trunk erect and knees bent so multiple muscle groups work together in a synchronized manner.
- Avoid twisting. Twisting your spine can lead to serious injury.
- The best height for lifting vertically is approximately 2 feet off the ground and close to the lifter's center of gravity.

Body mechanics are the coordinated effort of the musculoskeletal and nervous systems to maintain balance, posture, and body alignment during lifting, bending, moving, and performing activities of daily living (ADLs). Body mechanics also facilitate body movement so a person can carry out a physical activity without using excessive muscle energy.

PATIENT-CENTERED CARE

Ultimately it is the patient's choice to increase his or her mobility and activity level. Consider the patient's knowledge, cultural beliefs, and circumstances surrounding the loss of independent activity when developing a plan of care. Care planned with the patient motivates and encourages the patient to participate. For example, taking a few minutes to assess a patient's knowledge and providing information about the complications of immobility may be all that is needed to elicit his or her cooperation in ambulating after surgery. It is also important to assess the patient's cultural and ethnic beliefs to incorporate appropriate interventions that match individual beliefs. For instance, some patients have a fear of becoming addicted to a narcotic (opioid) after one dose. Yet pain is preventing them from increasing their mobility. Knowing that the patient has a fear of opioids, individualize the plan of care and explain the safe and proper use of opioids for pain control. In addition, taking into consideration the circumstances surrounding the loss of independent activity and mobility is crucial in developing a plan of care that is realistic and attainable. Consider the example of a patient who has recently undergone surgery and who is expected to ambulate a prescribed number of feet on the second postoperative day. The nurse knows that this patient has a long history of pulmonary disease. This information prompts the nurse to alter the patient's plan of care based on this activity limitation to achieve a reasonable level of mobility and activity.

SAFETY

Nurses care for patients who have conditions resulting in immobility or who require limitations in activity imposed by their treatment plan. As a result, nursing has an important role in safely positioning and moving patients effectively to reduce the risks of immobilization. Positioning patients to maintain correct body alignment is essential to prevent complications. These complications include pressure ulcers (see Chapter 17), which can develop in 24 hours and require months of time and thousands of dollars to correct; and contractures, which can occur within a few days when muscles, tendons, and joints become less flexible because of lack of mobility and incorrect alignment. For example, plantar flexion contracture or footdrop occurs when the force of gravity pulls an unsupported, weakened foot into a plantar-flexed position and calf muscles and heel cords shorten, complicating future attempts at walking. Pillows placed under the knees or an elevated knee gatch can produce knee and hip contractures and increase pressure on the sacrum and thus the risk for pressure ulcers. A sagging mattress increases the risk of hip contractures. These knee and hip contractures can cause future gait and posture problems, making mobility more difficult.

Some patients are at higher risk for complications from improper positioning and have increased risk of injury during transfer. Patients with alterations in bone formation or joint mobility, impaired muscle development, and central nervous system (CNS) damage may experience motor impairment, proprioceptive loss, or cognitive dysfunction, all of which affect mobility. The application of proper body mechanics, alignment, and the use of transfer and positioning techniques assist the patient in achieving an optimal level of independence without resultant injury to the health care provider.

EVIDENCE-BASED PRACTICE TRENDS

Sedlak C and others: Development of the National Association of Orthopaedic Nurses guidance statement on safe patient handling and movement in the orthopaedic setting, *Orthop Nurs* 28(2S):S2, 2009.

Musculoskeletal disorders are the most prevalent and debilitating occupational health hazards among nurses. There has been little improvement in the incidence of musculoskeletal injuries in health care workers. In 1989 4.2 lost-workday injury cases per 100 were reported; in 2000 there were 4.1 cases per 100 (Baptiste and others, 2006; Bureau of Labor Statistics, 2003). Because the risk of injury continues for nurses and their patients, the American Nurses Association (ANA) developed position statements calling for the use of assistive equipment and devices to reposition and transfer patients to promote a safe health care environment (ANA, 2003; 2007). A task force was developed to identify high-risk tasks related to moving and lifting patients. Evidence-based practice trends were identified to develop solutions for safe patient handling (Sedlak and others, 2009).

The use of assistive equipment and continued use of proper body mechanics significantly reduce the risk of musculoskeletal injuries (ANA, 2007). In addition, OSHA recommends that manual lifting of patients be minimized in all cases and eliminated when possible (OSHA, 2009). Many facilities are moving toward limited lift policies that minimize patient handling by nurses (Miami Valley Hospital, 2007; UC Davis Health System, 2005). Instead, many agencies are using lift devices to reduce on-the-job injuries (Pelczarski, 2007; Sedlak and others, 2009). By becoming knowledgeable about safe, efficient lifting techniques and proper use of assistive equipment and devices, nurses can safely transfer patients without causing injury to themselves or patients.

SKILL 15.1 TRANSFER TECHNIQUES

- **Nursing Skills Online: Safety Module, Lesson 3**

Video Clips

Transferring is a nursing skill to help the dependent patient or the patient with restricted mobility attain positions to regain optimal independence as quickly and safely as possible. Physical activity maintains and improves joint motion, increases strength, promotes circulation, relieves pressure on skin, and improves urinary and respiratory functions. It also benefits the patient psychologically by increasing social activity and mental stimulation and providing a change in environment (Lampinen and others, 2006). Thus mobilization plays a crucial role in the patient's rehabilitation.

One of the major concerns during transfer is the safety of the patient and the nurse. The nurse prevents self-injury by using correct posture, minimal muscle strength, and effective body mechanics and lifting techniques. You must consider any special problems during a patient's transfer to avoid injury such as in a fall. For example, a patient who has been immobile for several days or longer may be weak or dizzy or may develop orthostatic hypotension (a drop in blood pressure) when transferred. As a rule of thumb, use a transfer belt and obtain assistance when transferring patients if there is any doubt about safe transfer.

ASSESSMENT

1. Review medical records to assess physiological capacity of a patient to transfer and need for special adaptive techniques. Assess the following:
   a. Muscle strength (legs and upper arms). *Rationale: Immobile patients have decreased muscle strength, tone, and mass, which affects the ability to bear weight or raise the body.*

b. Joint mobility and contracture formation. *Rationale: Immobility or inflammatory processes (e.g., arthritis) may lead to contracture formation and impaired joint mobility.*

c. Paralysis or paresis (spastic or flaccid). *Rationale: Patient with CNS damage may have bilateral paralysis (requiring transfer by swivel bar, sliding bar, mechanical lift) or unilateral paralysis, which requires belt transfer to strong side. Weakness (paresis) requires stabilization of knee while transferring. Support flaccid arm with sling during transfer.*

d. Bone continuity. *Rationale: Patients with trauma to one leg or hip may be nonweight bearing during a transfer. Amputees may use sliding board to transfer.*

2. Assess presence of weakness, dizziness, or postural hypotension. *Rationale: Determines patient's risk of fainting or falling during transfer. The move from a supine to a vertical position redistributes about 500 mL of blood; immobile patients may have decreased ability for autonomic nervous system to equalize blood supply, resulting in orthostatic hypotension (Phipps and others, 2007).*

3. Assess level of endurance by noting level of fatigue during activity and measuring vital signs. *Rationale: Estimates patient's ability to participate in transfer. Vital sign changes such as increased pulse and respiration may indicate activity intolerance (see Chapter 6).*

4. Assess patient's proprioceptive function (awareness of posture and changes in equilibrium), including ability to maintain balance while sitting in bed or on side of bed and tendency to sway or position self to one side. *Rationale: Determines stability of patient's balance for transfer and risk of falling.*

5. Assess sensory status, including central and peripheral vision, adequacy of hearing, and presence of peripheral sensation loss. *Rationale: Determines influence of sensory loss on ability to make transfer. Visual field loss decreases patient's ability to see in direction of transfer. Peripheral sensation loss decreases proprioception. Patients with visual and hearing losses need transfer techniques adapted to deficits.*

> **SAFETY ALERT** Patients with hemiplegia may "neglect" one side of the body (inattention to or unawareness of one side of the body or environment), which distorts perceptions of the visual field.

6. Assess patient for pain (e.g., joint discomfort, muscle spasm) and measure level of pain using a scale from 0 to 10. Offer prescribed analgesic 30 minutes before transfer. *Rationale: Pain reduces patient's motivation and ability to be mobile. Pain relief before transfer enhances patient participation.*

7. Assess patient's cognitive status, including ability to follow verbal instructions, short-term memory, and recognition of physical deficits and limitations to movement. *Rationale: Determines patient's ability to follow directions and learn transfer techniques.*

> **SAFETY ALERT** Patients with head trauma or cerebrovascular accident (CVA) may have perceptual cognitive deficits that create safety risks. If patient has difficulty in comprehension, simplify instructions by providing one step at a time and maintain consistency.

8. Assess patient's level of motivation such as eagerness versus unwillingness to be mobile. *Rationale: Altered psychological states reduce patient's desire to engage in activity.*

9. Assess previous mode of transfer (if applicable). *Rationale: Determines mode of transfer and assistance required to provide continuity of care. Use transfer (gait) belts with patients who need assistance (Nelson and others, 2009).*

10. Assess for conditions such as neuromuscular deficits, visual loss, motor weakness, fear of falling, or calcium loss from long bones. *Rationale: Increases patient's risk of falling and incurring injury.*

PLANNING

Expected Outcomes focus on maintaining body alignment and achieving safe transfer without injury.

1. Patient dangles legs or sits without dizziness, weakness, or orthostatic hypotension.
2. Patient transfers with minimal or no assistance.
3. Patient transfers without injury.
4. Patient tolerates increased activity.
5. Patient can bear more weight with increased endurance.
6. Patient is more motivated to be mobile.

Delegation and Collaboration

The skill of transfer techniques can be delegated to nursing assistive personnel (NAP). Instruct the NAP by:

- Explaining how to adapt transfer technique for specific patient's limitations.
- Explaining what to observe and report back to the nurse such as patient's ability to assist.

Equipment

- Transfer belt, sling, or lap board (as needed)
- Nonskid shoes, pillow, bath blanket
- Slide board (friction-reducing board)
- Stretcher
- *Option:* Mechanical/hydraulic lift, stand assist lift device
- Chair with arms or wheelchair

IMPLEMENTATION *for* TRANSFER TECHNIQUES

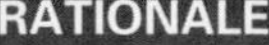

STEPS	RATIONALE
1. See Standard Protocol (inside front cover).	
2. Assist patient to sitting position on side of bed.	
a. With patient in supine position, raise head of bed 30 degrees and place bed in low position.	Decreases amount of work needed by patient and nurse to raise patient to sitting position. Low bed position prevents fall while sitting.
b. Turn patient onto side facing you on side of bed on which patient will be sitting.	Prepares patient to move to side of bed and protects from falling.
c. Stand opposite patient's hips. Turn diagonally to face patient and far corner of foot of bed.	Places nurse's center of gravity nearer patient. Reduces twisting of nurse's body because nurse is facing direction of movement.
d. Place feet apart in a wide base of support with foot closer to head of bed in front of other foot (see illustration).	Increases balance and allows nurse to transfer weight as patient is brought to sitting position on side of bed.
e. Place arm nearer head of bed under patient's shoulders, supporting head and neck.	Maintains alignment of head and neck as nurse brings patient to sitting position.
f. Place other arm over and around patient's thighs (see illustration).	Supports hip and prevents patient from falling backward during procedure.
g. On the count of three, have patient push down on mattress with upper arm (left arm in illustration) and move patient's lower legs and feet over side of bed. Pivot toward rear leg, allowing patient's upper legs to swing downward (see illustration).	Decreases friction and resistance. Weight of patient's legs when off bed allows gravity to lower legs, and weight of legs assists in pulling upper body into sitting position.

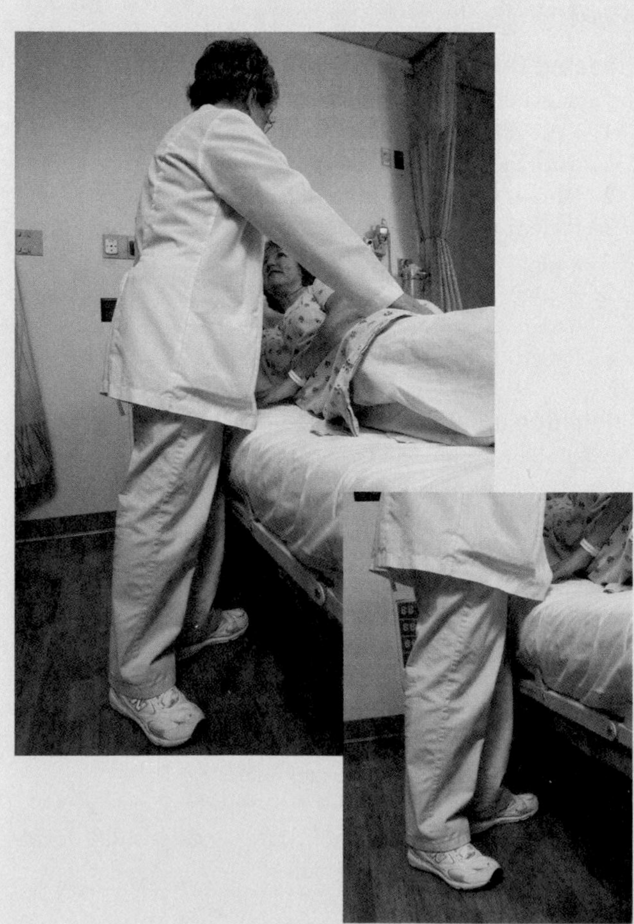

STEP 2d Proper foot placement.

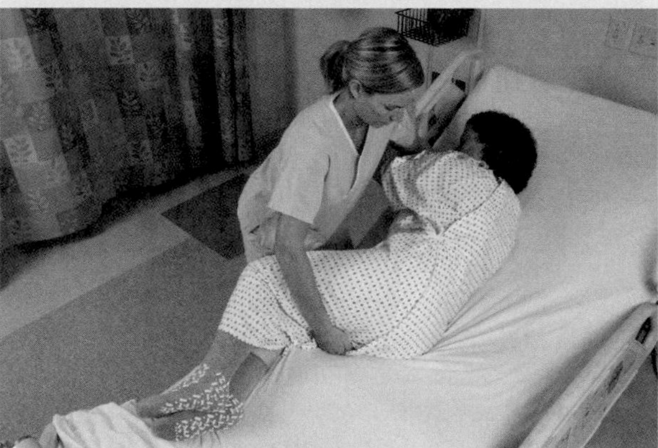

STEP 2f Nurse places arm over patient's thighs.

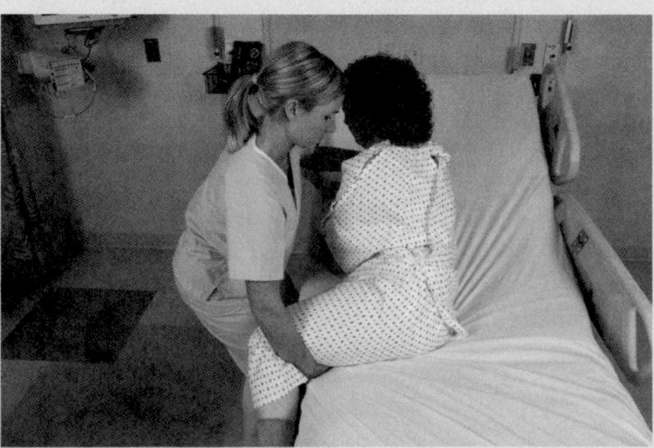

STEP 2g Nurse shifts weight to rear leg and elevates patient.

STEPS	RATIONALE
h. At same time shift weight to rear leg and elevate patient.	Allows nurse to transfer weight in direction of motion.

> **SAFETY ALERT** Remain in front until patient regains balance and continue to provide physical support to weak or cognitively impaired patient.

STEPS	RATIONALE
3. ***Transferring patient from bed to chair.***	
a. Determine if patient can bear weight. (1) Full weight bearing, nurse assistance not needed: nurse stands by to assist. (2) Partial weight bearing and patient is cooperative: use the bariatric transfer or pivot techniques that follow.	Determines degree of risk during transfer and technique required to safely assist patient.
b. If patient has partial weight bearing with upper body strength and caregiver must lift more than 35 pounds of patient's weight, use a bariatric transfer aid with minimum of two or three caregivers (see illustration).	The use of mechanical lift devices is strongly recommended to transfer a patient to reduce risk of musculoskeletal injury (Nelson and others, 2009).

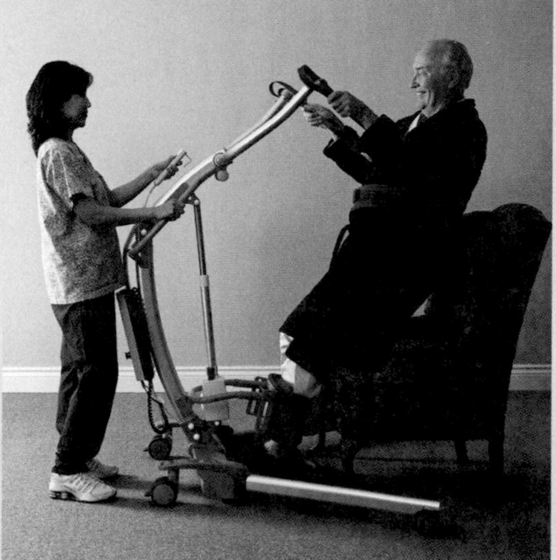

STEP 3b Stand-assist lift device.

> **SAFETY ALERT** If patient demonstrates weakness or paralysis of one side of the body, place chair on patient's strong side.

STEPS	RATIONALE
c. If patient has partial weight bearing, is cooperative and able to stand, and has upper body strength, use stand-and-pivot technique.	
(1) Place chair with arms in position at 45-degree angle to bed on patient's strong side. Assist patient to sitting position on side of bed (see Steps 2a to 2h). Allow patient to sit on side of the bed (dangling) for a few minutes before transferring to chair. Ask if patient feels dizzy. Do not leave patient unattended during dangling. Provide patient his or her glasses.	Facilitates transfer to patient's stronger side. Dangling or allowing a patient to sit on the side of the bed before transfer helps equilibrate blood pressure, reducing the risk of dizziness or fainting when standing.
(2) Apply transfer belt or other transfer aids. Patient's arm should be in sling if flaccid paralysis is present.	Transfer belt allows nurse to maintain stability of patient during transfer and reduces risk of falling (Nelson and others, 2009).

Continued

STEPS	RATIONALE
(3) Assist patient in applying stable nonskid shoes. Have patient place weight-bearing or strong leg forward, with weak foot back.	Nonskid soles decrease risk of slipping during transfer. Always have patient wear shoes during transfer; bare feet or wearing only socks increases risk of falls. Patient will stand on stronger, or weight-bearing, leg.
(4) Spread your feet apart, flex hips and knees, and align your knees with patient's knees (see illustration).	Ensures balance with wide base of support. Flexion of knees and hips lowers center of gravity to object to be raised; aligning knees with patients allows for stabilization of knees when patient stands.
(5) Grasp transfer belt at patient's side.	Provides movement of patient at center of gravity. Never lift patients by or under arms. This method has been found to be physically stressful for the nurse and uncomfortable for patients.
(6) Rock patient up to standing position on count of three while straightening hips and legs and keeping knees slightly flexed. Have patient push up with hands and knees (see illustration). While rocking the patient back and forth, make sure that your body weight is moving in the same direction as the patient's to ensure that you and the patient are moving in the same direction simultaneously.	Rocking motion gives patient's body momentum and requires less muscular effort to lift patient.
(7) Support the paralyzed or weak limb with your knee to stabilize the patient.	Maintain stability of patient's weak or paralyzed leg.
(8) Pivot and turn patient toward chair; pivot on your foot farther from chair. (See right foot in illustration for Step 3c(6)).	Maintains support of patient while allowing adequate space for patient to move.

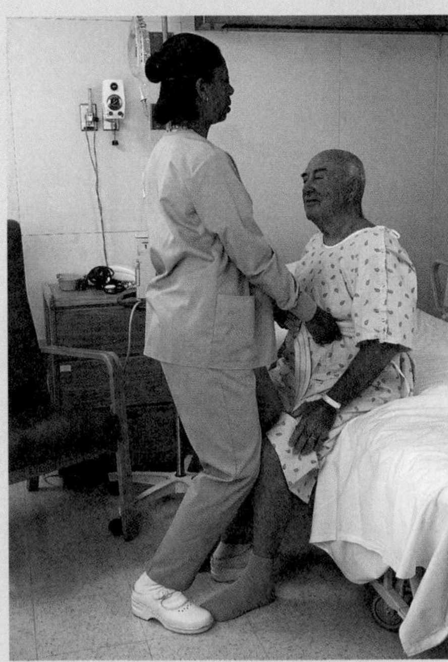

STEP 3c(4) Nurse flexes hips and knees, aligns knees with patient's knee, and grasps transfer belt.

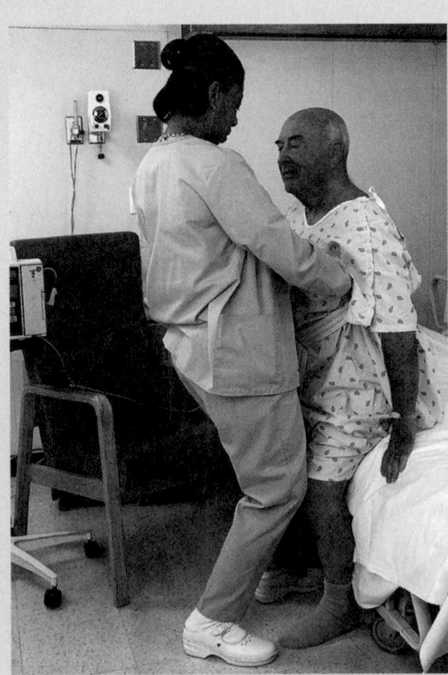

STEP 3c(6) Nurse rocks patient to standing position.

STEPS	RATIONALE
(9) Instruct patient to feel back of chair against legs and to use armrests on chair for support. Have patient ease into chair (see illustration).	Increases patient stability.
(10) Flex hips and knees while lowering patient into chair (see illustration).	Prevents injury to nurse from poor body mechanics.
(11) Help patient shift to back of chair. Assess patient for proper alignment for sitting position. Provide support for paralyzed extremities. Lap board or sling will support flaccid arm. Stabilize leg with bath blanket or pillow.	Prevents injury to patient from poor body alignment.
(12) Proper alignment for sitting position: head is erect, and vertebrae are in straight alignment. Body weight is evenly distributed on buttocks and thighs. Thighs are parallel and in horizontal plane. Both feet are supported on floor, and ankles are comfortably flexed. A 2.5- to 5-cm (1- to 2-inch) space is maintained between edge of seat and popliteal space on posterior surface of knee.	Prevents stress on intravertebral joints. Prevents increased pressure over bony prominences and reduces damage to underlying musculoskeletal system.
(13) Praise patient's progress, effort, and performance. Place call light in reach.	Support and encouragement provide incentive for patient perseverance. Patient needs call light to ask for assistance as needed.

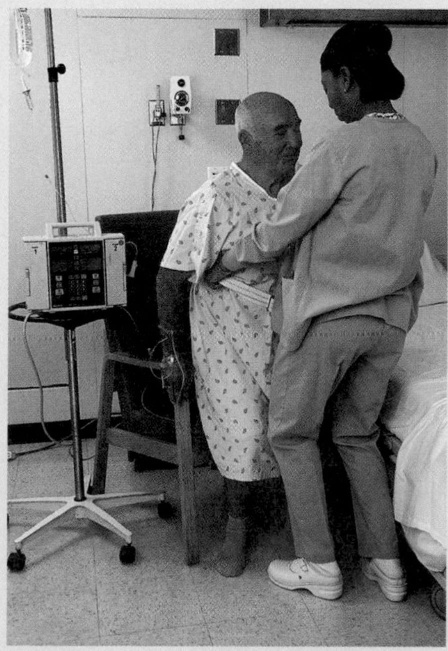

STEP 3c(9) Patient uses armrests for support.

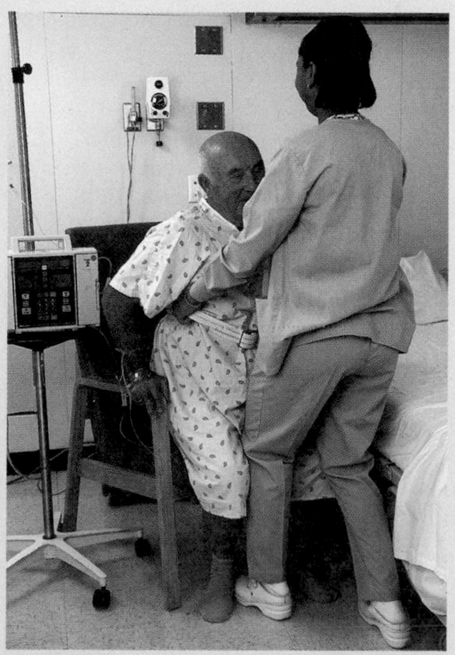

STEP 3c(10) Nurse eases patient into chair.

Continued

STEPS	RATIONALE
4. *Perform lateral transfer from bed to stretcher using slide board or friction-reducing board (see illustration).*	The three-person lift for horizontal transfer from bed to stretcher is not recommended and, in fact, is discouraged (Baptiste and others, 2006; OSHA, 2009). Physical stress can be decreased significantly by the use of a slide board or friction-reducing board. The patient is more comfortable with this method.
a. Determine if patient can assist.	Determines degree of risk during transfer and technique required to safely assist patient.
(1) Patient is able to assist by moving laterally, nurse assistance not needed; nurse stands by to assist.	
(2) Patient is partially or not at all able to move laterally; requires uses of a friction-reducing device.	
b. Determine number of staff required to laterally transfer patient safely (less than 200 pounds nurse can transfer using friction-reducing device, greater than 200 pounds use device with three caregivers).	During lateral transfer of a patient who has limited ability to assist, a caregiver should use a lift team when the patient weighs over 200 pounds. If any caregiver is required to lift more than 35 pounds of a patient's weight, the patient is considered fully dependent, and an assist device is used (Nelson and others, 2009).
c. Place bed at working height. Lower head of bed as much as patient can tolerate.	Maintains alignment of spinal column.
d. Cross patient's arms on chest.	Prevents injury to arms during transfer.
e. To place slide board under patient, position two nurses on side of bed to which patient will be turned. Position third nurse on the other side of bed.	Distributes weight equally among nurses.
f. Fanfold the drawsheet on both sides of patient.	Provides strong handles to grip the drawsheet without slipping.
g. On the count of three, turn patient onto side toward the two nurses. Turn patient as one unit with a smooth, continuous motion.	Maintains body in alignment, preventing stress on any part of the body.
h. Place slide board under drawsheet (see illustration).	Prevents friction from contact of skin with board.
i. Gently roll patient back onto slide board.	
j. Line up stretcher with bed. Lock brakes on stretcher and bed.	Ensures that stretcher or bed does not move during transfer.
k. Two nurses position themselves on the side of the stretcher while the third nurse positions self on the side of the bed without the stretcher.	

SAFETY ALERT A nurse may also be positioned at the head of patient's bed to protect and support patient's head and neck if he or she is weak or unable to assist.

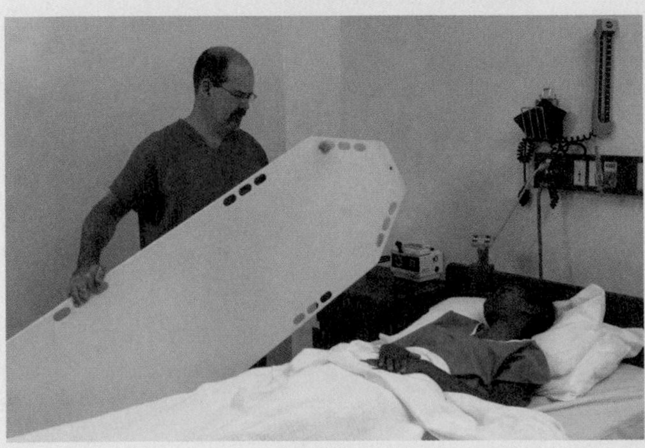

STEP 4 Slide board.

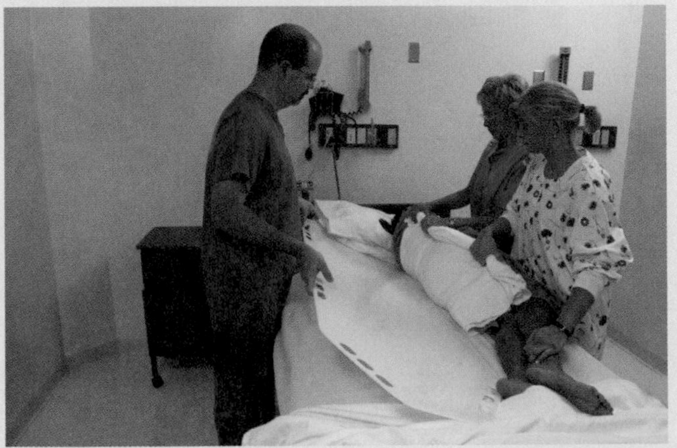

STEP 4h Placing slide board under drawsheet.

STEPS	RATIONALE
l. Fanfold drawsheet; on the count of three the two nurses pull drawsheet with patient onto stretcher while the third nurse holds the slide board in place (see illustration).	The slide board remains stationary, provides a slippery surface to reduce friction, and allows patient to transfer easily to the stretcher.

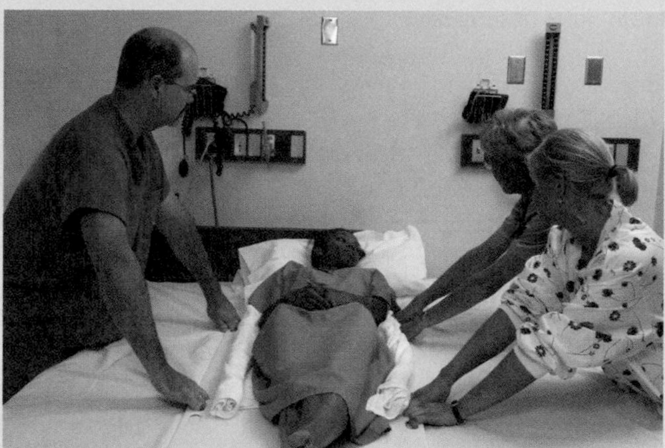

STEP 4l Transfer of patient to stretcher using slide board.

STEPS	RATIONALE
m. Position patient in center of stretcher. Raise head of stretcher if not contraindicated. Raise side rails of stretcher.	Provides for patient comfort and safety.
5. ***Use mechanical/hydraulic lift to transfer patient from bed to chair.***	Research supports the use of mechanical lifts to prevent musculoskeletal injuries (Nelson and others, 2009; Sedlak and others, 2009). The use of ceiling-mounted lifts is becoming a more popular choice because of the availability of the lift in each patient's room.
a. Determine if patient can bear weight and is cooperative.	Determines degree of risk during transfer and technique required to assist patient.
(1) Unable to bear weight and uncooperative patient requires use of full body sling lift and two caregivers.	
b. Bring lift to bedside. (Before using lift, be thoroughly familiar with its operation.)	Ensures safe elevation of patient off bed.
c. Position chair near bed and allow adequate space to maneuver lift.	Prepares environment for safe use of lift and subsequent transfer.
d. Raise bed to high position with mattress flat. Lower side rail. Have a nurse stand on each side of patient's bed.	Allows nurses to use proper body mechanics. Maintains patient safety.
e. Roll patient onto side.	Positions patient for use of lift sling.
f. Place hammock or canvas strips under patient to form sling. With two canvas pieces, lower edge fits under patient's knees (wide piece), and upper edge fits under patient's shoulders (narrow piece). Hooks should face away from patient's skin. Place sling under patient's center of gravity and greatest portion of body weight.	Two types of seats are supplied with mechanical/hydraulic lift: hammock style is better for patients who are flaccid, weak, and need support; canvas strips can be used for patients with normal muscle tone.
g. Roll patient to opposite side and pull hammock (strips) through.	Completes positioning of patient on mechanical/hydraulic sling.
h. Roll patient supine onto canvas seat.	Sling should extend from shoulders to knees (hammock) to support patient's body weight equally.
i. Remove patient's glasses if appropriate.	Swivel bar is close to patient's head and could break eyeglasses.

Continued

STEPS	RATIONALE
j. Place horseshoe bar or base of lift under side of bed (on side with chair).	Positions lift efficiently and promotes smooth transfer.
k. Lower horizontal bar to sling level by releasing hydraulic valve. Lock valve.	Positions hydraulic lift close to patient. Locking valve prevents injury to patient.
l. Attach hooks on strap (chain) to holes in sling. Short chains or straps hook to top holes of sling; longer chains hook to bottom of sling.	Secures hydraulic lift to sling.
m. Elevate head of bed. Fold patient's arms over chest.	Positions patient in sitting position. Prevents injury to patient's arms.
n. Pump hydraulic handle using long, slow, even strokes until patient is raised off bed (see illustration).	Ensures safe support of patient during elevation.
o. Use steering handle to pull lift from bed and maneuver to chair. Have a nurse move on each side of patient.	Moves patient from bed to chair. Nurses' positions reduce risk of fall from sling.
p. Roll base of lift around chair.	Positions lift in front of chair in which patient is to be transferred.
q. Release check valve slowly (turn to left), and lower patient into chair (see illustration).	Safely guides patient into back of chair as seat descends.
r. Close check valve as soon as patient is down and straps can be released.	If valve is left open, boom may continue to lower and injure patient.
s. Remove straps and mechanical/hydraulic lift.	Prevents damage to skin and underlying tissues from canvas or hooks.
t. Check patient's sitting alignment and correct if necessary.	Prevents injury from poor posture.
6. See Completion Protocol (inside front cover).	

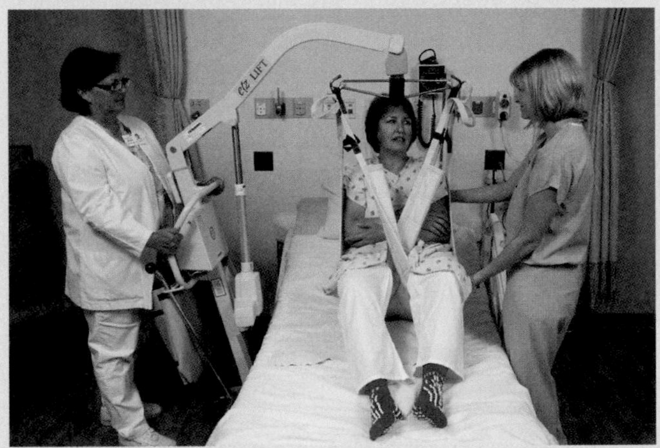

STEP 5n Patient lifted in hydraulic lift above bed.

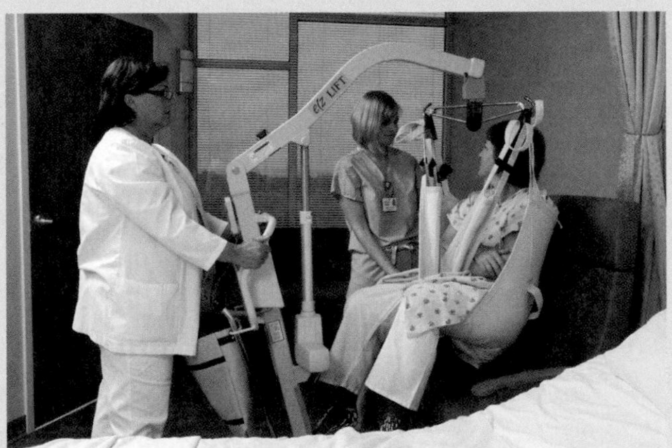

STEP 5q Use of hydraulic lift to lower patient into chair.

EVALUATION

1. Monitor vital signs. Ask if patient feels dizzy or fatigued.
2. Note patient's behavioral response to transfer.
3. Ask if patient experienced pain during transfer.
4. Observe patient's body alignment following transfer.

Unexpected Outcomes and Related Interventions

1. Patient is unable to comprehend and follow directions for transfer.
   a. Reassess continuity and simplicity of instruction.
   b. Add caregivers in transfer technique.
2. Patient sustains injury on transfer.
   a. Stay with patient and notify physician or health care provider immediately.
   b. Provide necessary supportive care until patient is stable.
   c. Evaluate incident that caused injury (e.g., assessment inadequate, change in patient status, improper use of equipment, insufficient number of caregivers to assist).
   d. Complete occurrence report according to agency policy.
3. Patient's level of weakness does not permit active transfer (e.g., unable to stand for time required to move to chair).
   a. Increase number of nursing personnel to assist during transfer.

b. Increase bed activity and exercise to heighten tolerance.

Recording and Reporting

- Record procedure, including pertinent observations: weakness, ability to follow directions, weight-bearing ability, balance, ability to pivot, number of personnel needed to assist, and amount of assistance (muscle strength) required.
- Report transfer ability and assistance needed to next shift or other caregivers. Report progress or remission to rehabilitation staff (physical therapist, occupational therapist).

Sample Documentation

0800 Transferred patient from bed to chair with gait belt and assistance of one. Cooperative and able to stand erect with encouragement.

0815 Requested to return to bed. Stated, "I'm so tired; I just can't sit up any longer." Needed assistance of two with transfer back to bed. Knees buckled and legs were shaking during attempt to stand. Vital signs remained within patient's baseline.

Special Considerations

Pediatric

- Whenever possible, transporting child by stretcher, stroller, or wheelchair outside confines of room increases environmental stimuli and provides social contact with others (Hockenberry and Wilson, 2007).

Geriatric

- A major health concern that threatens the function of the older adult is the risk of falls. Concern increases when the older adult is admitted to the hospital. Assess patient for the risk for falls on admission and implement a protocol to prevent falls (Phipps and others, 2007) (see Chapter 4).

Home Care

- Assess special transfer equipment needed for home setting. Assess home environment for hazards.
- Family caregiver should practice transfer in hospital to achieve success before taking patient home. Alternatively, patient (if living alone) should practice transfer skills in bed that will be used at home. Patient should learn to transfer to chair with arms for ease of rising and sitting.
- Home should be free of hazards (e.g., throw rugs, electric cords, slippery floors). If wheelchair is used, access must be possible through all doors, and space for transfer must be available in bedroom and bathroom.

PROCEDURAL GUIDELINE 15.1
Wheelchair Transfer Techniques

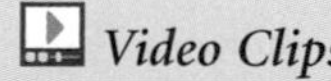
Video Clips

Transferring a patient from a bed to a wheelchair encompasses many of the same principles discussed in Skill 15.1. The following procedural guideline focuses on the safety precautions that need to be considered when using a wheelchair. Several additional steps must be taken to maintain safety of the patient and nurse to prevent injury when transferring from or to a wheelchair (Pierson and Fairchild, 2008). Check wheelchair locks, foot plates, and wheels for proper functioning before use.

Delegation and Collaboration

The skill of transferring a patient to or from a wheelchair can be delegated to nursing assistive personnel (NAP). Instruct the NAP by:

- Assisting and supervising when moving patients who are transferring for the first time after prolonged bed rest, extensive surgery, critical illness, or spinal cord trauma.
- Explaining the patient's mobility restrictions, changes in blood pressure, or sensory alterations that may affect safe transfer.
- Reminding NAP to back a wheelchair into or out of an elevator to avoid tipping.

Equipment

- Transfer belt
- Nonskid shoes
- Wheelchair

Procedural Steps

1. **See Standard Protocol (inside front cover).**
2. ***Transferring a patient from a bed to a wheelchair (patient is weight bearing and able to cooperate (Pierson and Fairchild, 2008).***
   a. Adjust the height of the bed to the level of the seat of the wheelchair if possible.
   b. Position the wheelchair at a 45-degree angle next to the same side of the bed as the patient's strong side.
   c. Face the wheelchair toward the foot of the bed midway between the head and foot of the bed.
   d. Lock the wheelchair. Locks are located above the rims of the wheels. Push handle forward to lock. Raise the foot plates.
   e. Sit patient up on side of the bed (see Skill 15.1).
   f. Place transfer belt on patient and assist patient to move to the edge of the mattress.

Continued

PROCEDURAL GUIDELINE 15.1
Wheelchair Transfer Techniques—cont'd

Video Clips

g. Position yourself slightly in front of patient to guard and protect patient throughout the transfer.
h. Coordinate transfer to chair with patient by counting to three (see Skill 15.1, Steps 3c(1-13).
i. Lower foot plates and place patient's feet on them.
j. Unlock wheelchair. Pull lock toward you to release.
k. Ensure that patient is positioned well back in the seat and ready to use wheelchair.

3. *Transferring a patient from a wheelchair to bed*
   a. Adjust the height of the bed to the level of the seat of the wheelchair if possible.
   b. Position the wheelchair at a 45-degree angle next to the bed.
   c. Face the wheelchair toward the foot of the bed midway between the head and foot of the bed.
   d. Lock the wheelchair. Locks are located above the rims of the wheels. Push handle forward to lock.
   e. Raise the foot plates and place the transfer belt on patient (if not already in place).
   f. Assist patient to move to the front of the wheelchair.
   g. Position yourself slightly in front of patient to guard and protect patient throughout the transfer.
   h. Coordinate transfer to the bed by having patient stand and then pivot to the side of the bed. Then have patient sit on the side of the mattress (see Skill 15.1).
   i. With patient sitting on side of the bed, place your arm nearest the head of the bed under the person's shoulders while supporting the head and neck. Take your other arm and place it under the person's knees. Bend your knees and keep your back straight.
   j. Tell patient to help lift the legs when you begin to move. On a count of three, standing with a wide base of support, raise patient's legs as you pivot his or her body and lower the shoulders onto the bed. Remember to keep your back straight.
4. **See Completion Protocol (inside front cover).**
5. Monitor vital signs as needed. Ask if patient feels dizzy or fatigued.
6. Note patient's behavioral response to transfer.

SKILL 15.2 MOVING AND POSITIONING PATIENTS IN BED

- **Nursing Skills Online: Safety Module, Lesson 3**

Video Clips

Correct positioning of patients is crucial for maintaining body alignment and comfort; preventing injury to the musculoskeletal and integumentary systems; and providing sensory, motor, and cognitive stimulation. A patient with impaired mobility, decreased sensation, impaired circulation, or lack of voluntary muscle control can develop damage to the musculoskeletal and integumentary systems while lying down. You must minimize this risk by maintaining unrestricted circulation and correct body alignment while moving, turning, or positioning patients. The term *body alignment* refers to the conditions of the joints, tendons, ligaments, and muscles in various body positions. When the body is aligned, whether standing, sitting, or lying, no excessive strain is placed on these structures. Body alignment means that the body is in line with the pull of gravity and contributes to body balance. Without this balance the center of gravity is displaced, which increases the force of gravity and predisposes the patient to falls and injuries. You achieve body balance when a wide base of support exists, the center of gravity falls within the base of support, and you can draw a vertical line from the center of gravity through the base of support (Fig. 15-1).

ASSESSMENT

1. Assess patient's body alignment and level of comfort while patient is lying down. *Rationale: Provides baseline for later comparisons. Determines ways to improve position and alignment.*
2. Assess for risk factors that may contribute to complications of immobility:
   a. *Paralysis:* Hemiparesis resulting from CVA. *Rationale: Paralysis impairs movement and muscle tone.*
   b. *Impaired mobility:* Traction, arthritis, hip fracture, joint surgery, or other contributing disease processes. *Rationale: Conditions result in decreased range of motion (ROM).*

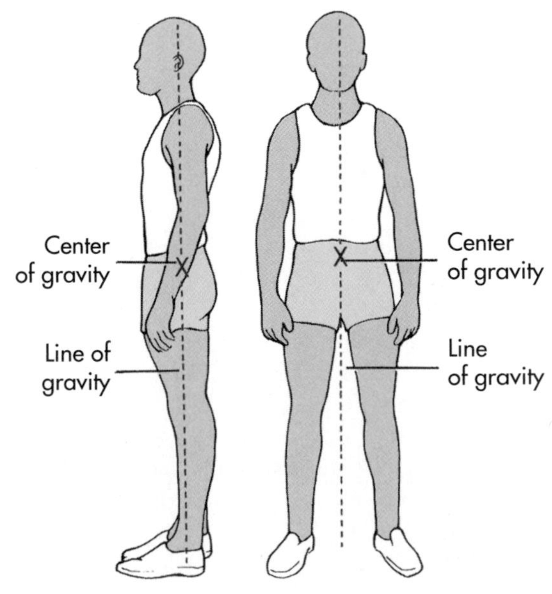

FIG 15-1 Body alignment when standing.

c. *Impaired circulation:* Arterial insufficiency. *Rationale: Decreased circulation predisposes patient to pressure ulcers.*

d. *Age:* Very young or older adult. *Rationale: Premature and young infants require frequent turning because their skin is fragile. Normal physiological changes associated with aging predispose older adults to greater risks for developing complications of immobility.*

e. *Sensation:* Decreased from CVA, paralysis, neuropathy. *Rationale: Because of poor awareness of body part or reduced sensation, patient is unable to protect and position body part from pressure.*

4. Assess patient's level of consciousness. *Rationale: Determines need for special aids or devices. Patients with altered levels of consciousness may not understand instructions nor be able to help during positioning.*
5. Assess patient's physical ability to help with moving and positioning, which may be affected by disease process, strength, ROM, and coordination. *Rationale: Enables nurse to use patient's mobility, strength, and coordination. Determines need for additional help, which ensures patient and nurse safety.*
6. Assess for presence of tubes, incisions, and equipment (e.g., traction). *Rationale: Alters positioning procedure, type of positions to use, and approach used for instruction.*
7. Assess motivation of patient and ability of family members to participate in moving and positioning patient in bed in anticipation of discharge to home. *Rationale: Indicates if instruction is needed.*
8. Check physician's or health care provider's orders before positioning patient. *Rationale: Some positions may be contraindicated in certain situations (e.g., spinal cord injury; hip fracture; respiratory difficulties; certain neurological conditions; presence of incisions, drains, or tubing).*

PLANNING

Expected Outcomes focus on safe mobility, self-care, and prevention of complications.

1. Patient retains ROM
2. Patient's skin shows no evidence of breakdown (see Chapter 25).
3. Patient experiences increased comfort.
4. Patient experiences increased level of independence in completing ADLs.

Delegation and Collaboration

The skills of moving and positioning patients in bed and maintaining correct body alignment can be delegated to nursing assistive personnel (NAP). Instruct the NAP by:

- Explaining any moving and positioning restrictions unique to patient (e.g., avoid prone position, patient has one-sided weakness).
- Designating specific times throughout the shift that NAP must reposition patient.
- Providing information about patient's individual needs for body alignment (e.g., patient with spinal cord injury).

Equipment

- Pillows, drawsheet
- Friction-reducing device
- Therapeutic boots/splints (optional)
- Trochanter rolls
- Sandbags
- Hand rolls

IMPLEMENTATION *for* MOVING AND POSITIONING PATIENTS IN BED

STEPS	RATIONALE
1. See Standard Protocol (see inside front cover).	
SAFETY ALERT Before placing bed in flat position, account for all tubing drains and equipment to prevent dislodgment or spillage if caught in mattress or bed frame as bed is lowered.	
2. Assist patient in moving up in bed.	This task is not a one-person task unless patient can fully assist (Nelson and others, 2009).
a. Can patient assist?	Determines degree of risk in repositioning patient and technique required to safely assist patient.
(1) Fully able to assist, nurse assistance not needed; nurse stands by to assist.	
(2) Partially able to assist; patient can assist using positioning cues or aids (e.g., drawsheet or friction-reducing device).	
b. ***Assist moving up in bed using a drawsheet (two to three nurses assist).***	
(1) Place patient supine with head of bed flat. A nurse stands on each side of bed.	Enables nurse to assess body alignment. Reduces pull of gravity on patient's upper body.

Continued

STEPS	RATIONALE
(2) Remove pillow from under head and shoulders and place it at head of bed.	Prevents striking patient's head against head of bed.
(3) Turn patient side to side to place drawsheet under patient, extending from shoulders to thighs.	Supports patient's body weight and reduces friction during movement.
(4) Return patient to supine position.	Even distribution of weight makes lift easier.
(5) Fanfold the drawsheet on both sides, with each nurse grasping firmly near patient.	Provides strong handles to grip drawsheet without slipping.

SAFETY ALERT Protect patient's heels from shearing force by having a third nurse lift heels while moving patient up in bed.

STEPS	RATIONALE
(6) Nurses place their feet apart with forward-backward stance. Flex knees and hips. On the count of three, shift weight from front to back leg and move patient and drawsheet to desired position in bed (see illustration).	Facing direction of movement ensures proper balance. Shifting weight reduces force needed to move load. Flexing knees lowers nurses' center of gravity and uses thighs instead of back muscles.

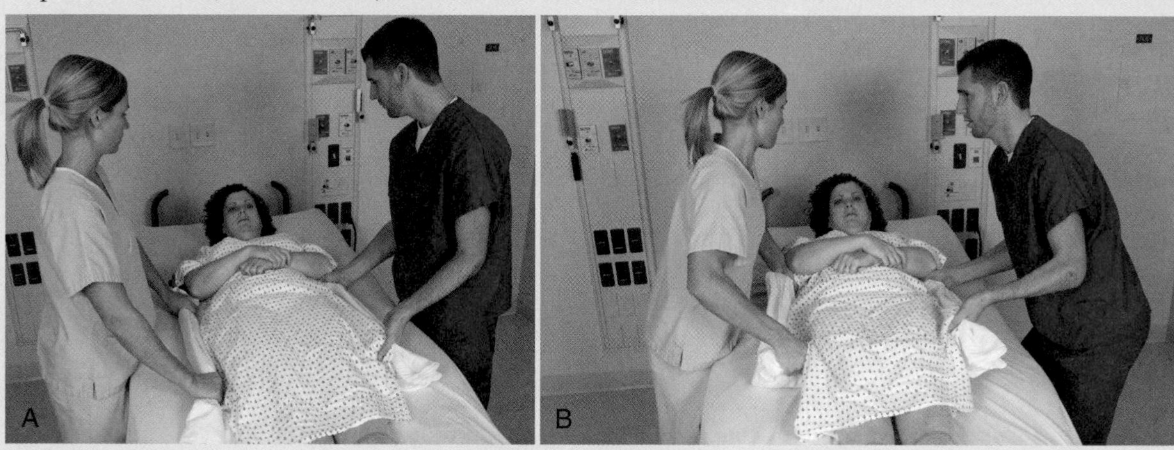

STEP 2b(6) **A** and **B,** Moving immobile patient up in bed with drawsheet.

STEPS	RATIONALE
c. ***Assist moving up in bed using a friction-reducing device (two to three nurses assist).***	Patients under 200 pounds require two to three nurses; patients over 200 pounds require three nurses (Nelson and others, 2009).
(1) Position patient as in Steps 2b(1-3).	Supine position on drawsheet prepares patient for placement of friction-reducing device.
(2) Place friction-reducing device under drawsheet by having patient turn side to side.	Prevents friction from contact of skin with board.
(3) Move patient up in bed by having two nurses grasp drawsheet and one hold onto friction-reducing device. Follow Steps 2b(5 and 6), moving patient up in bed.	The slide board remains stationary, provides a slippery surface to reduce friction, and allows the patient to move easily up in bed.
3. Position patient in one of the following positions using correct body alignment. Protect pressure areas. Begin with patient lying supine and move up in bed following either Steps 2b or 2c.	Prevents injury to musculoskeletal system.
a. ***Position patient in supported Fowler's position (see illustration).***	

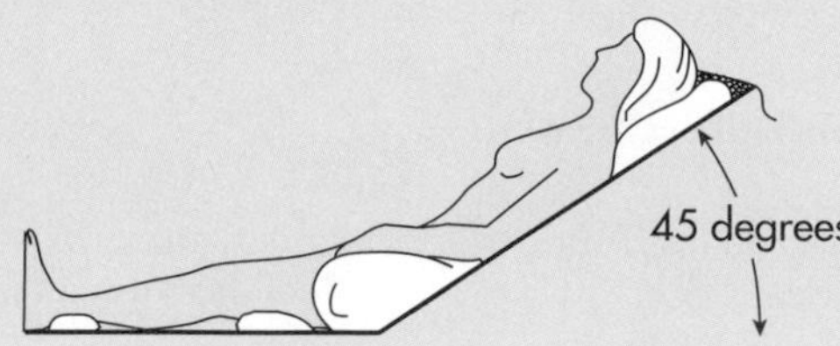

STEP 3a Fowler's position.

STEPS	RATIONALE
(1) With patient lying supine, elevate head of bed 45 to 60 degrees if not contraindicated.	Increases comfort, improves ventilation, and increases patient's opportunity to socialize or relax.
(2) Rest head against mattress or on small pillow.	Prevents flexion contractures of cervical vertebrae.
(3) Use pillows to support arms and hands if patient does not have voluntary control or use of hands and arms.	Prevents shoulder dislocation from effect of downward pull of unsupported arms, promotes circulation by preventing venous pooling, and prevents flexion contractures of arms and wrists.
(4) Position small pillow at lower back.	Supports lumbar vertebrae and decreases flexion of vertebrae.
(5) Place small pillow or roll under thighs. Support calves with pillows.	Prevents hyperextension of knee and occlusion of popliteal artery from pressure from body weight. Heels should not be in contact with bed to prevent prolonged pressure of mattress on heels. This is sometimes referred to as "floating" heels.
b. Position hemiplegic patient in supported Fowler's position.	
(1) Elevate head of bed 45 to 60 degrees. Adjust head of bed according to patient's condition. For example, those with increased risk of pressure ulcers remain at 30-degree angle (semi-Fowler's) (Chapter 25).	Increases comfort, improves ventilation, and increases patient's opportunity to relax.
(2) Position patient in Fowler's position as straight as possible.	Counteracts tendency to slump toward affected side. Improves ventilation and cardiac output; decreases intracranial pressure. Improves patient's ability to swallow and helps to prevent aspiration of food, liquids, and gastric secretions.
(3) Position head on small pillow with chin slightly forward. If patient is totally unable to control head movement, avoid hyperextension of the neck.	Prevents hyperextension of neck. Too many pillows under head may cause or worsen neck flexion contracture.
(4) Provide support for involved arm and hand by placing arm away from patient's side and supporting elbow with pillow.	Paralyzed muscles do not automatically resist pull of gravity as they do normally. As a result, shoulder subluxation, pain, and edema may occur.
(5) Take a rolled blanket (trochanter roll) and place firmly alongside patient's legs.	Ensures proper alignment. Prevents external rotation of hips, which contributes to contractures.
(6) Support feet in dorsiflexion with therapeutic boots or splints (see illustration).	Prevents plantar flexion contractures or footdrop by positioning patient's ankle in neutral dorsiflexion. Foot is positioned so heel is aligned in the opening of the splint to prevent pressure. Other therapeutic boots or splints are manufactured with thick padding to cushion the heel and prevent pressure ulcers.

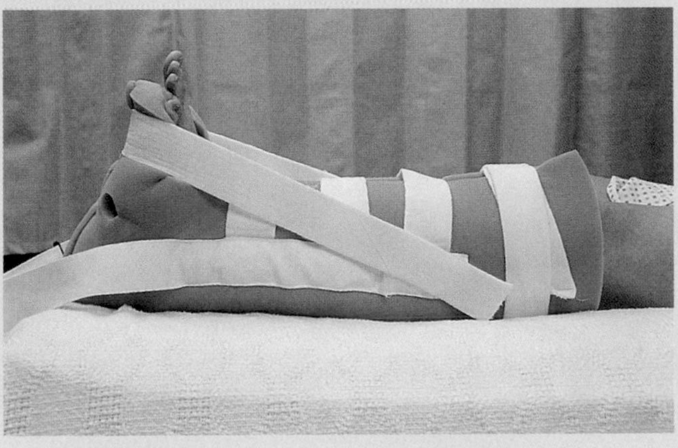

STEP 3b(6) Foot boot with lower leg extension

Continued

STEPS	RATIONALE
c. ***Position patient in supported supine position.***	
(1) Place small rolled towel under lumbar area of back.	Provides support for lumbar spine.
(2) Place pillow under upper shoulders, neck, or head.	Maintains correct alignment and prevents flexion contractures of cervical vertebrae.
(3) Place trochanter rolls or sandbags parallel to lateral surface of patient's thighs.	Reduces external rotation of hip.
(4) Place patient's feet in therapeutic boots or splints.	Maintains feet in dorsiflexion. Prevents plantar flexion contractures or footdrop.
(5) Place pillows under pronated forearms, keeping upper arms parallel to patient's body (see illustration).	Reduces internal rotation of shoulder and prevents extension of elbows. Maintains correct body alignment.
(6) Place hand rolls in patient's hands. Consider physical therapy referral for use of hand splints.	Reduces extension of fingers and abduction of thumb. Maintains thumb slightly adducted and in opposition to fingers.
d. ***Position hemiplegic patient in supine position.***	
(1) Place folded towel or small pillow under shoulder or affected side.	Decreases possibility of pain, joint contracture, and subluxation. Maintains mobility in muscles around shoulder to permit normal movement patterns.
(2) Keep affected arm away from body with elbow extended and palm up. Position affected hand in one of recommended positions for either flaccid or spastic hand. (Alternative is to place arm out to side, with elbow bent and hand toward head of bed.)	Maintains mobility in arm, joints, and shoulder to permit normal movement patterns. (Alternative position counteracts limitation of ability of arm to rotate outward at shoulder [external rotation]. External rotation must be present to raise arm over head without pain.)
(3) Place folded towel under hip of involved side.	Diminishes effect of spasticity in entire leg by controlling hip position.
(4) Flex affected knee 30 degrees by supporting it on pillow or folded blanket.	Slight flexion breaks up abnormal extension pattern of leg. Extensor spasticity is most severe when patient is supine.
(5) Support feet with soft pillows at right angle to leg.	Maintains foot in dorsiflexion and prevents footdrop. Pillows prevent stimulation to ball of foot by hard surface, which has tendency to increase muscle tone in patient with extensor spasticity of lower extremity.
e. ***Position patient in prone position, using two nurses.***	In certain patients with pulmonary conditions such as acute respiratory distress syndrome, the use of the prone position can help improve oxygenation.
(1) With head of bed flat and one nurse standing on each side of bed, roll patient to one side while placing arm on side to be turned alongside of body.	Prepares patient for positioning.

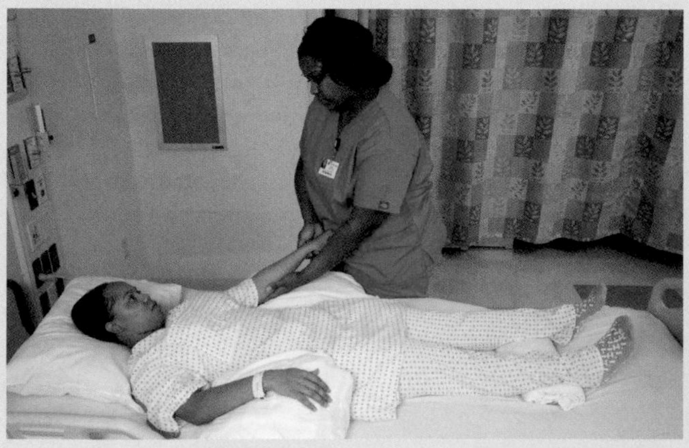

STEP 3c(5) Supported supine position with pillows in place.

STEPS	RATIONALE
(2) Roll patient over arm positioned close to body, with elbow straight and hand under hip. Position on abdomen in center of bed.	Positions patient correctly so alignment can be maintained.
(3) Turn patient's head to one side and support head with small pillow.	Reduces flexion or hyperextension of cervical vertebrae.
(4) Place small pillow under patient's abdomen below level of diaphragm.	Reduces pressure on breasts of some female patients and decreases hyperextension of lumbar vertebrae and strain on lower back. Improves breathing by reducing mattress pressure on diaphragm.
(5) Support arms in flexed position level at shoulders.	Maintains proper body alignment. Support reduces risk of joint dislocation.
(6) Support lower legs with pillow to elevate toes (see illustration).	Prevents footdrop. Reduces external rotation of legs. Reduces mattress pressure on toes.

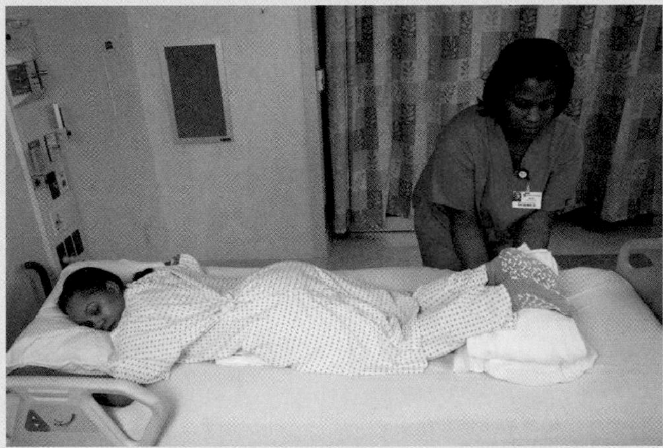

STEP 3e(6) Prone position with pillows supporting lower legs.

STEPS	RATIONALE
f. ***Position patient in 30-degree lateral (side-lying) position (one nurse).***	
(1) Lower head of bed completely or as low as patient can tolerate.	Provides position of comfort for patient and removes pressure from bony prominences on back.
(2) Position patient in supine position on side of bed opposite direction toward which patient is to be turned. Move upper trunk, supporting shoulders first, followed by moving lower trunk, supporting hips. Raise side rails and move to opposite side of bed.	Provides room for patient to turn to side.
(3) Prepare to turn patient onto side. Flex patient's knee that will not be next to mattress. Place one hand on patient's knee and one hand on patient's shoulder.	Use of leverage makes turning to side easy.
(4) Roll patient onto side toward you.	Rolling decreases trauma to tissues. In addition, patient is positioned so leverage on hip makes turning easy.
(5) Place pillow under patient's head and neck.	Maintains alignment. Reduces lateral neck flexion. Decreases strain on sternocleidomastoid muscle.
(6) Bring dependent shoulder blade forward.	Prevents patient's weight from resting directly on shoulder joint.
(7) Position both arms in slightly flexed position. Support upper arm by pillow level with shoulder; support the other arm with mattress.	Decreases internal rotation and adduction of shoulder. Supporting both arms in slightly flexed position protects joint and improves ventilation because chest is able to expand more easily.

Continued

STEPS	RATIONALE
(8) Place your hands under patient's hips and bring dependent hip slightly forward so angle from hip to mattress is approximately 30 degrees.	The 30-degree lateral position reduces pressure on trochanter.
(9) Place small tuck-back pillow behind patient's back. (Make by folding pillow lengthwise. Smooth area is slightly tucked under patient's back.)	Provides support to maintain patient on side.
(10) Place pillow under semiflexed upper leg level at hip from groin to foot (see illustration).	Flexion prevents hyperextension of leg. Maintains leg in correct alignment. Prevents pressure on bony prominences.

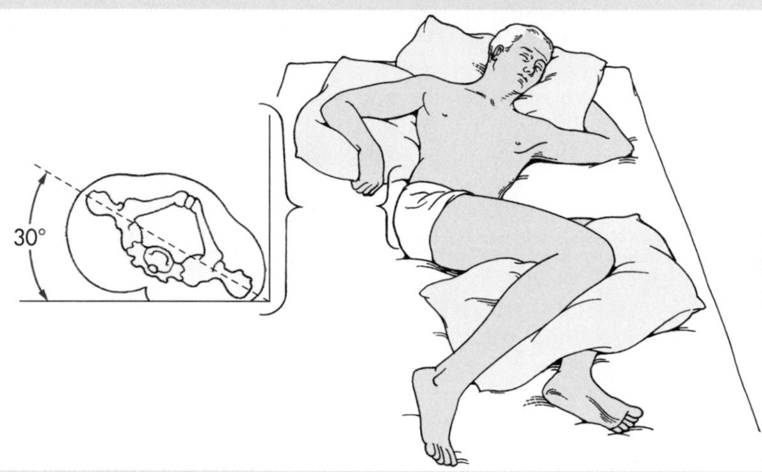

STEP 3f(10) 30-degree lateral position with pillows in place.

STEPS	RATIONALE
(11) Place sandbags parallel to plantar surface of dependent foot.	Maintains dorsiflexion of foot.
g. ***Position patient in Sims' (semiprone) position (one nurse).***	
(1) Position patient in supine position on side of bed opposite direction toward which patient is to be turned. Move upper trunk, supporting shoulders first; move lower trunk, supporting hips. Raise side rails and move to opposite side of bed.	Prepares patient for position.
(2) Move to other side of bed and turn patient on side. Position in lateral position, lying partially on abdomen, with dependent shoulder lifted out and arm placed at patient's side.	Patient is rolled only partially on abdomen.
(3) Place small pillow under patient's head.	Maintains proper alignment and prevents lateral neck flexion.
(4) Place pillow under flexed upper arm, supporting arm level with shoulder.	Prevents internal rotation of shoulder. Maintains alignment.
(5) Place pillow under flexed upper legs, supporting leg level with hip.	Prevents internal rotation of hip and adduction of leg. Flexion prevents hyperextension of leg. Reduces mattress pressure on knees and ankles.
(6) Place sandbags parallel to plantar surface of foot.	Maintains foot in dorsiflexion. Prevents plantar flexion contractures or footdrop.
h. ***Logroll the patient (three nurses).***	

SAFETY ALERT A nurse supervises and aids the NAP when there is an order to logroll a patient. Patients who have suffered from a spinal cord injury or are recovering from neck, back, or spinal surgery often need to keep the spinal column in straight alignment to prevent further injury.

STEPS	RATIONALE
(1) Place patient in supine position on side of bed opposite direction to be turned.	Prepares patient for turning onto side.
(2) Place small pillow between patient's knees.	Prevents tension on spinal column and adduction of hip.
(3) Cross patient's arms on chest.	Prevents injury to arms.
(4) Position two nurses on the side toward which patient is to be turned and one nurse on the side where pillows are to be placed (see illustration).	Distributes weight equally between nurses during turning.
(5) Fanfold the drawsheet along side of patient that will be turning.	Provides strong handles to grip the drawsheet without slipping.
(6) With one nurse grasping drawsheet at lower hips and thighs and the other nurse grasping drawsheet at patient's shoulders and lower back, roll patient as one unit in a smooth, continuous motion on the count of three (see illustration).	This maintains proper alignment by moving all body parts at the same time, preventing tension or twisting of the spinal column.
(7) Nurse on opposite side of the bed places pillows along length of patient for support (see illustration).	Maintains patient in side-lying position.
(8) Gently lean patient as a unit back toward the pillows for support.	Ensures continued straight alignment of spinal column, preventing injury.
4. See Completion Protocol (inside front cover).	

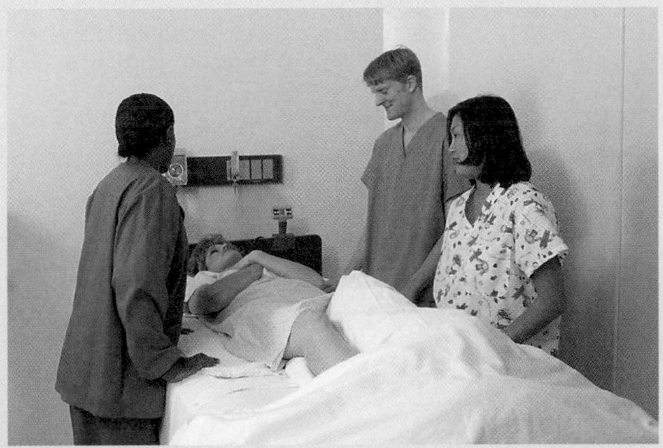

STEP 3h(4) Preparing patient for logroll.

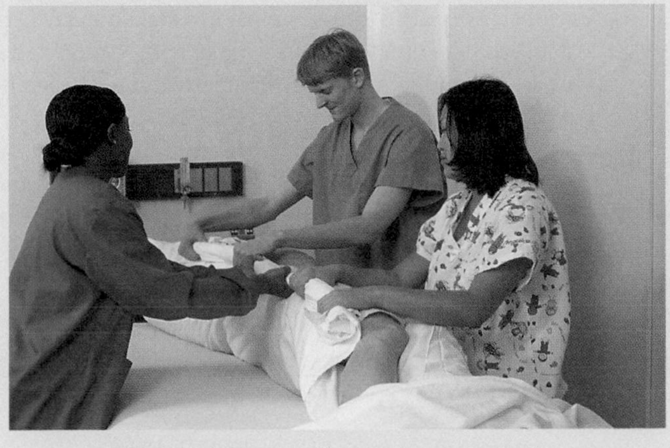

STEP 3h(6) Logrolling patient onto side.

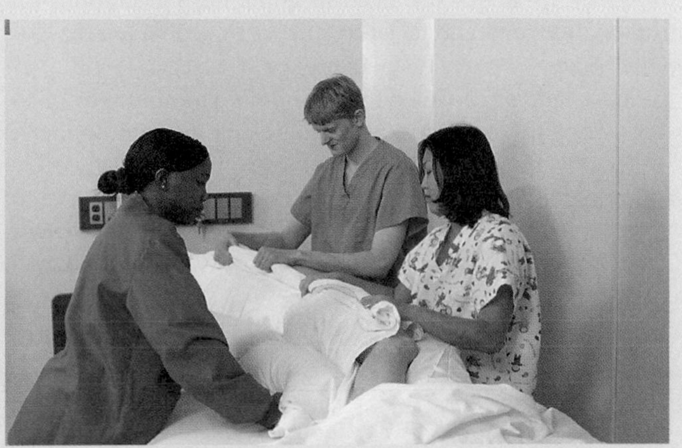

STEP 3h(7) Place pillows along patient's back for support.

EVALUATION

1. Evaluate patient's body alignment and position. Patient's body should be supported by adequate mattress, and vertebral column is without observable curves.
2. Evaluate patient's level of comfort. (Pain scale is an option.)
3. Measure ROM (see Chapter 7).
4. Observe for areas of erythema or breakdown involving skin.
5. Observe patient attempt self-care activities (e.g., bathing, eating).

Unexpected Outcomes and Related Interventions

1. Joint contractures develop or worsen.
   a. Offer ROM exercises to affected and immobilized areas (see Chapter 16).
2. Skin shows localized areas of erythema and breakdown.
   a. Increase frequency of repositioning.
   b. Place a turning schedule in location easily visible for all care providers.
3. Patient avoids moving.
   a. Medicate with analgesia as ordered by physician or health care provider to ensure patient's comfort before moving.
   b. Allow pain medication to take effect before proceeding.

Recording and Reporting

- Record transfer or positioning change and observations (e.g., condition of skin, joint movement, patient's ability to assist with positioning) in flow sheet or nurses' notes.
- Report observations at change of shift.
- Report skin or joint complications to physician or health care provider.

Sample Documentation

0900 Patient reports feeling of pressure over coccyx area. Coccyx slightly reddened. Positioned prone with assist of three caregivers. Pillows placed to support lower legs; small pillow positioned under head and below diaphragm. Patient denies discomfort or pain.

1000 Patient turned to left-lateral position. No further redness noted on coccyx area. Patient resting comfortably without report of pain or discomfort.

Special Considerations

Pediatric

- Encourage children to be as active as their condition and restrictive devices allow. Use developmentally appropriate toys or items that stimulate activity and participation in care.
- Children who are unable to move need passive exercise and movement (see Chapter 16).

Geriatric

- Reposition older adult patients at least every 1 to 2 hours and maintain a regular program of ROM exercises (Meiner and Lueckenotte, 2006).

Home Care

- Assess ability and motivation of patient and family caregivers to participate in moving and positioning patient in bed.
- Assess home to determine compatibility of environment with assistive devices (e.g., over-bed trapeze, Hoyer lift, hospital bed).

REVIEW QUESTIONS

Case Study for Questions 1 and 2

Mr. Clark is a 37-year-old man who suffered a spinal cord injury in a motor vehicle accident. He is admitted on the nurse's shift. He has sustained multiple deep lacerations on his face and trunk and facial fractures of maxillary and zygomatic bones. He rates his pain at 9 on a scale of 0 to 10.

1. Mr. Clark is scheduled for a computed tomography (CT) scan of the head and spine following an auto accident. He now reports pain at a level of 7 on a 0 to 10 scale. He weighs 210 pounds and refuses to allow the nurse to move him onto the stretcher. What interventions would the nurse select to successfully get Mr. Clark to the procedure? Select all that apply:
   1. Administer pain medication as ordered.
   2. Use two nurses to move patient to stretcher and explain procedure to patient.
   3. Prepare to have three nurses assist with transfer and explain procedure to patient.
   4. Tell him that it is a physician's order and must be carried out.
2. Mr. Clark has returned from the CT scan. The physician or health care provider has ordered him to be turned and positioned every 1 to 2 hours until he is taken to surgery to stabilize his spinal fracture. What is the safest technique to use to move him from side to side? Fill in the blank and give rationale.
3. A patient has been on bed rest for several days. When he tries to sit on the side of the bed, he becomes dizzy and nauseated. These are most likely symptoms of which of the following?
   1. Rebound hypertension
   2. Orthostatic hypotension
   3. Dysfunctional proprioception
   4. CNS rebound hypotension

4. A patient who weighs 104.5 kg (230 pounds) is being transferred from his bed to a chair. The patient is on partial weight bearing as a result of bilateral reconstructive knee surgery. Which of the following is the best technique for transfer?
   1. Friction-reducing device
   2. Bariatric transfer aid
   3. Three-person carry
   4. Stand-and-pivot using two nurses
5. An adolescent has been admitted with an unstable spinal cord injury sustained from a motor vehicle accident. The patient needs to be taken to the operating room. What is the most appropriate method to move this patient to a stretcher for transport?
   1. Use a step-by-step method: move the trunk, the hips, and finally the legs.
   2. Logroll the patient, place a slide board, and slide the patient to the stretcher as one unit maintaining body alignment.
   3. Allow the patient to stand and transfer to the stretcher.
   4. Use a mechanical lift device to transfer to the stretcher.
6. A patient is 1 day after abdominal surgery. He is refusing to move from the bed to the chair. What should the nurse assess first in determining appropriateness of transfer?
   1. Level of pain
   2. Any equipment connected to his body
   3. Patient's weight
   4. Patient's ability to follow directions
7. The nurse is transferring a patient from bed to chair. The patient has been on prolonged bed rest. Which one of the following should the nurse do first?
   1. Apply a transfer belt.
   2. Use the under-axilla method to assist the patient to a sitting position.
   3. Provide the patient with his or her glasses.
   4. Allow the patient to dangle at the side of the bed for a few minutes.
8. Two NAPs ask for the nurse's assistance to transfer a 56.8 kg (125-pound) patient from the bed to the stretcher. The patient is unable to assist. What is the best response?
   1. "As long as we use proper body mechanics, no one will get hurt."
   2. "The patient only weighs 56.8 kg (125 pounds). You do not need my assistance."
   3. "The three-man lift technique is recommended to ensure your safety and that of the patient."
   4. "Use the slide board; it's more comfortable for the patient and will lessen the chance of injury to us."
9. Place the following steps in sequence that promotes safe transfer of a patient from a wheelchair to a bed.
   1. Position wheelchair at a 45-degree angle next to the bed.
   2. Assist patient to move to the front of wheelchair.
   3. Raise the footplates and apply transfer belt.
   4. Lock the wheelchair. Push forward to lock.
   5. Position yourself slightly in front of the patient to guard and protect the patient throughout the transfer.
   6. Have patient stand and pivot to side of bed.
   7. Adjust the height of the bed to the level of the seat of the wheelchair.
10. Which of the following patients would benefit most from positioning in a 30-degree lateral position on the right side?
   1. A patient who has shortness of breath
   2. A patient who has signs of a stage I pressure ulcer on the left trochanter
   3. A patient who has hemiplegia on the right side
   4. A patient who is prone to orthostatic hypotension

REFERENCES

American Nurses Association: Position statement on elimination of manual patient handling to prevent work-related musculoskeletal disorders, June 2003. http://www.nursingworld.org.readroom/position/workplac/pathand.htm.

American Nurses Association: Nursing's legislative and regulatory initiatives for the 110th congress: workplace health and safety, Department of Government Affairs, 2007, http://www.anapoliticalpower.org.

Baptiste A and others: Friction-reducing devices for lateral patient transfers: a clinical evaluation, *AAOHN J* 54(4):173, 2006.

Bureau of Labor Statistics: Occupational industries and illnesses: industry data, 2003, http://stats.bls.gov/bls/occupation.htm.

Hockenberry MJ, Wilson D: *Wong's nursing care of infants and children*, ed 8, St Louis, 2007, Mosby.

Lampinen P and others: Activity as a predictor of mental well-being among older adults, *Aging Ment Health* 10(5):454, 2006.

Meiner S, Lueckenotte A: *Gerontologic nursing*, ed 3, St Louis, 2006, Mosby.

Miami Valley Hospital: Lift team case study, June 2007, http://www.miamivalleyhospital.com/.

Nelson A and others: *Safe patient handling and movement*, New York, 2009, Springer.

Occupational Health and Safety Administration: *Technical manual*, TED 01-00-015 [TED 1-0.15A], 2009, August 16, 2010, http://www.osha.gov/dts/osta/otm/otm_toc.html.

Pelczarski K: Take a proactive approach to bariatric patient needs, *Materials Management Magazine* June 2007.

Phipps W and others: *Medical-surgical nursing: health and illness perspectives*, ed 8, St Louis, 2007, Mosby.

Pierson M, Fairchild S: *Principles and techniques of patient care*, ed 4, St Louis, 2008, Saunders.

Sedlak C and others: Development of the National Association of Orthopaedic Nurses guidance statement on safe patient handling and movement in the orthopaedic setting, *Orthop Nurs* 28(2S):S2, 2009.

UC Davis Health System: New team gives nurses a lift in handling patients, March 2005, http://www.ucdmc.ucdavis.edu.

United States Department of Labor, Occupational Safety and Health Administration (OSHA): Guidelines for nursing homes: ergonomics for the prevention of musculoskeletal disorders, Washington, DC, 2003, OSHA.

CHAPTER

16

Exercise and Mobility

evolve WEBSITE

http://evolve.elsevier.com/Perry/nursinginterventions

Mobility is the capacity for movement, with movement providing a means of personal contact, sensation, exploration, pleasure, and control (Touhy, 2008). No matter the age, health care providers feel that engaging in some degree of physical activity is better than leading a sedentary life (Struck and Ross, 2006). The benefits of physical activity include increased energy, improved sleep, better appetite, less pain, and improved self-esteem. Therefore it is useful to incorporate active exercise into activities of daily living (ADLs) whenever possible (Box 16-1). Nurses make every effort to promote and maintain patients' functional mobility and are in a unique position to influence patients' participation in these health-promoting activities.

Three elements essential for mobility include: (1) the ability to move based on adequate muscle strength, control, coordination, and range of motion (ROM); (2) the motivation to move; and (3) the absence of barriers in the environment. Bed rest is a medical intervention in which a patient is restricted to bed for one of the following purposes: (1) decreasing oxygen requirements of the body, (2) reducing pain, or (3) allowing rest and recovery. Older adults' mobility can be impaired because of illness, loss of muscle strength and flexibility, and clothing that hinders their mobility (such as knee-length clothing that can get caught in a wheelchair) (Touhy, 2008). Consider all of these factors when incorporating activity into a patient's plan of care.

PATIENT-CENTERED CARE

Patients in pain are less mobile if they fear that activity will increase their pain or if the pain is limiting their ROM. When assessing a patient's level of pain, be aware that culture and gender can affect a patient's response. For example, Mexican men are less likely to report pain because of a perception that expressing pain is not machismo (Tran and Garcia, 2009). In contrast, Mexican women are likely to seek health care as soon as they feel pain. Nurses must be careful to examine verbal and nonverbal cues of all patients in evaluating pain (see Chapter 13). They must understand how to communicate effectively with patients so they can explain the benefits of mobility and the increased risks of complications to them if they are immobile. Include family members in any discussions so they can reinforce the importance of activity.

SAFETY

Caution patients about the risk for orthostatic hypotension during exercise. Signs and symptoms of orthostatic hypotension include dizziness, light-headedness, nausea, tachycardia, pallor, and fainting. In these patients moving to the dangling position (see Skill 16.2) may cause a gravity-induced drop in blood pressure, creating a risk for falling. When a patient stands, blood shifts from the thorax to the pelvis and lower extremities because of gravity. A drop in blood pressure results from the redistribution of blood (Phipps and others, 2007). To help prevent orthostatic blood pressure, advise patients to exercise calf muscles and to sit on the edge of the bed for 1 minute before standing up (Mayo Clinic, 2009).

To prevent injury to both patient and caregiver, use of safe patient handling techniques is essential. Nurses must work together with patients and members of the health care team to develop safe practices. The techniques for transferring a patient should be based on the patient's physical and cognitive status and medical condition (Nelson and others, 2007). Some researchers caution that assistive devices (e.g., slide board) alone are not enough and that nurses should take the word *lift* out of their vocabulary (Barnes, 2007). When nurses and patients work together to plan the best transfer approach,

BOX 16-1 EXAMPLES OF INCORPORATING EXERCISE INTO ACTIVITIES OF DAILY LIVING

Upper Body
- *Nodding head "yes":* Neck flexion
- *Shaking head "no":* Neck rotation
- *Reaching to bedside stand for book:* Shoulder extension
- *Scratching back:* Shoulder hyperextension
- *Brushing or combing hair:* Shoulder hyperextension
- *Eating, bathing, and shaving:* Elbow flexion and extension
- *Writing and eating:* Fingers and thumb flexion, extension, and opposition

Lower Body
- *Walking:* Hip flexion, extension, and hyperextension; knee flexion and extension; ankle dorsiflexion; plantar flexion
- *Moving to side-lying position:* Hip flexion, extension, and abduction; knee flexion and extension
- *Moving from side-lying position:* Hip extension and adduction; knee flexion and extension
- *While sitting, lifting knees up and straightening legs:* Strengthens muscles used for walking

all parties are empowered to participate and ensure that the care provided is acceptable and appropriate for the patient. Table 16-1 lists techniques designed to minimize caregiver injuries.

Immobility and lack of physical exercise can have profound effects on patients and their quality of life. Patients at risk for developing coronary heart disease, the leading cause of death in the United States, are most affected by physical inactivity (Gillespie, 2006). Older adults benefit from physical activity by improving strength and flexibility. Caution patients of all ages to avoid the "no pain, no gain" approach to exercise. To safely engage in an exercise program, educate patients in terms of appropriate frequency, intensity, and time and type of exercise; this can be referred to as the *exercise prescription* (Gillespie 2006). In addition, also discuss the importance of collateral issues of fluid intake, heart monitoring, risk factors, and rest periods to ensure safety in exercise.

EVIDENCE-BASED PRACTICE TRENDS

Struck BD, Ross KM: Health promotion in older adults: prescribing exercise for the frail and home bound, *Geriatrics* 61(5):22, 2006.

Balance training, ROM and stretching exercises, strength training, and aerobic exercise have been recommended as components of exercise for older adults. If an older adult is homebound, research has shown that walking, transfers, and performing ADLs are beneficial. Exercise has also been cited as a means for preventing fractures in older adults who have suffered a stroke (Struck, 2006). Exercise can improve balance, reduce falls, and improve bone density, thus reducing the risk of fractures. Many health benefits are associated with physical activity, and you should encourage people of all ages to participate. As people become more attached to their technology such as DVDs and computers, often more time is spent sitting. Nurses must take the time to highlight the benefits of physical activity and the associated health benefits.

TABLE 16-1 PREVENTING LIFT INJURIES IN HEALTH CARE WORKERS

ACTION	RATIONALE
When planning to move a patient, arrange for adequate help. If your institution has a lift team, use it as a resource.	A lift team is properly trained in techniques to prevent injury.
Use patient handling equipment and devices (e.g., adjustable-height beds, ceiling-mounted lifts, friction-reducing slide sheets, air-assisted devices)	These devices have shown promise in reducing a caregiver's muscular strain during patient handling.
Encourage patient to assist as much as possible.	Promotes patient's abilities and strength while minimizing caregiver workload.
Keep back, neck, pelvis, and feet aligned. Avoid twisting.	Twisting increases risk of injury.
Flex knees and keep feet about a shoulder width apart.	A broad base of support increases stability.
Position self close to patient (or object being lifted).	Reduces horizontal reach and stress on back.
Use arms and legs (not back).	Leg muscles are stronger, larger muscles capable of greater work without injury.
The person with the heaviest load coordinates efforts of a lift team by counting to three.	Simultaneous lifting minimizes the load for any one lifter.
Perform manual lifting as last resort and only if it does not involve lifting most or all of a patient's weight (Nelson and Baptiste, 2006).	Lifting is a high-risk activity that causes significant biochemical and postural stressors.

PROCEDURAL GUIDELINE 16.1
Range of Motion

ROM refers to the amount of movement that a person has at each joint (Tseng and others, 2007). ROM exercises may be active, passive, or active assisted. They are active if the patient is able to perform the exercise independently and passive if the exercises are performed for the patient by the caregiver. In every aspect of ADL, the nurse must encourage the patient to be as independent as possible. The nurse encourages and supervises active and passive ROM exercises every day. Incorporate active ROM exercises into the patient's ADLs (Table 16-2). You can easily incorporate passive ROM exercises into bathing and feeding activities. Always collaborate with the patient to develop a schedule for ROM activities.

Delegation and Collaboration

The skill of performing ROM exercises may be delegated to nursing assistive personnel (NAP). However, patients with spinal cord or orthopedic trauma usually require exercise by nurses or physical therapists. Instruct the NAP by:

- Explaining how to adapt skill for specific patient such as which joints need passive versus active ROM.
- Reviewing what to observe and report back to the nurse such as pain or fatigue during ROM.

Equipment

- No mechanical or physical equipment needed; clean gloves (if drainage or skin lesions present).

Procedural Steps

1. Review patient's chart for physical assessment findings, physician or health care provider orders, medical diagnosis, medical history, and progress.
2. Obtain data on patient's baseline joint function.
   a. Observe patient's ability to perform ROM exercises during ADLs.
   b. Observe for limitations in joint mobility, redness or warmth over joints, joint tenderness, deformities, or crepitus produced by joint motion.
3. Determine patient's or caregiver's readiness to learn. Explain all rationales for ROM exercises and describe and demonstrate exercises to be performed.
4. Assess patient's level of comfort (on a pain scale of 0 to 10) before exercises.

SAFETY ALERT Consider premedicating patient 30 minutes before ROM exercises begin if necessary.

TABLE 16-2 INCORPORATING ACTIVE RANGE-OF-MOTION EXERCISES INTO ACTIVITIES OF DAILY LIVING

JOINT EXERCISED	ACTIVITY OF DAILY LIVING	MOVEMENT
Neck	Nodding head yes	Flexion
	Shaking head no	Rotation
	Moving right ear to right shoulder	Lateral flexion
	Moving left ear to left shoulder	Lateral flexion
Shoulder	Reaching to turn on overhead light	Flexion, extension
	Reaching to bedside stand for book	Extension
	Applying deodorant	Abduction
	Combing hair	Flexion
Elbow	Eating, bathing, shaving, grooming	Flexion, extension
Wrist	Eating, bathing, shaving, grooming	Flexion, extension, abduction, adduction
Fingers and thumb	All activities requiring fine motor coordination (e.g., writing, eating, hobbies)	Flexion, extension, abduction, adduction, opposition
Hip	Walking	Flexion, extension
	Moving to side-lying position	Flexion, extension, abduction
	Moving from side-lying position	Extension, adduction
	Rolling feet inward	Internal rotation
	Rolling feet outward	External rotation
Knee	Walking	Flexion, extension
	Moving to and from side-lying position	Flexion, extension
Ankle	Walking	Dorsiflexion, plantar flexion
	Moving toe toward head of bed	Dorsiflexion
	Moving toe toward foot of bed	Plantar flexion
Toes	Walking	Extension, flexion
	Wiggling toes	Abduction, adduction, extension, flexion

PROCEDURAL GUIDELINE 16.1
Range of Motion—cont'd

5. **See Standard Protocol (inside front cover).**
6. Use gloves if wound drainage or skin lesions are present.
7. Assist the patient to a comfortable position, preferably sitting or lying down.
8. When performing active-assisted or passive ROM exercises (Table 16-3), support joint by holding distal and proximal areas adjacent to joint, cradling distal portion of extremity, or using cupped hand to support joint (see illustrations).
9. Complete exercises in head-to-toe sequence. Repeat each movement 5 times during exercise period. Inform patient how these exercises are performed and how they can be incorporated into ADLs (see Table 16-2).

SAFETY ALERT If new resistance is noted within a joint, do not force joint motion. Consult with health care provider or physical therapist.

10. Observe patient performing ROM activities.
11. Measure joint motion as needed.
12. Ask patient to rate any discomfort on a pain scale of 0 to 10.
13. **See Completion Protocol (inside front cover).**

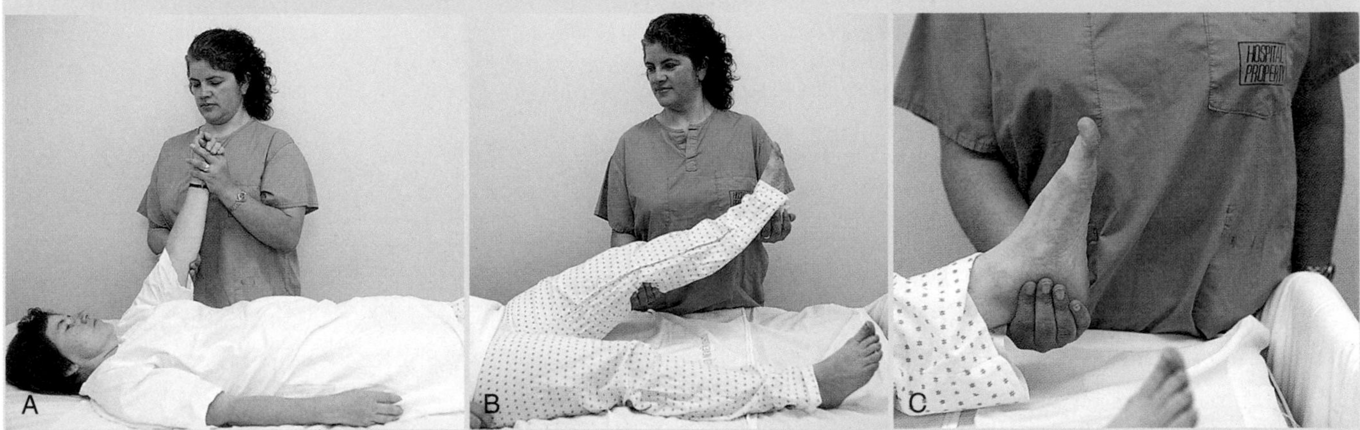

STEP 8 A, Support joint by holding distal and proximal areas adjacent to joint. **B,** Support joint by cradling distal portion of extremity. **C,** Use cupped hand to support joint.

TABLE 16-3 RANGE-OF-MOTION EXERCISES

BODY PART	TYPE OF JOINT	TYPE OF MOVEMENT	RANGE (DEGREES)	PRIMARY MUSCLES
Neck, cervical spine	Pivotal	*Flexion:* Bring chin to rest on chest.	45	Sternocleidomastoid
		Extension: Return head to erect position.	45	Trapezius
		Hyperextension: Bend head back as far as possible.	10	Trapezius
		Lateral flexion: Tilt head as far as possible toward each shoulder.	40-45	Sternocleidomastoid
		Rotation: Turn head as far as possible in circular movement.	180	Sternocleidomastoid, trapezius
Shoulder	Ball and socket	*Flexion:* Raise arm from side position forward to position above head.	45-60	Coracobrachialis, deltoid, pectoralis major
		Extension: Return arm to position at side of body.	180	Latissimus dorsi, teres major, triceps brachii
		Hyperextension: Move arm behind body, keeping elbow straight.	45-60	Latissimus dorsi, teres major, deltoid

Continued

TABLE 16-3 RANGE-OF-MOTION EXERCISES—cont'd

BODY PART	TYPE OF JOINT	TYPE OF MOVEMENT	RANGE (DEGREES)	PRIMARY MUSCLES
Shoulder (*Continued*)		*Abduction:* Raise arm to side to position above head with palm away from head.	180	Deltoid, supraspinatus
		Adduction: Lower arm sideways and across body as far as possible.	320	Pectoralis major
		Internal rotation: With elbow flexed, rotate shoulder by moving arm until thumb is turned inward and toward back.	90	Pectoralis major, latissimus dorsi, teres major, subscapularis
		External rotation: With elbow in full circle, move arm until thumb is upward and lateral to head.	90	Infraspinatus, teres major
		Circumduction: Move arm in full circle (circumduction is combination of all movements of ball-and-socket joint).	360	Deltoid, coracobrachialis, latissimus dorsi, teres major
Elbow	Hinge	*Flexion:* Bend elbow so that lower arm moves toward its shoulder joint and hand is level with shoulder.	150	Biceps brachii, brachialis, brachioradialis
		Extension: Straighten elbow by lowering hand.	150	Triceps brachii
Forearm	Pivotal	*Supination:* Turn lower arm and hand so that palm is up.	70-90	Supinator, biceps brachii
		Pronation: Turn lower arm so that palm is down.	70-90	Pronator teres, pronator quadratus
Wrist	Condyloid	*Flexion:* Move palm toward inner aspect of forearm.	80-90	Flexor carpi ulnaris, flexor carpi radialis
		Extension: Move fingers and hand posterior to midline.	80-90	Extensor carpi radialis brevis, extensor carpi radialis longus, extensor carpi ulnaris
		Hyperextension: Bring dorsal surface of hand back as far as possible.	80-90	Extensor carpi radialis brevis, extensor carpi radialis longus, extensor carpi ulnaris
		Abduction (radial deviation): Bend wrist laterally toward fifth finger.	Up to 30	Flexor carpi radialis, extensor carpi radialis brevis, extensor carpi radialis longus
		Adduction (ulnar deviation): Bend wrist medially toward thumb.	30-50	Flexor carpi ulnaris, extensor carpi ulnaris
Fingers	Condyloid hinge	*Flexion:* Make fist.	90	Lumbricales, interosseus volaris, interosseus dorsalis
		Extension: Straighten fingers.	90	Extensor digiti quinti proprius, extensor digitorum communis, extensor indicis proprius
		Hyperextension: Bend fingers back as far as possible.	30-60	Extensor digitorum
		Abduction: Spread fingers apart.	30	Interosseus dorsalis
		Adduction: Bring fingers together.	30	Interosseus volaris
Thumb	Saddle	*Flexion:* Move thumb across palmar surface of hand.	90	Flexor pollicis brevis
		Extension: Move thumb straight away from hand.	90	Extensor pollicis longus, extensor pollicis brevis

TABLE 16-3 RANGE-OF-MOTION EXERCISES—cont'd

BODY PART	TYPE OF JOINT	TYPE OF MOVEMENT	RANGE (DEGREES)	PRIMARY MUSCLES
Thumb (*Continued*)		*Abduction:* Extend thumb laterally (usually done when placing fingers in abduction and adduction).	30	Abductor pollicis brevis and longus
		Adduction: Move thumb back toward hand.	30	Adductor pollicis obliquus, adductor pollicis transversus
		Opposition: Touch thumb to each finger of same hand.	—	Opponens pollicis, opponens digiti minimi
Hip	Ball and socket	*Flexion:* Move leg forward and up.	90-120	Psoas major, iliacus, sartorius
		Extension: Move leg back, beside other leg.	90-120	Gluteus maximus, semitendinosus, semimembranosus
		Hyperextension: Move leg behind body.	30-50	Gluteus maximus, semitendinosus, semimembranosus
		Abduction: Move leg laterally away from body.	30-50	Gluteus medius, gluteus minimus
		Adduction: Move leg back toward medial position and beyond if possible.	30-50	Adductor longus, adductor brevis, adductor magnus
		Internal rotation: Turn foot and leg toward other leg.	90	Gluteus medius, gluteus minimus, tensor fasciae latae
		External rotation: Turn foot and leg away from other leg.	90	Obturatorius internus, obturatorius externus, quadratus femoris, piriformis, gemellus superior and inferior, gluteus maximus
		Circumduction: Move leg in circle.	120-130	Psoas major, gluteus maximus, gluteus medius, adductor magnus
Knee	Hinge	*Flexion:* Bring heel back toward back of thigh.	120-130	Biceps femoris, semitendinosus, semimembranosus, sartorius
		Extension: Return leg to floor.	120-130	Rectus femoris, vastus lateralis, vastus medialis, vastus intermedius
Ankle	Hinge	*Dorsal flexion:* Move foot so toes are pointed upward.	20-30	Tibialis anterior
		Plantar flexion: Move foot so toes are pointed downward.	45-50	Gastrocnemius, soleus
Foot	Gliding	*Inversion:* Turn sole of foot medially.	10 or less	Tibialis anterior, tibialis posterior
		Eversion: Turn sole of foot laterally.	10 or less	Peroneus longus, peroneus brevis
Toes	Condyloid	*Flexion:* Curl toes downward.	30-60	Flexor digitorum, lumbricalis pedis, flexor hallucis brevis
		Extension: Straighten toes.	30-60	Extensor digitorum longus, extensor digitorum brevis, extensor hallucis longus
		Abduction: Spread toes apart.	15 or less	Abductor hallucis, interosseus dorsalis
		Adduction: Bring toes together.	15 or less	Adductor hallucis, interosseus plantaris

SKILL 16.1 CONTINUOUS PASSIVE MOTION MACHINE

Continuous passive motion (CPM) machines are designed to exercise many different joints, including the hip, ankle, shoulder, wrist, and fingers. Orthopedic surgeons routinely order a knee CPM machine after surgery for a total knee arthroplasty (replacement). CPM may be initiated on the day of surgery or the first postoperative day, according to the individual surgeon's preference. CPM machines are also often used in outpatient physical therapy or home health settings (Fig. 16-1). In addition, CPM is now being looked at as a therapy for burn patients in the prevention and treatment of scar tissue contractures (Long, 2008).

It is beneficial to discuss with a patient the diversional activities that may be used during CPM before beginning treatment. The purpose of the CPM machine is to mobilize the knee joint to prevent contracture, muscle atrophy, venous stasis, and thromboembolism. Passive movement of the joint can replace more strenuous exercises during the first few postoperative days. The benefits of CPM include stimulating circulation in synovial fluids; accelerating venous blood flow, which improves cartilage nutrition and reduces edema; decreasing postoperative pain factors; and lowering the risk for deep vein thrombosis (DVT) (Long, 2008).

The electronically controlled CPM machine flexes and extends the knee to a prescribed degree and at a set speed as ordered by the surgeon. A typical initial setting is 20 to 30 degrees of flexion and full extension (0 degrees) at 2 cycles per minute; however, this setting varies according to the patient's condition and surgeon's preference (Ignatavicius and Workman, 2009).

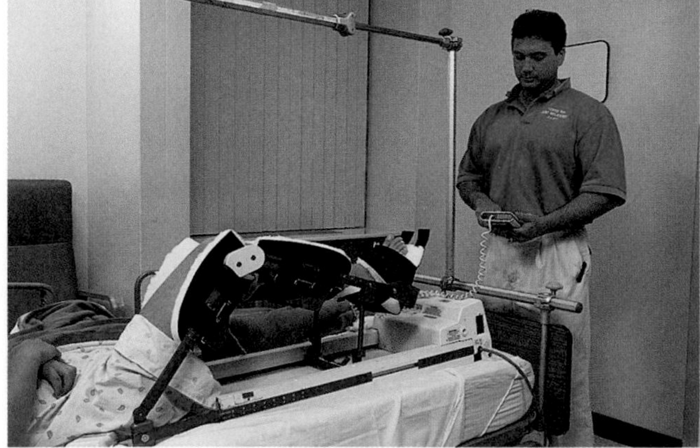

FIG 16-1 Use of continuous passive motion machine on knee.

ASSESSMENT

1. Check the electrical cord and equipment function of the machine. *Rationale: All electrical equipment in health care settings is routinely checked for safety. Routine observation of electrical cord and functioning of equipment each time it is used ensures electrical safety.*
2. Assess the setup of the machine before placing on bed: check the stability of the frame, flexion/extension controls, speed controls, and on/off switch. *Rationale: Ensures that all pieces of the equipment are operational and will prevent damage to the patient's knee.*
3. Assess patient's comfort on a pain scale of 0 to 10 before and during use. *Rationale: Establishes baseline to determine if the patient will be able to tolerate the CPM at the ordered flexion and extension.*
4. Assess patient's baseline heart rate and blood pressure. *Rationale: Provides baseline to measure exercise tolerance.*
5. Assess patient's ability and willingness to learn about the CPM machine. *Rationale: Determines readiness to learn, reduces anxiety, and promotes patient participation.*
6. Assess condition of skin at points where machine rubs/contacts leg and foot. *Rationale: Determines baseline for skin integrity.*
7. Assess patient's ROM before therapy begins (see Procedural Guideline 16.1). *Rationale: Provides baseline to use as a measure for evaluating effect of CPM.*

PLANNING

Expected Outcomes focus on improving joint ROM and maintaining physical mobility and skin integrity.

1. Patient increases length of time in CPM machine as ordered with no evidence of increased heart rate or increased blood pressure.
2. Patient denies discomfort during or after CPM exercise.
3. Patient increases flexion 6 to 7 degrees daily.
4. Patient maintains intact skin throughout use of CPM.

Delegation and Collaboration

Assessment of the patient's condition should not be delegated. Care of the patient during CPM may be delegated to nursing assistive personnel (NAP). Instruct the NAP by:

- Explaining the need to immediately report if the patient reports pain.

Equipment

- CPM machine and sheepskin liner for the CPM machine
- Clean gloves

IMPLEMENTATION for CONTINUOUS PASSIVE MOTION MACHINE

STEPS	RATIONALE
1. **See Standard Protocol (inside front cover).**	
2. Provide analgesia as ordered 20 to 30 minutes before CPM.	Assists patient in tolerating exercise.
3. Identify patient using two identifiers (e.g., name and birthday or name and account number, according to facility policy).	Ensures correct patient. Complies with The Joint Commission standards and improves patient safety (TJC, 2010).
4. Demonstrate machine functioning before placing patient's leg into the device.	Reduces anxiety and increases patient cooperation.
5. Stop the machine in full extension. Place sheepskin on CPM machine.	This position allows correct fit of patient's leg. Ensures that all exposed hard surfaces are padded to prevent rubbing and chafing of patient's skin.
6. If possible, two nurses place patient's leg in the machine, being sure to support above, below, and at knee.	Prevents damage or injury to patient or nurse.
7. Adjust CPM machine to patient by lengthening and shortening appropriate section of the CPM frame.	Ensures a proper fit.
8. Center patient's leg in the machine.	Avoids pressure on the lateral and medial aspects of the knee joint.
9. Align patient's knee joint (bend of the knee) with the machine knee hinge; position patient's knee 2 cm (0.8 inch) below knee joint line of CPM machine.	This is extremely important because, if the patient's new knee is not properly aligned, the knee may be damaged.
10. Adjust the foot support to approximately 20 degrees of dorsiflexion to prevent footdrop.	Footdrop is an abnormal condition caused by damage of the perineal nerve that can cause abnormal gait.
11. When patient's leg is in correct position, secure the Velcro straps across lower extremity (thigh) and top of foot (see illustration).	Correct placement of the thigh and foot straps prevents friction and skin breakdown.

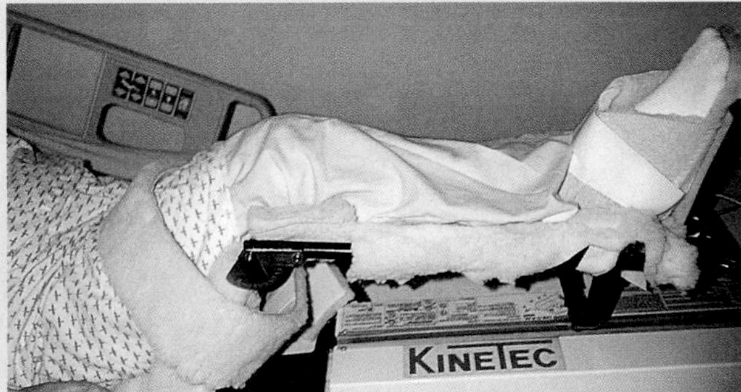

STEP 11 Patient's extremity correctly placed and secured to continuous passive motion machine.

STEPS	RATIONALE
12. Start CPM machine. Watch at least two full cycles of prescribed flexion and extension.	Ensures that CPM machine is fully operational at the preset flexion and extension modes.
13. Make sure that patient is comfortable. Provide patient with the on/off switch. Instruct to use only if CPM machine seems to be malfunctioning.	Allows patient to stop the machine if the degree of flexion/extension or speed changes, creating intolerable discomfort.
14. **See Completion Protocol (inside front cover).**	

EVALUATION

1. In the home, ask patient to keep a log of when the CPM machine is in use, with times and dates.
2. Observe patient at the initial onset of an increase in the flexion of the machine.
3. Measure heart rate or blood pressure during CPM operation and when stopped.
4. Ask patient to rate comfort level on a pain scale of 0 to 10.
5. Measure joint ROM achieved with CPM machine.
6. Observe skin every 2 hours for signs of breakdown.

Unexpected Outcomes and Related Interventions

1. Patient cannot increase flexion.
   a. Increase activities throughout the day to improve muscle strength (e.g., ambulation, physical therapy exercises).
   b. Give "time-out" periods throughout the day to rest the leg.
   c. Consider need for analgesia before CPM.
   d. Sit patient in chair and have gravity assist with increasing knee flexion.
2. Patient experiences increased pain when in CPM machine.
   a. Reassess efficacy of current analgesia and obtain new orders.
   b. Release leg out of CPM machine until pain subsides.
   c. Determine cause of increased pain.
3. Patient develops reddened areas on heel from foot support.
   a. Readjust foot in CPM machine at least every 2 hours.
   b. Provide additional padding to the foot support.

Recording and Reporting

- Record joint exercised, degree of joint motion, time of CPM machine use, pain and need for analgesia, any joint abnormalities, and patient's activity tolerance.
- Report immediately any resistance to ROM; increased pain with CPM; and swelling, heat, or redness in joint.

Sample Documentation

0930 Medicated with two Tylenol with codeine No. 3 tabs PO before initiation of CPM.

1000 Functional CPM applied to left leg; able to tolerate 0 degrees extension and 40 degrees flexion at slow speed. Skin dry and intact without evidence of breakdown. Tolerates slow flexion/extension with minimal c/o pain, 2 on scale 0/10.

Special Considerations

Geriatric

- Older adults who have chronic illnesses may need rehabilitation care to continue CPM because they are not able to manage the equipment in their home.
- Older adults have increased risk of skin breakdown because of decreased elasticity and increased fragility of the skin. Pressure from the CPM machine increases the risk of pressure ulcer development on the pressure points, especially the heel (Meiner and Lueckenotte, 2006).

Home Care

- Home care physical therapist may assist patient/family in continuing CPM in the home.
- Be sure patient/family have specific instructions regarding use of the CPM device; length of time for each session; expected outcomes; and what to do if patient experiences increased pain, patient is unable to tolerate the CPM sessions, or the equipment malfunctions.

PROCEDURAL GUIDELINE 16.2
Applying Elastic Stockings and Sequential Compression Device

There are many reasons why a patient may develop a DVT. Some common risk factors include injury to a vein from a broken bone or surgery, immobility caused by a cast or sitting a long time, inherited clotting disorders, obesity, smoking, and family history (Harvard Health Publications, 2009). Three factors (commonly referred to as Virchow's triad) contribute to DVT development: hypercoagulability of the blood, venous wall damage, and blood flow stasis (Monohan and others, 2007). Prevention is the best approach for DVTs, which can include anticoagulant medications such as warfarin (Coumadin); however, movement of the extremities and wearing compression stockings or foot pumps are equally important. Elastic stockings help reduce blood stasis and venous wall injury by promoting venous return and limiting venous dilation, which decreases the risk of endothelial tears. Sequential compression devices (SCDs) pump blood into deep veins, thus removing pooled blood and preventing venous stasis. Another device, venous plexus foot pumps, promotes circulation by mimicking the natural action of walking (Fig. 16-2).

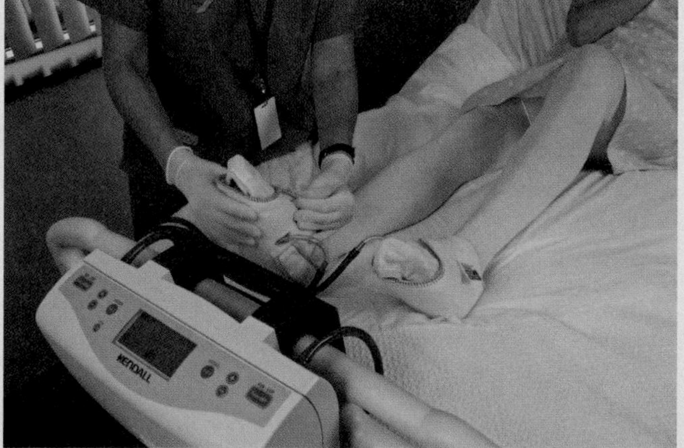

FIG 16-2 Venous plexus foot pump with bedside controls. (Courtesy Tyco Healthcare Group LP.)

Delegation

The skill of applying elastic stockings and SCDs may be delegated to nursing assistive personnel (NAP). The nurse initially determines the size of elastic stockings and assesses the patient's lower extremities for any signs and symptoms of DVTs or impaired circulation. Instruct the NAP by:

- Explaining the need to remove the SCD sleeves before allowing the patient to get out of bed.

PROCEDURAL GUIDELINE 16.2
Applying Elastic Stockings and Sequential Compression Device—cont'd

Equipment

- Tape measure
- Powder or cornstarch (optional)
- Elastic support stockings
- SCD motor, disposable SCD sleeve(s), tubing assembly

Procedural Steps

1. Assess patient for risk factors in Virchow's triad:
   a. Hypercoagulability (i.e., clotting disorders, fever, dehydration)
   b. Venous wall abnormalities (i.e., orthopedic surgery, varicose veins, atherosclerosis)
   c. Blood stasis (i.e., immobility, obesity, pregnancy)
2. Observe for contraindications for use of elastic stockings or SCDs:
   a. Dermatitis or open skin lesions
   b. Recent skin graft
   c. Decreased arterial circulation in lower extremities as evidenced by cyanotic, cool extremities and/or gangrenous conditions affecting the lower limb(s)
3. Assess condition of patient's skin and circulation to the legs (i.e., presence of pedal pulses, edema, discoloration of skin, temperature, lesions, cuts).
4. Obtain physician's or health care provider's order.
5. **See Standard Protocol (inside front cover).**
6. Identify patient using two identifiers (e.g., name and birthday or name and account number, according to facility policy).
7. Explain procedure and reason for applying elastic stockings and SCDs.
8. Position patient in supine position. Elevate head of bed to comfortable level. Use tape measure to measure patient's leg to determine proper elastic stocking and SCD size.
9. *Option:* Apply a small amount of powder or cornstarch to legs provided patient does not have sensitivity to either.
10. Apply elastic stocking:
    a. Turn elastic stocking inside out by placing one hand into the sock, holding toe of sock with other hand, and pulling (see illustration).
    b. Place patient' s toes into foot of elastic stocking, making sure that sock is smooth (see illustration).
    c. Slide remaining portion of sock over patient's foot, making sure that the toes are covered. Make sure that foot fits into the toe and heel position of the sock. Sock will now be right side out (see illustration).

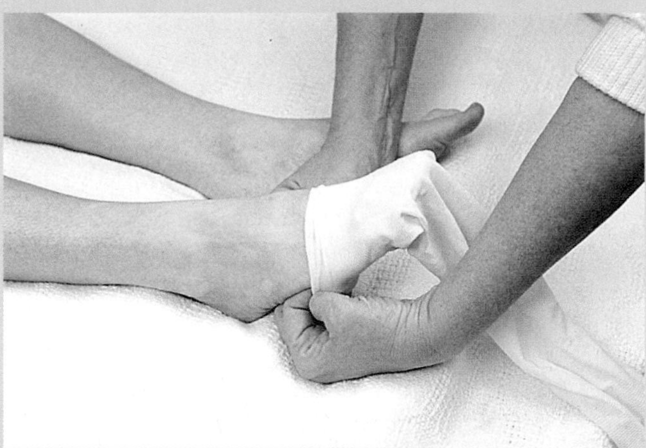

STEP 10b Place toes into foot of stocking.

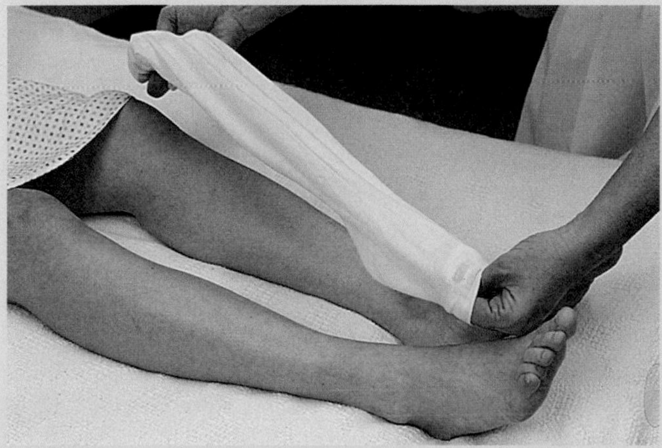

STEP 10a Turn stocking inside out; hold toe and pull through.

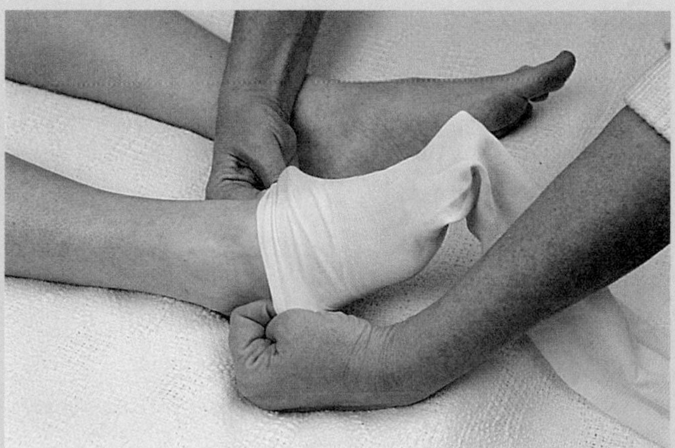

STEP 10c Slide remaining portion of sock over foot.

Continued

PROCEDURAL GUIDELINE 16.2
Applying Elastic Stockings and Sequential Compression Device—cont'd

- **d.** Slide sock up over patient's calf until sock is completely extended. Be sure that sock is smooth and that no ridges or wrinkles are present (see illustration).
- **e.** Instruct patient not to roll socks partially down.

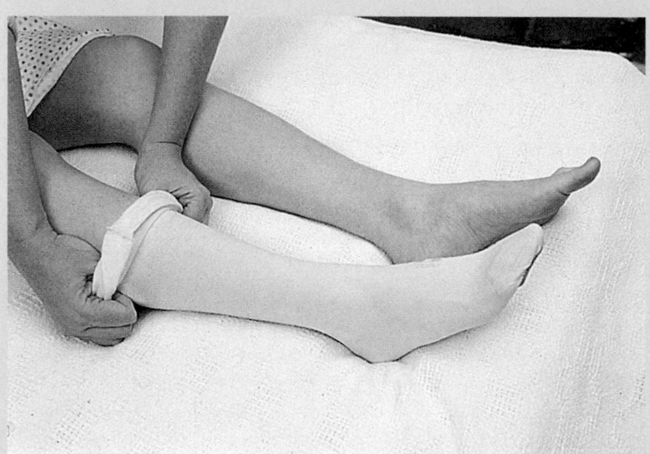

STEP 10d Slide sock up leg until completely extended.

11. Apply SCD sleeve(s):
- **a.** Remove SCD sleeves from plastic cover; unfold and flatten.
- **b.** Arrange SCD sleeve under patient's leg according to leg position indicated on inner lining of sleeve.
- **c.** Place patient's leg on SCD sleeve. Back of ankle should line up with ankle marking on inner lining of sleeve.
- **d.** Position back of knee with popliteal opening on the sleeve (see illustration).

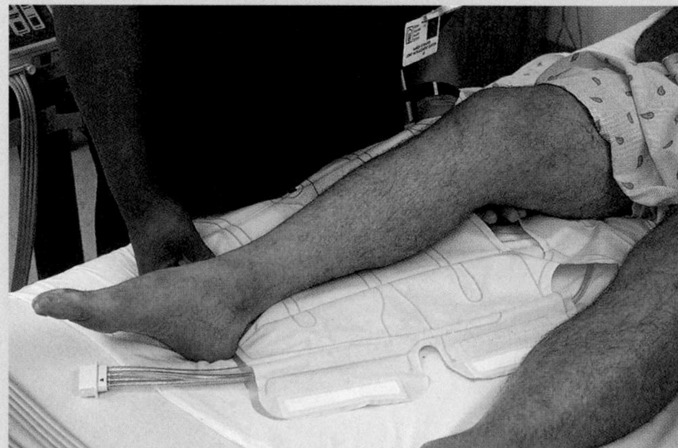

STEP 11d Position back of patient's knee with the popliteal opening.

- **e.** Wrap SCD sleeve securely around patient's leg. Check fit of SCD sleeve by placing two fingers between patient's leg and sleeve (see illustration).

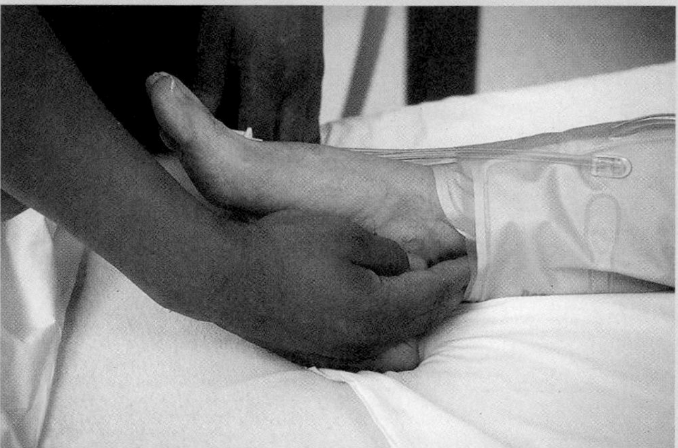

STEP 11e Check fit of sequential compression device sleeve.

12. Attach SCD sleeve connector to plug on mechanical unit. Arrows on connector line up with arrows on plug from mechanical unit (see illustration).

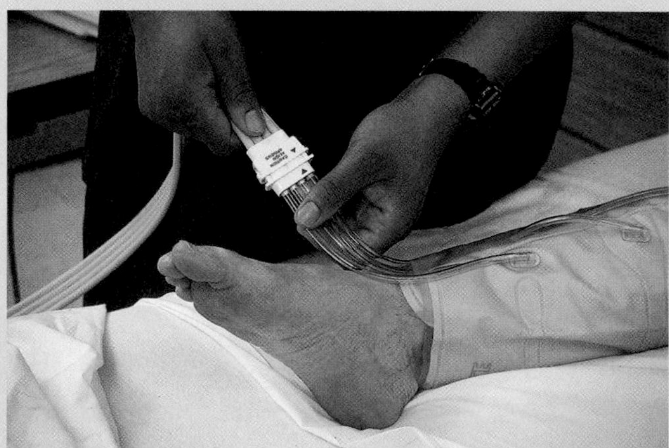

STEP 12 Align arrows when connecting to mechanical unit.

13. Turn mechanical unit on. Green light indicates that unit is functioning. Monitor functioning SCD through one full cycle of inflation and deflation.

14. **See Completion Protocol (inside front cover).**

15. Remove elastic stockings or SCD sleeves at least once per shift (e.g., long enough to inspect skin for irritation or breakdown).

SKILL 16.2 ASSISTING WITH AMBULATION

In the normal walking posture the head is erect; the cervical, thoracic, and lumbar vertebrae are aligned; the hips and knees have slight flexion; and the arms swing freely. Illness, surgery, injury, and prolonged bed rest can reduce activity tolerance and affect balance so assistance is required. Temporary or permanent damage to the musculoskeletal or nervous system may require use of an assistive device such as a cane, crutches, or walker (see Skill 16.3). Patients with altered cardiovascular or respiratory function or prolonged bed rest may experience difficulty with ambulation evidenced by chest pain, altered vital signs, dyspnea, orthostatic hypotension, or fatigue. For this reason it is important to monitor a patient during ambulation.

ASSESSMENT

1. Assess patient's most recent activity experience, including distance ambulated and tolerance of activity. *Rationale: This facilitates realistic planning and identifies degree of assistance needed.*
2. Determine the best time to ambulate, considering other scheduled activities such as bathing. *Rationale: Rest is necessary after activities that require exertion and after meals. Ambulating 30 minutes after analgesic administration improves patient's tolerance.*
3. Check the availability of hand rails on the walls for patient's safety.
4. Assess patient's motivation and ability to understand instructions and cooperate. *Rationale: Comparing this activity with patient plans for the home environment often enhances motivation.*
5. Assess patient's ability to bear weight. Evaluate patient's balance and determine if his or her weight is an issue in ambulation. *Rationale: Determines degree of assistance patient needs and/or need for assistive devices. For safety, another person may be needed initially to assist with patient ambulation. Allow the patient as much independence as possible.*
6. Assess risk for orthostatic hypotension by assessing medications that may alter stability, including antihypertensive or opioid medications. Check for history of patient falls. *Rationale: Drugs may cause hypotension, dizziness, or instability.*
7. Assess baseline resting vital signs before beginning ambulation. *Rationale: Comparison of postambulation vital signs to baseline determines patient's activity tolerance and whether patient is experiencing orthostatic hypotension.*

PLANNING

Expected Outcomes focus on developing activity and rest patterns that support increased tolerance of activity. It is essential that you individualize these to each patient's needs and abilities.

1. Patient ambulates without episode of injury.
2. Patient is able to ambulate without excessive fatigue or dizziness.
3. Patient maintains respirations, pulse, and blood pressure within 10% of resting values.
4. Patient maintains erect posture while standing and walking.

Delegation and Collaboration

The skill of assisting the patient with ambulation may be delegated to nursing assistive personnel (NAP). Instruct the NAP by:

- Explaining how to adapt skill for specific patient such as obtaining an intravenous (IV) pole for a patient with continuous IV fluids.
- Reviewing what to observe and report back to nurse (e.g., the distance patient was able to ambulate without fatigue).

Equipment

- Robe
- Nonskid footwear
- Portable IV pole (if needed)
- Transfer (gait) belt

IMPLEMENTATION *for* ASSISTING WITH AMBULATION

STEPS	RATIONALE
1. **See Standard Protocol (inside front cover).**	
2. Remove SCD if present.	Prevents patient from becoming tangled in cord.
3. Encourage patient to move slowly at own pace, maintain erect posture, and look straight ahead.	Reduces risk of losing balance, tripping, or falling.

Continued

STEPS	RATIONALE
4. Follow Skill 15.1, Step 2, for assisting patient to side of bed. With patient sitting, wait a few minutes and ask if he or she feels dizzy. Have patient dangle legs on side of bed and take a few deep breaths until balance is gained. Have patient move legs and feet while dangling (see illustration).	Allows a few minutes for circulation to equilibrate. Prevents orthostatic hypotension and potential injuries (Mayo Clinic, 2009). Pumping feet plantar/dorsiflexion increases venous return to the heart and brain.
5. Decide with patient how far to ambulate. Assist patient with putting on shoes or slippers with nonskid soles.	Determines mutual goal. Shoes or slippers provide stable walking support.
6. Ask if patient feels dizzy or light-headed. If patient appears light-headed, recheck blood pressure.	Allows nurse to detect orthostatic hypotension before ambulation begins.
7. Apply transfer (gait) belt around patient's waist. Be sure belt is snug but not too tight.	Transfer belt allows nurse to maintain stability of patient during ambulation and reduces risk of falling.
8. Assist patient to stand at the bedside. Encourage to stand fully erect with shoulders back and looking ahead (not at the floor).	Standing at bedside allows patient opportunity to stabilize before ambulating.
9. If patient is unstable, seat him or her in chair or return to bed immediately. Consider need for additional help. If patient is very heavy, unstable, or fearful, use a sit-to-stand lift.	Provides added stability. Lift provides maximum safety for both patient and caregiver if patient is unstable.
10. If patient has an IV line, place the IV pole on the same side as the site of infusion and instruct patient to hold and push the pole while ambulating.	
11. If a Foley catheter is present, patient or nurse carries the bag below the level of the bladder and prevents tension on the tubing.	Prevents reflux of urine from the bag back into bladder.
12. Stand on patient's strong side. Take a few steps, supporting patient with one arm grasping the gait belt and the other under the elbow of the flexed arm (see illustration). *Option:* Use ambulation lift/ceiling lift with gait harness for more dependent patients who are now walking for first time after being in bed.	This provides balance and facilitates lowering patient to the floor if he or she is unable to continue because of weakness or dizziness.

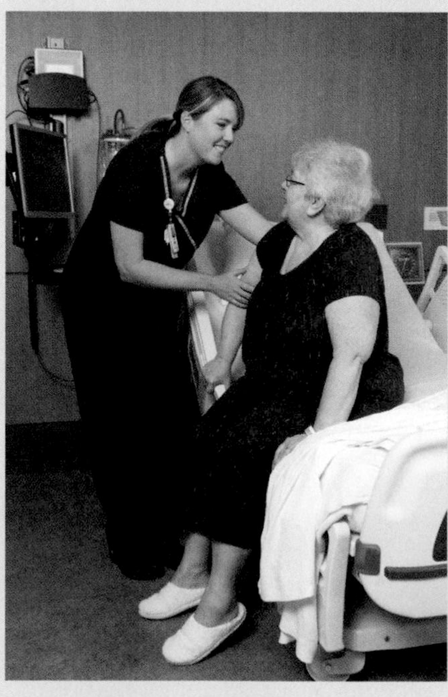

STEP 4 Patient dangling.

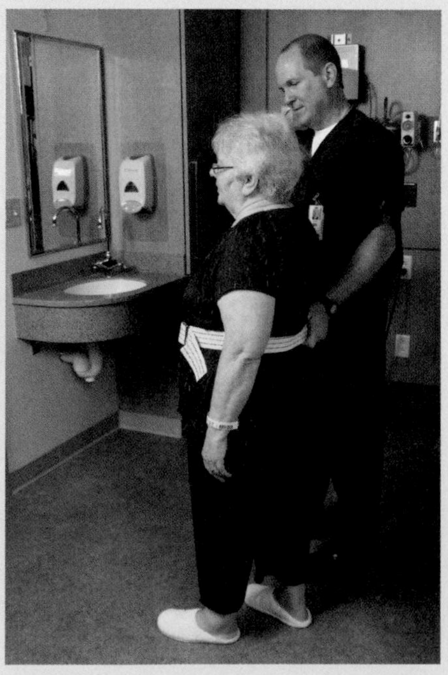

STEP 12 Nurse grasps transfer belt firmly.

STEPS	RATIONALE
13. When ambulating in a hallway, position patient between yourself and the wall. Encourage patient to use hand rails if available (see illustration).	The wall provides stable support for patients who start to fall away from nurse.

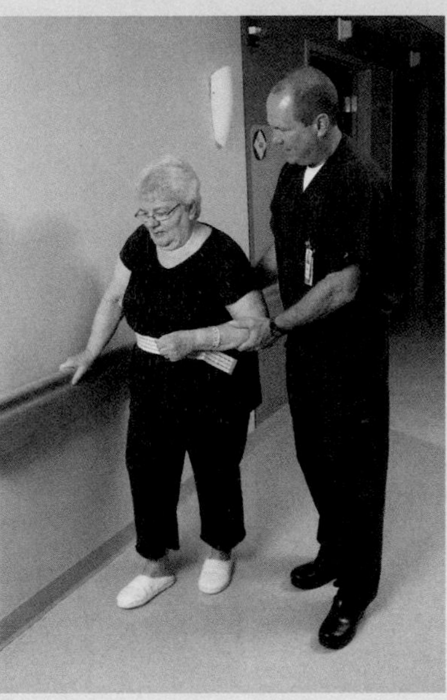

STEP 13 Nurse positions patient for use of handrail.

14. See Completion Protocol (inside front cover).

EVALUATION

1. Observe ambulation and tolerance of ambulation, noting the frequency of rest periods.

2. Compare patient's heart rate, respiratory rate, and blood pressure with baseline values immediately after ambulation and again after 5 minutes of rest.

3. Observe patient's body alignment and balance while standing and walking.

Unexpected Outcomes and Related Interventions

1. Vital signs are altered: pulse more than 10% to 20% over resting rate or greater than 120 beats per minute; systolic blood pressure shows orthostatic changes; or dyspnea, labored breathing, and wheezing are present. Patient reports feelings of excessive fatigue or weakness.
   a. Plan activity after adequate rest period.
   b. Pace activity to proceed more slowly and allow time to stop and rest at regular intervals. Sitting periodically may be helpful.
   c. Assistive devices such as a cane or walker may decrease energy required (see Skill 16.3).
2. Patient starts to fall.
   a. Call for help.
   b. Put both arms around patient's waist or grasp gait belt tightly (Fig. 16-3, *A*).
   c. Stand with feet apart for a broad base of support (see Fig. 16-3, *B*).
   d. Extend one leg and let patient slide against it to the floor. *Caution:* If patient is heavy, do not risk personal injury.
   e. Bend knees and lower your body as patient slides to the floor (see Fig. 16-3, *C*).
   f. Stay with patient until assistance arrives to help lift patient to wheelchair.

Recording and Reporting

- Record and report distance ambulated, patient's tolerance, and any changes in vital signs.

Sample Documentation

1300 Ambulated 100 feet in hall with assistance of one. Gait steady. States, "I am so tired. I don't know if I can make it back to my room." BP 160/82, HR 120, RR 20. Placed in wheelchair.

1305 Back in bed with assistance. BP 145/78, HR 92, RR 12. Denies dizziness.

Special Considerations

Geriatric

- Older patients are often fearful of falling when ambulatory, especially if they have fallen previously. This fear causes a person to move less often, which causes greater problems in his or her gait. Encouragement, reassurance, and assistance from family or caregiver decrease anxiety. Older adults may need more time in the morning to resume activity.

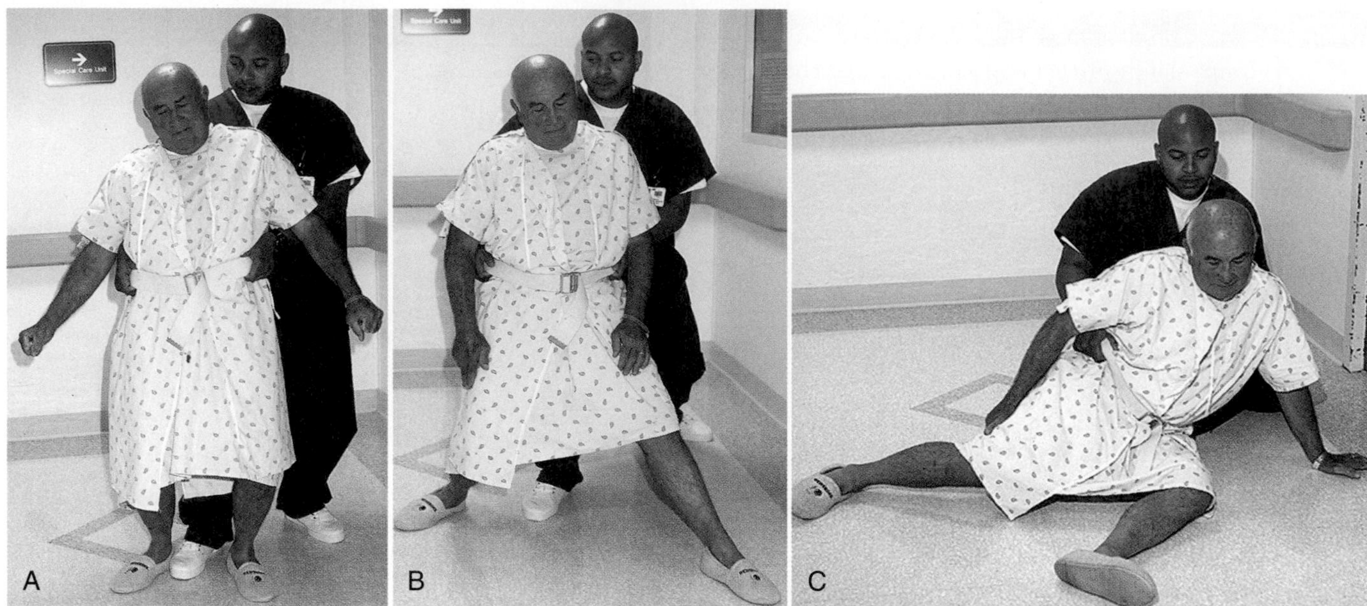

FIG 16-3 **A,** Stand with feet apart to provide broad base of support. **B,** Extend one leg and let patient slide against it to the floor. **C,** Bend knees to lower body as patient slides to floor.

SKILL 16.3 TEACHING USE OF CANES, CRUTCHES, AND WALKERS

Assistive devices (i.e., canes, crutches, and walkers) are recommended for patients who cannot bear full weight on one or more joints of the lower extremities. Other indications for their use are instability, poor balance, or pain in weight bearing. It is important for the nurse to know the patient's weight-bearing status, any specific movement precautions, and type of device ordered by the physician or health care provider. The nurse collaborates with the physical therapist to help the patient use the assistive device correctly and safely. The wrong weight-bearing status or improper movement can cause further damage to the injured extremity (Phipps and others, 2007).

Nonweight-bearing status requires the patient to support weight on the assistive device and the unaffected limb. The affected leg is kept off the floor at all times. Partial or touch-down weight bearing is similar to that for nonweight bearing, but either limb can be advanced initially. Partial weight bearing more closely approximates normal walking, except that less weight is placed on the affected limb. Total weight bearing allows the patient to distribute equal weight between each limb with minimal weight on the assistive device. Muscle-strengthening exercises such as knee-and-foot extension (kicking leg straight out while sitting in a chair) or hip flexion (marching while sitting in a chair) and walking in parallel bars help the patient increase strength and confidence before using an assistive device.

An assistive device should be kept in good working condition. Often patients bring assistive devices with them to the hospital. As a home health nurse you need to teach patients and family caregivers how to check the condition of their devices routinely. Rubber tips on the ends of assistive devices prevent slipping. Be sure that the tips are not cracked; otherwise they need replacing. Examine the condition of an assistive device to be sure that there are no bent parts, missing screws, or worn hand grips.

Teach the patient to lift rather than slide a device to reduce the possibility of catching the tips, which could cause the user to lose balance, trip, or fall. Personnel should attend to patients when using an assistive device until they are assured that the patient's understanding and strength are sufficient for safe solo ambulation. Observing unaccompanied patients on their walks may reveal a need for attendance and/or additional or continued reminders about the proper way to stand, the amount of weight permitted, or the distance covered. Talk to the patient about risks for falls. Let patients who have a fear of falling know that they can regain confidence with practice.

CANES

Canes primarily increase the person's security and balance by broadening the base of support. They also absorb or take the body weight when necessary for mobility during partial weight-bearing periods. There are three types of commonly used canes: the standard crook, tripod, and quad cane. The standard crook provides the least support, and the quad canes are useful for patients who have a partial or complete paralysis. Instruction for use of cane-assisted ambulation is required to assess the patient's balance, strength, and confidence. When canes are used unilaterally, they are most often used on the person's strong side and are advanced forward with the injured or affected limb.

CRUTCHES

Frequently you see persons using one or two crutches as aids for ambulation. Crutches remove weight from one or both legs. They are used when a person needs to transfer more weight to their arms than is possible with canes. The user's proficiency varies with factors such as age, condition, degree or extent of injury, and musculoskeletal functions. Crutches may be a temporary aid for persons with sprains, in a cast, or following surgical treatments. They may be used routinely and continuously for those with congenital or acquired musculoskeletal anomalies, neuromuscular weakness, or paralysis.

WALKERS

Constructed of aluminum or metallic alloys, walkers are lightweight aids strong enough to withstand prolonged use. Heights and weights are adjustable for individual needs. The use of a walker provides great stability and security. Before using a walker, the patient should understand the correct way to stand and advance the walker, the specific amount of weight bearing permitted, and how to use and care for the walker.

ASSESSMENT

1. Review patient's chart, including medical history, previous activity level, and current activity order, including type of gait. *Rationale: Reveals patient's current and previous health status.*
2. Assess patient's physical readiness: vital signs; presence of confusion; and orientation to time, place, and person. *Rationale: Baseline vital signs offer a means of comparison after exercise. Level of orientation or confusion may reveal risk for fall.*
3. Assess ability to bear weight, ROM, and muscle strength or the presence of foot deformities. *Rationale: Determines if assistance is needed for patient to ambulate safely.*
4. Assess patient for any visual, perceptual, or sensory deficits. *Rationale: Determines if patient can use assistive device safely.*
5. Assess environment for potential threats to patient safety (e.g., bed brake, bed position, objects in pathway). Make sure that floor is dry and area is well lit. *Rationale: Provides for a safe, clutter-free environment.*
6. Assess patient for discomfort. *Rationale: Determines if patient needs prescribed analgesic before exercise.*
7. Assess patient's understanding of technique of ambulation to be used. *Rationale: Allows patient to verbalize concerns.*
8. Assess patient's fall risks (e.g., vision, elimination problems, gait problems, or loss of sensation) (see Chapter 4). *Rationale: Determines if patient has other conditions that need to be addressed before attempting ambulation.*

PLANNING

Expected Outcomes focus on improving mobility, minimizing activity intolerance, preventing risk for injury, minimizing fatigue, and improving patient's knowledge.

1. Patient demonstrates correct use of assistive device, gait pattern, and weight-bearing status.
2. Patient rates discomfort or fatigue as 4 or less on a scale of 0 to 10 during ambulation.
3. Patient performs activities with return of vital signs to baseline 3 to 5 minutes after rest.
4. Patient independently performs all ADLs using assistive device safely.

Delegation and Collaboration

Teaching the patient the use of assistive devices should not be delegated. The skill of ambulating with assistive devices may be delegated to nursing assistive personnel (NAP). Instruct the NAP by:

- Explaining how to adapt skill for specific patients such as weight-bearing status.
- Reviewing what to observe and report back to nurse such as episodes of dizziness or fatigue.

Equipment

- Ambulation device (cane, crutches, walker)
- Well-fitting, nonskid flat shoes or slippers
- Robe; well-fitting pants or dress
- Transfer (gait) belt

IMPLEMENTATION *for* TEACHING USE OF CANES, CRUTCHES, AND WALKERS

STEPS	RATIONALE
1. **See Standard Protocol (inside front cover).**	
SAFETY ALERT Make sure that surface patient will walk on is clean, dry, and well lit. Remove objects that obstruct the pathway.	
2. Prepare patient for procedure.	
a. Explain reasons for exercise and demonstrate specific gait technique to patient or family caregiver.	Teaching and demonstration enhance learning, reduce anxiety, and encourage cooperation.

Continued

STEPS	RATIONALE
SAFETY ALERT Be extremely cautious if the patient has IV tubing or a Foley catheter. Obtain an IV pole with wheels that can be pushed as the patient walks. Urinary catheter drainage bags must stay below the level of the bladder; thus a second person may be needed to assist.	
b. Decide with patient how far to ambulate.	Determines mutual goal.
c. Schedule ambulation around patient's other activities. Apply patient's glasses (if worn).	Helps minimize patient fatigue. Ensures patient can see walking path.
d. Begin from side of bed with bed in low position or from a chair. Help patient put on well-fitting, flat shoes or nonskid slippers.	Reduces risk of injury.
3. Apply transfer (gait) belt. Gait belt encircles patient's waist. Assist patient to standing position and observe balance.	Providing constant contact by nurse reduces risk of fall or injury.
4. While standing next to patient's side, have patient take a few steps. When using a cane, stand next to patient's weak side with the device on the strong side. In the case of a walker and crutches, grasp the gait belt and stand behind and to the side of patient. If patient has weakness or paralysis, stand on his or her strong side.	Position of the nurse offers stability. Nurse can pull patient toward strong side in case of a loss of balance.
5. Take a few steps forward with patient, assessing patient's strength and balance.	Ensures that patient has satisfactory strength and balance to continue.
6. If patient becomes weak or dizzy, return him or her to bed or chair, whichever is closer.	Prevents patient from falling to floor.
7. Make sure that the assistive device is the appropriate height and has rubber tips.	Rubber tips increase surface tension and reduce the risk of the device slipping.
8. ***Cane (same steps are taught for standard or quad cane)***	
a. Have patient hold cane on strong side 10 to 15 cm (4 to 6 inches) to side of foot. Cane extends from greater trochanter to floor while cane is held 15 cm (6 inches) from foot (Hoeman, 2007). Allow approximately 15- to 30-degree elbow flexion.	Offers most support when on stronger side of body. Cane and weaker leg work together with each step. If cane is too short, patient has difficulty supporting weight and is bent over and uncomfortable. As weight is taken on by hands and affected leg is lifted off floor, complete extension of elbow is necessary.
b. Place cane forward 15 to 25 cm (6 to 10 inches), keeping body weight on both legs.	Distributes body weight equally.
c. Move involved leg forward, even with the cane (see illustration).	Body weight is supported by cane and strong leg.
d. Advance strong leg 15 to 25 cm (6 to 10 inches) past cane.	Aligns patient's center of gravity. Returns patient body weight to equal distribution.
e. Move involved leg forward, even with strong leg.	
f. Repeat these steps. Once comfortable, have patient advance cane and weak leg together.	
9. ***Crutches***	
a. Crutch measurement includes three areas: patient's height, distance between crutch pad and axilla, and angle of elbow flexion. Measurements may be taken with patient standing or lying down. Make sure shoes are on before performing measurements.	Measurement promotes optimal support and stability. Radial nerves that pass under axilla are superficial. If crutch is too long, it places pressure on axilla. Injury to nerve causes paralysis of elbow and wrist extensors, commonly called crutch palsy. If crutch is too long, shoulders are forced upward, and patient cannot push body off the ground. If ambulation device is too short, patient is bent over and uncomfortable.

STEPS	RATIONALE

SAFETY ALERT Instruct patient to report any tingling or numbness in upper torso. This may mean that crutches are being used incorrectly or that they are the wrong size.

(1) *Standing:* Position crutches with crutch tips at point 15 cm (6 inches) to side and 15 cm (6 inches) in front of patient's feet. Position crutch pads 5 cm (2 inches) below axilla (Hoeman, 2007). Two or three fingers should fit between top of crutch and axilla (see illustration).	Provides broad base of support.
(2) *Supine:* Crutch pad is approximately 5 cm (2 inches) or 2 to 3 fingerwidths under axilla, with crutch tips positioned 6 inches (15 cm) lateral to patient's heel (Hoeman, 2007) (see illustration).	
(3) Verify elbow flexion with a goniometer (see illustration). Adjust the handgrip so patient's elbow is flexed 15 to 20 degrees.	Low handgrips cause radial nerve damage. High handgrips cause patient's elbow to be sharply flexed, decreasing strength and stability of arms.

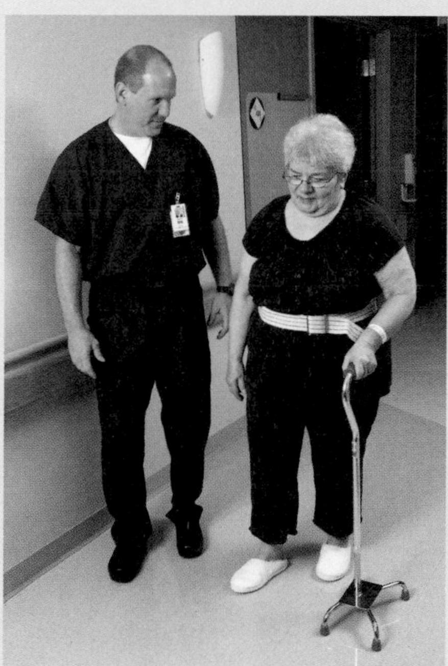

STEP 8c Patient moves involved leg forward even with the cane.

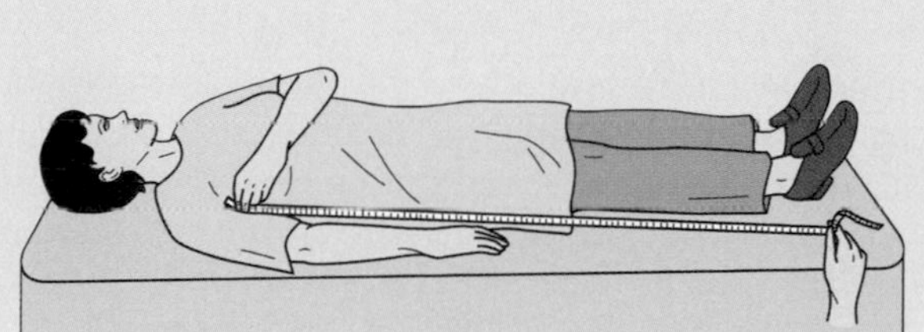

STEP 9a(2) Measuring length of crutch.

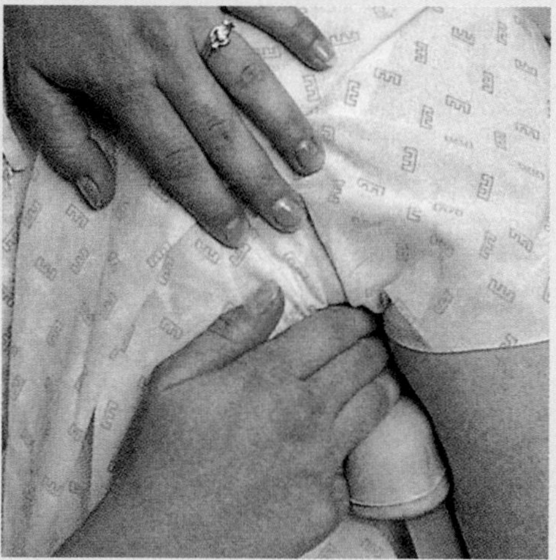

STEP 9a(1) Crutch pad is 2 to 3 fingerwidths under axilla.

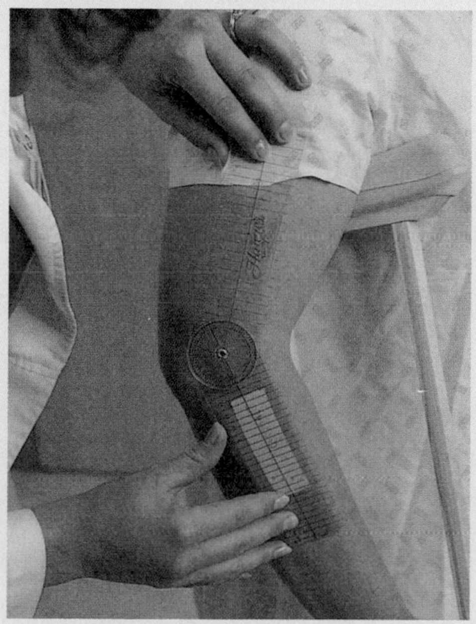

STEP 9a(3) Goniometer determines elbow flexion.

Continued

STEPS	RATIONALE
b. To use crutches, patient supports self with hands and arms. Therefore strength in arm and shoulder muscles, ability to balance body in upright position, and stamina are necessary. Type of crutch gait depends on amount of weight patient is able to support with one or both legs.	
c. Have patient stand up from a sitting position.	
(1) Move to edge of chair, with strong leg slightly under chair seat.	
(2) Place both crutches in the hand on the involved side. If chair has armrests and is heavy and solid enough to avoid tipping, patient uses one armrest and both crutches for bracing while rising. (If the chair is lightweight, patient should use both armrests for even bracing.)	Patients can lose balance or tip chairs with uneven or one-sided pressure.
(3) Push down on the crutch hand rests while raising the body to a standing position. Switch one crutch to strong side.	
d. Assist with prescribed crutch gait (darkened areas in illustrations indicate moving foot).	
(1) *Four-point gait:*	
(a) Begin in tripod position (see illustration) with crutches placed 15 cm (6 inches) in front and 15 cm (6 inches) to side of each foot. Posture should be erect head and neck, straight vertebrae, and extended hips and knees.	Most stable of crutch gaits, provides at least three points of support at all times. Requires weight bearing on both legs. Often used for paralysis, as in spastic children with cerebral palsy (Hockenberry and Wilson, 2007). May also be used for arthritic patients. Tripod improves balance by providing wider base of support.

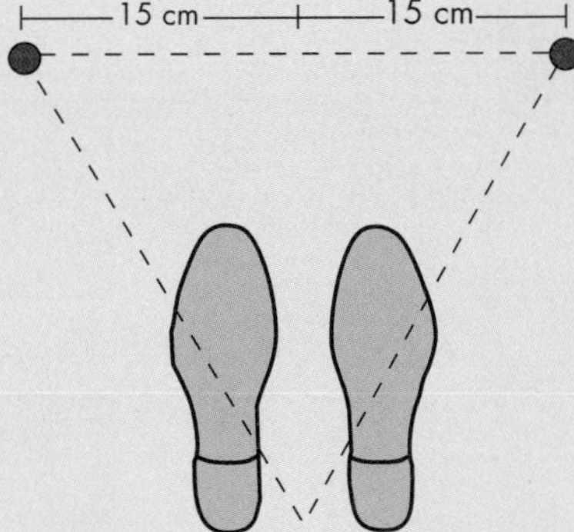

STEP 9d(1)(a) Tripod position.

STEPS	RATIONALE
(b) Move right crutch forward 4 to 6 inches (10 to 15 cm) (see illustration).	Crutch and foot position are similar to arm and foot position during normal walking.
(c) Move left foot forward to level of left crutch (see illustration).	
(d) Move left crutch forward 4 to 6 inches (see illustration).	
(e) Move right foot forward to level of right crutch (see illustration).	
(f) Repeat sequence.	
(2) *Three-point gait:*	Requires patient to bear all weight on one foot. Weight is placed on strong leg and then on both crutches. Involved leg does not touch ground during early phase of three-point gait. Useful for patients with broken leg or sprained ankle. Tripod provides wide base of support.
(a) Begin in tripod position with weight placed on strong leg (see illustration).	
(b) Advance both crutches and involved leg (see illustration).	
(c) Move stronger leg forward (see illustration).	
(d) Repeat sequence.	

STEPS	RATIONALE
(3) *Two-point gait:* **(a)** Begin in tripod position (see illustration) with partial weight bearing on both feet. **(b)** Move left crutch and right foot forward (see illustration). **(c)** Move right crutch and left foot forward (see illustration). **(d)** Repeat sequence.	Requires at least partial weight bearing on each foot. Is faster than the four-point gait. Requires more balance because only two points support body at one time (Hoeman, 2007). Tripod provides wide base of support. Crutch movements are similar to arm movement during normal walking.

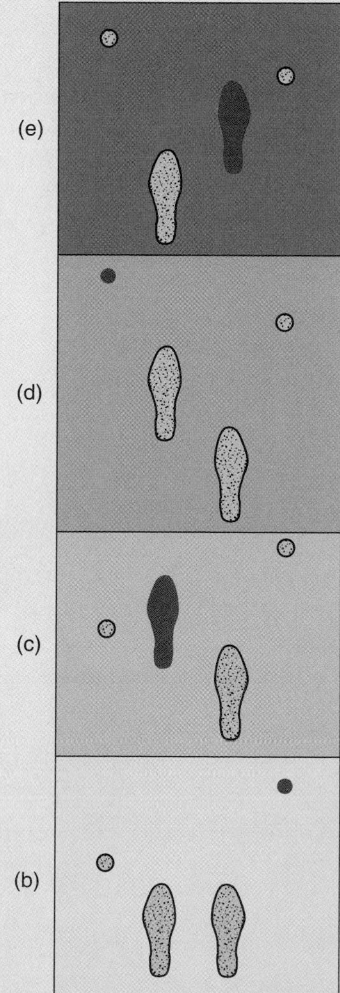

STEP 9d(1)(b-e) Four-point gait. Solid feet and crutch tips show foot and crutch tip movement in each of the four phases (read from bottom to top). Right tip moves forward (b). Left foot moves toward left crutch (c). Left crutch tip moves forward (d). Right foot moves toward right crutch (e).

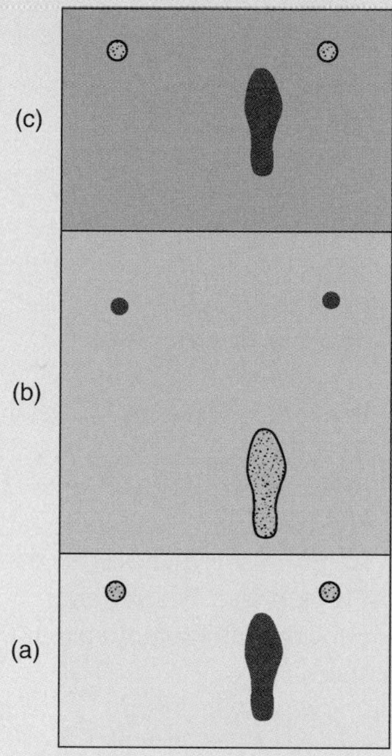

STEP 9d(2)(a-c) Three-point gait with weight borne on unaffected right leg. Solid foot and crutch tips show weight bearing in each phase (read bottom to top).

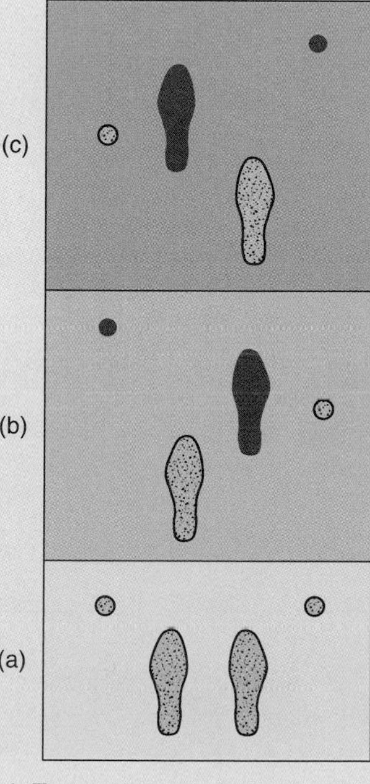

STEP 9d(3)(a-c) Two-point gait. Solid areas indicate weight-bearing leg and crutch tips (read bottom to top).

Continued

STEPS	RATIONALE
(4) *Swing-to gait:*	Frequently used by patients whose lower extremities are paralyzed or who wear weight-supporting braces on their legs. This is the easier of the two swinging gaits. It requires the ability to bear body weight partially on both legs.
(a) Begin in tripod position with partial weight bearing on both feet.	
(b) Move both crutches forward.	
(c) Lift and swing legs to crutches, letting crutches support body weight.	
(d) Repeat two previous steps.	
(5) *Swing-through gait:*	
(a) Start in tripod position with partial weight bearing on both feet.	Requires that patient have the ability to sustain partial weight bearing on both feet.
(b) Move both crutches forward.	Increases base of support so, when the body swings forward, patient is moving the center of gravity toward the additional support provided by crutches.
(c) Lift and swing legs through and beyond crutches. Repeat sequence.	
(6) *Climbing stairs with crutches, nonweight bearing, one leg:*	
(a) Begin in tripod position.	Improves patient's balance by providing wider base of support.
(b) Patient transfers body weight to crutches (see illustration).	Prepares patient to transfer weight to unaffected leg when ascending first stair.
(c) Advance strong leg onto the step (see illustration).	Crutch adds support to affected leg. Patient then shifts weight from crutches to unaffected leg.
(d) Align both crutches with the strong leg on the step (see illustration).	Maintains balance and provides wide base of support.
(e) Repeat sequence until patient reaches top of stairs.	Improves patient's balance by providing wider base of support.
(7) *Descending stairs with crutches, nonweight bearing, one leg:*	

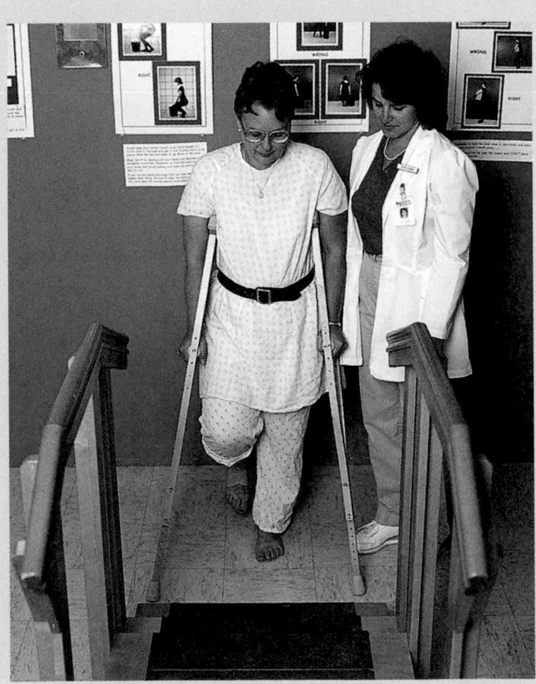

STEP 9d(6)(b) Transfer body weight to crutches.

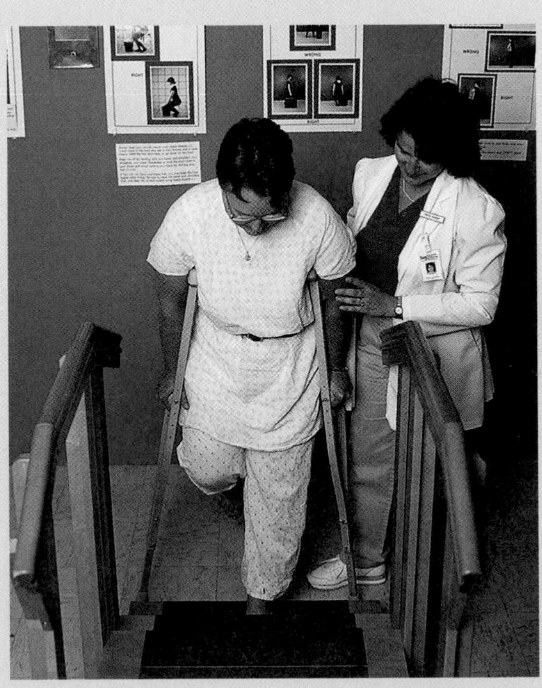

STEP 9d(6)(c) Advance unaffected leg to stair.

STEPS	RATIONALE
(a) Begin in tripod position.	Prepares patient to release support of body weight maintained by crutches.
(b) Transfer body weight to strong leg.	Maintains patient's balance and base of support.
(c) Move crutches to stair below and instruct patient to transfer body weight to crutches and move involved leg forward.	
(d) Move strong leg to stair below and align with crutches.	
(e) Repeat sequence until patient reaches bottom step.	The nonweight-bearing patient should be able to balance on one leg before transferring both crutches to the same hand.
(8) *Sitting in a chair:*	
(a) Transfer both crutches to the same hand and transfer weight to crutches and unaffected leg. Feel back of chair against legs.	Provides stable base of support.
(b) Grasp arm of chair with free hand and extend affected leg out while lowering into chair (see illustration).	
10. *Walker*	
a. When patient relaxes the arms at the side of their body, the top of the walker should line up with the crease on the inside of the wrist. Elbows should be flexed about 15 to 30 degrees when standing with walker, with hands on handgrips.	Walkers without wheels must be picked up and moved forward. Patient must have sufficient strength to be able to move walker. A four-wheeled walker, which does not have to be picked up, is not as stable and may cause injury.
b. Assist patient in ambulating.	
(1) Have patient stand in center of walker and grasp handgrips on upper bars.	Patient balances self before attempting to walk. Position provides broad base of support between walker and patient. Patient then moves center of gravity toward the walker. It is necessary to keep all four feet of the walker on the floor to prevent tipping the walker.

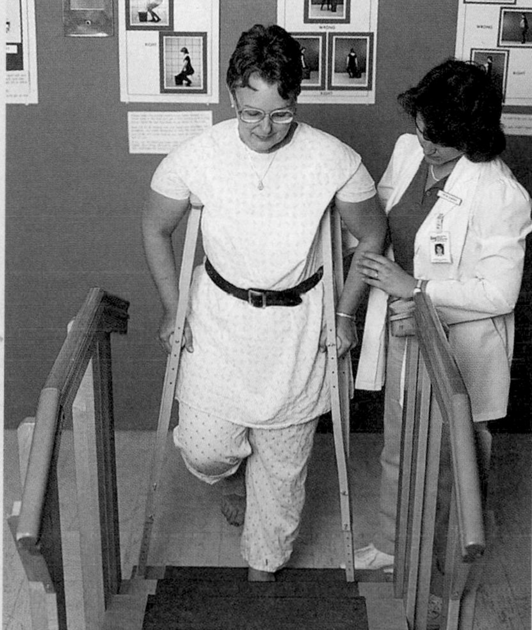

STEP 9d(6)(d) Align crutches with unaffected leg.

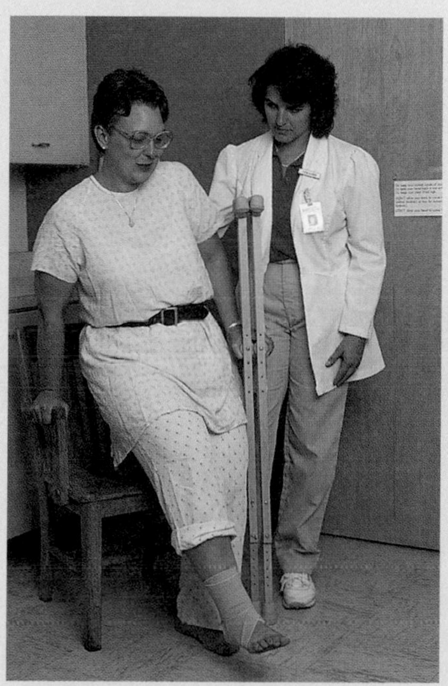

STEP 9d(8)(b) Grasp arm of chair with free hand.

Continued

STEPS	RATIONALE
(2) Lift walker, moving it 15 to 20 cm (6 to 8 inches) forward, making sure that all four feet of walker stay on the floor. Take a step forward with either foot. Follow through with the other foot (see illustration). *If patient has one-sided weakness:* After patient advances the walker, instruct him or her to step forward with the weaker leg, support self with the arms, and follow through with the strong leg. *If patient is unable to bear full weight on the involved leg:* After patient advances walker, have him or her swing the stronger leg through while supporting weight on hands. Instruct patient not to advance the lower extremity past the front bar of the walker.	Moving 15 to 20 cm (6 to 8 inches) simulates normal distance of steps. Providing constant contact of all four walker feet with the floor reduces the risk of injury or fall. Advancing with weaker extremity allows patient to have maximal support of walker.

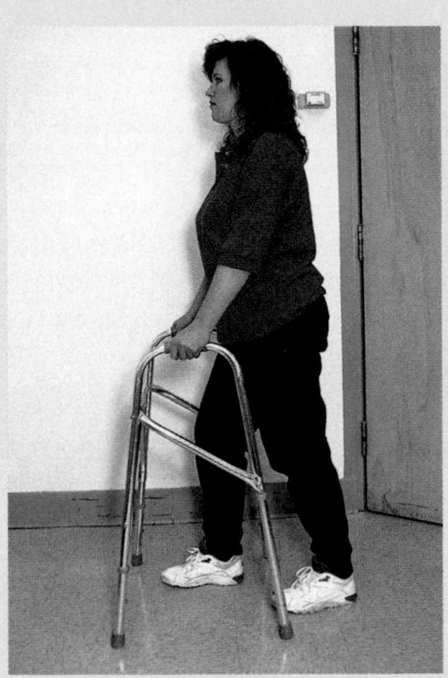

STEP 10b(2) Lift walker, move it 6 to 8 inches, take step forward.

STEPS	RATIONALE
11. Have patient take a few steps with the assistive device being used. If patient is hemiplegic (one-sided paralysis) or has hemiparesis (one-sided weakness), stand next to his or her strong side. Support patient by placing arm closest to patient on gait belt.	Ensures that patient has satisfactory strength and balance to continue.
12. Take a few steps forward with patient. Assess for strength and balance.	Allows patient to rest.
13. If patient becomes weak or dizzy, return to bed or chair, whichever is closer.	
14. **See Completion Protocol (inside front cover).**	

EVALUATION

1. Observe patient using assistive device.
2. Inspect hands and axillae for redness, swelling, or skin irritation caused by using assistive device.
3. Ask patient to rate level of discomfort or fatigue if present after ambulating.
4. Monitor patient for postural hypotension, increased heart rate, decreased blood pressure, increased respirations, or shortness of breath during and after ambulation.
5. Ask patient/family about the ease with which ADLs are performed using assistive device.

Unexpected Outcomes and Related Interventions

1. Patient is unable to ambulate correctly.
   a. Reassess patient for correct fit of assistive device.
   b. Have added assistance nearby to ensure safety.
   c. Reassess comfort level.
   d. Reassess muscle strength in uninvolved extremities. Alternative device may be necessary.
   e. Obtain physical therapy referral for gait training.
2. Patient becomes dizzy and light-headed.
   a. Call for assistance.
   b. Have patient sit or lie down on nearest chair or bed.
   c. Assess patient's vital signs.
   d. Allow patient to rest thoroughly before resuming activity.
   e. Ask if patient is ready to continue.

Recording and Reporting

- Record type of gait patient used, weight-bearing status, amount of assistance required, tolerance of activity, and distance walked in progress notes. Document instructions given to patient and family.
- Immediately report any injury sustained during attempts to ambulate, alteration in vital signs, or inability to ambulate.

Sample Documentation

0900 Ambulated 20 feet correctly using quad cane, standby assist of one, and partial weight bearing on right lower extremity. Requested pain pills. Rates pain in right knee at 6 (scale 0 to 10). Returned to bed.

0930 Resting quietly in bed. Rates pain in right knee at 2 (scale of 0 to 10).

Special Considerations

Pediatric

- For rehabilitation of a small child who has not yet learned to walk or who is unsteady, special crutches with three or four legs provide the needed stability to allow the child to maintain an upright posture and learn to walk (Hockenberry and Wilson, 2007).

Geriatric

- The older adult with arthritis may require additional time in the morning before resuming activities.

Home Care

- Instruct patient on how to use the ambulation aid on various terrains (e.g., carpet, stairs, rough ground, inclines).
- Instruct patient on how to maneuver around obstacles such as doors and how to use the aid when transferring (e.g., to and from a chair, toilet, tub, and car).
- Instruct patient and family caregiver in proper way to check that assistive device is functioning.
- Attach a "saddle bag" to patient's walker to carry objects; caution patient not to overfill to prevent forward tipping of walker.

REVIEW QUESTIONS

Case Study for Questions 1 and 2

A woman was recently released from the hospital after suffering a heart attack. The patient lives in a single family home with her husband and two cats. She gets short of breath and feels unsteady at times when walking and will require the use of an assistive device short-term for the first time in her life. When the home health nurse visits, the patient expresses that she wants to be as mobile as possible but has her concerns about her ability to manage an assistive device.

1. It is determined that the patient will benefit from use of a cane. On what will initial teaching by the nurse for the patient focus? Select all that apply.
   1. Using the cane on her dominant side
   2. Ensuring that walking surface is clean and dry
   3. Instructing patient to walk barefoot
   4. Avoiding flexion of elbow when ambulating
2. The patient's husband is concerned for his wife's safety during ambulation. The nurse gives him suggestions to help his wife be as mobile as possible in a safe manner. What should the nurse instruct the husband to do?
   1. Give his wife an opioid analgesic just before ambulating.
   2. Encourage his wife to bend forward when walking.
   3. Schedule daily activities so there is time between them.
   4. Have his wife hold her breath when rising to a standing position.
3. The nurse is presenting a health promotion program on exercise and mobility to a group of older adults who reside in single-family homes in their communities. The older adults are on fixed incomes and are concerned that they have no options for exercise. Which activity does the nurse suggest?
   1. Join a local fitness club.
   2. Form a walking group.
   3. Organize a book-readers club.
   4. Invest in home exercise equipment.
4. The patient has returned to the nurse's unit following total knee replacement surgery. What should the nurse do as he begins to apply the CPM?
   1. Inject analgesic medication directly into the patient's knee.
   2. Position the machine's knee hinge 10 cm (4 inches) above the patient's knee.
   3. Support the patient's leg above, below, and at the knee.
   4. Instruct the patient to expect to feel severe discomfort during the therapy.

5. The nurse is assisting a patient to the side of the bed and recognizes that the patient is experiencing orthostatic hypotension. Which of the following signs and symptoms alert the nurse to this condition? Select all that apply.
   1. Pallor
   2. Bradycardia
   3. Nausea
   4. Dizziness
   5. Irritability
6. The nurse teaches a patient ROM exercises for the shoulder. For abduction, how high is the patient taught to raise the arm?
   1. 120 degrees
   2. 140 degrees
   3. 180 degrees
   4. 220 degrees
7. A child with cerebral palsy can experience difficulty with movement, loss of balance, and lack of muscle control. Which gait does the nurse instruct the parents of a child with cerebral palsy to use for crutch walking?
   1. Four-point
   2. Three-point
   3. Two-point
   4. Swing-to
8. Which of the following actions prevents injury when the nurse is lifting a patient? Select all that apply.
   1. Keep knees in locked position.
   2. Avoid twisting.
   3. Move the patient without assistance.
   4. Use arms and legs, not the back.
   5. Encourage patient to help if able.
9. Which situation is a contraindication for the use of elastic stockings?
   1. Prior use of stockings within 3 months
   2. Recent skin graft to the lower leg
   3. Increased circulation of lower extremities
   4. Immobility for more than 1 week
10. Place the following steps for climbing stairs with crutches in the correct order from first to last step.
    1. Align crutches with unaffected leg on step.
    2. Stand in tripod position.
    3. Advance unaffected leg onto step.
    4. Transfer body weight to crutches.

REFERENCES

Barnes AF: Erasing the word 'lift' from nurses' vocabulary when handling patients, *Br J Nurs* 16(18):1144, 2007.

Gillespie HO: Exercise. In Edelman C, Mandle C, editors: *Health promotion throughout the lifespan*, ed 5, St Louis, 2006, Mosby.

Harvard Health Publications: On the alert for deep-vein blood clots, *Harvard Heart Lett* 19(9):4, 2009.

Hockenberry MJ, Wilson D: *Wong's nursing care of infants and children*, ed 8, St Louis, 2007, Mosby.

Hoeman S: *Rehabilitation prevention, intervention, and outcomes*, ed 4, St Louis, 2007, Mosby.

Ignatavicius D, Workman L: *Medical surgical nursing: critical thinking for collaborative care*, ed 6, St Louis, 2009, Mosby.

Long F: A healing machine, *Rehabil Manage Interdiscip J Rehabil* 21(5):34, 2008.

Mayo Clinic: Orthostatic hypotension (postural hypotension): lifestyle and home remedies, 2009, http://www.mayoclinic.com/health/orthostatic-hypotension/DS00997/DSECTION=lifestyle-and-home-remedies.

Meiner SE, Lueckenotte AG: *Gerontologic nursing*, ed 3, St Louis, 2006, Mosby.

Monohan WJ and others: *Phipps/medical-surgical nursing, health and illness perspectives*, ed 8, St Louis, 2007, Mosby.

Nelson A, Baptiste AS: Evidence-based practices for safe patient handling and movement, *Orthop Nurs* 25(6):366, 2006.

Nelson A and others: Safer patient handling, *Nurs Manage* 38(3):26, 2007.

Phipps W and others: *Medical-surgical nursing: concepts and clinical practice*, ed 8, St Louis, 2007, Mosby.

Struck BD, Ross KM: Health promotion in older adults: prescribing exercise for the frail and home bound, *Geriatrics* 61(5):22, 2006.

The Joint Commission (TJC): *2010 National Patient Safety Goals,* Oakbrook Terrace, Ill, 2010, The Commission, http://www.jointcommission.org/PatientSafety/NationalPatientSafetyGoals, accessed February 14, 2010.

Touhy TA: Mobility. In Ebersole P and others, editors: *Toward healthy aging: human needs & nursing response*, ed 7, St Louis, 2008, Mosby.

Tran PD, Garcia K: An international study of health knowledge, behaviors, and cultural perceptions of young Mexican adults, *Hispanic Health Care Int* 7(1):5, 2009.

Tseng CN and others: Effects of a range-of-motion exercise program, *J Adv Nurs* 57(2):181, 2007.

CHAPTER

17

Traction, Cast Care, and Immobilization Devices

evolve WEBSITE

http://evolve.elsevier.com/Perry/nursinginterventions

Trauma or disease that affects the musculoskeletal system requires immobilization, stabilization, and support to the involved body part. Traction, casts, and immobilization devices are examples of methods used to accomplish these purposes to enhance the healing process.

These devices are prescribed to correct or improve deformities or joint contractures. They are also used to treat a joint dislocation; reduce, immobilize, and align a fracture (Box 17-1); and prevent and manage muscle spasms. By controlling spasms and overriding bones, these devices can prevent further soft tissue damage. Finally, preoperative and postoperative positioning and alignment, skeletal lengthening, and rest of a diseased joint can be managed using one or more of these devices.

Traction involves a pulling force applied through weights to a part of the body while a second force, called countertraction, pulls in the opposite direction. Age, condition of the patient, and purpose of the traction determine the amount of weight on the pulling force. In straight or running traction the traction force pulls against the long axis of the body while the patient's body supplies countertraction. In balanced-suspension skeletal traction (BSST), the amount of force in the traction is equal to the amount of force in the countertraction. A sling or hammock and a system of weights attached to an over-bed frame support the affected part while weight is attached to the pin or wire traversing the femoral bone.

Although there are many types of traction for different parts of the body, there are six general principles of traction care: (1) maintain the established line of pull, (2) maintain traction equipment, (3) maintain countertraction, (4) maintain continuous traction unless ordered otherwise, (5) maintain correct body alignment, and (6) prevent friction and pressure on the skin (Whiteing, 2008).

A second treatment method for immobilization involves the use of a cast. Applied externally, a cast immobilizes injured or deformed musculoskeletal tissues in proper position to promote healing. Therefore tissue structures must be in optimal position for healing when the cast is applied. An advantage of using a cast is that it permits early ambulation and in some cases partial weight bearing.

A third treatment device used with musculoskeletal injury or disorder is the orthotic device. These devices immobilize a body part, prevent deformity, protect against injury, relieve pain and muscle spasm, maintain position until healing is complete, and assist with function. Immobilization devices are applied externally to the body and are available in many variations ranging from arm slings to back braces and finger splints. They are made from a variety of materials such as rubber, leather, metal, and plastics.

PATIENT-CENTERED CARE

When a patient has had a musculoskeletal injury, patient-centered care focuses on minimizing pain, managing stabilization and immobilization devices to minimize tissue injury, and recognizing how the injury affects the patient's well-being. Routine monitoring ensures that you can identify pain early and find ways to make patients more comfortable.

When traction or other orthopedic devices are applied, it is normal for patients to feel anxious about whether the procedure will be painful. Using a calm, confident approach in your care will help minimize anxiety.

Skeletal traction is a type of traction applied by a physician under sterile conditions and used for treatment of fractures. It involves placing a pin or wire through the bone. Weights are then attached to the device using ropes and pulleys. When

BOX 17-1 TYPES OF FRACTURES

Closed fracture: Skin intact over fracture
Open or compound fracture: Skin punctured by bone ends
Comminuted: Having three or more bone fragments
Compression: Bone that is crushed (e.g., vertebra)
Depressed: Bone fragments pushed inward
Displaced: Two edges of fracture that have moved out of alignment
Impacted: Bone ends pushed into each other
Longitudinal: Fracture that runs parallel with bone
Oblique: Fracture that slants across bone
Pathologic: Results from minor stress applied to pathologically weakened bone
Segmental: Segment of bone fractured and detached
Spiral: Around the bone
Transverse: Across the bone

assisting with application of traction, it is helpful to tell the patient to expect slight tension. This helps to minimize anxiety and discomfort as the traction is applied.

When assisting with application of a cast, explain the procedure to the patient, including how you will position him or her and how it will feel. Let the patient know that it is normal to experience some dampness and warmth under the cast during the application process and a sensation of heat as it dries. Remind patients that they may experience itching when they have a cast, but that scratching can lead to infection. Be sure that your care includes medication to control itching.

When a patient first begins to use a brace/splint, it is helpful for him or her to know that initially it seems awkward; but with practice it feels more comfortable, and there is more ease of movement. Remind the patient that assistance may be needed to apply and remove the brace/splint. With orthopedic injuries the treatment may lead to some degree of immobility and restriction. Lack of ability to function in a normal role (e.g., parent, homemaker, breadwinner) may lead to feelings of frustration or even depression.

SAFETY

Proper and timely monitoring of all immobilization and stabilization devices will help to prevent the occurrence of skin and nerve damage. Skin traction noninvasively applies pull to an affected body structure by straps attached to the skin around the structure. However, there is a risk for pressure from the traction itself. Thus it is important to monitor the patient's skin and underlying tissues for signs of pressure.

The swelling from soft tissue trauma of a fracture creates pressure that affects circulation and neurological function. In addition, pressure exerted from tightly applied circumferential bandages, casts, or braces may result in neurovascular deficits. Cool skin temperature, pale skin color, diminished pulses, and prolonged capillary refill are evidence of decreased perfusion. Ashen-gray appearance of skin and nail beds in African American patients may indicate a deficit instead of the pallor seen in Caucasian patients. Sensory complaints such as pain, numbness, tingling, and motor changes such as weakness or inability to move the extremity distal to the pressure may indicate a developing neurovascular problem. As a nurse you must monitor for the Five P's: **Pain, Pallor, Paralysis, Paresthesia, Pulselessness.** Pain on passive motion is often the first clinical manifestation when neurovascular deficit is developing. Promptly report the development of compromised neurovascular status to the patient's health care provider.

Pin site infection with skeletal traction can occur at the entry point through the skin. The pin site provides a point of entry for microorganisms to enter the soft tissues and bone. Meticulous skin care prevents the development of pin site infection.

EVIDENCE-BASED PRACTICE TRENDS

Holmes SB, Brown SJ: Skeletal pin site care: National Association of Orthopaedic Nurses guidelines for orthopaedic nursing, *Orthop Nurs* 24(2):99, 2005.

Skeletal pin site care has been based on tradition with very little research to support the practice. Holmes and Brown (2005) reviewed the research literature and subsequently made four recommendations for skeletal pin site care. First, pins located in areas with considerable soft tissue are at greater risk for infection and require meticulous care. Second, after the first 48 to 72 hours (when drainage may be heavy), provide pin site care daily or weekly for sites with mechanically stable bone-pin interfaces. Third, chlorhexidine, 2-mg/mL, solution is the most effective cleansing solution for pin site care. Finally teach patients and/or their families pin site care before discharge from the hospital or the clinic setting. Have patients demonstrate pin care and provide written instructions that include signs and symptoms of infection and what to do when infection occurs.

SKILL 17.1 CARE OF THE PATIENT IN SKIN TRACTION

Skin traction is the application of a pulling force directly to the skin and soft tissue that indirectly pulls on the skeletal system. Skin traction immobilizes a fracture and relieves muscle spasms and pain; continuous application is required to achieve that goal. Skin traction usually provides temporary immobilization until the fracture can be repaired surgically by open reduction and internal fixation (ORIF) or skeletal traction can be implemented. Furthermore, skin traction maintains alignment and reduces contractures and dislocations. Patients need written physician's orders for specific traction weights, bed position, and turning regimen.

There are several types of skin traction. The most common type of adult skin traction is Buck's extension. It is applied to one or both legs using straps or a commercially prepared foam boot with Velcro straps (Fig. 17-1). Dunlop's traction is another form of skin traction. Dunlop's traction is applied to the forearm to treat fractures of the humerus (Fig. 17-2).

Cervical traction using a head halter involves a halter with a cutout for the ears and face (Fig. 17-3). The halter cradles the chin and has straps leading to a bar attached to ropes, pulleys, and weights. Cervical traction immobilizes arthritic conditions of the cervical vertebrae, not fractures. It can be removed periodically.

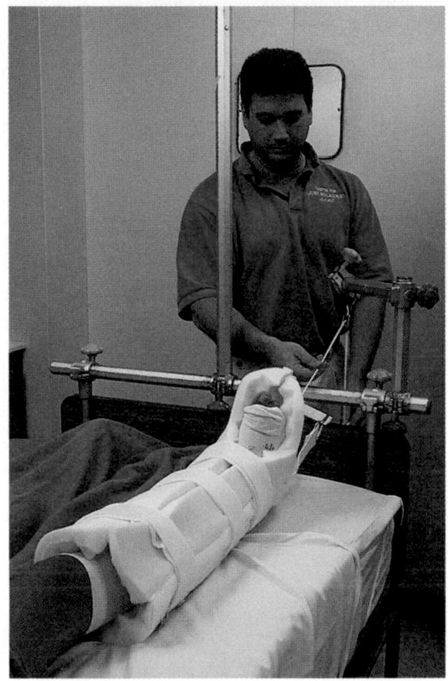

FIG 17-1 Buck's extension.

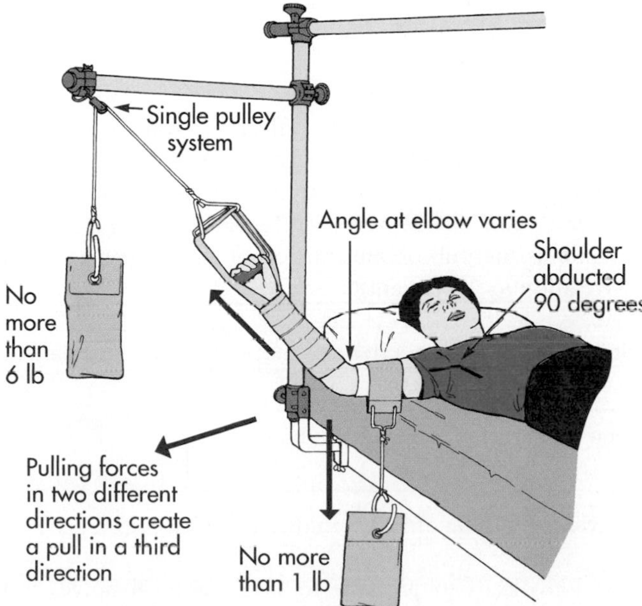

FIG 17-2 Dunlop's traction. (From Folcik MA, Carini-Garcia G, Birmingham JJ: *Traction: assessment and management*, St Louis, 1994, Mosby.)

The more weight applied to the traction, the greater the chance of skin breakdown. No more than 7 pounds is used for Buck's extension traction. Cervical traction may use 7 to 10 pounds. Skin problems such as ulcers, dermatitis, burns, or abrasions prevent the use of skin traction because of the danger of exacerbation. Older patients and patients with diabetes are at increased risk of skin breakdown.

When caring for a patient in skin traction, initially and regularly monitor patients for correct maintenance of the traction device and proper musculoskeletal alignment. Hospital policy may specify a frequency of checks, which needs to be at least every 4 to 8 hours. Traction maintenance involves monitoring the weights, the direction of pull, the ropes and pulleys, and all connections (Box 17-2).

ASSESSMENT

1. Assess patient's knowledge of the reason for traction. *Rationale: Determines concerns, fears, and need for further teaching.*
2. Assess integrity and condition of skin before traction application. *Rationale: Establishes baseline for skin integrity. Intact skin and local tissue have increased ability to tolerate the pulling forces of traction.*
3. Assess patient's overall health condition, including degree of mobility, ability to perform activities of daily living (ADLs), and current medical conditions. *Rationale: Determines patient's ability to tolerate traction, self-care ability, and anticipated need for assistance.*
4. Assess patient's position in bed: supine, perpendicular to the ends of the bed, with the affected limb in proper body alignment. *Rationale: Ensures that the pull of the traction is at the proper angle in relation to the patient's body.*

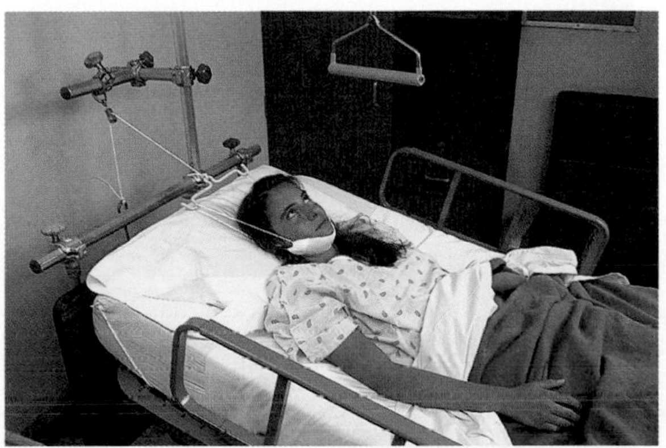

FIG 17-3 Cervical traction.

BOX 17-2 TRACTION ASSESSMENT (THE FOUR P'S)

Pounds: Is the correct weight in place and hanging freely?
Pressure: Is each clamp and connection tight?
Pull: Is the direction of pull aligned with the long axis of the bone?
Pulleys: Is the rope riding over the pulley and gliding smoothly?

5. Assess patient's level of pain using a scale of 0 to 10 and determine need for analgesics before procedure begins. *Rationale: Analgesics decrease patient's discomfort while skin traction is being applied, and assessment also serves as the baseline for later comparison.*
6. Assess neurovascular status of extremity distal to the traction, including skin color, temperature, capillary refill, presence of distal pulses, sensation, and patient's ability to move digits. *Rationale: Provides necessary baseline information for early detection of neurovascular deficit.*

PLANNING

Expected Outcomes focus on improving patient's mental status, skin integrity, comfort level, neurovascular status, and mobility.

1. Patient experiences reduced anxiety levels as evidenced by a decrease in symptoms of apprehension, irritability, and/or helplessness.
2. Skin under traction boot or elastic wrap remains intact, without redness or breakdown.
3. Patient participates in ADLs as much as possible within limitations.
4. Patient verbalizes an increased sense of comfort with a rating of 3 or lower on a scale of 0 to 10 after repositioning and administration of analgesics.
5. Patient is free of neurovascular deficit following application of circumferential dressing or boot.
6. Patient maintains correct body alignment.
7. Patient moves all extremities independently by date of discharge.

Delegation and Collaboration

Neurovascular assessment of the patient's condition cannot be delegated. The skill of assisting with application of skin traction may be delegated to nursing assistive personnel (NAP) who have had specific training. Instruct the NAP about the following:

- How to adapt skill for specific patient
- To inform the nurse if patient demonstrates any change in skin condition or complains of discomfort

Equipment

- Overhead frame for attachment of traction
- Traction bar
- Cross clamp and pulley
- Buck's traction boot or moleskin and elastic bandages
- 1- to 7-pound weights
- Spreader bar

IMPLEMENTATION *for* CARE OF THE PATIENT IN SKIN TRACTION

STEPS	RATIONALE
1. **See Standard Protocol (inside front cover).**	
2. Discuss procedure with patient.	Decreases patient anxiety.
3. Identify patient using two identifiers (e.g., name and birthday or name and account number, according to facility policy). Compare identifiers with information on patient's medication administration record (MAR) or medical record.	Ensures correct patient. Complies withThe Joint Commission standards and improves patient safety (TJC, 2010).
4. Administer analgesic for acute pain and muscle relaxant for spasms in advance of traction application.	Allows drugs to reach peak effect at time of traction application, thereby reducing pain and resultant muscle spasm. Analgesics do not effectively reduce muscle spasm pain.
5. Position patient supine and nearly flat with no more than 30 degrees of elevation, with the affected leg halfway between the edge and the middle of the bed.	Maintains the pull of the traction at the proper angle in relation to the patient's body.
6. Wash affected leg (or legs) gently and pat dry. Do not shave legs.	Shaving may create micro nicks that could become inflamed under traction straps.

SAFETY ALERT Do not place skin traction over irritated, damaged, or broken skin.

STEPS	RATIONALE
7. Apply foam boot, moleskin, or elastic bandages to affected leg, proceeding from distal to proximal.	Prevents trapping of blood in distal region.
a. Ensure that boot fits snugly.	Too tight leads to pressure to skin, peroneal nerve, and vasculature structures. Too loose leads to slipping and lack of traction force.

STEPS	RATIONALE
b. Seat heel properly in traction boot. Do not pad at heel.	Prevents pressure on patient's heel.
c. Do not apply traction boot over sequential pneumatic compression devices. Instead use foot pumps.	Causes pressure on tissues and renders compression device ineffective.

SAFETY ALERT Skin traction that is too tight puts pressure on nerves and vascular structures, putting the patient at risk for an irreversible neurovascular deficit. Skin traction that is too loose will slip.

STEPS	RATIONALE
8. Attach weight to boot gradually and gently at the end of the bed. Physician determines exact amount of weight to be applied and position to be maintained.	Traction is established slowly to avoid involuntary muscle spasms or pain for patient. Weight should create enough pull to overcome muscle spasms but not cause marked increase in pain.

SAFETY ALERT When applying Buck's extension, avoid pressure to the peroneal nerve at the neck of the fibula. Decreased sensation in the web space between the great and second toes and an inability to dorsiflex the foot and extend the toes may indicate pressure to the nerve. Be alert to pressure over bony prominences around the ankle or the back of the heel.

STEPS	RATIONALE
9. Inspect traction setup, making sure that: • Knots are secure. • Ropes are in pulleys and not frayed. • Weights are hanging freely, not caught on bed or resting on floor. • Bedclothes are not interfering with traction apparatus. Check the four *Ps* of traction maintenance (see Box 17-2).	Routine observation of these checkpoints is necessary to maintain appropriate amount of tension and effective immobilization.
10. Before physician leaves, assess patient's position and ask about additional permissible positions for patient and bed. Patient is primarily on back but may be allowed to turn to unaffected side for brief periods (10 to 15 minutes).	Positioning on side permits back care and relief of pressure to tissues.
11. Evaluate neurovascular status of extremity distal to the traction, including skin color and temperature, capillary refill, presence of distal pulses, sensation, and patient's ability to move digits.	Altered circulation, sensation, or motion indicates potential problems that can result in permanent neurovascular damage.

SAFETY ALERT If tissues distal to skin traction are cold or cool or if capillary refill is greater than 3 seconds, compare with unaffected extremity. If deficit is related to traction, wrap extremity, remove traction, and report neurovascular compromise.

STEPS	RATIONALE
12. Release and reapply traction boot every 4 to 8 hours and provide skin care according to physician's orders.	Permits visualization of skin and opportunity to provide skin care.
13. See Completion Protocol (inside front cover).	

EVALUATION

1. Evaluate patient's anxiety level for symptoms of apprehension, irritability, and/or helplessness.
2. Inspect skin tissues for signs of pressure, color changes, edema, or tenderness.
3. Observe patient for correct alignment.
4. Evaluate patient's ability to perform ADLs.
5. Ask patient to rate discomfort on a scale of 0 to 10 and to report muscle spasms.
6. Evaluate neurovascular status every 30 minutes × 2, then every 2 hours for 24 hours, and every 4 hours thereafter (see agency policy).
7. Observe patient's use of trapeze and unaffected limbs to reposition self correctly.

Unexpected Outcomes and Related Interventions

1. Patient complains of increased pain after traction is applied.
   a. Take the traction off (if allowed by physician), reposition patient, and reapply the traction. If not allowed, loosen traction slightly to prevent a tourniquet effect and reassess neurovascular status.
   b. Administer analgesics as prescribed.
   c. Realign body and/or limb.
   d. If increased pain continues or pain occurs on passive motion, notify physician of possible neurovascular deficit.
2. Patient has reddened areas on leg or heel under Buck's traction boot.
   a. Obtain physician order to remove foam boot for 1 hour to relieve pressure.
   b. Apply foam boot securely (you should be able to insert one finger between patient's skin and Buck's traction boot). Recheck correct tightness frequently.
   c. Increase frequency of skin checks to every hour.
   d. Apply protective barrier agent (e.g., Aloe Vista or Sween cream) to affected limb for protection against skin breakdown.
   e. Ensure that heels do not rest on bed or pillow.

Recording and Reporting

- Record pain assessment and assessment of skin integrity beneath traction, nursing interventions, and length of time patient is in or out of specific traction in nurses' notes.
- Record neurovascular assessments on flow sheet or nurses' notes.
- Report any neurovascular deficits to appropriate health care provider immediately.

Sample Documentation

0900 Buck's traction boot applied to patient's left leg and attached to a 5-pound weight. No complaints of pain, tingling, or numbness. Bilateral pedal pulses strong, equal, and regular. Capillary refill 3 seconds in nail beds of toes bilaterally; able to move or flex toes; skin warm, dry, and pink to lower left leg. Side rails up, bed down, brakes locked, call light within reach, and weights hanging freely. Knots tied, rope in pulley. In supine position with left leg in proper alignment.

Special Considerations

Pediatric

- Infants and young children are unable to remain still and in alignment.

Geriatric

- Some patients may have keratoses, rashes, or other lesions that could become irritated in skin traction.
- The presence of long-standing conditions of musculoskeletal tissues such as arthritis or gout can increase the risk for inflamed tissues and skin breakdown.
- Older and chronically ill patients have increased need for position changes as a result of limitations from osteoporosis, osteomalacia, weakened muscles, or increased risk of skin breakdown.
- Older adult's skin heals more slowly and is more fragile, less elastic, and thinner than when they were younger (Ebersole and others, 2008). Use pressure relief devices to reduce the risk of impaired skin integrity (see Chapter 25).

Home Care

- When the patient is discharged home, instruct family caregivers about home traction, mode of ambulation, and any limitations.
- Teach family caregivers how to maintain integrity of traction by inspecting at least daily: weights hang freely; traction ropes rest in groove of pulley and hang freely, not caught on bed or resting on floor.

SKILL 17.2 CARE OF THE PATIENT IN SKELETAL TRACTION AND PIN SITE CARE

Skeletal traction immobilizes fractures of the femur below the trochanter, fractures of the cervical spine, and some fractures of the bones of the arm or ankle. It also immobilizes the head of the femur in the case of acetabular fractures. Slow healing requires longer periods of traction (6 to 8 weeks) to promote bone repair. Skeletal traction is used less frequently with newer surgical repair procedures.

Skeletal traction involves puncturing the skin at the site where the pin enters and exits. In the case of external fixation or halo traction, the device attaches to the bone through the skin. Skeletal traction immobilizes patients until the bone heals. Prolonged immobilization influences nursing care, which focuses on supporting ADLs, maintaining traction, and preventing fat emboli and complications of immobility such as skin breakdown and pulmonary emboli.

A common form of skeletal traction is BSST, which is usually used for a fractured femur (Fig. 17-4). BSST relieves muscle spasms, realigns the fracture fragments, and promotes callus formation. Callus formation is the development of new supportive bone around the injured site. BSST temporarily stabilizes the patient's condition while waiting for surgical insertion of an internal fixation device such as a plate, screw, or nail. Balanced suspension involves a sling attached to splints around the leg and a Steinmann pin or Kirschner wire supplying the traction (Fig. 17-5). Sufficient weight to overcome the quadriceps and hamstring muscle spasms may be 30 to 40 pounds.

Other common forms of skeletal traction are sidearm traction (with a pin drilled through the lower humerus) and external fixation (used for comminuted fractures with soft tissue injury, skull and facial fractures, and pelvic bones). For cervical spine fractures, Crutchfield or Gardner-Wells tongs are inserted into the skull. Halo traction is frequently used for neurologically intact patients, stabilizing the spinal vertebra and preventing further injury to the spinal cord (Fig. 17-6).

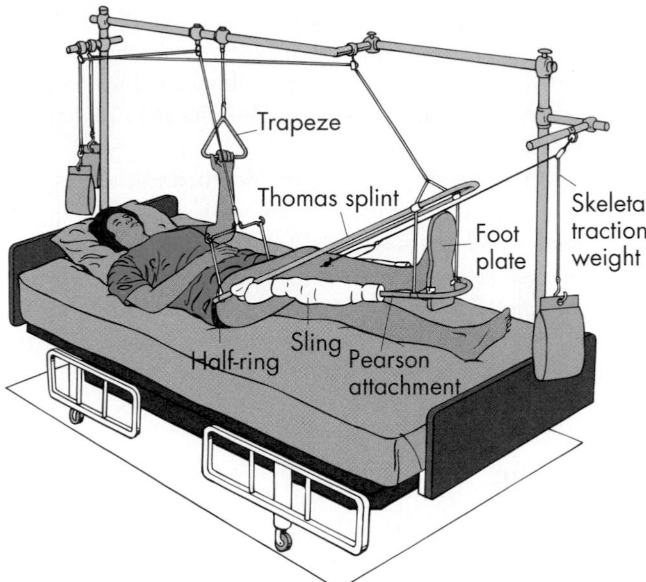

FIG 17-4 Balanced-suspension skeletal traction. Traction in long axis of right thigh is applied by means of Kirschner wire through proximal portion of tibia. Limb is supported by Thomas splint beneath thigh and Pearson attachment beneath leg. Foot plate attachment prevents footdrop. Weights apply countertraction to upper end of Thomas splint and suspend its lower end. By using the left arm and leg as shown, patient can shift position of the hips without change in amount of traction.

External fixation is a form of skeletal traction that consists of a frame or apparatus to hold pins placed into or through bones above and below a fracture site. External fixation devices promote early ambulation and use of other joints while maintaining immobilization of affected bones. A variety of external fixation frames are used for skull and facial fractures, ribs, bones of the extremities, and pelvic bones (Fig. 17-7).

All skeletal traction involves placement of a device through the skin, called a *pin site*. Pin site care reduces the risk for pin tract infections. Procedures for pin site care must be kept current with evidence-based guidelines. Some institutions have policies outlining pin site care. Hydrogen peroxide is no longer advocated because it is potentially damaging to healthy

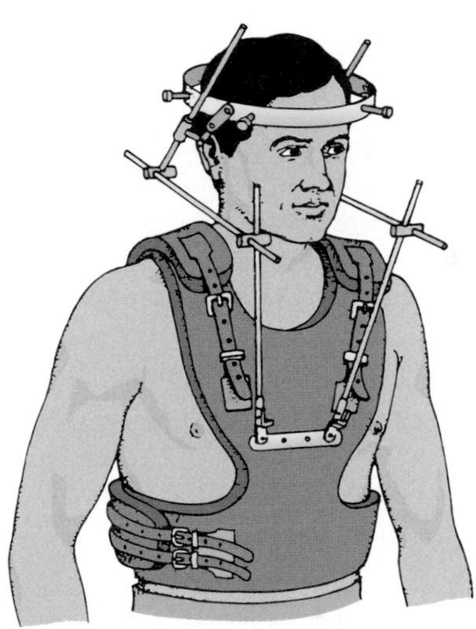

FIG 17-6 Halo traction. (Redrawn from Beare PG, Myers JL: *Principles and practice of adult health nursing,* ed 3, St Louis, 1998, Mosby.)

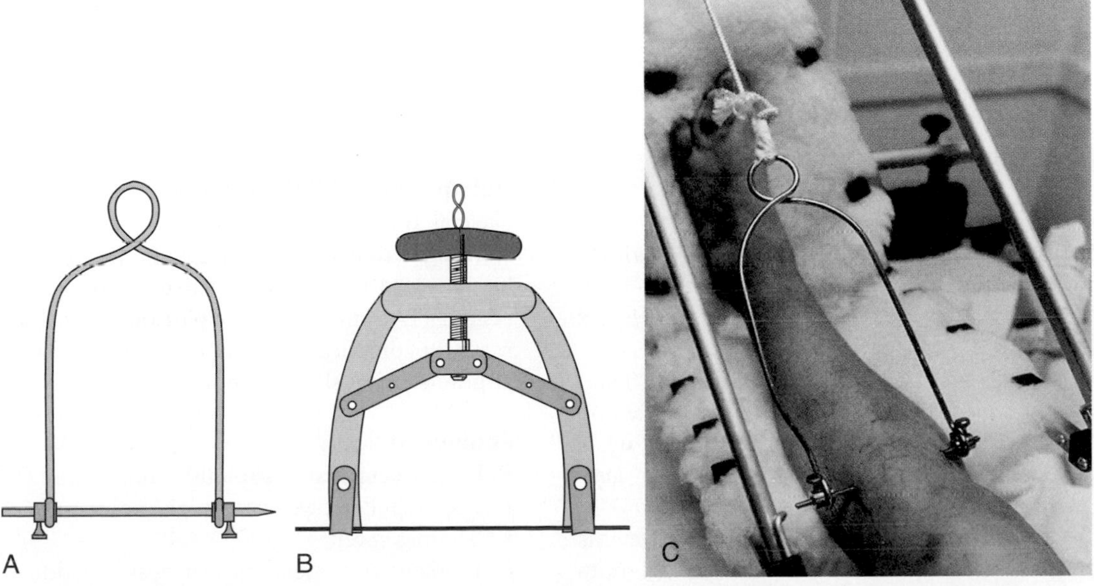

FIG 17-5 A, Steinmann pin and holder. **B,** Kirschner wire and tractor. **C,** Steinmann pin placed in tibial plateau for treatment of distal femoral fracture. (**C,** From Phipps W and others: *Medical surgical nursing: concepts and clinical practice,* ed 6, St Louis, 1995, Mosby.)

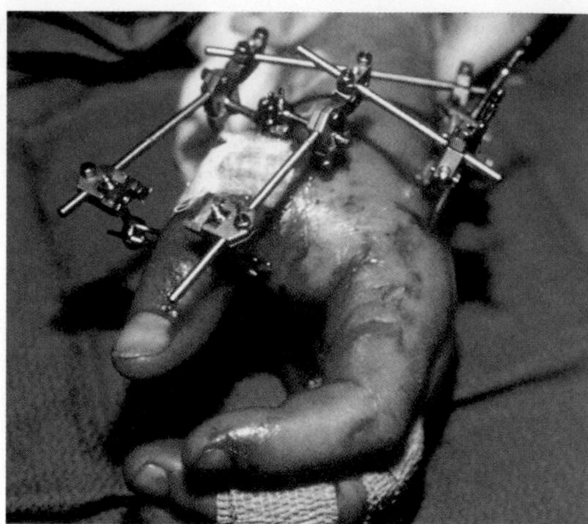

FIG 17-7 External fixator.

skin around the pin and causes corrosion to the pins. Chlorhexidine, 2-mg/mL solution, is possibly the most effective cleansing solution for pin site care (Holmes and Brown, 2005). Some agencies require specific physician's orders to specify frequency of pin site care and the cleansing agent to use. Skeletal pin site care guidelines were established by a panel of experts and published by the National Association of Orthopaedic Nurses (see Evidence-Based Practice Trends, p. 402).

ASSESSMENT

1. Assess patient's knowledge of the reason for traction, including nonverbal behavior and responses. *Rationale: Determines concerns, anxiety, and need for further teaching.*
2. Inspect integrity and condition of skin over bony prominences (e.g., use Braden Scale to assess risk for pressure ulcers) and under devices in use. Consider need for special bed or mattress (see Chapter 25). *Rationale: Provides baseline status of dependent tissues at risk for pressure ulcer formation.*
3. Assess for proper alignment of extremity. *Rationale: Ensures that the pull of the traction is at the proper angle in relation to the patient's body.*
4. Assess patient's degree of mobility, ability to perform ADLs, and current medical conditions. *Rationale: Determines patient's health state as a baseline for future reference.*
5. Assess patient's level of pain using a scale of 0 to 10 and determine the need for analgesics before procedure begins. *Rationale: Decreases patient's discomfort while applying traction and serves as a baseline for later comparison.*
6. Following application, assess traction setup: weights hanging freely, ordered amount of weight applied, ropes moving freely through pulleys, all knots tight in ropes and away from pulleys. *Rationale: Ensures accurate function of traction.*
7. Assess neurovascular status of extremity distal to the traction, including skin color, temperature, capillary refill, presence of distal pulses, sensation, and patient's ability to move digits. *Rationale: Provides necessary baseline information and detects neurovascular deficits that would occur below the level of the injury.*
8. Assess patient's ability to reposition and participate in ADLs. *Rationale: Determines patient's ability to change position and reduce risks for hazards of immobility.*
9. Following application, assess pin sites for redness, edema, discharge, or odor. *Rationale: Identifies signs and symptoms associated with infection.*
10. Assess respiratory rate, rhythm, depth, and chest expansion. *Rationale: Pulmonary embolus can occur in the patient who has associated spinal cord injury or who is on prolonged bed rest. Fat embolus syndrome (FES) can occur with long bone fracture. Halo vests are not recommended for patients with respiratory insufficiency because of the restricted chest expansion.*

PLANNING

Expected Outcomes focus on patient's anxiety level, skin integrity, self-care abilities, comfort and mobility level, neurovascular status, infection risks, and pulmonary status.

1. Skeletal deformity is reduced, alignment is maintained, and injury is healed.
2. Patient verbalizes decreased anxiety.
3. Skin over bony prominences or under halo vest remains intact, without redness or breakdown.
4. Patient performs ADLs independently to all unaffected areas.
5. Patient verbalizes a sense of comfort (3 or below on a scale of 0 to 10) after repositioning and administration of analgesics.
6. Patient is free of neurovascular deficit following application of traction.
7. Skin around pin sites remains free of redness, swelling, or drainage.

Delegation and Collaboration

Skeletal traction is applied by the physician. The skill of assisting with insertion of skeletal pins and pin site care may be delegated to nursing assistive personnel (NAP) who are adequately trained in principles of surgical asepsis. Assessment for complications, including infection or inflammation at pin insertion site, may not be delegated.

Equipment

Balanced-suspension skeletal traction (see Fig. 17-4)

- Ropes, pulleys, weights, weight holders
- Thomas splint
- Pearson attachment with sheepskin padding
- Foot plate
- Trapeze
- Clean gloves

Halo traction (see Fig. 17-6)
- Halo ring with four pins
- Molded vest jacket
- Vertical metal bars connecting ring to jacket
- Tracheostomy tray (for emergency resuscitation)
- Allen wrench (allows removal of screws for resuscitation)

Pin site care supplies
- Sterile cotton-tipped applicators
- Prescribed cleansing agent. Preferred agent is chlorhexidine, 2 mg/mL solution (Holmes and Brown, 2005). Sterile normal saline solution, sterile water, or Betadine solution may be used (check agency policy)
- Antiseptic ointment (check agency policy)
- Split 2 × 2–inch gauze dressings
- Clean gloves

IMPLEMENTATION *for* CARE OF THE PATIENT IN SKELETAL TRACTION AND PIN SITE CARE

STEPS	RATIONALE
1. See Standard Protocol (inside front cover).	
2. Discuss procedure with patient.	Decreases patient anxiety.
3. Identify patient using two identifiers (e.g., name and birthday or name and account number, according to facility policy). Compare identifiers with information on patient's medication administration record (MAR) or medical record.	Ensures correct patient. Complies with The Joint Commission standards and improves patient safety (TJC, 2010).
4. Initial traction setup:	
a. Position patient per physician's order. Support limb to be placed in traction. Do not move distal portion unnecessarily. Patient will likely be placed in supine position with head of bed slightly elevated.	Ensures proper alignment during and after traction application. Movement can cause severe pain or additional trauma.
b. Physician will wear sterile gloves and gown while cleaning skin over pin site and injecting local anesthetic.	Anesthetic desensitizes area where pin site will be made. Patient feels pressure during drilling but should feel no pain. Procedure requires surgical asepsis.
c. Burr holes may be drilled in the outer layer of the skull for placement of tongs in a halo traction.	
d. Talk with patient during the drilling procedure.	Distraction reduces patient anxiety.
e. Assist (usually by holding spreader bar or splint) while physician continues to use drill to insert pins needed for traction. Support area of joints not at injury site. Do not move distal portion unnecessarily.	Movement can cause severe pain and additional trauma.
f. Once traction setup is applied, attach weights and gently lower until rope is taught.	Reduces spasms and discomfort.
5. Inspect traction setup, making sure that: • Knots are secure and foot plate is in place. • Ropes are in pulleys and not frayed. • Weights are hanging freely, not caught on bed or resting on floor. • Bedclothes are not interfering with traction apparatus (see Box 17-2).	Routine observation of these checkpoints is necessary to maintain appropriate amount of tension and effective immobilization. Foot plate prevents footdrop.
6. Evaluate neurovascular status and peripheral tissue perfusion of distal aspects of involved extremities compared with corresponding body part every 2 hours for the first 24 hours and then according to agency policy.	Swelling within the muscle compartment is most likely to develop in the first 24 hours after injury. This provides any evidence of increased pressure and the development of compartment syndrome (Judge, 2007).

SAFETY ALERT Irreversible tissue death from ischemia occurs within 4 to 12 hours.

Continued

STEPS	RATIONALE
7. Provide pin site care according to hospital policy or physician's orders.	
a. Remove gauze dressings from around pins and discard in receptacle. Remove and discard gloves. Perform hand hygiene.	
b. Inspect sites for redness, purulent drainage, or inflammation.	Signs indicate infection. Clear drainage or crusting may be expected.
c. Prepare supplies.	
d. Clean each pin site with prescribed cleansing solution by placing moistened sterile applicator close to the pin and cleaning away from the insertion site. Dispose of applicator. Use a clean applicator for each swipe.	Removes infectious material without contaminating pin site. Touching one pin site with material used on another pin site increases risk of transmission of microorganisms.
e. Repeat the process for each pin site.	
f. Using a sterile applicator, apply a small amount of topical antibiotic ointment to pin site if this is the physician's order or hospital policy.	May reduce development of infection.
g. Cover with a sterile 2 × 2–inch split gauze dressing or leave site open to air as prescribed or according to hospital policy.	
8. See Completion Protocol (inside front cover).	
9. Provide routine traction care.	Massage to compromised tissues increases tissue breakdown.
a. Inspect skin (bony prominences, heels, elbows, sacrum, and areas under appliances) for signs of pressure. Use pressure relief devices as appropriate (Chapter 25). Try to reposition any areas under pressure, if possible. Do not massage areas of pressure if there is tenderness, reactive hyperemia (see Chapter 25), or areas of skin breakdown.	
10. Provide nonpharmacological and pharmacological pain relief as indicated (see Chapter 13).	When analgesics reach their peak effect, nonpharmacological pain-relief measures may be more effective.
11. Encourage the use of unaffected extremities for ADLs and active and passive exercises (see Chapter 16). Encourage use of trapeze bar for repositioning in bed.	Prevents muscle atrophy and maintains muscle tone for later ambulation.
12. For elimination provide a fracture pan if necessary (see Chapter 19).	Smaller bedpan is more comfortable for and easier to place under patient.

EVALUATION

1. Inspect body part that is in traction for alignment.
2. Monitor neurovascular status and peripheral tissue perfusion every 2 hours for the first 24 hours and every 4 to 12 hours thereafter (see agency policy). This includes inspecting color and temperature of distal area, observation for edema, and measurement of capillary refill (normally color returns in 3 seconds.
3. Observe behaviors reflecting patient's anxiety level in response to traction and immobilization.
4. Inspect skin overlying dependent areas and around the site for evidence of breakdown.
5. Ask patient to rate participation in ADLs and use of unaffected extremities.
6. Have patient rate level of pain and discomfort from muscle spasms.
7. Monitor respiratory status for fat embolism syndrome, atelectasis, and pulmonary embolism every shift (see Chapter 6).
8. Observe for local and systemic indications of infection, including purulent drainage and inflammation at pin sites, fever, elevated white blood cell count, continuous dull aching pain, redness, or warmth in extremity (possible osteomyelitis [i.e., bone infection]).

Unexpected Outcomes and Related Interventions

1. Patient has severe edema, marked increase in pain, or inability to actively move joint or increased pain on passive movement, indicating compartment syndrome.
   a. Prompt management is critical. Consult with physician or health care provider.
   b. Elevate extremity.
   c. Reduce or eliminate compression caused by therapeutic devices.
2. Signs of infection or osteomyelitis, including fever, elevated white blood cell count, and general malaise, develop. This is especially a concern with open fractures and extensive soft tissue injury.
   a. Cultures of drainage may be indicated to identify infecting organism. (Health care provider's order is required; see agency policy) (see Chapter 8).
   b. Consult with physician or health care provider. Orders may include irrigation of the site with antibiotic solution and/or intravenous (IV) antibiotics.
   c. Encourage fluid intake and provide comfort measures for fever.
3. Nerve damage develops from pressure or trauma to nerves, depending on type of traction in place. For example, peroneal nerve: footdrop may develop with inability to evert and dorsiflex foot; radial or median nerve at wrist: inability to approximate thumb and fingers (radial) and numbness and tingling of thumb, index, middle fingers (medial) with wrist drop.
   a. Eliminate pressure if possible according to type of traction in place.
   b. Notify physician or health care provider.
4. FES (more common in fractures of pelvic and long bones) with symptoms of hypoxia, restlessness, mental changes, tachycardia, tachypnea, dyspnea, low blood pressure, and occasionally petechial rash over upper chest and neck.
   a. This is a life-threatening emergency—50% of persons with fat emboli die.
   b. Notify physician or health care provider and initiate major resuscitation efforts.

Recording and Reporting

- Record in nurses' notes type of traction, site to which traction is applied, amount of weights, and patient's response.
- Record in nurses' notes site care performed and appearance of sites.
- Record on flow sheet specific routine assessments and frequency of assessment.

Sample Documentation

0700 BSST in place with 20-pound weight to left femur. Knots secure, ropes in pulleys, weights hanging freely. Neurovascular assessment to left foot—color pink, temperature warm, no numbness or tingling, wiggles toes on command, capillary refill 2 seconds. Reports pain at 2 on scale of 0 to 10. Lateral pin site dry, medial pin site draining small amount clear fluid (¼-inch diameter circle). No odor. No redness.

0900 Medial pin site drainage changed to yellow drainage (1-cm [½-inch] diameter circle). Pin site cultured. Reports pain of 6 on scale of 0 to 10. Physician notified of pin site drainage.

Special Considerations

Pediatric

- Blood loss from a fracture in a child poses a greater danger because the blood volume in a child is 70% to 85% of total body weight and only about 60% in the adult (Hockenberry and Wilson, 2007).
- Caregivers and parents work together to develop strategies to combat boredom of child in traction. Counseling regarding possibility of regressive type of behaviors lessens the parents' anxiety. Interference with schoolwork is remedied by obtaining work from school as soon as the child is able to perform tasks.
- Assure children that someone will be there to assist them while they are in traction.

Geriatric

- Older adults are at increased risk for impaired skin integrity when they are immobilized and not repositioned frequently. This risk results from a decreased amount of subcutaneous fat and skin that is less elastic, thinner, drier, and more fragile than that of a younger adult (Ebersole and others, 2008).
- Older and chronically ill patients have increased need for position changes to prevent the complications of immobility and those resulting from limitations imposed by osteoporosis, osteomalacia, or weakened muscles. Severe varicose veins prevent the use of skin traction in the older patient because of the risk of skin breakdown.

Home Care

- Following removal of skeletal traction, teach patient to ambulate slowly within medical guidelines, gradually increasing length of time out of bed and distance walked.
- Teach patient to notify physician of undesirable signs such as marked increase in pain, muscle spasms, and increased numbness, indicating reinjury or insufficient healing.
- Teach family members how to apply skin traction correctly if it is prescribed for home use following the removal of the skeletal traction.
- Instruct patients in home safety methods to prevent further injuries.

SKILL 17.3 CARE OF THE PATIENT DURING CAST APPLICATION

A cast immobilizes an injured extremity to protect it from further injury, provides alignment of a fracture by holding the bone fragments in reduction and alignment during the healing process, and promotes comfort. In addition, it maintains a limb in alignment to prevent or correct structural abnormalities. Casts are used in many different ways (Fig. 17-8). The use and type of application materials required depend on the anatomical area of injury.

Casts are made of one of two types of materials, plaster of Paris or synthetic material. The type of cast material selected depends on the number of cast changes anticipated and the type of musculoskeletal injury. Plaster of Paris is composed of open-weave cotton roll or strip covered with calcium sulfate crystals. When moistened with water, this material molds easily during application; but drying may require 24 to 72 hours, depending on the size of the cast. During drying the cast must be exposed to air, well supported on firm surfaces, handled with palms (not fingertips) to avoid indentations such as fingerprints, and turned regularly so it dries evenly. Weight bearing is delayed until the cast is completely dry. Lifting the cast by supporting the joints above and below the casted area prevents injury to underlying soft tissues. This type of cast is heavier than a synthetic cast.

Synthetic casting materials are composed of open-weave fiberglass tape covered with a polyurethane resin that is activated by water. This cast sets very quickly, in approximately 15 minutes, and can withstand pressure or weight bearing after 20 minutes. It forms a lightweight, sturdy cast that is both radiolucent and waterproof. Different colors of this casting material are also available, ranging from fluorescent pink and green to navy blue and purple. Colors are often more appealing to children and aid in maintaining the appearance of the cast. These casts are more expensive than plaster casts.

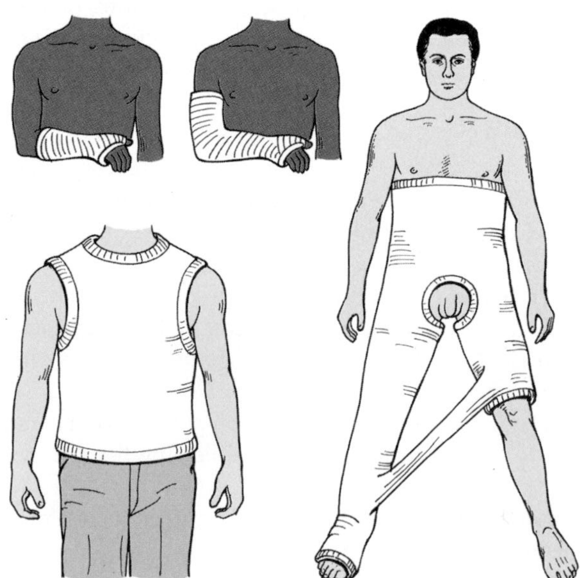

FIG 17-8 Types of casts. *Top left,* short arm cast. *Top center,* long arm cast. *Bottom left,* plaster body jacket cast. *Far right,* one and one-half hip spica cast.

This skill includes assessment parameters before, during, and after cast application, including peripheral neurovascular status. It also discusses assisting with cast application. It is important to follow guidelines for care after application with respect to pressure against cast and weight bearing.

ASSESSMENT

1. Assess factors that may affect wound healing such as diabetes, poor nutritional status, or steroid medication use. *Rationale: When there is a risk of slower healing, additional nutritional supplements may be required.*
2. Assess patient's ability to cooperate and level of understanding concerning the casting procedure. *Rationale: Sudden movement during procedure could cause injury.*
3. Inspect condition of the skin that will be under the cast. Specifically note any areas of skin breakdown, rashes present, or incisional wound. *Rationale: Provides baseline for skin condition. Open lesions may prohibit casting.*
4. Assess neurovascular status of the area to be casted. Specifically note alteration of motor and sensory function, skin color, temperature, and capillary refill. Compare with opposite extremity or surrounding tissues. Pay particular attention to tissues distal to cast. *Rationale: Changes in neurovascular status may occur after casting, possibly further compromising already injured tissues. It is important to note the baseline neurovascular status so these changes, if they occur, are accurately assessed and compared with the baseline data.*
5. Assess patient's pain status using a scale of 0 to 10. *Rationale: Using a pain rating scale provides baseline data to determine efficacy of nursing measures.*
6. Consult with physician to determine the extent to which patient will be able to use the casted body part. *Rationale: Determines extent to which self-care will be impaired.*

PLANNING

Expected Outcomes focus on skin integrity, comfort, self-care, mobility, prevention of neurovascular complications, and maintenance of cast integrity.

1. Patient's exposed skin distal to cast is warm and pink, with capillary refill less than 3 seconds.
2. Patient exhibits no elevated temperature or other signs of infection.
3. Pulses distal to the cast are palpable, strong, and regular.
4. Cast remains clean, without indentations or fraying, until removal.
5. Patient has edema of 1+ or less and demonstrates less than 25% decrease in active range of motion (ROM) of affected extremity after cast application.

6. Patient verbalizes pain of 3 or less (scale of 0 to 10) after analgesic administration 20 to 30 minutes before the procedure.
7. Patient requires minimal assistance with ADLs after an extremity is casted.
8. Patient describes the steps of proper cast care.

Delegation and Collaboration

A complete assessment of the patient before cast applications may not be delegated to nursing assistive personnel (NAP). However, the skill of assisting with cast application may be delegated. Instruct the NAP about the following:

- The method to assist in positioning for specific patient with mobility restrictions

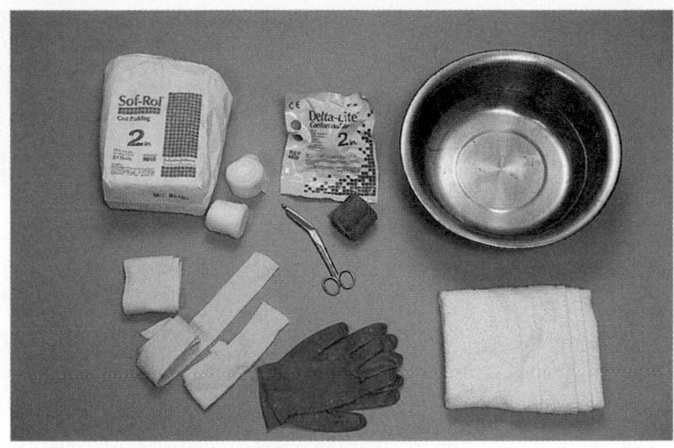

FIG 17-9 Casting materials.

Equipment (May Be on Cast Cart) (Fig. 17-9)

- Plaster cast
- Plaster rolls: 2, 3, 4, or 6 inch
- Padding material (felt, sheet wadding, Webril, stockinette, or gore lining)
- Clean gloves, apron, or protective cover
- Plastic-lined bucket or basin
- Water warmed at time of application
- Cart, chair, and fracture table scissors
- Paper or plastic sheets
- Synthetic cast
- Synthetic rolls: 2, 3, or 4 inch
- Pail with water to dampen rolls
- Padding materials (nylon stockinette and synthetic padding)
- Cast cutter (to trim edge of cast if needed)

IMPLEMENTATION *for* CARE OF THE PATIENT DURING CAST APPLICATION

STEPS	RATIONALE
1. See Standard Protocol (inside front cover).	
2. Discuss procedure with patient.	Decreases patient anxiety.
3. Identify patient using two identifiers (e.g., name and birthday or name and account number, according to facility policy). Compare identifiers with information on patient's medication administration record (MAR) or medical record.)	Ensures correct patient. Complies with The Joint Commission standards and improves patient safety (TJC, 2010).
4. Administer analgesic before cast application: oral (PO), 30 to 40 minutes before; intramuscular (IM), 20 to 30 minutes before; IV, 2 to 5 minutes before.	Reduces pain during cast application. Provides optimal analgesic effect.
5. Use latex-free gloves if there is risk of an allergic reaction.	Synthetic cast can leave gluelike resin on hands. Prevents exposure to allergen (First national guideline on latex allergy, 2008).
6. Assist health care provider or certified technician in positioning patient and injured extremity as desired, depending on type of cast to be used and area to be casted.	The parts to be casted must be supported and in optimal alignment.
7. Prepare skin that will be enclosed in the cast. Change any dressing (if present), and cleanse the skin with mild soap and water.	Assists in maintaining skin integrity.

SAFETY ALERT Patients with skin damage or skin lesions may not be candidates for casting.

Continued

STEPS	RATIONALE
8. Assist with application of padding material around body part to be casted (see illustration). Avoid wrinkles or uneven thicknesses.	Decreases complications to the skin and prevents pressure points under the cast.
9. Hold body part or parts to be casted or assist with preparation of casting materials.	Support of body part may require application of slight manual traction.
a. *Plaster cast:* Mark the end of the roll by folding one corner of the material under itself. Hold plaster roll under water in a plastic-lined bucket or basin until bubbles stop; squeeze slightly and hand roll to person applying the cast.	Once dampened, the end of the casting tape is sometimes difficult to find. Dampened plaster rolls are unrolled and molded to fit the extremity or body part to be casted.
b. *Synthetic cast:* Submerge cast roll in lukewarm water for 10 to 15 seconds. Squeeze to remove excess water. You can use a water bottle to apply water judiciously to the casting material.	The polyurethane prepolymer is activated by the application of water (Smith, Hart, and Tsai, 2005).
10. Continue to hold the body parts as necessary as the cast is applied (see illustration) or supply additional rolls of casting tape as needed. When wrapping is complete, gently compress with hands (see illustration).	Manual traction maintains the necessary alignment. Thickness determines strength of the plaster cast. Compression promotes bonding of cast layers.
11. Provide walking heel, brace, bar, or other material to stabilize the cast as requested by the health care provider. Use an abduction bar or wooden post to stabilize a spica cast.	Ambulation may be permitted with partial weight bearing on the affected extremity after cast has dried. Braces incorporated into a cast assist in joint motion and mobility.

SAFETY ALERT Do not use abduction bar on spica cast as a handle for positioning the patient.

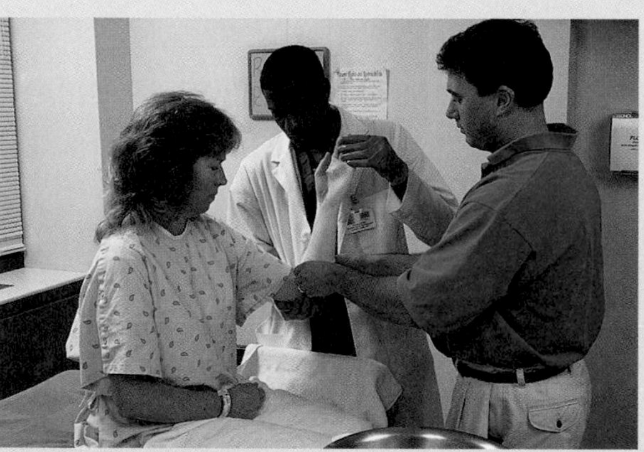

STEP 8 Padding under cast is smooth.

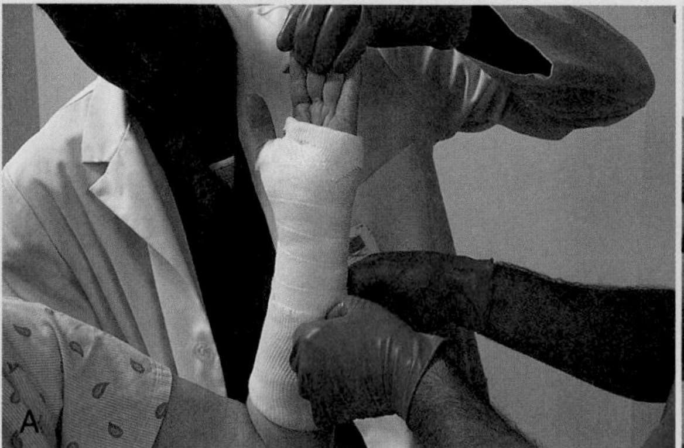

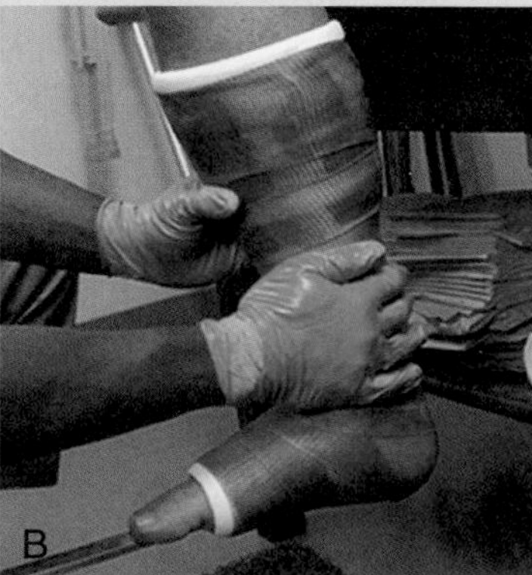

STEP 10 A, Support extremity during cast application. **B,** Applying synthetic cast roll.

STEPS	RATIONALE
12. Assist with "finishing" the cast by folding the edge of the stockinette down over the cast to provide a smooth edge. Unroll a dampened plaster roll over the stockinette to hold it in place. Cushion any rough edges of cast with tape or moleskin.	Smooth edges decrease the chance for skin irritation or tissue injury.
13. Using scissors, trim the cast around fingers, toes, or the thumb as necessary. Remove and discard gloves and perform hand hygiene.	The cast should not restrict joint movement or constrict circulation.
14. Depending on the tissue to be casted:	
a. Elevate to heart level the casted tissues on two to three cloth-covered pillows or in a sling. Avoid complete encasing of the cast. Air dry. If ice is ordered, place to side of cast to prevent indentation to top.	Pillows prevent indentations, which could harden and cause underlying pressure. Elevation enhances venous return and decreases edema. Covering the cast delays drying. Plaster gives off heat from a chemical reaction when drying. Encasing cast restricts air movements and impedes drying.
b. When applying a sling, ensure that the sling supports but does not encase the cast.	
15. Inform patient to notify health care provider of any alteration in sensation, numbness, tingling, unusual pain, pain on passive motion, or inability to move fingers or toes in affected extremity.	Edema within a casted extremity causes pressure on nerves, blood vessels, and muscle tissues. This leads to neurovascular deficit, compartment syndrome, and necrosis of tissues.
16. Using palms of hands to support casted areas, assist patient with transfer to stretcher or wheelchair for return to unit or preparation for discharge. Use additional personnel to transfer patient safely, especially with patient in a spica or other large body cast.	Avoids indentations in cast that could cause pressure areas on underlying skin. Use pillows, restraints, and side rails to maintain principles of safe transport.

SAFETY ALERT Patient with wet large-limb or wet spica cast requires three people to assist in turning and transfer. Proper assistance prevents undue pressure on cast and prevents patient injury.

STEPS	RATIONALE
17. Have patient turn every 2 to 3 hours. Do not rest heel of cast on bed or pillow.	Avoids indentation and prevents continuous pressure to one area.
18. See Completion Protocol (inside front cover).	

EVALUATION

1. Inspect exposed skin and assess circulation to distal extremity by checking capillary refill by pressing on toe or finger (Fig. 17-10).

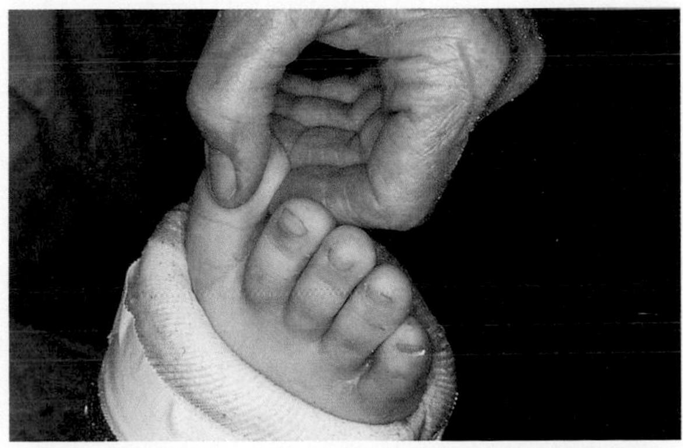

FIG 17-10 Inspecting toe to assess capillary refill.

2. Palpate the temperature of tissues around the casted area for warmth and assess for hot spots, which could indicate underlying localized infection.
3. Palpate any accessible pulses distal to the cast.
4. Inspect alignment of the limb and condition of the cast.
5. Observe for edema of tissues distal to the cast for signs of vascular compromise (whitish, bluish, or ashen-gray coloration).
6. Observe patient for signs of pain or anxiety (hyperventilation, tachycardia, blood pressure elevation).
7. Observe patient perform ADLs and ROM.
8. Observe patient or family caregiver perform cast care.

Unexpected Outcomes and Related Interventions

1. Patient experiences impaired physical mobility related to the cast.
   a. Assist patient with ROM exercises every 3 to 4 hours.
   b. Teach isometric exercises.

2. Patient reports increased severity in pain after application of the cast.
   a. Reposition casted extremity or the patient. Adjust elevation of pillows as necessary.
   b. Apply ice bags along sides of cast. Do not place heavy ice bags on top of damp cast because of risk of indentation.
   c. Administer analgesics as ordered to maintain patient's comfort level.
   d. Increase frequency of neurovascular checks.
   e. Assess tightness of the cast by checking with two fingers around the edges and checking with patient. Cast should be snug but not tight.
   f. If pain continues, notify health care provider.
3. Patient develops compartment syndrome with severe pain unrelieved by analgesics; change in neurovascular status such as numbness, tingling, pain on passive motion, or decreased movement in distal skin and tissues; bluish color to distal parts; marked edema; diminished or absent pulse in area distal to casted extremity (pulselessness develops late in the syndrome); or capillary refill over 3 seconds.
   a. Elevate cast.
   b. Consult immediately with health care provider.
   c. Prepare to bivalve cast using a cast cutter. Cut through underlying wadding and padding.

Recording and Reporting

- Record cast application, condition of skin, status of circulation (e.g., temperature, sensation), and motion of distal part.
- Record instructions given to patient and family.

BOX 17-3 CAST CARE INSTRUCTIONS

The First 24 Hours

- Follow physician's instructions.
- Keep the cast and extremity above the level of the heart for at least 48 hours by propping your cast up on firm pillows. Elevation reduces swelling.
- Put ice next to the fractured area for 24 hours, but be sure to enclose the ice in a plastic bag to keep the cast dry. Do not place ice on the top of a damp cast.
- Move the parts of your body above and below the cast regularly to aid circulation and relieve stiffness. Massaging the joints and extremities gently around the cast also improves circulation.
- Your cast needs at least 24 hours to completely dry if it is plaster and possibly 72 hours for a large cast. Avoid handling it as much as possible. When you do have to move the cast such as when you change your body position, use only the palms of your hands and support the cast under your joints. You want to avoid putting indentations in the cast that will put pressure on the skin inside.
- Use a fan placed 46 to 61 cm (18 to 24 inches) from the cast to aid its drying in the first 24 hours. Be sure to expose the whole cast for drying and do not cover it with linen for the first 24 hours.
- Never insert any object into your cast for any purpose (e.g., do not try to scratch under cast when it itches).

How to Care for Your Cast

Plaster

- Do not get the cast wet because it will lose its strength. If cast does become wet, dry immediately. Use a towel to blot moisture off the cast and then dry it with a hair dryer set on low. When your cast does not feel cold and damp, it is dry.
- To keep the cast clean and dry, cover it with plastic when bathing, using the toilet (if it is a spica cast), or going out in rain or snow.
- Use a damp cloth and scouring powder to clean soiled spots on the cast. Be sure to brush away plaster crumbs or other objects from the edges of the cast but do not remove or rearrange any padding. Do not break off or trim cast edges.

Synthetic

- If you have a fiberglass cast without wounds or incisions under it, you may be able to continue a more normal lifestyle (e.g., bathing) if your doctor approves. A fiberglass cast can become wet.
- Washing or rinsing inside your fiberglass cast may reduce odor and irritation and improve the overall skin condition of the cast area. You may use a spray nozzle at a sink or a flexible shower head to rinse inside your cast with warm water.
- You must dry the cast thoroughly after wetting. Lightly towel off excess water and use a hair dryer on cool or low setting to dry inside cast. Do not cover the cast while it is drying.

Skin Care

- Skin care is very important during the time a cast is worn. Routinely look at the skin condition around the cast each day for signs of redness or friction. Also, look for areas of cracks in the cast.
- Do not insert objects under the cast because you could scrape the skin or add pressure and cause an infection or sore under the cast.
- You may use powders and lotions only outside the cast so the skin stays clean and soft. Powder inside a cast can cake and cause sore areas.

Activity

- Do not walk on a leg cast for the first 48 hours. If you are allowed to walk on it, be sure to walk on the walking heel.
- If your arm is in a cast, be sure to use your sling for support and comfort.

Contact Your Doctor If:

- You have pain, burning, or swelling.
- You feel a blister or sore developing inside the cast.
- You experience numbness or persistent tingling.
- Your cast becomes badly soiled.
- Your cast breaks, cracks, or develops soft spots.
- Your cast becomes too loose.
- You develop skin problems at the cast edges.
- You develop a fever or foul odor under the cast.
- You have any questions regarding your treatment.

- Report abnormal or untoward findings from neurovascular checks; report signs and symptoms of compartment syndrome immediately.

Sample Documentation

0900 Left long arm synthetic cast applied, and left arm placed in shoulder sling by physician. Capillary refill of left index finger is 2 seconds. Skin warm, dry, and intact. Able to move all fingers of left hand, fingers warm to touch, nail beds pink, no swelling noted. Complains of pain at 5 (scale of 0 to 10).

0910 Tylox 1 tab administered PO. Left long arm cast and sling readjusted.

0945 Left long arm cast intact with sling. Capillary refill of left index finger unchanged. Moves all fingers of left hand, denies any numbness or tingling present, fingers warm to touch. No edema noted. Reports pain decreased to 1 (scale of 0 to 10).

Special Considerations

Pediatric

- Teach caregivers to protect plaster cast from moisture and ensure that synthetic casts are dried thoroughly if damp. Protect lower-extremity casts with plastic wrap during urination or defecation.
- Monitor children closely to ensure that they do not place objects beneath the cast to scratch. Use medication, ice pack, and/or a hair dryer set to cool setting to control itching (Hockenberry and Wilson, 2007).
- Recognize that babies and young children demonstrate pain by restlessness and crying.

Geriatric

- Lightweight synthetic casts are less restrictive and have the advantage of lighter weight for older adults, helping them maintain better balance.
- Tactile sensory receptors do not transmit sensations as rapidly, leading to reduced sensation in older adults (Ebersole and others, 2008).
- Older adults with age-related decreases in muscle strength may have difficulty ambulating with a cast.

Home Care

- See Box 17-3.

PROCEDURAL GUIDELINE 17.1
Care of the Patient During Cast Removal

When caring for patients with casts, it is also important to understand the techniques for cast removal, which consist of removing the cast and padding, followed by skin care to the affected area. The cast is removed by use of a cast saw. The saw is noisy, but the procedure is painless because the saw vibrates and thus will not cut the skin. However, it is necessary, to prepare the patient adequately for cast removal. A small child or confused adult may require gentle restraint during removal to avoid any injury. Careful removal of a synthetic cast (with gore lining) is important to prevent burns that may result from the heat generated by the vibrating saw. After cast removal the patient may experience tenderness, soreness, muscle weakness and atrophy, and a build-up of dead skin cells.

Delegation and Collaboration

The skill of cast removal may be delegated to nursing assistive personnel (NAP) who have had specific training. Instruct the NAP about the following:

- Proper positioning methods for specific patients
- Skin care required following cast removal

Equipment

- Cast saw
- Plastic sheets or paper
- Cold water enzyme wash
- Skin lotion
- Basin and water
- Washcloth and towels
- Scissors
- Eye protection (goggles, glasses) for health care provider and patient

Procedural Steps

1. **See Standard Protocol (inside front cover).**
2. Assist with positioning of patient
3. Describe the physical sensations to expect during cast removal (vibration of cast saw and generation of heat) (see illustration).

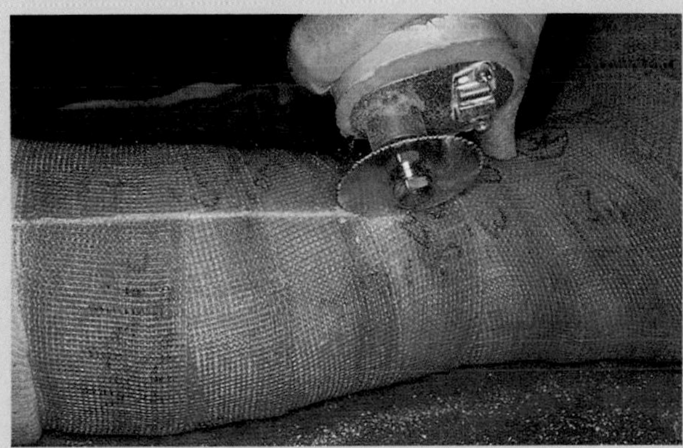

STEP 3 Vibration of cast cutter generates heat.

Continued

PROCEDURAL GUIDELINE 17.1
Care of the Patient During Cast Removal—cont'd

4. Describe the expected appearance of the extremity. Skin under cast is often scaly with dead cells that slough off. Muscle atrophy occurs from disuse.
5. Describe and demonstrate the loud noise of the cast saw.
6. Apply eye goggles or protective glasses to self and patient.
7. Stay with patient and explain progress of procedure as cast and underlying padding are removed (see illustration).
8. Inspect tissues underlying the cast after removal.
9. If skin is intact, apply cold water enzyme wash (if available) to skin and leave on for 15 to 20 minutes. Use oil or mild soap and water to soften crust. Do not scrub skin.
10. Gently wash off enzyme wash or soap and water. If possible, immerse tissues in basin or tub to assist in dead cell removal.
11. Pat extremity dry. Apply generous coat of lotion to patient's skin.
12. **See Completion Protocol (inside front cover).**

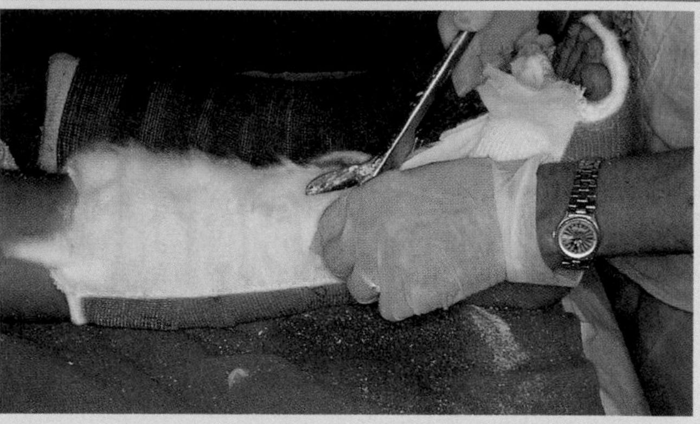

STEP 7 Removing padding beneath cast.

13. After cast removal, explain and provide written skin care procedures for patient before discharge (Box 17-4).
14. Obtain physician's order to perform active and passive ROM and clarify level of activity allowed.
15. Instruct patient to observe for swelling and continue to elevate the extremity to control it.

BOX 17-4 CARE AFTER CAST REMOVAL

Skin Care

- Apply enzyme wash solution such as Woolite or Delicare and leave in place for at least 20 minutes. The enzymes in the solution loosen dead cells and help emulsify fatty or crusty lesions but cause no skin irritation.
- After 20 minutes immerse the area in warm water and gently wash away the debris. Do not rub or scrub the skin areas but gently swab them with a soft cloth.
- Rinse with clear warm water and pat dry.
- Apply a moisturizing skin lotion or a little oil, gently massaging it in to help maintain the integrity of the cells.
- Repeat these steps in 24 to 48 hours, after which the area should need no special care.

Relieving Edema

- Apply cloth-covered ice bags if the edema is marked. Do not place ice directly on skin.
- Elevate the affected tissues for the next 24 hours or when swelling occurs.

Managing Tenderness, Weakness, Discomfort

- Take prescribed analgesic every 3 to 4 hours to build a therapeutic blood level and continue the medication for 24 to 48 hours.
- Immerse the part or the entire body in warm water and gently exercise muscles under water.
- Begin to reuse affected tissues and muscles slowly to avoid pain. Explain that usually it takes twice as long as the part was in a cast to regain full function.
- Perform prescribed muscle exercises with 5 to 10 repetitions every 4 hours while awake to aid in regaining muscle strength. If muscle soreness persists, continue intake of prescribed nonnarcotic analgesic. Soak in warm water before exercise. Soreness should lessen as muscle regains strength. Consult with therapist to prescribe appropriate exercises to increase mobility and strength.

SKILL 17.4 CARE OF THE PATIENT WITH AN IMMOBILIZATION DEVICE—BRACE, SPLINT, OR SLING

Immobilization devices increase stability, support a weak extremity, or reduce the load on weight-bearing structures such as hips, knees, or ankles. A splint immobilizes and protects a body part. Temporary splints reduce pain and prevent tissue damage from further motion immediately after an injury such as a fracture or sprain. Air splints, Thomas splints, and improvised splints from material on hand are examples of temporary splints applied in emergency situations. Upper-extremity fractures are sometimes managed using splints such as hand and digital splints or sugar-tong splints. Slings support splints, casts, or injured upper extremities. They are available commercially or can be made for almost any body part. Velcro or buckle closures permit these devices to be adjusted to fit a body part of almost any size and shape. The abduction splint (Fig. 17-11), used after hip replacement surgery, maintains the patient's legs in an abducted position.

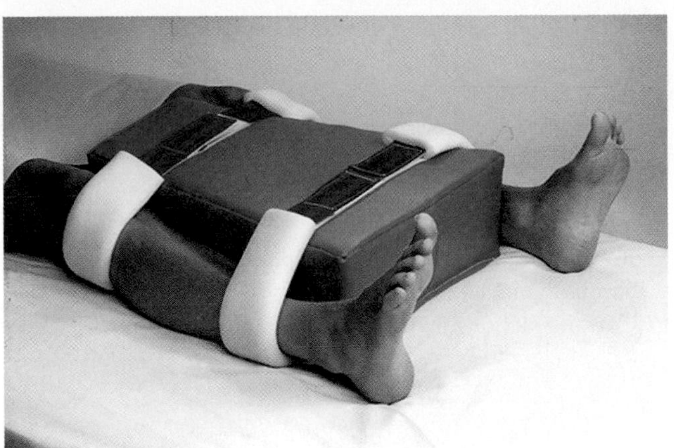

FIG 17-11 Abduction pillow.

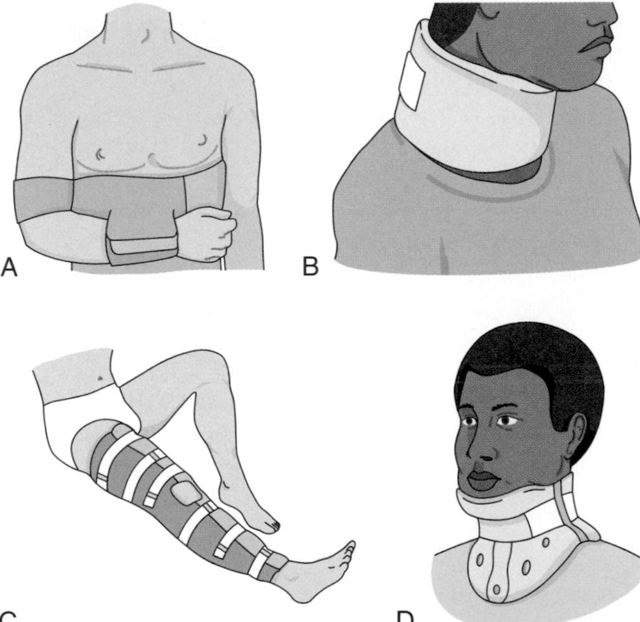

FIG 17-12 Examples of immobilizers. **A,** Shoulder immobilizer. **B,** Soft cervical collar. **C,** Knee immobilizer. **D,** Hard cervical collar. (Redrawn from Beare PG, Meyers JL: *Principles and practice of adult health nursing,* ed 3, 1998, Mosby.)

This permits the patient to be turned without changing the position of the healing limb and prevents dislocation of the hip prosthesis. The device is easily removed for nursing care such as skin care, dressing changes, or neurovascular assessments. A posterior splint with elastic wraps is sometimes used to support an extremity.

Cloth and foam splints, known as *immobilizers,* provide long-term immobilization (Fig. 17-12). Immobilizers treat sprains and dislocations that do not require complete and continuous immobilization in a cast or traction. They are often used following orthopedic surgery. Other common types of immobilizers include cervical collars (soft or hard), belt-type shoulder immobilizers, and vinyl wrist forearm splints. Molded splints made of plastic provide support to patients with chronic injuries or diseases such as arthritis. They maintain the body part in a functional position to prevent contractures and muscle atrophy during the period of disuse. A splint goes into place and is removed quickly and easily when the skin or a wound is assessed.

Braces support weakened structures during weight bearing. For this reason they are made of sturdy materials such as leather, metal, and molded plastic. Chest and abdominal braces such as the Milwaukee and Boston braces immobilize the thoracic and lumbar vertebral column to treat scoliosis (curvature of the spine). The brace does not correct the curve but instead prevents its progression. Lumbar braces support lumbar and sacral tissues after spinal surgery or fusion. Leg braces hold the thigh, leg, and foot in functional positions for weight bearing and ambulation. Both short- and long-leg braces support weak leg muscles, aid in control of involuntary muscle movement, and maintain surgical correction during the postoperative healing process.

ASSESSMENT

1. Review patient's medical history; previous and current activity level; and description of the condition requiring bracing, splinting, or a sling. *Rationale: Reveals patient's current and previous health status and purpose for brace/splint.*
2. Determine patient's previous experience with braces, splints, or slings. *Rationale: Reveals patient's baseline knowledge and need for instruction.*
3. Assess patient's understanding of reason for brace/splint/sling and its care, application, and schedule of wear. *Rationale: Determines need for further teaching.*
4. Inspect area of skin to be in contact with support device. *Rationale: Provides baseline to monitor patient for skin breakdown. Immobile and older patients are particularly vulnerable.*
5. Obtain assessment of patient's level of pain on a scale of 0 to 10. *Rationale: Provides baseline to determine if immobilization device affects comfort.*
6. Refer to occupational or physical therapy consultation to determine type of brace to be used, desired position, and amount of activity and movement permitted. *Rationale: Provides direction in proper use of brace.*
7. Assess patient's additional need for an assistive device such as a cane, walker, or crutches (see Chapter 16). *Rationale: Patient may need an assistive device to provide support and promote balance during ambulation.*

PLANNING

Expected Outcomes focus on maintaining skin integrity, improving patient's knowledge, and preventing risk for injury.

1. Patient's skin remains intact without circulatory impairment.
2. Patient/significant other verbalizes purpose, correct application, and care of the device.
3. Patient does not report an increase in pain on a scale of 0 to 10 during device application.

4. Skin distal to brace/splint/sling is intact, warm to touch, without signs of pressure, and with normal sensation.
5. Patient uses the device correctly, including schedule of wear, activity limitations, and positioning.

Delegation and Collaboration

Assessment of the patient's condition should not be delegated; however, the skill of caring for the patient wearing a brace, splint, or sling may be delegated to nursing assistive personnel (NAP). Instruct the NAP about the following:

- Correct application of the brace/splint and positioning of any ties or straps
- Schedule of wear and activities permitted while in the brace
- To alert the nurse if patient complains of pain, rubbing, or pressure from the brace or splint or if a change occurs in patient's skin condition

Equipment

- Brace/splint/commercially prepared sling or triangular bandage and safety pin
- Cotton shirt or gown

IMPLEMENTATION *for* CARE OF THE PATIENT WITH AN IMMOBILIZATION DEVICE—BRACE, SPLINT, OR SLING

STEPS	RATIONALE
1. See Standard Protocol (inside front cover).	
2. Identify the patient using two identifiers (e.g., name and birthday or name and account number, according to facility policy).	Ensures correct patient. Complies with The Joint Commission standards and improves patient safety (TJC, 2010).
3. Explain reasons for brace, splint, or sling and demonstrate how device works.	Teaching and demonstration enhance learning, reduce anxiety, and encourage cooperation
4. Assist patient to a comfortable position: apply upper-extremity braces/splints/slings with patient sitting upright; apply lower-extremity braces with patient lying down.	Facilitates correct, aligned placement of brace.
5. Prepare skin that will be enclosed in brace/splint/sling by cleaning skin with soap and water; rinse, pat dry, and change any dressings (if present). If applying a back brace, put a thin cotton shirt or gown on patient. Ensure that there are no wrinkles to cause pressure.	This protects skin and keeps brace clean. Smooth cotton clothing between the brace and skin protects the skin from irritation and absorbs moisture.
6. Inspect device for wear, damage, or rough edges.	Decreases potential for skin breakdown and maintains correct alignment.
7. Apply brace/splint as directed by physician, orthotist, physical therapist, or occupational therapist. If securing splint with elastic bandage:	Proper application of the brace/splint is important to avoid skin breakdown, pressure ulcers, neurovascular compromise, calluses, or worsening of the deformity.
a. Apply even tension as bandage is wrapped from distal to proximal.	Prevents trapping of blood distal to immobilization device.
b. Prevent padding from gathering or bunching.	Prevents irritation to underlying tissues.
8. Apply sling using triangular bandage:	
a. Position one end of the bandage over the shoulder of the unaffected arm.	
b. Take the remaining bandage and place the material against the chest, then under and over the affected arm, cradling the arm.	
c. Position the pointed end of the triangle toward the elbow.	Position cradles the arm.
d. Tie the two ends of the triangle at the side of the neck.	Prevents skin irritation and pressure to back of the neck
e. Fold the pointed end of the sling at the elbow in the front and secure with a safety pin, closing the end of the sling.	

STEPS	RATIONALE
f. Be sure the sling supports the limb comfortably without interfering with circulation.	
9. Teach patient prescribed schedule of wear and activities while in brace/splint/sling as directed by physician, physical therapist, or occupational therapist.	Proper use of brace/splint/sling facilitates healing and mobility and reduces pain and stress.
10. Reinforce instruction regarding signs of skin breakdown, pressure, or rubbing to report.	Brace/splint/sling may need to be adjusted. Changes may also be required because of growth or atrophy, when muscles regain or lose strength, or after reconstructive surgery.
11. Teach patient how to care for the brace/splint/sling:	To maintain integrity of the brace/splint/sling.
a. When not in use, store metal braces upright in a safe but easily accessible location.	To prevent deformity or bending of the brace.
b. Store splints of molded materials away from heat.	To prevent melting and deformation of the splint.
c. Treat any leather material with leather preservative.	To prevent drying or cracking.
d. Keep brace clean, dry, and in good working order.	Plastic parts are cleaned with a damp cloth and thoroughly dried. Metal joints are cleaned with a pipe cleaner and oiled weekly. Remove rust with steel wool and clean metal parts with a solvent.
12. Assist patient in ambulating with brace/splint/sling in place.	Determines if patient is able to ambulate safely.
13. Have patient or family caregiver apply and remove the brace/splint/sling.	Promotes patient independence; demonstration confirms level of learning skill.
14. See Completion Protocol (inside front cover).	

EVALUATION

1. Inspect exposed skin and check capillary refill by pressing on toe or finger.
2. Palpate the temperature of tissues distal to the immobilization device.
3. Palpate any accessible pulses distal to the immobilization device.
4. Inspect alignment of the limb.
5. Observe for edema of tissues distal to the immobilization device.

Unexpected Outcomes and Related Interventions (see also Skill 17.3)

1. Patient reports increased severity in pain after application of the device.
   a. Reposition extremity.
   b. Administer analgesics as ordered to maintain patient's comfort level.
   c. Increase frequency of neurovascular checks.

Recording and Reporting

- Record application of and type of device, condition of skin, status of circulation (e.g., temperature, sensation) and motion of distal part, and instructions given to patient and family.
- Report abnormal or untoward findings from neurovascular checks.

Sample Documentation

0900 Splint applied to left wrist. Skin warm, dry, and intact. Able to move all fingers of left hand, fingers warm to touch, nail beds pink, no swelling noted. Complains of pain at 3 (scale of 0 to 10).

Special Considerations

Pediatric

- Monitor children closely to ensure that they do not remove immobilization device.
- Recognize that babies and young children demonstrate pain by restlessness and crying.

Geriatric

- Lightweight immobilization devices are less restrictive.
- Tactile sensory receptors do not transmit sensations as rapidly, leading to reduced sensation in older adults (Ebersole and others, 2008).

Home Care

- Remind to inspect skin daily for pressure or friction areas.
- Remind to inspect cast daily for cracks or changes in alignment.

REVIEW QUESTIONS

Case Study for Questions 1 and 2

Emma Hill is a 6-year-old first grader who fell off a set of swings at school and broke her left radius and ulna.

1. To assist in caring for her short-arm plaster cast, the nurse recommends to Emma's mother that she do which of the following?
   1. Completely cover the cast with plastic wrap to keep it clean.
   2. Cushion any sharp edges of the cast with tape or moleskin.
   3. Scrape rough edges off the cast with a blunt knife.
   4. Blow dry the cast following a shower.
2. Emma's arm has been casted for the past 6 weeks. It is now time to remove her cast. The nurse is assisting with the removal of the cast. Place the following steps in appropriate order for removal of the cast:
   - **a.** Describe the vibration of the cast saw and the feeling of warmth that the saw causes.
   - **b.** Assist with positioning Emma.
   - **c.** Inspect the tissues underlying the cast.
   - **d.** Gently wash intact skin with cold water enzyme.
   1. A, B, C, D
   2. B, A, C, D
   3. A, B, D, C
   4. B, A, D, C
3. Jessica Breland, an 88-year-old widow, fell at home and fractured her right hip. She has been admitted to the emergency department for evaluation and treatment. The physician ordered Buck's extension skin traction to her right leg until an ORIF can be performed. The nurse gathers the traction boot and equipment to set up the traction. When applying the traction boot, the nurse performs the following nursing actions. Select all that apply.
   1. Shave the affected leg.
   2. Ensure that the boot fits snugly.
   3. Pad the heel of the traction boot.
   4. Attach weight to the boot gradually and gently at the end of the bed.
   5. Reassess neurovascular status of the extremity proximal to the traction.
4. In the first 24 hours following application of skeletal traction, how often should the nurse perform neurovascular assessment distal to the traction? (short answer)

   ____
5. A patient develops severe pain and swelling in the tissues beneath his cast. The toes on the casted foot are cold, and capillary refill to the toes is over 6 seconds. Which of the following actions should the nurse complete and in what order should they be completed?
   - **a.** Elevate the casted leg for 15 minutes in anticipation of the symptoms subsiding.
   - **b.** Lower the casted leg for 15 minutes in anticipation of the symptoms subsiding.
   - **c.** Apply warm compresses to sides of cast for 15 minutes in anticipation of the symptoms subsiding.
   - **d.** Prepare to cut a window in the cast to allow visualization of the skin.
   - **e.** If pain is not relieved, notify physician.
   - **f.** Administer acetaminophen (Tylenol No. 3).
   - **g.** Prepare the equipment to bivalve the cast.
   1. A, C, G
   2. B, D, F
   3. C, G, E
   4. F, E, D
   5. A, E, G
6. Joshua David fell out of a tree stand and fractured his back. Following surgery to fuse the vertebrae, he is in a back brace. Which of the following directions should the nurse provide Mr. David for the use and care of the brace?
   1. Place no clothing between the brace and skin.
   2. Inspect the brace for wear, damage, or rough edges daily.
   3. Clean the metal joints with a small steel brush and apply emollient cream to joints weekly.
   4. Clean the plastic parts of the molded brace with ammonia and dry thoroughly weekly.
7. The nursing care plan for the patient who has a Steinmann pin inserted for skeletal traction includes assessing for possible infection. Which of the following signs is most likely to indicate infection?
   1. Crusting
   2. Ashen skin color
   3. Clear drainage from pin sites
   4. Erythema at pin site
8. During rounds the nurse inspects the patient's balanced suspension skeletal traction setup. Which of the following nursing actions are correct?
   1. Add weight to the traction if it does not seem to be exerting enough force.
   2. Adjust position of the weights if the weights are not hanging freely at the end of the bed.
   3. Alter the line of pull of the ropes to ensure that they are at a 45-degree angle.
   4. Alter a slipped Steinmann pin back into place.
9. A patient who sustained multiple fractures in a motor vehicle accident has been admitted to the hospital. He is placed in balanced skeletal traction of the left leg. In developing his plan of care, which precautions should the nurse include?
   1. Avoid using an overhead trapeze.
   2. Remove weights when moving him up in bed.
   3. Maintain alignment of the injured limb with the trunk.
   4. Release the traction for 15 minutes every 8 hours.

10. When a patient complains of severe itching under his cast, which instructions should the nurse give him?
   1. "Scratching can cause skin breaks and infection. I'll get you some medication for the itching."
   2. "Go ahead and scratch if you're able to reach your fingers down the cast."
   3. "Itching is part of the healing process and you should not interfere with it."
   4. "I'll get you a tongue blade to use to scratch. Do not use your fingernails."

REFERENCES

Ebersole P and others: *Geriatric nursing and healthy aging*, ed 3, St Louis, 2008, Mosby.

First national guideline on latex allergy, *Occup Health* 60(6):37, 2008.

Hockenberry MJ, Wilson D: *Wong's nursing care of infants and children*, ed 8, St Louis, 2007, Mosby.

Holmes SB, Brown SJ: Skeletal pin site care: National Association of Orthopaedic Nurses guidelines for orthopaedic nursing, *Orthop Nurs* 24(2):99, 2005.

Judge NL: Neurovascular assessment, *Nurs Stand* 21(45):39, 2007.

Smith GD, Hart RG, Tsai TM: Fiberglass cast application, *J Emerg Med* 23(3):347, 2005.

The Joint Commission (TJC): *2010 National Patient Safety Goals*, Oakbrook Terrace, Ill, 2010, The Commission, http://www.jointcommission.org/PatientSafety/NationalPatientSafetyGoals/, accessed February 14, 2010.

Whiteing NL: Fractures: pathophysiology, treatment, and nursing care, *Nurs Stand* 23(2):49, 2008.

CHAPTER

18

Urinary Elimination

evolve WEBSITE

http://evolve.elsevier.com/Perry/nursinginterventions

Video Clips

Nursing Skills Online

A basic human function is urinary elimination, which may be compromised by a wide variety of illnesses and conditions. It is the role of the nurse to assist the patient as needed in such activities as emptying the bladder when walking to a bathroom and/or sitting on a toilet is not possible; intervening when the bladder does not empty by inserting and maintaining a urinary catheter; implementing measures to minimize risk for infection when urinary drainage tubes are used; and, in the case of renal impairment, performing peritoneal dialysis.

PATIENT-CENTERED CARE

Urinary elimination is a natural and private process. When a patient is no longer able to access a toilet independently or the bladder empties inadequately, nursing intervention is required. Patients with altered urinary elimination require both physiological and psychological support. Physiological support may include invasive procedures such as the insertion of a catheter into the bladder or simply assisting patients using a urinal or bedpan. Of equal importance is supporting patients if they experience embarrassment, fear, and/or apprehension associated with meeting their elimination needs. Urinary elimination is a very intimate and private bodily function; thus it is essential that the nurse acknowledge these feelings and respect patient privacy and dignity as much as possible. A good nurse is competent in performing technical skills and sensitive to patients' psychological needs.

SAFETY

The urinary tract is normally a sterile environment. It is of great importance to minimize the risk for introducing pathogens into the urinary tract. The risk for infection increases whenever the urinary tract is compromised such as during catheterization. In addition, patients with indwelling urinary catheters develop bacteriuria at a rate of 3% to 10% per day for every day with a catheter (Parker and others, 2009a). Thus persons with catheters are at great risk for developing serious and potentially life-threatening infections. Nursing care must include measures to minimize infection such as using aseptic technique when inserting urinary catheters; maintaining a closed urinary drainage system; providing catheter care that uses principles of asepsis; and, above all, removing urinary catheters as soon as medically indicated.

EVIDENCE-BASED PRACTICE TRENDS

Parker D and others: Evidence-based report card: nursing interventions to reduce the risk of catheter-associated urinary tract infection. Part 1. Catheter selection, *J Wound Ostomy Continence Nurs* 36(1):23, 2009.

Willson and others: Evidence-based report card: nursing interventions to reduce the risk of catheter-associated urinary tract infection. Part 2. Staff education, monitoring, and care techniques, *J Wound Ostomy Continence Nurs* 36(2):137, 2009.

In 2009 the Centers for Medicare and Medicaid Services (CMS) enacted policies that addressed expensive and potentially preventable conditions. One of those conditions included the use of indwelling urinary catheters in acute care settings (CMS, 2008). A major focus of these policies was to prevent catheter-associated complications such as catheter-associated urinary tract infection (CAUTI). Evidenced-based nursing interventions are an essential component of preventing these expensive and potentially life-threatening infections. Interventions with some evidence of effectiveness include using antimicrobial catheters for short-term indwelling catheterization, daily cleansing of the urethral meatus with soap and water or perineal cleanser, and maintaining a closed urinary drainage system. Interventions that have not been proven to be effective include regular catheter irrigations, placement of an antiseptic solution in the drainage bag, frequent changes of the drainage bag, and special drainage bags with filters or two chambers. There is some research to support that the prompt removal of catheters and education of nursing staff about good catheter care reduce the incidence of CAUTI. There is a need for ongoing investigation of the optimal insertion techniques and care of patients with both short- and long-term indwelling catheters.

PROCEDURAL GUIDELINE 18.1 Assisting with Use of a Urinal

Video Clips

A urinal is a container used to hold urine when access to a toilet is restricted because of such things as immobility related to musculoskeletal injury or other illnesses that prevent access to a toilet. Although men are typically the ones to use urinals, specially designed urinals are available for women. The female urinal has a larger opening at the top with a defined rim that helps position the urinal close against the genitalia (Fig. 18-1).

Delegation and Collaboration

The skill of assisting a patient with a urinal may be delegated to nursing assistive personnel (NAP). Instruct the NAP by:

- Explaining any special need/adaptations such as how much help the patient needs in positioning the urinal.
- Instructing personnel to provide personal hygiene as necessary after urination.
- Instructing to report immediately any changes in urine color, clarity, and odor; development of incontinence (involuntary loss of urine); patient reports of dysuria, which could indicate an infection; and any changes in the frequency and amount of urine output.
- Explaining the procedure to the patient and family to promote understanding and participation in care.

Equipment

- Clean gloves
- Urinal
- Graduated container (used for measuring volume if on intake and output [I&O])
- Toilet tissue (women)
- Supplies for diagnostic urine tests and specimen collection (see Chapter 8)
- Washbasin
- Washcloths, towels, and soap (as needed for patient hand and perineal hygiene)

Procedural Steps

1. Assess patient's normal urinary elimination habits, including any episodes of incontinence.
2. Determine the ability of patient to place and remove the urinal.
3. Determine if a urine or stool specimen is to be collected.
4. **See Standard Protocol (inside front cover).**
5. Provide privacy by closing curtains around bed and door of room.
6. Assist patient into appropriate position: male patient: on side or back, sitting with head of

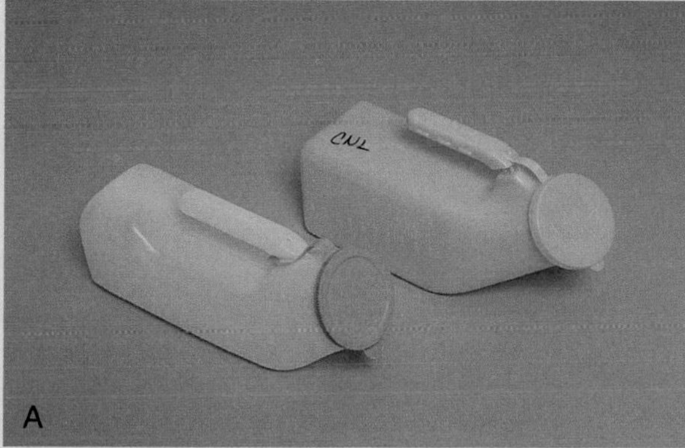

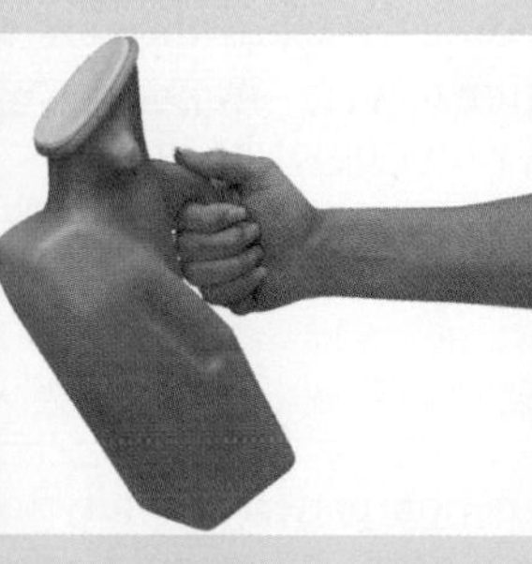

FIG 18-1 Male **(A)** and female **(B)** urinals. (Courtesy of Briggs Medical Service Company.)

Continued

PROCEDURAL GUIDELINE 18.1
Assisting with Use of a Urinal—cont'd

bed elevated, or a standing position. Always determine mobility status and risk for orthostatic hypotension before having a patient stand to void. Position a female patient supine.

7. If possible, patient should hold urinal. If a male patient needs assistance, position penis completely in urinal and hold urinal in place or assist patient in holding urinal. Ensure that the urinal is placed dependent of the flow of urine. Assist a female patient in positioning the urinal against the perinea. The patient may need help keeping the urinal against the perinea and dependent of the flow of urine. Place an absorbent pad under a patient's buttocks to protect bed linens from accidental spills.
8. If possible, give the patient privacy by covering with the bed linens and placing the call device within reach. Leave patient if possible, ensuring that they are in a safe and comfortable position.
9. After patient has finished voiding, remove urinal and assess characteristics of the urine for color, clarity, odor, and amount. Assist patient with washing and drying penis or genitalia.
10. Empty and cleanse urinal. Return urinal to patient for future use.
11. **See Completion Protocol (inside front cover).**

SKILL 18.1 APPLYING A CONDOM-TYPE EXTERNAL CATHETER

- **Nursing Skills Online: Urinary Catheterization Module, Lessons 1 and 3**

The external catheter, also called a *condom catheter* or *penile sheath*, is a soft, pliable condom-like sheath that fits over the penis, providing a safe and noninvasive way to contain urine. Most external catheters are made of soft silicone that aids in reducing friction and are clear to allow for easy visualization of skin under the catheter. Latex catheters are still available and used by some patients. It is important to verify that a patient does not have a latex allergy before applying this type of catheter.

Condom-type external catheters are held in place by an adhesive coating on the internal lining of the sheath, a double-sided self-adhesive strip, brush-on adhesive applied to the penile shaft, or an external strap or tape. They may be attached to a small-volume (leg) drainage bag or a large-volume (bedside) urinary drainage bag, both of which need to be kept lower than the level of the bladder. The condom-type external catheter is suitable for incontinent patients who have complete and spontaneous bladder emptying. Condom-type external catheters come in a variety of styles and sizes. For the best fit and correct application it is important to refer to the manufacturer's guidelines. Condom-type external catheters are associated with less risk for urinary tract infection (UTI) than indwelling catheters; thus they are an excellent option for the male with urinary incontinence (Saint and others, 2006). For men who cannot be fitted for a condom-type external catheter, there are other externally applied catheters.

ASSESSMENT

1. Assess urinary elimination patterns, ability to empty the bladder effectively, and degree of incontinence. *Rationale: Incontinent patients are at risk for skin breakdown and thus are candidates for condom catheters.*
2. Assess mental status of patient and patient's knowledge of the purpose of an external catheter. *Rationale: Reveals need for patient instruction. Teaching can include self-application.*
3. Assess condition of penis. *Rationale: Provides a baseline to compare changes in condition of skin after application of the condom catheter.*
4. Use manufacturer's measuring guide to measure the diameter of the penis in a flaccid state. The penile shaft should be at least 2 cm (0.8 inches) in length. *Rationale: Measurement of the penile shaft aids in determining appropriate catheter size.*
5. Assess for latex allergy. *Rationale: Influences choice of condom material.*

PLANNING

Expected Outcomes focus on promoting dryness and preventing continual exposure of skin to urine.

1. Patient is continent with condom catheter intact.
2. Penile shaft is free of skin irritation, breakdown, or swelling.
3. Patient can explain the purpose of the procedure and what to expect.

Delegation and Collaboration

The skill of applying a condom catheter may be delegated to nursing assistive personnel (NAP), depending on agency policy. Instruct the NAP to:

- Follow manufacturer's guidelines for applying and securing the condom catheter.
- Monitor urine output and record I&O if applicable.
- Immediately report pain, swelling, redness, skin irritation, or breakdown of the glans penis or penile shaft.

Equipment

- Condom catheter kit (condom sheath of appropriate size, securing device (internal adhesive, strap or tape),

skin preparation solution (per manufacturer's recommendations)
- Skin protectant
- Urinary collection bag with drainage tubing or leg bag and straps
- Basin with warm water and soap
- Towels and washcloth(s)
- Bath blanket
- Clean gloves
- Scissors, hair guard, or paper towel

IMPLEMENTATION *for* APPLYING A CONDOM-TYPE EXTERNAL CATHETER

STEPS	RATIONALE
1. **See Standard Protocol (inside front cover).**	
2. Identify patient using two identifiers (e.g., name and birthday or name and account number, according to facility policy).	Ensures correct patient. Complies with The Joint Commission standards and improves patient safety (TJC, 2010).
3. Prepare urinary drainage collection bag and tubing (large-volume drainage bag or leg bag). Clamp off drainage bag port. Secure collection bag to bed frame; bring drainage tubing up between side rails and bed frame. Be sure that you do not pull tubing when side rails are raised.	Provides easy access to drainage equipment after applying catheter. Positioning keeps drainage bag below level of patient's bladder.
4. Assist patient into supine position, thighs slightly apart, with a bath blanket over upper torso and sheets folded over the lower extremities; expose only genitalia for procedure.	Promotes comfort; draping prevents unnecessary exposure of body parts.
5. Provide perineal care (see Procedural Guideline 10.1), Dry thoroughly before applying device. In the uncircumcised male ensure that the foreskin has been replaced before applying the condom catheter. Do not apply barrier cream.	Prevents skin breakdown from exposure to secretions. Removes any residual adhesives. Perineal care minimizes skin irritation and promotes adhesion of the new external catheter. Barrier creams prevent the sheath from adhering to the penile shaft (Pomfret, 2006).
6. If prescribed, apply skin protectant to penis and allow drying.	Skin protectant reduces the risk of skin irritation from catheter adhesives and moisture. The protectant increases the adherence of the condom catheter to the skin.
7. Clip hair at base of penis as necessary before application of the condom catheter. Some manufacturers provide a hair guard that is placed over the penis before applying the device. After application the hair guard is removed. An alternative to a hair guard is to tear a hole in a paper towel, place it over the penis, and remove after application of the device.	Hair adheres to condom and is pulled during condom removal or may get caught in the adhesive as external catheter is applied.

SAFETY ALERT The pubic area should not be shaved because it may increase risk for skin irritation (Pomfret, 2006).

STEPS	RATIONALE
8. Apply condom catheter. With nondominant hand grasp penis along shaft. With dominant hand hold rolled condom sheath at tip of penis with the head of the penis in the cone. Smoothly roll sheath onto penis. Allow 2.5 to 5 cm (1 to 2 inches) of space between tip of glans penis and end of condom catheter (see illustration).	Excessive wrinkles or creases in an external catheter sheath after application may mean that the patient needs a smaller size (Robinson, 2006).

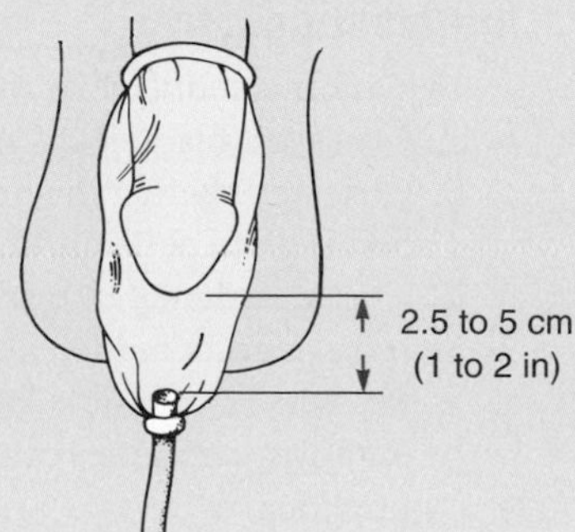

STEP 8 Condom catheter.

Continued

STEPS	RATIONALE
9. Apply appropriate securing device as indicated in the manufacturer's guidelines. **a.** Self-adhesive condom catheters: apply catheter as in Steps 7 and 8; then apply gentle pressure on penile shaft for 10 to 15 seconds to secure catheter. **b.** Spiral wrap penile shaft with supplied strip of elastic adhesive. Strip should be spiral wrapped and not overlap itself (see illustration). The elastic strip should be snug, not tight.	Condom must be secured firmly so it is snug and stays on but not tight enough to cause constriction of blood flow. Application of gentle pressure ensures adherence of adhesive with penile skin.

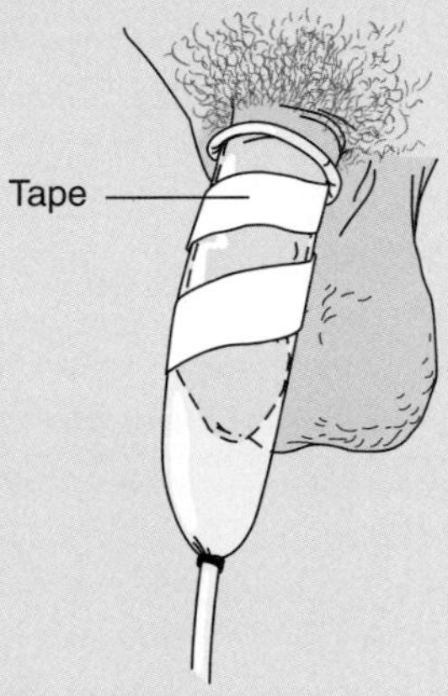

STEP 9b Tape applied in spiral fashion.

SAFETY ALERT Do not apply standard adhesive tape, Velcro, or elastic strips around the penis; this could interfere with circulation and cause necrosis of the penis.

STEPS	RATIONALE
10. Connect drainage tubing to end of condom catheter. Be sure that condom is not twisted. Catheter can be connected to a large-volume bag or leg bag.	Allows urine to be collected and measured. Keeps patient dry. Twisted condom obstructs urine flow, causing urine pooling, skin irritation, and weakening and deterioration of the adhesive and causing the catheter to come off. (Pomfret, 2006).
11. Place excess coiling of tubing on bed and secure to bottom sheet.	Prevents looping of tubing and promotes free drainage of urine.
12. Assist patient to a safe and comfortable position. Lower bed and place side rails accordingly.	Promotes patient comfort and safety.

SAFETY ALERT If applying a condom catheter with outer securing strip, check the strip on the penis 20 minutes after application to ensure that the band is not too tight.

13. See Completion Protocol (inside front cover).

EVALUATION

1. Observe urinary drainage.
2. Inspect penis with condom catheter in place within 30 minutes after application. Assess for swelling and discoloration. Ask patient if there is any discomfort.
3. Inspect skin on penile shaft for signs of breakdown or irritation at least daily when removing condom catheter and providing perineal care and before reapplying condom catheter.
4. Determine patient's understanding of the procedure.

Unexpected Outcomes and Related Interventions

1. Urination is reduced in amount or frequency.
   a. Check for bladder distention.
   b. Observe whether urine is pooling at tip of condom, bathing the penis in urine; reapply as necessary.
   c. Check for kinks in tubing or condom catheter.
2. Skin on penis is reddened, ulcerated, or denuded.
   a. Reassess for possible latex allergy.
   b. Remove condom catheter and notify health care provider.

   c. Do not reapply until penis and surrounding skin are free from irritation.
3. Condom catheter does not stay on.
   a. Ensure that catheter tubing is anchored and that patient understands to not pull or tug on catheter.
   b. Reassess condom catheter size. Refer to manufacturer's guidelines for sizing.
   c. Observe whether condom catheter outlet is kinked and urine is pooling at tip of condom, bathing the penis in urine; reapply as necessary and avoid catheter obstruction.
   d. Assess need for another brand of condom catheter (i.e., self-adhesive versus one with spiral wrap).
4. Penile swelling or discoloration occurs.
   a. Remove condom catheter.
   b. Notify health care provider.
   c. Reassess current condom catheter size and type.

Recording and Reporting

- Record condom application; condition of penis, skin, and scrotum; urinary output and voiding pattern; and patient response to external catheter application.
- Report penile erythema, rashes, and/or skin breakdown.

Sample Documentation

0900 Incontinent of small volumes of urine multiple times. Applied self-adhesive size large condom catheter and attached to leg drainage bag. Skin of penis intact without erythema or edema. Scrotum and groin without erythema, breakdown, or rash. Patient tolerated procedure well.

1300 Condom catheter intact. No erythema or skin breakdown. 400 mL of clear yellow urine in drainage bag.

Special Considerations

Pediatric

- Condom catheters are uncommon in children. When used in adolescents, take precautions to minimize embarrassment.

Geriatric

- Evaluate patients with neuropathy carefully before application of a condom catheter and assess penile skin at more frequent intervals, at least twice daily.
- Condom catheters are not recommended in patients with prostatic obstruction.

Home Care

- Teach patient and family caregivers appropriate assessments such as signs and symptoms of UTI, signs of skin irritation, or poor-fitting catheter sheath.
- Teach patient and caregivers about the option to use a small-volume drainage bag (leg bag) during the day and a large-volume (bedside) drainage bag at night.
- Loose-fitting clothing may be needed to accommodate the catheter and drainage system.
- Ensure that patient and caregiver understand correct steps in applying the condom catheter and how to empty the drainage bag. Manufacturers often supply educational materials for the patient.

PROCEDURAL GUIDELINE 18.2
Bladder Scan

A bladder scanner is a noninvasive device that measures the volume of urine in the bladder by creating an ultrasound image of the bladder from which calculations are made to report accurate urine volumes (DeGennaro and others, 2006, Oh-Oka and Fujisawa, 2007). Use the bladder scanner to assess bladder volume whenever inadequate bladder emptying is suspected such as after the removal of indwelling urinary catheters, in the evaluation of new-onset incontinence, when bladder distention is suspected, and to assess voiding after urologic surgery. The most common use for the bladder scan is to measure postvoid residual (PVR). PVR is the volume of urine in the bladder after a normal voiding. To be most accurate, PVR must be measured within 10 minutes of voiding (Newman and Wein, 2009), with a volume less than 50 mL considered normal. Two or more PVR measurements greater than 100 mL require further investigation (Neumann and Wein, 2009). If a bladder scanner is not available, obtain a PVR by measuring urine emptied from the bladder after straight catheterization (see Skill 18.2).

Delegation and Collaboration

In some settings the use of the bladder scanner may be delegated to nursing assistive personnel (NAP) (see agency policy). The nurse, in collaboration with the health care provider, determines the timing and frequency of bladder scan measurement and interprets the measurements obtained. Instruct the NAP to:

- Follow the manufacturer's recommendations for the use of the device.
- Measure PVR volumes within 10 minutes after assisting patient to void.
- Report and record bladder scan volumes.

Equipment

- Bladder scanner
- Ultrasound gel
- Alcohol pads
- Paper towels

Continued

PROCEDURAL GUIDELINE 18.2
Bladder Scan—cont'd

Procedural Steps

1. **See Standard Protocol (inside front cover).**
2. Assess the I&O record to determine urine output trends and check the plan of care to verify correct timing of the bladder scan measurement.
3. Identify patient using two identifiers (i.e., name and birthday or name and account number, according to facility policy).
4. If the measurement is for PVR, ask patient to void and measure voided urine volume.
5. Assist patient to the supine position with the head slightly elevated. Raise bed to appropriate working height. If side rails are raised, lower side rail on working side.
6. Expose patient's lower abdomen.
7. Turn on the scanner per manufacturer's guidelines.
8. Set the gender designation per manufacturer's guidelines. Women who have had a hysterectomy should be designated as male on the scanner.
9. Wipe the scanner head with an alcohol pad and allow to air dry.
10. Palpate the patient's symphysis pubis (pubic bone). Apply a generous amount of ultrasound gel (or, if available, a bladder scan gel pad) to the midline abdomen 2.5 to 4 cm (1 to 1.5 inches) above the symphysis pubis. The ultrasound gel ensures adequate transmission and thus accurate measurement.
11. Place the scanner head on the gel, ensuring that the scanner head is oriented per the manufacturer's guidelines.
12. Apply light pressure, keep the scanner head steady, and point the scanner head slightly downward toward the bladder. Press and release the scan button.
13. Verify accurate aim (refer to manufacturer's guidelines). Complete the scan and print the image (if needed) (see illustration).

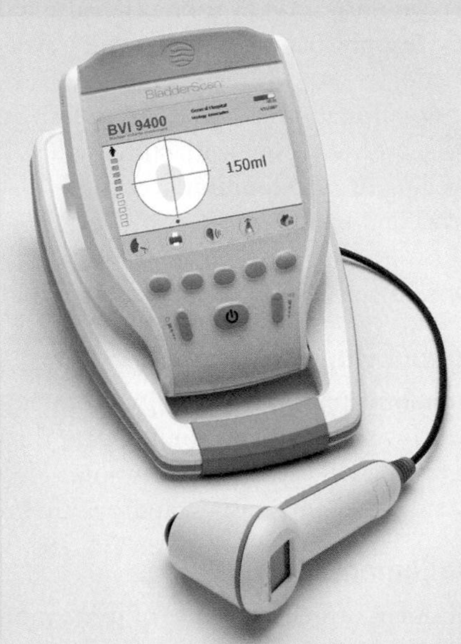

STEP 13 Bladder scan image. (Courtesy Verathon Inc.)

14. Remove ultrasound gel from patient's abdomen with a paper towel.
15. Remove ultrasound gel from scanner head and wipe with alcohol pad; let air dry.
16. **See Completion Protocol (inside front cover).**

SKILL 18.2 INSERTION OF A STRAIGHT OR INDWELLING CATHETER

- **Nursing Skills Online: Urinary Catheterization, Lessons 1 and 2**

Urinary catheterization is the placement of a tube into the bladder to remove urine. This is an invasive procedure that requires a medical order and in institutional settings aseptic technique (Lo and others, 2008; Nazarko, 2008). Urinary catheterization may be short term (2 weeks or less) or long term (more than 1 month) (Parker and others, 2009a). Conditions that require use of urinary catheters include the need to monitor urine output, relief of urinary obstruction, postoperative care, or a bladder that inadequately empties as a result of a neurological condition. Excessive accumulation of urine in the bladder increases the risk for UTI and can cause backward flow of urine up the ureters to the kidneys, causing kidney damage. Urinary incontinence, an involuntary leakage of urine, may require indwelling catheterization if the leaking urine interferes with wound healing. Intermittent catheterization is used to measure PVR when a bladder scanner is not available (see Procedural Guideline 18.2).

The steps for inserting an indwelling and a single-use straight catheter are the same. The difference lies in the inflation of a balloon to keep the indwelling catheter in place and the presence of a closed drainage system. Urinary catheters are made with one to three lumens (Fig. 18-2). Single-lumen catheters (see Fig. 18-2, *A)* are used for intermittent catheterization (i.e., the insertion of a catheter for one-time bladder emptying). Double-lumen catheters, designed for indwelling catheters, provide one lumen for urinary drainage while a second lumen is used to inflate a balloon that keeps the catheter in place (see Figure 18-2, *B*). Triple-lumen catheters (see Fig. 18-2, *C)* are used for continuous bladder irrigation (CBI) or to instill medications into the bladder. One lumen drains the bladder, a second lumen is used to inflate the balloon, and

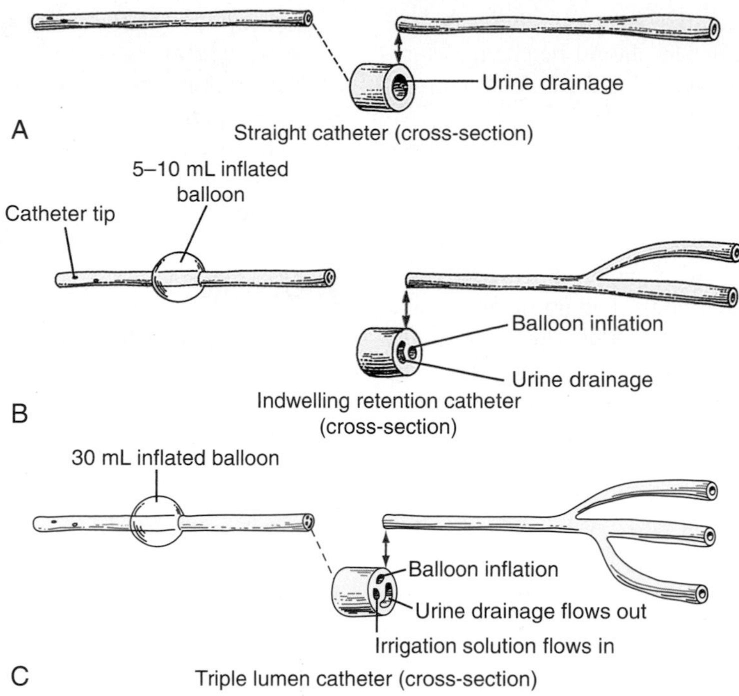

FIG 18-2 A, Straight catheter (cross-section). **B,** Indwelling retention catheter (cross-section). **C,** Triple-lumen catheter (cross-section).

a third lumen delivers fluid from an irrigation bag into the bladder.

A health care provider chooses a catheter on the basis of factors such as latex allergy, history of catheter incrustation, and susceptibility for infection. Indwelling catheters are made of latex or silicone. Some have special coatings that reduce urethral irritation and incrustation (Gray, 2006). Antimicrobial catheters are coated with silver or an antibiotic. These coated catheters have been shown to reduce the incidence of CAUTI for short-term use, but to date there are insufficient data to support their use in long-term catheter users (Johnson and others, 2006; Drekonja and others, 2008; Schumm and Lam, 2008; Parker and others, 2009b). Straight or intermittent catheters are made of rubber (softer and more flexible) or polyvinyl chloride. Patients that self-catheterize have a large selection of catheters: some with special coatings that do not require lubrication and others that are self-contained systems consisting of a lubricated catheter and packaged with a connected drainage bag.

The size of a urinary catheter is based on the French (Fr) scale, which reflects the internal diameter of the catheter. Most adults with an indwelling catheter should have a size 14 to 16 Fr to minimize trauma and risk for infection. Larger-catheter diameters increase the risk for urethral trauma (Parker and others, 2009b). However, larger sizes are often needed in special circumstances such as after urological surgery. Smaller sizes such as a 5 to 6 Fr for infants and an 8 to 10 Fr for children are needed.

Indwelling catheters come in a variety of balloon sizes from 3 mL (for a child) to 30 mL for CBI. The size of the catheter and balloon is usually printed on the catheter port (Fig. 18-3). The recommended balloon size for an adult is a 5-mL balloon. Long-term use of larger balloons has been associated with irritation and trauma to the bladder wall (Newman, 2009). In addition, a larger balloon (30 mL) increases the volume of urine that pools below the level of the catheter lumen and increases the risk of infection (Gray, 2006).

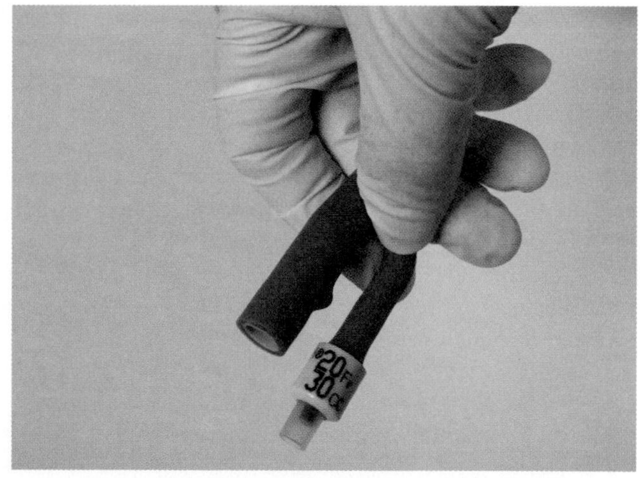

FIG 18-3 Size of catheter and balloon printed on catheter.

For patients requiring long-term catheterization (i.e., urinary retention or critical illness), catheter changes should be individualized, not routine (Green and others, 2008; Willson and others, 2009). Catheters should be changed for leaking or blockage and before obtaining a sterile specimen for urine culture (Smith and others, 2008). Avoid long-term catheterization because of its association with UTI (Green and others, 2008) and remove catheters as soon as a patient can void.

An indwelling catheter is attached to a urinary drainage bag to collect the continuous flow of urine. Always hang the bag below the level of the bladder on the bed frame or a chair so urine will drain down, out of the bladder. The bag should never touch the floor. When a patient ambulates, carry the bag below the level of the bladder. The only exception to this rule is when a catheter is attached to a specially designed drainage bag (belly bag) that is worn across the abdomen. A one-way valve on this bag prevents the back flow of urine into the bladder.

ASSESSMENT

1. Review patient's medical record, including health care provider's order and nurses' notes. Note previous catheterization, including catheter size, response of patient, and time of last catheterization. *Rationale: Identifies purpose of inserting catheter such as for measurement of residual urine or specimen collection, previous catheter size, and potential difficulty with catheter insertion.*
2. Assess patient's knowledge and prior experience with catheterization. *Rationale: Reveals need for patient instruction and/or support.*
3. Review the medical record for any pathological condition that may impair passage of catheter (e.g., enlarged prostate gland in men, urethral strictures). *Rationale: Obstruction of the urethra may prevent passage of the catheter into the bladder.*
4. Ask patient and check chart for allergies. *Rationale: Identifies allergy to antiseptic, tape, latex, and lubricant. Povidone-iodine allergies are common; if patient is unaware of allergy, ask instead if allergic to shellfish.*
5. Assess patient's weight, level of consciousness, developmental level, ability to cooperate, and mobility. *Rationale: Determines positioning for catheterization and indicates how much assistance is needed to properly position patient, ability of patient to cooperate during the procedure, and level of explanation needed.*
6. Assess patient's gender and age. *Rationale: Determines catheter size.*
7. Ask patient the time of last voiding and/or check I&O flow sheet. *Rationale: Determines time of last void and indicates if urinary retention is likely.*
8. Assess the bladder for fullness by palpating it over symphysis pubis or by using the bladder scanner (see Procedural Guideline 18.2). *Rationale: A full bladder with an inability to void or voiding small amounts frequently indicates a need to insert a catheter. Palpation of a full or overfull bladder causes pain and/or urge to void.*
9. Inspect perineal region, observing for perineal landmarks, erythema, drainage, or discharge and odor. *Rationale: Determines the visibility of the urethra and need for cleansing the perineum.*

PLANNING

Expected Outcomes focus on emptying the bladder and promoting patient comfort.

1. Patient's bladder is not palpable.
2. Patient verbalizes absence of a sensation of discomfort or bladder fullness.
3. Patient has a urine output of at least 30 mL/hr of clear, light yellow urine in urinary drainage bag.

Delegation and Collaboration

The insertion of an indwelling or straight urinary catheter may be delegated in some settings (see agency policy). Otherwise instruct nursing assistive personnel (NAP) to:

- Assist the nurse with positioning patient and directing the light source.
- Report any changes in the color, amount, and odor of the urine and if the indwelling catheter leaks or causes pain.

Equipment

- Catheter kit containing the following sterile items. (Note: Catheter kits vary.)
  - Straight catheterization kit: single-lumen catheter, drapes (one fenestrated), gloves, lubricant, cleansing solution incorporated in an applicator or to be added to cotton balls, and specimen container
  - Indwelling catheterization kit: drapes (one fenestrated), gloves, lubricant, antiseptic cleansing solution incorporated in an applicator or to be added to cotton balls, specimen container, and a prefilled syringe with sterile water (to inflate balloon). Some kits contain a catheter with attached drainage bag; others contain only a catheter; others have no catheter.)
  - Sterile drainage tubing and bag (if not included in indwelling catheter insertion kit)
  - Device to secure catheter (catheter strap or other device)
  - Extra sterile gloves and catheter (optional)
  - Clean gloves
  - Basin with warm water, washcloth, towel, and soap for perineal care
  - Flashlight or other additional light source
  - Bath blanket, waterproof absorbent pad
  - Measuring container for urine

IMPLEMENTATION *for* INSERTION OF A STRAIGHT OR INDWELLING CATHETER

STEPS	RATIONALE
1. See Standard Protocol (inside front cover).	
2. Check patient's plan of care for size and type of catheter.	Ensures that patient receives the correct size and type of catheter.
3. Identify patient using two identifiers (e.g., name and birthday or name and account number, according to facility policy).	Ensures correct patient. Complies with The Joint Commission standards and improves patient safety (TJC, 2010).
4. Position patient. Arrange for extra nursing personnel to assist with positioning as needed.	Some patients may not be able to assume the needed positioning for the procedure independently.
a. *Position female* patient dorsal recumbent (on back with knees flexed) and ask patient to relax thighs. Drape with bath blanket so only the perineum is exposed (see illustration).	Exposes perineum, allows hip joints to be rotated externally, and minimizes the risk for contamination by fecal material (Cochran, 2007).
b. *Alternate female position*: position side-lying (Sims') with upper leg flexed at knee and hip. Ensure that rectal area is covered with drape to reduce risk of contamination. Support patient with pillows if necessary to maintain position.	Alternate position is more comfortable if patient cannot abduct leg at the hip joint (e.g., if patient has arthritic joints or contractures).
c. *Position male* patient supine with legs extended and thighs slightly abducted. Cover upper body with small sheet or towel. Cover legs with separate sheet so only genitals are exposed (see illustration).	Aids in visualization of penis.
5. Cleanse patient's perineal area with soap and water, rinse, and dry (see Procedural Guideline 10.1). Identify the urinary meatus. Place waterproof pad under patient. Remove and discard gloves. Perform hand hygiene.	Perineal hygiene minimizes risk for fecal contamination (Lever, 2007).
6. Position light to illuminate perineum or have assistant available to hold light source to visualize urinary meatus.	Helps to illuminate the perineum.
7. Remove gloves and perform hand hygiene.	

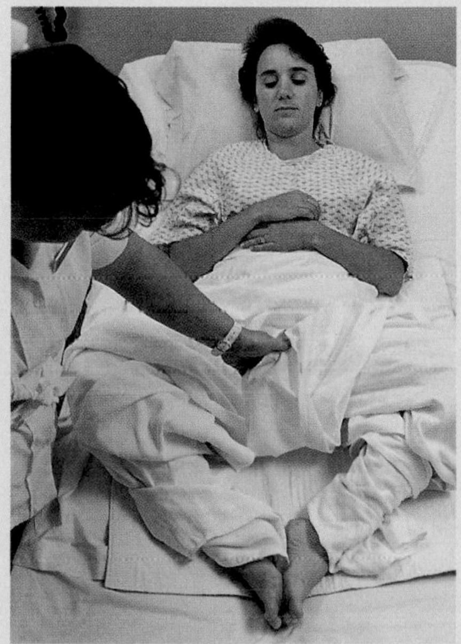

STEP 4a Draping female patient with blankets.

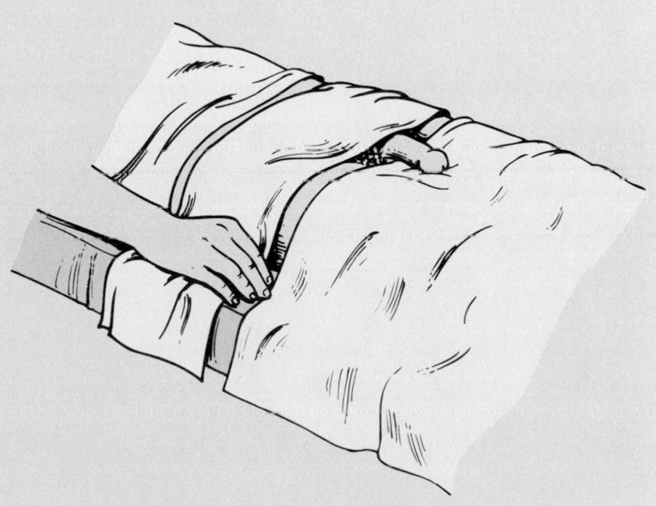

STEP 4c Draping male patient with blankets.

Continued

STEPS	RATIONALE
8. Open outer wrapping of catheterization kit. Place inner wrapped catheter kit tray on clean surface such as a bedside table or if possible between patients' open legs. Patient size and positioning dictate exact placement.	Provides easy access to supplies during catheter insertion.
9. Open inner sterile wrap using sterile technique (see Chapter 5).	The sterile wrap serves as a sterile field.
a. Indwelling catheterization open system: Open the separate package that contains the drainage system bag, check to make sure that clamp on drainage port is closed, and place drainage bag over edge of bottom bed frame and drainage tube up between mattress and side rail. Open outer package of catheter, maintaining sterility of inner wrapper.	Keeps the system sterile.
b. Indwelling catheterization closed system: Open the package containing the drainage bag with preattached catheter and check to make sure that the clamp on the drainage port is closed. Place bag near end of bed. Keep sterile catheter on sterile field. Some kits may have a drainage bag with a preattached catheter as part of the catheterization tray (see Step 12).	Closed systems have a catheter preattached to drainage tubing and bag, which helps maintain a sterile system.
c. Straight catheterization: All needed supplies are in the sterile tray. The tray that contains supplies can be used for urine collection.	
10. Put on sterile gloves.	
11. Drape perineum, keeping gloves sterile.	The sterile drapes provide a sterile field over which the nurse works during catheterization.
a. ***Drape female:***	Outer surface of drape covering hands remains sterile. Sterile drape against sterile gloves maintains sterility of gloves and workspace.
(1) Pick up square drape and unfold without touching unsterile surfaces. Allow top edge of drape to form cuff over both hands. Place drape with the shiny side down on bed between patient's thighs. Slip cuffed edge just under buttocks as you ask patient to lift the hips. Take care not to touch contaminated surfaces with sterile gloves.	
(2) Pick up fenestrated sterile drape. Allow drape to unfold without touching unsterile surfaces. Allow top edge of drape to form cuff over both hands. Drape over perineum, exposing the labia (see illustration).	

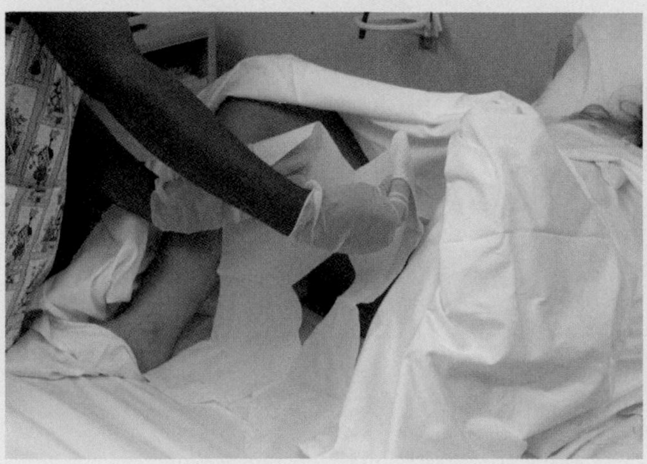

STEP 11a(2) Place sterile fenestrated drape (with opening in center) over perineum with labia exposed.

STEPS	RATIONALE
b. ***Drape male:*** Pick up square drape and allow unfolding without touching unsterile surfaces; place over thighs with shiny side down, just below penis. Allow top edge of drape to form cuff over both hands and place fenestrated drape with opening centered over penis (see illustration).	
c. In some kits the sterile gloves may be below the square sterile drape. In this case the square drape is picked up from the tray by the edges and allowed to unfold without touching unsterile surfaces. The top edge is then folded away from the patient to form a cuff over both hands and carefully placed (see Steps 11 a(1) and b). Next, put on sterile gloves and place fenestrated drape (see Steps 11a(1) and b).	The sequence of supplies in a kit varies. Use supplies in order of use to prevent contamination of underlying supplies.
12. Arrange supplies on sterile field, maintaining sterility of gloves. Place sterile tray with cleaning solution (premoistened swab sticks or cotton balls, forceps, and solution) lubricant, catheter, and prefilled balloon inflation syringe (indwelling catheterization only) on the sterile drape close to the perineum.	Provides easy access to supplies during catheter insertion and helps to maintain aseptic technique. Appropriate placement is determined by size of patient and position during catheterization.
a. Open package of sterile antiseptic solution. Pour solution over sterile cotton balls. Some kits may contain a package of premoistened swab sticks. Open the end of the package for easy access.	
b. Open sterile specimen container if specimen is to be obtained (see Skill 8.1).	
c. For indwelling catheterization, open inner sterile wrapper of catheter. If part of the kit, remove tray with catheter and attached drainage bag and place on sterile drape. Make sure that clamp on drainage port of the bag is closed.	

SAFETY ALERT The practice of testing the inflation balloon of an indwelling catheter is no longer common. Early inflation/deflation of the balloon can lead to the formation of ridges in the balloon, potentially causing trauma on insertion. It is essential to check the manufacturer's instructions before inserting an indwelling catheter.

STEPS	RATIONALE
13. Open packet of lubricant and squeeze out on catheter tray or sterile field. Lubricate catheter by dipping catheter into water-soluble gel 2.5 cm to 5 cm (1 to 2 inches) for women and 12.5 to 17.5 cm (5 to 7 inches) for men (see illustration).	Lubrication minimizes trauma to the urethra and discomfort during catheter insertion. Female urethra is shorter.

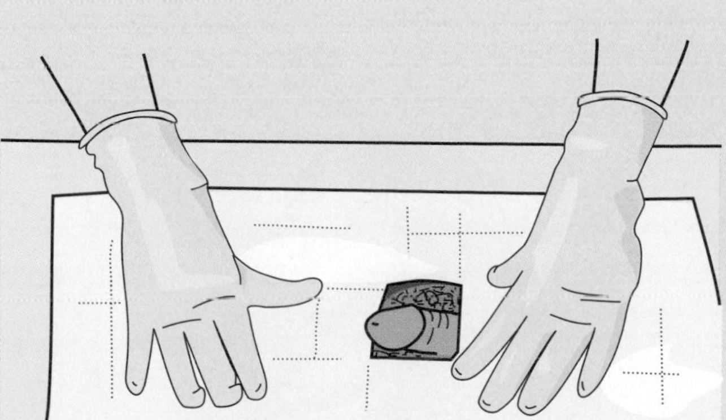

STEP 11b Draping male.

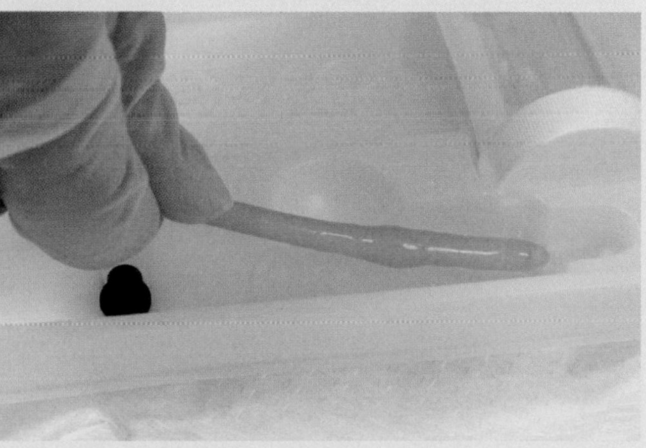

STEP 13 Lubricating catheter.

Continued

STEPS	RATIONALE
14. Cleanse urethral meatus.	
a. *Cleansing female*:	
(1) Separate labia with fingers of nondominant hand (now contaminated) to fully expose urinary meatus. (2) Maintain position of nondominant hand continuously until catheter has been inserted. (3) Use the forceps to hold one cotton ball or one swab stick at a time. Clean labia and urinary meatus from clitoris toward anus. Use a new cotton ball/swab stick for each area cleansed. Cleanse by wiping the far labial fold, the near labial fold, and directly over center of urethral meatus (see illustration).	Reduces risk of introducing microorganisms into sterile bladder. Front to back cleansing is cleaning from area of least contamination toward highly contaminated area. Dominant hand remains sterile. Closure of the labia during cleansing means that the area is now contaminated and requires the cleaning procedure to be repeated.
b. *Cleansing male*:	
(1) With nondominant hand (now contaminated) retract foreskin (if uncircumcised) and gently grasp penis at shaft just below glans. Hold shaft of penis at right angle to body. This hand remains in this position for remainder of procedure. (2) Using uncontaminated dominant hand, cleanse meatus with cotton balls/swab sticks using circular strokes, beginning at the meatus and working outward in a spiral motion. (3) Repeat three times using clean cotton ball/swab stick each time (see illustration).	When grasping shaft of penis, avoid pressure on dorsal surface to prevent compression of urethra.
15. Hold catheter 7.5 cm to 10 cm (3 to 4 inches) from tip. Hold end of catheter loosely coiled in palm of dominant hand. If catheter is not attached to a drainage bag, make sure to position urine tray so end of catheter can be placed there once insertion begins.	Holding catheter near tip allows for easier manipulation during insertion. Coiling the catheter in the palm prevents distal end from striking a nonsterile surface.

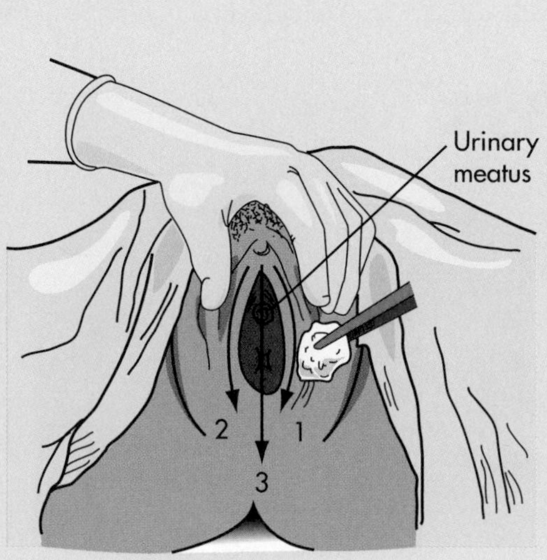

STEP 14a(3) Cleansing female perineum.

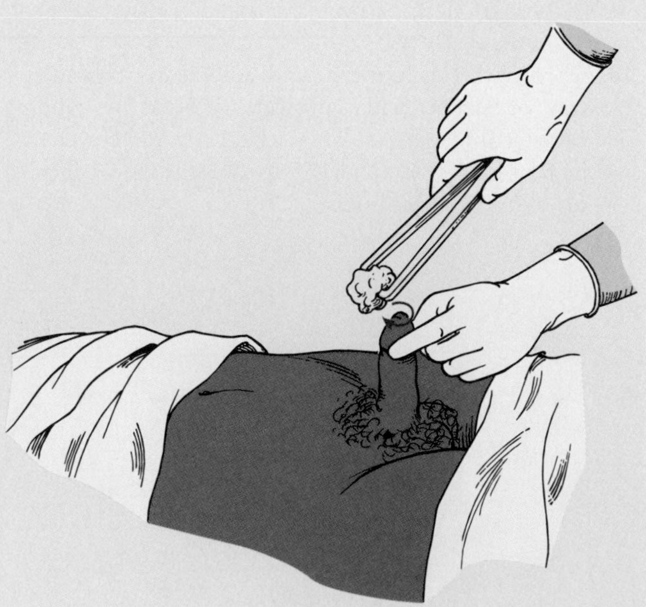

STEP 14b(3) Cleansing male urinary meatus.

STEPS	RATIONALE
16. Insert catheter.	
a. *Female patient:*	
(1) Ask patient to bear down gently and insert catheter through meatus (see illustration).	Bearing down may help visualize urinary meatus and promotes relaxation of external urinary sphincter, aiding in catheter insertion.
(2) Advance catheter slowly a total of 5 to 7.5 cm (2 to 3 inches) or until urine flows out end of catheter.	
b. *Male patient:*	
(1) Gently apply upward traction to penis as it is held in a 90-degree angle from body.	It is normal to meet resistance at the prostate. When resistance is met, hold catheter firmly against sphincter without forcing. After a few seconds sphincter may relax, and catheter can be advanced (Senese and others, 2006b).
(2) Ask patient to bear down as if to void and then slowly insert catheter through the meatus (see illustration).	
(3) Advance catheter 17 to 22.5 cm (7 to 9 inches) or until urine flows out end of catheter.	

SAFETY ALERT Do not force catheter insertion. If you encounter resistance or pain during the insertion of a catheter, stop the progression of the catheter immediately. Ask the patient to take slow deep breaths to promote relaxation while the catheter is slowly advanced in the urethra (Senese and others, 2006b).

STEPS	RATIONALE
17. Allow bladder to empty fully unless institution policy restricts maximum volume of urine drained (see agency policy).	Retained urine may serve as reservoir for growth of microorganisms.
18. Collect urine specimen as needed.	
a. Fill specimen container to desired level (20 to 30 mL) by holding end of catheter in dominant hand over cup.	
b. Label specimen according to agency policy and send to laboratory immediately.	Fresh urine specimen ensures more accurate findings.
19. Straight catheterization: When urine stops flowing, withdraw catheter slowly and smoothly until removed.	
20. Measure urine and record.	Monitor output as a baseline assessment.

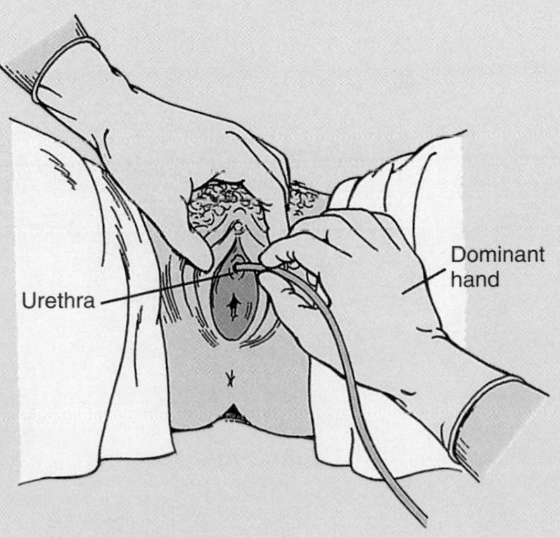

STEP 16a(1) Inserting catheter into female urinary meatus.

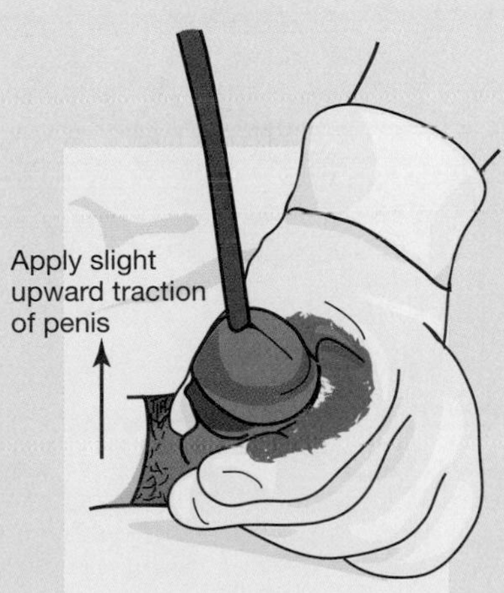

STEP 16b(2) Inserting catheter into male urinary meatus.

Continued

STEPS	RATIONALE
21. Indwelling catheterization	
a. *Female patient*	
(1) As soon as urine appears, advance catheter another 2.5 to 5 cm (1 to 2 inches). Do not force catheter if resistance is met.	Indicates that catheter tip is in bladder or lower urethra. Advancement ensures correct catheter placement (Senese and others, 2006a).
(2) Release labia but maintain secure hold of catheter with nondominant hand.	
b. *Male patient*	
(1) After catheter is inserted through the meatus and urine appears, advance catheter to bifurcation of drainage and balloon inflation port (see illustration).	Further advancement of catheter to bifurcation of drainage and balloon inflation port ensures proper placement (Senese and others, 2006b).
(2) Lower penis and hold catheter securely in nondominant hand.	
22. Inflate catheter balloon with amount of fluid designated by manufacturer.	Indwelling catheter balloons should not be underinflated because underinflation causes balloon distortion and potential bladder damage (Newman, 2009).
a. Continue to hold catheter with nondominant hand.	By moving catheter slightly back into bladder, pressure on bladder neck is avoided.
b. With free dominant hand, attach prefilled syringe in injection port at end of catheter.	
c. Slowly inject total amount of fluid (see illustration).	
d. After inflating catheter balloon, release catheter from nondominant hand. Gently pull catheter until resistance is felt. Then advance it slightly. If not previously connected, attach catheter to drainage bag.	

SAFETY ALERT If a patient complains of sudden pain during inflation of a catheter balloon, stop injection, withdraw fluid from balloon, advance catheter further, and reinflate balloon. The balloon may be inflating in the urethra.

23. Secure indwelling catheter with catheter strap or other securing device. Leave enough slack to allow leg movement. Attach the securing device just below the catheter bifurcation.	Securing the catheter reduces the risk of urethral erosion or accidental catheter removal. Attaching the securing device at the catheter bifurcation prevents occlusion of the catheter (Gray, 2008).

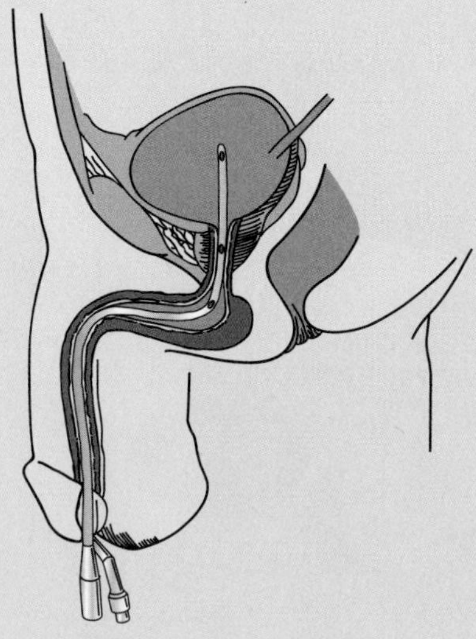

STEP 21b(1) Correct catheter insertion to the bifurcation of the drainage and balloon inflation port in male patient.

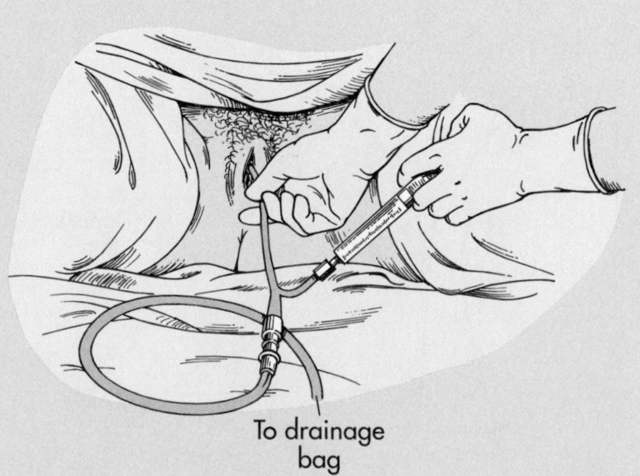

STEP 22c Inflating the balloon (indwelling catheter).

STEPS	RATIONALE
a. *Female:* Secure catheter to inner thigh, allowing enough slack to prevent tension (see illustration).	

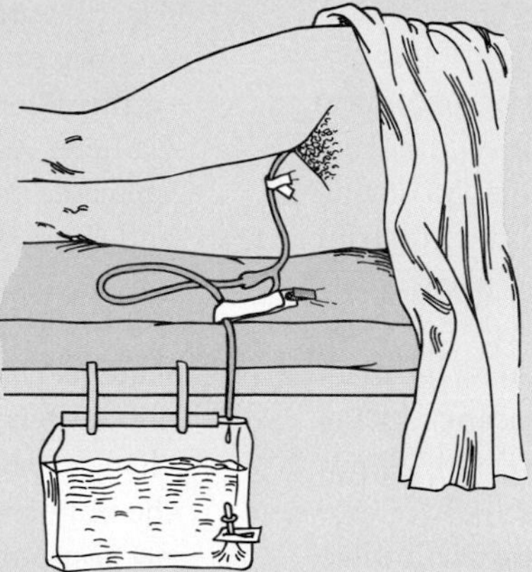

STEP 23a Securing the female indwelling catheter.

STEPS	RATIONALE
b. *Male:* Secure to upper thigh or lower abdomen. If retracted, replace foreskin over the glans penis.	
24. Clip drainage tubing to edge of mattress. Position drainage bag lower than bladder by attaching to bed frame. Do not attach to side rails of bed.	Keeping the drainage bag below the level of the bladder reduces the risk for CAUTI (Lo and others 2008, Parker and others, 2009b). Placing on side rails could result in bag being raised above bladder.
25. Check to make sure that there is no obstruction to urine flow. Coil excess tubing on bed and fasten to bottom sheet with clip or other securing device.	
26. See Completion Protocol (inside front cover).	

EVALUATION

1. Palpate bladder and observe amount, color, and clarity of urine.
2. Evaluate patient's level of comfort.
3. Observe character and amount of urine in drainage tubing and bag or collection container.

Unexpected Outcomes and Related Interventions

1. Patient complains of discomfort during inflation of balloon.
   a. Stop inflation immediately; allow inflation fluid to return to syringe.
   b. Advance another 2.5 cm (1 inch) and retry inflation.
   c. If patient still complains of pain, remove catheter and report to health care provider.
2. Catheter goes into vagina.
   a. Leave catheter in vagina.
   b. Recleanse urinary meatus. Using another catheter kit or another sterile catheter, insert catheter into meatus.
   c. Remove catheter in vagina after successful insertion of second catheter in bladder.
3. Sterility is broken during catheterization by nurse or patient.
   a. Replace gloves if contaminated and start over.
   b. If patient touches sterile field but equipment remains sterile, avoid touching that part of sterile field.
   c. If equipment is contaminated, replace it with sterile items or start over again with new kit.
4. Patient complains of bladder discomfort, and the catheter is patent as evidenced by adequate urine flow.
   a. Notify health care provider.

Recording and Reporting

- Record and report the reason for catheterization, type and size of catheter inserted, amount of fluid used to inflate balloon, specimen collection (if applicable), characteristics and amount of urine, patient's response to procedure, and any education.
- Record on I&O flow sheet record.

Sample Documentation

0800 Patient C/O lower abdominal fullness and inability to void; lower abdomen tender and distended. 16-Fr/5-mL balloon catheter inserted without difficulty; 700 mL of clear yellow urine returned. Balloon inflated with 10 mL sterile solution. Specimen sent for urinalysis and culture. After catheterization patient denies discomfort or pain.

Special Considerations

Pediatric

- When caring for an infant or young child, explain procedures to parents. Describe procedure to child at level the child is able to understand (Hockenberry and Wilson, 2007).
- Children and adolescents experience some discomfort during catheterization. Assistance and gentle holding may be necessary, especially with younger children. Most children prefer to have the parents remain with them during the procedure. Ask adolescents if they would like a parent to remain with them.
- Catheterization in infants and children may be made easier by use of an adequate amount of lubricant containing 2% lidocaine (Xylocaine) (Hockenberry and Wilson, 2007).
- Teaching young children to blow into a straw or pinwheel can aid in relaxing pelvic muscles (Hockenberry and Wilson, 2007).
- In uncircumcised infant boys it is not possible to fully retract the foreskin.

Geriatric

- The urethral meatus of an older woman may be difficult to identify because of urogenital atrophy.
- Symptoms of a UTI in the older adult may be difficult to recognize and may only be indicated by a change in mental status or fever (Smith and others, 2008).
- Older adults have an increased risk for UTI related to increased prevalence of chronic disease such as diabetes and prostatic hypertrophy and a higher prevalence of incontinence (Robichard and Blondeau, 2008).
- The presence of a urinary catheter and its drainage tubing and bag can interfere with already compromised mobility of the older adult.
- Catheter use in older adults has been associated with increased mortality (Holroyd and others, 2007; Srulevich and Chopra, 2008).

Home Care

- Patients who are at home may use a leg bag during the day and switch to a larger-volume bag at night. If a patient changes from a large-volume bag to a leg bag, instruct in the importance of handwashing and cleansing of the connection ports with alcohol before changing bags (Senese and others, 2006a and b).
- Teach patients and family caregivers how to properly position the drainage bag; empty the urinary drainage bag; and observe urine color, clarity, odor, and amount.
- Educate patients and/or caregivers about the signs of UTI and troubleshooting techniques for a leaking catheter.
- Arrange for home delivery of catheter supplies, always ensuring that there is at least one extra catheter, insertion kit, and drainage bag in the home.

SKILL 18.3 REMOVAL OF AN INDWELLING CATHETER

- **Nursing Skills Online: Urinary Catheterization, Lesson 5**

Removal of indwelling catheters is an important intervention to reduce risk of CAUTI (Green and others, 2008; Parker and others, 2009b). When removing the catheter, it is important to ensure that the catheter balloon is fully deflated to minimize trauma to the urethra. There is some evidence to support removal of short-term catheters at midnight (Griffiths, 2007). The practice of clamping a catheter before removal is not clearly supported by evidence that it will improve bladder function after removal (Johanna Briggs Institute, 2006).

All patients should have their voiding monitored after catheter removal for at least 24 to 48 hours by using a voiding record or bladder diary. The bladder diary should record the time and amount of each voiding, including any incontinence. You can use a bladder scanner to monitor bladder functioning by measuring PVR (see Procedural Guideline 18.2). Abdominal pain and distention, a sensation of incomplete emptying, incontinence, constant dribbling of urine, and voiding in very small amounts can indicate inadequate bladder emptying that requires intervention.

The risk of CAUTI increases with the use of an indwelling catheter (Parker and others, 2009a). Symptoms of infection can develop 2 to 3 or more days after catheter removal. Patients need to be informed of the risk for infection, prevention measures, and signs and symptoms that need to be reported to the primary care provider.

ASSESSMENT

1. Review patient's medical record, including health care provider's order and nurses' notes. Note length of time catheter has been in place. *Rationale: Catheters in place for more than a few days are more likely to cause urethral irritation and buildup of incrustation.*
2. Assess patient's knowledge and prior experience with catheter removal. *Rationale: Reveals need for patient instruction and/or support.*
3. Assess urine color, clarity, odor, and amount. Note any urethral discharge or the presence of incrustation. *Rationale: May be an indicator of inflammation or UTI and a source of pain during catheter removal.*
4. Determine size of catheter inflation balloon. *Rationale: Determines size of syringe required to deflate balloon.*

PLANNING

Expected Outcomes focus on patient comfort, adequate bladder emptying, and patient's learning about early detection of UTI.

1. Patient voids at least 150 mL with each voiding no more than 6 to 8 hours after catheter removal.
2. Patient verbalizes feeling of comfort after catheter is removed.
3. Patient identifies signs and symptoms of UTI.

Delegation and Collaboration

Assessment of the patient's condition should not be delegated to nursing assistive personnel (NAP); however, the skill of removing a urinary catheter may be delegated. Instruct the NAP to:

- Report characteristics of urine (color, odor, and amount) before and after catheter removal.
- Report how the patient tolerated the procedure, the exact time the catheter was removed, and the time and amount of subsequent voiding.
- Record urine volume on the I&O record.

Equipment

- Clean gloves, basin with warm water, washcloth, towel, and soap for perineal care
- 10-mL syringe or larger without a needle or (size depends on volume of solution used to inflate the balloon)
- Waterproof pad
- Toilet, bedside commode, urine "hat," urinal, or bedpan

IMPLEMENTATION *for* REMOVAL OF AN INDWELLING CATHETER

STEPS	RATIONALE
1. **See Standard Protocol (inside front cover).**	
2. Check the size and type of catheter on the patient's plan of care.	Ensures that the correct syringe size for balloon deflation is available.
3. Identify patient using two identifiers (i.e., name and birthday or name and account number, according to facility policy).	Ensures correct patient. Complies with The Joint Commission standards and improves patient safety (TJC, 2010).
4. Position patient supine and place waterproof pad under buttocks. Pad can lie on male's thighs. Cover with bath blanket, exposing only perineal area. If soiled, perform perineal hygiene (see Procedural Guideline 10.1).	Position provides access to catheter and promotes patient dignity as much as possible.
5. Remove catheter-securing device.	
6. Remove gloves, perform hand hygiene and apply clean gloves.	
7. Move syringe plunger up and down to loosen and then withdraw plunger 0.5 mL from end of syringe. Insert hub of syringe into inflation valve (balloon port). Allow balloon fluid to drain into syringe by gravity. Make sure that entire amount of fluid is removed by comparing removed amount to volume needed for inflation.	A partially inflated balloon causes trauma to urethral wall as catheter is removed. Removed fluid may be less than amount inserted because of balloon leakage.

SAFETY ALERT All silicone catheter balloons should be deflated using gravity to avoid the formation of creases or ridges that could cause urethral trauma (Cochran, 2007). Do not cut balloon inflation valve to drain water.

STEPS	RATIONALE
8. Pull catheter out smoothly and slowly. Examine it to ensure that it is whole. Catheter should slide out very easily. Do not use force. If you note any resistance, repeat Step 7 to remove remaining water. Notify health care provider if balloon does not deflate completely.	Nonwhole catheter means that pieces of catheter may still be in bladder. Notify health care provider immediately.
9. Wrap contaminated catheter in waterproof pad. Unhook collection bag and drainage tubing from bed.	
10. Reposition patient as necessary. Provide perineal hygiene if needed.	Promotes patient comfort and safety.
11. Empty, measure, and record urine present in drainage bag.	Records urinary output.

Continued

STEPS	RATIONALE
12. See Completion Protocol (inside front cover).	
13. Encourage patient to maintain or increase fluid intake (unless contraindicated).	Maintains normal urinary output.
14. Initiate voiding record or bladder diary. Instruct patient to tell you when the need to empty the bladder occurs and that all urine needs to be measured. Make sure that patient understands how to use the collection container.	Evaluates bladder function.
15. Explain that many patients experience mild burning, discomfort, or small-volume voiding with first voiding, which soon subsides.	Burning is result of urethral irritation from catheter.
16. Inform patient to report any signs of UTI.	Increases likelihood of timely treatment.
17. Ensure easy access to toilet, commode, bedpan, or urinal. Place urine "hat" on toilet seat if patient is using toilet. Place call bell within easy reach.	

EVALUATION

1. Observe time (less than 6 to 8 hours) and amount of first voiding (at least 150 mL).
2. Monitor voiding for 24 to 48 hours using a voiding record or bladder diary.
3. Ask patient to describe comfort level.
4. Ask patient to list signs and symptoms of UTI.

Unexpected Outcomes and Related Interventions

1. Water from inflation balloon does not return into syringe.
   a. Reposition patient; ensure that catheter is not pinched or kinked.
   b. Remove syringe. Attach new syringe and allow enough time for passive emptying.
   c. Attempt to empty balloon by gently pulling back on the syringe plunger.
2. Patient exhibits one or more of the following: fever; painful urination; cloudy, foul-smelling urine; abdominal pain; flank pain; frequent small-volume voiding; hematuria.
   a. Assess for bladder distention.
   b. Monitor vital signs and urine output.
   c. Report findings to health care provider; signs and symptoms may indicate a UTI.
3. Patient is unable to void after catheter removal, having had adequate fluid intake. Bladder is distended.
   a. Assist to normal position for voiding.
   b. Provide privacy.
   c. Perform bladder ultrasound (see Procedural Guideline 18.2) to assess residual urine. Notify health care provider if volume is greater that 100 mL.

Recording and Reporting

- Record and report time catheter was removed; teaching related to increasing fluid intake and signs and symptoms of UTI; and time, amount, and characteristics of first voiding.
- Record intake and voiding times and amounts on voiding record or bladder diary as indicated.

Sample Documentation

0600 No. 16-Fr/5-mL balloon catheter removed without difficulty. Patient instructed to report any symptoms of a UTI; encouraged to increase fluids and save urine for measurement.

0800 Voided 100 mL of clear yellow urine. No complaints of dysuria.

Special Considerations

Pediatric

- Do not force catheter out of bladder if resistance is met. When excessive tubing has been inserted in the bladder, there have been occurrences of knotting of the tubing (Hockenberry and Wilson, 2007).

Geriatric

- Older adults may exhibit atypical signs and symptoms of UTI such as a change in mental status attributed to delirium (in addition to confusion, agitation, lethargy).

Home Care

- Include family caregivers in the plan of care. Some may need extra support when learning how to take care of someone who now needs regular help with toileting.

PROCEDURAL GUIDELINE 18.3
Care of an Indwelling Catheter

- **Nursing Skills Online:** Urinary Elimination, Lesson 5

Indwelling urinary catheters are one of the most common sources for hospital-acquired infection, and CAUTI carries significant risk for chronic and life-threatening infection (Parker and others, 2009b). If an indwelling catheter is required, there are some measures you can take to reduce infection risk such as keeping a closed drainage system, keeping the drainage bag below the level of the bladder, using silicone or hydrogel catheters for long-term use or silver catheters for short-term use, and routine meatal care (Parker and others, 2009b). Daily meatal care and care after any episodes of fecal soiling have the potential to significantly decrease CAUTI risk (Tsuchida and others, 2008).

Delegation and Collaboration

Routine catheter care may be delegated to nursing assistive personnel (NAP) and is often incorporated into perineal care. Instruct the NAP to:

- Report characteristics of urine output from the catheter, including color, odor, and amount.
- Report the condition of catheter (leaks, secretions, or incrustation at catheter insertion site) and perineum (presence of inflammation, discharge, contamination from fecal discharge).

Equipment

- Soap
- Washcloth and towel
- Basin with warm water
- Clean gloves
- Bath blanket
- Waterproof pad

Procedural Steps

1. Assess the urethral meatus and surrounding tissues for inflammation, swelling, secretions, or incrustations at the catheter insertion site.
2. Assess color, clarity, and odor of urine.
3. Assess for any complaints of pain or discomfort in lower abdomen.
4. Monitor patient's temperature and fluid intake.
5. Check medical order for catheter removal.
6. Assess patient's understanding of catheter care.
7. **See Standard Protocol (inside front cover).**
8. Position female patients in dorsal recumbent position and male patients supine. Place waterproof pad under buttocks. Cover with bath blanket, exposing only catheter and perineal area. Provide perineal care as needed (see Procedural Guideline 10.1).
9. Remove catheter tubing from the securing device.
10. With nondominant hand:
    a. *Female:* Gently retract labia to fully expose urethral meatus and catheter.
    b. *Male:* Retract foreskin if not circumcised and hold penis at shaft just below glans.
    c. Grasp the catheter with two fingers to stabilize catheter near the meatus.
11. Using a clean washcloth, soap, and water, take the dominant hand and wipe in a circular motion along the length of the catheter for about 10 cm (4 inches) starting at the meatus and moving away. Avoid placing tension on or pulling on the exposed catheter tubing. Make sure to remove all traces of soap.
12. Replace the catheter securing device as necessary (see Skill 18.2).
13. Check drainage tubing and bag to ensure that:
    a. Tubing is coiled and secured onto bed linen.
    b. Tubing is not looped or positioned above level of bladder.
    c. Tubing is not kinked or clamped.
    d. Drainage bag is positioned on lower bed frame with urine flowing freely from tubing (see Skill 18.2).
14. Empty collection bag as necessary or at least every 8 hours.
15. **See Completion Protocol (inside front cover).**

SKILL 18.4 SUPRAPUBIC CATHETER CARE

A suprapubic catheter is a urinary drainage tube inserted surgically into the bladder through the abdominal wall above the symphysis pubis (Fig. 18-4). The catheter may be sutured to the skin, secured with an adhesive material, or retained in the bladder with a fluid-filled balloon similar to an indwelling catheter.

Suprapubic catheters are placed when there is blockage of the urethra (e.g., enlarged prostate, urethral stricture, after urological surgery) and in situations when a long-term urethral catheter causes irritation or discomfort or interferes with sexual functioning.

ASSESSMENT

1. Assess urine in drainage bag for amount, clarity, color, odor, and sediment. *Rationale: Abnormal findings may indicate potential complications such as infection, decreased urinary output, and catheter occlusion.*

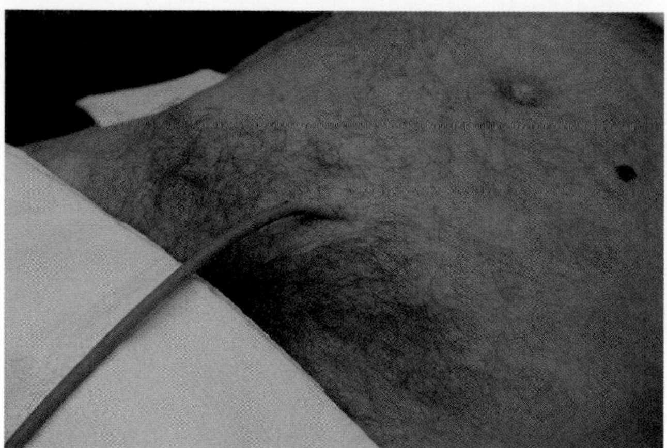

FIG 18-4 Suprapubic catheter without dressing.

2. Assess catheter insertion site for inflammation, pain, erythema, edema, and drainage. *Rationale: If insertion site is new, slight inflammation may be expected as part of normal wound healing but can also indicate infection.*
3. Assess for elevated temperature and chills. *Rationale: Indicates UTI or site infection.*
4. Assess site where catheter is secured on abdomen for signs of irritation. *Rationale: Repeated taping can cause skin irritation and breakdown.*
5. Check for allergies. *Rationale: Patient may be sensitive to tape, latex, or antiseptic solution.*
6. Assess patient's and/or caregiver's knowledge of purpose of catheter and its care. *Rationale: Determines level of instruction/support required.*

PLANNING

Expected Outcomes focus on maintaining flow of urine, patient comfort, and prevention of infection.

1. Catheter is patent, and output is 30 mL or greater per hour.
2. Catheter insertion site is free of signs of infection: erythema, edema, discharge, or tenderness.
3. Patient remains afebrile.
4. Patient verbalizes no pain or discomfort at insertion site.

Delegation and Collaboration

The care of a newly placed suprapubic catheter cannot be delegated to nursing assistive personnel (NAP); however, the skill of caring for an established suprapubic catheter may be delegated (refer to agency policy). Instruct the NAP to:

- Report if the patient has any discomfort related to the suprapubic tube.
- Empty the drainage bag, document urinary output on the I&O record and report any change in the amount and character of the urine.
- Report any signs of redness or drainage around catheter insertion site, any foul odors, or elevated temperature.

Equipment

- Gloves: sterile and clean
- Sterile gauze for cleaning site
- Sterile cotton tip applicator
- Cleansing agent (sterile saline)
- Sterile drain (split) gauze
- Tape
- Velcro tape holder or tube stabilizer (optional)
- Washcloth, towel, soap, water

IMPLEMENTATION *for* SUPRAPUBIC CATHETER CARE

STEPS	RATIONALE
1. **See Standard Protocol (inside front cover).**	
2. Identify patient using two identifiers (e.g., name and birthday or name and account number, according to facility policy).	Ensures correct patient. Complies with The Joint Commission standards and improves patient safety (TJC, 2010).
3. Remove dressing around catheter; discard gloves. Perform hand hygiene.	
4. Prepare supplies and cleansing agent for applying a dry, sterile dressing (see Skill 26.1). Established catheters are often cleansed with mild soap and water (see agency policy).	The newly inserted catheter insertion site is a surgical incision and should be treated like other incisions.
5. Inspect insertion site and patency of catheter.	Reveals how catheter is held in place. With newly established catheters, sutures should be clearly seen wrapped around catheter and secured to skin. Urine should be seen draining in tubing.

STEPS	RATIONALE
6. Perform site care.	
a. Newly established catheters	
(1) Apply sterile gloves.	
(2) Without creating tension, hold catheter erect with nondominant hand while cleaning. Cleanse in circular motion, starting near catheter insertion site and continuing in outward widening circles for approximately 5 cm (2 inches) (see illustration).	Moves from area of least contamination to area of most contamination. Tension on catheter may cause discomfort or damage to wall of bladder or cause the catheter to slip out of place.
(3) With fresh, moistened gauze, gently cleanse base of catheter, moving up and away from site of insertion (proximal to distal).	Removes microorganisms and any drainage that adheres to tubing.
(4) With sterile gloved hand, apply drain dressing (split gauze) around catheter and tape in place (see illustration).	
b. Long-term/established catheters	
(1) Without creating tension, hold catheter erect with nondominant hand while cleaning. Cleanse with soap and water in circular motion, starting near catheter insertion site and continuing in outward widening circles for approximately 5 cm (2 inches).	Sterile gloves are not needed with an established suprapubic catheter because there is no longer a surgical wound.
(2) With a fresh washcloth or gauze, gently cleanse base of catheter, moving up and away from site of insertion (proximal to distal).	
(3) If indicated, apply drain dressing (split gauze) around catheter and tape in place.	
7. Secure catheter to abdomen with tape or Velcro multipurpose tube holder to reduce tension on insertion site.	Secures catheter and reduces risk of excessive tension on suture and/or body seal.
8. Coil excess tubing on bed and secure it to dressing. Keep drainage bag below level of bladder at all times.	Prevents kinking and backflow of urine from the tubing into the bladder.
9. See Completion Protocol (inside front cover).	

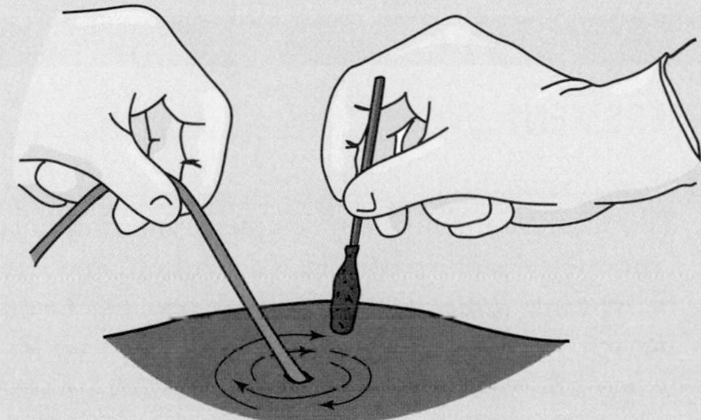

STEP 6a(2) Cleansing around suprapubic catheter, avoiding tension on catheter.

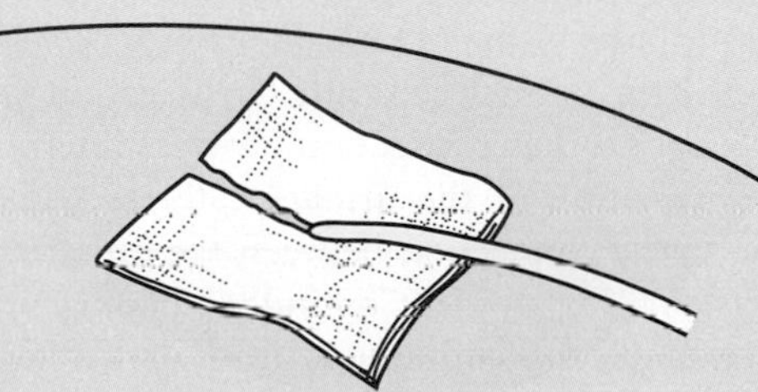

STEP 6a(4) Split drain dressing for suprapubic catheter.

EVALUATION

1. Monitor suprapubic catheter urine output.
2. Observe catheter insertion site for erythema, edema, discharge, or tenderness.
3. Monitor for signs of infection (e.g., fever, elevated white blood cell count) and observe patient's urine for clarity, sediment, or unusual odor.
4. Ask patient to rate any discomfort or pain related to the catheter on a scale of 0 to 10.

Unexpected Outcomes and Related Interventions

1. Patient complains of lower abdominal pain and/or distention; urine flow slows or stops. Catheter suspected to be obstructed (blood clots or sediment form; tip of catheter in bladder is positioned against bladder wall).
   a. Check catheter and drainage tubing for kinks.
   b. Ensure that the patient is not lying on the catheter or drainage tubing.
   c. Reposition the patient and observe for any increase in urine flow.
   d. Notify health care provider. In some cases you may need to irrigate the catheter, which requires an order.
2. Patient develops symptoms of a UTI or catheter site infection.
   a. Increase fluids to at least 1500 mL/day (if not contraindicated).
   b. Monitor vital signs and I&O; observe amount, color, consistency of urine; assess site.
   c. Administer antiinfective as prescribed.
3. Urine leaks around catheter.
   a. Check catheter and drainage tubing for kinks or for other causes of occlusion.
   b. Monitor vital signs; assess urine for signs of infection.
   c. Change dressing frequently; protect skin from moisture.
   d. Notify health care provider.
4. Catheter becomes dislodged.
   a. Apply sterile gauze to site.
   b. Apply pressure if bleeding.
   c. Reassure patient.
   d. Notify health care provider immediately.

Recording and Reporting

- Record and report character of urine and type of dressing change, including assessments of insertion site and patient's comfort level with the catheter and dressing change.
- Record urine output on I&O flow sheet. In a situation in which there is both a suprapubic and a urethral catheter, record outputs from each catheter separately.

Sample Documentation

0800 Suprapubic catheter drained 100 mL of clear yellow urine. Dressing with small amount of dark brown drainage removed from suprapubic catheter site. No redness, edema, or drainage at the site. Insertion site cleansed and dressed with drain dressing. Denies any pain at insertion site.

Special Considerations

Home Care

- Patients and family caregivers should learn how to cleanse and apply a dressing (if applicable) using a clean technique.
- Teach patients and/or caregivers how to properly position the drainage bag; empty the urinary drainage bag; and observe urine color, clarity, odor, and amount.
- Arrange for home delivery of catheter supplies, always ensuring that there is at least one extra catheter and drainage bag in the home.
- Teach patients and/or caregivers signs of catheter obstruction, UTI, and wound infection.

SKILL 18.5 PERFORMING CATHETER IRRIGATION

Urinary catheter irrigations are performed on an intermittent or continuous basis to maintain catheter patency. There are two types of irrigation: closed catheter irrigation and open irrigation. Closed catheter irrigation provides intermittent or continuous irrigation of the urinary catheter without disrupting the sterile connection between the catheter and the drainage system (Fig. 18-5). Continuous bladder irrigation (CBI) is an example of a continuous infusion of a sterile solution into the bladder, usually using a three-way irrigation closed system with a triple-lumen catheter. CBI is frequently used following genitourinary surgery to keep the bladder clear and free of blood clots or sediment.

Open catheter irrigation is used for intermittent irrigation of the catheter and bladder. The skill involves breaking or opening the closed drainage system at the connection between the catheter and the drainage system. Strict asepsis is required throughout the procedure to minimize contamination and subsequent development of a UTI. Both open and closed irrigation can be used to instill medication into the bladder.

ASSESSMENT

1. Verify in the medical record:
   a. The order for method (continuous or intermittent) and type (sterile saline or medicated solution) and amount of irrigant. *Rationale: An order is required to initiate therapy. Frequency and volume of solution used for irrigation may be in the order or standardized as part of agency policy. Each type of irrigation requires different equipment.*
   b. Type of catheter in place. *Rationale: Single- and double-lumen catheters are used with open irrigation. Triple-lumen catheters are used for both intermittent and continuous closed irrigation.*

2. Palpate bladder for distention and tenderness. *Rationale: Bladder distention indicates that flow of urine may be blocked from draining.*

3. Assess patient for abdominal pain or spasms, sensation of bladder fullness, or catheter bypassing (leaking).

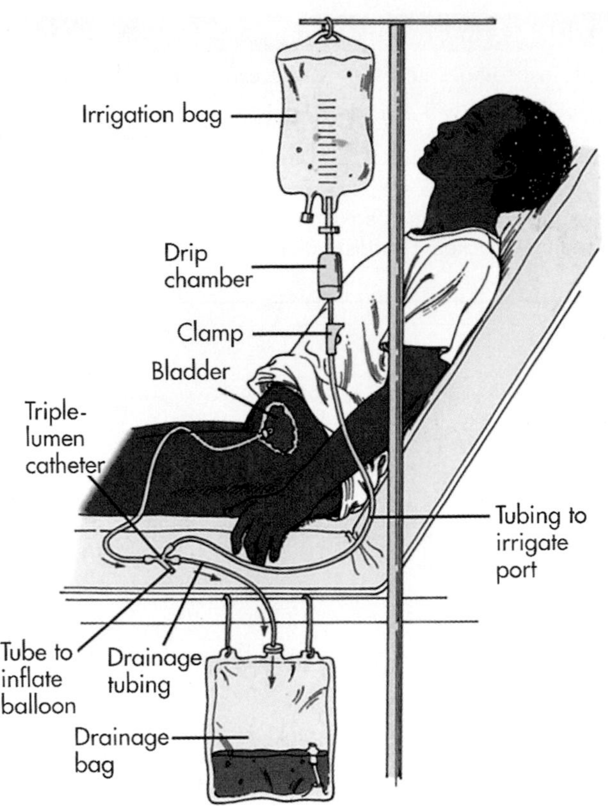

FIG 18-5 Continuous bladder irrigation setup.

Rationale: May indicate overdistention of the bladder caused by blockage of the catheter. Offers baseline to determine if therapy is successful.

4. Observe urine for color; amount; clarity; and presence of mucus, clots, or sediment. *Rationale: Indicates if patient is bleeding or sloughing tissue, which would require increased irrigation rate or frequency of catheter irrigation.*
5. Monitor I&O. *Rationale: During a CBI the amount of fluid draining from the bladder should exceed the amount of fluid infused into the bladder. If output does not exceed solution infused, you should suspect catheter obstruction (i.e., blood clots, kinked tubing).*
6. Assess patient's knowledge regarding purpose of performing catheter irrigation. *Rationale: Reveals need for patient instruction/support.*

PLANNING

Expected Outcomes focus on continuous urine flow and patient comfort.

1. Urine output is greater than volume of irrigating solution instilled.
2. Patient's urine output has decreased blood clots and sediment. (NOTE: Urine is bloody following bladder/urethral surgery, gradually becoming lighter and blood tinged in 2 to 3 days.)
3. Patient reports relief of bladder pain or spasms.
4. Patient remains afebrile and free of lower abdominal pain and cloudy and/or foul-smelling urine.

Delegation and Collaboration

The skill of catheter irrigation cannot be delegated to nursing assistive personnel (NAP). Instruct the NAP to:

- Report if the patient complains of pain or discomfort or leakage of fluid around the catheter.
- Monitor and record I&O; report immediately any decrease in urine output.

Equipment

Closed intermittent irrigation

- Antiseptic swabs
- Sterile irrigation solution at room temperature as prescribed
- Sterile container
- Sterile 30- to 60-mL irrigation syringe (piston type)
- Syringe to access system: Luer-Lok syringe for needleless access port (per manufacturer's indications)
- Screw clamp or rubber band (used to temporarily occlude catheter as irrigant is instilled)

Closed continuous irrigation

- Antiseptic swabs
- Bag of sterile irrigation solution at room temperature as prescribed
- Irrigation tubing with clamp to regulate irrigation flow rate
- Y connector (optional) to connect irrigation tubing to double-lumen catheter
- Intravenous (IV) pole (closed continuous or intermittent)

Open intermittent irrigation

- Antiseptic swabs
- Sterile irrigation solution at room temperature as prescribed
- Disposable sterile irrigation kit that contains solution container, collection basin, drape, gloves, 30- to 60-mL irrigation syringe (piston type)
- Sterile catheter plug

IMPLEMENTATION *for* PERFORMING CATHETER IRRIGATION

STEPS	RATIONALE
1. **See Standard Protocol (inside front cover).**	
2. Identify patient using two identifiers (i.e., name and birthday or name and account number, according to facility policy). Compare identifiers with information on patient's MAR or medical record.	Ensures correct patient. Complies with The Joint Commission standards and improves patient safety (TJC, 2010).

Continued

STEPS	RATIONALE
3. Position patient supine and expose catheter junction (catheter and drainage tubing).	Position provides access to catheter and promotes patient dignity as much as possible.
4. Remove catheter securing device.	

> **SAFETY ALERT** During catheter irrigation be sure that the drainage tubing from the indwelling catheter is patent (not clamped or obstructed). If irrigation solution continues to infuse rapidly and drainage from the bladder is blocked, overdistention can result in extreme discomfort and bladder damage or rupture.

STEPS	RATIONALE
5. ***Closed continuous irrigation***	
a. Close clamp on tubing.	
b. Hang bag of irrigating solution on IV pole.	
c. Insert (spike) tip of sterile irrigation tubing into designated port of irrigation solution bag using aseptic technique (see illustration).	Prevents transmission of microorganisms.
d. Open tubing clamp and allow solution to flow (prime) through tubing, keeping end of tubing sterile. Once fluid has completely filled the tubing, close the clamp and recap end of tubing.	Priming the tubing with fluid prevents introduction of air into the bladder.
e. Using aseptic technique, remove cap and connect tubing securely to drainage port of Y connector on double/triple–lumen catheter.	Prevents transmission of microorganisms.
f. Calculate drip rate and adjust rate at roller clamp. If urine is bright red or has clots, increase irrigation rate until drainage appears pink (according to ordered rate or agency protocol).	Continuous drainage is normal. It assists with prevention of clotting in presence of active bleeding in bladder and flushes clots out of bladder.
g. Observe for outflow of fluid into the drainage bag. Empty catheter drainage bag as needed.	Discomfort, bladder distention, and possibly injury can occur from overdistention of the bladder when bladder irrigant cannot flow from the bladder adequately. Bag fills rapidly and may need to be emptied every 1 to 2 hours.
h. Compare urine output with infusion of irrigation solution every hour.	Determines urinary output and ensures that irrigant is draining freely.
6. ***Closed intermittent irrigation***	
a. Pour prescribed sterile irrigation solution into sterile container.	Fluid is instilled through catheter in a bolus, flushing the system. Fluid drains out after irrigation is complete.
b. Draw prescribed volume of solution into syringe using aseptic technique (usually 30 to 50 mL). • Place sterile cap on tip of needleless syringe	
c. Clamp catheter tubing below soft injection port with screw clamp (or fold catheter tubing onto itself and secure with rubber band).	Occluding catheter tubing below the point of injection allows the irrigating solution to enter the catheter and flow upward toward the bladder.
d. Using circular motion, cleanse catheter port (specimen port) with antiseptic swab.	Prevents the transmission of microorganisms.
e. Insert tip of needleless syringe using twisting motion into port.	Ensures that syringe tip enters port.
f. Inject solution using slow, even pressure.	Gentle instillation of solution minimizes trauma to the bladder mucosa.
g. Withdraw syringe.	
h. Remove clamp (or rubber band) and observe outflow of solution. Some medicated solutions may need to dwell in the bladder for a prescribed period of time, requiring the catheter to be clamped temporarily.	Some irrigation solutions require time in the catheter and bladder to exert therapeutic effect. You should never leave clamped drainage tubing and bag unattended.

STEPS	RATIONALE
7. *Open intermittent irrigation*	
a. Open sterile irrigation tray: Establish sterile field (see Chapter 5) and pour required amount of sterile solution into sterile solution container. Replace cap on large container of solution. Add sterile irrigation syringe (piston type) to field.	Maintains a sterile field.
b. Position sterile drape under catheter.	Creates sterile field on which the nurse can work and prevents soiling of bed linen.
c. Aspirate prescribed volume of irrigation solution into irrigating syringe (usually 30 mL). Place syringe in sterile solution container until ready to use.	Maintains sterility of irrigating syringe.
d. Move sterile collection basin close to patient's thigh.	
e. Wipe connection point between catheter and drainage tubing with antiseptic wipe before disconnecting.	Reduces transmission of microorganisms.
f. Disconnect catheter from drainage tubing, allowing any urine to flow into sterile collection basin; cover open end of drainage tubing with sterile protective cap and position tubing so it stays coiled on top of bed with the end on the sterile drape.	Maintains sterility of inner aspects of catheter lumen and drainage tubing. Reduces potential for infection by way of microorganism contamination.
g. Insert tip of syringe into lumen of catheter and gently push plunger to instill solution (see illustration).	Gentle fluid instillation minimizes risk of trauma to bladder.

SAFETY ALERT When irrigating a catheter using the open method, do not force the irrigation. Catheter may be completely occluded and needs to be changed.

STEPS	RATIONALE
h. Remove syringe, lower catheter, and allow solution to drain into basin. Drainage solution amount should be equal to or greater than amount instilled. If ordered, repeat instilling solution and drain until drainage is clear of clots and sediment.	If clot has been removed, solution drains freely into basin.

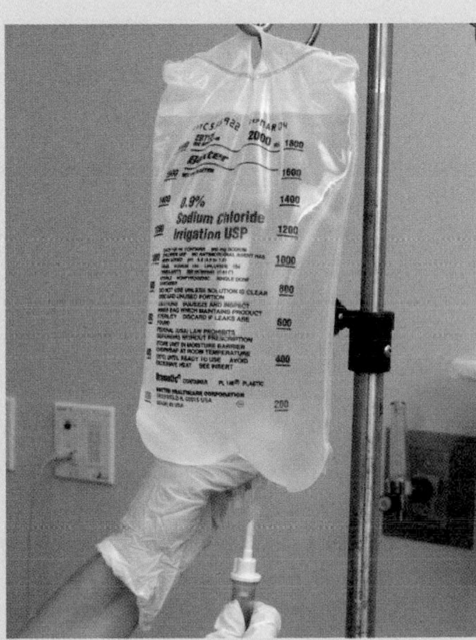

STEP 5c Spiking bag of sterile irrigation solution for continuous bladder irrigation.

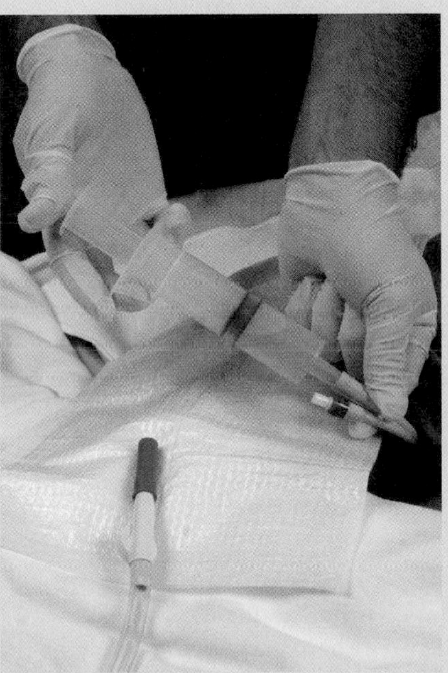

STEP 7g Gentle instillation of sterile irrigation solution irrigates catheter.

Continued

STEPS	RATIONALE
i. After irrigation is complete, remove protector cap from urinary drainage tubing adapter, cleanse adapter with antiseptic wipe, and reinsert adapter into lumen of catheter.	
8. Anchor catheter (see Skill 18.2).	
9. See Completion Protocol (inside front cover).	

EVALUATION

1. Measure actual urine output by subtracting total amount of irrigation fluid infused from total volume drained.
2. Review I&O flow sheet to verify that hourly output into drainage bag is in appropriate proportion to irrigating solution entering bladder. Expect more output than fluid instilled because of urine production.
3. Observe for catheter patency; inspect urine for blood clots and sediment, tubing not kinked or occluded.
4. Assess patient comfort.
5. Assess for signs and symptoms of infection.

Unexpected Outcomes and Related Interventions

1. Irrigation solution does not infuse or is slower than previously set.
   a. Examine drainage tubing for clots, sediment, or kinks.
   b. Notify health care provider if solution is retained, patient complains of severe pain, or bladder is distended.
2. Drainage output is less than amount of irrigation solution infused.
   a. Examine drainage tubing for clots, sediment, or kinks.
   b. Inspect urine for presence of or increase in blood clots and sediment.
   c. Evaluate patient for pain and distended bladder.
   d. Notify health care provider.
3. Bright-red bleeding with irrigation (CBI) drip wide open.
   a. Assess for hypovolemic shock (vital signs, skin color and moisture, anxiety level).
   b. Leave irrigation drip wide open and notify health care provider.
4. Patient experiences pain with irrigation.
   a. Examine drainage tubing for clots, sediment, or kinks.
   b. Evaluate urine for presence of or increase in blood clots and sediment.
   c. Evaluate for distended bladder.
   d. Notify health care provider.

Recording and Reporting

- Record amount and type of solution used as irrigant, amount infused, amount returned as drainage, and characteristics of output.
- Report catheter occlusion, sudden bleeding, infection, or increased pain.
- Record I&O.

Sample Documentation

0800 Lower abdomen soft and flat. CBI with normal saline infusing at 60 mL/hr. Catheter draining bright-red urine with moderate-size dark bloody clots. Patient denies any pain.

Special Considerations

Home Care

- Patients and/or family caregivers can learn to perform catheter irrigations with adequate support, demonstration/return demonstration, and written instructions.
- Teach patients and/or family caregivers to observe urine color, clarity, odor, and amount.
- Arrange for home delivery and storage of catheter/irrigation supplies.
- Teach patients and/or family caregivers signs of catheter obstruction, UTI.

REVIEW QUESTIONS

1. The nurse is applying an external condom-type catheter. Which nursing intervention helps minimize the risk of trauma and infection?
   1. Apply the condom sheath so the end of the catheter is 7.5 to 12.5 cm (3 to 5 inches) from the tip of the penis.
   2. Shave the pubic area so hair does not adhere to the condom or is pulled during removal.
   3. Provide perineal hygiene before applying the condom-type catheter.
   4. Apply tape to the condom sheath to keep it securely in place.

Case Study for Questions 2 and 3

A female patient receiving opioid pain medicine has not been able to void for the past 6 hours. She now complains of lower abdominal pain and fullness. A bladder scan is done and reads 750 mL, and an order for an indwelling catheter is obtained.

2. Which of the following lists of steps for insertion of this patient's indwelling catheter are in the correct order?
   a. Insert and advance catheter.
   b. Lubricate catheter.
   c. Inflate catheter balloon.
   d. Cleanse urethral meatus.

e. Drape the patient with the sterile square and fenestrated drapes.
f. When urine appears, advance another 2.5 to 5 cm (1 to 2 inches).
g. Prepare sterile field and supplies.
h. Gently pull catheter until resistance is felt.
i. Attach drainage tubing.

1. g, d, e, b, a, f, c, h, i
2. e, g, b, d, a, f, c, h, i
3. g, e, b, d, f, a, c, h, i
4. d, e, g, b, a, f, h, c, i

3. What would the nurse include next in this patient's plan of care after the insertion of the indwelling catheter?
   1. Irrigate the catheter with sterile water every shift.
   2. Hang the collection bag on the side rail, below the level of the bladder.
   3. Cleanse the urinary meatus with an antiseptic solution daily.
   4. Attach the drainage tubing to the bed, avoiding dependent loops.
4. The nurse is preparing to remove an indwelling urinary catheter. Which nursing interventions should the nurse implement? Select all that apply.
   1. Attach a 5-mL syringe to the inflation port.
   2. Allow the balloon to drain into the syringe by gravity.
   3. Initiate a voiding record/bladder diary.
   4. Pull catheter quickly.
   5. With steady force, pull back on the syringe plunger.
5. Which nursing interventions are appropriate in the care of a patient with a new suprapubic catheter? Select all that apply.
   1. Using sterile technique, cleanse the skin close to the catheter using a circular motion.
   2. Wipe away any drainage on the catheter by wiping down the catheter toward the skin.
   3. Inspect the insertion site for any sutures, erythema, edema, discharge, or tenderness.
   4. Secure catheter to abdomen with tape or a tube holder device.
   5. Apply tension to the catheter when cleansing the site and tubing.

Case Study for Questions 6 and 7

An older man recently had urologic surgery and has an order for CBI, with the goal to keep the urine pink. When assessing the three-way indwelling urinary catheter and CBI, the nurse finds very little urine in the drainage bag, and the patient is complaining of lower abdominal pain and a sensation of bladder fullness.

6. What would be an initial nursing action?
   1. Increase the rate of the CBI.
   2. Assess the catheter drainage tubing for kinking.
   3. Encourage fluid intake.
   4. Remove the catheter.
7. What would be the most likely cause of the decreased urine output?
   1. Blood clots from surgery
   2. Occlusion from bacteria biofilm
   3. Decreased fluid intake
   4. Defective urinary catheter
8. The nurse is assisting a male patient with a urinal. Place the following steps in the proper order.
   1. Apply clean gloves.
   2. Place urinal between the legs with penis in urinal.
   3. Rinse the urinal and return to patient.
   4. Explain the procedure to the patient.
   5. Close bedside curtains and door of room.
9. What is an initial step when preparing to irrigate an indwelling urinary catheter using open intermittent technique?
   1. Cleanse the catheter (specimen) port with an antiseptic swab.
   2. Prime the irrigation tubing, ensuring that no air is present in the tubing.
   3. Clamp the catheter below the soft injection port with screw clamp or fold catheter over on itself and secure with a rubber band.
   4. Wipe connection point between catheter and drainage tubing with antiseptic wipe.

REFERENCES

Centers for Medicare & Medicaid Services (CMS): *Hospital-acquired conditions (present on admission indicator)*, 2008, http://www.cms.hhs.gov/HospitalAcqCond/06_Hospital-Acquired_Conditions.asp, accessed August 21, 2009.

Cochran S: Care of the indwelling urinary catheter: is it evidenced based? *J Wound Ostomy Continence Nurs* 34(3):282, 2007.

DeGennaro M and others: Reliability of bladder volume measurement with bladder scan in paediatric patients, *Scand J Urol Nephrol* 40(5):370, 2006.

Drekonja DM and others: Antimicrobial urinary catheters: a systemic review, *Expert Rev Med Devices* 5(4):495, 2008.

Gray M: Expert review: best practices in managing the indwelling catheter, *Perspectives* 25(1):1, 2006.

Gray M: Securing the indwelling catheter, *Am J Nurs* 108(12):44, 2008.

Green L and others: Guide to the elimination of catheter-associated urinary tract infections. In *APIC text of infection control and epidemiology*, Washington, DC, revised 2008, Association for Professionals in Infection Control and Epidemiology Inc.

Griffiths R, Fernandez R: Strategies for the removal of short-term indwelling urethral catheters in adults. *Cochrane Database of Syst Rev* 2:CD004011, 2007.

Holroyd JM and others: The relationship of indwelling urinary catheters to death, length of hospital stay, functional decline, and nursing home admission in hospitalized older medical patients, *J Am Geriatr Soc* 55(2):227, 2007.

Hockenberry MJ, Wilson D: *Wong's nursing care of infants and children*, ed 8, St Louis, 2007, Mosby.

Johanna Briggs Institute: Removal of short-term catheters, *Best Pract* 10(3):1, 2006.

Johnson JR and others: Systematic review: antimicrobial urinary catheters to prevent catheter-associated urinary tract infection in hospitalized patients, *Ann Intern Med* 144(2):116, 2006.

Lever R: The evidence for urethral meatal cleansing, *Nurs Stand* 21(41):39, 2007.

Lo DS and others: A compendium of strategies to prevent healthcare-associated infections in acute care hospitals, *Infect Control Hosp Epidemiol* 29(Suppl 1):s12, 2008.

Nazarko L: Reducing the risk of catheter-related urinary tract infection, *Br J Nurs* 17(16):1002, 2008.

Newman DK, Wein AJ: *Managing and treating urinary incontinence*, ed 2, Baltimore, 2009, Health Professions Press.

Oh-Oka H, Fujisawa M: Study of low bladder volume measurement using 3-dimensional ultrasound scanning device: improvement in measurement accuracy through training when bladder volume is 150 mL or less, *J Urol* 177(2):595 2007.

Parker D and others: Catheter-associated urinary tract infections fact sheet, *J Wound Ostomy Continence Nurs* 36(2):156, 2009a.

Parker D and others: Evidenced-based report card: nursing interventions to reduce the risk of catheter-associated urinary tract infection, *J Wound Ostomy Continence Nurs* 36(1):23, 2009b.

Pomfret I: Penile sheaths: a guide to selection and fitting, *J Commun Nurs* 20(11):14, 2006.

Robichard S, Blondeau JM: Urinary tract infections in older adults: current issues and new therapeutic options, *Geriatr Aging* 11(1):582, 2008.

Robinson J: Continence: sizing and fitting a penile sheath, *Br J Community Nurs* 11(10):420,422,424, 2006.

Saint S and others: Condom versus indwelling urinary catheters: a randomized trial, *J Am Geriatr Soc* 54:1055, 2006.

Senese V and others: Clinical practice guidelines female urethral catheterization, *Urol Nurs* 26(4):314, 2006a.

Senese V and others: Clinical practice guidelines male urethral catheterization, *Urol Nurs* 26(4):315, 2006b.

Schumm K, Lam TBL: Types of urethral catheters for management of short-term voiding problems in hospitalized adults, *Neurourol Urodynamics* 27(8):738, 2008.

Smith PW and others: SHEA/APIC guideline: infection prevention and control in the long-term care facility, *Am J Infect Control* 36:504, 2008.

Srulevich M, Chopra A: Voiding disorders in long-term care, *Ann Longterm Care* 16(12):1, 2008.

The Joint Commission (TJC): *2010 National Patient Safety Goals*, Oakbrook Terrace, Ill, 2010, The Commission, http://www.jointcommission/PatientSafety/NationalPatientSafetyGoals, accessed June 2010.

Tsuchida T and others: Relationship between catheter care and catheter-associated urinary track infection at Japanese general hospitals: a prospective observational study, *Int J Nurs Stud* 45(3):352, 2008.

Willson M and others: Evidenced-based report card: nursing interventions to reduce the risk of catheter-associated urinary tract infection. Part 2: Staff education, monitoring, and care techniques, *J Wound Ostomy Continence Nurs* 36(2):137, 2009.

CHAPTER

19

Bowel Elimination and Gastric Intubation

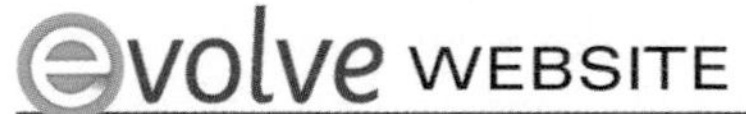

http://evolve.elsevier.com/Perry/nursinginterventions
Video Clips
Nursing Skills Online

Regular elimination of bowel waste products is essential for normal body functioning. Because bowel function depends on the balance of physical and psychological factors, elimination patterns and habits vary among individuals. When patients' functional status changes or they become ill, they may require assistance to maintain or regain their normal elimination habits. These include bedpan use or enema administration. To manage patients' bowel elimination problems, you need to understand normal elimination and factors that promote, impede, or alter elimination such as constipation, diarrhea, and fecal incontinence.

Disorders of the bowel requiring direct nursing intervention include diarrhea, constipation, and bowel incontinence. Left unrecognized, constipation progresses to fecal impaction, in which stool blocks the intestinal lumen. Stasis of bowel contents produces abdominal distention and pain. In some cases liquid stool passes around the impaction, which is frequently misinterpreted as diarrhea. If a patient is constipated, you will likely administer enemas or digitally remove impacted stool (Kyle, 2009).

When patients undergo surgery or experience an alteration in gastrointestinal (GI) peristalsis, the insertion of a nasogastric (NG) tube is needed for gastric decompression. Gastric decompression reduces nausea and vomiting by keeping the stomach empty. When a patient has absent or decreased gastric peristalsis, it is important to keep the stomach empty.

PATIENT-CENTERED CARE

Bowel elimination is a very private activity. It is important to show respect for a patient's privacy, provide necessary comfort and hygiene measures, and attend to the patient's emotional needs when performing required skills. Assist immobilized patients with the elimination process by helping them on and off bedpans.

Emotional factors affect bowel elimination. Anxiety, fear, and anger may accelerate peristalsis, resulting in diarrhea and gaseous distention. Other emotional factors (e.g., depression) and physical factors (e.g., reduced mobility, changes in diet) often cause decreased peristalsis, resulting in increased reabsorption of water from the stool and subsequent constipation.

Be aware of the patient's cultural practices. Providing gender-congruent care is important, but for some cultures this intervention is not enough. For example, Hindus and Muslims have distinct hygiene practices. The left hand is designated for unclean procedures such as practices associated with bowel elimination (Galanti, 2008; Giger and Davidhizar, 2008). Use the right hand to touch the patient and assist with other aspects of care and use the left for handling the bedpan and perineal cleansing following bowel elimination.

SAFETY

When assisting patients with bowel elimination or inserting an NG tube for gastric decompression, safe nursing practices are essential. Safe patient handling techniques, used when positioning a patient for removal of a fecal impaction or administering an enema are essential. It is important that the patient understand the need to maintain the position and try to relax. Sudden movement increases the risk of injury from the rectal tube. Patients with poor sphincter control cannot retain an enema; positioning the patient on the bedpan eases enema administration, contains enema fluid, and prevents the patient from moving suddenly when the enema fluid leaks out.

When removing a fecal impaction, there are additional safety issues. If your patient has a history of cardiac dysrhythmias, there is a risk for procedural-associated bradycardia because of stimulation of the sacral branch of the vagus nerve. This procedure is often contraindicated in cardiac patients. However, if it is absolutely necessary, monitor your patient's heart rate before and during the procedure.

Placement of an NG tube for gastric decompression has multiple safety implications with regard to placing, maintaining, and removing the tube (see Skill 19.3); however, there are other implications. For example, pressure of the tube against the patient's nares increases the risk for skin breakdown. Thus meticulous skin care around the nares and nose is needed. Because of the tube's location in the nose, patients mouth-breathe, causing the oral mucosa to dry. Frequent and meticulous oral hygiene minimizes oral discomfort and the risk of damage to the oral mucosa.

EVIDENCE-BASED PRACTICE TRENDS

Gevirtz C: Controlling pain: Managing opioid-induced constipation, *Nursing 2008* (July):55, 2008.

Constipation is a symptom, not a disease. To relieve constipation, changes in lifestyle such as increased dietary fiber, increased fluids, moderate exercise, and elimination of laxative use are helpful. There is increasing evidence that eating low-fat foods and foods containing dietary fiber and bulk reduces the patient's risk of colorectal cancers, fecal incontinence, and digestive diseases. In addition, opioid medications, commonly used for chronic pain, cause constipation. These patients commonly require a stool-softening agent and, if tolerated, a high-fiber diet to manage opioid-induced constipation (Gevirtz, 2008).

Constipation and fecal incontinence are especially troublesome in older adults. The signs of constipation usually include infrequent bowel movements (less than every 3 days), difficulty in evacuating feces, inability to defecate, and hard feces. Helping patients and their families select different foods may reduce the incidence of these problems. Unless contraindicated, encourage the patient to drink 2000 to 3000 mL of fluids daily. A high-fiber diet (25 to 30 g/day) reduces constipation. As fiber passes through the colon, it acts as a sponge; as a result, bulkier and softer stools are formed. In addition, the waste moves through the body more easily and results in more regular bowel movements, thus reducing constipation and incontinence.

Management of fecal incontinence requires a complete understanding of the causes. The presence of diarrhea is frequently associated with incontinence episodes. Continual seepage of diarrhea may also occur with an impaction, and a digital rectal examination verifies the presence of the impaction. Diarrhea is often caused by diet or antibiotic use, which alters the normal flora in the GI tract. Diarrhea is controlled by supplementing coarse bran rather than refined fiber to slow intestinal transit time and increase the bulk of the fecal contents.

PROCEDURAL GUIDELINE 19.1
Providing a Bedpan

Video Clips

A patient restricted to bed uses a bedpan for bowel elimination. Two types of bedpans are available (Fig. 19-1). The regular and most commonly used bedpan has a curved, smooth upper end and a tapered lower end. A fracture pan, designated for patients with body or leg casts or patients restricted from raising their hips (e.g., after a total joint replacement), slips easily under a patient. The upper end (wide end) of a regular bedpan fits under the patient's buttocks toward the sacrum, with the lower end (tapered end) fitting just under the upper thighs.

Delegation and Collaboration

The skill of providing a bedpan can be delegated to nursing assistive personnel (NAP). Instruct the NAP about the following:

- Correct positioning guidelines for patients with mobility restrictions or for those who have therapeutic equipment such as wound drains, intravenous (IV) catheters, or traction
- To provide perineal and hand hygiene for patient as necessary after using the bedpan

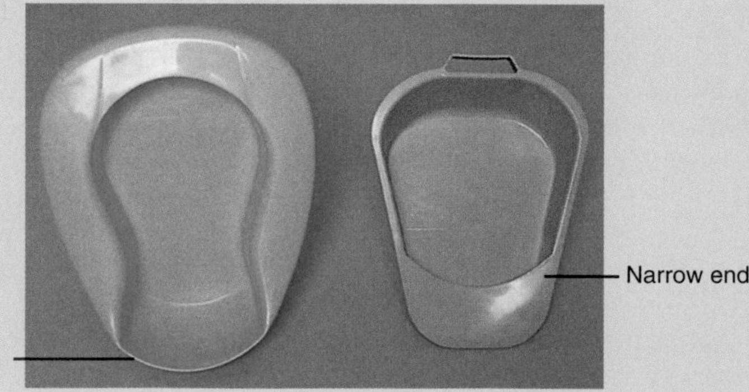

FIG 19-1 Types of bed pans. *Left,* Regular bedpan, *Right,* Fracture bedpan.

PROCEDURAL GUIDELINE 19.1
Providing a Bedpan—cont'd

Equipment

- Clean gloves
- Bedpan (regular or fracture) (see Fig. 19-1)
- Toilet tissue
- Specimen container (if necessary) or plastic specimen bag clearly labeled with date, patient's name, and identification number
- Washbasin, washcloths, towels, and soap
- Waterproof, absorbent pads (if necessary)
- Clean drawsheet (if necessary).

Procedural Steps

1. **See Standard Protocol (inside front cover)**
2. Assess patient's normal elimination habits: routine pattern, character of stool, effect of certain foods/fluids and eating habits on bowel elimination, effect of stress and level of activity on normal bowel elimination patterns, current medications, and normal fluid intake.
3. Auscultate for bowel sounds and palpate lower abdomen for distention.
4. Assess patient to determine level of mobility, including ability to sit upright and lift hips or turn.
5. Assess patient's level of comfort. Especially note presence of rectal or abdominal pain or hemorrhoids or skin irritation surrounding anus.
6. Determine if a specimen is needed.
7. For a patient's comfort, place metal bedpan under warm, running water for a few seconds and dry. Be careful that pan is not too hot.
8. Raise side rail on opposite side of bed.
9. Raise bed horizontally according to nurse's height.
10. Have patient assume supine position.

SAFETY ALERT Observe for presence of drains, IV fluids, and traction. These devices may impede a patient from assisting with the procedure and may also require more staff to assist placing the patient on a bedpan.

11. ***Place patient who can assist on bedpan.***
    - **a.** Raise patient's head 30 to 60 degrees.
    - **b.** Remove upper bed linens just enough so they are out of the way but do not expose patient. Place bedpan in accessible location.
    - **c.** Instruct patient on how to flex knees and lift hips upward.
    - **d.** Place hand closest to patient's head palm up under patient's sacrum to assist lifting. Ask patient to bend knees and raise hips. As patient raises hips, use other hand to slip regular bedpan under patient (see illustration). Be sure that open rim of bedpan is facing toward foot of bed. Do not shove bedpan under patient's hips.
    - **e.** *Optional:* If using a fracture pan, slip it under patient as hips are raised. Be sure that narrow rim of bedpan is facing toward foot of bed.

SAFETY ALERT Use a fracture pan if the patient had a total hip replacement. An abduction pillow must be placed between the legs when turning to prevent dislocation of the new joint.

12. ***Place patient who is immobile or has mobility restrictions on bedpan.***
    - **a.** Lower head of bed flat or raise head slightly (if tolerated by medical condition).

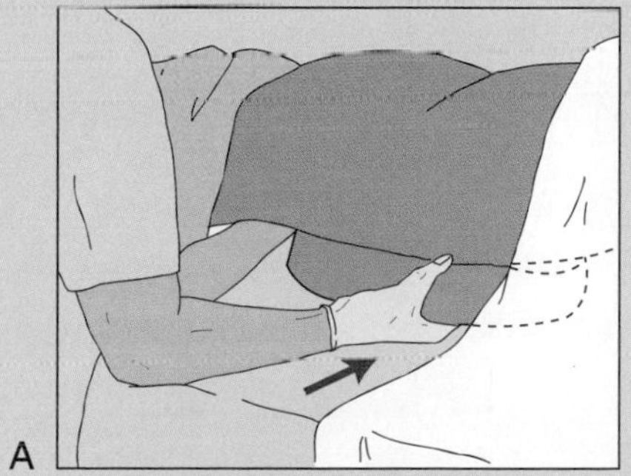

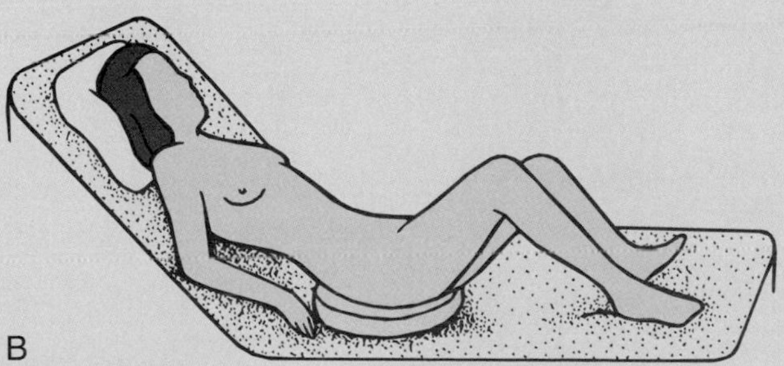

STEP 11d A, Placement of bedpan under patient hips. **B,** Correct positioning for patient on bedpan.

Continued

PROCEDURAL GUIDELINE 19.1
Providing a Bedpan—cont'd

b. Remove top linens as needed to turn patient while minimizing exposure.
c. Assist patient with rolling onto one side, with backside toward you.
d. Place regular bedpan firmly against patient's buttocks and down into mattress. Be sure open rim of bedpan is facing toward foot of bed (see illustrations).
e. Keeping one hand against bedpan, place other hand around patient's far hip. Ask patient to roll back onto bedpan. Do not force bedpan under patient.
f. Raise patient's head 30 degrees or to level of comfort (unless contraindicated). Have patient bend knees or raise knee gatch (unless contraindicated).

13. Maintain patient's comfort and safety. Cover patient for warmth.
14. Keep call bell and toilet tissue within easy reach for patient and place bed in lowest position with upper side rails raised.
15. Remove and discard gloves.
16. Allow patient to be alone but monitor status and respond promptly.
17. *Remove bedpan.*
    a. Position patient's bedside chair close to working side of bed.
    b. Maintain privacy; determine if patient is able to wipe own perineal area. If nurse must wipe perineal area, use several layers of toilet tissue or disposable washcloths. For female patients, cleanse from mons pubis toward rectal area.
    c. Deposit contaminated tissue in bedpan. However, if you need to measure intake and output (I&O) or need a specimen, discard contaminated tissue in the toilet. Allow patient to perform hand hygiene after wiping perineal area.
    d. *For mobile patient:* Ask patient to flex knees, placing body weight on lower legs, feet, and upper torso; lift buttocks up from bedpan. At same time place hand farthest from patient on side of bedpan and place other hand (closest to patient) under sacrum to assist in lifting. Have patient lift hips and remove bedpan. Place bedpan on draped bedside chair and cover.
    e. *For immobile patient:* Lower head of bed. Assist patient with rolling onto side and off of bedpan. Hold bedpan flat and steady while patient is rolling off; otherwise spillage will occur. After patient is completely lifted off bedpan, place it on bedside chair and cover.
18. Change any soiled linens, remove gloves, and return patient to comfortable position.
19. **See Completion Protocol (inside front cover).**
20. Obtain specimen as ordered. Empty bedpan into toilet or in special receptacle in appropriate utility room. Spray faucet attached to most institution toilets allows bedpan to be rinsed thoroughly. Remove gloves and perform hand hygiene.
21. Observe and record the appearance and characteristics of stool, including color, odor, consistency, frequency, amount, shape, and constituents.
22. Observe skin integrity in the perineal and perianal area.

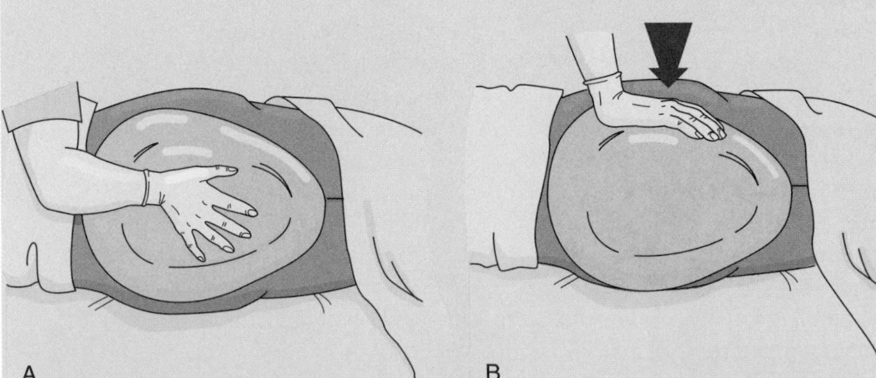

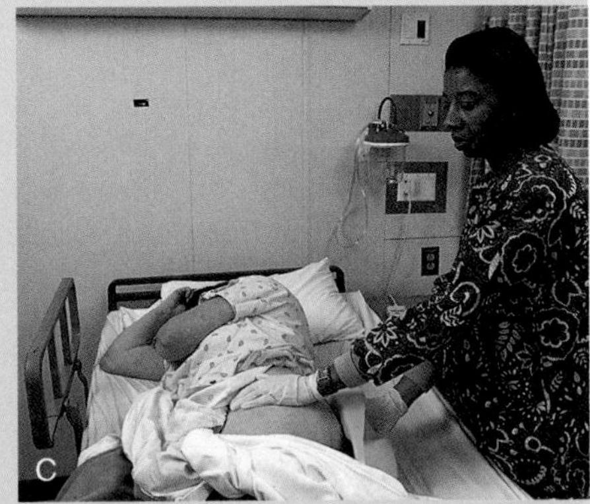

STEP 12d A, Position patient on one side and place bedpan firmly against buttocks. **B,** Push down on bedpan and toward patient. **C,** Nurse places the bedpan in position. (**A** and **B,** From Sorrentino SA: *Mosby's textbook for nursing assistants,* ed 7, St Louis, 2008, Mosby.)

SKILL 19.1 REMOVING FECAL IMPACTION

Fecal impaction, the inability to pass a hard collection of stool, occurs in all age-groups. Physically and mentally incapacitated persons and institutionalized older adults are at greatest risk. Many of these residents receive laxatives and stool softeners, which alters their elimination patterns and contributes to impactions and ultimately fecal incontinence (Schnelle and others, 2009). Fecal impaction occurs when there is a history of constipation. Constipation is defined as infrequent stools. However, a consensus definition of functional constipation includes two or more of the following factors for at least 3 months: (1) straining with defecation at least one fourth of the time, (2) lumpy or hard stools (or both) at least one fourth of the time, (3) sensation of incomplete evacuation at least one fourth of the time, or (4) two or fewer bowel movements in a week (Kyle, 2009). A variety of interventions (e.g., diet and exercise) normally successfully relieve constipation and reduce the risk for impaction.

Symptoms of fecal impaction include constipation, rectal discomfort, anorexia, nausea, vomiting, abdominal pain, diarrhea (leaking around the impacted stool), and urinary frequency. Prevention is the key to managing fecal impaction. However, once it occurs, digital removal of the stool is the only alternative. Digital removal of an impaction is embarrassing and uncomfortable for the patient. Excessive rectal manipulation may cause irritation to the mucosa and subsequent bleeding or vagus nerve stimulation, which can produce a reflex slowing of heart rate. The skill is performed when the administration of enemas (e.g., oil retention) or suppositories is not successful at removing impacted stools.

ASSESSMENT

1. Ask patient about normal and current bowel elimination pattern, including frequency and characteristics of stool, use of laxatives, enemas, and other medications; level of regular exercise; urge to defecate but inability to do so; presence of hemorrhoids; abdominal discomfort, especially when attempting to defecate; feelings of incomplete emptying; and sensations of bloating, cramping, or excessive gas. *Rationale: This information is valuable in determining contributing factors and preventive measures.*
2. Inspect patient's abdomen for distention. *Rationale: Observation initially identifies any distended or asymmetrical areas, which are further investigated on auscultation or palpation.*
3. Auscultate all four quadrants for presence of bowel sounds. *Rationale: Hypoactive bowel sounds may result from partial obstruction of the GI tract as with constipation or masses. Hyperactive bowel sounds may be present as a result of intestinal irritation as with diarrhea, partial obstruction of GI tract, or before defecation.*
4. Palpate patient's abdomen for distention, discomfort, or masses. *Rationale: Symptoms are related to accumulation of feces in intestinal tract. When severe constipation occurs, a palpable mass may be felt.*
5. Observe the anal area for signs of irritation from passing stool or hemorrhoids. *Rationale: Indicates possible straining on defecation.*
6. Measure patient's current vital signs and comfort level on a scale of 0 to 10. *Rationale: Establishes a baseline for detecting slowing in heart rate from vagus nerve stimulation during digital stimulation.*
7. Observe consistency of stool, seepage of liquid stool, or continual passage of small amounts of hard stool. Remove gloves and perform hand hygiene. *Rationale: Seepage of stool is symptomatic of an impaction high in colon. Patient may be able to pass small pieces of hard stool or have episodes of passing small amounts of liquid stool (Leung and Rao, 2009).*
8. Determine if patient is receiving anticoagulant therapy. *Rationale: Procedure may be contraindicated. Irritation and manipulation of the rectum often cause rectal bleeding, which will be more prolonged with anticoagulation.*
9. Check patient's record for health care provider's order for digital removal of impaction. *Rationale: A health care provider's order is necessary because of possible vagus nerve stimulation.*

PLANNING

Expected Outcomes focus on removal of the impaction and prevention of patient injury.

1. Patient's rectum is free of stool.
2. Patient's vital signs remain normal during and after procedure.
3. Patient is free of rectal or abdominal discomfort.
4. Anal area is free of tissue damage.

Delegation and Collaboration

The skill of removing an impaction cannot be delegated to nursing assistive personnel (NAP). Instruct the NAP about the following:

- Assisting the RN in positioning patient for the procedure
- What to observe for (e.g., color and consistency of any evacuated stool, rectal bleeding or bloody mucus) and report back to nurse
- Providing frequent perineal care to patient

Equipment

- Clean gloves
- Water-soluble local anesthetic lubricant (NOTE: Some institutions require use of water-soluble lubricant without anesthetic when nurse performs procedure.)
- Waterproof, absorbent pads
- Bedpan
- Bedpan cover (optional if available)
- Bath blanket
- Washbasin, washcloths, towels, and soap
- Vital sign equipment

IMPLEMENTATION *for* REMOVING FECAL IMPACTION

STEPS	RATIONALE
1. **See Standard Protocol (inside front cover).**	
2. Identify patient using two identifiers (e.g., name and birthday or name and account number, according to facility policy).	Ensures correct patient. Complies with The Joint Commission standards and improves patient safety (TJC, 2010).
3. Obtain assistance to help change patient's position if necessary.	Promotes safe patient handling and good body mechanics.
4. Lower side rail on patient's right side. Keeping far side rail raised, assist patient to left side-lying position with knees flexed and back toward nurse.	Promotes patient safety. Provides access to rectum.
5. Drape patient's trunk and lower extremities with bath blanket and place waterproof pad under patient's buttocks.	Maintains patient's sense of privacy and prevents unnecessary exposure of body parts.
6. Place bedpan next to patient.	
7. Lubricate gloved index and middle fingers of dominant hand with anesthetic lubricant.	Reduces discomfort and permits smooth insertion of finger into anus and rectum.
8. Instruct patient to take slow deep breaths during procedure; gradually and gently insert gloved index finger and feel anus relax around the finger. Then insert middle finger.	Slow deep breaths may help to relax patient. Gradual insertion of index finger helps to dilate anal sphincter.
9. Gradually advance fingers slowly along rectal wall toward umbilicus.	Allows you to reach impacted stool high in rectum.
10. Gently loosen fecal mass by moving fingers in a scissors motion to fragment fecal mass. Work fingers into hardened mass.	Loosening and penetrating mass allows nurse to remove it in small pieces, resulting in less discomfort to patient.
11. Work stool downward toward end of rectum. Remove small sections of feces and discard into bedpan.	Prevents need to force finger up into rectum and minimizes trauma to mucosa.
12. Observe patient's response and periodically assess heart rate and look for signs of fatigue.	Vagal stimulation slows heart rate and may cause dysrhythmias. Procedure may exhaust patient.

SAFETY ALERT Stop procedure if heart rate drops, rhythm changes, or rectal bleeding occurs.

STEPS	RATIONALE
13. Continue to clear rectum of feces and allow patient to rest at intervals.	Rest improves patient's tolerance of procedure.
14. After removal of impaction, provide perineal hygiene (see Chapter 10).	Promotes patient comfort and sense of cleanliness.
15. Remove bedpan and dispose of feces.	Reduces transmission of microorganisms.
16. If needed, assist patient to toilet or clean bedpan. (Procedure may be followed by enema or cathartic.)	Removal of impaction stimulates defecation reflex.
17. **See Completion Protocol (inside front cover).**	

EVALUATION

1. Perform rectal examination for stool and observe anal and perianal area for irritation or skin breakdown.
2. Obtain vital signs and compare to baseline values. Continue to monitor patient for bradycardia for 1 hour.
3. Auscultate for bowel sounds.
4. Palpate abdomen to determine if it is soft and not tender.
5. Ask patient to rate comfort level on a scale of 0 to 10.

Unexpected Outcomes and Related Interventions

1. Patient experiences bradycardia, decrease in blood pressure, and decrease in level of consciousness as a result of vagus nerve stimulation.
   a. Stop procedure and measure vital signs.
   b. Notify health care provider immediately.
   c. Remain with patient and monitor vital signs and level of consciousness.
2. Patient has seepage of liquid fecal material after removal of impaction.
   a. Assess patient for continuing impaction.
   b. Contact health care provider. A suppository or an enema is often needed to remove hardened feces higher in the rectum.
   c. Increase fluids (if allowed), fiber in diet, and activity level to increase peristaltic activity.

3. Patient has trauma to the rectal mucosa as evidenced by blood on the gloved finger.
   a. Stop procedure if bleeding is excessive.
   b. If bleeding continues, notify physician or health care provider for further treatment measures.

Recording and Reporting

- Record patient's tolerance to procedure, amount and consistency of stool removed, vital signs, pain level on a scale of 0 to 10, and adverse effects.
- Report any changes in vital signs or adverse effects to nurse in charge or health care provider.

Sample Documentation

1600 Ten pieces, ranging from 1-2 cm, of hard, dark brown, lumpy stool removed from rectum without rectal bleeding, pain, or fatigue. Pulse 80-88 strong and regular. Normal bowel sounds present in all four quadrants. No abdominal distention or complaints of pain.

Special Considerations

Pediatric

- Digital removal of stool is not recommended in pediatrics (Hockenberry and Wilson, 2007).

Geriatric

- Many older adults are especially prone to dysrhythmias and other problems related to vagal stimulation; monitor heart rate and rhythm closely.
- At least 28% of older adults are constipated as a result of insufficient dietary bulk, inadequate fluid intake, laxative abuse, diminished muscle tone and motor function, decreased defecation reflex, mental or physical illness, and presence of tumors (Ebersole and others, 2008).
- For older adults, instituting a diet adequate in dietary fiber (6 to 10 g/day) adds bulk, weight, and form to stool and improves defecation (Ebersole and others, 2008).
- Consider development of regular toileting routine that includes responding to the urge to defecate.

Home Care

- Consider having patient or family member keep a week's diary of meals and fluid intake. Determine if dietary pattern contributes to constipation. Recommend a diet adequate in fiber that includes patient's food choices.
- Have patient or family caregiver maintain a weekly bowel diary.
- Individualized bowel programs developed following a stroke, brain, or spinal cord injury help reduce the occurrence of constipation and subsequent impaction.

SKILL 19.2 ADMINISTERING AN ENEMA

- **Nursing Skills Online: Bowel Elimination Module, Lesson 2**

Video Clips

An enema is the instillation of a solution into the rectum and sigmoid colon to promote defecation by stimulating peristalsis. They are used to treat constipation or empty the bowel before diagnostic procedures or abdominal surgeries. Preoperative enemas are common for some surgeries. Teach your patients not to rely on enemas to maintain bowel regularity because they do not treat the cause of irregularity or constipation. Frequent enemas disrupt normal defecation reflexes, resulting in dependence on them for elimination.

Cleansing enemas promote complete evacuation of feces from the colon. They act by stimulating peristalsis through infusion of a large volume of solution or through irritation of the colon mucosa. Each solution influences the movement of fluids in the colon. When "enemas until clear" is ordered in preparation for surgery or diagnostic testing, the water expelled may be colored but should not contain solid fecal material. When administering "enemas until clear," patients usually receive only three consecutive enemas to prevent fluid and electrolyte imbalance (check agency policy).

Medicated enemas contain pharmacological agents to reduce dangerously high serum potassium levels (e.g., sodium polystyrene sulfonate [Kayexalate] enema) or to reduce bacteria in the colon before bowel surgery (e.g., neomycin enema).

A carminative enema such as the Harris or return-flow enema relieves accumulated flatus. Always administer a small amount (100 to 200 mL) of enema solution into the patient's rectum and colon. As the container is lowered, the solution flows back through the enema tubing to the container. Flatus also returns. You can slowly repeat raising and lowering the container numerous times to reduce flatus and increase peristalsis.

The volume or type of fluid that breaks up the fecal mass stretches the rectal wall and initiates the defecation reflex. Common types of enemas include:

- *Tap water (hypotonic) enema* should not be repeated after first installation because water toxicity or circulatory overload can develop. *Normal saline* is safest. Infants and children can tolerate only normal saline because of their predisposition to fluid imbalance. A *hypertonic solution* (e.g., commercially prepared Fleet enema) is useful for patients who cannot tolerate large volumes of fluid. Only 120 to 180 mL (4 to 6 ounces) is usually effective.
- *Harris flush enema* is a return-flow enema that helps to expel intestinal gas. Fluid alternately flows into and out of the large intestine. This stimulates peristalsis in the large intestine and assists in expelling gas.
- *Soapsuds enema* is pure castile soap added to either tap water or normal saline, depending on patient's condition and frequency of administration. Use *only* castile pure soap. Recommended ratio of pure soap to

solution is 5 mL (1 teaspoon) to 1000 mL (1 quart) warm water or saline. Add soap to enema bag *after* water is in place to reduce excessive suds.
- *Oil-retention enema* uses an oil-based solution. The colon absorbs a small volume, which allows the oil to soften stool for easier evacuation.
- *Carminative solution* provides relief from gaseous distention. An example is MGW solution, which contains 30 mL of magnesium, 60 mL of glycerin, and 90 mL of water.

ASSESSMENT

1. Review health care provider's order for enema and clarify reason for enema administration. *Rationale: Order by health care provider is required for hospitalized patient. The order states the type of enema and how many enemas patient will receive.*
2. Determine patient's level of understanding of purpose of enema. *Rationale: Allows nurse to provide adequate instruction.*
3. Inspect abdomen for distention and auscultate for bowel sounds. *Rationale: Provides baseline to evaluate response to enema.*
4. Assess medical record for presence of increased intracranial pressure; cardiac disease; glaucoma; or recent abdominal, rectal, or prostate surgery. *Rationale: Conditions contraindicate use of enemas.*
5. Assess last bowel movement, normal versus recent bowel elimination pattern, presence of hemorrhoids, mobility, and presence of abdominal pain or cramping. *Rationale: Determines factors indicating need for enema and influences type of enema used. Also establishes baseline for bowel function. Hemorrhoids may obscure the rectal opening and cause discomfort or bleeding with evacuation.*

PLANNING

Expected Outcomes focus on establishing a normal pattern of bowel elimination and normal consistency of stools.

1. Stool is evacuated.
2. Enema return is clear.
3. Abdomen is soft and nondistended.

Delegation and Collaboration

The skill of enema administration can be delegated to nursing assistive personnel (NAP). Instruct the NAP about the following:

- How to properly position patients with therapeutic equipment such as drains, IV catheters, or traction
- How to properly position patients with mobility restrictions
- Informing the nurse immediately about the presence of blood in the stool or around rectal area, any change in vital signs, abdominal pain, abdominal cramping, or distention

Equipment

- Clean gloves
- Water-soluble lubricant
- Waterproof absorbent underpads
- Toilet tissue
- Bedpan, bedside commode, or access to toilet
- Washbasin, washcloths, towel, and soap
- Bath blanket
- IV pole

Enema bag administration

- Enema container (Fig. 19-2)
- Tubing and clamp (if not already attached to container)
- Appropriate-size rectal tube (adult: 22 to 30 Fr.; child 12 to 18 Fr)
- Correct volume of warmed (tepid) solution (adult: 750 to 1000 mL; adolescent: 500 to 700 mL; school-age child: 300 to 500 mL; toddler: 250 to 350 mL; infant: 150 to 250 mL)

Prepackaged enema

- Prepackaged enema container with rectal tip (Fig. 19-3)

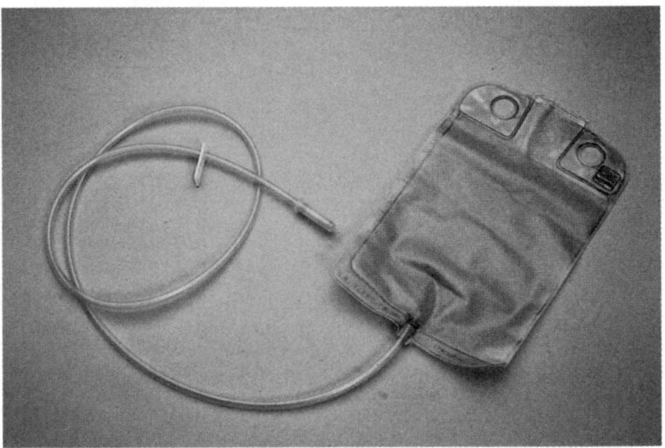

FIG 19-2 Enema bag with tubing.

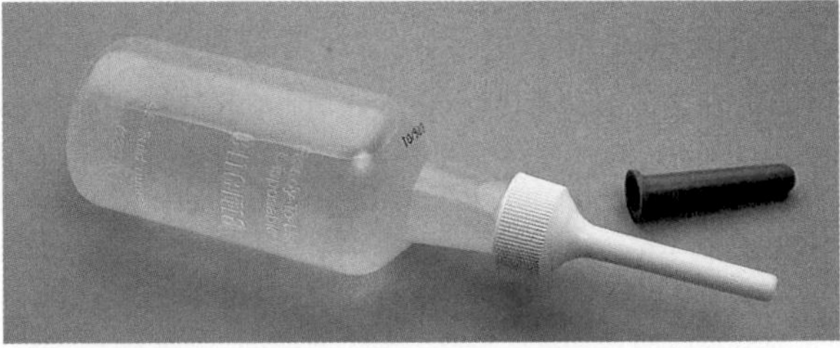

FIG 19-3 Prepackaged enema container with rectal tip and cap.

IMPLEMENTATION *for* ADMINISTERING AN ENEMA

STEPS	RATIONALE
1. **See Standard Protocol (inside front cover).**	
2. Check accuracy and completeness of each medication administration record (MAR) with health care provider's written medication or procedure order. Check patient's name, type of enema, and time for administration. Compare MAR with label of enema solution.	The order sheet is the most reliable source and only legal record of drugs or procedure the patient is to receive. Ensures that patient receives correct medication.
3. Identify patient using two identifiers (e.g., name and birthday or name and account number, according to facility policy). If medicated enema is to be given, compare identifiers with information on patient's MAR or medical record.	Ensures correct patient. Complies with The Joint Commission standards and improves patient safety (TJC, 2010).
4. Assist patient into left side-lying (Sims') position with right knee flexed. Encourage patient to remain in position until procedure is completed. Children are also positioned in dorsal recumbent position.	Allows enema solution to flow downward by gravity along natural curve of sigmoid colon and rectum, thus improving retention of solution.

SAFETY ALERT Patients with poor sphincter control require placement of a bedpan under the buttocks. Administering enema with patient sitting on toilet is unsafe because curved rectal tubing can abrade rectal wall.

STEPS	RATIONALE
5. Place waterproof pad absorbent side up under hips and buttocks.	Prevents soiling linen.
6. Cover patient with bath blanket, exposing only rectal area and allowing anus to be visualized clearly.	Provides warmth, reduces exposure of body parts, and allows patient to feel more relaxed and comfortable. Provides access to anus.
7. Separate buttocks and examine perianal region for abnormalities, including hemorrhoids, anal fissure, and rectal prolapse.	Findings influence nurse's approach to insertion of enema tip. Rectal prolapse contraindicates an enema. Hemorrhoids can obscure anal opening.
8. Place bedpan or commode in easily accessible position. If patient will be expelling contents into toilet, ensure that toilet is available and place patient's slippers and bathrobe in easily accessible location.	Bedpan is used if patient unable to get out of bed.
9. Administer enema.	
a. ***Administer prepackaged disposable enema.***	
(1) Remove plastic cap from tip of container. Tip may already be lubricated. Apply more water-soluble lubricant if needed.	Lubrication provides for smooth insertion of tip without rectal irritation or trauma.
(2) Gently separate buttocks and locate anus. Instruct patient to relax by breathing out slowly through mouth.	Breathing out promotes relaxation of external rectal sphincter. Presence of hemorrhoids obscures location of anus.
(3) Expel any air from enema container.	Air entering colon from the enema container causes further distention and discomfort.

Continued

STEPS	RATIONALE
(4) Insert lubricated tip of container gently into anal canal toward umbilicus (see illustration). *Adult:* 7.5 to 10 cm (3 to 4 inches) *Adolescent:* 7.5 to 10 cm (3 to 4 inches) *Child:* 5 to 7.5 cm (2 to 3 inches) *Infant:* 2.5 to 3.5 cm (1 to 1½ inches)	Gentle insertion prevents trauma to rectal mucosa.
(5) Roll plastic bottle from bottom to tip until all of solution has entered rectum and colon. Instruct patient to retain solution for 2 to 5 minutes until urge to defecate.	Hypertonic solutions require only small volumes to stimulate defecation. Intermittent squeezing results in return of solution to bottle.
b. Administer enema in standard enema bag.	
(1) Add warmed solution to enema bag: Warm tap water as it flows from faucet, place saline solution in basin of warm water before adding saline solution to enema bag, and check temperature of solution by pouring small amount of solution over inner wrist.	Hot water can burn intestinal mucosa. Cold water can cause abdominal cramping and is difficult to retain.
(2) If soap suds enema is ordered, add castile soap after the water.	Prevents suds in enema bag.
(3) Raise container, release clamp, and allow solution to flow long enough to fill tubing.	Removes air from tubing.
(4) Reclamp tubing.	
(5) Lubricate 6 to 8 cm (2½ to 3 inches) of tip of tubing with lubricant.	Eases tube insertion through anus.
(6) Gently separate buttocks and locate anus. Instruct patient to relax by breathing out slowly through mouth.	Breathing out promotes relaxation of external anal sphincter.
(7) Insert tip of rectal tube slowly by pointing tip in direction of patient's umbilicus. Length of insertion varies (see Step 9a(4)).	Careful insertion prevents trauma to rectal mucosa from accidental lodging of tube against rectal wall. Forceful insertion beyond recommended length can cause bowel perforation.

SAFETY ALERT If tube does not pass easily, do not force. Consider allowing a small amount of fluid to infuse and trying to slowly reinsert tube. The instillation of fluid may relax the sphincter and provide added lubrication.

STEPS	RATIONALE
(8) Hold tubing in rectum constantly until end of fluid instillation.	Bowel contraction can cause expulsion of rectal tube.
(9) Open regulating clamp and allow solution to enter slowly with container at patient's hip level.	Rapid infusion can stimulate evacuation of tubing and cause cramping.
(10) Raise height of enema container slowly to appropriate level above anus: 30 to 45 cm (12 to 18 inches) for high enema; 30 cm (12 inches) for regular enema (see illustration); 7.5 cm (3 inches) for low enema. Instillation time varies with volume of solution administered (e.g., 1 L may take 10 minutes). Hang container on IV pole.	Allows for continuous, slow instillation of solution. Raising container too high causes rapid infusion and possible painful distention of colon. High pressure can cause rupture of bowel in infant.

SAFETY ALERT Temporary cessation of infusion minimizes cramping and promotes ability to retain all the solution. Lower container or clamp tubing if patient complains of abdominal cramping or if fluid escapes around rectal tube.

STEPS	RATIONALE
(11) Instill all solution and clamp the tubing. Tell patient that the procedure is completed and that you will be removing the rectal tube.	Prevents entrance of air into rectum. Patients may misinterpret the sensation of removing the tube as loss of control.
10. Place layers of toilet tissue around tube at anus and gently remove tubing.	Provides for patient's comfort and cleanliness.
11. Explain to patient that feeling of distention is normal. Ask patient to retain solution as long as possible until urge to defecate occurs. This usually takes only a few minutes. Stay at bedside. Have patient lie quietly in bed if possible. (For infant or young child gently hold buttocks together for a few minutes.)	Solution distends bowel. Length of retention varies with type of enema and patient's ability to contract rectal sphincter. Longer retention promotes more effective stimulation of peristalsis and defecation.
12. Assist patient to bathroom or commode if possible. If using the bedpan, assist to as near the normal position for evacuation as possible.	Normal squatting position promotes defecation.
13. Observe character of stool and solution passed (caution patient against flushing toilet before inspection).	Determines if enema was effective.
14. Assist patient as needed to wash anal area with warm soap and water.	Fecal contents can irritate skin. Hygiene promotes patient's comfort.
15. See Completion Protocol (inside front cover).	

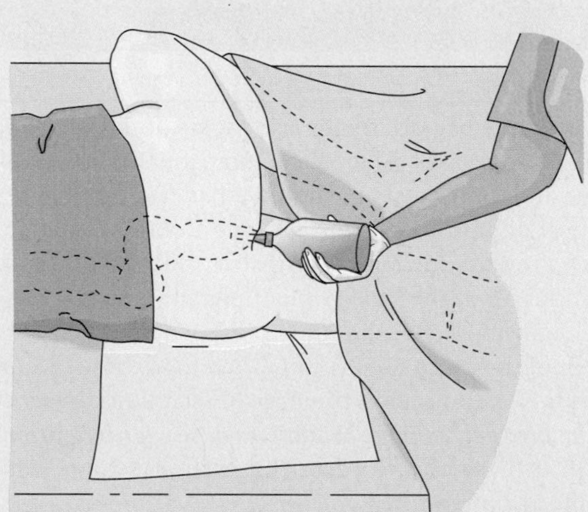

STEP 9a(4) With patient in left lateral Sims position, insert the tip of the commercial enema into the rectum. (From Sorrentino SA: *Mosby's textbook for nursing assistants,* ed 6, St Louis, 2006, Mosby.)

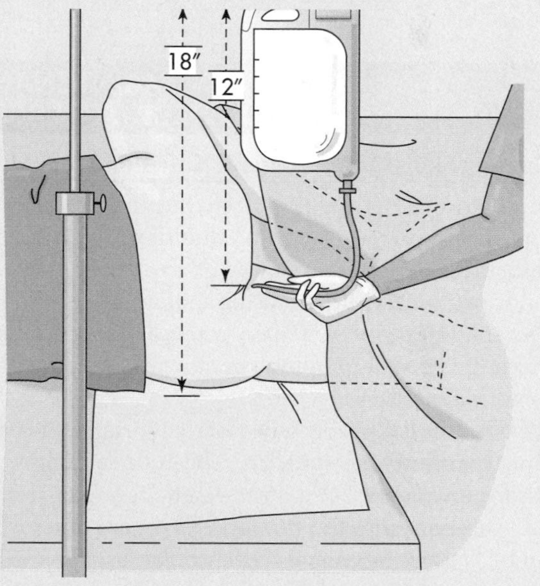

STEP 9b(10) The IV pole is positioned so the enema bag is 30 cm (12 inches) above the anus and approximately 45 cm (18 inches) above the mattress (depending on patients' size). (Adapted from Sorrentino SA: *Mosby's textbook for nursing assistants,* ed 7, St Louis, 2008, Mosby.)

EVALUATION

1. Ask patient if abdominal discomfort was relieved.
2. Inspect color, consistency, and amount of stool; odor; and characteristics of fluid passed.
3. Assess for abdominal distention.

Unexpected Outcomes and Related Interventions

1. Patient is unable to hold enema solution.
   a. If this occurs during instillation, slow rate of infusion.
   b. Position on bedpan while administering the solution.
2. Severe cramping, bleeding, or sudden severe abdominal pain occurs and is unrelieved by temporarily stopping or slowing flow of solution.
   a. Stop enema.
   b. Notify health care provider.
3. With an order for "enemas until clear," after three enemas the water is highly colored or contains solid fecal material.
   a. Notify health care provider.

Recording and Reporting

- Record the time, type, and volume of enema administered; patient's signs and symptoms; response to enema; and results, including color, amount, and appearance of stool.
- Report failure of patient to defecate or any adverse reactions.

Sample Documentation

2000 Last bowel movement 5 days ago. Complains of abdominal fullness and rectal pressure. Abdomen distended, firm; 1000-mL soap suds enema given with "mild" abdominal cramping during administration. Solution returned with large amount of dark-brown, soft-formed stool.

2100 States, "I feel better now." Abdomen soft, nondistended. Resting in bed with side rails up × 2.

Special Considerations

Pediatric

- The use of oral stool softeners is the initial recommended treatment of constipation in children.

Geriatric

- Older adults may tire more quickly and are at greater risk for fluid and electrolyte imbalances; use caution when administering enemas "until clear."
- Teach older adults and their caregivers dietary and activity measures to avoid constipation.
- Older adults may have difficulty in retaining enema solution.

Home Care

- Assess patient's and family caregiver's ability and motivation to administer enema in the home and provide instruction as needed.
- Assess patient's ability to manipulate equipment to self-administer enema.
- Instruct patient and family caregiver not to exceed number and volume of enemas.

SKILL 19.3 INSERTION, MAINTENANCE, AND REMOVAL OF A NASOGASTRIC TUBE FOR GASTRIC DECOMPRESSION

- **Nursing Skills Online: Enteral Nutrition Module, Lesson 2**

At times normal peristalsis is altered temporarily, either following major surgery or from conditions affecting the GI tract. Because peristalsis is slowed or absent, a patient cannot eat or drink fluids without causing abdominal distention. The temporary insertion of a nasogastric (NG) tube into the stomach serves to decompress the stomach, keeping it empty until normal peristalsis returns.

An NG tube is a pliable tube inserted through the patient's nasopharynx into the stomach. The tube is hollow, which allows for the removal of gastric secretions and the introduction of solutions into the stomach. There are times when an NG tube is used for enteral feedings, but a softer small-bore feeding tube is preferred for feeding purposes (see Chapter 12). The Levin and Salem sump tubes are the most common for stomach decompression. The Levin tube is a single-lumen tube with holes near the tip (Fig. 19-4). You connect the tube to a drainage bag or an intermittent suction device to drain stomach secretions. The Salem sump tube is preferable for stomach decompression. The tube has two lumina: one for removal of gastric contents and one to provide an air vent, which prevents suctioning of gastric mucosa into eyelets at the distal tip of the tube. A blue "pigtail" is the air vent that connects with the second lumen (Fig. 19-5). When the main lumen of the sump tube is connected to suction, the air vent permits free, continuous drainage of secretions. ***Never clamp off the air vent, connect to suction, or use for irrigation.*** The health care provider orders the suction setting, which is usually low intermittent.

NG tube insertion uses clean technique. The procedure is uncomfortable, with patients experiencing a burning sensation as the tube passes through the sensitive nasal mucosa. One of the greatest nursing care challenges is keeping the patient comfortable because the tube is a constant irritation to mucosa. Routinely assess the condition of the naris and

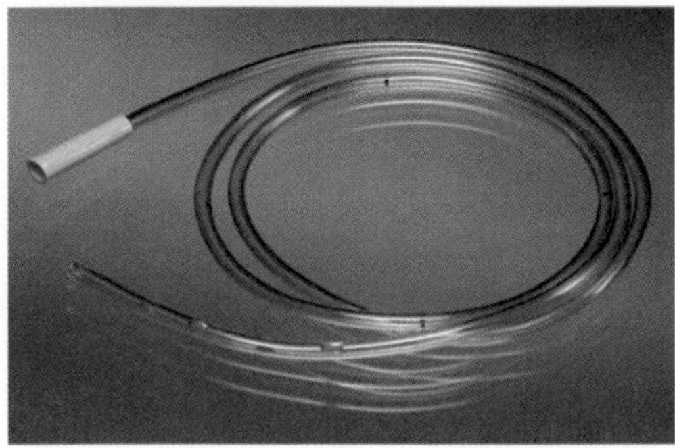

FIG 19-4 Levin tube. (Courtesy Bard Medical, Covington, Ga.)

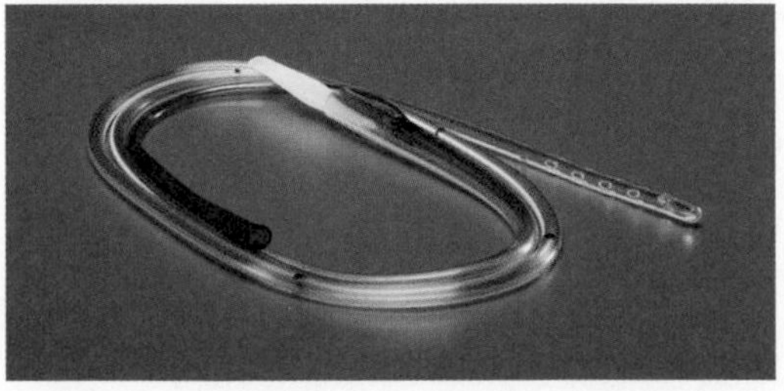

FIG 19-5 Salem sump tube. (Copyright © 2010 Covidien. All rights reserved. Used with permission of Covidien.)

mucosa for inflammation and excoriation. Supportive care includes changing soiled tape or fixation devices, keeping the naris lubricated and clean, and providing frequent mouth care to minimize dehydration from mouth breathing.

ASSESSMENT

1. Inspect condition of patient's nasal and oral cavity. *Rationale: Determines need for special nursing hygiene measures after tube placement.*
2. Ask if patient has had history of nasal surgery or congestion and allergies and note if deviated nasal septum is present. *Rationale: Alerts nurse of potential obstruction. Insert tube into uninvolved nasal passage. Procedure may be contraindicated if surgery is recent.*
3. Auscultate for bowel sounds. Palpate patient's abdomen for distention, pain, and rigidity. *Rationale: Bowel sounds are generalized, so most often they can be assessed by listening in one place (Seidel and others, 2011). This documents baseline for any abdominal distention, gastrointestinal ileus, or general GI function and later serves as comparison once tube is inserted.*
4. Assess patient's level of consciousness and ability to follow instructions. *Rationale: Determines patient's ability to assist in procedure.*

> **SAFETY ALERT** If patient is confused, disoriented, or unable to follow commands, obtain assistance from another staff member to insert the tube.

5. Determine if patient had previous NG tube and which naris was used. *Rationale: Patient's previous experience complements any explanations and prepares patient for NG tube placement.*
6. Verify order for type of NG tube to be placed and whether tube is to be attached to suction or drainage bag. *Rationale: Requires an order from health care provider. Adequate decompression depends on NG suction.*

PLANNING

Expected Outcomes focus on decompression of the stomach, comfort, adequacy of fluid volume, and prevention of complications related to NG intubation.

1. Abdomen is soft without distention.
2. Patient's level of comfort improves or remains the same.
3. NG tube remains patent.
4. Patient's nasal mucosa is moist and intact.

Delegation and Collaboration

The skill of inserting and maintaining an NG tube cannot be delegated to nursing assistive personnel (NAP). Instruct the NAP about the following:

- When to measure and record the drainage from an NG tube
- How often to provide oral hygiene
- Selected comfort measures such as positioning or offering ice chips if allowed
- How to anchor the tube to the patient's gown during routine care to prevent accidental displacement

Equipment

- 14 or 16 Fr NG tube (smaller-lumen catheters are not used for decompression in adults because they must be able to remove thick secretions)
- Water-soluble lubricating jelly
- pH test strips (measure gastric aspirate acidity)
- Tongue blade
- Flashlight
- Emesis basin
- Asepto bulb or catheter-tipped syringe
- 2.5-cm (1-inch) wide hypoallergenic tape or commercial fixation device
- Safety pin and rubber band
- Clamp, drainage bag, or suction machine or pressure gauge if wall suction is to be used
- Towel
- Glass of water with straw
- Facial tissues
- Normal saline
- Tincture of benzoin (optional)
- Suction equipment
- Clean gloves

IMPLEMENTATION *for* INSERTION, MAINTENANCE, AND REMOVAL OF A NASOGASTRIC TUBE FOR GASTRIC DECOMPRESSION

STEPS	RATIONALE
1. **See Standard Protocol (inside front cover).**	
2. Identify patient using two identifiers (e.g., name and birthday or name and account number, according to facility policy).	Ensures correct patient. Complies with The Joint Commission standards and improves patient safety (TJC, 2010).

Continued

STEPS	RATIONALE
3. Place patient in high-Fowler's position. Place pillows behind head and shoulders. Raise bed to horizontal level comfortable for nurse.	Promotes patient's ability to swallow during procedure.
4. Place bath towel over patient's chest; give facial tissues to patient. Place emesis basin within reach.	Prevents soiling patient's gown. Tube insertion through nasal passages may cause tearing and coughing with increased salivation.
5. Wash bridge of nose with soap and water or alcohol swab.	Removes oils from nose to allow tape to adhere.
6. Stand on patient's right side if right-handed, left side if left-handed.	Allows easiest manipulation of tubing.
7. Instruct patient to relax and breathe normally while occluding one naris. Then have him or her repeat action for other naris. Select nostril with greater airflow.	Tube passes more easily through naris that is more patent.
8. Measure distance to insert tube:	
a. *Traditional method:* Measure distance from tip of nose to earlobe to xiphoid process (see illustration).	Tube extends from naris to stomach; distance varies with each patient.
b. *Hanson method:* First mark 50-cm (20-inch) point on tube and then measure traditionally. Tube insertion is a midway point between 50 cm (20 inches) and traditional mark.	
9. With a small piece of tape placed around tube, mark length that you will insert.	Indicates amount of tube to be inserted.
10. Curve 10 to 15 cm (4 to 6 inches) of end of tube tightly around index finger and release.	Aids insertion and decreases stiffness of tube.
11. Lubricate 7.5 to 10 cm (3 to 4 inches) of end of tube with water-soluble lubricating gel.	Minimizes friction against nasal mucosa and aids insertion of tube. Water-soluble lubricant is less toxic than oil-soluble lubricant if aspirated.
12. Alert patient when procedure will begin.	Decreases patient anxiety and increases patient cooperation.
13. Initially instruct patient to extend neck back against pillow; insert tube slowly through naris with curved end pointing downward (see illustration).	Facilitates initial passage of tube through naris and maintains clear airway for open naris.

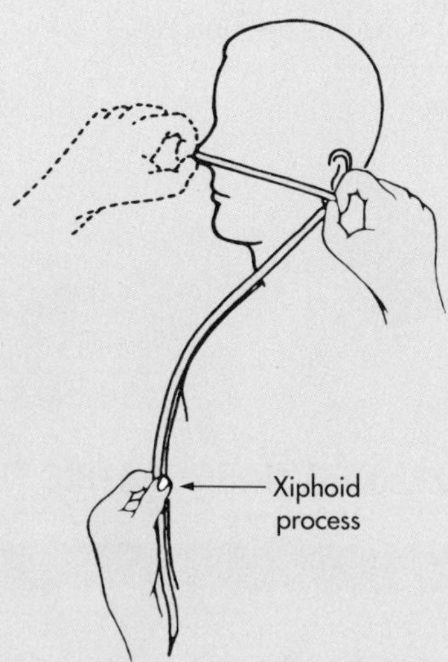

STEP 8a Technique for measuring distance to insert nasogastric tube.

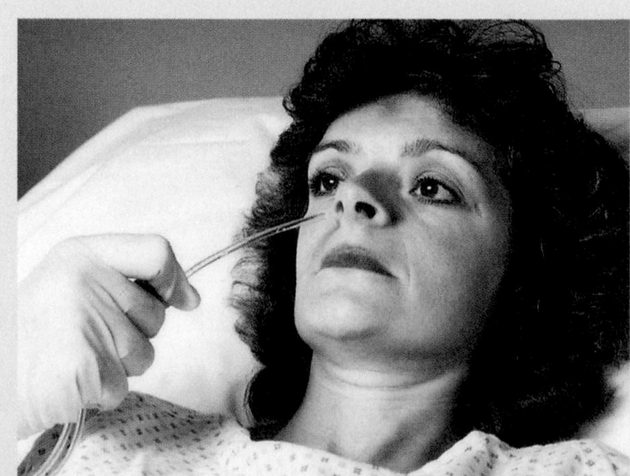

STEP 13 Insert nasogastric tube with curved end pointing downward.

STEPS	RATIONALE
14. Continue to pass tube along floor of nasal passage, aiming down toward ear. When you feel resistance, apply gentle downward pressure to advance tube (do not force past resistance).	Minimizes discomfort of tube rubbing against upper nasal turbinates. Resistance caused by posterior nasopharynx. Downward pressure helps tube curl around corner of nasopharynx.
15. If you meet continued resistance, try to rotate tube and see if it advances. If still resistant, withdraw tube, allow patient to rest, lubricate tube again, and insert into other naris.	Forcing against resistance causes trauma to mucosa. Allowing patient to rest helps relieve anxiety.

SAFETY ALERT If unable to insert tube in either naris, stop procedure and notify health care provider.

STEPS	RATIONALE
16. Continue insertion of tube until just past nasopharynx by gently rotating tube toward opposite naris.	
a. Once past nasopharynx, stop tube advancement, allow patient to relax, and provide tissues.	Relieves patient's anxiety; tearing is natural response to mucosal irritation, and excessive salivation may occur because of oral stimulation.
b. Explain to patient that next step requires that patient swallow. Give patient glass of water unless contraindicated.	Sipping water aids passage of NG tube into esophagus.
17. With tube just above oropharynx, instruct patient to flex head forward, take a small sip of water, and swallow. Advance tube 2.5 to 5 cm (1 to 2 inches) with each swallow of water. If patient is not allowed fluids, instruct to dry swallow or suck air through straw. Advance tube with each swallow.	Flexed position closes off upper airway to trachea and opens esophagus. Swallowing closes epiglottis over trachea and helps move tube into esophagus. Swallowing water reduces gagging or choking. Remove water from stomach by suction after insertion.
18. If patient begins to cough, gag, or choke, withdraw slightly and stop tube advancement. Instruct patient to breathe easily and take sips of water.	Cough reflex is initiated when tube accidentally enters larynx. Withdrawal of the tube reduces risk of laryngeal entry. Small sips of water frequently reduce gagging. Give water cautiously to reduce the risk of aspiration.

SAFETY ALERT If vomiting occurs, assist patient in clearing airway. Perform oral suctioning as needed.

STEPS	RATIONALE
19. If patient continues to cough during insertion, pull tube back slightly.	Tube may enter larynx and obstruct airway.
20. If patient continues to gag and cough or complains that tube feels as though it is coiling behind throat, check back of oropharynx using flashlight and tongue blade. Withdraw tube until tip is back in oropharynx if coiled. Then reinsert with patient swallowing.	Tube may coil around itself in the back of the throat and stimulate gag reflex.
21. After patient relaxes, continue to advance tube with swallowing until you reach tape or mark on tube, which signifies that tube is in the desired distance. Temporarily anchor tube to patient's cheek with piece of tape until tube placement is verified.	Tip of tube needs to be within stomach to decompress properly. Anchoring tube prevents accidental displacement while tube placement is verified.
22. Verify tube placement: Check agency policy for recommended methods of checking tube placement.	
a. Ask patient to talk.	Patient is unable to talk if NG tube has passed through vocal cords.
b. Inspect posterior pharynx for presence of coiled tube.	Tube is pliable and can coil up in back of the pharynx instead of advancing into esophagus.

Continued

STEPS	RATIONALE
c. Attach Asepto or catheter-tipped syringe to end of tube. Aspirate gently back on syringe to obtain gastric contents, observing color (see illustration).	Observation of gastric contents is useful to determine initial tube placement (Metheny and others, 2007). Contents are usually cloudy and green but are sometimes off-white, tan, bloody, or brown in color. Other common aspirate colors include yellow or bile stained (duodenal placement) or possibly saliva-appearing (esophagus).

SAFETY ALERT Aspiration of pale yellow fluid from a newly inserted tube is a signal of possible placement in the respiratory tract; placement of tube is always confirmed by radiography (Metheny and others, 2007).

STEPS	RATIONALE
d. Use gastric (Gastroccult) pH test paper to measure aspirate for pH with color-coded pH paper. Be sure that paper range of pH is at least from 1 to 11 (see illustration).	Gastric aspirates have decidedly acidic pH values, preferably 4 or less, compared with intestinal aspirates, which are usually greater than 4, or respiratory secretions, which are usually greater than 5.5.
e. Obtain x-ray film examination of chest and abdomen.	Radiography is the gold standard for verification of initial placement of the tube. This must be done before any medication or liquid is administered (Metheny and others, 2007).
f. If tube is not in stomach, advance another 2.5 to 5 cm (1 to 2 inches) and repeat Steps 22a to 22d to check initial tube position and verify with radiography.	Tube must be in stomach to provide decompression.
23. Anchor tube.	
a. Clamp end of tube or connect tube to drainage bag or suction machine after properly inserted.	Use gravity for drainage bag. Intermittent suction is most effective for decompression. Patient going to operating room often has tube clamped.
b. Tape tube to nose; avoid putting pressure on naris.	Prevent tissue necrosis. Tape anchors tube securely.
(1) Cut a strip of tape about 10 cm (5 inches) and split down the middle halfway.	
(2) Apply small amount of tincture of benzoin to lower end of nose and allow drying before taping tube to nose (optional).	Benzoin prevents loosening of tape if patient perspires or has oily skin.
(3) Apply tape to nose, leaving split end free. Be sure that top end of tape over nose is secure.	
(4) Carefully wrap two split ends of tape around tube in opposite directions (see illustration).	

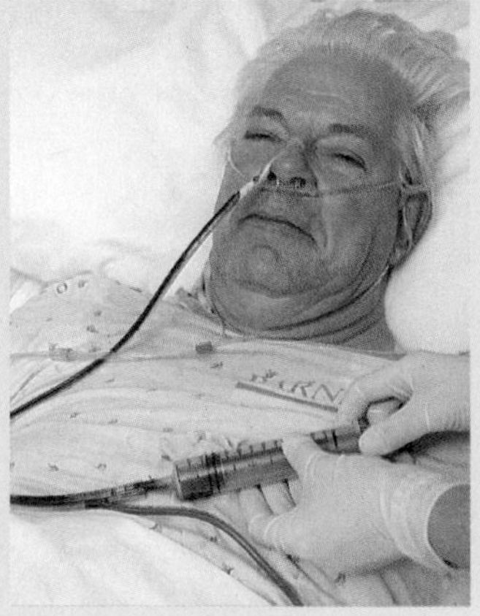

STEP 22c Aspiration of gastric contents.

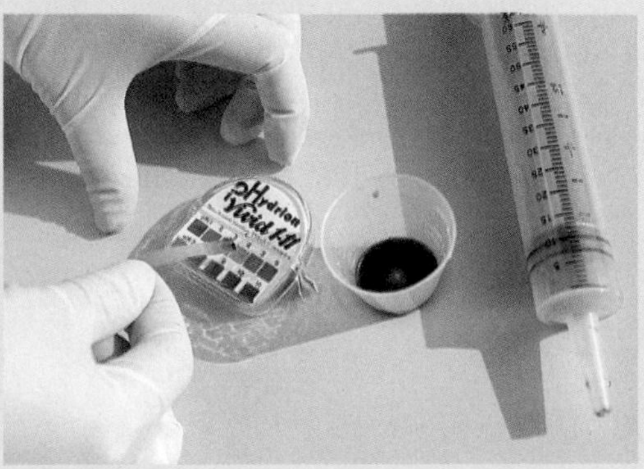

STEP 22d Checking pH of gastric contents.

STEPS	RATIONALE
(5) Alternative: Apply tube fixation device using shaped adhesive patch (see illustration).	
c. Fasten end of NG tube to patient's gown by looping rubber band around tube in slipknot. Pin rubber band to gown.	Reduces pressure on naris if tube moves. Provides slack for movement without dislodging the NG tube.
d. When using a Salem sump tube, keep pigtail above level of stomach.	Prevents siphoning action that clogs the tube.
e. Unless health care provider orders otherwise, elevate head of bed 30 degrees.	Helps prevent esophageal reflux and minimizes irritation of tube against posterior pharynx.
f. Explain to patient that sensation of tube decreases somewhat with time.	Helps patient to adapt to continued sensory stimulus.
24. Once placement is confirmed:	
a. Place a mark, either a red ink mark or tape, on tube to indicate where tube exits nose.	The mark on tube is a guide to indicate if tube remains in correct position.
b. Alternative: Measure length of tube from naris to connector.	
c. Document length of tube in patient's record.	Information assists in determining tube placement.

SAFETY ALERT Never reposition an NG tube of a gastric surgical patient since positioning can rupture the suture line.

STEPS	RATIONALE
25. Attach NG tube to suction as ordered.	Suction setting is usually ordered low intermittent, which decreases gastric irritation from NG tube.

SAFETY ALERT If lumen of tube is narrow and secretions are thick, NG will not drain as desired. Irrigate tube (see Step 26). Consult with health care provider for higher suction setting if unable to irrigate tube because of thick secretions.

STEPS	RATIONALE
26. ***NG tube irrigation:***	
a. 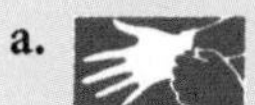 Perform hand hygiene.	Reduces transmission of microorganisms.
b. Check for tube placement in stomach (see Step 22). Then temporarily clamp tube or reconnect to connecting tube and remove syringe.	Prevents accidental entrance of irrigating solution into lungs.
c. Use same syringe to draw up 30 mL of normal saline.	Use of saline minimizes loss of electrolytes from stomach fluids.

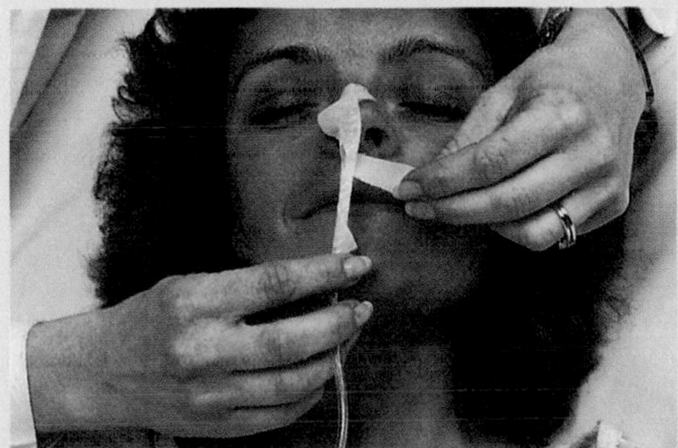

STEP 23b(4) Tape is crossed over and around nasogastric tube.

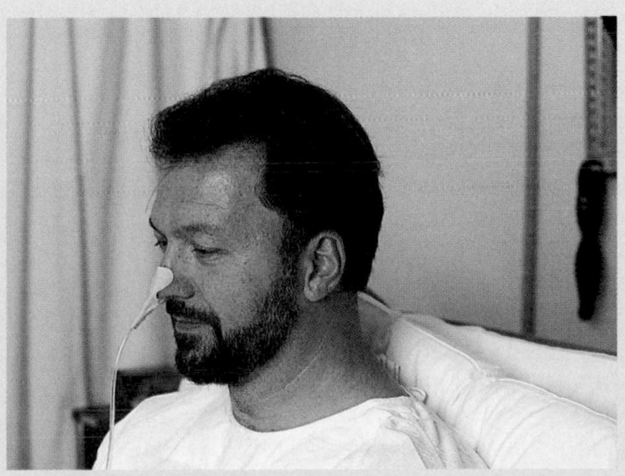

STEP 23b(5) Patient with tube fixation device.

Continued

STEPS	RATIONALE
d. Clamp NG tube. Disconnect from connection tubing and lay end of connection tubing on towel.	Reduces soiling of patient's gown and bed linen.
e. Insert tip of irrigating syringe into end of NG tube. Remove clamp. Hold syringe with tip pointed at floor and inject saline slowly and evenly. Do not force solution.	Position of syringe prevents introduction of air into vent tubing, which causes gastric distention. Solution introduced under pressure causes gastric trauma.

SAFETY ALERT Do not introduce saline through blue "pigtail" air vent of Salem sump tube.

STEPS	RATIONALE
f. If resistance occurs, check for kinks in tubing. Turn patient onto left side. Report repeated resistance to health care provider.	Tip of tube may lie against stomach lining. Repositioning on left side may dislodge tube away from the stomach lining. Buildup of secretions causes distention.
g. After instilling saline, immediately aspirate or pull back slowly on syringe to withdraw fluid. If amount aspirated is greater than amount instilled, record difference as output. If amount aspirated is less than amount instilled, record difference as intake.	Irrigation clears tubing; thus the stomach remains empty. Measure and document irrigation inserted in tube as intake.
h. Use an Asepto syringe to place 10 mL of air into blue pigtail of Salem sump tube.	Ensures patency of air vent.
i. Reconnect NG tube to drainage or suction. (Repeat irrigation if solution does not return.)	Reestablishes drainage collection; may repeat irrigation or repositioning of tube until NG tube drains properly.
27. ***Removal of NG tube:***	
a. Verify order to remove NG tube.	An order is required for procedure.
b. Explain procedure to patient and reassure that removal is less distressing than insertion.	Minimizes anxiety and increases cooperation. Tube passes out smoothly.
c. Perform hand hygiene.	Reduces transmission of microorganisms.
d. Turn off suction and disconnect NG tube from drainage bag or suction. Take irrigating syringe and insert 20 mL of air into lumen of NG tube. Remove tape or fixation device from bridge of nose and unpin tube from gown.	Have tube free of connections before removal. Clears gastric fluids from tube to prevent aspirating contents or soiling clothing and bedding.
e. Stand on patient's right side if right-handed, left side if left-handed.	Allows easiest manipulation of tube.
f. Hand patient facial tissue; place clean towel across chest. Instruct patient to take and hold breath.	Some patients wish to blow nose after tube is removed. Towel keeps gown from soil. Temporary airway obstruction occurs during tube removal.
g. Clamp or kink tubing securely and pull tube out steadily and smoothly into towel held in other hand while patient holds breath.	Clamping prevents tube contents from draining into oropharynx. Reduces trauma to mucosa and minimizes patient's discomfort. Towel covers tube, which is an unpleasant sight. Holding breath helps to prevent aspiration.
h. Inspect intactness of tube.	
i. Measure amount of drainage and note character of content. Dispose of tube and drainage equipment into proper container.	Provides accurate measure of fluid output. Reduces transfer of microorganisms.
j. Clean naris and provide mouth care.	Promotes comfort.
k. Position patient comfortably and explain procedure for drinking fluids if not contraindicated. Instruct patient to notify you if nausea occurs.	Sometimes patients are not allowed anything by mouth (NPO) for up to 24 hours. When fluids are allowed, orders usually begin with small amount of ice chips each hour, and amounts are increased as patient is able to tolerate more.
28. See Completion Protocol (inside front cover).	

EVALUATION

1. Observe amount and character of contents draining from NG tube. Ask if patient feels nauseated.
2. Auscultate for presence of bowel sounds, being sure to turn off suction. Palpate patient's abdomen periodically. Note any distention, pain, and rigidity.
3. Inspect condition of naris and nose.
4. Observe position of tubing.
5. Ask if patient feels sore throat or irritation in pharynx.

Unexpected Outcomes and Related Interventions

1. Patient's abdomen is distended and painful.
   a. Assess patency of tube. NG may not be in stomach or it may be kinked and not draining.
   b. Irrigate tube.
   c. Verify that suction is on as ordered.
2. Patient complains of sore throat from dry, irritated mucous membranes.
   a. Perform oral hygiene more frequently.
   b. Ask health care provider whether patient can suck on ice chips or throat lozenges or if a local anesthetic medication can be used.
3. Patient develops irritation or erosion of skin around naris.
   a. Provide frequent skin care to area.
   b. Tape tube on naris to avoid pressure.
   c. Consider switching tube to other naris.
4. Patient develops signs and symptoms of pulmonary aspiration: fever, shortness of breath, or pulmonary congestion.
   a. Perform complete respiratory assessment.
   b. Notify health care provider.
   c. Obtain chest x-ray film examination as ordered.

Recording and Reporting

- Record length, size, type of gastric tube inserted, and naris in which tube was introduced. Also record patient's tolerance of procedure, confirmation of tube placement, character of gastric contents, results of x-ray film, pH value, whether the tube is clamped or connected to drainage bag or to suction, and amount of suction supplied.
- Record difference between amount of normal saline instilled and amount of gastric aspirate removed on I&O sheet. Record amount and character of contents draining from NG tube every shift in nurses' notes or flow sheet.
- Record removal of tube "intact," patient's tolerance to procedure, and final amount and character of drainage.

Sample Documentation

1000 Inserted 16 Fr NG tube into left naris, advanced to 50-cm mark. Patient assisted with insertion by swallowing and states he is comfortable. 50 mL of light-green secretions aspirated, pH 4.0. Tube secured with tape and attached to low intermittent suction. Tube placement verified by x-ray. Bowel sounds absent.

Special Considerations

Pediatric

- For children consider the use of sedation before tube insertion (Hockenberry and Wilson, 2007).
- Consider the child's developmental stage and prepare child and family before initiating the procedure. Never surprise the child with this procedure (Hockenberry and Wilson, 2007).

Geriatric

- Check for ill-fitting dentures and remove them for patient's safety and comfort during the insertion.
- Oral and nasal mucosal drying is sometimes present. Adequately lubricate the tube for insertion.
- If patient wears a hearing aid, be sure that the aid is in place during preprocedure explanation and insertion of the tube so patient is able to hear any instructions.

REVIEW QUESTIONS

Case Study for Questions 1 and 2

John Jefferson is a 30-year-old with severe vomiting and abdominal pain. He has a preliminary diagnosis of pancreatitis. The health care provider ordered a series of laboratory tests and abdominal scans. However, before the scan the health care provider wants an NG tube inserted for gastric decompression.

1. During the nursing history Mr. Johnson tells the nurse that he broke his nose playing college football 9 years ago. Based on this information, what is the next step?
   1. Add extra lubricant to the tube during insertion.
   2. Assess patency of each naris.
   3. Call the health care provider for an order for local anesthetic.
   4. Tell Mr. Johnson that the prior injury will prevent the tube insertion.
2. Once the tube is inserted and verified with an x-ray film, which of the following aspirates indicates that the tube is properly placed in the stomach?
   1. Clear aspirate with pH 6.7
   2. Light brown aspirate with pH 4.8
   3. Green aspirate with pH 3.2
   4. Yellow aspirate with pH 5.5
3. While receiving a soaps suds enema, a patient complains of abdominal cramping. Which of the following techniques help relieve this sensation? Select all that apply.
   1. Ask the patient to hold his or her breath.
   2. Ask the patient to breathe slowly.
   3. Lower the fluid container.
   4. Raise the fluid container.

4. When a patient is suspected of having hardened feces from prolonged constipation, which of the following type of enemas would the nurse anticipate administering?
   1. Kayexalate
   2. Oil retention
   3. Soap suds
   4. Tap water
5. A patient comes to the clinic complaining of abdominal discomfort. Which of the following signs might suggest functional constipation?
   1. Diarrhea and abdominal distention
   2. Hard stools and reduced fluid intake
   3. Lumpy, hard stools and absent bowel sounds
   4. Straining with defecation and sensation of incomplete evacuation
6. One risk associated with digital removal of impacted stool is stimulation of the vagus nerve. When this nerve is stimulated, what can occur?
   1. Reflex bradycardia
   2. Reflex tachycardia
   3. Reflex urination
   4. Reflex vomiting
7. When measuring length of insertion for an NG tube, which is the correct measure?
   1. Corner of mouth to earlobe to xiphoid process
   2. Tip of nose to earlobe to xiphoid process
   3. 50 cm (20 inches) from tip of tube
   4. Tip of nose to umbilicus
8. The patient has had an NG tube for 2 days and is complaining about abdominal pain and severe nausea. The NG output has decreased over the past 3 hours, and the nurse is concerned that the tube is not draining properly. What is the nurse's next action?
   1. Irrigate the tube with saline and withdraw the instilled fluid.
   2. Notify the health care provider.
   3. Turn the patient to his left side to promote drainage.
   4. Withdraw the tube 5 to 7.5 cm (2 to 3 inches).
9. After removal of the NG tube, which of the following may indicate that the tube needs to be replaced? Select all that apply.
   1. Abdominal distention
   2. Decreased bowel sounds
   3. Lack of appetite
   4. Passage of flatus
10. A new nurse on the unit is caring for a patient with a Salem sump NG tube. Which of the following indicates that the nurse needs additional education to care for this patient? Select all that apply.
    1. Nurse auscultates for bowel sounds.
    2. Nurse measures gastric output.
    3. Nurse prepares to irrigate the blue pigtail.
    4. Nurse prepares to attach the blue pigtail to portable suction.

REFERENCES

Ebersole P and others: *Toward a healthy aging: human needs and nursing response*, ed 7, St Louis, 2008, Mosby.

Galanti GA: *Caring for people from different cultures*, ed 4, Philadelphia, 2008, University of Pennsylvania Press.

Gevirtz C: Controlling pain: Managing opioid-induced constipation, *Nursing 2008* (July):55, 2008.

Giger JN, Davidhizar RE: *Transcultural nursing: assessment and intervention*, ed 5, St Louis, 2008, Mosby.

Hockenberry MJ, Wilson D: *Wong's nursing care of infants and children*, ed 8, St Louis, 2007, Mosby.

Kyle G: Constipation. Part 1: Causes and assessment, *Pract Nurs* 29(12):611, 2009.

Leung FW, Rao SSC: Fecal incontinence in the elderly, *Gastroenterol Clin North Am* 38:503, 2009.

Metheny NS and others: Complications related to feeding tube placement, *Curr Opin Gastroenterol* 23:187, 2007.

Schnelle JF and others: Prevalence of constipation symptoms in focally incontinent nursing home residents, *J Am Gerontol Soc* 57:647, 2009.

Seidel HM and others: *Mosby's guide to physical examination*, ed 7, St Louis, 2011, Mosby.

The Joint Commission (TJC): *2010 National Patient Safety Goals,* Oakbrook Terrace, Ill, 2010, The Commission, http://www.jointcommision.org/PatientSafety/NationalPatientSafetyGoals, accessed July 2010.

CHAPTER

20

Ostomy Care

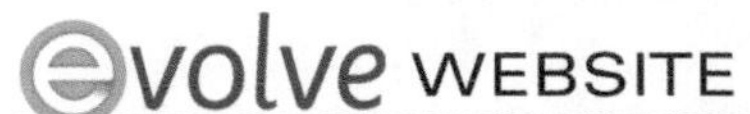

http://evolve.elsevier.com/Perry/nursinginterventions
Video Clips
Nursing Skills Online

Certain diseases or conditions require surgical intervention to create an opening into the abdominal wall for fecal or urinary elimination. Some of these conditions include cancer, inflammatory bowel disease, infections such as diverticulitis that lead to perforation of the colon, neurologic disease, or trauma. The opening is called a *stoma* and is constructed from a section of colon or small intestine. The output from the stoma is called the *effluent.*

An opening in the large intestine or colon is called a *colostomy*; the fecal effluent varies in consistency, depending on where the opening in the colon is created. A colostomy in the descending or sigmoid colon (Fig. 20-1) generally results in a stool similar to that normally passed through the rectum. If the opening is in the ascending or transverse colon, the effluent varies from thick liquid to semiformed stool. An opening in the ileal portion of the small intestine is called an *ileostomy* (Fig. 20-2); the fecal effluent is watery-to-thick liquid and contains some digestive enzymes. Fecal ostomies are either temporary or permanent, depending on the underlying condition and the surgical procedure performed.

A urostomy or ileal conduit (Fig. 20-3) is surgically created by transplanting the ureters into a closed-off portion of the intestinal ileum. One end of the conduit is sutured closed, and the ureters are implanted through the mucosa. The other end is brought out on the abdominal wall, and a stoma is formed for urine to exit the body. This ostomy is permanent. The patient with a colostomy, ileostomy, or ileal conduit has no sensation or control over the time or frequency of the output and wears a pouch to collect the effluent. With a descending colostomy it is possible that, with dietary measures or a process called *irrigation*, the bowel movement may be regulated so the person would be able to wear a small pouch or a stoma cap over the stoma that would contain gas or small amounts of stool.

PATIENT-CENTERED CARE

Before ostomy surgery a physician or certified ostomy care nurse or an enterostomal therapy [ET] nurse will meet with a patient to mark a stoma site, talk to the patient about the surgery, and answer any concerns or questions. Evaluating the patient's abdomen while lying, sitting, and standing allows the nurse and the patient to find an optimal location and avoid having a stoma that is difficult to pouch (ASCRS/WOCN, 2007). This is especially important for patients who will have an incontinent urostomy. These patients have a risk for urine leakage and skin irritation. Poor stoma placement causes undue hardship and has a negative impact on the patient's psychological and emotional health (AUA/WOCN, 2009).

With any ostomy requiring a pouching system, a secure seal to prevent leakage of the effluent and protect the skin around the stoma (peristomal skin) is vital to helping patients resume normal activities and accept the changes in their bodies as a result of the surgery. In addition to the stress of illness and surgical recovery, patients with ostomies face body image changes, fear of social rejection, and concern about sexual function and intimacy; and they need help with personal care. It is very important to provide an effective pouching system to facilitate the emotional adjustment to the ostomy (Li, 2009). Do not act offended by the odor or appearance of the effluent in the pouch. A negative reaction from caregivers reinforces the patient's feelings that this alteration in bodily function makes them personally and socially unacceptable, but a supportive nurse can make the initial period of adjustment easier (Krouse and others, 2007). Encourage the patient who has cared for an ostomy independently to resume self-care as soon as possible. Respect the patient's routine of care even if it differs from usual care in the facility.

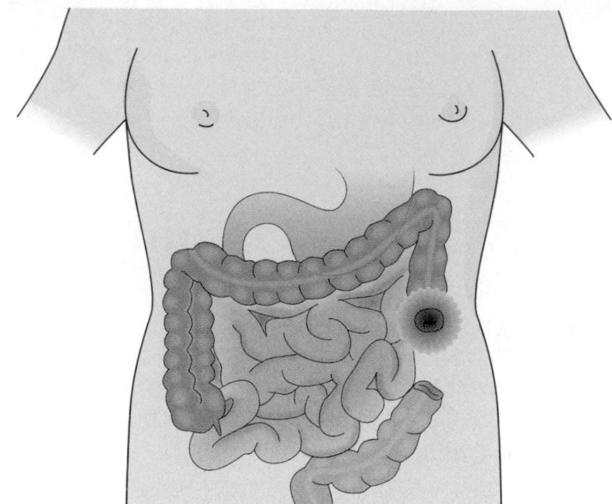

FIG 20-1 Sigmoid colostomy.

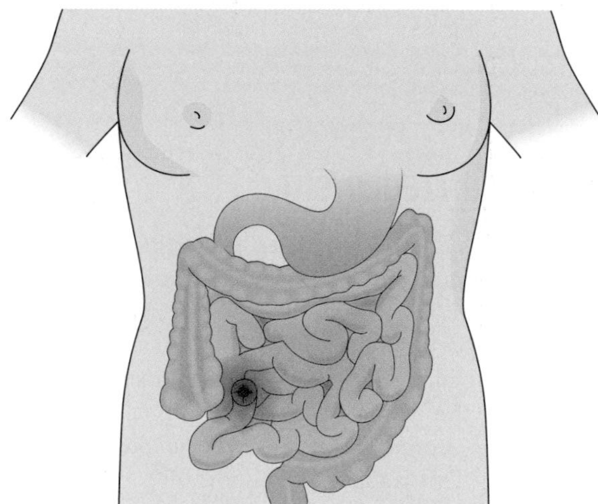

FIG 20-2 Ileostomy.

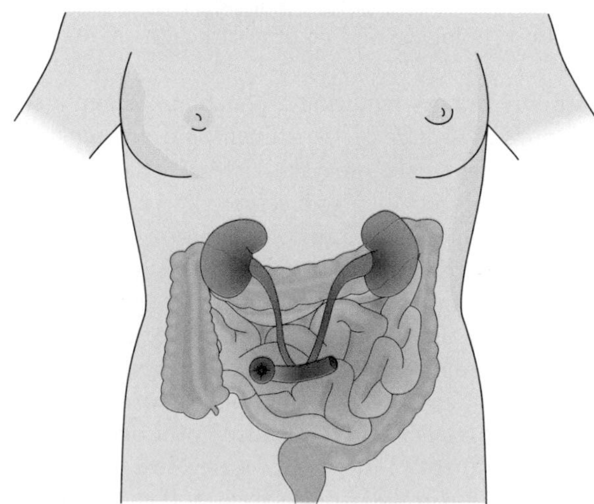

FIG 20-3 Urostomy (ileal conduit).

In any culture the presence and care of an ostomy presents unique challenges. New ostomies require monitoring and observation, and patients from other cultures often find this more invasive and embarrassing. Most cultures consider bowel and urinary secretions unfit for public display. Typically Asians, Africans, Hispanics, Hindus, Muslims, Arabic, Orthodox Jewish, and Amish groups avoid exposure of the lower torso, which is needed for ostomy care (Black, 2009). When caring for patients with ostomies from these cultures, it is helpful to assign gender-congruent caregivers if possible and allow presence of a family member if requested by the patient.

As you communicate with the patient during any care procedure, be sensitive and avoid communicating anything that the patient may interpret as disrespect or disgust. As always, prepare adequately for the procedure; seek necessary assistance; and maintain a calm, professional demeanor.

SAFETY

Safety is a concern when determining proper stoma placement. Proper stoma placement reduces the risk of poor stomal healing, skin irritation, and impaired skin integrity related to drainage. Proper placement also enhances patient self-management of stoma care. When a stoma is properly placed, the patient can visualize the stoma, cleanse the stoma and peristomal site, and easily remove and reapply the new appliance (ASCRS/WOCN, 2007; AUA/WOCN, 2009).

During the immediate postoperative period assess the new stoma to determine that the opening on the appliance accommodates postoperative stomal edema and abdominal distention. If not, the stoma is deprived of circulation and can become necrotic.

Safe hygiene practices are very important for patients who have ostomies. When caring for a patient with a colostomy, it is important to observe the same hygiene measures that you would use for any patient using the bathroom. The patient should be allowed to wash his or her hands before and after participating in the care. Although a new stoma is created surgically, care of the stoma and surrounding skin is not a sterile procedure. Make sure to position the patient comfortably to observe the care and learn what the nurse is teaching.

EVIDENCE-BASED PRACTICE TRENDS

Polle SW and others: Body image, cosmesis, quality of life, and functional outcome of hand-assisted laparoscopic versus open restorative proctocolectomy: long-term results of randomized trials, *Surg Endosc* 21(8):1301, 2007.

Richbourg L, Fellows J: Ostomy pouch wear time in the United States, *J Wound Ostomy Continence Nurs* 35(5):504, 2008.

WOCN guidelines: *Basic ostomy care for health care providers and patients*, Mount Laurel, NJ, 2007, The Association.

The primary changes in ostomy care are related to improvements in surgical techniques for fecal and urinary diversions. The development of the continent ileostomy and urostomy reservoirs has progressed to the development of a variety of ileal reservoirs for bowel and urinary effluent that are controlled using the patient's urinary or anal sphincter. Laparoscopic surgery is now done for abdominal and pelvic procedures and stoma creation. Laparoscopic surgery decreases postoperative recovery time and use of analgesics and improves body image (Polle and others, 2007).

Stoma care is improved because pouching systems are now more effective and adhesive technology more advanced. These improvements include a wider variety of sizes and shapes of skin barriers, depths of convexity from shallow to deep, and degrees of flexibility. The current trend is to apply the pouch to clean, dry skin without other skin preparations, paste, or adhesives unless the patient has a specific problem keeping the pouch intact (WOCN, 2007). The adhesives on the skin barriers are pressure and heat sensitive; thus have the patient apply gentle pressure with the hand over the skin barrier for several minutes to facilitate the adherence of the barrier to the skin. There are new and improved accessory products such as rings or seals for managing abdominal contours that are uneven or peristomal skin that is not intact. Some pouches have effective gas filters that allow for flatus to escape slowly from the pouch through a charcoal filter. This filter absorbs odor and does not allow leakage of liquid effluent through the filter. All of the ostomy companies now have pouches with integrated closures. An integrated closure is made from a Velcro-like product and eliminates the need for a clip to close the bottom of the pouch. It requires less manual dexterity to empty the pouch A pouch may be worn for 3 to 7 days, depending on the contours of the stoma and the abdomen, the condition of the peristomal skin, and the personal preference of the person with an ostomy. A recent study of over 500 subjects across the United States found that the average wear time was 4.8 days (Richbourg and Fellows, 2008).

SKILL 20.1 POUCHING A BOWEL DIVERSION

- **Nursing Skills Online: Bowel Elimination/Ostomy Module, Lessons 1, 3, 4** *Video Clips*

Immediately after a fecal surgical diversion, it is necessary to place a pouch over the newly created stoma to contain effluent when the stoma begins to function. The pouch keeps the patient clean and dry, protects the skin from drainage, and provides a barrier against odor. It is best to use a "cut-to-fit," transparent pouching system that covers the peristomal skin without constricting the stoma and allows for visibility of the stoma.

In the immediate postoperative period the stoma may be edematous, and the abdomen distended. These symptoms resolve over a 4- to 6-week period after surgery, but during this time it is necessary to revise the pouching system to meet the changing size of the stoma and the changes in body contours.

There are many types of pouching systems, but all have a protective layer that adheres to the skin called a *skin barrier* and a pouch. A one-piece pouching system (Fig. 20-4, *A*) has the two parts integrated together. A two-piece system (Fig. 20-4, *B*) has a separate skin barrier and pouch that snaps in place. The flush or retracted stoma may require a convex wafer (Fig. 20-5) for successful pouching. This type of skin barrier provides gentle pressure on the peristomal skin to push the stoma through the opening in the wafer. You apply the pouch to the skin barrier by attaching it to a flange (a plastic ring) on the barrier. You must use the skin barrier with flange with the corresponding size pouch from the same manufacturer so the two pieces fit together properly to avoid leakage between the skin barrier and the pouch. Some pouching systems have precut openings in the barrier for the stoma, whereas others need to be custom cut to size for the patient's stoma measurement. It is important to understand how to use each of these different pouching systems before applying them on patients. The websites for the companies that make ostomy supplies have both patient and health care provider instructions that are helpful in understanding how to use the pouching systems.

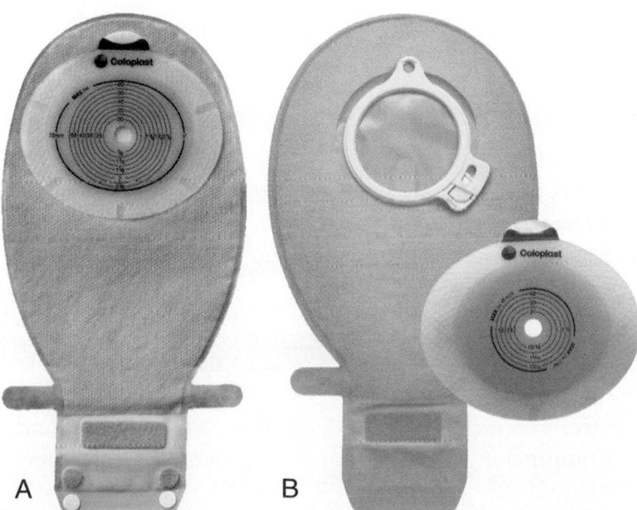

FIG 20-4 **A,** One-piece pouch with Velcro closure. **B,** Two-piece pouching system with separate skin barrier and attachable pouch. (**A** and **B** Courtesy Coloplast, Minneapolis, Minn.)

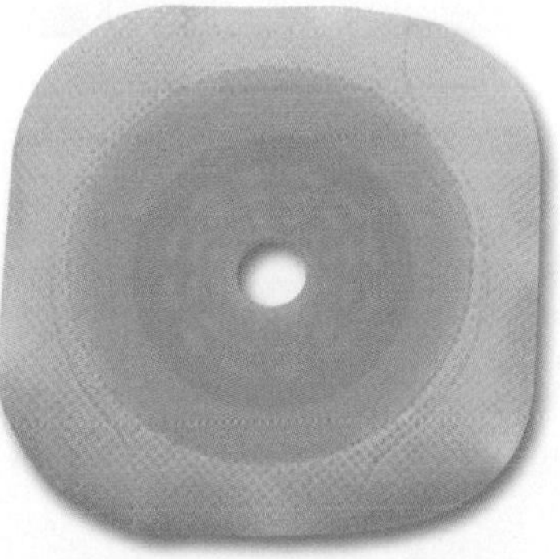

FIG 20-5 Convex skin barrier wafer. (Courtesy Hollister Inc., Libertyville, Ill.)

ASSESSMENT

1. Observe existing skin barrier and pouch for leakage and note the length of time in place. The pouch should be changed every 3 to 7 days, not daily. *Rationale: Assesses effectiveness of pouching system for determining frequency of change. If an ostomy pouch is leaking, change it. Taping or patching it to contain effluent leaves the skin exposed to chemical or enzymatic irritation.*
2. Observe amount of effluent in the pouch and empty the pouch if it is more than ⅓ to ½ full by opening the clip or integrated Velcro-like closure and draining it into a container for measurement of the output. *Rationale: Decreases the weight of the pouch and the chance of the pouch loosening or spilling when changing it.*
3. Observe stoma for color, swelling, trauma, and condition of the peristomal skin. If you cannot observe effluent, remove pouch by gently pushing skin away from the adhesive barrier. Properly dispose of soiled pouch and save any clamp. Assess type of stoma and whether it is budded (protruding above the skin surface [Fig. 20-6, *A*]), flush with the skin surface, or retracted (below the skin surface [Fig. 20-6, *B*]). Clear pouches permit viewing of a stoma without their removal. *Rationale: Stoma characteristics aid in determining the appropriate pouching system.*
4. Observe the abdominal contour and note the presence of scars or incisions. *Rationale: Determines type of pouching system needed. Abdominal contours, scars, or incisions affect the type of system and how the system adheres to the patient's skin.*
5. Observe patient's readiness to learn by willingness to look at stoma and ask questions. If patient is apprehensive about touching or looking at stoma, encourage him or her to observe the pouch change procedure initially. Whenever possible, consult the ostomy care nurse. *Rationale: Determines patient's readiness to learn and facilitates self-management or home care.*

A B

FIG 20-6 A, Budded stoma. **B,** Retracted stoma. (**A** and **B** Courtesy Jane Fellows.)

PLANNING

Expected Outcomes focus on maintaining integrity of stoma and peristomal skin, promoting normal elimination, and promoting patient's ability to manage ostomy.

1. Stoma is moist and reddish pink. Skin is intact and free of burning or irritation; sutures are intact.
2. Stoma drains moderate amount of liquid or soft stool and flatus in pouch.
3. Patient or family caregiver observe and return demonstrate pouching change.
4. Patient asks questions about procedure and may attempt to assist with pouch change.

Delegation and Collaboration

The skill of pouching a new bowel diversion cannot be delegated to nursing assistive personnel (NAP). In some agencies care of an established ostomy (4 to 6 weeks after surgery) can be delegated. Instruct the NAP about the following:

- Expected appearance of the stoma; the amount, color, and consistency of drainage from the ostomy
- Special equipment needed to complete procedure
- Changes in patient's stoma and surrounding skin integrity that should be reported

Equipment

- Pouch, clear drainable one-piece or two-piece, cut-to-fit or precut size
- Pouch closure device such as a clip if needed
- Measuring guide
- Adhesive remover (optional)
- Clean gloves
- Washcloth
- Towel or disposable waterproof barrier
- Basin with warm tap water
- Scissors

IMPLEMENTATION *for* POUCHING A BOWEL DIVERSION

STEPS	RATIONALE
1. **See Standard Protocol (inside front cover).**	
2. Identify the patient using two identifiers (e.g., name and birthday or name and account number, according to facility policy).	Ensures correct patient. Complies with The Joint Commission standards and improves patient safety (TJC, 2010).
3. Position patient semireclining or supine during assessment and pouching. (NOTE: Some patients with established ostomies prefer to stand.) If possible, provide patient a mirror for observation.	Position ensures there are fewer skin wrinkles, which allows for ease of application of pouching system.

STEPS	RATIONALE
4. Place towel or disposable waterproof barrier under patient and across patient's lower abdomen.	Protects bed linen.
5. If not removed during assessment, remove used pouch and skin barrier gently by pushing skin away from barrier. An adhesive remover may be used to facilitate removal of skin barrier. Dispose of pouch.	Reduces skin trauma. Improper removal of pouch and barrier can cause peristomal skin irritation or breakdown.
6. Cleanse peristomal skin gently with warm tap water using a washcloth; do not scrub skin. Minor bleeding from a stoma is normal during cleansing. Pat the skin dry.	Avoid soap. It leaves residue on skin, which interferes with pouch adhesion (WOCN, 2007). Pouch does not adhere to wet skin.
7. Measure stoma (see illustration). Expect size of stoma to change for first 4 to 6 weeks following surgery.	Allows for proper fit of pouch that will protect peristomal skin.
8. Trace pattern of stoma measurement on adhesive backing of pouch (see illustration).	Prepares for cutting opening in the pouch.
9. Cut opening in pouch (see illustration).	Customizes pouch to provide appropriate fit over stoma.
10. Remove protective backing from adhesive (see illustration).	

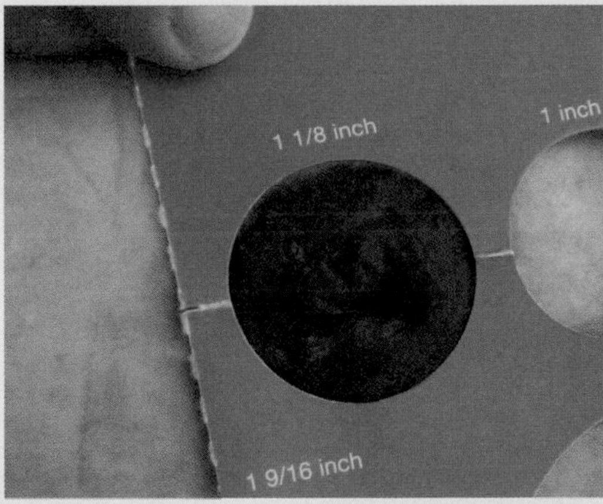

STEP 7 Measure stoma. (Courtesy Coloplast, Minneapolis, Minn.)

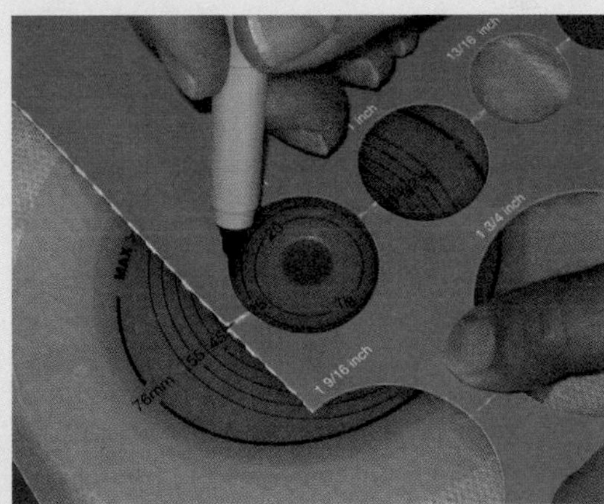

STEP 8 Trace measurement. (Courtesy Coloplast, Minneapolis, Minn.)

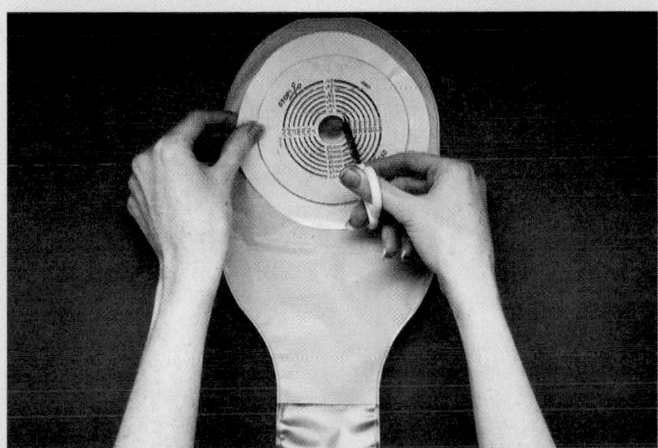

STEP 9 Cut-to-fit, one-piece drainable ostomy pouch. (© 2010 Convatec Inc. Reprinted with permission.)

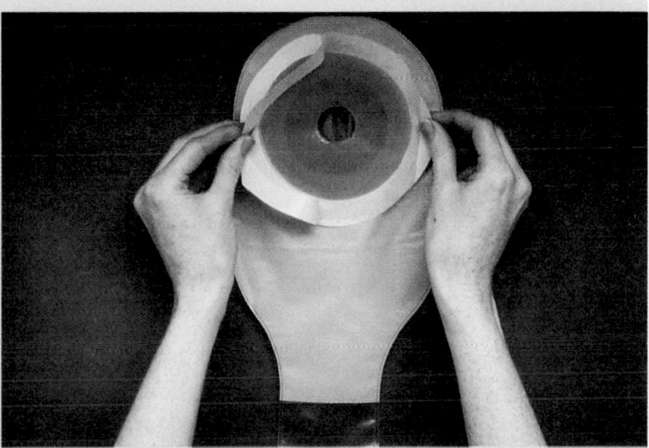

STEP 10 Removing the backing paper for the barrier on a one-piece pouch. (© 2010 Convatec Inc. Reprinted with permission.)

Continued

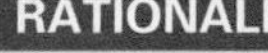

STEPS	RATIONALE
11. Apply one-piece pouch (see illustration).	
a. Press adhesive backing of pouch smoothly against skin, starting from bottom and working up around sides.	Ensures smooth, wrinkle-free seal.
b. Hold firmly into place around stoma and outside edges. Bottom of pouch points toward patient's knees when sitting.	
c. Teach patient to hold hand over pouch to apply heat to secure seal. Hold for about 1 to 2 minutes.	Pouch adhesives are heat activated and will hold more securely at body temperature.
12. If using a two-piece barrier wafer and pouch:	
a. Apply the barrier to the skin first (see illustration) and then attach the pouch.	
b. Snap on pouch and maintain finger pressure.	
13. For both types of pouches, gently tug on end of pouch in a downward fashion. Close end of pouch with clip or integrated closure.	Ensures pouch is secure. Closure contains effluent.
14. See Completion Protocol (inside front cover).	

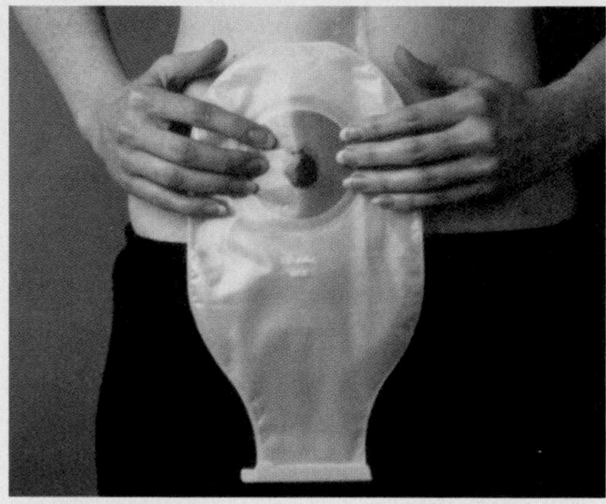

STEP 11 Patient applying a one-piece pouch. (© 2010 Convatec Inc. Reprinted with permission.)

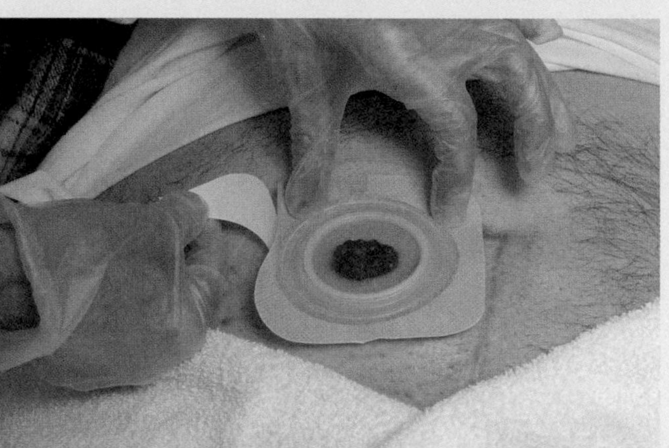

STEP 12a Application of barrier-paste flange for two-piece pouch.

EVALUATION

1. Observe appearance of stoma, peristomal skin, abdominal contours, and suture line during pouch change.
2. Observe patient's and family member's or significant other's willingness to view stoma and ask questions about the procedure. Have them perform a return demonstration.

Unexpected Outcomes and Related Interventions

1. Skin around the stoma is blistered or bleeding, or a rash is noted. May be caused by allergic reaction to one of the products used, yeast rash, or exposure of the skin to fecal effluent caused by undermining of the skin barrier.
   a. Remove pouch carefully.
   b. Consult ostomy nurse.
2. Necrotic stoma is manifested by purple or black color, dry rather than moist texture, failure to bleed when washed gently, or presence of tissue sloughing.
   a. Report to health care provider/nurse.
   b. Consult with ostomy nurse.
3. Patient refuses to look at stoma or participate in care.
   a. Explore patient's feelings and enlist family support.
   b. Consult ostomy nurse.
   c. Knowledge and acceptance by staff facilitate understanding and adjustment.

Recording and Reporting

- Record type of pouch and skin barrier applied, amount and appearance of effluent in pouch, size and appearance of stoma, and condition of peristomal skin. Record patient/family level of participation and teaching that was done and response to teaching.

- Report any of the following to nurse and/or health care provider: abnormal appearance of stoma, suture line, peristomal skin, or volume and character of output.

Sample Documentation

1600 Ileostomy stoma, round, ½ inch in diameter, slightly swollen, red in color. Peristomal skin intact. Draining 900 mL of dark-brown liquid stool. Bowel sounds present in all quadrants. Two-piece ostomy system intact, without leakage. ET scheduled to begin instruction today. Patient has not viewed stoma as yet.

Special Considerations

Pediatric

- Select pediatric pouches designed especially for neonates, infants, and children, which are smaller and have a more skin-sensitive adhesive on the barrier.
- Children and adolescents may have ostomy surgery for conditions such as cancer, inflammatory bowel disease, and trauma.
- Neonates often have multiple stomas on their tiny abdomens that are the result of corrective bowel surgeries. Select a cut-to-fit pouch that allows multiple stoma openings in skin barrier yet still fits on neonate's tiny abdomen.
- If caring for a preterm infant, be aware that the peristomal skin is not fully developed; as a result, you should not use skin sealants and adhesive removers because they damage the epithelium.

Geriatric

- Evaluate older adult's cognitive status for understanding of ostomy self-care instructions.
- Some older patients have impaired manual dexterity or limited vision; make adaptations for this while teaching. For patients who are unable to custom cut the size of their skin barriers, consider having barriers precut by ostomy equipment supplier or using a precut two-piece system.
- Financial concerns about cost of ostomy supplies and reimbursement are an important issue for patients on fixed income.

Home Care

- Evaluate patient's home toileting facilities and ability to position self to empty pouch directly into the toilet.
- Patient may shower without covering pouch.
- Instruct patient and family that ostomy care does not require any sterile supplies.
- Family caregivers do not need to wear gloves when providing care.
- Patients should avoid placing pouches in extremely hot or cold locations because temperature affects barrier and adhesive materials.

SKILL 20.2 POUCHING AN INCONTINENT UROSTOMY

Because urine flows continuously from an incontinent urinary diversion, a urinary pouch is usually placed over the opening immediately after surgery. Placement of the pouch is more challenging than with a fecal diversion because urine flow keeps the skin moist. In the immediate postoperative period urinary stents extend out from the stoma (Fig. 20-7). The surgeon places these stents into the ureters to keep them from becoming stenosed or closed at the site where the ureters are attached to the conduit. The stents are removed during the hospital stay or at the first postoperative visit with the surgeon. The stoma of a urinary diversion is normally red and moist. It is made from a portion of the intestinal tract, usually the ileum. It should protrude above the skin. An ileal conduit is usually located in the right lower quadrant. While the patient is in bed, the pouch may be connected to a bedside drainage bag to decrease the need for frequent emptying. When the patient goes home, the bedside drainage bag may be used at night to avoid having to get up to empty the pouch. Each type of urostomy pouch (Fig. 20-8) comes with a connector for the bedside drainage bag. Incorrect pouch placement, large volumes of urine in the pouch, or a urinary pouch without an antireflux valve promotes reflux and the risk of infection. You can reduce the risk of reflux by attaching the urinary pouch to straight drainage when high urinary output is expected. A patient must understand the importance of draining the pouch frequently and using clean technique during stomal and skin care.

FIG 20-7 Urostomy stoma with stents in place. (Courtesy Jane Fellows.)

ASSESSMENT

1. Observe existing skin barrier and pouch for leakage of urine and length of time in place. The pouch should be changed every 3 to 7 days, not daily. *Rationale: Assesses effectiveness of pouching system and determines frequency for changing pouch.*

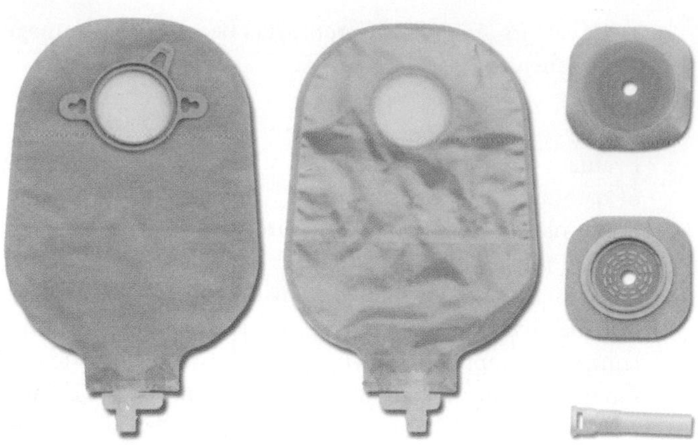

FIG 20-8 Urostomy pouching system with adapter to connect pouch to bedside drainage bag. (Courtesy Hollister Inc., Libertyville, Ill.)

2. Observe amount of urine in the pouch and empty it if it is more than ⅓ to ½ full by opening the tap at the end of the pouch and draining it into a container for measurement. *Rationale: Decreases the weight of the pouch and chance of it loosening or spillage when changing it. Urine output provides information about renal status.*
3. Observe stoma for color, swelling, trauma, and healing of the peristomal skin. Assess type of stoma. Clear pouches permit viewing of stoma without their removal. If pouch is not clear, remove pouch by gently pushing skin away from the adhesive barrier. Properly dispose of soiled pouch and save any clamps. *Rationale: Stoma characteristics are one of the factors to consider in selecting an appropriate pouching system. Convexity in the skin barrier is often necessary with a flush or retracted stoma.*
4. Observe patient's readiness to learn by willingness to look at stoma and ask questions. If patient is apprehensive about touching or looking at stoma, encourage him or her to observe the pouch change procedure initially. Whenever possible, consult the ostomy care nurse. *Rationale: Assesses patient's reaction to stoma and readiness to begin learning self-care.*

PLANNING

Expected Outcomes focus on maintaining integrity of stoma and peristomal skin, condition of stents, and normal urine output, and on promoting patient's ability to manage ostomy.

1. Stoma is moist and reddish pink with stents protruding from it in the postoperative period. Skin is intact and free of irritation; sutures are intact.
2. Urine drains freely from stents or stoma. Urine is yellowish with mucus shreds and is without foul odor. The urine may be pink or contain small blood clots after surgery.
3. Volume of output is within acceptable limits (30 mL/hr).
4. Patient and family caregiver observe and return demonstrate steps of procedure.
5. Patient asks questions about procedure and may attempt to assist with pouch change.

Delegation and Collaboration

The skill of pouching a new incontinent urostomy cannot be delegated to nursing assistive personnel (NAP). In some agencies care of an established urostomy (4 to 6 weeks or longer after surgery) can be delegated. Instruct the NAP about the following:

- Expected appearance of the stoma; amount, color, and consistency of urine from the ostomy
- Special equipment needed to complete procedure
- Changes in patient's stoma and surrounding skin integrity that should be reported

Equipment

- Urinary pouch (with antireflux flap) and skin barrier; clear, drainable one- or two-piece, cut-to-fit or precut size with appropriate adaptor for connection to bedside drainage bag (see Fig. 20-8)
- Measuring guide
- Bedside urinary drainage bag
- Clean gloves
- Washcloth
- Towel or disposable waterproof barrier
- Basin with warm tap water
- Scissors
- Adhesive remover
- Absorbent wick made from gauze rolled tightly in the shape of a tampon

IMPLEMENTATION *for* POUCHING AN INCONTINENT UROSTOMY

STEPS	RATIONALE
1. **See Standard Protocol (inside front cover).**	
2. Identify the patient using two identifiers (e.g., name and birthday or name and account number, according to facility policy)	Ensures correct patient. Complies with The Joint Commission standards and improves patient safety (TJC, 2010).
3. Position patient semireclining or supine. If possible provide patient a mirror for observation.	Position ensures there are fewer skin wrinkles, which allows for ease of pouch application.

STEPS	RATIONALE
4. 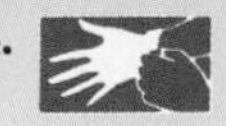 Place towel or disposable waterproof barrier under patient and one across patient's lower abdomen.	Protects bed linen because there will be a continuous flow of urine from the stoma. Maintains patient's dignity.
5. Remove used pouch and skin barrier (if not removed during assessment) by gently pushing skin away from barrier. If stents are present, *do not pull on them.*	Reduces risk of trauma to skin and risk of dislodging stents. Stents are necessary to keep the ureters patent during the immediate postoperative period.
6. Place rolled gauze at stoma opening. Maintain gauze at the stoma opening continuously during pouch measurement and change.	Rolled gauze contains the urine from the stoma site. The gauze forms a wick; using a wick at stoma opening keeps urine from leaking onto the skin and prevents peristomal skin from becoming wet with urine during pouching change procedure.
7. While keeping rolled gauze in contact with the stoma, cleanse peristomal skin gently with warm tap water using washcloth; do not scrub skin, and avoid using soap. Minor bleeding of the stoma during washing is normal. Pat the skin dry.	Soap leaves residue on skin, which interferes with pouch adhesion (WOCN, 2007). Pouch does not adhere to wet skin.
8. Measure stoma (see illustration, Skill 20.1, Step 7). Expect size of stoma to change for first 4 to 6 weeks following surgery.	Allows for proper fit of pouch that will protect peristomal skin.
9. Trace pattern on pouch/skin barrier on adhesive of pouch (see illustration, Skill 20.1, Step 8).	Prepares for cutting opening in the pouch.
10. Cut opening in pouch (see illustration, Skill 20.1, Step 9).	Customizes pouch to provide appropriate fit over stoma.
11. Remove protective backing from adhesive surface (see illustration, Skill 20.1, Step 10). Remove wick from stoma.	Prepares pouch for adhesion to the skin. Pouch adhesives are heat activated and hold more securely at body temperature.
12. Apply pouch (see illustration, Skill 20.1, Step 11). Press adhesive barrier firmly into place around stoma and outside edges. Have patient hold hand over pouch 1 to 2 minutes to apply heat to secure seal.	Pouch adhesives are heat activated to create a secure seal on skin.
13. Use adapter provided with pouches to connect pouch to bedside urinary bag.	Provides for collection and measurement of urine. Allows patient to rest without frequent emptying of the pouch.
14. See Completion Protocol (inside front cover).	

EVALUATION

1. Observe volume and character of urine and appearance of stoma, peristomal skin, abdominal contours, and suture line during pouch change.
2. Observe patient's and family member's or significant other's willingness to view stoma and ask questions about the procedure. Have patient return demonstrate pouch change.

Unexpected Outcomes and Related interventions

(see Skill 20.1)

1. There is no urinary output for several hours, or output is less than 30 mL/hr. Urine has foul odor.
   a. Notify health care provider.
   b. Determine patency of stents or stoma by observing urine flow.
   c. Obtain urine specimen if ordered by health care provider for culture and sensitivity to test for possible infection (see Skill 20.3).
2. Necrotic stoma is manifested by purple or black color, dry rather than moist texture, failure to bleed when washed gently, or presence of tissue sloughing.
   a. Report to health care provider/nurse.
   b. Document findings.

Recording and Reporting

- Record type of pouch and skin barrier applied, amount and appearance of urine emptied from pouch, size and appearance of stoma, and condition of peristomal skin.
- Record patient/family level of participation, teaching that was done, and response to teaching.
- Report any of the following to nurse and/or health care provider: abnormal appearance of stoma, suture line, or peristomal skin; or change in volume, color, or odor of urine output.

Sample Documentation

0800 Ileal conduit ostomy shiny, moist, and beefy red. 250-mL clear yellow urine with white mucus present in pouch. Peristomal skin intact. Suture line dry and approximated. Pouch changed with patient assisting. Patient correctly applied pouch.

Special Considerations

Pediatric

- In neonates urinary diversions are less common than fecal ostomies. Surgical repair of congenital urinary abnormalities usually occurs in stages and focuses initially on drainage of the upper urinary tract to preserve renal function.
- Select pediatric pouches designed especially for neonates, infants, and children, which are smaller and have a more skin-sensitive adhesive on the barrier.

Geriatric

- Evaluate older adult's cognitive status for understanding of ostomy self-care instructions.
- Some older patients have impaired manual dexterity or limited vision; make adaptations for this while teaching. For patients who are unable to custom cut the size of their skin barriers, consider having barriers precut by ostomy equipment supplier or using a precut two-piece system.
- Financial concerns about cost of ostomy supplies and reimbursement are an important issue for patients on fixed income.

Home Care (see Skill 20.1)

- Evaluate patient's home toileting facilities and ability to position self to empty pouch directly into the toilet.
- Patient may shower without covering pouch.
- Ostomy care does not require sterile supplies.
- Family caregivers do not need to wear gloves when providing care.
- At home patient can open pouch spout and connect it to straight drainage at night. Make sure that patient understands that adapter will be needed to connect pouch to the bedside drainage bag.

SKILL 20.3 CATHETERIZING A URINARY DIVERSION

Catheterization of a urinary diversion is the only way to obtain an accurate culture and sensitivity specimen for screening for infection. When it is necessary to obtain a urine specimen from a urinary diversion, the best method is to insert a sterile catheter into the stoma. Obtaining a specimen from urine in the pouch does not provide accurate results because of the risk for contamination. With the use of strict sterile asepsis, catheterization is relatively safe and easy. If a patient uses a two-piece pouch, you can remove the pouch from the skin barrier and replace it after the catheterization. If a patient uses a one-piece pouch, you have to remove the pouch to obtain the specimen and replace with a new pouch afterwards. To prevent trauma of tissues, you need to understand how the stoma and implanted ureters are constructed for a patient. Reflux of urine into the ureters can cause infection.

ASSESSMENT

1. Observe signs and symptoms of urinary tract infection such as elevated temperature, chills, foul-smelling urine, and elevated white blood cell count. *Rationale: Determines need to perform catheterization to obtain a sterile specimen from urinary diversion.*
2. Obtain health care provider's order for catheterization. *Rationale: Procedure and laboratory test requires health care provider's order.*
3. Assess patient's understanding of the need for procedure and how procedure is done. *Rationale: Determines willingness to cooperate and reduces patient's anxiety.*

PLANNING

Expected Outcomes focus on obtaining an uncontaminated urine specimen.

- Urine is obtained correctly.
- Laboratory results are accurate.

Delegation and Collaboration

The skill of catheterizing a urinary diversion cannot be delegated to nursing assistive personnel (NAP). Instruct the NAP to:

- Inform the nurse if patient complains of peristomal or back pain.
- Inform the nurse if there is a change in color, odor, or amount of urine or if there is blood in the urine.

Equipment

- Urinary catheterization supplies (may be contained in prepackaged sterile catheter kit or may need to be gathered separately):
  - 14- to 16-Fr sterile catheter
  - Water-soluble lubricant
  - Antiseptic swabs (e.g., chlorhexidine)
  - Sterile gloves
  - Sterile specimen container
- Absorbent gauze wick
- Gauze pad
- Bed protection barrier
- Towels
- Urinary diversion pouch if patient is using one-piece system (if using two-piece system, same pouch can be removed and replaced for procedure as long as skin barrier adhesive remains intact)
- Clean gloves

IMPLEMENTATION *for* CATHETERIZING A URINARY DIVERSION

STEPS	RATIONALE
1. See Standard Protocol (inside front cover).	
2. Identify the patient using two identifiers (e.g. name and birthday or name and account number, according to facility policy).	Ensures correct patient. Complies with The Joint Commission standards and improves patient safety (TJC, 2010).
3. If possible, position patient sitting and drape towel across lower abdomen.	Gravity facilitates flow of urine. Maintains patient's dignity. Towel absorbs urine.
4. Remove pouch. If patient uses two-piece system, remove pouch only but leave barrier attached to skin.	Access to stoma.
5. Remove and discard gloves. Perform hand hygiene. Open sterile catheterization set according to instructions or open needed equipment and place on sterile barrier. If not using catheterization kit, place gauze pad on sterile field and squeeze small amount of lubricant onto gauze.	Avoids contamination.
6. Apply sterile gloves.	
7. If needed, have patient hold absorbent wick over stoma while waiting.	Prevents leakage of urine on peristomal skin, linens, and clothing.
8. Cleanse surface of stoma with antiseptic swabs using circular motion from center outward. Using new swab each time; repeat twice. Allow antiseptic to dry.	Removes surface bacteria.
a. If patient has stents in place, use antiseptic swab to cleanse the ends of the stents and place the stents in the sterile cup. Allow urine to drip into the cup until an adequate amount for a specimen has been obtained. Then go directly to Step 13.	
9. Lubricate tip of catheter with water-soluble lubricant.	Lubricant facilitates passage of catheter through stoma.
10. Remove lid from specimen container. Place distal end of catheter into specimen container. Hold catheter in container with nondominant hand.	The conduit is for passage of urine, and only a small volume of urine is obtained.
11. With your dominant hand, gently insert catheter into stoma. Do not force catheter; redirect course as needed. Use gentle but firm pressure similar to regular catheterization of urethra. Have patient cough or turn slightly to facilitate flow of urine.	Use care to avoid trauma to conduit.
12. Maintain container below level of stoma. Have patient cough as needed. Urine may flow around and through catheter. This is acceptable, but only urine from catheter is desired. Normally wait 5 minutes; if no urine is in container, pinch catheter and remove; direct any urine "trapped" in catheter into cup.	Facilitates drainage of urine. Culture and sensitivity studies only require 3 to 5 mL of urine.
13. After withdrawing catheter, place absorbent pad over stoma.	Keeps skin dry.
14. Apply lid to specimen container.	Prevents accidental spillage.
15. Reapply new urostomy pouch or reattach pouch if patient uses a two-piece system.	Pouch is necessary to contain urine.
16. Remove gloves; perform hand hygiene. Label and send specimen to laboratory at once.	Avoids transmission of infection. Labeling ensures acceptance of specimen by laboratory and processing. Allowing urine to sit for long periods at room temperature affects laboratory results.
17. See Completion Protocol (inside front cover).	

EVALUATION

1. Refer to laboratory report and compare results of culture and sensitivity with normal expected findings. Remember that mucus is a normal finding in the urine of a patient with an ileal or colon conduit. If specimen is contaminated, a second specimen will be needed.

Unexpected Outcomes and Related Interventions

1. Unable to obtain urine.
   a. Reposition patient.
   b. Push fluids and try again later.
2. Skin or stoma reveals complications.
   a. Provide appropriate care.
   b. Consult with ostomy care nurse or health care provider.

Recording and Reporting

- Record time specimen was collected; patient's tolerance of procedure; and appearance of urine, skin, and stoma.
- Report results of laboratory test to nurse in charge or health care provider.

Sample Documentation

0700 Ileal conduit stoma catheterized for sterile urine specimen. 150 mL cloudy urine with a foul odor obtained. Specimen sent to the laboratory. Peristomal skin intact; stoma is shiny, moist, and red.

REVIEW QUESTIONS

Case Study for Questions 1 and 2

The nurse is assigned to care for Tiffany Jones, a 28-year-old woman who was admitted to the hospital with abdominal pain. She was diagnosed with Crohn's disease when she was 16 and has had numerous hospital admissions and tried many medications, but now she will need surgery to remove part of her intestine and will have an ileostomy.

1. When Tiffany returns from surgery, the nurse assesses the stoma. She should expect the stoma to:
   1. Be red and moist
   2. Be just below the skin level
   3. Have a stents protruding from it
   4. Be pink and dry
2. When teaching Tiffany about care at home, how often should the nurse recommend that she change or empty her ostomy pouch?
   1. Change daily
   2. Empty when it is $\frac{1}{3}$ to $\frac{1}{2}$ full
   3. Empty every 4 to 6 hours
   4. Change every 10 days
3. A patient with a total colectomy and new ileostomy notices that the bowel movement is always liquid and asks when it will be formed like it was before surgery. How should the nurse respond?
   1. Tell the patient that it will be formed after complete recovery from the surgery.
   2. Tell the patient to eat foods that are constipating until the bowel movement is a firm consistency.
   3. Tell the patient that this is a normal output for an ileostomy.
   4. Tell the patient to reduce fluid intake and it will become more formed.
4. From the following list, select the most important task to be done before surgery to promote successful patient adjustment to an ostomy.
   1. Give the patient a chance to empty a pouch.
   2. Make sure that the patient has a nutrition consultation.
   3. Schedule stoma site marking with a qualified ostomy nurse.
   4. Administer a barium enema.
5. To obtain a urine specimen for culture and sensitivity from a patient with a urostomy, which of the following should be done?
   1. Catheterize the stoma.
   2. Take the specimen from a clean pouch.
   3. Take a specimen before changing the pouch
   4. Attach the pouch to a bedside drainage bag and take the specimen through the port in the tubing.
6. The nurse is changing the pouch on a urostomy. Place the following steps in the correct order.
   1. Cut opening in the pouch.
   2. Dispose of used pouch and soiled equipment.
   3. Maintain gentle finger pressure around barrier for 1 to 2 minutes.
   4. Cleanse skin around stoma with warm tap water.
   5. Wick stoma with a rolled gauze.
   6. Press adhesive barrier firmly but gently on the skin.
7. A patient has a new colostomy. Which of the following statements is true for this patient? Select all that apply.
   1. The patient will be able to take a shower.
   2. Someone else will always have to change his or her pouch.
   3. The skin around the stoma will always be red and itchy.
   4. The pouch will be emptied only once a day.
   5. The pouch can only be changed once a week.
   6. The pouches are disposable.
   7. A rash or skin breakdown around the stoma is not normal and requires treatment.
8. An ostomy stoma should be measured with each pouch change because it may change size:
   1. For several months after surgery
   2. For the first few days after surgery
   3. For as long as the patient has a stoma
   4. In the first 4 to 6 weeks after surgery

9. To which factor is patient adjustment to an ostomy most closely related?
   1. Age
   2. Level of education
   3. Support of spouse, family, significant others
   4. Manual dexterity
10. A patient with a new ostomy begins crying as the nurse helps her change her pouch for the first time. What should the nurse do?
    1. Tell her that no one will know that she has an ostomy.
    2. Allow her to express her grief over this change in her body.
    3. Request a psychiatric consultation.
    4. Reassure her that it could be worse if the surgeon had not removed all the cancer.

REFERENCES

American Society of Colon and Rectal Surgeons Committee Members; Wound Ostomy Continence Nurses Society Committee Members (ASCRS/WOCN): ASCRS and WOCN Joint Position Statement on the value of preoperative stoma marking for patients undergoing fecal ostomy surgery, *J Wound Ostomy Continence Nurs* 34(6):627, 2007.

American Urological Association; Wound Ostomy Continence Nurses Society (AUA/WOCN): AUA and WOCN Joint Position Statement on the value of preoperative stoma marking for patients undergoing creation of an incontinent urostomy, *J Wound Ostomy Continence Nurs* 36(3):267, 2009.

Black P: Cultural and religious beliefs in stoma care nursing, *Br J Nurs* 18(13):790, 2009.

Krouse R and others: Quality of life outcomes in 599 cancer and noncancer patients with colostomies, *J Surg Res* 138(1):79, 2007.

Li CC: Sexuality among patients with a colostomy, *J Wound Ostomy Continence Nurs* 36(3):288, 2009.

Polle SW and others: Body image, cosmesis, quality of life, and functional outcome of hand-assisted laparoscopic versus open restorative proctocolectomy: long-term results of randomized trials, *Surg Endosc* 21(8):1301, 2007.

Richbourg L, Fellows J: Ostomy pouch wear time in the United States, *J Wound Ostomy Continence Nurs* 35(5):504, 2008.

The Joint Commission (TJC): *2010 National Patient Safety Goals*, Oakbrook Terrace, Ill, 2010, The Commission, http://www.jointcommision.org/PatientSafety/NationalPatientSafetyGoals, accessed July 2010.

WOCN guidelines: *Basic ostomy care for health care providers and patients,* Mount Laurel, NJ, 2007, The Association.

CHAPTER 21

Preparation for Safe Medication Administration

evolve WEBSITE

http://evolve.elsevier.com/Perry/nursinginterventions
Nursing Skills Online

Safe and accurate medication administration is one of your most important responsibilities. A nurse is responsible for having a full understanding of medication therapy and the related nursing implications. The nursing process is a useful framework for administering medications. Assessment and planning involve identifying factors that influence the way you administer medications and provide patients with instruction on self-administration. Nursing diagnoses communicate problems related to drug therapy and direct interventions for appropriate nursing care. Implementation includes administering medications correctly and safely and, in many cases, teaching patients how to self-administer medications. Evaluation involves monitoring patients' responses to medications and measuring learning. This chapter includes basic information for safely preparing to administer medications. Subsequent chapters address administration of nonparenteral medications and injections.

PATIENT-CENTERED CARE

Regardless of the health care setting, nurses are responsible for administering medications, evaluating the effects of the medications on the patient's health status, and teaching the patient about medications and their side effects. You are also responsible for ensuring that patients follow medication regimens and evaluating their administration techniques. In the acute care setting you will spend much time administering medications to patients. Safe techniques are essential. Before discharge you make sure that patients or family caregivers are adequately prepared to administer medications in the home. This requires thorough instruction and having patients and family caregivers explain their medication schedules.

A nurse's responsibility when administering medications safely must include effective communication with staff, pharmacy, patients, and family caregivers. Consider factors that influence patient's abilities to communicate effectively such as anxiety, pain, hearing, or culture. Therapeutic communication is essential to nursing practice.

Culturally a patient's values and beliefs affect medication response. A patient's level of education, prior experience with medication therapy, and the family's influence on actions significantly influence medication compliance. For example, in Japan it is not acceptable to verbalize complaints about stomach problems; thus it is common for these patients to not report nausea, vomiting, and bowel changes related to medication use. Some cultures' use of herbal and homeopathic remedies alters the response to a medication. Ethnicity needs to be considered when medications are prescribed and administered.

SAFETY

Because medication administration is essential to nursing practice. You need to know your patients' medication history and any drug allergies. In addition, you need to be knowledgeable about the actions and effects of the medications you give to patients. To safely and accurately administer medications, you need to have an understanding of pharmacokinetics, growth and development, nutrition, and mathematics.

PHARMACOKINETICS

When administering medications, know the mechanism of action, the therapeutic effects of the drugs, the purpose of the medication for the specific patient, and the desired effect. Equally important is knowledge of possible side effects and adverse reactions.

Pharmacokinetics is the study of how drugs enter the body (absorption), reach the site of action (distribution), are metabolized, and are excreted from the body. Absorption describes how a drug enters the body and passes into body fluids and tissues. Absorption influences the route of drug administration. Distribution is the way drugs move to the sites of action in the body. Metabolism refers to the chemical reactions by which a medication is broken down (e.g., in the liver) until it becomes chemically inactive. Excretion is the process of drug elimination from the body through the gastrointestinal tract, kidneys, or other body secretions (Skidmore-Roth, 2010).

DRUG ACTIONS

Mechanism of Action

When giving a drug to a patient, you can expect a predictable chemical reaction that changes the physiological activity of the body. This occurs as the medication bonds chemically at a specific site in the body called a *receptor site*. The reactions are possible only when the receptor site and the chemical fit together like a key in a lock. When the chemical fits well, the chemical response is good. These drugs are called agonists (Skidmore-Roth, 2010). Some drugs attach at the receptor site but do not produce a new chemical reaction. These drugs are called *antagonists*. Other drugs attach and produce only a small response or prevent other reactions from occurring. These drugs are called *partial agonists*.

Understanding pharmacokinetics enables you to make the decisions necessary to ensure that drugs are given by the appropriate route and to recognize and act based on the nature and extent of drug actions, interactions, and adverse actions. In addition, this knowledge helps in planning drug administration schedules. For example, knowing when the peak action of an analgesic occurs allows you to administer the drug at a time when you anticipate that the patient's pain will increase (e.g., before ambulation). Most agencies have standard administration schedules (see Appendix B, Abbreviations and Equivalents). For example, most schedules allow you to administer a drug one half hour before or after the scheduled time without concern for altering the effectiveness of the medication. Some medications are ordered for administration as needed (prn) within certain parameters prescribed by the physician.

Pharmacokinetics affects how much of a drug dose reaches the site of action. These processes are influenced by factors such as body surface area, body water content, body fat content, and body protein stores. When certain medications such as antibiotics are prescribed, the goal is to achieve a constant drug blood level within a safe therapeutic range. The patient and nurse must follow regular dosage schedules and administer prescribed doses at correct intervals. Knowledge of the following time intervals of drug action helps you to anticipate the effect of a drug:

1. *Onset of action:* The time interval between when a drug is given and the first sign of its effect
2. *Peak action:* The time it takes for a drug to reach its highest effective concentration
3. *Duration of action:* The time period from onset of drug action to the time when a response is no longer seen
4. *Plateau:* Blood serum concentration reached and maintained after repeated, fixed doses
5. *Therapeutic range:* The range of plasma concentration that produces the desired drug effect without toxicity

Laboratory tests monitor the therapeutic level of a drug in the body. Test results allow physicians to modify drug dosages to achieve a constant desired blood level. A blood sample is drawn to identify the peak serum level of a drug, which varies according to the specific drug involved. The lowest serum level is known as the trough level. Blood samples for peak and trough levels are usually drawn just before the next scheduled dose of medication. Coordinate blood sampling with the laboratory to obtain the most accurate peak and trough levels.

Therapeutic Effects

A therapeutic effect is the intended or desired physiological response of a medication. A single medication may have many therapeutic effects. For example, aspirin creates analgesia, reduces inflammation and fever, and slows blood clotting. Other drugs have more limited therapeutic effects. For example, an antihypertensive medication lowers blood pressure.

Side Effects and Adverse Reactions

Medications can produce unpredictable and unexplainable responses. A side effect is a predictable and unavoidable secondary effect produced at a usual therapeutic dose. Some side effects may be harmless, whereas others cause injury. For example, a common side effect of codeine phosphate is constipation, which can be managed with a change in diet and fluid intake. If side effects are serious enough to outweigh the beneficial effects of the therapeutic action of a drug, the prescriber may discontinue the drug. Patients often stop taking medications because of side effects such as anorexia, drowsiness, or dry mouth. Report any side effects to a physician or pharmacist so they can determine the symptoms are not more serious adverse reactions.

Adverse Reactions

Adverse reactions are unintended, undesirable, and often unpredictable drug effects. Some reactions occur immediately, whereas others develop more slowly over time. An example of an adverse reaction is a patient becoming comatose after taking a drug. When adverse responses to medications occur, the prescriber discontinues the medication immediately. Adverse reactions can range from mild to toxic effects. Prompt recognition and reporting of adverse reactions can prevent serious injury to patients.

Toxic effects Toxic medication effects develop after prolonged intake of high doses of medication, ingestion of drugs intended for external application, or when a drug builds up in the blood because of impaired metabolism or excretion. Toxic effects may be lethal, depending on the action of a drug. For example, morphine, an opioid analgesic, relieves pain by depressing the central nervous system (CNS). However, toxic levels of morphine cause severe respiratory depression and death.

Idiosyncratic reactions Medications may cause unpredictable effects such as an idiosyncratic reaction. In this case a patient overreacts or underreacts to a drug. Predicting which patients will have an idiosyncratic response is impossible. For example, lorazepam (Ativan), an antianxiety medication, when given to an older adult may worsen anxiety and cause agitation and delirium.

Allergic reactions Allergic reactions are also unpredictable responses to medications. Taking a medication the first time may cause an immunological response. When this occurs, the drug acts as an antigen, causing the production of antibodies. With repeated administration the patient develops an allergic response to the drug, its chemical preservatives, or a metabolite of it.

The antibodies create a mild or severe reaction, depending on the patient and the drug. Among the different classes of drugs, antibiotics cause a high incidence of allergic reactions. Table 21-1 summarizes common allergy symptoms. Severe, or anaphylactic, reactions are characterized by sudden constriction of bronchiolar muscles, edema of the pharynx and larynx, and severe wheezing and shortness of breath. The patient may become severely hypotensive, necessitating emergency resuscitation measures.

It is common practice for hospitalized patients with known drug allergies to have their allergy information recorded in a clearly identifiable place. This allows all caregivers to be aware of the patient's allergies. In many institutions this information is recorded on the front of the patient's medical record on an eye-catching sticker. Patients also wear a wristband that contains the name of the medications to which the patient is allergic. Patient allergies must be recorded on the patient's medication administration record (MAR). Patients cared for in other settings (e.g., home) and who have a known history of an allergy to a medication should wear an identification bracelet or medal that alerts all health care providers to the allergy in case the patient is unconscious when receiving medical care.

TABLE 21-1 COMMON ALLERGIC REACTIONS

SYMPTOM	DESCRIPTION
Angioedema	An acute, painless, dermal, subcutaneous, or submucosal swelling involving the face, neck, lips, larynx, hands, feet, or genitalia
Eczema (rash)	Small, raised vesicles that are usually reddened; often distributed over the entire body
Pruritus	Itching of the skin; accompanies most rashes
Rhinitis	Inflammation of mucous membranes lining the nose, causing swelling and a clear watery discharge
Urticaria (hives)	Raised, irregularly shaped skin eruptions with varying sizes and shapes; eruptions have reddened margins and pale centers
Wheezing	Constriction of smooth muscles surrounding bronchioles that decreases diameter of airways; occurs primarily on inspiration because of severely narrowed airways; development of edema in pharynx and larynx further obstructs airflow

Medication Interactions

When one medication modifies the action of another, a medication interaction occurs. A medication can enhance or reduce the action of other medications and alter the way in which the body absorbs, metabolizes, or eliminates the drug. When two drugs have a synergistic effect, the effect of the two medications combined is greater than the effect of one drug given separately. Alcohol is a CNS depressant that has a synergistic effect with antihistamines, antidepressants, and opioid analgesics.

A drug interaction may be desirable. Often a physician orders combination drug therapy to create a drug interaction for therapeutic benefit. For example, a patient with moderate hypertension may receive several drugs such as diuretics and vasodilators, which act together to keep blood pressure at a desirable level.

Medication Tolerance and Dependence

Medication tolerance occurs over time. A patient receives the same medication for long periods of time and then requires higher doses to produce the same desired effect. Patients taking various pain medications may develop tolerance over time. It may take a month or even longer for tolerance to occur.

Medication tolerance is not the same as medication dependence. Two types of medication dependence exist: psychological (or addiction) and physical. In psychological dependence the patient desires the medication for a benefit other than the intended effect. Physical dependence implies that a patient will suffer withdrawal effects if the medication is stopped abruptly. When patients receive medications for a short term such as for postoperative pain, dependence is rare.

Medication Misuse

Misuse of medication includes overuse, underuse, erratic use, and contraindicated use of medications. Patients of all ages misuse medications. Older adults are at greatest risk because of polypharmacy. Some people use medications for purposes other than their intended effect because of peer pressure, curiosity, or the pursuit of pleasure. Problems are not limited to illegal street drugs. The incidence of prescription and over-the-counter (OTC) drug misuse and abuse is also on the rise. The most commonly abused prescription medications include opioids, stimulants, tranquilizers, and sedatives. Common OTC medications that patients misuse or abuse include cough syrup and cold medication (USDHHS SAMHSA, 2008). You are ethically and legally responsible to understand the problems of persons using medications improperly. When caring for patients with suspected medication abuse or dependence, be aware of your values and attitudes about the willful use of harmful substances. Do not let your personal values interfere with understanding the patient's needs and concerns.

ADMINISTERING MEDICATIONS

Nursing Skills Online: Safe Medication Administration Module, Lesson 1

You are not solely responsible for medication administration. The prescriber (e.g., physician or advanced practice nurse [APN]) and pharmacist also help to ensure that the right medication gets to the right patient. You are accountable for knowing what medications are ordered, understanding their therapeutic effects, recognizing undesired effects, and administering medication correctly.

Medication Orders

A physician's order is required for all medications to be administered by a nurse (except in states where Nurse Practice Acts allow APNs and nurse practitioners to prescribe). A physician's order sheet is in written or electronic form. The physician writes the date, time, and medication order, including:

1. The name of the medication, which may be either the trade name (e.g., Percocet) or the generic name (e.g., oxycodone)
2. The dose (e.g., 5 mg)
3. The route (e.g., by mouth [PO])
4. The frequency (e.g., every 4 hours [q4h])
5. Orders for medications to be given prn (as needed) also include the reason they are to be given (e.g., for pain)
6. The signature of the prescriber

Verbal and telephone orders are optional forms of orders when written or electronic communication between the prescriber and nurse is not possible. When you receive a verbal or telephone order, you enter the order on the physician's order sheet. The name of the prescriber and your signature are included. The prescriber will countersign the order at a later time, usually within 24 hours after making the order (see agency policy). Box 21-1 provides guidelines for safely taking verbal or telephone orders for medications.

BOX 21-1 GUIDELINES FOR TELEPHONE ORDERS AND VERBAL ORDERS

- Clearly identify patient's name, room number, and diagnosis. Read back all orders to physician or health care provider (TJC, 2010).
- Use clarification questions to avoid misunderstandings.
- Write "TO" (telephone order) or "VO" (verbal order), including date and time, name of patient, and complete order; sign the name of the physician or health care provider and nurse.
- Follow agency policies; some institutions require documentation of the "read-back" or require two nurses to review and sign telephone or verbal orders.
- Physician or health care provider co-signs the order within the time frame required by the institution (usually 24 hours; verify agency policy).

There are five common types of medication orders. The type of order is based on the frequency and/or urgency of medication administration. Types of medication orders include standing orders; prn orders; and single (one-time) orders, which also include stat orders and now orders.

You carry out a *standing order* until the health care provider cancels it by another order or until a prescribed number of days elapse. A standing order sometimes indicates a final date or number of doses. Many institutions have a policy for automatically discontinuing standard orders.

Medications can be ordered to be given only when a patient requires or requests it. This is a prn order. You must assess a patient thoroughly to determine whether the patient needs the medication. Sometimes a different type of therapy is more appropriate. A prn order usually has minimum intervals set for the time of administration. This means that you cannot give the drug any more frequently than what is prescribed.

Single (one-time) orders are common for preoperative medications or medications given before diagnostic examinations. The medication is ordered to be given only once at a specified time. A stat order means that you give a single dose of a medication immediately and only once. Stat orders are used for emergencies when the patient's condition changes suddenly. A now order is more specific than a one-time order. It is used when a patient needs a medication quickly but not as soon as a stat order. When you receive a now order, you have as long as 90 minutes to give the drug (see agency policy). Nursing students cannot take medication orders.

The Joint Commission (2009b) now discourages the use of range orders for prn medications. An example of a range order is morphine sulfate 2 to 6 mg IV push q2-4h prn for pain. Range orders are often unclear and a source of medication errors. The Joint Commission recommends that organizations develop practice guidelines to define how range orders can be implemented (TJC, 2009a).

Communication and Transcription of Orders

After new medication orders are written, the drugs must be obtained from the pharmacy. Usually the copy of the physician's order sheet is sent to the pharmacy. The pharmacist is responsible for preparing the correct medications and delivering them to the nursing unit. Pharmacists also assess the medication plan and ensure that orders are valid.

Medication Errors

The Joint Commission (2009a) defines a medication error as any preventable event that may cause inappropriate medication use or jeopardize patient safety. Medication errors include inaccurate prescribing; administration of the wrong medication, route, and time interval; and administering extra doses or failing to administer a medication. Hospital delivery systems have a system of checks that help prevent medication errors. *Conscientious adherence to the six rights of medication administration is your best way to prevent errors.*

When an error occurs, acknowledge it immediately and then assess the patient. You have an ethical and professional obligation to report the error to the patient's physician, the nurse manager, and any other persons indicated by the institution policy regarding errors. Appropriate follow-up may include administering an antidote, withholding a subsequent dose, and monitoring the effects of the medication. The patient's record should include a notation that indicates what was given, who was notified, the observed effects of the medication, and follow-up measures taken.

You are also responsible for completing a report describing the incident. Most institutions have a policy or protocol for reporting adverse events. This report provides an objective analysis of what went wrong. It provides information for the risk management team to identify factors contributing to errors and develop ways to avoid similar errors in the future.

EVIDENCE-BASED PRACTICE TRENDS

Chang Y, Mark B: Antecedents of severe and nonsevere medication errors, *J Nurs Scholarsh* 41(1):70, 2009.

The Institute of Medicine report initiated the development of strategies to prevent medical errors and specifically reduce medication errors (Box 21-2). Chang and Mark (2009) identified differences between severe and nonsevere medication errors by reviewing work dynamics; hours each nurse worked; communication between nurses and physicians; nurses' expertise; nurse education; patient age, health status, and number of hospitalizations; and medication support services. They found that with a higher percentage of BSN-prepared nurses, there was a reduced incidence of severe medication errors, and the more experienced nurses reported more nonsevere errors. Nursing implications include targeting error prevention strategies to specific types of medication errors.

DISTRIBUTION SYSTEMS

Systems for storing and distributing medications vary. Institutions providing nursing care have special areas for stocking and dispensing medications. Medication storage areas must be locked when unattended.

Unit-Dose System

The unit-dose system uses portable carts containing a drawer with a 24-hour supply of medications for each patient. The unit dose is the ordered dose of medication that the patient receives at one time. Each medication form is wrapped separately. The cart also contains limited amounts of prn and stock medications for special situations. The medication cart can be pushed from room to room to facilitate administration of medications at routine times. The cart is kept locked when not attended. In some settings the medications are kept in a locked cabinet in the patient's room.

Automated Medication Dispensing Systems

Automated medication dispensing systems (AMDSs) are variations of unit-dose and floor stock systems. The systems within the health care agency are networked with each other and with other computer systems in the agency (e.g., the computerized medical record). AMDSs control the dispensing of all medications, including narcotics. Each nurse has a security code, allowing access to the system. If your agency uses a system that requires bioidentification, you have to place

BOX 21-2 STEPS TO TAKE TO PREVENT MEDICATION ERRORS

- Prepare medications for only one patient at a time.
- Follow the six rights of medication administration.
- Be sure to read labels at least three times (comparing MAR with label): when removing medication from storage, before taking to patient's room, before giving medication.
- Use at least two patient identifiers (e.g., patient name on name band, account number, or patient stating name) when administering medications.
- Do not allow any other activity to interrupt your administration of medication to a patient (e.g., phone calls, discussions with other staff).
- Double-check all calculations and verify with another nurse.
- Do not interpret illegible handwriting; clarify with prescriber.
- Question unusually large or small doses.
- Document all medications as soon as they are given.
- When you have made an error, reflect on what went wrong and ask how you could have prevented the error.
- Evaluate the context or situation in which a medication error occurred. This helps to determine if nurses have the necessary resources for safe medication administration.
- When repeated medication errors occur within a work area, identify and analyze the factors that may have caused the errors and take corrective action.
- Attend in-service programs on the medications you commonly administer.
- Follow agency policies and protocols during medication administration; do not take short cuts.

your finger on a screen to access the computer. Once logged onto the AMDS, you select the patient's name and medication profile. Then you select the medication, dosage, and route from a list on the computer screen. The system opens the medication drawer or dispenses the medication to the nurse, records the event, and charges it to the patient. If the system is connected to the patient's medical record, information about the medication (e.g., name, dose, time) and the name of the nurse who retrieved the medication from the AMDS is recorded in the patient's medical record. Some systems require nurses to scan bar codes before recording this information in the patient's computerized medical record. AMDS and bar code scanning reduce the chance of medication errors (Chang and Mark, 2009; Foote and Coleman, 2008; Ross, 2008).

MEDICATION ADMINISTRATION RECORD

A MAR is a form used to verify that the right medications are being administered at the correct times. The process of verification of medications varies among health care agencies. During the transcription process the nurse and pharmacist check all medication orders for accuracy and thoroughness several times, and the prescriber's complete order is placed on the appropriate medication form, the MAR. The MAR includes the patient's name, room, and bed number and the names, doses, frequencies, and routes of administration for each medication. If the MAR is handwritten, a registered nurse (RN) completes or updates the MAR. Some agencies use a computer to generate the MAR. Use the MAR printout to record medications given. When the MAR is electronic, it is viewed on a computer screen. Regardless of the type of MAR your agency uses, be sure that you refer to the MAR each time you prepare a medication and have it available at the patient's bedside when administering medications. It is essential that you verify the accuracy of every medication you give to the patient with the patient's orders. If the medication order is incomplete, incorrect, or inappropriate or if there is a discrepancy between the written order and what is on the MAR, consult with the prescriber. Do not give the medication until you are certain that you are able to follow the six rights of medication administration. When you give the wrong medication or an incorrect dose, **you** are legally responsible for the error.

THE SIX RIGHTS OF MEDICATION ADMINISTRATION

Preparing and administering medications require accuracy and your full attention. The six rights is a traditional checklist to promote accuracy in drug administration.

Right Medication

The Joint Commission includes medication reconciliation as a national patient safety goal for 2010 (TJC, 2010). When a patient enters a hospital setting, a complete list of the patient's current medications must be reviewed and documented with the patient involved. You will also compare the medications the health care provider orders with those on the patient's list. When the patient is transferred to another service or health care setting, you once again must reconcile the patient's current list of medications.

The Joint Commission (2009a) published a list of unacceptable abbreviations that have been found to increase the incidence of errors in medication administration (Table 21-2). You are responsible for using correct abbreviations and

TABLE 21-2 PROHIBITED AND ERROR-PRONE ABBREVIATIONS*

DO NOT USE	PROBLEM	USE INSTEAD
U (unit)	Mistaken for "0" (zero), the number "4" (four), or "cc"	Write "unit"
IU (international unit)	Mistaken for IV (intravenous), the number 10 (ten), or unit	Write "international unit"
q.d. or QD (daily)	Mistaken for qid	Write "daily"
Q.O.D., QOD, q.o.d., qod (every other day)	Mistaken for qd (daily) or qid (four times daily) if "o" is poorly written	Write "every other day"
Trailing zero (e.g., 1.0 mg)†	Decimal point is missed	Write X mg (e.g., 1 mg)
Lack of leading zero (e.g., .1 mg)	Decimal point is missed	Write 0.X mg (e.g., 0.1 mg)
MS	Can mean both morphine sulfate or magnesium sulfate	Write "morphine sulfate" or write "magnesium sulfate"
MSO_4 and $MgSO_4$	Confused for one another	Write "morphine sulfate" or write "magnesium sulfate"

Data from The Joint Commission: The official "Do Not Use" list, Oakbrook Terrace, Ill, 2009, TJC, http://www.jointcommission.org/PatientSafety/DoNotUseList/accessed September 22, 2010. ©The Joint Commission, 2009. Reprinted with permission.

*Applies to all orders and medication-related documentation that is handwritten (including free-text computer entry or on preprinted forms).

†*Exception*: A "trailing zero" may be used only where required to show precision of a reported value (e.g., laboratory test results), studies that report the size of lesions, or catheter and tube sizes. A "trailing zero" cannot be used in medication orders or medication-related documentation.

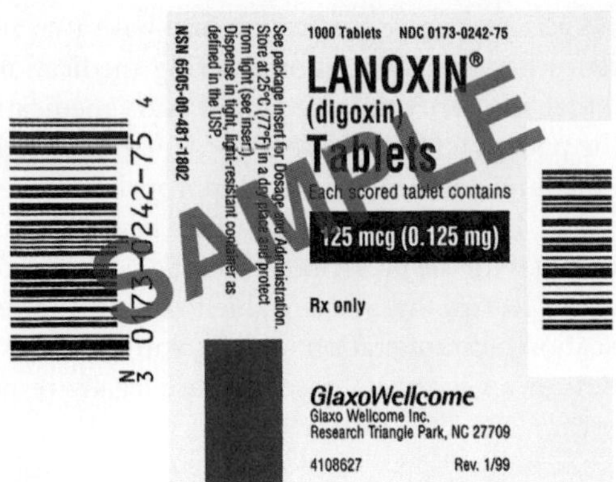

FIG 21-1 Sample drug label. (Reproduced with permission of Glaxo Wellcome, Inc., Research Triangle Park, NC.)

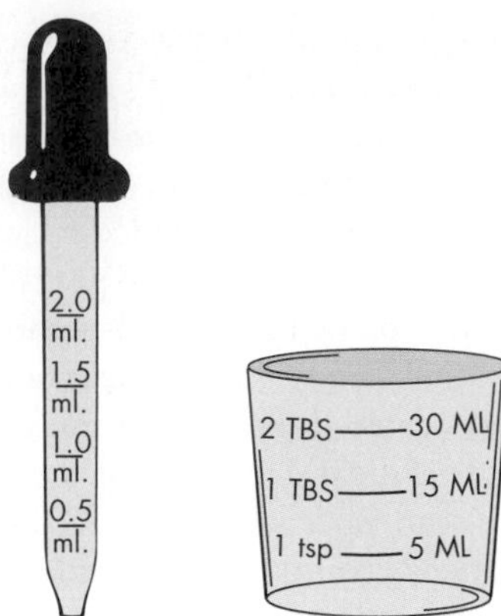

FIG 21-2 Scaled dropper for pediatric use and cup to measure oral liquids. (From Clayton BD, Stock YN: *Basic pharmacology for nurses*, ed 14, St Louis, 2010, Mosby.)

verifying that the order was accurately transcribed. Many institutions have a policy that requires RNs on a specific shift to verify the accuracy of MAR forms printed for each patient each day. Whenever new orders are handwritten on the MAR, the RN adding the orders must verify that they are accurately added to the MAR. When verification is complete, you initial and sign the order.

During medication administration, you compare the label of the medication (Fig. 21-1) with the MAR three times: (1) when removing the medication from the storage bin; (2) before placing the medication in the medicine cup or before taking the medication to the patient's room; and (3) again at the bedside before giving the medication to the patient. If the medication is ordered by trade name and dispensed from the pharmacy by generic name, verify that there is no discrepancy.

If a patient questions a medication, stop and recheck to be certain that there is no mistake. In most cases the medication order has been changed or the drug is manufactured by a different company than the patient has been using at home. However, attention to a patient's question is how errors are identified and prevented.

Right Dose

When a medication is prepared in a dose other than is the dose ordered, the chance of errors increases. After calculating the dose of a high-risk medication such as insulin or warfarin (Coumadin), compare the calculation with one done independently by a second nurse. This is especially important if it is an unusual calculation or involves a potentially toxic drug.

After calculating dosages, use appropriate measuring devices to prepare medications. Liquid preparations can be measured using a medicine cup marked in milliliters or a syringe for oral use. Some pediatric medications come with a scaled dropper (Fig. 21-2).

Right Patient

Your patient must be identified using two patient identifiers. Neither of the identifiers can be the patient's room number or his or her physical complaint (TJC, 2009a). Check the MAR against the patient's identification bracelet and ask the patient to state his or her full name. In some agencies a nurse also compares the medical record number on the MAR with the identification bracelet. Some agencies use a wireless bar code scanner to identify the right patient. This system requires you to scan a personal bar code that is commonly placed on your name tag first. Then you scan a bar code on the single-dose medication package. Finally, you scan the patient's armband. This information is then stored in a computer for documentation purposes. This system helps eliminate medication errors because it provides another step to ensure that the right patient receives the right medication (Chang and Mark, 2009).

Right Route

The prescriber's order must designate a route of administration (Table 21-3). If the route of administration is missing or if the specified route is not the recommended route, you must consult the prescriber immediately. When injections are administered, use only preparations intended for parenteral use. Injection of a liquid intended for oral use can produce local complications such as sterile abscess or fatal systemic effects. Medication companies label parenteral medications "for injectable use only."

Right Time

Each agency has routine time schedules for medications ordered at standard intervals. For example, medications to be given three times a day (tid) may be routinely scheduled for 0800, 1400, and 2000; or 0900, 1300, and 1900, depending on agency policy. A drug may also be ordered every 8 hours (q8h), which is also three times a day. The medication ordered q8h needs to be given around the clock (ATC) to maintain adequate therapeutic levels and would, for example, be given at 0800, 1600, and 2400. Generally the standard is for all routinely ordered medications to be given within 30 minutes before or after the scheduled time. Nursing judgment may allow some variance, depending on the medication involved.

TABLE 21-3 ROUTES OF MEDICATION ADMINISTRATION

ROUTE	DESCRIPTION OF MEDICATION
Oral	
Solid Forms	
Caplet	Solid dosage form for oral use; shaped like a capsule and coated for ease of swallowing
Capsule	Medication encased in a gelatin shell
Tablet	Powdered medication compressed into hard disk or cylinder
Enteric coated	Tablet that is coated so it does not dissolve in stomach; meant for intestinal absorption
Liquid Forms	
Elixir	Clear fluid containing water and alcohol; designed for oral use; usually has sweetener added
Syrup	Medication dissolved in a concentrated sugar solution
Extract	Concentrated medication form made by removing the active portion of medication from its other components
Aqueous solution	Substance dissolved in water and syrups
Topical	
Ointment (salve or cream)	Semisolid, externally applied preparation, usually containing one or more medications
Lotion	Semi-liquid suspension often used to cool, protect, or clean skin
Transdermal patch	Medicated disk or patch absorbed through the skin over a designated period of time (e.g., 24 hours)
Parenteral	
Solution	Sterile preparation that contains water with one or more dissolved compounds
Powder	Sterile particles of medication that are dissolved in a sterile solution (e.g., water, normal saline) before administration
Body Cavity	
Intraocular disk	Medicated disk (similar to a contact lens) that is inserted into the patient's eye; medication absorbed over a designated period of time
Suppository	Solid dosage form mixed with gelatin and shaped in the form of a pellet for insertion into a body cavity (rectum or vagina); melts when it reaches body temperature, allowing medication to be absorbed

A medication may also be ordered for special circumstances. A preoperative medication may be ordered stat (to be given immediately); now, which means as soon as available, usually within an hour; or on call, which means that the operating or procedure room personnel will notify the nurse when it is the appropriate time. A drug may be ordered before meals (ac) or after meals (pc).

Right Documentation

To ensure the right documentation, first make sure that the information on your patient's MAR corresponds exactly with the prescriber's order and the label on the medication container. Do not give medications that have illegible or incomplete orders. Verify inaccurate orders before giving medications. It is better to give the correct medication at a later time than to give your patient the wrong medication. Record the administration of each medication on the MAR as soon as you give it. Never document that you have given a medication until you have actually given it. Document the name of the medication, the dose, the time of administration, and the route. Also document the site of any injections you give. Document the patient's response to the medication in the nurses' notes. Accurate documentation prevents medical errors.

Medication Preparation

It is legally advisable to administer only the medications that you prepare. Administering a medication prepared by another nurse increases the opportunity for error. The nurse who gives the wrong medication or an incorrect dose is legally responsible for the error. The importance of checking similar names and verifying for the correct drug cannot be overemphasized.

Interpreting Medication Labels

Medication labels include several basic pieces of information: the trade name of the drug in large letters, the generic name in smaller letters, the form of the drug, the dosage, the expiration date, the lot number, and the name of the manufacturer. The trade name given by the manufacturer often suggests the action of the drug, and the generic name is the chemical name (Fig. 21-3).

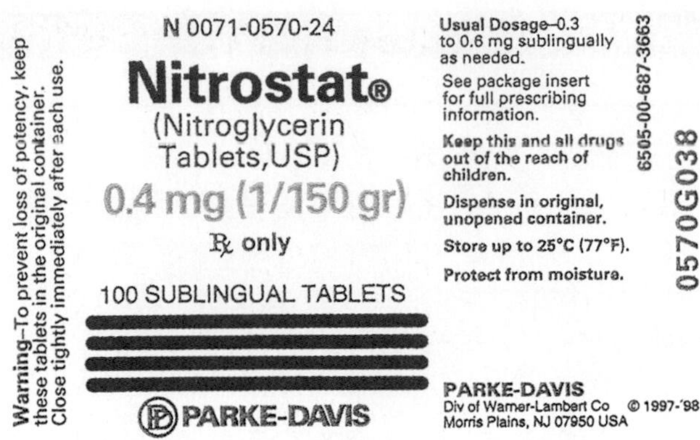

FIG 21-3 Interpreting a drug label. (Reproduced with permission of Warner-Lambert Company.)

Clinical Calculation

To administer medications safely, use your mathematics skills to safely calculate medication dosages and mix solutions. This is important because you will not always dispense medications in the unit of measure in which they are ordered. Medication companies package and bottle certain standard equivalents. For example, the patient's health care provider orders 250 mg of a medication that is available only in grams. You are responsible for converting available units of volume and weight to the desired doses. Therefore be aware of approximate equivalents in all major measurement systems. An example follows:

The order reads: vancomycin 1 g IV.

The pharmacy supplies vancomycin in 500-mg vials.

Because the dose on the medication label is in milligrams, conversion should be from grams to milligrams; 1 g = 1000 mg.

SYSTEMS OF MEASUREMENT

The proper administration of medication depends on your ability to compute drug dosages accurately and measure medications correctly. A careless mistake in placing a decimal point or adding a zero to a dosage can lead to a fatal error. The prescriber and patient depend on you to check the dosage before giving a drug. The metric system is the most common system used in the measurement of medications.

Metric System

As a decimal system, the metric system is the most logically organized of the measurement systems. Each basic unit of measure is organized into units of 10. Multiplying or dividing by 10 forms secondary units. In multiplication the decimal point moves to the right; in division the decimal moves to the left. To convert grams to milligrams you multiply by 1000 or move the decimal point three places to the right (0.5 g = 500 mg). Conversely, to convert milligrams to grams you divide by 1000 or move the decimal point three places to the left (500 mg = 0.5 g).

The basic units of measure in the metric system are the meter (length), liter (volume), and gram (weight). For drug calculations you will use primarily volume and weight units. In the metric system small or large letters designate the basic units:

Gram: g or gm

Liter: l or L

Small letters are abbreviations for subdivisions of major units:

Milligram: mg

Milliliter: mL

TABLE 21-4 EQUIVALENTS OF MEASUREMENT

METRIC	HOUSEHOLD
1 mL	15 drops (gtt)
5 mL	1 teaspoon (tsp)
15 mL	1 tablespoon (tbsp)
30 mL	2 tablespoons (tbsp)
240 mL	1 cup (c)
480 mL (approximately 500 mL)	1 pint (pt)
960 mL (approximately 1 L)	1 quart (qt)
3840 mL (approximately 5 L)	1 gallon (gal)

Household Measurements

Household measures are familiar to most people, but these measures are not recommended for medication administration because of the variability in the size of household utensils. Included in household measures are drops, teaspoons, tablespoons, and cups for volume and ounces and pounds for weight. Before the actual administration of medication, you may need to convert units within a system or between systems and calculate drug dosages (Table 21-4).

Solutions

Solutions are used for injections, irrigations, and infusions. A solution is a given mass of solid substance dissolved in a known volume of fluid or a given volume of liquid dissolved in a known volume of another fluid. Solutions are available in units of mass per units of volume (e.g., g/mL, g/L). You can also express a concentration of a solution as a percentage. A 10% solution is 10 g of solid dissolved in 100 mL of solution.

Dosage Calculations

Dosage calculations are necessary when the dose on the medication label differs from the dosage ordered. There are several dosage calculation methods. The most common methods are ratio-proportion or use of a formula (Box 21-3). Dimensional analysis is a method for dosage calculation that involves simple multiplication and division and not algebra (Box 21-4).

Example 1

When the dose ordered has the same label as the dose available:

BOX 21-3 FORMULA METHOD

$\frac{D}{H} \times V$ = Amount to give

D is the desired dose or the dose ordered by the physician for the patient (e.g., 250 mg of penicillin PO 4 times daily).
H is the drug dose on hand or available for use. The dose is on the drug label (e.g., penicillin tablets of 250 mg each).
V is the volume (liquid) or vehicle (number of tablets, capsules) that delivers the available dose.
NOTE: The desired dose **(D)** and the on-hand dose **(H)** must be in the same unit of measurement. If they are in different units, you must perform conversions before completing the formula.

BOX 21-4 DIMENSIONAL ANALYSIS

Use the following steps to solve medication problems using dimensional analysis:

1. Identify the unit of measure that you need to administer. For example, if you are giving a pill, you will usually be giving a tablet or a capsule; for parenteral or oral medications, the unit is milliliters.
2. Estimate the answer in your mind.
3. Place the name or appropriate abbreviation for *x* on the left side of the equation (e.g., *x* tab, *x* mL).
4. Place available information from the problem in a fraction format on the right side of the equation. Place the abbreviation or unit that matches what you are going to administer (determined in Step 1) in the numerator.
5. Look at the medication order and add other factors into the problem. Set up the numerator so it matches the unit in the previous denominator.
6. Cancel out like units of measurement on the right side of the equation. You should end up with only one unit left in the equation, and it should match the unit on the left side of the equation.
7. Reduce to the lowest terms if possible and solve the problem or solve for *x*. Label your answer.
8. Compare your estimate from Step 1 with your answer in Step 2.

Dose ordered: 0.5 g
Tablets available: 0.25 g per tablet

Step 1. The starting factor is 0.5 g.
The answer label is tablets (i.e., how many tablets should be given).

Step 2. Formulate the conversion equation:
The equivalent needed is 1 tablet = 0.25 g.

$$\frac{0.5\text{ g}}{1} \times \frac{1\text{ tab}}{0.25\text{ g}} = \text{tabs}$$

Cancel labels (g).
NOTE: If properly written, all labels except the answer label will cancel.

Step 3. Solve the equation:
Reduce the numerical values and multiply the numerators and denominators.

$$\frac{{}^{2}\cancel{0.5\text{ g}}}{1} \times \frac{1\text{ tab}}{\cancel{0.25\text{ g}}} = 2\text{ tabs}$$

Example 2

When the dose ordered has a different label than the dose available:

Dose ordered: 0.5 g
Tablets available: 250 mg per tablet

Step 1. The starting factor is 0.5 g.
The answer label is tablets (i.e., how many tablets should be given).

Step 2. Formulate the conversion equation:
The equivalents needed are 1 g = 1000 mg and 1 tab = 250 mg.

$$\frac{0.5\text{ g}}{1} \times \frac{1000\text{ mg}}{1\text{ g}} \times \frac{1\text{ tab}}{250\text{ mg}} = \text{tabs}$$

Cancel labels (g, mg).

Step 3. Solve the equation:
Reduce the values and multiply the numerators and denominators.

$$\cancel{0.5\text{ g}} \times \frac{\overset{4}{\cancel{1000\text{ mg}}}}{\underset{2}{\cancel{1\text{ g}}}} \times \frac{1\text{ tab}}{\cancel{250\text{ mg}}} = \frac{4}{2} = 2\text{ tabs}$$

Example 3

When the dose ordered is available in a liquid form:

Dose ordered: Cephalexin (Keflex) 250 mg PO
Available: 125 mg per 5 mL

Step 1. The starting factor is 250 mg.
The answer label is mL.

Step 2. Formulate the conversion equation:
The equivalent needed is 125 mg = 5 mL.

$$\frac{250\text{ mg}}{1} \times \frac{5\text{ mL}}{125\text{ mg}} = \text{mL}$$

Cancel labels (mg).

Step 3. Solve the equation:
Reduce and multiply.

$$\frac{{}^{2}\cancel{250\text{ mg}}}{1} \times \frac{5\text{ mL}}{\cancel{125\text{ mg}}} = 10\text{ mL}$$

NURSING PROCESS

Nurses use the nursing process to integrate medication therapy into patient care. As a nurse your role extends beyond simply giving drugs to a patient. You are responsible for monitoring patients' responses to medications, providing education to the patient and family about the medication regimen, and informing the physician when medications are effective, ineffective, or no longer necessary.

Assessment

Begin your assessment with the patient's medical history, which provides any indications or contraindications for medication therapy. Certain diseases or illnesses place patients at risk for adverse medication effects. For example, if a patient has a gastric ulcer, forms of aspirin increase the chance of bleeding. Long-term health problems require specific medications. This knowledge helps you anticipate the medications that your patient requires.

Include an assessment of patient allergies. Many medications have ingredients found in food sources. For example, if your patient is allergic to shellfish, he or she may be sensitive to products containing iodine such as Betadine or dyes used in radiological testing. When assessing for medication allergies, you must differentiate between actual allergic reactions, which can be life threatening, and drug intolerances, which are uncomfortable side effects. In an acute care setting patients with allergies wear identification bands that list each medication allergy. All allergies and the types of reactions are noted on the patient's admission notes, medication records, and history and physical examination.

Your assessment also involves identifying all medications that the patient takes every day at home, including prescriptions, OTC preparations, and herbal supplements. Determine how long the patient has taken each medication, current dosage schedule, and whether the patient has had any adverse effects to any of the medications. The patient should know the name, purpose, dosage, route, and side effects of medications and supplements that are being taken. Often patients take many medications and carry a list that includes this information. Patients have different levels of understanding. One patient may describe a diuretic as a "water pill," whereas another describes it as a drug to minimize swelling and lower blood pressure. Still another may describe it as "the little white pill I take in the morning." By assessing the patient's level of knowledge, you determine the need for teaching. If a patient is unable to understand or remember pertinent information, it may be necessary to involve a family member.

Complete appropriate assessments, which may include but are not limited to vital signs, laboratory data, or nature and severity of symptoms. If data contraindicate medication administration, hold the drug and notify the prescriber.

Planning

During planning, organize nursing activities to ensure the safe administration of medications. Current evidence shows that distractions or hurrying during medication preparation administration increases the risk of medication errors (Fowler and others, 2009). Suggestions to reduce distraction include gathering all equipment needed before preparing medications; asking other nurses to answer patient call bells during medication preparation, and wearing some identifying clothing to indicate that medications are being prepared (Kreckler and others, 2008). The following are general goals of medication administration:

1. Patient achieves therapeutic effect of the prescribed medication.
2. Patient complications related to the prescribed medication are absent.
3. Patient and/or family understand medication therapy.
4. Patient and family self-administer medication safely (when appropriate).

Implementation

Nursing interventions focus on safe and effective drug administration. This includes careful medication preparation, accurate and timely administration, and patient education.

Preadministration Activities

1. Identify the medication action, purpose, side effects, and nursing implications for administering and monitoring. Ensure that the medication order has not expired.
2. Calculate medication doses accurately and use appropriate measuring devices. Verify that the dose prescribed is appropriate for the patient situation.
3. Give medications within 30 minutes before or after the scheduled time to maintain a therapeutic level. NOTE: Medications ordered stat should be given immediately. Preoperative medications may be ordered on call and are given when the operating or procedure room personnel notify the nurse of the appropriate time. Certain medications such as insulin should be given at a precise interval before a meal. Others should be given with meals or on an empty stomach.
4. Use good hand-hygiene technique. Avoid touching tablets and capsules. Use sterile technique for parenteral medications. Wear clean gloves when administering parenteral medications and certain topical medications.
5. Administer only medications that you personally prepare. Do not ask another person to administer medications that you prepare. Keep medications secure (Fig. 21-4). Do not administer medications prepared by someone else.
6. When preparing medications, be sure that the label is clear and legible and that the drug is properly mixed, has not changed in color, clarity, or consistency, and has not expired.
7. Keep tablets and capsules in their wrappers and open them at the patient's bedside. This allows you to review each

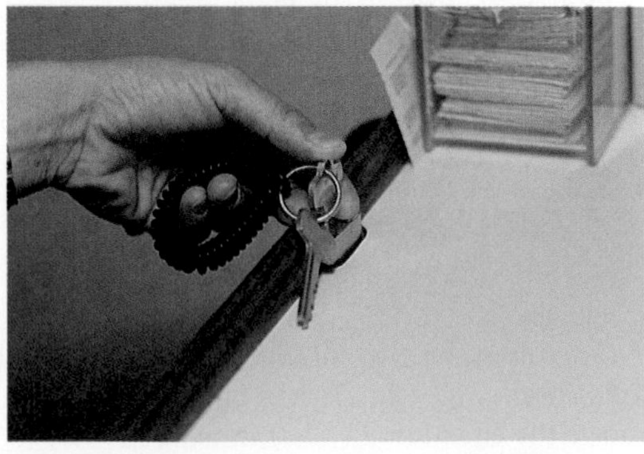

FIG 21-4 Medication carts must be kept locked when unattended, and the key kept by an authorized person.

medication with the patient. If a patient refuses medication, there is no question about which one is withheld.

Drug Administration

1. Follow the six rights for medication administration.
2. Inform the patient of the name, purpose, action, and common side effects of each medication. Evaluate the patient's knowledge of the medication and provide appropriate teaching.
3. Stay with the patient until the medication is taken. Provide assistance as necessary. Do not leave medication at the bedside without a prescriber's order. For example, some patients may take their own vitamins or birth control pills while in the hospital.
4. Respect the patient's right to refuse medication. If the medication wrapper is intact, the medication may be returned to the patient's storage bin. When medication is refused, determine the reason for this and take action accordingly. For example, if the patient has unpleasant side effects, it may be possible to eliminate them by giving the pills with food or using a different time schedule.

Postadministration Activities

1. Record medications immediately after administration (see agency policy). Include the drug name, dose, route, time, and your signature.
2. Document data pertinent to the patient's response. This is especially important when giving drugs ordered prn.
3. If a medication is refused, document that it was not given, the reason for the refusal, and when the physician was notified.

Evaluation

1. Monitor for evidence of therapeutic effects, side effects, and adverse reactions. This includes monitoring physical response (e.g., heart rhythm, blood pressure, urine output, or laboratory results).
2. When a medication is given for relief of symptoms, ask patient to report if symptoms have diminished or been relieved.
3. Observe injection sites for bruises, inflammation, localized pain, numbness, or bleeding.
4. Evaluate patient's understanding of medication therapy and ability to self-administer medication.

PATIENT AND FAMILY TEACHING

A well-informed patient is more likely to take medications correctly. However, many patients have limited health literacy, meaning that they do not understand how to read medication labels or calculate doses. Provide an individualized approach to teaching, using visual aids, instructional booklets, or even video tapes. When teaching patients about their medications, include persons identified as being significant to the patient's recovery. This may include family members, partners, or home care providers. Specific nursing interventions are appropriate in the home setting (Box 21-5).

Teaching Patients About Side Effects

All medications have side effects. You are responsible for teaching the patient and family members about side effects associated with each prescribed medication. If you do not inform patients properly about medications or if your patients have problems with health literacy, it is possible that they will take their medications incorrectly or they will not take their medications at all. You need to adapt your approaches for patients with low health literacy so they will understand instruction. Because medications can have many side effects, teaching the patient about all of them can be overwhelming. Remember that patient learning is a continual process. When beginning to teach a patient about a new medication, evaluate each of the side effects. Then teach the patient about the ones that are most likely to occur and occur early after administration. For example, some antibiotics cause hypersensitivity reactions, hepatotoxicity, nephrotoxicity, and platelet dysfunction. Hypersensitivity reactions are likely to occur shortly after taking a few doses of an antibiotic. The other side effects tend to occur after long-term antibiotic administration. Teach patients about side effects in terms of things that they can see, feel, touch, or hear. For example, thrombocytopenia, a reduction in the number of platelets in the blood, can be a medication side effect. The patient cannot see, feel, touch, or hear thrombocytopenia. However, thrombocytopenia can cause bleeding. Teach the patient how to look for evidence of bleeding. Be sure to teach the patient what to do about side effects when they are discovered.

Medications and the Patient's Activities of Daily Living

Evaluate the patient's activities of daily living and the effect they will have on his or her ability to comply with medication schedules. When medications are initiated in the acute care setting, they are often given ATC. In the community or home it may not be reasonable for patients to administer medications according to this schedule. In collaboration with the prescriber or the pharmacist, teach the patient and family members how to adjust medication schedules that are consistent with the patient's lifestyle. Include what to do for missed doses.

Evaluating Teaching Effectiveness

Evaluating the effectiveness of teaching ensures that the patient can administer medications in a safe manner. One method of evaluating patient understanding is to create medication cards with the generic and trade names of the medication on the front of the card and all pertinent medication information on the back of the card. You can flash the card in front of the patient and ask him or her to read the names of the medication. Another method is to have patients read labels on prepared medications. Remember that medication bottles often have fine print and are difficult to read for the patient with impaired vision. If the patient correctly identifies the name of the medication, ask him or her the following questions:

BOX 21-5 HOME CARE

1. During each home visit, assess all of the patient's prescription and nonprescription medications. Review information about medications, including desired effect, dose, frequency, and adverse effects.
2. Assess patient's health literacy by determining ability to understand what is read and complete simple medication calculations. If health literacy is poor, ensure that information is presented at a level the patient can understand and arrange for help from family, friends, and/or home health nurses.
3. Teach the complications and interactions of all food, OTC, and herbal medications to patients and their caregivers.
4. Collaborate with social workers to identify community resources for financial assistance with pharmaceutical needs.
5. Monitor and evaluate the effectiveness of the prescribed medications:
   a. Note changes in physical and functional status (e.g., vital signs, sleeping, elimination).
   b. Note changes in mental status (e.g., level of alertness, memory).
   c. Monitor blood levels as needed.
   d. Communicate potential problems to health care provider.
6. Monitor urinary output status of patients because changes in renal excretion may require a decrease or increase in medication dosage.
7. For patients who have difficulty remembering when to take medications, make a chart that lists the times to take each medication or prepare a special container that organizes and stores medications according to when the patient needs to take them.
8. Reduce the chance of medication error by labeling or color-coding medication bottles.
9. Keep an accurate record of the homebound patient's weight, especially the older adult, because many medication dosages are calculated by body weight.
10. Teach medication safety in the home environment by instructing patients to do the following:
    a. Keep medications in original, labeled containers.
    b. Dispose of outdated medications in a sink or toilet only; never dispose of them in the trash within reach of children.
    c. Never "share" drugs with friends or family members.
    d. Always finish a prescribed medication; do not save it for a future illness.
    e. Read labels carefully and follow all instructions.
11. Instruct patients with arthritis or debilitating illness who have difficulty opening child-proof containers to request nonchild-proof containers from their health care providers.

Data from Ebersole P and others: *Toward healthy aging: human needs and nursing response*, ed 7, St Louis, 2008, Mosby; and Kairuz T and others: Identifying compliance issues with prescription medications among older people: a pilot study, *Drugs Aging* 25(2):153, 2008.

- Why are you taking this medication?
- How often do you take this medication?
- What side effects can occur with this medication?
- If this side effect occurs, what are you going to do about it?

Be sure to also assess the patient's sensory, motor, and cognitive functions. Impairments may affect the patient's ability to safely self-administer medications; and family members, friends, or home health aides may need to assist with medication administration. Many self-help devices are also available for purchase (e.g., pill boxes with times displayed and electronic dispensers).

SPECIAL HANDLING OF CONTROLLED SUBSTANCES

As a nurse you are responsible for following legal regulations when administering controlled substances (medications with potential for abuse). Violations of the Controlled Substances Act may result in fines, imprisonment, and loss of license. Health care institutions have policies for the proper storage and distribution of controlled substances, including opioids (Box 21-6). Many agencies use computerized systems for medication access and distribution (Fig. 21-5).

BOX 21-6 STORAGE AND ACCOUNTABILITY FOR CONTROLLED SUBSTANCES

- All controlled substances are stored in a locked cabinet or container (see Fig. 21-4).
- Authorized nurses carry a set of keys or computer entry code for the cabinet.
- An inventory record is kept to record all controlled substances used, including patient's name, date, name of medication, and time of medication administration.
- Before any medication is removed from the cabinet, the number actually available is compared with the number indicated on the controlled substance record. If incorrect, the discrepancy must be rectified before proceeding.
- If any part of a dose of a controlled substance is discarded, a second nurse witnesses disposal of the unused portion, and the record is signed by both nurses.
- At change of shift one nurse going off duty counts all controlled substances with a nurse coming on duty. Both nurses sign the record to indicate that the count is correct. (Computerized storage has eliminated this process.)
- Discrepancies in controlled substance counts are reported immediately.

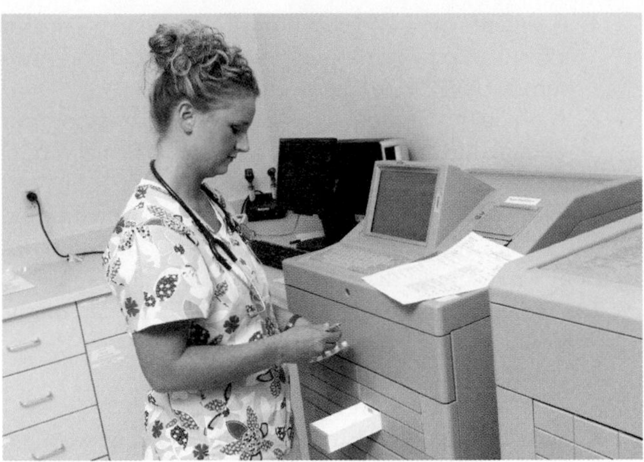

FIG 21-5 Computerized system for medication distribution.

Special Considerations

Pediatric

Children vary in age; weight; and ability to absorb, metabolize, and excrete medications. Children's doses are lower than those of adults, and caution is needed in preparing medications. Medication may or may not be prepared and packaged in doses appropriate for children. Preparing appropriate doses often requires calculation based on body weight (Hockenberry and Wilson, 2009). A child's parents may be helpful in determining the best way to give a child medication.

Geriatric

Individuals older than age 65 are the largest users of prescription and OTC medication (Ebersole and others, 2008). Because of physiological changes associated with the aging process, special nursing interventions are needed to promote safe and effective medication administration. Nursing interventions include spacing medication times to not interfere with meals; if the older adult has difficulty swallowing a large pill, substituting liquid medication if possible; providing memory aids in large print; and observing the older adult opening and preparing his or her medication safely. Be aware of the following patterns related to medication use:

- *Polypharmacy.* Polypharmacy happens when a patient uses two or more medications to treat the same illness, when a patient takes two or more medications from the same chemical class, or when the patient uses two or more medications with the same or similar actions to treat different illnesses (Ebersole and others, 2008; Sidhu and others, 2007). Polypharmacy also occurs when a patient mixes nutritional supplements or herbal products with medications. To decrease the risks associated with polypharmacy, work with your patient's prescribers to make sure that the patient's medication regimen is as simple as possible.
- *Self-prescribing.* Older adults often attempt to seek relief from a variety of problems with OTC preparations, folk medicines, and herbs.
- *Misuse of drugs.* Misuse by older adults includes overuse, underuse, erratic use, and contraindicated use.
- Noncompliance. Deliberate misuse of medication is considered to be noncompliance. Older adults alter doses because of ineffectiveness, unpleasant side effects, and lack of financial resources.

REVIEW QUESTIONS

1. The nurse uses a current drug index to look up a pain medication and finds that the onset of action of the drug is 30 minutes, it peaks in 60 minutes, and the duration of action is 3 hours. The patient asks the nurse to administer this medication so it will be most effective when the patient participates in a strenuous hour-long physical therapy session later in the day. When should the nurse give this medication to the patient?
   1. Stat
   2. Fifteen minutes before the physical therapy session
   3. An hour before the physical therapy session
   4. Just before the patient begins the physical therapy session
2. The nurse finds the following new medication order written in a patient's hospital chart: "3/17/09 0800 furosemide 40 mg twice a day." What should the nurse do first?
   1. Enter the order in the hospital computer.
   2. Administer the medication.
   3. Contact the prescriber.
   4. Review the order with a pharmacist.
3. List the six rights of medication administration.
4. On admission to the medical unit, the nurse is doing a medication reconciliation of the patient's current medication. She finds that the patient is taking 8 different medications, all for management of arthritis pain. Of what is this an example?
   1. Medication dependence
   2. Medication tolerance
   3. Polypharmacy
   4. A desirable medication interaction
5. The physician's order for a medication states: "Percocet 1 or 2 tabs BID and prn." The physician is very busy, does not like to be bothered, and is known for being difficult to work with. What should the nurse do?
   1. Consult a pharmacist to interpret the order.
   2. Call the physician and have the order verified.
   3. Administer the medication twice a day and as the patient needs.
   4. Talk to the unit secretary on the floor who is good at reading the physician's handwriting.

6. The patient has an order for 1 tbsp of Robitussin for a cough. Converting this to the metric system, what dose would the nurse give to the patient?
   1. 5 mL
   2. 10 mL
   3. 15 mL
   4. 30 mL
7. A patient is to receive cephalexin, 500 mg PO. The drawer of the automated medication dispensing system (AMDS) opens. There are five tablets, each labeled 250 mg cephalexin in the drawer. What should the nurse give to the patient?
   1. ½ tablet
   2. 1 tablet
   3. 1½ tablets
   4. 2 tablets
8. The nurse has to give the following medications to her patients. To which patient should she give medications first?
   1. A patient who is to receive 325 mg of aspirin who has a history of coronary artery disease
   2. A patient who needs 2 tablets of acetaminophen/hydrocodone (Vicodin) who is rating his incisional pain at an 8 on a pain scale of 0 to 10
   3. A patient who is to get captopril (Capoten) 25 mg for a history of hypertension whose current blood pressure is 125/72 mm Hg
   4. A patient who is receiving trimethoprim/sulfamethoxazole (Bactrim DS) for a urinary tract infection
9. An older adult states that she cannot see her medication bottles clearly to determine when to take her prescription. What should the nurse do? Select all that apply.
   1. Provide a dispensing container for each day of the week.
   2. Provide larger, easier-to-read labels.
   3. Tell the patient what is in each container.
   4. Have the family administer the medication.
10. The nurse receives a telephone order to administer 20 mEq of potassium by mouth to her patient stat. What does she need to do first?
   1. Read back the order to the prescriber to verify.
   2. Prepare 20 mEq of potassium by mouth and administer it.
   3. Contact the pharmacist to see if the medication can be prepared in the pharmacy.
   4. Ask the prescriber to come to the unit and write the order before administering the medication.

REFERENCES

Chang Y, Mark B: Antecedents of severe and nonsevere medication errors, *J Nurs Scholarsh* 41(1):70, 2009.

Ebersole P and others: *Toward healthy aging: human needs and nursing response*, ed 7, St Louis, 2008, Mosby.

Foote SO, Coleman JR: Medication administration: the implementation process of bar-coding for medication administration to enhance medication safety, *Nurs Econ* 26(3):207, 2008.

Fowler S and others: Bar-code technology for medication administration: medication errors and nurse satisfaction, *Medsurg Nurs* 18(2):103, 2009.

Hockenberry MJ, Wilson D: *Wong's essentials of pediatric nursing*, ed 8, St Louis, 2009, Mosby.

Kreckler S and others: Interruptions during drug rounds: an observational study, *Br J Nurs* 17(21):1329, 2008.

Ross J: Collaboration—integrating nursing, pharmacy and information technology into a barcode medication administration system implementation, *Caring: Connecting, Sharing, & Advancing Healthcare Informatics* 23(1):1, 2008.

Sidhu AK: Polypharmacy and the elderly: a review of the literature, *Nurs J Singapore* 34(4):11, 2007.

Skidmore-Roth L: *Mosby's drug guide for nurses*, ed 4, St Louis, 2010, Mosby.

The Joint Commission: *2009 National patient safety goals: hospital program*, Oakbrook Terrace, Ill, 2009a, TJC, http://www.jointcommission.org/PatientSafety/NationalPatientSafetyGoals/09_hap_npsgs.htm.

The Joint Commission: *2009 Critical access hospital and hospital national patient safety goals*, Oakbrook Terrace, Ill, 2009b, TJC, http://www.jointcommission.org/PatientSafety/NationalPatientSafetyGoals/09_hap_npsgs.htm.

The Joint Commission (TJC): *2010 National Patient Safety Goals*, Oakbrook Terrace, Ill, 2010, The Commission, http://www.jointcommision.org/PatientSafety/NationalPatientSafetyGoals, accessed July 2010.

United States Department of Health and Human Services Substance Abuse and Mental Health Services Administration (USDHHS SAMHSA): *The NSDUH Report: nonmedical use of pain relievers in substate regions*, 2004-2006, 2008, http://www.oas.samhsa.gov/2k8/pain/substate.cfm.

CHAPTER

22

Administration of Nonparenteral Medications

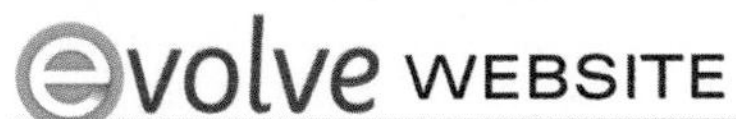

http://evolve.elsevier.com/Perry/nursinginterventions
Video Clips
Nursing Skills Online

Nonparenteral medications include those that are not given by injection such as oral medications, eyedrops, and eardrops. The route chosen depends on the properties and desired effects of the medication and the physical and mental condition of the patient. The oral route (by mouth) is the easiest and most desirable way to administer medications. Each route has advantages and disadvantages (Table 22-1). There are many reasons why you may find it necessary to recommend a change from one route to another. When this occurs, you are responsible for consulting with the health care provider for an order or conferring with a pharmacist to safely meet the patient's needs.

Topical administration of medications involves applying drugs directly to skin, mucous membranes, or tissue membranes. You apply medications to the skin by painting, spraying, or spreading medication over a localized area. Transdermal patches (adhesive-backed medicated disks) applied to the skin provide a continuous release of medication over several hours or days. Topical administration avoids puncturing the skin and lessens tissue injury and risk of infection that may occur with injections.

Medications applied to membranes such as the cornea of the eye or rectal mucosa are absorbed quickly because of the vascularity of the membrane. When drug concentrations are high, systemic effects can occur. For example, bradycardia and hypotension may occur after instillation of ophthalmic beta blockers such as timolol (Timoptic). Mucous and tissue membranes differ in their sensitivity to medications. For example, the cornea of the eye is extremely sensitive to chemicals. Patients commonly experience burning sensations during administration of eyedrops and nose drops. Medications generally are less irritating to vaginal or rectal mucosa.

PATIENT-CENTERED CARE

An excellent time to provide patient education is during medication administration. Most patients discharged from hospitals are placed on new medications, and they often continue previously ordered medications. The goal of patient education is to improve patient adherence to medication regimens. The problem is that studies show 34.9% to 80% of patients fail to adhere to their regimens (Kilbourne and others, 2005; Sorensen and others, 2005). Poor adherence can lead to serious complications, side effects, and even death. Patients often fail to adhere to medication regimens for three reasons: patient issues, medication issues, and provider issues (Shearer, 2009). Patient issues include cognitive impairment, depression, physical limitation, social and financial issues, and lack of knowledge. Medication issues include multiple medications and medication discrepancies. Provider issues include inappropriate prescriptions, poor instruction, and lack of provider knowledge about adherence. Simply explaining medications and offering printed information are not enough. Studies show that it is important to discuss not only the purpose of medications, but also their specific benefits, expected effects, and how to plan daily drug schedules. In

TABLE 22-1 NONPARENTERAL ROUTES OF ADMINISTRATION

ROUTE	ADVANTAGES	DISADVANTAGES
Inhalation	Directly acts on lung tissues and provides rapid relief of respiratory distress	It is difficult for some patients to hold or manipulate canister correctly. Patients must be taught how to use equipment.
Mucous membranes: eyes, ears, nose; vaginal, rectal	Local application to involved site; limited side effects; rectal route an alternative when oral route not available	Insertion of vaginal or rectal products may cause embarrassment. Rectal suppositories are contraindicated with rectal surgery or active rectal bleeding.
Oral (swallowed)	Easy, comfortable, economical; may produce local or systemic effects	Some drugs are destroyed by gastric secretions. Cannot be given if patient is NPO, is unable to swallow, is nauseated, has gastric suction, or is unconscious or confused and unwilling to cooperate. They may irritate lining of GI tract, discolor teeth, or have unpleasant taste.
Skin: topical application or transdermal patches	Provides primarily local effect; painless; limited side effects; transdermal application provides systemic effects and bypasses the liver and its first-pass effects	Extensive topical applications may be bulky or cause difficulty in maneuvering. They may leave oily or pasty substance on skin; may soil clothing. Systemic absorption can be unreliable. Allergies to the adhesive in transdermal patches may develop.

Modified from Lilley LL, Harrington S, Snyder JS: *Pharmacology and the nursing process,* ed 5, St Louis, 2007, Mosby.
NPO, Nothing by mouth; *GI,* gastrointestinal.

addition, repetition of information is important, especially when caring for older adults and patients with cognition problems (e.g., changes in consciousness, inability to attend because of symptoms). Be sure to involve family caregivers in education sessions since they may be the ones administering medications. Also involve pharmacists in medication instruction because they can often simplify medication schedules and offer further insight about the importance of adherence (Lakey and others, 2009).

SAFETY

The physical environment where you prepare medications contributes to medication errors. Often the most critical drug calculations, judgments, and medication preparations are made in noisy, dimly lit, and chaotic areas of a nursing unit (Simmons, Graves, and Flynn, 2009). Be aware of the conditions in the area where you prepare medications. Because we rely on visual stimulation to make critical decisions, both artificial light and natural light are important to safety. Always have sufficient lighting when locating equipment, reading labels, calculating doses, and preparing medications. Increased noise and disruptions increase your cognitive workload, thus making it difficult to perform safely (Simmons and others, 2009). For example, construction noise, foot traffic, monitoring machines, telephones, and hallway conversations are just some of the factors that decrease your ability to concentrate and attend properly to medication administration. In some agencies policies have been established for nurses who are in medication preparation areas. They cannot be approached or interrupted during the medication preparation process. Pape and others (2005) conducted a study using colored vests to signal to all staff on a nursing unit that the nurse wearing the vest was involved in medication administration. The results showed a drop in medication errors.

EVIDENCE-BASED PRACTICE TRENDS

Shearer J: Improving oral medication management in home health agencies, *Home Healthcare Nurse* 27(3):184, 2009.

Medication management is a primary reason for home health care. In a study involving 204 home health agencies, nurses were surveyed to identify which evidence-based practices were seen to improve patients' ability to manage oral medications. They included use of reminder strategies (e.g., cueing strategies such as alarm clock use, selecting the location of medications, and written notes on refrigerators or cabinet doors), use of phone follow-up intervention by home health nurses, repetition of patient medication education during future home care visits, and use of medication simplification strategies for patients taking multiple medications. Medication simplification strategies included removing or discarding old or expired medications, using a single pharmacy for each patient, using nondrug alternatives so fewer medications are prescribed, coordinating doses with the patient's established daily routines, using long-acting/sustained-release (SR) alternatives to reduce the number of medications, decreasing multiple medications for a single health condition, and discontinuing or substituting cautionary medications.

SKILL 22.1 ADMINISTERING ORAL MEDICATIONS

• **Nursing Skills Online: Nonparenteral Medication Administration, Lesson 1** *Video Clips*

Patients usually are able to ingest or self-administer oral medications with few problems. However, situations may arise that contraindicate patients receiving medications by mouth, including the presence of gastrointestinal (GI) alterations, the inability of a patient to swallow food or fluids, and the use of gastric suction. An important precaution to take when administering any oral preparation is to protect patients from aspiration.

Aspiration is a life-threatening condition that occurs when food, fluid, or medication intended for GI administration accidentally enters the respiratory tract. You can protect patients from aspiration by evaluating their ability to safely swallow (see Skill 12.2). Properly positioning the patient also helps in preventing aspiration. Unless contraindicated, position the patient in a seated high-Fowler's position when administering oral medications. The side-lying position is also used when the patient's swallow, gag, and cough reflexes are intact. A patient who has difficulty swallowing should be evaluated by appropriate personnel (e.g., speech therapist) before receiving oral medications. When a feeding tube is present, always verify the correct tube placement before giving medications to prevent aspiration (see Skill 12.4).

Absorption of an oral medication after it is ingested depends largely on its form or preparation. Solutions and suspensions that are already in a liquid state (Fig. 22-1) are absorbed more readily than tablets or capsules. Oral medications are absorbed more easily when administered between meals and when the stomach is not filled with food, which slows absorption. When effective absorption in the stomach is required, give drugs at least 1 hour before or 2 hours after meals or antacids.

Some drugs are not absorbed until reaching the small intestine. Enteric coatings on some tablets resist being dissolved by gastric juices and prevent digestion in the upper GI tract. The coating protects the stomach lining from irritation by the medication. Eventually the drug is absorbed in the intestine. Do *not* crush or dissolve enteric-coated medications before administration. The website of the Institute for Safe Medication Practices, http://www.ismp.org/Tools/doNotCrush.pdf, contains a complete list of medications that cannot be crushed.

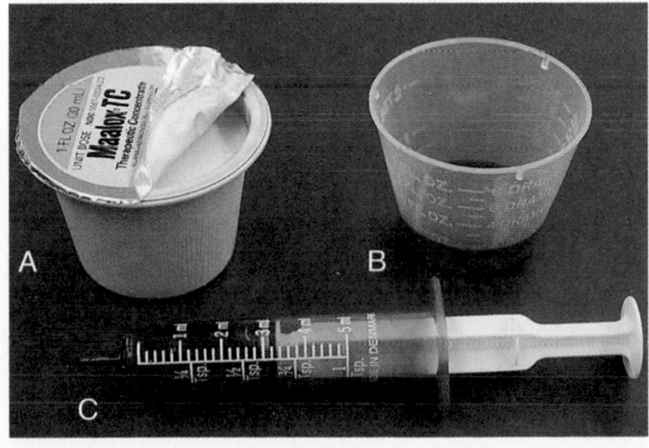

FIG 22-1 A, Liquid medication in a single-dose package. **B,** Liquid measured in a medicine cup, **C,** Oral medicine in syringe.

ASSESSMENT

1. Check accuracy and completeness of each medication administration record (MAR) with health care provider's medication order. Check patient's name, drug name and dosage, route of administration, and time for administration. Recopy or reprint any portion of printed MAR that is difficult to read. *Rationale: The health care provider's order is the most reliable source and only legal record of drugs patient is to receive. Ensures that patient receives the right medications (Eisenhauer and others, 2007, Furukawa and others, 2008).*
2. Review pertinent information related to medication, including action, purpose, normal dose and route, side effects, time of onset and peak action, and nursing implications. *Rationale: Allows you to anticipate effects of drug and observe patient's response.*
3. Assess for any contraindications to oral medication, including being on NPO status, inability to swallow, nausea/vomiting, bowel inflammation, reduced peristalsis, recent GI surgery, gastric suction, and decreased level of consciousness (LOC). Notify the health care provider if any contraindications are discovered. *Rationale: Alterations in GI function can interfere with drug absorption, distribution, and excretion. Giving oral medication to patients with impaired swallowing or decreased LOC increases their risk of aspiration.*
4. Assess risk for aspiration using a dysphagia screening tool if available (see Skill 12.2) Note patient's ability to swallow and assess cough and gag reflexes. *Rationale: Patients with dysphagia are at risk for aspirating oral medication.*
5. Assess patient's medical history, history of allergies, medication history, and diet history. List any drug allergies on each page of the MAR. When allergies are present, patient should wear an allergy bracelet. *Rationale: These factors influence how drugs act, and information reveals any previous problems with medication administration.*
6. Gather and review physical assessment findings and laboratory data that influence drug administration such as vital signs and results of renal and liver function tests. *Rationale: Data may lead to holding a medication or reveal that a certain drug is contraindicated.*
7. Assess patient's knowledge about health and medication use. *Rationale: Determines patient's need for medication education and guidance needed to achieve appropriate drug adherence.*

8. Assess patient's preferences for fluids and determine if medications can be given with these fluids. Maintain fluid restrictions as prescribed. *Rationale: Some fluids interfere with medication absorption. Offering fluids during drug administration is an excellent way to increase patient's fluid intake. Fluids ease swallowing and facilitate absorption from the GI tract. However, fluid restrictions must be maintained.*

PLANNING

Expected Outcomes focus on safe, accurate, and effective drug therapy.

1. Patient experiences desired medication effect within period of onset of medication.
2. Patient denies any GI discomfort or symptoms of alterations.
3. Patient explains purpose of medication and drug dosage schedule.

Delegation and Collaboration

In acute care settings administration of oral medication cannot be delegated to nursing assistive personnel (NAP). In some long-term care settings, trained and certified nursing assistants (CNAs) administer certain nonopioid, nonparenteral medications to stable patients. Instruct the NAP about the following:

- Potential side effects of medications and reporting their occurrence

Equipment

- Medication administration record (MAR)
- Automated, computer-controlled drug dispensing system, or medication cart
- Disposable medication cups
- Glass of water, juice, or preferred liquid and drinking straw
- Device for crushing or splitting tablets (optional)
- Paper towel
- Clean gloves (if handling an oral medication)

IMPLEMENTATION *for* ADMINISTERING ORAL MEDICATIONS

STEPS	RATIONALE
1. See Standard Protocol (inside front cover).	
2. Prepare medications.	
a. Plan preparation to avoid interruptions, keep door to medication room closed, do not take phone calls; follow agency policy.	Interruptions contribute to medication administration errors (Biron and others, 2009).
b. Arrange medication tray and cups in medication preparation area or move medication cart to position outside patient's room.	Organization of equipment saves time and reduces error.
c. Access automated dispensing system or unlock medicine drawer or cart.	Unauthorized access to medications is prevented when dispensing systems are locked.
d. Prepare medications for *one patient at a time*. Follow the six rights of medication administration. Keep all pages of MARs or computer printouts for one patient together.	Prevents preparation errors.
e. Select correct drug from stock supply, unit-dose drawer, or automated dispensing system. Compare name of medication on the label with MAR or computer printout. Exit the automated dispensing system after removing drug.	Reading label and comparing it against transcribed order reduce errors. *This is the first check for accuracy.*
f. Check or calculate drug dose as needed. Double-check any calculation.	Double-checking pharmacy calculations reduces risk of error. Some agencies require nurses to check calculations of certain medications such as insulin with another nurse.
g. Check expiration date on all medications. Return all outdated drugs to pharmacy.	Medications used past expiration date may be inactive or harmful to patient.
h. To prepare unit-dose tablets or capsules, place packaged tablet or capsule directly into medicine cup without removing wrapper (see illustration). Give medications only from containers with labels that are clearly marked and legible.	Wrapper identifies drug name and dose, which can facilitate teaching.

STEPS	RATIONALE
i. To prepare tablets or capsules from a floor stock bottle, pour required number into bottle cap and transfer medication to medication cup. Do not touch medication with fingers. Return extra tablets or capsules to bottle.	Avoids contamination of medications and avoids waste. Floor stock bottles are common in long-term care settings for over-the-counter (OTC) drugs such as laxatives and nonopioid analgesics.
j. When using a blister pack, "pop" medications through foil or paper backing into a medication cup.	Long-term care agencies use blister packs, which provide about a 1-month supply of prescription drugs for a patient. Each "blister" usually contains a single dose. Blister packs are prepared by a pharmacist or pharmaceutical company.
k. If it is necessary to break a medication to give half the dose, use a clean, gloved hand to break the tablet or cut with a clean pill-cutting device (see illustration). Only break tablets prescored by the manufacturer (line transverses the center of the tablet).	Reduces contamination of the tablet. Tablets that are not prescored cannot be broken into equal halves, resulting in an inaccurate dose. A cutting device results in a more even split of a tablet (ISMP, 2006).
l. Place all tablets or capsules that patient will receive in one medicine cup, except for those requiring preadministration assessments (e.g., pulse rate, blood pressure).	Serves as a reminder to complete appropriate assessment and facilitates withholding drugs (if necessary).

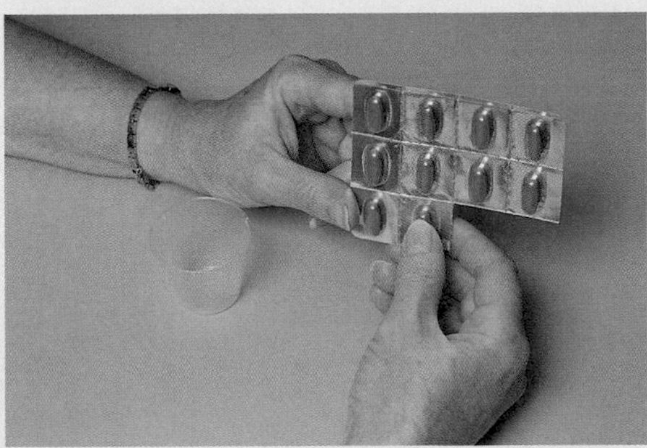

STEP 2h Place tablet into medicine cup without removing wrapper.

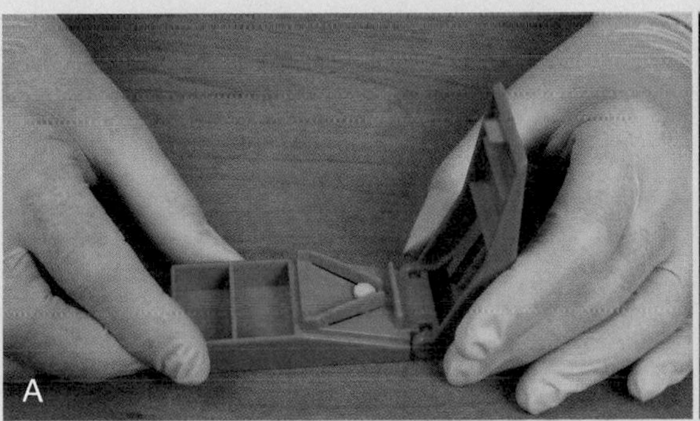

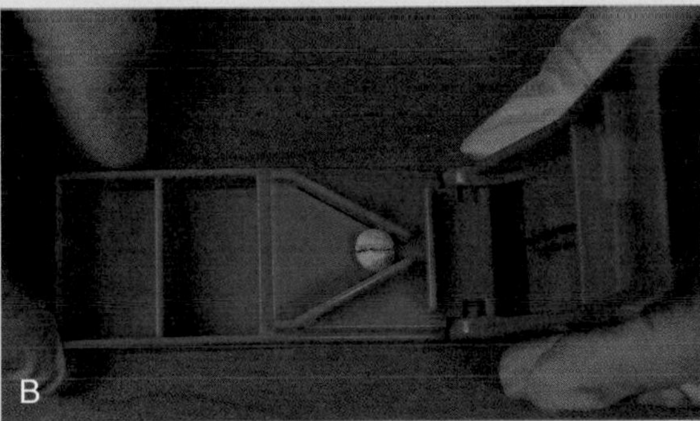

STEP 2k Tablet is placed in pill-cutting device **(A)** and cut in half **(B)**.

Continued

STEPS	RATIONALE
m. If patient has difficulty swallowing, crush each medication separately. In one such device, place medicine in between the two cups and then grind and crush (see illustration). Mix ground tablet in small amount (teaspoon) of soft food (custard or applesauce).	Large tablets are often difficult to swallow. Ground tablet mixed with palatable soft food is usually easier to swallow.
n. Prepare liquids.	
(1) Thoroughly mix by shaking gently before administering. If drug is in a unit-dose container with the correct volume, shaking is not needed.	Mixing liquid suspensions just before pouring ensures that the correct amount of medication, and not just the solvent, is measured for the dose.
(2) If drug is in a multidose bottle, remove cap from container and place it upside down on the work surface. Check and discard medications that are cloudy or have changed color.	Prevents contamination of inside of cap.
(3) Hold bottle with label against palm of hand while pouring.	Any spilled liquid will not soil or obscure label.
(4) Place medication cup at eye level on countertop or, when necessary, in hand, and fill to desired level on scale (see illustration). Scale should be even with fluid level at its surface or base of meniscus, not edges.	Ensures accurate measurement.
(5) Wipe lip of bottle with paper towel. Recap the bottle.	Prevents contamination of contents of bottle and prevents bottle cap from sticking.
(6) If giving less than 10 mL of liquids, prepare medication in an oral dosing syringe (see Fig. 22-1, *C*). Do not use a hypodermic syringe or a syringe with a needle or syringe cap.	Allows more accurate measurement of small amounts. If hypodermic syringes are used, the medication may accidentally be given parenterally. If the needle or syringe cap is not removed, it may dislodge and become aspirated during administration of oral drugs.
o. When administering controlled drugs such as opioids, check the controlled drug record for previous drug count and compare with supply available. Controlled drugs may be stored in a computerized locked cart (see Chapter 21).	Controlled substance laws require careful monitoring of dispensed opioids. In most facilities co-signature by a registered nurse (RN) is required when students administer controlled drugs.
p. Before going to patient's room, compare MAR with labels on prepared drugs for drug name and patient name (see illustration).	Reading labels a second time reduces errors. *This is the second check for accuracy.*

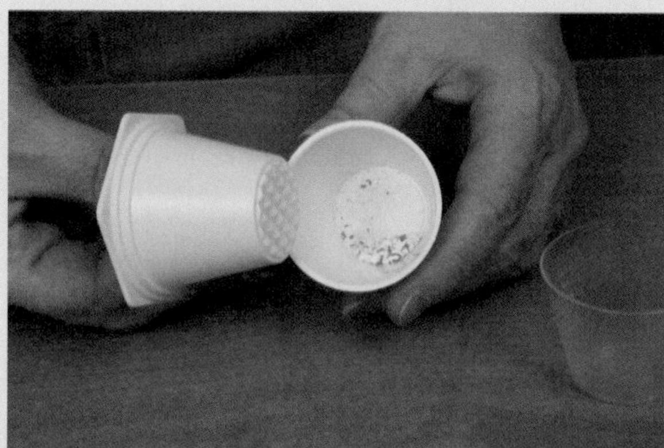

STEP 2m Crushing a tablet with pill-crushing device.

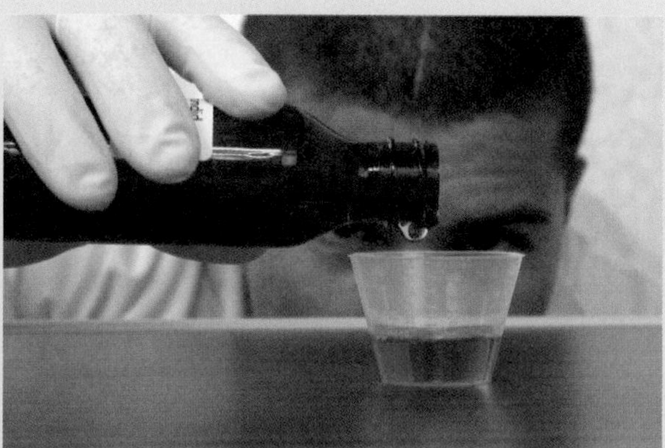

STEP 2n(4) Measuring liquid medication. Look at meniscus at eye level. (From Lilley LL and others: *Pharmacology and the nursing process*, ed 6, St Louis, 2011, Mosby.)

STEPS	RATIONALE

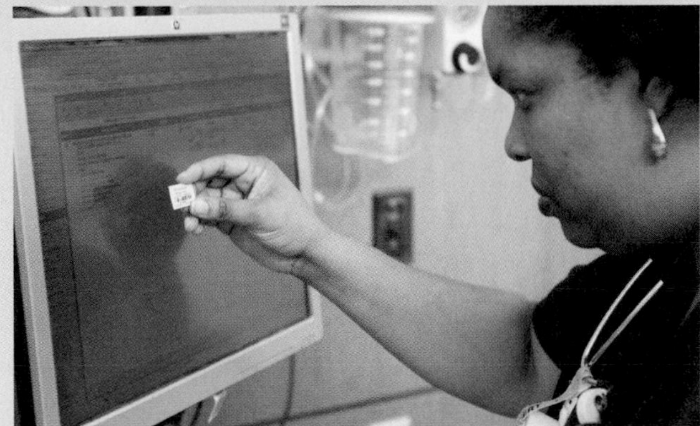

STEP 2p The nurse compares the medicine administration record to the medication label.

STEPS	RATIONALE
(1) Return stock containers or unused unit-dose medications to shelf or drawer. Label medication cups and poured medications with patient's name before leaving medication preparation room. Do not leave drugs unattended.	Ensures that correct medications are prepared for correct patient.
3. Administer medications.	
a. Take medications to patient at correct time, within 30 minutes before or after prescribed time (see agency policy). Give stat and single-order medications at the exact time. During administration apply the six rights of medication administration.	Promotes intended therapeutic effect.
b. At the patient's bedside compare the MAR or computer printout with the names of medications on the medication labels and patient name.	*This is the third check for accuracy* and ensures that the patient receives the correct medication.
c. Identify patient using two identifiers (e.g., name and birthday or name and account number, according to facility policy). Compare identifiers with information on patient's MAR or medical record.	Ensures correct patient. Complies with The Joint Commission standards and improves patient safety (TJC, 2010).
d. Perform necessary preadministration assessment (e.g., blood pressure, pulse) for specific medications. Ask patient if he or she has allergies.	Determines whether specific medications should be withheld at that time. Confirms patient's allergy history.
e. Discuss the purpose of each medication, action, and possible adverse effects. Allow patient to ask any questions about drugs.	Patient has the right to be informed, and patient's understanding of each medication improves adherence with drug therapy.
f. Assist patient to sitting or side-lying position if patient is unable to sit.	Position decreases risk of aspiration during swallowing.

SAFETY ALERT If in doubt about patient's ability to swallow, check swallow, cough, and gag reflexes (see Skill 12.2). If these reflexes are impaired or if the patient is unable to swallow pills without choking, withhold the medication, keep the patient NPO, and notify the health care provider. It may be necessary to ask the health care provider to consider administering the drug in another form (crushed, oral liquid, suppository, or by injection).

STEPS	RATIONALE
g. *For tablets*: Patient may wish to hold solid medications in hand or cup before placing in mouth. Offer water or juice to help patient swallow medications.	Patient becomes familiar with medications by seeing each drug. Choice of fluid can improve fluid intake.

Continued

STEPS	RATIONALE
h. *For orally disintegrating formulations (tablets or strips):* Remove medication from blister packet just before use. Do not push the tablet through the foil. Place medication on top of patient's tongue and caution against chewing the medicine.	Orally disintegrating formulations begin to dissolve when placed on the tongue. Water is not needed. Careful removal from packaging is needed because the tablets and strips are thin and fragile (Uko-Ekpenyong, 2006).
i. *For sublingually administered medications*: Have patient place medication under tongue and allow it to dissolve completely (see illustration). Caution patient against swallowing tablet or saliva.	Drug is absorbed through blood vessels of undersurface of tongue. If swallowed, drug is destroyed by gastric juices or rapidly detoxified by liver, preventing therapeutic blood level.

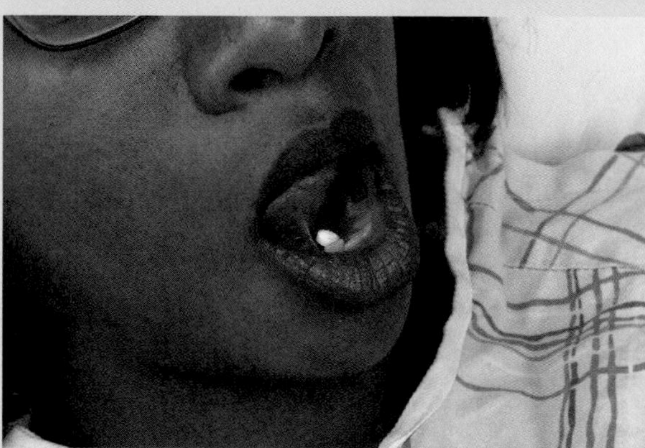

STEP 3i Proper placement of sublingual tablet in sublingual pocket.

STEPS	RATIONALE
j. *For buccal administered medication:* Have patient place medication in mouth between mucous membranes of cheek and gums until it dissolves.	Buccal drugs act locally or systemically as they are swallowed in saliva.
k. *For powdered medications:* Mix with liquids at bedside and give to patient to drink.	When prepared in advance, powdered drugs thicken; and some even harden, making swallowing difficult.
l. *For crushed medications mixed in food:* Give each medication separately in teaspoon of food.	
m. Caution patient against chewing or swallowing lozenges.	Lozenges act through slow absorption through oral mucosa, not gastric mucosa.
n. If patient is unable to hold medications, place medication cup to the lips and gently introduce each drug into the mouth, one at a time. A spoon can also be used to place the pill in the patient's mouth. Do not rush or force medications.	Administering a single tablet or capsule eases swallowing and decreases risk for aspiration.

SAFETY ALERT If a tablet or capsule falls to the floor, discard it and repeat preparation. Drug is contaminated.

STEPS	RATIONALE
o. Stay until patient completely swallows each medication or takes it by prescribed route. Ask patient to open mouth if you are uncertain whether medication was swallowed.	Nurse is responsible for ensuring that patient receives ordered dose. If left unattended, patient may not take dose or may save drugs, causing health risk.

SAFETY ALERT If patient is to receive a combination of oral tablets, capsules, and sublingual or buccal drugs, administer tablets/capsules first. Have patient take sublingual and buccal medications last. Do not give liquids until oral-disintegrating, buccal, or sublingual medication is completely dissolved.

STEPS	RATIONALE
p. For highly acidic medications (e.g., aspirin), offer patient a nonfat snack (e.g., crackers) if not contraindicated by patient's condition.	Reduces gastric irritation. The fat content of foods may delay drug absorption.

4. See Completion Protocol (inside front cover).

EVALUATION

1. Return within appropriate time to determine patient's response to medications, including therapeutic effects, side effects or allergy, and adverse reactions. Sublingual/buccal medications act in 15 minutes; most oral medications act in 30 to 60 minutes.
2. Ask patient or family member to identify drug name and explain purpose, action, dosage schedule, and potential side effects of drug.

Unexpected Outcomes and Related Interventions

1. Patient exhibits adverse effects (e.g., side effect, toxic effect, allergic reaction).
   a. Withhold further doses and assess vital signs.
   b. Notify the health care provider and pharmacy.
   c. Symptoms such as urticaria, pruritus, rhinitis, and wheezing may indicate emergency medications for allergic reaction.
2. Patient is unable to explain drug information.
   a. Further assess the patient's or family caregiver's knowledge of medications and guidelines for drug safety.
   b. Provide further instruction as necessary.
3. Patient refuses medication.
   a. Assess why patient is refusing medication (e.g., nausea, disagreement with treatment plan, side effects).
   b. Educate patient about the purpose of the medication and the potential effects of not taking the drug.
   c. Do not force the patient to take medications.
   d. Notify health care provider.
   e. Record information taught, refusal of medication, and patient's stated reason.
4. Administration error occurs (wrong drug, dose, patient, route, or time).
   a. Evaluate patient for untoward effects according to the drug action and side effects.
   b. Acknowledge error immediately.
   c. Take measures to counteract the effects of the error if necessary (e.g., keep patient on bed rest, administer ordered antidotes, hold other medications if ordered).
   d. Notify health care provider.
   e. Complete medication error form as required by the agency. These reports can assist in preventing similar errors in the future.

Recording and Reporting

- Record drug, dose, route, and time administered on MAR immediately *after* administration, not before. Include initials or signature. Record patient teaching and validation of understanding in nurses' notes.
- If drug is withheld, record reason in nurses' notes. Follow facility policy for marking held medications on the MAR. Most agencies require that the nurse circle the time the drug normally would have been given on the MAR or computer printout.
- Report adverse effects/patient response and/or withheld drugs to nurse in charge or health care provider.

Sample Documentation

NOTE: Documentation of medications is usually done on the MAR. Other documentation occurs only if a problem is noted.

0900 Apical pulse 50 beats/min and regular; c/o nausea; skin cool and moist to touch. Digoxin held, health care provider notified.

Special Considerations

Pediatric

- Liquid medications are safer to swallow to avoid aspiration of small pills.
- Pediatric doses are usually calculated based on body weight.
- Children will refuse bitter or distasteful oral medicines. Mix the drug with a small amount (about 1 teaspoon) of a sweet-tasting substance such as jam, applesauce, sherbet, or fruit puree. Do not use honey in infants because of the risk of botulism. Offer the child juice or an ice pop after medication administration. Do not place medication in an essential food item such as milk or formula; the child may refuse the food at a later time.
- Measure small amounts of liquid medications using a plastic calibrated syringe. Amounts less than a teaspoon are impossible to measure accurately with a molded medicine cup (Hockenberry and Wilson, 2007).

Geriatric

- Physiological changes of aging influence how oral medications are distributed, absorbed, and excreted. Common changes include dry mouth; delayed esophageal clearance and impairing swallowing; reduction in gastric acidity and stomach peristalsis; reduced liver function, resulting in altered drug metabolism; and reduced renal function and colon motility, slowing drug excretion.
- Give with a full glass of water (unless restricted) to aid passage of the drug. Give patient time to swallow.
- Patients may have several health problems or chronic conditions that require the use of multiple drugs, often prescribed by different health care providers. Polypharmacy creates a high risk for drug interactions and adverse reactions. Assess for potential drug interactions.
- When instructing patients about their medication regimen, include the patient's spouse or another family caregiver.
- If possible, provide a written medication schedule for patient to follow at home. Use large print in written materials if vision is impaired.

Home Care

- Instruct patient about specific drug regimen (purpose, action, dose, dosage intervals, side effects, food to avoid or take with drugs).
- When measuring liquid medications at home, patients should use kitchen measuring spoons or measuring spoons designed for medications, not eating utensil spoons that may vary in volume.

SKILL 22.2 ADMINISTERING MEDICATIONS THROUGH A FEEDING TUBE

- **Nursing Skills Online: Enteral Nutrition Module, Lesson 5**

Patients who have enteral feeding tubes are unable to receive food or medication by mouth. Chapter 12 describes the clinical indications and nursing care implications for nasogastric (NG), nasointestinal, gastrostomy, and jejunostomy tubes. Preferably medications administered by enteral tubes should be in liquid form. If a medication is not available in a liquid, you will need to prepare an oral medication tablet or capsule by crushing or dissolving it. However, you cannot crush sublingual, SR, chewable, long-acting, or enteric-coated medications. Check with a pharmacist about whether you can crush or dissolve a medication. Always verify the position of an enteral tube before administering any medication (see Skill 12.4).

If a medication is to be administered through an NG tube inserted for decompression, consult the health care provider because the tube must be clamped for 30 minutes to an hour after instillation of the medication. In most cases do not give medications into NG/intestinal tubes that are inserted for decompression of the stomach.

ASSESSMENT

1. Check accuracy and completeness of each MAR with health care provider's medication order. Check patient's name, drug name and dosage, route of administration, and time for administration. Recopy or reprint any portion of printed MAR that is difficult to read. *Rationale: The health care provider's order is the most reliable source and only legal record of drugs patient is to receive. Ensures that patient receives the right medications (Eisenhauer and others, 2007; Furukawa and others, 2008).*
2. Review pertinent information related to medication, including action, purpose, normal dose and route, side effects, time of onset and peak action, and nursing implications. *Rationale: Allows you to anticipate effects of drug and observe patient's response.*
3. Assess for any contraindications to patient receiving medication enterally, including presence of bowel inflammation or reduced peristalsis, recent GI surgery, presence of gastric suction that cannot be temporarily turned off. *Rationale: Alterations in GI function interfere with drug distribution, absorption, and excretion. Patients with GI suction do not benefit from the medication because it may be suctioned from GI tract before it can be absorbed.*
4. Assess patient's medical history: history of allergies, medication history, and diet history. If you identify contraindications for a medication, withhold and inform health care provider. *Rationale: History may reveal past problems with medication tolerance and response. Historical data allow you to anticipate how certain drugs might act.*
5. In the case of a postoperative patient, review postoperative orders for type of enteral tube care. *Rationale: Manipulation and irrigation of tube or instillation of medication may be contraindicated.*
6. Gather and review physical assessment data (e.g., bowel sounds, abdominal distention) and laboratory data (e.g., renal and liver function) that may influence drug administration. *Rationale: Physical examination findings or laboratory data may contraindicate drug administration.*
7. Assess for potential drug-food interactions. *Rationale: Some drugs such as phenytoin (Dilantin), warfarin (Coumadin), and fluoroquinolone antimicrobials may require that tube feeding be stopped for an hour before and 2 hours after the dose (McKenry and others, 2006).*
8. Check with the pharmacy for availability of liquid preparations for patient's medications. An order from the health care provider may be needed to change the dosage form.

PLANNING

Expected Outcomes focus on administration of appropriate medication; avoidance of tube clogging; and safe, accurate, and effective drug therapy.

1. Patient experiences desired medication effect within period of onset of medication.
2. Patient's feeding tube remains patent after medication administration.
3. Patient does not aspirate during or after medication administration.

Delegation and Collaboration

The skill of administering medications by enteral feeding tubes cannot be delegated to nursing assistive personnel (NAP). Instruct the NAP to:

- Keep the head of the bed elevated for 15 to 30 minutes after medication administration.
- Report the occurrence of potential side effects of medications as identified by the nurse.

Equipment

- Medication administration record (MAR)
- 60-mL syringe, catheter tip for large-bore tubes, Luer-Lok tip for small-bore tubes
- Gastric pH test strip (scale of 0 to 11)
- Graduated container
- Medication to be administered
- Pill crusher if medication in tablet form
- Water
- Tongue blade or straw to stir dissolved medication
- Clean gloves
- Stethoscope (for evaluation)

IMPLEMENTATION *for* ADMINISTERING MEDICATIONS THROUGH A FEEDING TUBE

STEPS	RATIONALE
1. If the medication is not compatible with the feeding solution, stop the feeding 15 to 30 minutes before medication administration.	Facilitates absorption of medication (Monahan and others, 2007).
2. Perform hand hygiene. Prepare medications for instillation into feeding tube (see Skill 22.1). Liquid medication is preferable. Check label of medication against MAR two times. Fill graduated container with 50 to 100 mL of tepid water.	*This includes the first and second checks for accuracy.* Preparation process ensures that right patient receives right medication. Tepid water prevents abdominal cramping, which can occur with cold water.

SAFETY ALERT Whenever possible, use liquid medications instead of crushed tablets. If you have to crush tables, flush the tubing before and after medication administration to prevent the drug from adhering to the inside of the tube. Never add crushed medications directly to a tube feeding.

STEPS	RATIONALE
a. *Tablets:* Crush each tablet into a fine powder, using a pill-crushing device. If a pill-crushing device is not available, place tablet between two medication cups and grind with a blunt instrument. Dissolve each tablet in separate cup of 30 mL of warm water.	Fine powder dissolves more readily, reducing chance of occluding feeding tube.
b. *Capsules:* Ensure that contents of capsule (granules or gelatin) can be expressed from the covering (check with pharmacist). Open capsule or pierce gel cap with sterile needle and empty contents into 30 mL of warm water (or solution designated by drug company). Gel caps dissolve in warm water, but this may take 15 to 20 minutes.	Dissolved medication does not occlude feeding tube.
3. Take medications to patient at correct time, within 30 minutes before or after prescribed time (see agency policy). Give stat and single-order medications at the exact time ordered. During administration apply the six rights of medication administration.	Promotes intended therapeutic effect.
4. See Standard Protocol (inside front cover).	
5. At patient's bedside again compare the MAR or computer printout with the names of medications on the medication labels. Ask patient if he or she has allergies.	*This is the third check for accuracy* and ensures that the patient receives correct medication. Confirms patient's allergy history.
6. Identify the patient using two identifiers (e.g., name and birthday or name and account number, according to facility policy). Compare identifiers with information on patient's MAR or medical record.	Ensures correct patient. Complies with The Joint Commission standards and improves patient safety (TJC, 2010).
7. Discuss the purpose of each medication, action, and possible adverse effects. Allow patient to ask any questions about drugs.	Patient has the right to be informed, and patient's understanding of each medication improves adherence with drug therapy.
8. Elevate head of bed to 45 degrees (unless contraindicated) or sit the patient up in a chair (ASPEN, 2009). Position in reverse Trendelenburg's position if spinal injury is present.	Reduces risk of aspiration, keeping head above stomach.
9. If a continuous enteric tube feeding is infusing, adjust the infusion pump to hold the tube feeding.	Feeding solution should not infuse while residuals are checked or while medications are administered.
10. Check placement of feeding tube (see Skill 12.4) by observing gastric contents and checking pH of aspirate contents. A properly obtained pH value of 0 to 4.0 is a good indication of gastric placement (Metheny, 2006).	Ensuring tube placement reduces the risk of introducing fluids into the respiratory tract.

Continued

STEPS	RATIONALE
11. Check for gastric residual volume (GRV). Draw up 30 mL of air into 60-mL syringe and connect to feeding tube. Flush tube with air, then pull back slowly to aspirate gastric contents (see illustration) (see Chapter 12). Determine GRV using either the scale on the syringe or the graduate container. Return aspirated contents to stomach unless the GRV exceeds 200 mL (twice) or 250 mL (once) (or as defined by agency policy). In the case of a nasointestinal tube, GRV should be less than 10 mL. When GRV is excessive, hold the medication and contact the health care provider for orders.	GRV categories have been identified in studies as significant when patients have two or more GRVs of at least 200 mL or one or more GRVs of at least 250 mL (Metheny and others, 2008). Large residuals indicate delayed gastric emptying.
12. Irrigate the tubing.	
a. Pinch or clamp the enteral tube and remove the syringe. Draw up 30 mL of water into the syringe. Reinsert tip of syringe into the tube, release clamp, and flush tubing. Clamp tube again and remove the syringe.	Pinching the tubing or using a valve prevents leakage or spillage of stomach contents. Flushing ensures that the tube is patent.
b. Some enteral tubes are connected to continuous feeding tubing with a stopcock apparatus such as a Lopez valve that contains a medication port (see illustration). Attach the tip of a syringe to the medication port on the stopcock; turn the "off" setting of the stopcock away from the patient and toward the infusion tubing. Flush the feeding tube and set stopcock "off" again toward the medication port. Remove the syringe.	
13. Remove bulb or plunger from syringe and reinsert syringe into tip of feeding tube.	Removal of bulb or plunger prepares syringe for delivery of medication.
14. Administer first dose of liquid or dissolved medication by pouring into syringe (see illustration). Allow to flow by gravity.	

SAFETY ALERT If medication does not flow freely, raise the height of the syringe to increase the rate of flow or try having the patient change position slightly because the end of the feeding tube may be against gastric or intestinal mucosa. If still not flowing, try a gentle push with bulb or plunger of the syringe.

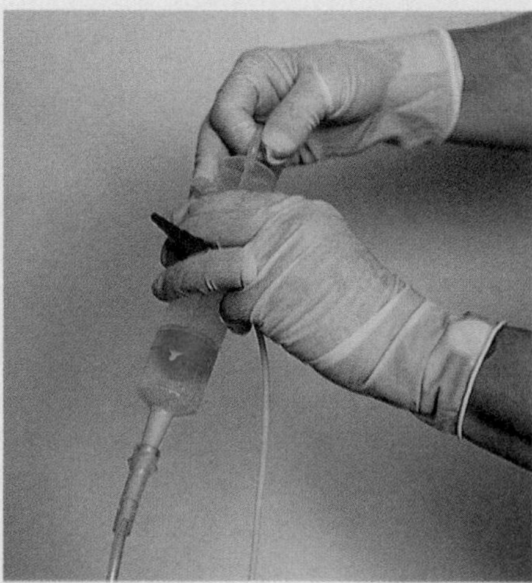

STEP 11 Aspirate stomach contents for residual volume.

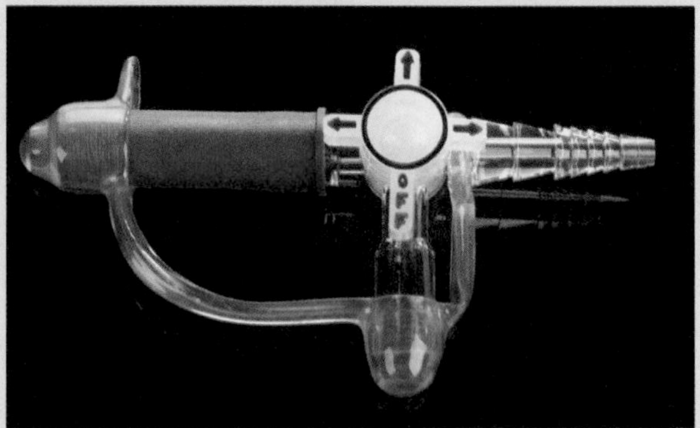

STEP 12b Lopez valve with medication port. (Courtesy ICU Medical Inc, San Clemente, Calif.)

STEPS	RATIONALE

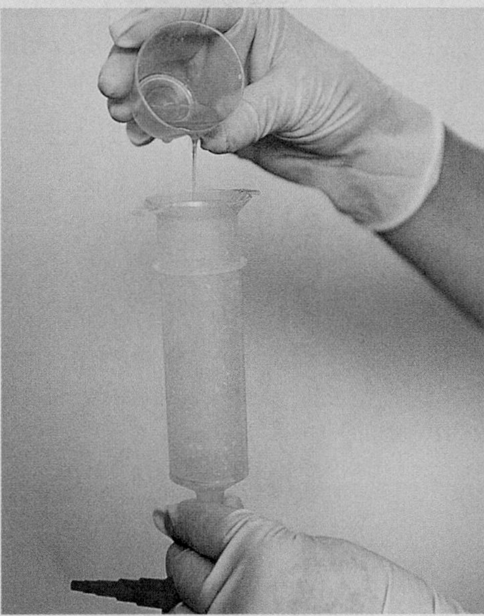

STEP 14 Pour liquid medication into syringe.

STEPS	RATIONALE
a. If giving only one dose of medication, flush with 30 mL of water after administration.	Maintains patency of enteral tube and ensures that medication passes through tube to stomach.
b. To administer more than one medication, give each separately and flush between medications with 15 to 30 mL of water.	Allows for accurate identification of medication if a dose is spilled. In addition, some medications may be incompatible (Lilley and others, 2007).
c. Follow last medication with 30 to 60 mL of water.	Avoids tube clogging with medication and ensures that medication enters stomach.
15. Clamp the proximal end of feeding tube if a tube feeding is not being administered and cap end of tube.	Prevents air from entering the stomach between medication doses.
16. When continuous tube feeding is being administered by an infusion pump, follow medication administration Steps 1 to 13. If the medicines are not compatible with the feeding solution, hold the feeding for an additional 30 to 60 minutes.	Allows for adequate absorption of medication and avoids potential drug-food interaction between medication and enteral feeding.
17. Assist patient to a comfortable position and keep the head of the bed elevated for at least 1 hour (per agency policy).	Promotes adequate passage of the medication through the stomach and reduces risk of aspiration (Ignatavicius and Workman, 2010).
18. See Completion Protocol (inside front cover).	

EVALUATION

1. Return within 30 minutes to evaluate patient's response to medications.
2. Observe tube patency before and after medication administration.
3. Monitor patient for signs of aspiration such as dyspnea, choking, gurgling speech, or congested breath sounds during and after medication administration.

Unexpected Outcomes and Related Interventions

1. Patient is unable to receive medication because of blocked enteral tube.
   a. For newly inserted tube, notify health care provider and obtain x-ray film confirmation of positioning.
   b. Attempt to gently flush tube with large-bore syringe and warm water to clear clog. (Avoid using a small-bore syringe because this exerts large amounts of pressure and may rupture tube.)
   c. If irrigation is not effective, obtain an order for a pancrelipase tablet (such as Viokase) and follow manufacturer's guidelines for tube irrigation. In addition, a declogging stylus may be used (see agency policy).
   d. Tube may have to be removed, and a new one inserted.
2. Patient shows signs of aspiration such as respiratory distress, changes in vital signs, and decreased oxygen saturation.
   a. Stop the administration of all fluids/medications through the feeding tube.

b. Elevate the head of the bed and stay with the patient. Have another staff member notify the patient's health care provider.
c. Assess vital signs, oxygen saturation, and breath sounds.
3. Patient exhibits adverse effects (side effect, toxic effect, allergic reaction).
a. Withhold further doses and assess vital signs.
b. Notify health care provider and pharmacy.
c. Prepare for possible administration of emergency medications for allergic reaction.

Recording and Reporting

- Record in nurses' notes check for tube placement, GRV, and pH of aspirate.
- Record drug, dose, route, and time administered on MAR immediately *after* administration, not before. Include initials or signature. Record patient teaching and validation of understanding in nurses' notes.
- Record total amount of water used for medication administration on proper intake/output (I&O) form.
- Report adverse effects, patient response, and/or withheld drugs to nurse in charge or health care provider.

Sample Documentation

NOTE: Documentation for medications via feeding tube is usually done on the MAR. Fluids given without medications must be recorded as intake on I&O. Other documentation occurs only if a problem is noted.

1300 Unable to administer medication because of clogged feeding tube, despite attempts to irrigate with 60 mL of tap water. Health care provider notified; medications and tube feeding held pending placement of new tube.

Special Considerations

Geriatric

- Assess patient for use of medications that may affect the pH of gastric secretions such as H_2-receptor antagonists or antacids. H_2-receptor antagonists reduce volume of gastric acid secretion and the acid content of secretions, thus causing the pH value to be higher or more basic (Metheny, 2006).

Home Care

Teach patient or family caregiver:
- How to store medications and tube feeding supplements.
- How to check placement of tube before administering any medication.
- Importance of not giving medication and to notify the health care provider if there is any doubt concerning the placement of the tube.
- About importance of consistent irrigation of feeding tube before, during, and after medications are given.
- Provide the patient or primary caregiver with resources to determine which medications can be crushed, which medications should not be crushed, and how to obtain liquid formulations of the medications.

SKILL 22.3 APPLYING TOPICAL MEDICATIONS TO THE SKIN

- **Nursing Skills Online: Nonparenteral Medication Administration, Lesson 2** *Video Clips*

Topical administration of medications involves applying drugs locally to skin, mucous membranes, or tissues. Topical drugs such as lotions, patches, pastes, and ointments primarily produce local effects; but they can also create systemic effects if absorbed through the skin. Systemic effects are more likely to occur if the skin is thin, drug concentration is high, contact with the skin is prolonged, or the drug is applied to broken skin. To protect from accidental exposure, apply topical drugs using gloves and applicators. Skin encrustations and dead tissue harbor microorganisms and block contact of medications with the affected tissue or membrane. Simply applying new medications over previously applied drugs does little to prevent infection or provide a therapeutic benefit. Always cleanse the skin or a wound thoroughly before applying a dose of a topical drug. Apply each type of medication, whether an ointment, lotion, or patch, in a specific way to ensure proper penetration and absorption.

ASSESSMENT

1. Check accuracy and completeness of each MAR with health care provider's medication order. Check patient's name, drug name and dosage, route of administration, and time for administration. Recopy or reprint any portion of printed MAR that is difficult to read. *Rationale: The health care provider's order is the most reliable source and only legal record of drugs patient is to receive. Ensures that patient receives the right medications (Eisenhauer and others, 2007; Furukawa and others, 2008).*
2. Review pertinent information related to medication, including action, purpose, normal dose and route, time of onset and peak action, side effects, and nursing implications. *Rationale: Allows you to anticipate effects of drug and observe patient's response.*
3. Assess condition of skin or membrane where medication is to be applied (see Chapter 7). You can do this just before applying the medication. If there is an open wound, apply clean gloves. First wash site thoroughly with mild, nondrying soap and warm water; rinse; and dry. Remove any previously applied medication or debris. Also remove any blood, secretions, excretions, or other body fluids. Assess for symptoms of skin irritation such as pruritus or burning. *Rationale: Provides baseline to determine change in condition of skin after therapy. Topical agents can lessen or aggravate these symptoms.*

> **SAFETY ALERT** Do not administer topical medications to the skin or membranes if integrity is altered unless indicated by health care provider.

4. Assess patient's medical history, history of allergies (including latex or topical agent), and medication history. Ask if patient has had a reaction to a cream or lotion applied to the skin. *Rationale: Allergic contact dermatitis is relatively common and can worsen existing dermatological condition. Latex allergy requires use of nonlatex gloves.*
5. Determine amount of topical agent required for application by assessing skin site, reviewing health care provider's order, and reading application directions carefully (a thin, even layer is usually adequate). *Rationale: An excessive amount of topical agent can chemically irritate the skin, negate the effectiveness of the drug, and/or cause adverse systemic effects such as decreased white blood cell (WBC) counts.*
6. Determine if patient or family caregiver is physically able to apply medication by assessing grasp, hand strength, reach, and coordination. *Rationale: This is necessary if patient is to self-administer drug in the home.*
7. Assess patient's knowledge of action and purpose of medication being given and willingness to adhere to drug regimen. *Rationale: Determines if patient or caregiver can administer drug in the home.*

PLANNING

Expected Outcomes focus on safe, accurate, and effective drug therapy.

1. With repeated application, patient's condition improves (e.g., relief of pain, inflammation or drainage).
2. Patient or family caregiver administers topical medication or patch correctly.
3. Patient or caregiver explains purpose of medication, dosage schedule, and possible side effects.

Delegation and Collaboration

The skill of administering most topical preparations, including patches, cannot be delegated to nursing assistive personnel (NAP). However, some agencies (e.g., long-term care) may allow NAP to apply some forms of topical agents to irritated skin or for the protection of the perineum during morning or perineal care. Check agency policies. Instruct the NAP about the following:

- The expected therapeutic and potential side effects to report to the nurse

Equipment

- Clean gloves (for intact skin) or sterile gloves (for nonintact skin)
- Cotton-tipped applicators or tongue blades (optional)
- Ordered medication (powder, cream, lotion, ointment, spray, patch)
- Basin of warm water, washcloth, towel, nondrying soap
- Sterile dressing, tape (if needed)
- Felt-tip pen
- Medication administration record (MAR)

IMPLEMENTATION *for* APPLYING TOPICAL MEDICATIONS TO THE SKIN

STEPS	RATIONALE
1. Prepare medications for application. Check label of medication against MAR two times (see Skill 22.1). Preparation usually involves taking bottle or tube of lotion, cream or ointment, or patch out of storage and then to patient room. Check expiration date on containers.	*This includes the first and second checks for accuracy.* Process for preparation ensures that right patient receives right medication.
2. Take medications to patient at correct time, within 30 minutes before or after prescribed time (see agency policy). Give stat and single-order medications at the exact time ordered. During administration apply the six rights of medication administration.	Promotes intended therapeutic effect.
3. **See Standard Protocol (inside front cover).**	
4. At patient's bedside again compare the MAR or computer printout with the names of medications on the medication labels. Ask patient if he or she has allergies.	*This is the third check for accuracy* and ensures that patient receives correct medication. Confirms patient's allergy history.
5. Identify patient using two identifiers (e.g., name and birthday or name and account number, according to facility policy). Compare identifiers with information on patient's MAR or medical record.	Ensures correct patient. Complies with The Joint Commission standards and improves patient safety (TJC, 2010).
6. Discuss the purpose of each medication, action, and possible adverse effects. Allow patient to ask any questions.	Patient has the right to be informed, and patient's understanding of each medication improves adherence with drug therapy.

Continued

STEPS	RATIONALE
7. If skin is broken, apply sterile gloves.	
8. ***Apply topical creams, ointments, and oil-based lotions.***	
a. Expose affected area while keeping unaffected areas covered.	Adequate visualization is necessary for application. Protects patient privacy.
b. Wash, rinse, and dry affected area before applying medication (see Assessment, Step 3).	Cleansing removes microorganisms resident in remaining debris.
c. If skin is excessively dry and flaking, apply topical agent while skin is still damp.	Retains moisture within skin layers.
d. Remove gloves and apply new clean or sterile gloves.	Sterile gloves are used when applying agents to open, noninfectious skin lesions. Changing gloves prevents cross-contamination of infected or contagious lesions and protects the nurse from drug effects.
e. Place required amount of medication in palm of gloved hand and soften by rubbing briskly between hands.	Softening of topical agent makes it easier to apply to skin.
f. Tell patient that skin will feel soothed by application but initially it might feel cold. Once medication is softened, spread it evenly over skin surface, using long, even strokes that follow direction of hair growth. Do not rub skin vigorously. Apply thickness as directed by manufacturer's instructions.	Ensures even distribution of medication. Technique prevents irritation of hair follicles.
g. Explain to patient that skin may feel greasy after application.	Ointments often contain oil.
9. ***Apply antianginal (nitroglycerin) ointment.***	
a. Remove previous dose paper. Fold used paper containing any residual medication with used sides together and dispose in biohazard trash container. Wipe off residual medication with a tissue.	Prevents overdose that can occur with multiple-dose papers left in place. Proper disposal protects others from accidental exposure to medication.
b. Write date, time, and nurse's initials on new application paper.	Label provides reference to prevent missing doses.
c. Antianginal (nitroglycerin) ointments are usually ordered in inches and can be measured on small sheets of paper marked off in 1.25-cm ½-inch) markings. Apply desired number of inches of ointment to paper measuring guide (see illustration).	Ensures correct dose of medication.

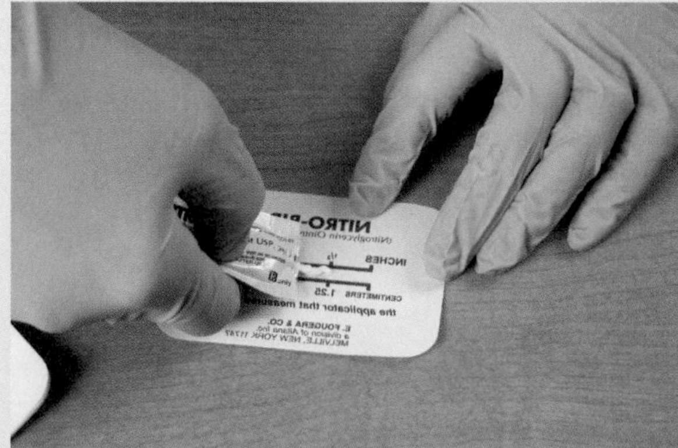

STEP 9c Ointment spread in inches over measuring guide.

> **SAFETY ALERT** Unit-dose packages are available. (Warning: One package equals 2.5 cm (1 inch); smaller amount should not be measured from this package.)

STEPS	RATIONALE
d. Select application site: Apply nitroglycerin to the chest area, back, abdomen, or anterior thigh (Lehne, 2007). Do not apply on hairy surfaces or over scar tissue.	Application on hairy surfaces or scar tissue may interfere with absorption.

STEPS	RATIONALE
e. Be sure to rotate application sites.	Minimizes skin irritation.
f. Apply ointment to skin surface by holding edge or back of paper measuring guide and placing ointment and paper directly on the skin (see illustration).	Minimizes chance of ointment covering gloves and later touching nurse's hands.

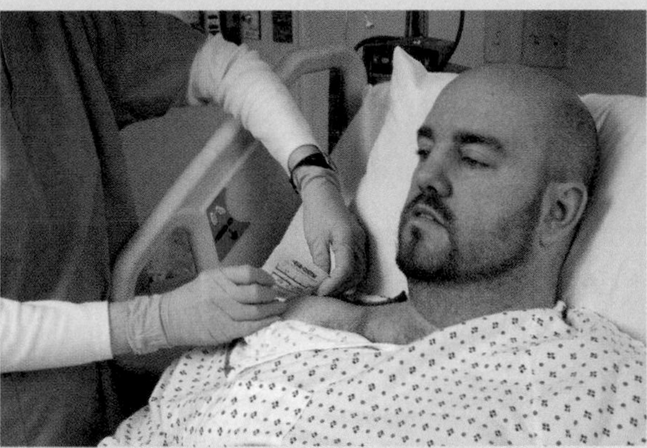

STEP 9f Nurse applies measuring guide with medication on patient's skin.

STEPS	RATIONALE
g. Do not rub or massage ointment into skin.	Medication is designed to absorb slowly over several hours; massaging may increase absorption.
h. Secure ointment and paper with a transparent dressing or strip of tape. Plastic wrap is another option.	Prevents staining of clothes or accidental removal of medication.
10. ***Apply transdermal patches (e.g., analgesic, nicotine, nitroglycerin, estrogen).***	
a. If an old patch is present, remove it and cleanse the area. Be sure to check between skin folds for patch.	Failure to remove old patches may result in overdose. Many patches are small, clear, or flesh-colored and can easily be hidden beneath skin folds. Cleansing removes traces of previous dose.
b. Dispose of old patch by folding in half with sticky sides together. Some agencies require the patch to be cut before disposal (see agency policy). Dispose in biohazard trash bag.	Proper disposal prevents accidental exposure to medication.
c. Date and initial the outer side of the new patch before applying it and note time of administration. Use a soft-tip or felt-tip pen.	Visual reminder prevents missing or extra doses. A ballpoint pen damages the patch and alters medication delivery.
d. Choose a new site that is clean, dry, and free of hair. Some patches have specific instructions for placement locations (e.g., Testoderm patches are placed on scrotum; a scopolamine patch is placed on back of the ear; never apply an estrogen patch to the breast tissue or waistline). Do not apply a patch on skin that is oily, burned, cut, or irritated in any way.	Ensures complete medication absorption.

SAFETY ALERT Never apply heat such as with a heating pad over a transdermal patch because this results in an increased rate of absorption with potentially serious adverse effects (ISMP, 2005).

STEPS	RATIONALE
e. Carefully remove the patch from its protective covering by pulling off the liner. Hold the patch by the edge without touching the adhesive.	Touching only the edges ensures that the patch will adhere and that the medication dose has not been changed. Removing the protective covering allows the medication to be absorbed through the skin.
f. Apply the patch, pressing firmly with the palm of one hand for 10 seconds. Make sure that it sticks well, especially around the edges. Apply overlay if provided with patch.	Adequate adhesion prevents loss of the patch, which results in decreased dose and effectiveness.

Continued

STEPS	RATIONALE
g. Do not apply patch to previously used site for at least 1 week.	Rotation of site reduces skin irritation from medication and adhesive.
h. Instruct patient that transdermal patches are never to be cut in half; a change in dose would require a prescription for a new strength of transdermal medication.	Cutting a transdermal patch in half would alter the intended medication delivery of the transdermal system, resulting in inadequate or altered drug levels.

SAFETY ALERT It is recommended to have a daily "patch-free" interval of 10 to 12 hours because tolerance develops if patches are used 24 hours a day every day (Lehne, 2007). Apply a new patch each morning, leave in place for 12 to 14 hours, and remove in the evening.

STEPS	RATIONALE
i. Instruct patient to always remove old patch before applying new one. Patients should not use alternative forms of medications when using patches. For example, patients should not smoke while using a nicotine patch. Patients should not apply nitroglycerin ointment in addition to the patch unless specifically ordered to do so by their health care provider.	Use of patch with an additional/alternative drug preparation can result in toxicity and other side effects.
11. ***Administer aerosol sprays (e.g., local anesthetic sprays).***	
a. Shake container vigorously. Read container label for distance recommended to hold spray away from area, usually 15 to 30 cm (6 to 12 inches).	Mixing ensures delivery of a fine, even spray. Proper distance ensures that fine spray hits skin surface. Holding container too close results in thin, watery distribution.
b. Ask patient to turn face away from spray or briefly cover face with towel when spraying neck or chest.	Prevents inhalation of spray.
c. Spray medication evenly over affected site (in some cases spray is timed for period of seconds).	Entire affected area of skin should be covered with thin spray.
12. ***Apply suspension-based lotion.***	
a. Shake container vigorously.	Mixes powder throughout liquid to form well-mixed suspension.
b. Apply small amount of lotion to small gauze dressing or pad and apply to skin by stroking evenly in direction of hair growth.	Method of application leaves protective film of powder on skin after water base of suspension dries. Technique prevents irritation of hair follicles.
c. Explain to patient that area will feel cool and dry.	Water evaporates to leave thin layer of powder.
13. ***Apply a powder.***	
a. Be sure that skin surface is thoroughly dry. With your nondominant hand fully spread apart any skin folds such as between toes or under axilla and dry with a towel.	Minimizes caking and crusting of powder. Fully exposes skin surface for application.
b. If area of application is near the face, ask patient to turn face away from powder or briefly cover face with towel.	Prevents inhalation of powder.
c. Dust skin site lightly with dispenser so area is covered with fine, thin layer. *Option:* Cover skin area with dressing if ordered by health care provider.	Thin layer of powder has slight lubricating properties to reduce friction and promote drying (Lilley and others, 2007).
14. See Completion Protocol (inside front cover).	

EVALUATION

1. Inspect condition of skin between applications.
2. Observe patient or family caregiver apply topical medication.
3. Ask the patient or family caregiver to name the medication and its purpose, dosage, schedule, and side effects.

Unexpected Outcomes and Related Interventions

1. Skin site appears inflamed and edematous with blistering and oozing of fluid from lesions, or patient continues to complain of pruritus and tenderness.
   a. Notify health care provider; additional or alternative therapies may be needed.

2. Patient is unable to explain information about topical application or does not administer as prescribed.
   a. Identify possible reasons for nonadherence and explore alternative approaches (e.g., family caregiver) or options.

Recording and Reporting

- Record drug, dose or strength, site of application, and time administered on MAR immediately after administration, not before. Include initials or signature. Record patient teaching and validation of understanding in nurses' notes.
- Describe condition of skin before each application in nurses' notes. Do not chart medication administration until after it is given.
- Report adverse effects/changes in appearance and condition of skin lesions to health care provider.

Sample Documentation

0930 Skin on the back of both hands and wrists is dry, red, and flaky. Complains of itching. Hydrocortisone cream 1% applied sparingly to affected areas as prescribed.
1000 Reported itching is relieved.

Special Considerations

Geriatric

- Changes in the skin of an older adult include increased wrinkling, dryness, flaking, and increased tendency to bruise. Handle fragile skin gently when applying topical medications.

Home Care

- Instruct patient on safe disposal techniques at home. Fold used patches with medication sides together and wrapped in newspaper before discarding. Used applicators or patches are placed into cardboard or plastic disposable containers. Children and pets may become ill if they ingest or handle used patches; careful disposal is necessary to ensure safety in the home.

SKILL 22.4 INSTILLING EYE AND EAR MEDICATIONS

- **Nursing Skills Online: Nonparenteral Medication Administration, Lessons 3 and 4** *Video Clips*

Common eye (ophthalmic) medications are in the form of drops and ointments, including OTC preparations such as artificial tears and vasoconstrictors (e.g., Visine and Murine). However, many patients receive prescribed ophthalmic drugs for eye conditions such as glaucoma and infections and following cataract extraction. In addition, there is a third type of delivery system, the intraocular disk. Medications delivered by disk resemble a contact lens, but the disk is placed in the conjunctival sac, not on the cornea, and it remains in place for up to 1 week.

The eye is the most sensitive organ to which you apply medications. The cornea is richly supplied with sensitive nerve fibers. Care must be taken to prevent instilling medication directly onto the cornea. The conjunctival sac is much less sensitive and thus a more appropriate site for medication instillation.

Any patient receiving topical eye medications should learn correct self-administration of the medication, especially patients with glaucoma, who must often undergo lifelong medication administration for control of their disease. You can easily instruct patients and family caregivers while administering medications. Family caregivers often administer eye medications when patients are unable to manipulate applicators and immediately after eye surgery, when a patient's vision is so impaired that it is difficult to assemble needed supplies and handle applicators correctly.

Ear (otic) medications are usually in a solution and instilled by drops. When administering ear medications, be aware of certain safety precautions. Internal ear structures are very sensitive to temperature extremes; administer eardrops at room temperature. Instilling cold drops can cause vertigo (severe dizziness) or nausea and debilitate a patient for several minutes. Although structures of the outer ear are not sterile, use sterile drops and solutions in case the eardrum is ruptured. Entrance of nonsterile solutions into the middle ear can cause serious infection. A final precaution is to avoid forcing any solution into the ear. Do not occlude the ear canal with a medicine dropper because this can cause pressure within the canal during instillation and subsequent injury to the eardrum. If you follow these precautions, instillation of ear drops is a safe and effective therapy.

ASSESSMENT

1. Check accuracy and completeness of each MAR with health care provider's medication order. Check patient's name, drug name and dosage, route (eye[s] or ear[s]) receiving medication, and time for administration. Recopy or reprint any portion of printed MAR that is difficult to read. *Rationale: The health care provider's order is the most reliable source and only legal record of drugs patient is to receive. Ensures that patient receives the right medications (Eisenhauer and others, 2007; Furukawa and others, 2008).*
2. Review pertinent information related to medication, including action, purpose, normal dose and route, side effects, time of onset and peak action, and nursing implications. *Rationale: Allows you to anticipate effects of drug and observe patient's response.*

3. Assess condition of external eye or ear structures (see Chapter 7). *Rationale: This may also be done just before drug instillation. Provides a baseline to determine later if local response to medications occurs. This also indicates the need to clean the area before drug application.*
4. Determine whether patient has symptoms of eye or ear discomfort or hearing or visual impairment. *Rationale: Certain eye medications can act to either lessen or increase symptoms. Occlusion of external ear canal by swelling, drainage, or cerumen can impair hearing acuity and is painful.*
5. Assess patient's medical history, history of allergies (including latex), and medication history. *Rationale: Factors influence how certain drugs act. Reveals patient's need for medication.*
6. Assess patient's LOC and ability to follow instructions. *Rationale: Patient must lie still during drug administration. Sudden movements can cause injury from dropper.*
7. Assess patient's knowledge regarding drug therapy and desire to self-administer medication. Assess patient's ability to manipulate and hold dropper. *Rationale: Findings indicate need for health teaching and/or involvement of family caregiver. Motivation influences teaching approach. Reflects patient's ability to learn to self-administer medication.*
8. Assess patient's ability to manipulate and hold dropper or ocular disks. *Rationale: Reflects patient's ability to self-administer drug.*

PLANNING

Expected Outcomes focus on relief of symptoms without unpleasant adverse reactions and on safe, accurate, and effective drug therapy.

1. Patient states that symptoms (e.g., irritation, dryness) are relieved.
2. Patient denies unpleasant side effects or adverse reactions.
3. Patient describes medication effects and technique of application.
4. Patient correctly demonstrates self-instillation of eyedrops or eardrops.

Delegation and Collaboration

- The skills of administering eyedrops/eardrops may not be delegated to nursing assistive personnel (NAP). Instruct the NAP about the following:
- Potential side effects of medications and how to report their occurrence, including hearing changes or vision impairment

Equipment

- Appropriate medication (eyedrops with sterile dropper, ointment tube, medicated intraocular disk, or eardrops)
- Clean gloves (for eyedrops and if ear has drainage)
- Medication administration record (MAR).

Eyedrops/ointment

- Facial tissue
- Warm water and washcloth
- Eye patch and tape (optional)

Eardrops

- Cotton-tipped applicator, cotton balls

IMPLEMENTATION *for* INSTILLING EYE AND EAR MEDICATIONS

STEPS	RATIONALE
1. Prepare medications for application. Check label of medication against MAR two times (see Skill 22.1).	*This includes the first and second checks for accuracy.* Ensures that right patient receives right medication.
a. Check expiration date on medication.	Medications used past expiration date may be inactive or harmful to patient.
b. Check drug dose or concentration. If the dose or concentration printed on package differs from what is ordered, calculate correct amount to give. Double-check the eye or ear to receive medication.	Double-checking pharmacy calculations and ordered route reduces risk of error.
2. Take medications to patient at correct time, within 30 minutes before or after prescribed time (see agency policy). Give stat and single-order medications at the exact time ordered. During administration apply the six rights of medication administration.	Promotes intended therapeutic effect.
3. **See Standard Protocol (inside front cover).**	
4. At the bedside again compare the MAR or computer printout with the names of medications on the medication labels. Ask patient if he or she has allergies.	*This is the third check for accuracy* and ensures that patient receives correct medication. Confirms patient's allergy history.

STEPS	RATIONALE
5. Identify patient using two identifiers (e.g., name and birthday or name and account number, according to facility policy). Compare identifiers with information on the patient's MAR or medical record.	Ensures correct patient. Complies with The Joint Commission standards and improves patient safety (TJC, 2010).
6. Discuss the purpose of each medication, action, and possible adverse effects. Allow patient to ask any questions. Explain procedure. Patients who self-instill medications may be allowed to give drops under nurse's supervision (check agency policy). Tell patients receiving eyedrops (e.g., mydriatics) that vision will be temporarily blurred and sensitivity to light may occur.	Patient has the right to be informed, and patient's understanding of each medication improves adherence with drug therapy. Patients often become anxious about medication being instilled into eye because of potential discomfort.

SAFETY ALERT Patient should not drive or attempt to perform any activity that requires acute vision or sensitivity to light until vision returns to normal.

STEPS	RATIONALE
7. *Instill eye medications.*	
a.  Ask patient to lie supine or sit back in chair with neck slightly hyperextended.	Position provides easy access to eye/ear for medication instillation and minimizes drainage of eye medication into tear duct.

SAFETY ALERT Do not hyperextend the neck of a patient with a cervical neck injury.

STEPS	RATIONALE
b. If crusting or drainage is present along eyelid margins or inner canthus, gently wash away. Soak any dried crusts with a warm, damp washcloth or cotton ball over eye for several minutes. Always wipe clean from inner to outer canthus (see illustration). Remove gloves and perform hand hygiene.	Cleansing eye from inner to outer canthus avoids introducing microorganisms into lacrimal ducts (Lilley and others, 2007). Soaking allows easy removal of crusts without applying pressure to eye.

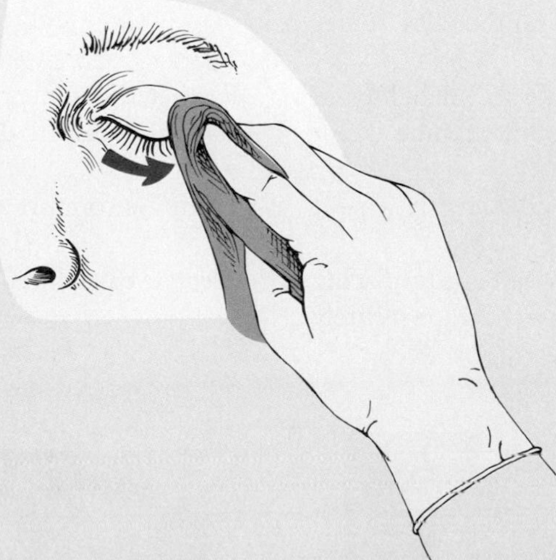

STEP 7b Cleanse eye, washing from inner to outer canthus, before administering drops or ointment.

STEPS	RATIONALE
c. Explain that there might be a temporary burning sensation from the drops.	Cornea is highly sensitive.
d. *Instill eyedrops.*	
(1) Hold a clean tissue in nondominant hand on patient's cheekbone just below lower eyelid.	Tissue absorbs medication that escapes eye.

Continued

STEPS	RATIONALE
(2) With tissue resting below lower lid, gently press downward with thumb or forefinger against bony orbit, exposing conjunctival sac. Never press directly against patient's eyeball.	Prevents pressure and trauma to eyeball and prevents fingers from touching eye.
(3) Ask patient to look at ceiling.	Action moves sensitive cornea up and away from conjunctival sac into which you instill medication. Reduces stimulation of blink reflex.
(4) Rest dominant hand gently on patient's forehead and hold filled medication eyedropper approximately 1 to 2 cm (½ to ¾ inch) above conjunctival sac.	Prevents accidental contact of eyedropper with eye and reduces risk of injury and transfer of microorganisms to dropper. Contact of eyedropper with eye contaminates the container (ophthalmic medications are sterile).
(5) Drop prescribed number of drops into conjunctival sac (see illustration).	The sac normally holds 1 or 2 drops. Applying drops into sac evenly distributes medication across eye.
(6) If patient blinks or closes eye, causing drops to land on outer lid margins, repeat procedure.	Therapeutic effect of drug is obtained only when drops enter conjunctival sac.
(7) When giving drops that may cause systemic effects, apply gentle pressure to patient's nasolacrimal duct with a clean tissue for 30 to 60 seconds over each eye, one at a time. Avoid pressure directly against patient's eyeball.	Prevents overflow of medication into nasal and pharyngeal passages. Minimizes absorption into systemic circulation.
(8) After instilling drops, ask patient to close eyes gently.	Helps to distribute medication. Squinting or squeezing eyelids forces medication from conjunctival sac.
e. ***Instill eye ointment.***	
(1) 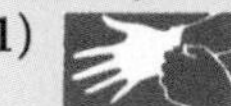 Ask patient to look up.	Moves the sensitive cornea up and away from the conjunctival sac and reduces stimulation of the blink reflex during ointment application.
(2) Holding applicator above lower lid margin, apply thin ribbon of ointment evenly along inner edge of lower eyelid on conjunctiva (see illustration) from inner canthus to outer canthus.	Distributes medication evenly across eye and lid margin.
(3) Have patient close eye and rub lid lightly in circular motion with a tissue if rubbing is not contraindicated.	Further distributes medication without traumatizing eye. Avoid pressure directly against patient's eyeball.
(4) If excess medication is on eyelid, gently wipe it from inner to outer canthus.	Promotes comfort and prevents trauma to eye.
8. If patient needs an eye patch, apply clean one by placing it over affected eye so entire eye is covered. Tape securely without applying pressure to eye.	Clean eye patch reduces chance of infection.

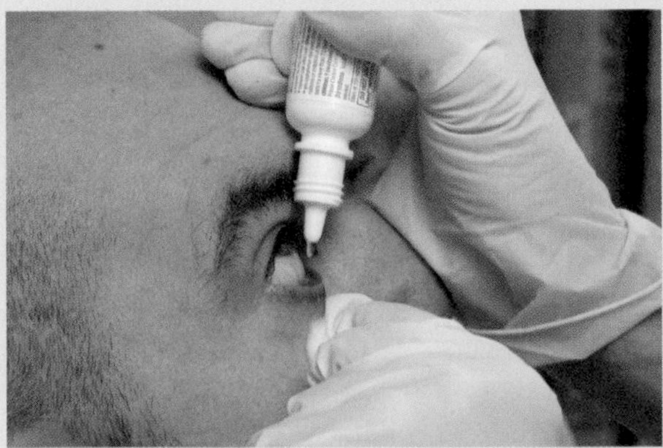

STEP 7d(5) Hold eyedropper over lower conjunctival sac.

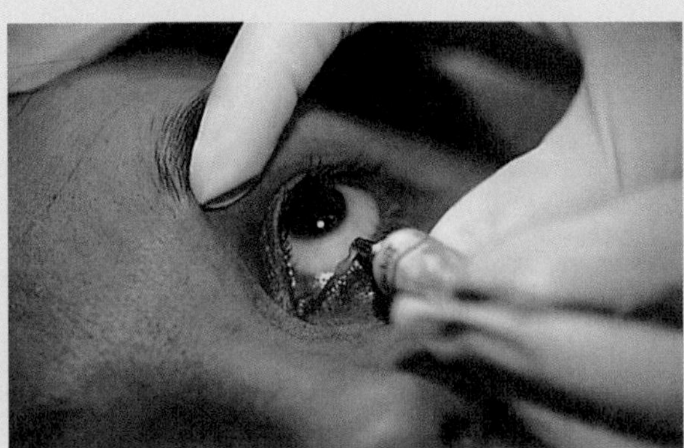

STEP 7e(2) Apply eye ointment along inside edge of lower eyelid on conjunctiva from inner to outer canthus.

STEPS	RATIONALE
9. *Apply intraocular disk.*	
a. Open package containing the disk. Gently press your fingertip against the disk so it adheres to your finger. Position the convex side of the disk on your fingertip. It may be necessary to moisten gloved finger with sterile saline.	Allows you to inspect disk for damage or deformity.
b. With your other hand, gently pull the patient's lower eyelid away from the eye. Ask patient to look up.	Prepares conjunctival sac for receiving medicated disk and moves sensitive cornea away.
c. Place the disk in the conjunctival sac so it floats on the sclera between the iris and lower eyelid (see illustration).	Ensures delivery of medication.
d. Pull patient's lower eyelid out and over the disk. You should not be able to see the disk at this time. Repeat if you can see the disk (see illustration).	Ensures accurate medication delivery.
10. *Remove intraocular disk.*	
a. Gently pull downward on the lower eyelid using the nondominant hand.	Exposes the disk.
b. Using the forefinger and thumb of your dominant hand, pinch the disk and lift it out of patient's eye (see illustration).	
11. If excess medication is on eyelid, gently wipe it from inner to outer canthus.	Promotes comfort and prevents trauma to eye.
12. If patient had eye patch, apply clean one by placing it over affected eye so entire eye is covered. Tape securely without applying pressure to eye.	Clean eye patch reduces chance of infection.
13. *Instill ear drops.*	
a. Apply only if drainage is present.	
b. Warm medication to room temperature by running warm water over the bottle (making sure not to damage the label or allow water to enter the bottle).	Ear structures are very sensitive to temperature extremes. Cold may cause vertigo and nausea.
c. Position patient on side (if not contraindicated) with ear to be treated facing up, or patient may sit in a chair or at the bedside. Stabilize patient's head with his or her hand.	Facilitates distribution of medication into ear.
d. Straighten ear canal by pulling pinna upward and outward (adult or child older than age 3) or down and back (child).	Straightening of ear canal provides direct access to deeper external ear structures. Anatomical differences in younger children and infants require different methods of positioning canal.

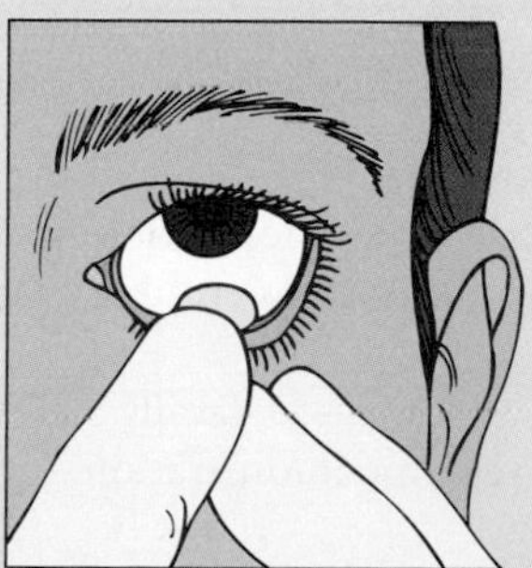

STEP 9c Place disk in conjunctival sac between iris and lower eyelid.

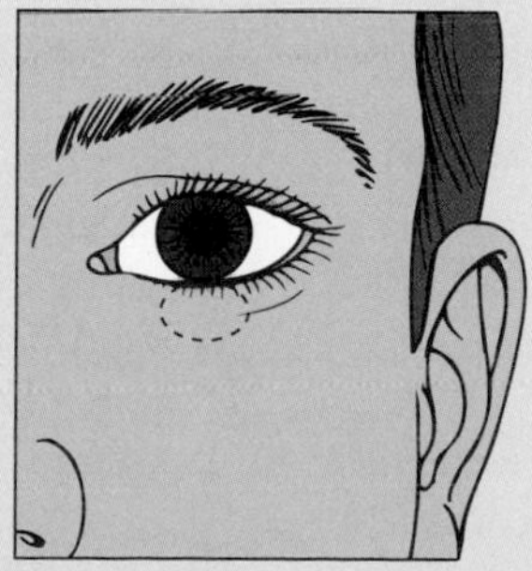

STEP 9d Gently pull lower eyelid over disk.

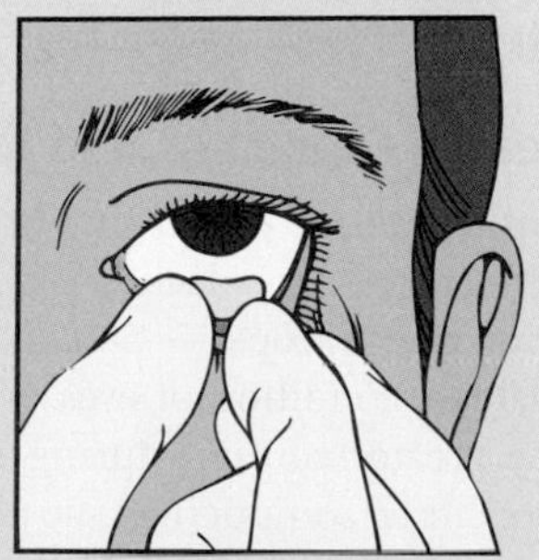

STEP 10b Carefully pinch disk to remove it from patient's eye.

Continued

STEPS	RATIONALE
e. If cerumen or drainage occludes outermost portion of ear canal, wipe out cerumen that you can see by gently using a cotton-tipped applicator. Take care not to force wax into canal (see illustration).	Cerumen and drainage harbor microorganisms and can block distribution of medication into canal. Occlusion blocks sound transmission.
f. Instill prescribed drops, holding dropper 1 cm (½ inch) above ear canal.	Avoiding contact prevents contamination of the dropper, which could contaminate the medication in the container.
g. Ask patient to remain in side-lying position for a few minutes. Apply gentle massage or pressure to tragus of ear with finger (see illustration).	Allows complete distribution of medication. Pressure and massage move medication inward.
h. If ordered, gently insert a portion of cotton ball into outermost part of canal. Do not press cotton into canal.	Prevents escape of medication when patient sits or stands.
i. Remove cotton after 15 minutes. Assist patient to comfortable position after drops are absorbed.	Allows time for drug distribution and absorption.
14. See Completion Protocol (inside front cover).	

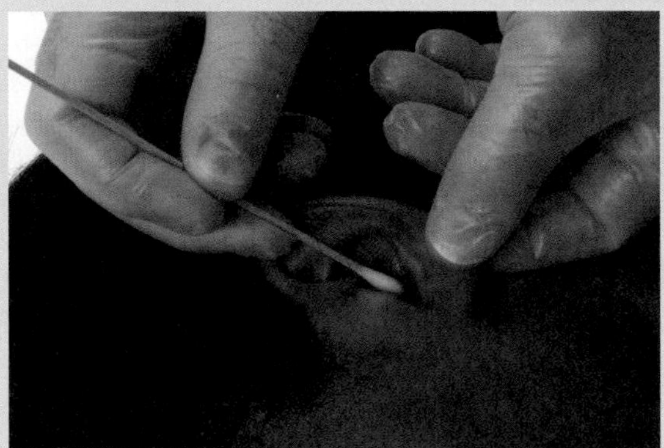

STEP 13e Always cleanse only outer canal. Do not push secretions into ear.

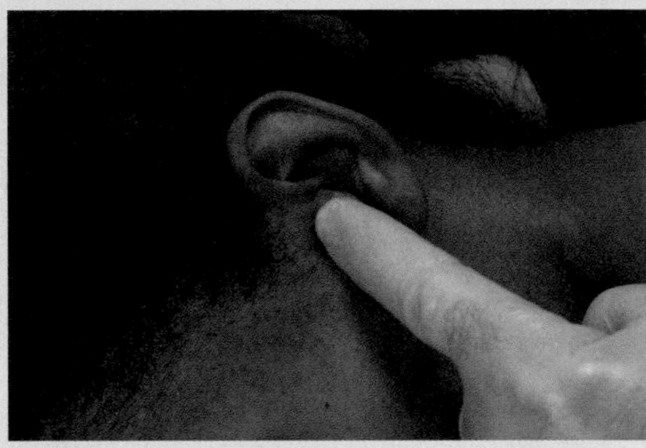

STEP 13g Nurse applies gentle pressure to tragus of ear after instilling drops.

EVALUATION

1. Observe effects of medication by evaluating desired changes (e.g., level of eye irritation, ear pain).
2. Note patient's response to instillation, observe for side effects, and ask if any discomfort was felt.
3. Ask patient to discuss purpose, action, and side effects of drug and technique of administration.
4. Observe patient demonstrate self-administration of next dose.

Unexpected Outcomes and Related Interventions

1. Patient complains of burning or pain or experiences local side effects (e.g., headaches, bloodshot eyes) after administration of eyedrops.
   a. Evaluate condition of eyes.
   b. Use greater caution during next instillation to instill drops into conjunctival sac and not onto the cornea.
   c. Notify health care provider.
2. Patient experiences systemic effects from eyedrops (e.g., increased heart rate and blood pressure from epinephrine or decreased heart rate and blood pressure from timolol. Local anesthetics and antibiotics can cause anaphylaxis.
   a. Hold further doses and notify health care provider immediately.
   b. Stay with patient and assess vital signs.
3. Ear canal remains inflamed, swollen, tender to palpation. Drainage is present.
   a. Notify health care provider.
4. Patient's hearing acuity continues to be reduced.
   a. Wax may be impacted. Ear irrigation can remove cerumen.
   b. Notify health care provider.
5. Patient is unable to explain drug information or steps for taking eyedrops/eardrops and/or has trouble manipulating dropper.
   a. Repeat instructions and include family caregiver as appropriate. Include return demonstration.

Recording and Reporting

- Record drug, dose or strength, site(s) of application (e.g., right eye, left, eye, both), and time administered on MAR

immediately after administration, not before. Include initials or signature. Record patient teaching and validation of understanding in nurses' notes.
- Record objective data related to condition of tissues involved (e.g., redness, drainage, irritation), any subjective data (e.g., pain, itching, altered vision or hearing) and patient's response to medications. Note evidence of any side effects experienced in nurses' notes.
- Report any side effects or continued complaints of visual or hearing deficits to nurse in charge or health care provider.

Sample Documentation

1300 Complaining of dry and irritated eyes; some yellowish drainage in lacrimal sac. Redness noted on both sclerae. Artificial tears 2 drops instilled into each eye after eyes cleansed.

1345 Patient states eyes feel less irritated. Able to read meal menu.

Special Considerations

Pediatric

- Infants often clench the eyes tightly to avoid eyedrops. Place the drops in the nasal corner where the lids meet as the infant lies supine. When the infant opens the eye, the medication will flow into the eye.
- Insert cotton pledgets loosely into ear canal to prevent medication from flowing out of the external ear canal. To prevent cotton from absorbing medication in ear, premoisten cotton with a few drops of medication (Hockenberry and Wilson, 2007).
- Ensure that parents and/or caregivers are aware of the proper method of administration (e.g., for children younger than 3 years gently pull the pinna of the ear downward and straight back).
- Restrain infants or young children in supine position with head turned to expose affected ear. Hold child in this position until the drug has time to be absorbed (Hockenberry and Wilson, 2007).
- Teach the signs of hearing loss and the need for frequent follow-ups to parents with children who have chronic otitis media.

Geriatric

- Many older adults accumulate cerumen in the ear. This should be removed by irrigation before administration of medication (see Chapter 11).

Home Care

- Have patients with chronic health problems consult their health care provider before using OTC eye medications. When using OTC medications, encourage patient to follow manufacturer's directions closely.
- Patients should not share eyedrops with other family members. Risk of infection transmission is high.

SKILL 22.5 USING METERED-DOSE INHALERS

- **Nursing Skills Online: Nonparenteral Medication Administration, Lesson 5**

Inhaled medications produce local effects (e.g., bronchodilators open narrowed bronchioles). However, because these medications are absorbed rapidly through the pulmonary circulation, some have the potential for producing systemic side effects (e.g., palpitations, tremors, and tachycardia). Patients who receive drugs by inhalation frequently suffer from chronic respiratory disease. Because they depend on these medications for disease control, they must learn about them and how to administer them safely. Inhalers and small-volume nebulizers (see Skill 22.6) are devices that deliver inhaled medications.

A metered-dose inhaler (MDI) is a small, handheld device that disperses medication into the airways through an aerosol spray or mist by activation of a propellant. Dosing is usually achieved with 1 or 2 puffs. Dry powder inhalers (DPIs) deliver inhaled medication in a fine powder formulation to the respiratory tract (see Procedural Guideline 22.1). Fig. 22-2 illustrates examples of MDIs and DPIs. The deeper passages of the respiratory tract provide a large surface area for drug absorption, and the alveolar-capillary network absorbs medication rapidly.

An MDI delivers a measured dose of a drug with each push of a canister. Approximately 5 to 10 pounds of pressure is needed to activate the aerosol. This is difficult for some older adults because hand strength diminishes with age. Because use of an MDI requires coordination during the breathing cycle, many patients spray only the back of their throats and fail to receive a full dose. The inhaler must be depressed to expel medication just as the patient inhales. This ensures that

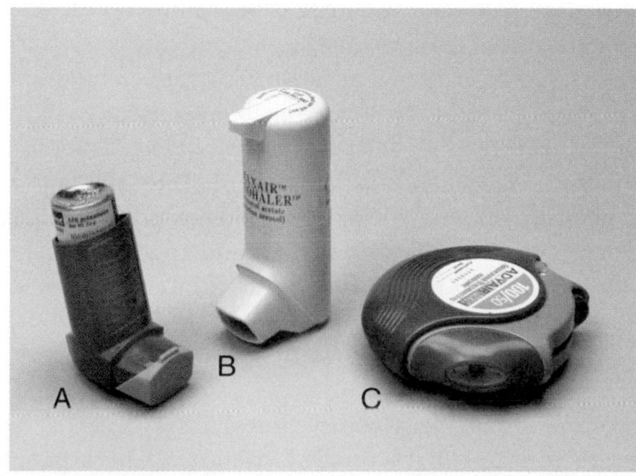

FIG 22-2 Types of inhalers **A,** Metered-dose inhaler (MDI). **B,** Breath-activated inhaler. **C,** Dry powder inhaler (DPI). (From Lilley LL and others: *Pharmacology and the nursing process,* ed 6, St Louis, 2011, Mosby.)

BOX 22-1 COMMON PROBLEMS WHEN USING AN INHALER

- *Not taking the medication as prescribed:* Taking either too much or too little.
- *Incorrect activation:* This usually occurs through pressing the canister before taking a breath. These actions should be done simultaneously so the drug can be carried down to the lungs with the breath.
- *Forgetting to shake the inhaler:* The drug is in a suspension; therefore particles may settle. If the inhaler is not shaken, it may not deliver the correct dose of the drug.
- *Not waiting long enough between puffs:* The whole process should be repeated when taking the second puff; otherwise an incorrect dose may be delivered, or the drug may not penetrate into the lungs.
- *Failure to clean the valve:* Particles may jam the valve in the mouthpiece unless it is cleaned occasionally. This is a frequent cause of failure to get 200 puffs from one inhaler.
- *Failure to observe whether the inhaler is actually releasing a spray:* If it is not, this should be checked with the pharmacist.

the medication reaches the lower airways. Poor coordination can be solved by the use of spacer devices (AeroChamber, InspirEase) or a breath-activated MDI such as the Maxair Auto-inhaler. A spacer device decreases the amount of medication deposited into the oropharyngeal mucosa. Some spacers have a one-way valve that activates on inhalation, thereby removing the need for good hand-breath coordination (Lehne, 2007). Box 22-1 summarizes common problems that occur when using an inhaler.

Patients who use MDIs need to know when a canister becomes empty. For years patients learned to measure the amount of medication remaining in a canister by floating it in a container of water. The angle of flotation was thought to indicate whether the canister was full, half-full, or empty. However, this method is not reliable because of differences in canister sizes and designs. In addition, exposing the neck of the actuation valve to water may cause damage. Research by Rubin and Durotoye (2005) found that patients used a variety of methods to determine if a canister was empty, but none of the methods were found to be reliable. Consequently most MDI canisters are used long past their intended duration. The researchers recommended that, when MDIs do not have built-in dose counters, instruction in dose counting (calculating the number of puffs used per day and how many days the inhaler should last) is vital for correct MDI use.

ASSESSMENT

1. Check accuracy and completeness of each MAR with health care provider's medication order. Check patient's name, drug name and dosage, the route of administration, and time for administration. Recopy or reprint any portion of printed MAR that is difficult to read. *Rationale: The health care provider's order is the most reliable source and only legal record of drugs patient is to receive. Ensures that patient receives the right medications (Eisenhauer and others, 2007; Furukawa and others, 2008).*
2. Review pertinent information related to medication, including action, purpose, normal dose and route, side effects, time of onset and peak action, and nursing implications. *Rationale: Allows you to anticipate effects of drug and observe patient's response.*
3. Assess patient's medical history, history of allergies, and medication history. *Rationale: Factors influence how certain drugs act. Reveals patient's need for medication.*
4. Assess respiratory pattern and auscultate breath sounds. *Rationale: Establishes baseline of airway status for comparison during and after treatment.*
5. Assess patient's ability to hold, manipulate, and depress canister and inhaler. *Rationale: Impairment of grasp or presence of tremors of hands interferes with patient's ability to depress canister within inhaler.*
6. Assess patient's readiness to learn: asks questions about medication, requests education in use of inhaler; is mentally alert; and participates in own care.
7. Assess patient's ability to learn: Patient should not be fatigued, in pain, or in respiratory distress; assess level of understanding of terms.
8. Assess patient's knowledge and understanding of disease and purpose and action of prescribed medications. *Rationale: May assist in assessing patient's potential for compliance with self-administration.*

PLANNING

Expected Outcomes focus on relief of symptoms; promoting knowledge for self-administration of inhalers; and safe, accurate, and effective drug therapy.

1. Patient correctly self-administers metered dose.
2. Patient describes proper time during respiratory cycle to inhale spray and number of inhalations for each administration.
3. Patient's breathing pattern improves, and airways become less restrictive with adequate gas exchange.
4. Patient lists side effects of medications and criteria for calling health care professional if dyspnea develops.

Delegation and Collaboration

The skill of administering MDIs should not be delegated to nursing assistive personnel (NAP). Instruct the NAP about the following:

- Potential side effects of medications and reporting their occurrence
- Signs of breathing difficulties (e.g., paroxysmal coughing, audible wheezing)

Equipment

- Inhaler device with medication canister (MDI or DPI) (see Fig. 22-2)

- Spacer device such as AeroChamber or InspirEase (optional)
- Facial tissues (optional)
- Medication administration record (MAR)
- Stethoscope
- Pulse oximeter (optional)

IMPLEMENTATION *for* USING METERED-DOSE INHALERS

STEPS	RATIONALE
1. Prepare medications for administration: Check label of inhaler against MAR two times (see Skill 22.1).	*This includes the first and second check for accuracy.* Ensures that right patient receives right medication.
a. Check expiration date on medication.	Medications used past expiration date may be inactive or harmful to patient.
2. Take medications to patient at correct time, within 30 minutes before or after prescribed time (see agency policy). Give stat and single-order medications at the exact time ordered. During administration apply the six rights of medication administration.	Promotes intended therapeutic effect.
3. See Standard Protocol (inside front cover).	
4. At patient's bedside compare name of medication on the label with MAR or computer printout. Ask patient if he or she has allergies.	Reading label and comparing it against transcribed order reduces errors. *This is the third check for accuracy.* Confirms patient's allergy history.

SAFETY ALERT If patient is to receive inhaled bronchodilators and inhaled corticosteroids at the same time, the bronchodilators should be given first to promote opening of the airways. After 5 minutes administer the second drug (Lilly and others, 2007).

STEPS	RATIONALE
5. Identify patient using two identifiers (e.g., name and birthday or name and account number, according to facility policy). Compare identifiers with information on patient's MAR or medical record.	Ensures correct patient. Complies with The Joint Commission standards and improves patient safety (TJC, 2010).
6. Discuss the purpose of each medication, action, and possible adverse effects. Allow patient to ask any questions. Explain what a metered dose is and how to administer. Warn about overuse of inhaler, including side effects.	Patient has the right to be informed, and patient's understanding of each medication improves adherence with drug therapy. Makes patient a participant and reduces anxiety in learning new skill.
7. Allow adequate time for patient to manipulate inhaler, canister, and spacer device (if provided). Explain and demonstrate how canister fits into inhaler.	Patient must be familiar with how to assemble and use equipment.

SAFETY ALERT If using an MDI that is new or has not been used for several days, push a "test spray" into the air to prime the device before using. This ensures that the MDI is patent and the metal canister is positioned properly.

STEPS	RATIONALE
8. *Explain steps for administering MDI, without spacer* (demonstrate when possible).	Simple step-by-step explanation allows patient to ask questions at any point during procedure.
a. Remove mouthpiece cover from inhaler after inserting MDI canister into the holder.	
b. Shake inhaler well for 2 to 5 seconds (five or six shakes).	Ensures mixing of medication in canister.
c. Hold inhaler in dominant hand.	
d. Instruct patient to position inhaler in one of two ways:	

Continued

STEPS	RATIONALE
(1) Place mouthpiece in mouth with opening toward back of throat, closing lips tightly around it (see illustration).	Directs aerosol towards airways.
(2) Position mouthpiece 2 to 4 cm (1 to 2 inches) in front of widely opened mouth (see illustration), with opening of inhaler aimed toward back of throat. Lips do not touch inhaler.	Directs aerosol spray toward airway. This is the best way to deliver the medication without a spacer.
e. Have patient take a deep breath and exhale completely.	Prepares airway to receive medication.
f. With inhaler positioned, have patient hold inhaler with thumb at the mouthpiece and index and middle fingers at the top. This is a three-point or bilateral hand position.	Hand position ensures proper activation of MDI (Lilly and others, 2007).
g. Instruct patient to tilt head back slightly and inhale slowly and deeply through the mouth for 3 to 5 seconds while depressing the canister fully.	Medication is distributed to airways during inhalation.
h. Have patient hold breath for about 10 seconds.	Allows the tiny drops of aerosol spray to reach deeper branches of airways.
i. Remove MDI from mouth before exhaling and exhale slowly through nose or pursed lips.	Keeps small airways open during exhalation.
9. *Explain steps to administer MDI using a spacer device* (demonstrate when possible).	
a. Remove mouthpiece cover from MDI and mouthpiece of spacer device.	Inhaler fits into end of spacer device.
b. Shake inhaler well for 2 to 5 seconds (five or six shakes).	Mixes medication in canister.
c. Insert MDI into end of spacer device.	Spacer device traps medication released from MDI; patient then inhales the drug from the device. The spacer improves delivery of correct dose of inhaled medication.
d. Instruct patient to place spacer device mouthpiece into mouth and close lips. Do not insert beyond raised lip on mouthpiece. Avoid covering small exhalation slots with the lips.	Medication should not escape through mouth.
e. Have patient breathe normally through spacer device mouthpiece (see illustration).	Allows patient to relax before delivering medication.
f. Instruct patient to depress medication canister, spraying one puff into spacer device.	Device contains the fine spray and allows patient to inhale more medicine.

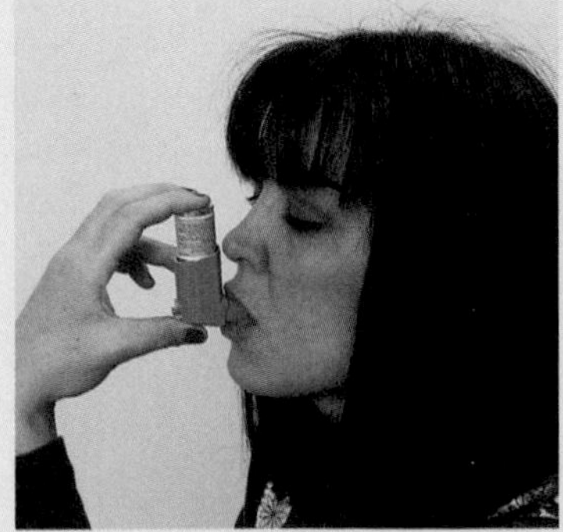

STEP 8d(1) Using metered-dose inhaler.

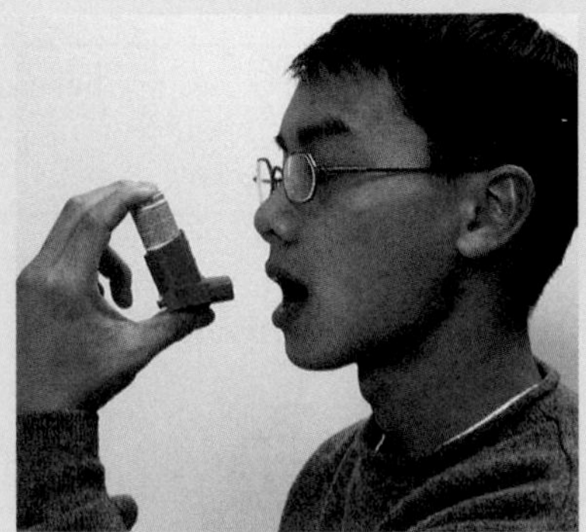

STEP 8d(2) Alternative technique for using metered-dose inhaler.

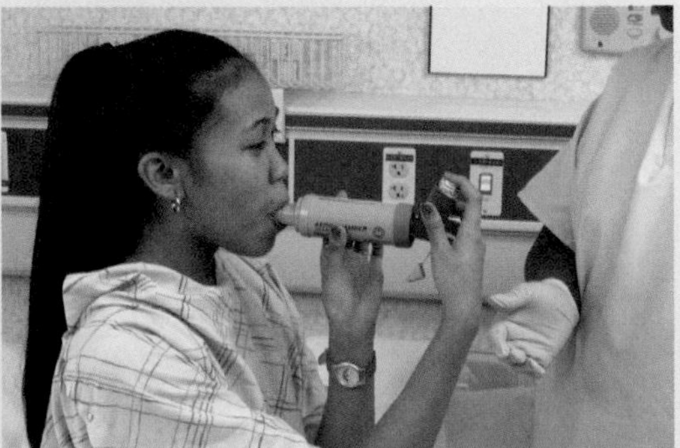

STEP 9e Using spacer device with metered-dose inhaler. (From Lilley LL and others: *Pharmacology and the nursing process*, ed 6, St Louis, 2011, Mosby.)

STEPS	RATIONALE
g. Patient breathes in slowly and fully (for 5 seconds).	Particles of medication are able to distribute to deeper airways.
h. Instruct patient to hold breath for 10 seconds.	Ensures full drug distribution.
10. Instruct patient to wait 20 to 30 seconds between inhalations (if same medication) or 2 to 5 minutes between inhalations (if different medication).	Drugs must be inhaled sequentially. Always administer bronchodilators before steroids so dilators can open airway passages (Lilley and others, 2007).
11. Instruct patient to not repeat inhalations before next scheduled dose.	Drugs are prescribed at intervals during the day to provide a constant drug level and minimize side effects. Beta-adrenergic MDIs are used either on an "as needed" basis or regularly every 4 to 6 hours.
12. Warn patients that they might feel a gagging sensation in throat caused by droplets of medication on pharynx or tongue.	This occurs if medication is sprayed or inhaled incorrectly.
13. About 2 minutes after a dose, instruct patient to rinse mouth out with warm water and spit the water out after use of the MDI.	Inhaled bronchodilators may cause dry mouth and taste alterations. Steroids may alter the normal flora of the oral mucosa and lead to development of fungal infection (Lilley and others, 2007).
14. For daily cleaning, instruct patient to remove medication canister, rinse the inhaler and cap with warm running water, and be sure that inhaler is completely dry before reuse. Do not get the valve mechanism of the canister wet.	Removes residual medication and reduces transmission of infection. Water damages the valve.
15. Ask if patient has any questions.	
16. **See Completion Protocol (inside front cover).**	

EVALUATION

1. Have patient explain and demonstrate steps in use and cleaning of inhaler.
2. Ask patient to explain drug schedule and dose of medication.
3. After medication instillation, assess patient's respirations, breath sounds, and peak flow measures if ordered.
4. Ask patient to describe side effects and criteria for calling health care provider.

Unexpected Outcomes and Related Interventions

1. Patient's breathing pattern is ineffective; respirations are rapid and shallow.
   a. Evaluate vital signs and respiratory status.
   b. Evaluate type of medication and/or patient's administration technique.
   c. Notify health care provider.
2. Patient experiences paroxysms of coughing.
   a. Evaluate patient's administration technique.
   b. Notify health care provider.
3. Patient needs a bronchodilator more than every 4 hours (this can signal respiratory problems).
   a. Notify health care provider to reassess type of medication.
   b. Evaluate patient's administration technique.
4. Patient has cardiac dysrhythmias (light-headedness, syncope).
   a. Evaluate cardiac and pulmonary status (see Chapter 7)
   b. Withhold all further doses of medication.
   c. Notify health care provider.
5. Patient is not able to self-administer medication correctly.
   a. Explore alternative delivery routes.
   b. Assess potential benefits of a spacer device.

Recording and Reporting

- Record drug, dose or strength, number of inhalations, and time administered on MAR immediately after administration, not before. Include initials or signature. Record patient teaching and validation of understanding in nurses' notes.
- Record in nurses' notes patient's response to the MDI (e.g., respiratory rate and pattern, breath sounds), evidence of side effects (e.g., arrhythmia, patient's feelings of anxiety), and patient's ability to use the MDI.
- Report any side effects of medication to health care provider.

Sample Documentation

0900 Coughing violently and reports difficulty breathing. Wheezing noted throughout all lung fields. R 32, P 98 and regular. Self-administered Albuterol per MDI (2 puffs) correctly with no verbal coaching. Reported relief from shortness of breath within 1 minute.

0915 Reports breathing more at ease, R 24, P 94 and regular. Wheezing remains in L upper lobe, R lung fields are clear.

Special Considerations

Pediatric

- A spacer is a benefit to young children because they have difficulty coordinating the activation of the inhaler and inhaling (Hockenberry and Wilson, 2007).
- Educate child and parent about the need to use inhaler during school hours. Help family find resources within the school or day care facility. Many school systems do not permit self-administration of MDIs. Follow school policy. A health care provider's order is required.

Geriatric

- An older adult may be unable to depress the medication canister because of weakened grasp. If there is difficulty with coordinating activation of the inhaler and inhalation, the use of a spacer device may be helpful.

Home Care

Teach patients how to count doses in an MDI. Failure to do so might result in a patient using an empty inhaler during an acute episode of a respiratory problem. To track doses:

- Note first day of use on a calendar.
- Note number of inhalations in the canister (e.g., 200 inhalations per MDI).
- Note number of inhalations used per day (e.g., 2 inhalations a day, 3 times a day, equals 6 inhalations a day).
- Divide the total number of inhalations in canister by the number of inhalations needed per day to determine number of days inhaler should last (e.g., 200/6 = 33 days of 3 times–a-day dosing).
- Mark on calendar the date inhaler will be empty; obtain a refill a few days before.
- Remind patients to carry prescribed inhalers with them at all times to use as immediate treatment in case of an acute asthma attack.

PROCEDURAL GUIDELINE 22.1
Using a Dry Powder Inhaler (DPI)

DPIs hold dry, powdered medication and create an aerosol when the patient inhales through a reservoir that contains a dose of medicine. In contrast with an MDI, the DPI has no propellant. DPIs require less manual dexterity; and, because the device is breath activated, there is no need to coordinate puffs with inhalation. Compared with MDIs, DPIs deliver more drug to the lungs (20% versus 10% of the total released) and less to the oropharynx (Lehne, 2007). A DPI does not require a spacer. Medication inside a DPI can clump if the patient lives in a humid climate. Some patients cannot inhale fast enough to administer the entire dose of the medication.

Delegation and Collaboration

The skill of administering DPI medications cannot be delegated to nursing assistive personnel (NAP). Instruct the NAP about the following:

- Potential side effects of medications and to report their occurrence
- Reporting paroxysmal coughing, audible wheezing, and patient's report of breathlessness or difficulty breathing

Equipment

- DPI (see Fig. 22-2, *C*)
- Stethoscope
- Washbasin or sink with warm water
- Medication administration record (MAR)
- Facial tissues (optional).

Procedural Steps

1. Check accuracy and completeness of each MAR with health care provider's medication order. Check patient's name, drug name and dosage, route of administration, and time for administration. Recopy or reprint any portion of printed MAR that is difficult to read.
2. Review pertinent information related to medication, including action, purpose, normal dose and route, side effects, time of onset and peak action, and nursing implications. *Rationale: Allows you to anticipate effects of drug and to observe patient's response.*
3. Assess patient's medical history, history of allergies, and medication and diet history.
4. Assess respiratory pattern and auscultate breath sounds.
5. Assess patient's knowledge of medication and readiness to learn (e.g., asks questions about medication, requests education in use of DPI; is mentally alert; participates in own care).
6. Assess patient's ability to learn: patient should not be fatigued, in pain, or in respiratory distress and should understand technical vocabulary terms.
7. Determine patient's ability to hold, manipulate, and activate the DPI.
8. If previously instructed in self-administration of inhaled medicine, assess patient's technique in using a DPI.
9. Prepare medication for instillation; check label on inhaler against MAR two times. *This is the first and second check for accuracy.*

PROCEDURAL GUIDELINE 22.1
Using a Dry Powder Inhaler (DPI)—cont'd

10. Take medications to patient at correct time. Most agencies require administration within 30 minutes before or after scheduled time (see agency policy). Stat and single-order medications are given at the exact time ordered. During administration apply the six rights of medication administration (see Chapter 21).
11. **See Standard Protocol (inside front cover).**
12. At patient's bedside again compare the MAR or computer printout with the names of medications on the medication labels. *This is the third check for accuracy.* Also ask patient if he or she has allergies.
13. Identify patient using two identifiers (e.g., name and birthday or name and account number, according to agency policy). Compare identifiers with information on patient's MAR or medical record (TJC, 2010).
14. Discuss the purpose of each medication, action, and possible adverse effects with patient. Allow patient to ask any questions about drugs.
15. If the DPI has an external counter, note the number indicated to determine doses remaining. Otherwise use the technique in Skill 22.5 for counting doses.
16. Prepare the DPI for administration. Some DPIs require loading the medication before administration, some require rotation of a lever to load the medication or the insertion of a capsule, and some require insertion of a disk into the inhaler device. Follow manufacturer's specific instructions.

SAFETY ALERT The patient's inhaled breath pulls the drug into the airway. DPIs may differ as to how fast the patient should inhale the medication; consult manufacturer's specific instructions. In addition, do not shake the DPI because powdered medication may spill out of the device.

17. Have patient place lips over the mouthpiece of the DPI and inhale quickly and deeply. Remove inhaler from mouth as soon as inhalation is complete but before exhalation. Instruct patient that he or she may not taste the powdered medication.
18. Have patient hold breath for 10 seconds or as long as possible and then exhale. Do not exhale into the DPI.
19. After using the DPI, have patient rinse mouth with warm water and spit it out to reduce throat irritation and prevent oral candidiasis.
20. Return the DPI to closed position or remove loaded capsule or disk if necessary. If an external counter is present, note the number, which should be one less than the number in Step 15.
21. **See Completion Protocol (inside front cover).**
22. Have patient demonstrate use of the DPI at next scheduled dose. Ask patient to discuss purpose, action, and side effects of medication.
23. Auscultate patient's breath sounds, evaluate respiratory rate, and ask if patient feels greater ease in breathing.
24. Record drug, dose or strength, route, number of inhalations, and time administered on MAR immediately after administration, not before. Include initials or signature. Record patient teaching and validation of understanding in nurses' notes.

SKILL 22.6 USING SMALL-VOLUME NEBULIZERS

Nebulization is a process of adding medications or moisture to inspired air by mixing particles of various sizes with air. Adding moisture to the respiratory system through nebulization improves clearance of pulmonary secretions. Medications such as bronchodilators, mucolytics, and corticosteroids are often administered by nebulization.

Small-volume nebulizers are machines that convert a drug solution into a mist that can be inhaled by a patient into the tracheobronchial tree. The droplets in the mist are much finer than those created by MDIs or DPIs. Inhalation of the nebulized mist is delivered via face mask or a mouthpiece held between the teeth. A nebulized medication is designed to create a local effect, but it can be absorbed into the bloodstream through the alveoli. As a result, systemic effects from the medications may occur.

ASSESSMENT

1. Check accuracy and completeness of each MAR with health care provider's medication order. Check patient's name, drug name and dosage, route of administration, and time for administration. Recopy or reprint any portion of printed MAR that is difficult to read. *Rationale: The health care provider's order is the most reliable source and only legal record of drugs patient is to receive. Ensures that*

patient receives the right medications (Eisenhauer and others, 2007; Furukawa and others, 2008).

2. Review pertinent information related to medication, including action, purpose, normal dose and route, time of onset and peak action, side effects, and nursing implications. *Rationale: Allows you to anticipate effects of drug and observe patient's response.*
3. Assess patient's medical history (e.g., history of cardiac disease), history of allergies, medication and diet history. *Rationale: Factors influence how certain drugs act. Reveals patient's need for medication and risk for side effects.*
4. Assess patient's grasp and ability to assemble, hold, and manipulate the nebulizer equipment. *Rationale: Any impairment of grasp or hand tremors interfere with ability to use nebulizer.*
5. Assess pulse, respirations, breath sounds, pulse oximetry, and peak flow measurement (if ordered). *Rationale: Provides baseline to determine effect of medication.*
6. Assess patient's knowledge of medication and readiness to learn (e.g., patient asks questions about medication, requests education in use of nebulizer, is mentally alert, participates in own care).

PLANNING

Expected Outcomes focus on safe, accurate, and effective drug therapy; relief of symptoms; and promoting knowledge of self-administration of small-volume nebulizer.

1. Patient's breathing pattern is effective.
2. Patient's gas exchange is adequate.
3. Patient is able to demonstrate self-administration of nebulized dose of medication correctly.
4. Patient is able to describe side effects of medication and criteria for calling health care provider.

Delegation and Collaboration

In many facilities a respiratory therapist performs the skill of administering medications by nebulizer. The nurse must be aware of the type and actions of the inhaled medication that the patient is receiving. The skill of administering medications by nebulizer cannot be delegated to nursing assistive personnel (NAP). Instruct the NAP about the following:

- Potential side effects of medications and to report their occurrence to the nurse
- Reporting paroxysmal coughing, ineffective breathing patterns, and other respiratory difficulties

Equipment

- Medication ordered and diluent (if needed)
- Medicine dropper or syringe
- Nebulizer bottle and tubing assembly
- Small-volume nebulizer machine (often called *handheld nebulizer* or simply *nebulizer*)
- Pulse oximeter
- Stethoscope
- Medication administration record (MAR)

IMPLEMENTATION *for* USING SMALL-VOLUME NEBULIZERS

STEP	RATIONALE
1. Prepare medications for administration: Check label of nebulized medication against MAR two times (see Skill 22.1).	*This includes the first and second check for accuracy.* Ensures that right patient receives right medication.
a. Check expiration date on medication	Medications used past expiration date may be inactive or harmful to patient.
2. Take medications to patient at correct time, within 30 minutes before or after prescribed time (see agency policy). Give stat and single-order medications at the exact time ordered. During administration apply the six rights of medication administration (see Chapter 21).	Promotes intended therapeutic effect.
3. **See Standard Protocol (inside front cover).**	
4. At patient's bedside compare name of medication on the label with MAR or computer printout. Ask patient if he or she has allergies.	Reading label and comparing it against transcribed order reduces errors. *This is the third check for accuracy.* Confirms patient's history of allergies.
5. Identify patient using two identifiers (e.g., name and birthday or name and account number, according to facility policy). Compare identifiers with information on patient's MAR or medical record.	Ensures correct patient. Complies with The Joint Commission standards and improves patient safety (TJC, 2010).
6. Discuss the purpose of each medication, action, and possible adverse effects. Allow patient to ask any questions. Explain procedure to patient during medication administration, including how to assemble nebulizer.	Patient has the right to be informed, and patient's understanding of each medication improves adherence with drug therapy. Makes patient a participant in care and minimizes anxiety. Enables patient to self-administer drug if physically able and motivated.

STEP	RATIONALE
7. Explain use of nebulizer and warn patient of possible drug side effects.	Helps to make patient more knowledgeable about treatment and medication.
8. Assemble nebulizer equipment per manufacturer's directions.	Assembly may vary slightly with different manufacturers. Proper assembly ensures safe delivery of medication.
9. Add prescribed medication using medicine dropper or syringe and diluent (if needed) to nebulizer cup.	Ensures proper dose and delivery of ordered medication.
10. Attach the top portion of the nebulizer cup and connect the mouthpiece or face mask to the cup.	
11. Connect the tubing to both the aerosol compressor and nebulizer cup.	
12. Have patient hold mouthpiece between lips with gentle pressure (see illustration).	

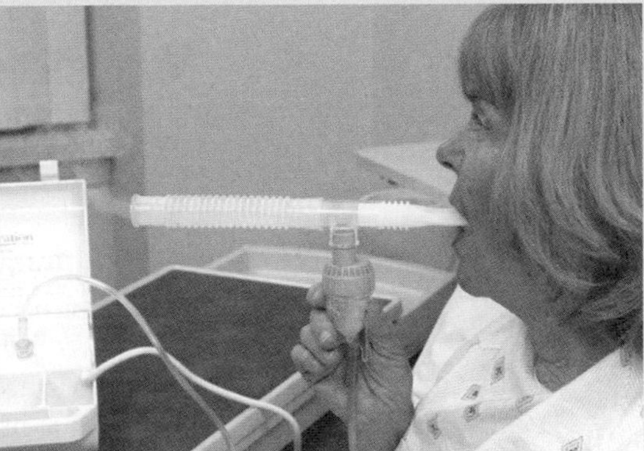

STEP 12 Nebulizer mouthpiece placed between patient's lips during treatment.

STEP	RATIONALE
a. If patient is an infant, child, or fatigued adult or unable to follow instructions, use a face mask.	Use of a face mask does not require patient to remember to hold mouthpiece correctly. Correct delivery ensures sufficient deposition of medication.
b. Use special adapters for patients with a tracheostomy.	Promotes greater deposition of medication in the airways.
13. Turn on the small-volume nebulizer machine and ensure that a sufficient mist is formed.	Verifies that equipment is working properly during delivery of medication.
14. Have patient take a deep breath, slowly, to a volume slightly greater than normal. Encourage a brief, end-inspiratory pause; then have patient exhale passively.	Improves effectiveness of medication.
a. If patient is dyspneic, encourage him or her to hold every fourth or fifth breath for 5 to 10 seconds.	Maximizes effectiveness of medication.
b. Remind patient to repeat the breathing pattern until the drug is completely nebulized. This usually takes about 10 minutes.	Maximizes effectiveness of medication.
(1) Some practitioners set a timed limit as the length of the treatment rather than waiting for the medication to completely nebulize.	
c. Tap the nebulizer cup occasionally during treatment and toward the end of the treatment.	Releases droplets that are clinging to the side of the cup, thus allowing for renebulization of the solution.
d. Monitor patient's pulse during procedure, especially if beta-adrenergic bronchodilators are used.	Enables nurse to observe for potential side effects of medications.

SAFETY ALERT Some respiratory medications can cause systemic effects such as restlessness, nervousness, and palpitations. Administer these medications with caution to patients with cardiac disease because of the possibility of hypertension, dysrhythmias, or coronary insufficiency. If severe bronchospasm occurs during treatment, discontinue drug immediately and notify health care provider.

Continued

STEP	RATIONALE
15. When medication is completely nebulized, turn off machine. Rinse the nebulizer cup per agency guidelines. Dry completely. Store tubing assembly per agency policy. For daily cleansing check agency policy.	Proper storage reduces transfer of microorganisms. In some agencies cleansing the nebulizer each day in soap and water is adequate.
16. If steroids are nebulized, instruct patient to rinse mouth and gargle with warm water after nebulizer treatment.	Removes medication residue from oral cavity and helps to prevent oral candidiasis, a possible adverse effect of inhaled steroid therapy.
17. After the nebulization have patient take several deep breaths and cough to expectorate mucus.	A nebulized medication is often ordered to open airways and promote expectoration of mucus.
18. See Completion Protocol (inside front cover),	

EVALUATION

1. Assess patient's respirations, breath sounds, cough effort, sputum production, and pulse oximetry; assess peak flow measures if ordered.
2. Have patient explain and demonstrate steps in use of nebulizer.
3. Ask patient to explain drug schedule.
4. Ask patient to describe side effects of medication and criteria for calling health care provider.

Unexpected Outcomes and Related Interventions

1. Patient's breathing pattern is ineffective; respirations are rapid and shallow; breath sounds indicate wheezing.
   a. Reassess type of medication and/or delivery method.
   b. Notify health care provider.
2. Patient experiences paroxysms of coughing. Aerosolized particles can irritate posterior pharynx.
   a. Reassess type of medication and/or delivery method.
   b. Notify health care provider.
3. Patient experiences cardiac dysrhythmias (syncope, lightheadedness), especially if receiving beta-adrenergics.
   a. Withhold all further doses of medication. Assess vital signs.
   b. Notify health care provider for reassessment of type of medication and delivery method.
4. Patient is unable to self-administer medication properly.
   a. Explore alternative delivery routes or devices.
   b. Determine feasibility of having family caregiver learn how to administer.
5. Patient is unable to explain technique and risks of drug therapy.
   a. Provide further instruction, including family caregivers if appropriate.

Recording and Reporting

- Record drug, dose or strength, length of treatment, route, and time administered on MAR immediately after administration, not before. Include initials or signature. Record patient teaching and validation of understanding and ability to self-administer medication in nurses' notes.
- Document patient's response to treatment.
- Report adverse effects/patient response and/or withheld drugs to nurse in charge or health care provider.

Sample Documentation

0900 Reports that he "has trouble catching my breath" after walking down hallway. Dyspnea noted, with R 32, P 95, and scattered wheezes throughout lung fields bilaterally. Budesonide 500 mcg given by nebulizer over 20 minutes.

0930 Postnebulizer R 26, P 100; wheezes decreased. States he is "breathing easier now."

Special Considerations

Pediatric

- Use a mask for the nebulizer treatment if child is too young to hold mouthpiece correctly for the duration of the treatment (Hockenberry and Wilson, 2007).
- Instruct child to breathe normally with mouth open to provide a direct route to the airways for the medication.
- Educate child and parent about the use of a nebulizer during school or day care hours. Help family find resources within the school or day care facility. Follow school policy regarding having the nebulizer and medication available for use during school hours. A health care provider's order may be necessary.

Geriatric

- Patients may have weakened grasp, hand tremors, or coordination problems that make it difficult to hold nebulizer. A family caregiver might be able to assist.

Home Care

- Rinse the nebulizer parts after each use with clear water and air dry. In addition, clean the parts daily with warm, soapy water; rinse; and allow to dry.
- Once a week the nebulizer parts should be soaked in a solution of vinegar and water (one part white vinegar to four parts water) for 30 minutes, rinsed thoroughly with clean water, and air dried. Nebulizer parts should never be stored until totally dried. Wet equipment encourages the growth of bacteria and mold (Lilley and others, 2007).

- Follow manufacturer's recommendations for maintenance of small-volume nebulizer machine, including changing the filters when they become discolored (grayish).
- Advise patients taking long-acting beta agonists, which are used for long-term control of symptoms, about possible adverse effects: nervousness, restlessness, tremor, headache, nausea, rapid or pounding heart rate, and dizziness. Emphasize that the drug should be taken only as ordered so a tolerance is not developed.

PROCEDURAL GUIDELINE 22.2
Administering Vaginal Medications

- **Nursing Skills Online:** Nonparenteral Medication Administration Module, Lesson 6

Female patients who develop vaginal infections often require topical application of antiinfective agents. Vaginal medications are available in foam, jelly, cream, or suppository form. Medicated irrigations or douches can also be given. However, their excessive use can lead to vaginal irritation.

Vaginal suppositories are oval shaped and come individually packaged in foil wrappers. They are larger and more oval than rectal suppositories. Fig. 22-3 shows a comparison with rectal suppositories. Storage in a refrigerator prevents the solid suppositories from melting. You insert a suppository into the vagina either with an applicator or a gloved hand. After insertion, body temperature causes the suppository to melt, and the medication is distributed. Foam, jellies, and creams are administered with an inserter or applicator. Patients often prefer administering their own vaginal medications, and you should give them privacy to do so. After instillation of the drug, a patient may wish to wear a perineal pad to collect excess drainage. Because vaginal medications are frequently given to treat infection, any discharge is often foul smelling. Follow good aseptic technique and offer the patient frequent opportunities for perineal hygiene (see Chapter 10).

Delegation and Collaboration

The skill of administering vaginal instillations cannot be delegated to nursing assistive personnel (NAP). Instruct the NAP about the following:

- Potential side effects of medications and to report their occurrence to the nurse
- Reporting a change in comfort level or new or increased vaginal discharge or bleeding to the nurse

Equipment

- Vaginal cream, foam, jelly, tablet, suppository, or irrigating solution
- Applicators (Fig. 22-4) (if needed)
- Clean gloves
- Tissues
- Towels and/or washcloths
- Perineal pad; drape or sheet
- Water-soluble lubricants
- Bedpan
- Irrigation or douche container (if needed)
- Medication administration record (MAR)

Procedural Steps

1. Check accuracy and completeness of each MAR with health care provider's medication order. Check patient's name, drug name and dosage, route of administration, and time for administration. Recopy or reprint any portion of printed MAR that is difficult to read. *This is the first and second check for accuracy.*
2. Review pertinent information related to medication, including action, purpose, normal dose and route, side effects, time of onset and peak action, and nursing implications.
3. Assess patient's medical history, history of allergies, and medication history.
4. During perineal care inspect condition of vaginal tissues (wearing gloves); note if drainage is present.
5. Ask if patient is experiencing any symptoms of pruritus, burning, discharge, or discomfort.

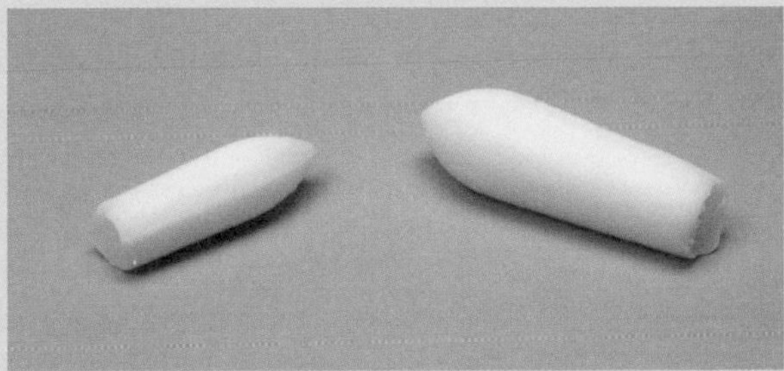

FIG 22-3 Vaginal suppositories *(right)* are larger and more oval than rectal suppositories *(left)*. (From Lilley LL and others: *Pharmacology and the nursing process,* ed 4, St Louis, 2004, Mosby.)

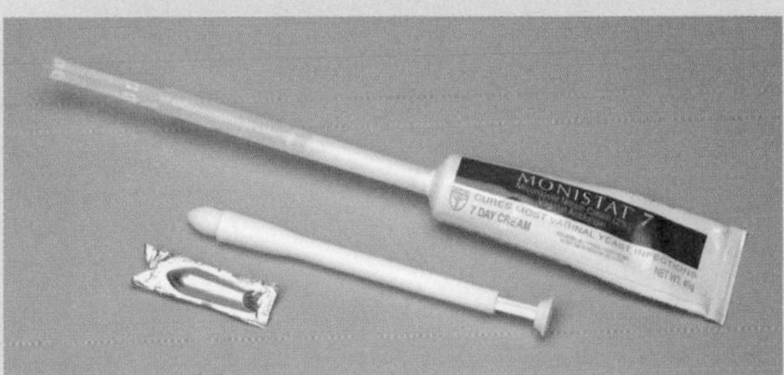

FIG 22-4 *From top:* Vaginal cream with applicator, applicator, and vaginal suppository. (From Lilley LL and others: *Pharmacology and the nursing process,* ed 6, St Louis, 2011, Mosby.)

Continued

PROCEDURAL GUIDELINE 22.2
Administering Vaginal Medications—cont'd

6. Assess patient's knowledge of medication, readiness to learn (e.g., patient asks questions about medication, requests education in use of suppository).
7. Assess patient's ability to insert suppository (cognitive level and hand coordination).
8. Have patient void to prevent accidental passing of urine during insertion.
9. Prepare suppository for administration. Check label on medication against MAR two times (see Skill 22.1).
10. Take medications to patient at correct time, within 30 minutes before or after prescribed time (see agency policy). During administration apply the six rights of medication administration.
11. **See Standard Protocol (inside front cover).**
12. At patient's bedside again compare the MAR or computer printout with the names of medications on the medication labels. *This is the third check for accuracy.* Also ask patient if he or she has allergies.
13. Identify patient using two identifiers (i.e., name and birthday or name and hospital number, according to agency policy). Compare identifiers with information on patient's MAR or medical record (TJC, 2010).
14. Discuss the purpose of each medication, action, and possible adverse effects. Allow patient to ask any questions. Explain procedure to patient and be specific if patient plans to self-administer medication.
15. Assist patient with lying in dorsal recumbent position. Patients with restricted mobility in knees or hips may lie supine with legs abducted.
16. Keep abdomen and lower extremities draped.
17. Be sure that vaginal orifice is well illuminated by room light. Otherwise position portable gooseneck lamp.
18. Inspect condition of external genitalia and vaginal canal (see Chapter 7).
19. Insert vaginal suppository:
    a. Remove suppository from foil wrapper and apply liberal amount of water-soluble lubricant to smooth or rounded end (see illustration). Be sure that suppository is at room temperature. Lubricate gloved index finger of dominant hand.

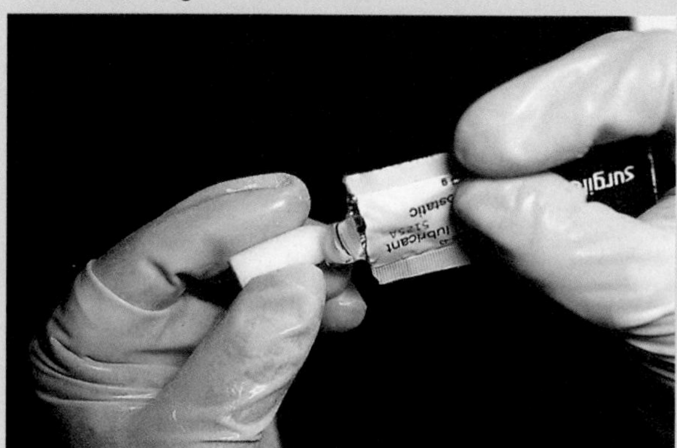

STEP 19a Lubricate tip of suppository.

    b. With nondominant gloved hand gently separate labial folds in the front-to-back direction.
    c. With dominant gloved hand insert rounded end of suppository along posterior wall of vaginal canal entire length of finger (7.5 to 10 cm [3 to 4 inches]) (see illustration).

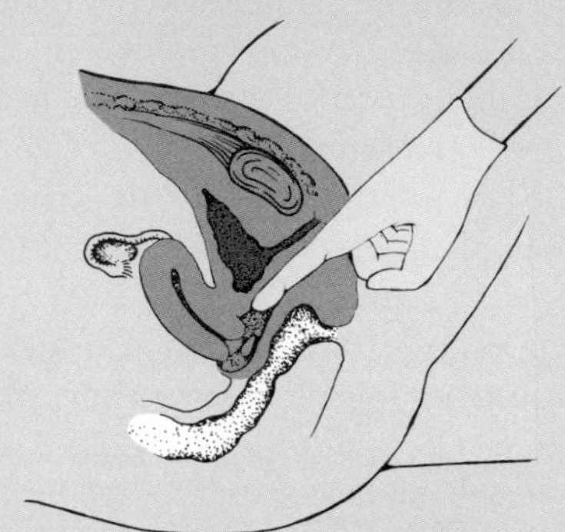

STEP 19c Vaginal suppository insertion.

    d. Withdraw finger and wipe away remaining lubricant from around orifice and labia with a tissue or cloth.
20. Apply cream or foam:
    a. Fill cream or foam applicator following package directions.
    b. With nondominant gloved hand gently separate labial folds. Insert applicator approximately 5 to 7.5 cm (2 to 3 inches). Push applicator plunger to deposit medication into vagina (see illustration).

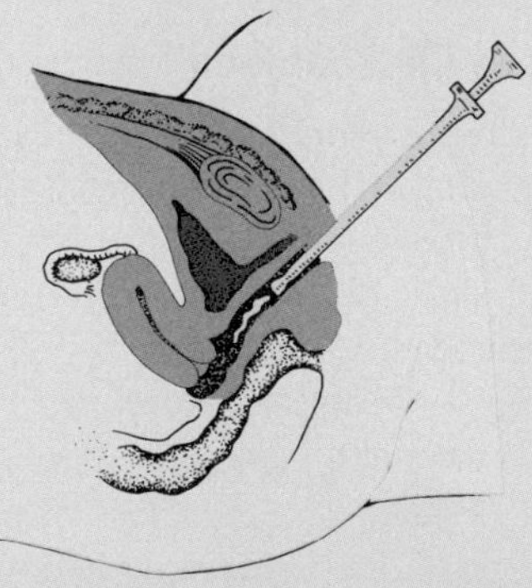

STEP 20b Applicator with cream inserted into vaginal canal.

    c. Withdraw applicator and place on paper towel. Wipe off residual cream from labia or vaginal orifice with a tissue or cloth.
21. Instruct patient who received suppository or cream to remain on her back for at least 10 minutes.
22. If using an applicator, wash with soap and warm water, rinse, and store for future use.
23. Offer perineal pad when patient resumes ambulation.
24. **See Completion Protocol (inside front cover).**

PROCEDURAL GUIDELINE 22.2
Administering Vaginal Medications—cont'd

25. Thirty minutes after administration, inspect condition of vaginal canal and external genitalia between applications. Assess vaginal discharge if present. Remove gloves and perform hand hygiene.
26. Question patient regarding continued pruritus, burning, discomfort, or discharge.
27. Ask patient to discuss purpose, action, and side effects of medication. Observe patient self-administer next dose.
28. Record drug, dose or strength, length of treatment, route, and time administered on MAR immediately after administration, not before. Include initials or signature. Record patient teaching and validation of understanding and ability to self-administer medication in nurses' notes.
29. Report to health care provider if patient states that symptoms do not disappear or that symptoms get worse.
30. Report adverse effects/patient response and/or withheld drugs to nurse in charge or physician.

PROCEDURE GUIDELINE 22.3
Administering Rectal Suppositories

Nursing Skills Online: Nonparenteral Medication Administration Module, Lesson 6

A rectal suppository is a thin, bullet-shaped form of medication that acts when it melts and is absorbed into the rectal mucosa. Rectal medications exert either a local effect on GI mucosa such as promoting defecation or systemic effects such as relieving nausea or providing analgesia. The rectal route is not as reliable as oral or parenteral routes in terms of drug absorption and distribution. However, the medications are relatively safe because they rarely cause local irritation or side effects. Rectal medications are contraindicated in patients with newly developed stomach pain (cause unknown); recent surgery on the rectum, bowel, or prostate gland; rectal bleeding or prolapse; and very low platelet counts (Lilley and others, 2007). In addition, patients with acute coronary conditions should not receive rectal suppositories because of the risk of vagal stimulation during insertion.

Rectal suppositories are thinner and more bullet shaped than vaginal suppositories (see Fig. 22-3). The rounded end prevents anal trauma during insertion. When administering a rectal suppository, place it past the internal anal sphincter and against the rectal mucosa. Improper placement can result in expulsion of the suppository before the medication dissolves and is absorbed into the mucosa. If a patient prefers to self-administer a suppository, give specific instructions so the medication is deposited correctly. Do not cut the suppository into sections to divide the dosage; the active drug may not be distributed evenly within the suppository, and the result may be an inaccurate dose (Lilley and others, 2007).

Delegation and Collaboration

The skill of rectal medication administration cannot be delegated to nursing assistive personnel (NAP). Instruct the NAP about the following:

- Reporting expected fecal discharge or bowel movement to the nurse
- Reporting occurrence of specific potential side effects of medications to the nurse
- Informing the nurse of any rectal discharge, pain, or bleeding

Equipment

- Rectal suppository
- Water-soluble lubricating jelly
- Clean gloves
- Tissue
- Drape
- Medication administration record (MAR)

Procedural Steps

1. Check accuracy and completeness of each MAR with health care provider's medication order. Check patient's name, drug name and dosage, route of administration, and time for administration. Recopy or reprint any portion of printed MAR that is difficult to read.
2. Review pertinent information related to medication, including action, purpose, normal dose and route, side effects, time of onset and peak action, and nursing implications.
3. Assess patient's medical history for rectal surgery or bleeding, cardiac problems, history of allergies, and medication history.
4. Ask patient if having symptoms of rectal irritation, pain, or bleeding.
5. Review any presenting signs and symptoms of GI alterations (e.g., constipation or diarrhea).
6. Assess patient's ability to hold suppository and position self to insert medication.

Continued

PROCEDURE GUIDELINE 22.3
Administering Rectal Suppositories—cont'd

7. Review patient's knowledge of purpose of drug therapy and interest in self-administering suppository.
8. Prepare suppository for administration. Check label on medication against MAR two times (see Skill 22.1). *This is the first and second check for accuracy.*
9. Take medications to patient at correct time, within 30 minutes before or after prescribed time (see agency policy). Give stat and single-order medications at the exact time ordered. During administration apply the six rights of medication administration.
10. **See Standard Protocol (inside front cover).**
11. At patient's bedside again compare the MAR or computer printout with the names of medications on the medication labels. *This is the third check for accuracy.* Also ask patient if he or she has allergies.
12. Identify patient using two identifiers (e.g., name and birthday or name and account number, according to agency policy). Compare identifiers with information on patient's MAR or medical record (TJC, 2010).
13. Discuss the purpose of each medication, action, and possible adverse effects. Allow patient to ask any questions. Explain procedure to patient. Be specific if patient plans on self-administering medication.
14. Assist patient in assuming a left side-lying Sims' position with upper leg flexed upward. Position exposes anus and relaxes anal sphincter.
15. If patient has mobility impairment, assist him or her to a left lateral position. Obtain assistance from another health care provider to help patient turn and use pillows under patient's upper arm and leg for support and comfort.
16. Keep patient draped with only anal area exposed.
17. Examine condition of anus externally and palpate rectal walls as needed (e.g., if impaction is suspected) (see Chapter 7). Dispose of gloves if they become soiled. Turn them inside out and dispose in trash receptacle.

SAFETY ALERT Do not palpate patient's rectum if patient has had rectal surgery. Generally a rectal suppository is contraindicated in the presence of active rectal bleeding or diarrhea (Lilley and others, 2007).

18. Apply clean gloves if previous gloves were soiled and discarded.
19. Remove suppository from foil wrapper and lubricate rounded end with water-soluble lubricant. Lubricate gloved index finger of dominant hand. If patient has hemorrhoids, use a liberal amount of lubricant and handle area gently.
20. Ask patient to take slow, deep breaths through mouth and relax anal sphincter.
21. Retract patient's buttocks with nondominant hand. With gloved index finger of dominant hand, insert suppository gently through anus, past internal sphincter, and against rectal wall, 10 cm (4 inches) in adults (see illustration) or 5 cm (2 inches) in infants and children.

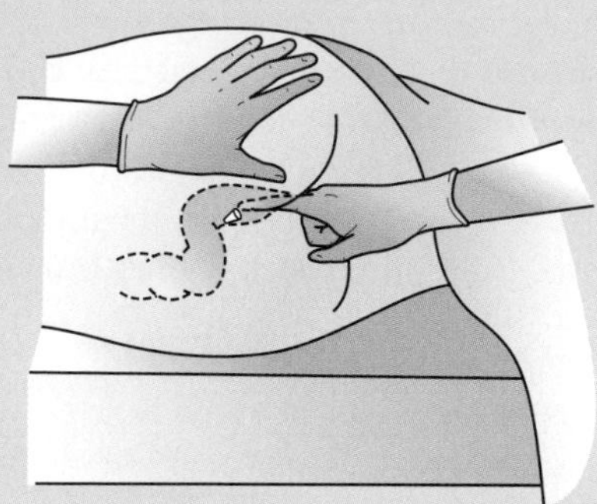

STEP 21 Inserting rectal suppository.

SAFETY ALERT Do not insert suppository into a mass of fecal material; this reduces effectiveness of medication.

22. Withdraw finger and wipe patient's anal area.
23. *Option:* A suppository may be given through a colostomy (not ileostomy) if ordered. Patient should lie supine. Use a small amount of water-soluble lubricant for insertion.
24. Ask patient to remain flat or on side for 5 minutes to prevent expulsion of suppository.
25. If suppository contains laxative or fecal softener, place call light within reach so patient can obtain assistance to reach bedpan or toilet.
26. If suppository was given for constipation, remind patient *not* to flush the commode after the bowel movement.
27. **See Completion Protocol (inside front cover).**
28. Return to bedside within 5 minutes to determine if suppository was expelled.
29. Ask if patient is experiencing any localized anal or rectal discomfort.
30. Evaluate patient for relief of symptoms for which medication was prescribed.
31. If patient is to self-administer medication, have him or her demonstrate administration at next dose.
32. Record drug, dose or strength, length of treatment, route, and time administered on MAR immediately after administration, not before. Include initials or signature. Record patient teaching and validation of understanding and ability to self-administer medication in nurses' notes.
33. Report adverse effects/patient response and/or withheld drugs to nurse in charge or health care provider.

REVIEW QUESTIONS

Case Study for Questions 1 and 2

Mrs. Schneider is a 55-year-old woman who has contact dermatitis on her right forearm. She is visiting the medicine clinic for her regular checkup. Mrs. Schneider is also hypertensive and takes a diuretic and a beta-adrenergic blocker.

1. The nurse in the clinic provides instruction to Mrs. Schneider on how to apply a topical cream for her dermatitis. Which of the following statements, if made by the patient, would indicate that she needs further instruction?
   1. I should wash, rinse, and dry my arm before applying the cream.
   2. If the skin seems dry, it helps to apply the cream when the skin is still damp.
   3. I should soften the cream in the palm of my hand before applying to the skin.
   4. I will spread the cream on the skin and rub it in vigorously so it will absorb.
2. The nurse practitioner taught Mrs. Schneider how to measure her own blood pressure at home. When should Mrs. Schneider measure her blood pressure in relationship to taking her antihypertensive medications?
3. The nurse is instructing a patient on the proper method for using an MDI with spacer. The patient is to receive a bronchodilator and a corticosteroid, 2 puffs each, 3 times a day. The two medications are prescribed for the same time each day. The patient takes the bronchodilator first. Which of the following steps for self-administering an MDI are incorrect in this patient's situation? Select all that apply.
   1. Shake inhaler well for 2 to 5 seconds (five or six shakes) and insert MDI into end of spacer.
   2. Place spacer device mouthpiece into mouth and close lips. Pass the mouthpiece into the back of the pharynx. Avoid covering small exhalation slots with the lips.
   3. Breathe normally through spacer device mouthpiece.
   4. Depress medication canister, spraying one puff into spacer device.
   5. Breathe in slowly and fully (for 5 seconds) and then hold breath for 10 seconds.
   6. Wait 30 seconds after the second puff of bronchodilator and then take the steroid.
4. The nurse should include which instruction when teaching the patient about using transdermal patches for chronic pain management?
   1. Apply the patch to the same spot each day for consistent dosing.
   2. If the patient experiences severe sedation, cut the patch in half for the next dose.
   3. If pain is not relieved, apply a second patch without removing the first one.
   4. Remove the old patch and cleanse the area before applying a new patch.
5. The nurse is caring for a patient who has an order for an acetaminophen (Tylenol) rectal suppository. Which of the following findings in the nurse's assessment would contraindicate administration?
   1. Rectal hemorrhoids
   2. Presence of a fever
   3. Rectal bleeding
   4. Diarrhea
6. A patient comes to the clinic and is told that he is receiving a new medication that switches him from an MDI to a DPI for delivery of an inhalant. Which of the following steps used in administering an MDI is not part of a DPI administration?
   1. Do not repeat an inhalation until next scheduled dose.
   2. Always count remaining doses.
   3. Hold your breath for 10 seconds after an inhalation.
   4. Be sure to coordinate a puff with inhalation.
7. When administering eardrops to a 5-year-old child, how should the nurse hold the child's ear?
   1. Pull the pinna down and back before administering the eardrops.
   2. Pull the pinna up and outward before administering the eardrops.
   3. Retract the tragus out from ear canal.
   4. Have child sit up and pull pinna forward.
8. Fill in the Blank. When administering a medication through a feeding tube, always flush the tubing with __________ mL of water after each medication. After the last medication flush the tubing with _________ mL of water.
9. When inserting a vaginal suppository, which of the following techniques is/are not correct? Select all that apply.
   1. Have the patient void before insertion.
   2. Have patient lie on left side.
   3. With dominant gloved hand insert suppository along posterior wall of vaginal canal entire length of finger (7.5 to 10 cm [3 to 4 inches]).
   4. With dominant glove hand insert the suppository 10 cm (4 inches) into the vaginal canal.
10. Short Answer: Describe the first two steps the nurse should follow before the administration of any nonparenteral medication.

REFERENCES

American Society for Parenteral and Enteral Nutrition (ASPEN): ASPEN Enteral Nutrition Practice Recommendations, *J Parenter Enteral Nutr* 22:122, 2009.

Biron AD and others: Work interruptions and their contribution to medication administration errors: an evidence review, *Worldviews Evid Based Nurs* 6(2):70, 2009.

Eisenhauer LA and others: Nurses' reported thinking during medication administration, *J Nurs Scholarsh* 39(1):82, 2007.

Furukawa MF and others: Adoption of health information technology for medication safety in U.S. hospitals, 2006, *Health Affairs* 27(3):865, 2008.

Garlapati RR and others: Indicators for the correct usage of intranasal medications: a computational fluid dynamics study, *Laryngoscope*, epub Aug 4, 2009.

Hockenberry MJ, Wilson D: *Wong's nursing care of infants and children*, ed 8, St Louis, 2007, Mosby.

Ignatavicius DD, Workman ML: *Medical-surgical nursing: critical thinking for collaborative care*, ed 6, Philadelphia, 2010, Saunders.

Institution for Safe Medication Practices (ISMP): New fentanyl warnings: more needed to protect patients, *ISMP Medication Safety Alert*, August 11, 2005, http://www.ismp.org/Newsletters, accessed August 31, 2009.

Institution for Safe Medication Practices (ISMP): Tablet splitting: do it only if you "half" to, and then do it safely, *ISMP Medication Safety Alert* 11(10), 2006, http://www.ismp.org/Newsletters, accessed August 28, 2009.

Kilbourne AM and others: How does depression influence diabetes medication adherence in older patients? *Am J Geriatr Psychiatry* 13(3):202, 2005.

Lakey SL and others: Assessment of older adults' knowledge of and preferences for medication management tools and support systems, *Ann Pharmacother* 43(6):1011, 2009.

Lehne RA: *Pharmacology for nursing care*, ed 6, Philadelphia, 2007, Saunders.

Lilley LL and others: *Pharmacology and the nursing process*, ed 5, St Louis, 2007, Mosby.

McKenry L and others: *Mosby's pharmacology in nursing*, ed 22, St Louis, 2006, Mosby.

Metheny NA: Preventing respiratory complications of tube-feeding: evidence-based practice, *Am J Crit Care* 15:360, 2006.

Metheny NA and others: Gastric residual volume and aspiration in critically ill patients receiving gastric feedings, *Am J Crit Care* 17(6):512, 2008.

Monahan F and others: *Phipps' medical-surgical nursing*, ed 8, St Louis, 2007, Mosby.

Pape TM and others: Innovative approaches to reducing nurses' distractions during medication administration, *J Contin Educ Nurs* 36(3):108, 2005.

Rubin DK, Durotoye L: How do patients determine that their metered dose inhaler is empty? *Chest* 126(4):1134, 2005.

Shearer J: Improving oral medication management in home health agencies, *Home Healthc Nurse* 27(3):184, 2009.

Simmons D, Graves K, Flynn E: Threading needles in the dark: the effect of the physical work environment on nursing practice, *Crit Care Nurs Q* 32(2):71, 2009.

Sorensen L and others: Medication management at home: medication-related risk factors associated with poor health outcomes, *Age Ageing* 34(6):626, 2005.

The Joint Commission (TJC): *2010 National Patient Safety Goals*, Oakbrook Terrace, Ill, 2010, The Commission, http://www.jointcommission.org/PatientSafety/NationalPatientSafetyGoals.

Uko-Ekpenyong G: Improving medication adherence with orally disintegrating tablets, *Nursing* 36(9):20, 2006.

CHAPTER

23

Administration of Parenteral Medications

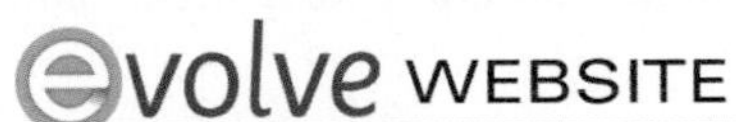

http://evolve.elsevier.com/Perry/nursinginterventions
Video Clips
Nursing Skills Online

The route of medication administration is the path by which a drug comes in contact with the body. *Parenteral* means administered in a manner other than through the digestive tract. Medications administered by the parenteral route enter body tissues and the circulatory system by injection. Injected medications are more quickly absorbed than oral medications; and parenteral routes are used when patients are vomiting, cannot swallow, and/or are restricted from taking oral fluids. There are four routes for parenteral administration:

1. *Subcutaneous (subcutaneous) injection:* Injection into tissues just under the dermis of the skin
2. *Intramuscular (IM) injection:* Injection into the body of a muscle
3. *Intradermal (ID) injection:* Injection into the dermis just under the epidermis
4. *Intravenous (IV) injection or infusion:* Injection into a vein

PATIENT-CENTERED CARE

Injections are invasive and involve some discomfort. Because risk of tissue or nerve damage exists, site selection is an important nursing concern. Prepare patients by explaining the procedure and use good communication techniques to distract them in a way to minimize discomfort. Additional ways to minimize the patient's discomfort when giving an injection include:

- Using sharp, beveled needles in the shortest length and smallest gauge possible.
- Changing the needle if liquid medication coats the shaft of the needle.
- Positioning and flexing patient's limbs to reduce muscular tension.
- Spraying vapocoolant on an injection site 15 seconds before injection or placing wrapped ice on the site for a minute before injection.
- Inserting the needle smoothly and quickly. Do not hesitate and slowly push the needle into tissue.
- Injecting the medication slowly but smoothly.
- Holding the syringe steady once the needle is in the tissue to prevent tissue damage.
- Withdrawing the needle smoothly at the same angle used for insertion.
- Gently applying an antiseptic pad (e.g., alcohol) or dry, sterile gauze pad to the site.
- Applying gentle pressure at the injection site.
- Rotating injection sites to prevent the formation of indurations and abscesses.

Research demonstrates that ethnicity, genetics, culture, and patient adherence and education influence drug response, pharmacokinetics, and pharmacodynamics (Ng and others, 2008). Knowledge about variations in therapeutic dose and adverse effects is essential in administering medications to different ethnic groups. Some patients experience a therapeutic response at a lower dose than recommended and require careful monitoring. For example, Japanese and Taiwanese patients require lower doses of lithium (Ng and others, 2008). You need skill in communicating with and educating diverse patient populations. For example, if a patient values patience and modesty, make your questions specific and take time when assessing their knowledge of drug effects. Cultural assessment also yields information about dietary preferences and use of tobacco, alcohol, and herbal remedies that affect drug action and response. Cultural context is essential in planning education for patients and families (Schim, 2007).

SAFETY

Patient safety in administering medication involves following the six rights of medication administration (see Chapter 21). When managing a patient's medications, communicate clearly with members of the health care team, assess and incorporate the patient's priorities of care and preferences, and use the best evidence when making decisions about patient care. Follow these guidelines to ensure safe medication administration:

- Be vigilant during medication administration. Avoid distractions while preparing an injection. Be sure that your patients receive the appropriate medications. Know why your patient is receiving each medication; know what you need to do before, during, and after medication administration; and evaluate the effectiveness of medications and any adverse effects after your patient takes medications.
- Verify that medications have not expired.
- Use at least two identifiers before administering medications and check against the medication administration record (MAR). Follow agency policy for patient identification.
- Clarify unclear medication orders and ask for help whenever you are uncertain about an order or calculation. Consult with your peers, pharmacists, and other health care providers and be sure that you have resolved all concerns related to medication administration before preparing and giving medications.
- Use technology (e.g., bar scanning, electronic MARs) that is available in your agency when preparing and giving medications. Follow all policies related to use of the technology and do not use "workarounds." A **workaround** bypasses a procedure, policy, or problem in a system. Nurses who use "workarounds" fail to follow agency protocols, policies, or procedures during medication administration in an attempt to get medications administered to patients in a more timely fashion.
- Use strict aseptic technique during medication preparation and administration.
- Educate patients about each medication they take while you are administering medications. Patients often are able to identify inappropriate medications. Make sure that you answer all of their questions before administering medications. Educate family caregivers if appropriate.
- Most of the time you cannot delegate medication administration. Ensure that you follow standards set by the nurse practice act of your state and guidelines established by your health care agency. Licensed practical nurses (LPNs) or licensed vocational nurses (LVNs) usually can administer medications via the oral (PO), subcutaneous, IM, and ID routes. Sometimes they can give medications intravenously if they have had special training and if the medications are not high-alert medications. Some states also allow certified medication assistants (CMAs) to administer some types of medications (e.g., oral medications) in long-term care facilities.

Needlestick Prevention

The most frequent route of exposure to bloodborne disease is from needlestick injuries (ANA, 2009; OSHA, 2009). These injuries occur when health care workers recap needles, mishandle IV lines and needles, or leave stray needles at a patient's bedside. The use of safer needle devices and implementation of education about needle safety may prevent 80% of needlesticks (ANA, 2009). The Needlestick Safety and Prevention Act is a federal law that mandates health care facilities to use safe needle devices to reduce the frequency of needlestick injury. Employers must update their exposure control plans and seek employees' input when evaluating and selecting safer medical devices (OSHA, 2009).

A sharp with engineered sharps injury protection (SESIP) is a device effective in preventing needlesticks. One type of SESIP is a blunt-end cannula (Fig. 23-1, *A*); another is a safety syringe equipped with a plastic guard or sheath that slips over the needle as it is withdrawn from the skin (see Fig. 23-1, *B*). The guard immediately covers the needle, eliminating the chance for a needlestick injury. A variety of other SESIP devices are found in IV line connection systems (see Chapter 28). Box 23-1 lists recommendations for health care workers to use to reduce their risk of needlestick injuries.

Special puncture- and leak-proof containers are available in health care agencies for the disposal of sharps. Containers are made so only one hand needs to be used when disposing of uncapped needles. Keeping the other hand well away from the container prevents accidental injury (Fig. 23-2). Never force a needle into a full needle-disposal receptacle.

EVIDENCE-BASED PRACTICE TRENDS

Cocoman A, Murray J: Intramuscular injection: a review of best practices for mental health nurses, *J Psychiatr Mental Health Nurs* 15(5):424, 2008.

Ramtahal J and others: Sciatic nerve injury following intramuscular injection: a care report and review of the literature, *J Neurosci Nurs* 38(4):238, 2006.

There is more evidence in the literature to address practice guidelines for the administration of IM injections. Site selection in the past was not evidence based, and needle selection

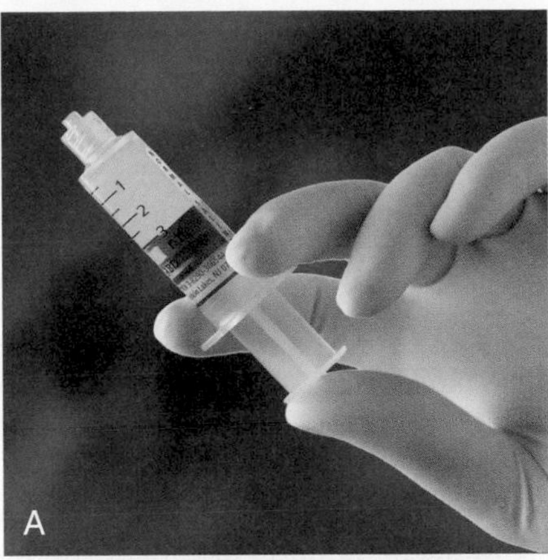

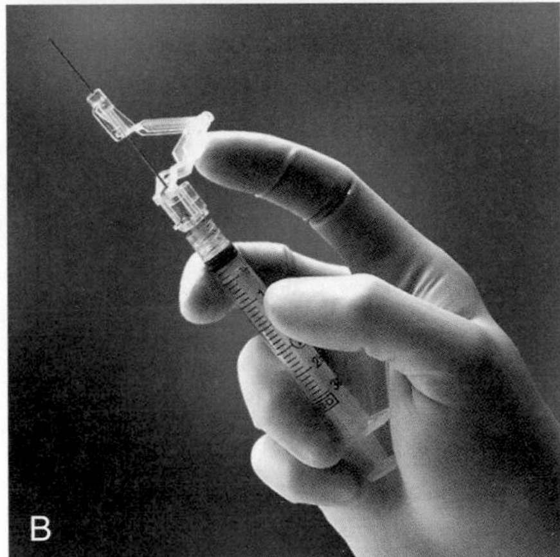

FIG 23-1 Needleless system. **A,** Blunt-end cannula. **B,** Safety syringe with guard.

was based on nursing preference. The literature identified the ventrogluteal site as best suited for IM injection. However, nurses were inconsistent in this practice because of difficulty in anatomically locating the site and their belief that the site was not as safe as the dorsogluteal. The rationale for use of the ventrogluteal site includes more prominent bony landmarks and greater muscle thickness, which reduce the risk of giving an IM injection subcutaneously. Research identifies that injuries such as fibrosis, nerve damage, abscess, and tissue necrosis are associated with all the common IM sites except the ventrogluteal site. There is now enough consensual evidence to develop evidence-based guidelines for administration of IM injections.

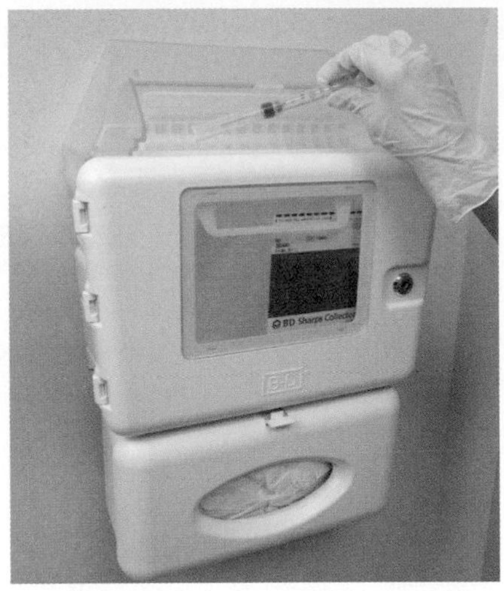

FIG 23-2 Sharps disposal using only one hand.

BOX 23-1 RECOMMENDATIONS FOR THE PREVENTION OF NEEDLESTICK INJURIES

1. Avoid using needles when effective needleless systems or engineered sharps injury protection (SESIP) devices are available.
2. Do not recap needles after medication administration.
3. Plan safe handling and disposal of needles before beginning a procedure that requires the use of a needle.
4. Immediately dispose of used needles, needleless systems, and SESIP into puncture- and leak-proof sharps disposal containers.
5. Maintain a sharps injury log (see agency policy).
6. Attend educational offerings regarding bloodborne pathogens and follow recommendations for infection prevention, including receiving the hepatitis B vaccine.
7. Report all needlestick and sharps-related injuries immediately, according to institutional policies.
8. Participate in the selection and evaluation of SESIP devices with safety features within your place of employment whenever possible.

Data from Occupational Safety and Health Administration (OSHA): *Bloodborne pathogens and needlestick injuries,* 2009, http://www.osha.gov/SLTC/bloodbornepathogens/index.html, accessed August 2009.

SKILL 23.1 PREPARING INJECTIONS: VIALS AND AMPULES

- **Nursing Skills Online: Injections Module, Lessons 1 and 2**

Syringes

Syringes are single use, disposable, and either Luer-Lok or non–Luer-Lok. They are packaged separately, in a paper wrapper or rigid plastic container. Syringes come with or without a sterile needle or with a needleless SESIP device. The parts of a syringe are shown in Fig. 23-3. Non–Luer-Lok syringes use needles or needleless devices that slip onto the tip. Luer-Lok syringes (Fig. 23-4, A) use standard needles or needleless devices that are twisted onto the tip and lock themselves in place. The Luer-Lok design prevents the accidental removal of the needle from the syringe.

Syringes come in a variety of sizes, ranging in capacity from 0.5 to 60 mL (see Fig. 23-4). When you select a syringe, choose the smallest syringe size possible to improve accuracy

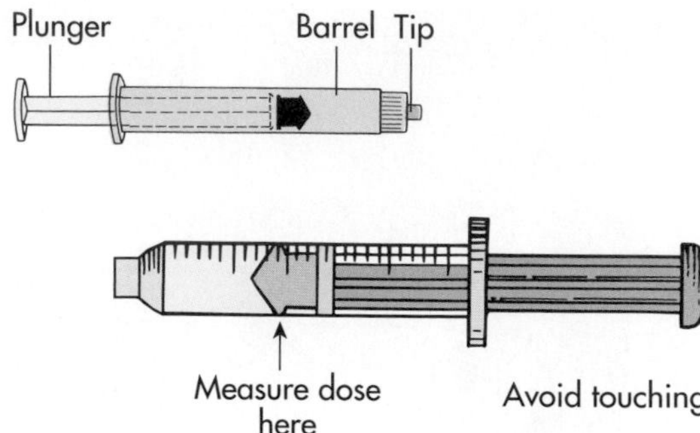

FIG 23-3 Parts of a syringe.

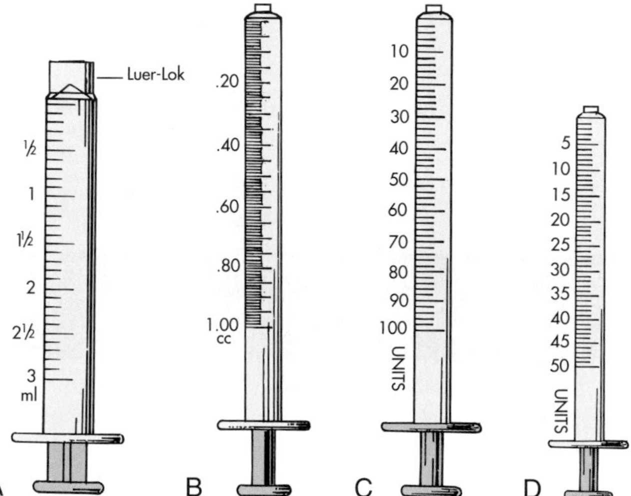

FIG 23-4 Types of syringes. **A,** 3-mL Luer-Lok syringe marked in 0.1 (tenths). **B,** Tuberculin syringe marked in 0.01 (hundredths) for doses of less than 1 mL. **C,** Insulin syringe marked in units (100). **D,** Insulin syringe marked in units (50) for low dose.

of medication preparation. In addition, avoid injecting a large volume of fluid into tissues. It is unusual to use a syringe larger than 5 mL for IM injections. A larger volume creates discomfort. Syringes are most commonly marked in a scale by tenths of a milliliter (see Fig. 23-4, *A*). You use tuberculin (TB) syringes to prepare small amounts of medications. You also use them for ID and subcutaneous injections (see Fig. 23-4, *B*). Insulin syringes (Fig. 23-4, *C* and *D*) hold 0.3 to 1 mL, come with preattached needles, and are calibrated in units. Most insulin syringes are U-100s, designed for use with U-100 strength insulin. Each milliliter of solution contains 100 units of insulin.

Needles

Some needles come attached to syringes. Others come packaged individually to allow flexibility in selecting the right needle for a patient. Needles are disposable, and most are made of stainless steel. A needle has three parts: the hub, which fits onto the tip of the syringe; the shaft, which connects to the hub; and the bevel, or slanted tip (Fig. 23-5). The needle hub, shaft, and bevel must remain sterile at all times. To prevent contamination, using gentle force place the needle onto a syringe with the cap intact.

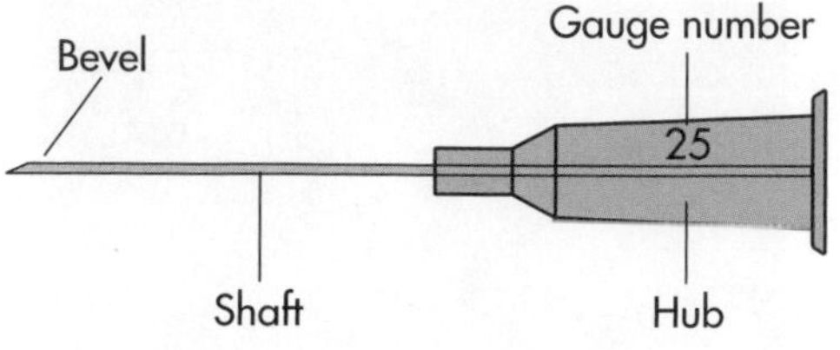

FIG 23-5 Parts of a needle.

The tip of a needle, or the bevel, is always slanted. The bevel creates a narrow slit when injected into tissue that quickly closes as the needle is removed to prevent leakage of medication, blood, or serum. Longer beveled tips are sharper and narrower, which minimizes discomfort from a subcutaneous or IM injection.

Most needles vary in length from $\frac{3}{8}$ to 3 inches. They are color coded for ease of selection. Use longer needles (1 to $1\frac{1}{2}$ inches) for IM injections and shorter needles ($\frac{3}{8}$ to $\frac{5}{8}$ inch) for subcutaneous injections. Choose the needle length according to the patient's size and weight and the type of tissue into which the medication is to be injected. Children and very small, thin adults generally require a shorter needle. The smaller the needle gauge, the larger the needle diameter. The selection of a gauge depends on the viscosity of fluid to be injected. For example, use a larger 22-gauge $1\frac{1}{2}$-inch needle for IM injections. Use a smaller 25-gauge $\frac{5}{8}$-inch needle for subcutaneous injections.

Disposable Injection Units

Single-dose, prefilled, disposable syringes are available for some medications. You do not need to prepare medication doses, except perhaps to expel portions of unneeded medication. However, it is important to check the medication and concentration carefully because prefilled syringes appear very similar. Prefilled unit-dose systems such as Tubex and Carpuject include reusable plastic syringe holders and disposable, prefilled, sterile, glass cartridge units (Fig. 23-6). To assemble, place the cartridge, Luer tip first, into the plastic syringe holder. Following manufacturer's instructions, turn the plunger rod to the left (counterclockwise) and the lock to the right (clockwise) until it "clicks." Finally remove the needle guard and advance the plunger to expel air and excess medication, as with a regular syringe. The cartridge may be used with SESIP needles.

Ampules and Vials

Ampules contain single doses of injectable medication in a liquid form. They are available in several sizes, from 1 to 10 mL or more. An ampule is made of glass with a constricted neck that is snapped off to allow access to the medication (Fig. 23-7, *A*). A colored ring around the neck indicates where the ampule is prescored to be broken easily. Medication is easily withdrawn from the ampule by aspirating the fluid with a filter needle and syringe. Filter needles must be used when preparing medication from a glass ampule to prevent glass particles from being drawn into the syringe (Alexander and others, 2009). *Do not* use a filter needle to administer a medication.

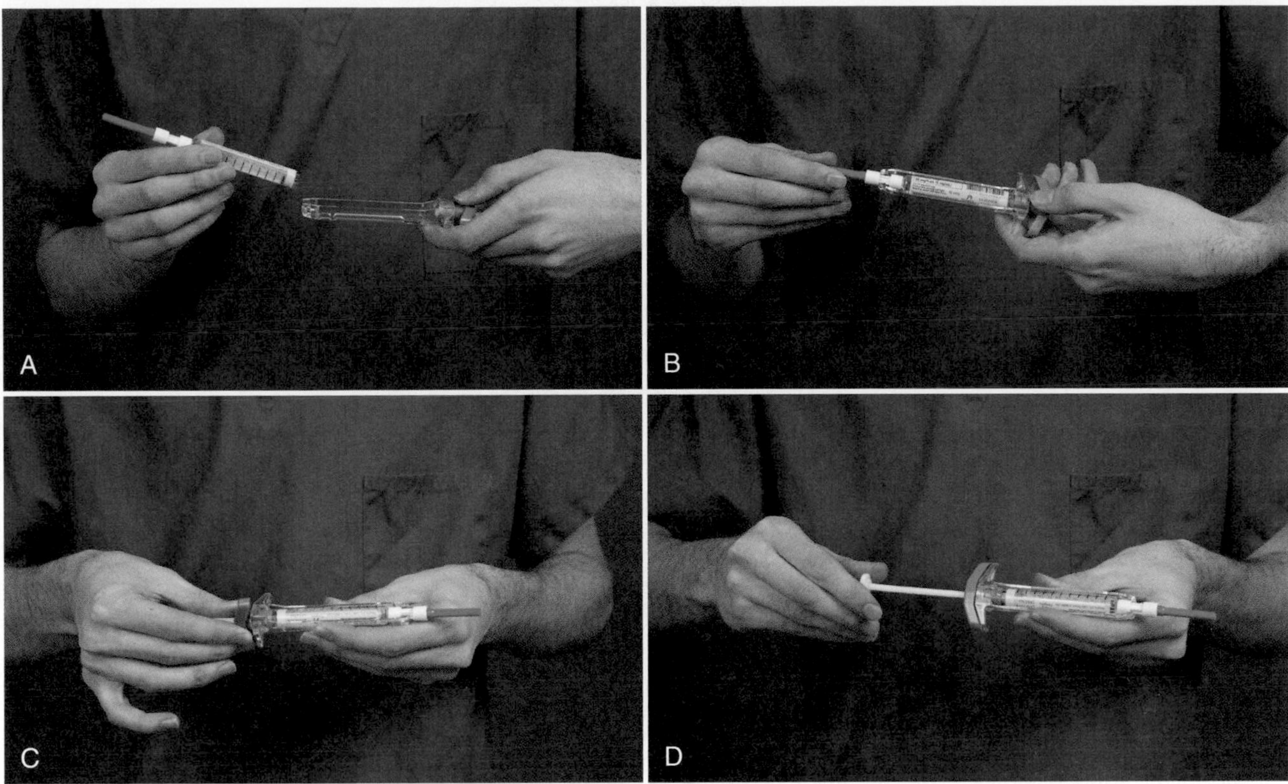

FIG 23-6 A to **D,** Carpuject syringe holder and needleless, prefilled, sterile cartridge.

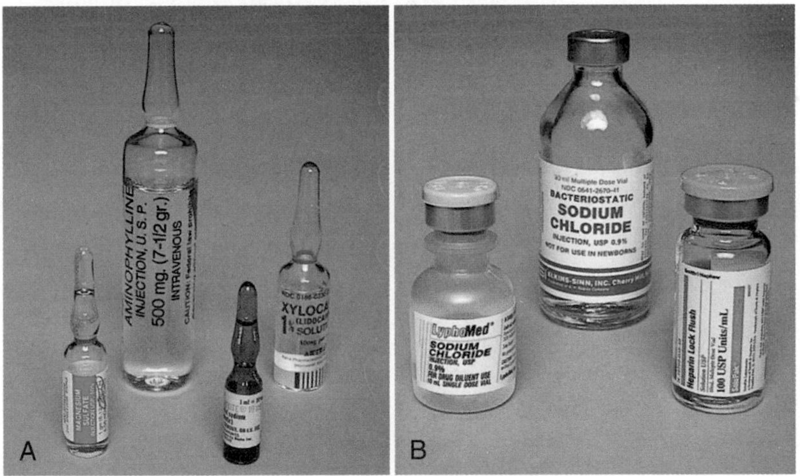

FIG 23-7 A, Medication in ampules. **B,** Medication in vials.

A vial is a single-dose or multidose plastic or glass container with a rubber seal at the top (see Fig. 23-7, *B*). After you open a single-dose vial discard it, regardless of the amount of medication used. A multidose vial contains several doses of medication and can be entered several times. When using a multidose vial, write the date that the vial is opened on the vial label. Verify with the agency how long an opened multidose vial may be used. Vials that exceed the time allowed by agency policy must be properly discarded.

A metal or plastic cap protects a rubber seal of the vial. Remove the cap when you first prepare the vial for use. Vials may contain liquid or dry forms of medications; medications that are unstable in solution are packaged in dry form. The vial label specifies the solvent or diluents used to dissolve the dry medication and the amount needed to prepare a desired medication concentration. Normal saline and distilled water are the most common solutions.

Some vials have two chambers separated by a rubber stopper. One chamber contains the diluent and the other chamber contains the dry medication. Before preparing the medication, push on the upper chamber to dislodge the rubber stopper and allow the powder and the diluent to mix. Unlike an ampule, a vial is a closed system. You must inject air into the vial to permit easy withdrawal of the solution. Some medications, even when in a vial, may need to be drawn up with a filter needle because of the nature of the drug.

Institutional policies and package inserts from the manufacturer indicate drugs that should be prepared with a filter needle.

Occasionally the prescriber orders an injectable medication that must be reconstituted because it comes in a powdered form. This frequently occurs for time-sensitive injectable medication, which must be administered within a specific time period to guarantee full drug effectiveness.

ASSESSMENT

1. Check accuracy and completeness of each MAR or computer printout with prescriber's written medication order. Check patient's name, drug name and dosage, route of administration, and time for administration. Recopy or reprint any portion of the MAR that is difficult to read. *Rationale: The prescriber's order is the most reliable source and only legal record of drugs patient is to receive. Ensures that patient receives the right medications. Handwritten MARs are a source of medication errors (Eisenhauer and others, 2007; Furukawa and others, 2008).*
2. Assess patient's medical and medication history and history of allergies. *Rationale: Determines possible contraindications for medication administration.*
3. Review medication reference information for action, purpose, side effects, and nursing implications. *Rationale: Allows you to administer drug properly and monitor patient's response.*
4. Assess patient's body build, muscle size, and weight if giving subcutaneous or IM medication. *Rationale: Determines type and size of syringe and needles for injection.*

PLANNING

Expected Outcomes focus on safe preparation of medication from ampules and vials.

1. Proper dose is prepared. No air bubbles are in syringe barrel.

Delegation and Collaboration

The skill of preparing injections cannot be delegated to nursing assistive personnel (NAP).

Equipment

Medication in an ampule

- Syringe, needle, and filter needle
- Small sterile gauze pad or unopened alcohol swab

Medication in a vial

- Syringe and two needles
- Needles:
  - Needleless blunt-tip vial-access cannula or needle for drawing up medication (if needed)
  - Filter needle if indicated
- Small sterile gauze pad or alcohol swab
- Diluent (e.g., 0.9% sodium chloride or sterile water if indicated)

Both

- SESIP safety needle for injection
- MAR or computer printout
- Medication in vial or ampule
- Puncture-proof container for disposal of syringes, needles, and glass

IMPLEMENTATION *for* PREPARING INJECTIONS: VIALS AND AMPULES

STEP	RATIONALE
1. See Standard Protocol (inside front cover).	
2. Prepare medications:	
a. If using a medication cart, move it outside patient's room.	Organization of equipment saves time and reduces error.
b. Unlock medicine drawer or cart or log onto computerized medication dispensing system.	Medications are safeguarded when locked in cabinet, cart, or computerized medication dispensing system.
c. Prepare medications for one patient at a time. Keep all pages of MARs or computer printouts for one patient together or look at only one patient's electronic MAR at a time.	Preventing distractions reduces medication preparation errors (LePorte and others, 2009; Wolf, 2007).
d. Select correct drug from stock supply or unit-dose drawer. Compare label of medication with MAR computer printout or computer screen.	Reading label and comparing it with transcribed order reduce errors. *This is the first check for accuracy.*
e. Check expiration date on each medication, one at a time.	Medications used past their expiration date are sometimes inactive, less effective, or harmful to patient.
f. Calculate drug dose as necessary. Double-check calculation. Ask another nurse to check calculations if needed.	Double-checking reduces risk of error.
g. If preparing controlled substance, check record for previous drug count and compare with supply available.	Controlled substance laws require careful monitoring of dispensed narcotics.
h. Do not leave drugs unattended.	Nurse is responsible for safekeeping of drugs.

STEP	RATIONALE
3. ***Prepare ampule.***	
a. Tap top of ampule lightly and quickly with finger until fluid moves from neck of ampule (see illustration).	Dislodges any fluid that collects above neck of ampule. All solution moves into lower chamber.
b. Place small gauze pad or unopened alcohol pad around neck of ampule (see illustration).	Protects fingers from trauma as glass tip is broken off. *Do not use opened alcohol swab to wrap around top of ampule because alcohol may leak into ampule.*
c. Snap neck of ampule quickly and firmly away from hands (see illustration).	Protects nurse's fingers and face from shattering glass.
d. Draw up medication quickly, using a filter needle long enough to reach bottom of ampule to access medication.	System is open to airborne contaminants. Filter needles filter out any fragments of glass (Alexander and others, 2009).
e. Hold ampule upside down or set it on a flat surface. Insert filter needle into center of ampule opening. Do not allow needle tip or shaft to touch rim of ampule.	Broken rim of ampule is considered contaminated. When ampule is inverted, solution dribbles out if needle tip, or shaft touches rim of ampule.
f. Aspirate medication into syringe by gently pulling back on plunger (see illustrations).	Withdrawal of plunger creates negative pressure within syringe barrel, which pulls fluid into syringe.

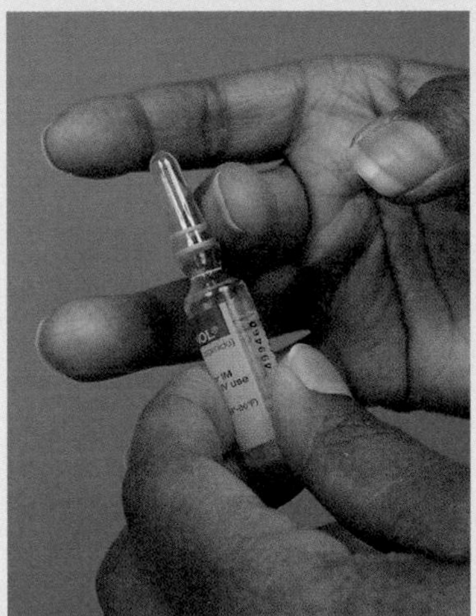

STEP 3a Tapping ampule moves fluid down neck.

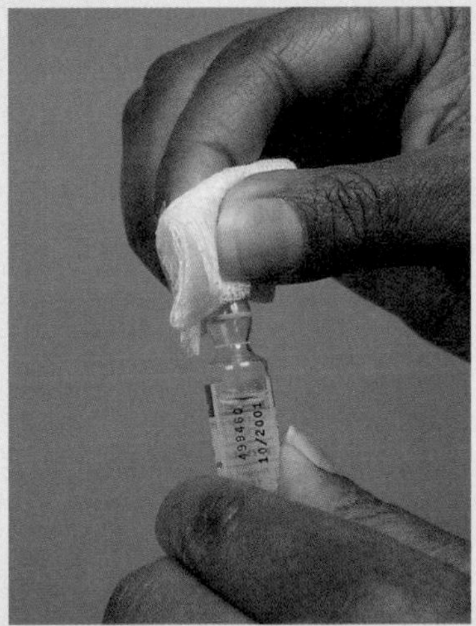

STEP 3b Gauze pad placed around neck of ampule.

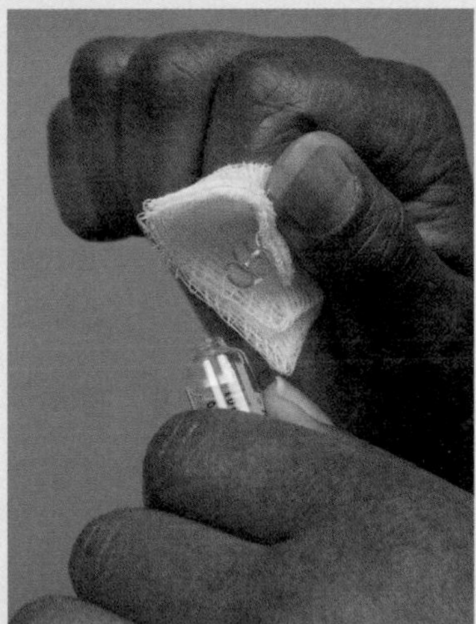

STEP 3c Neck snapped away from hands.

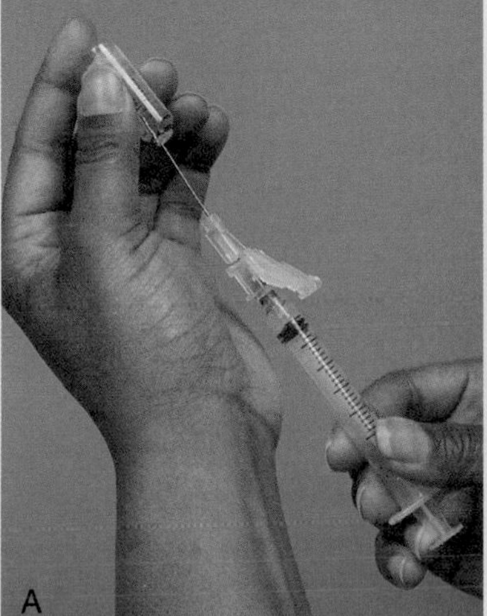

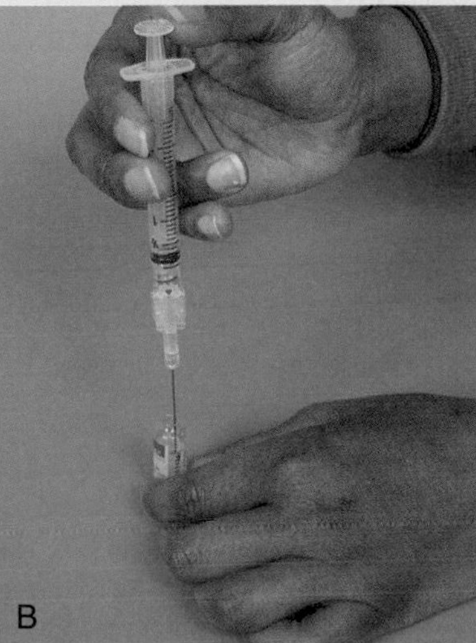

STEP 3f A, Medication aspirated with ampule inverted. **B,** Medication aspirated with ampule on flat surface.

Continued

STEP	RATIONALE
g. Keep needle tip under surface of liquid. Tip ampule to bring all fluid within reach of needle.	Prevents aspiration of air bubbles.
h. If you aspirate air bubbles, do not expel air into ampule.	Air pressure forces fluid out of ampule, and medication will be lost.
i. To expel excess air bubbles, remove needle from ampule. Hold syringe with needle pointing up. Tap side of syringe to cause bubbles to rise toward needle. Draw back slightly on plunger and push plunger upward to eject air. Do not eject fluid.	Withdrawing plunger too far removes it from barrel. Holding syringe vertically allows fluid to settle in bottom of barrel. Pulling back on plunger allows fluid within needle to enter barrel so you do not expel fluid. You then expel air at top of barrel and within needle.
j. If syringe contains excess fluid, use sink for disposal. Hold syringe vertically with needle tip up and slanted slightly toward sink. Slowly eject excess fluid into sink. Recheck fluid level in syringe by holding it vertically.	Safely disperses medication into sink. Position of needle allows you to expel medication without it flowing down needle shaft. Rechecking fluid level ensures proper dose.
k. Cover needle with its safety sheath or cap. Replace filter needle with regular SESIP needle.	Do not use filter needles for injection.
4. *Prepare vial containing a solution.*	
a. Remove cap covering top of unused vial to expose sterile rubber seal. If a multidose vial has been used before, cap is already removed. Firmly and briskly wipe surface of rubber seal with alcohol swab and allow it to dry.	Vial comes packaged with cap that cannot be replaced after seal removal. Not all drug manufacturers guarantee that caps of unused vials are sterile. Swabbing reduces transmission of microorganisms. Allowing alcohol to dry prevents it from coating needle and mixing with medication.
b. Pick up syringe and remove needle cap or cap covering needleless access device (see illustration). Pull back on plunger to draw amount of air into syringe equivalent to volume of medication to be aspirated from vial.	Injecting air into vial prevents buildup of negative pressure in vial when aspirating medication.

SAFETY ALERT Some medications and some agencies require use of filter needle when preparing medications from vials. Check agency policy or medication reference. If you use a filter needle to aspirate medication, you need to change it to a regular SESIP needle of the appropriate size to administer the medication (Alexander and others, 2009).

STEP	RATIONALE
c. With vial on flat surface, insert tip of needleless device or needle through center of rubber seal. Apply pressure to tip of needle during insertion.	Center of seal is thinner and easier to penetrate. Using firm pressure prevents coring of rubber seal, which could enter vial or needle.
d. Inject air into the air space of vial, holding on to plunger. Hold plunger with firm pressure; plunger sometimes is forced backward by air pressure within the vial.	Inject air before aspirating fluid to create vacuum needed to get medication to flow into syringe. Injecting into air space of vial prevents formation of bubbles and inaccurate dose.
e. Invert vial while keeping firm hold on syringe and plunger. Hold vial between thumb and index finger of nondominant hand. Grasp end of syringe barrel and plunger with thumb and forefinger of dominant hand to counteract pressure in vial.	Inverting vial allows fluid to settle in lower half of container. Position of hands prevents forceful movement of plunger and permits easy manipulation of syringe.
f. Keep tip of needle below fluid level.	Prevents aspiration of air.
g. Allow air pressure from vial to fill syringe gradually with medication (see illustration). If necessary, pull back slightly on plunger to obtain correct amount of solution.	Positive pressure within vial forces fluid into syringe.
h. When you obtain desired volume, position needle into air space of vial; tap side of syringe barrel carefully to dislodge any air bubbles. Eject any air remaining at top of syringe into vial.	Forcefully striking barrel while needle is inserted in vial may bend needle. Accumulation of air displaces medication and causes dose errors.

STEP	RATIONALE
i. Remove needleless access device or needle from vial by pulling back on barrel of syringe.	Pulling plunger rather than barrel would cause plunger to separate from barrel, resulting in loss of medication.
j. Hold syringe at eye level at 90-degree angle to ensure correct volume and absence of air bubbles. Remove any remaining air by tapping barrel to dislodge any air bubbles. Draw back slightly on plunger and push plunger upward to eject air. Do not eject fluid. Recheck volume of medication.	Holding syringe vertically allows fluid to settle in bottom of barrel. Pulling back on plunger allows fluid within needle to enter barrel so you do not expel fluid. You then expel air at top of barrel and within needle.
k. If you need to inject medication into patient's tissue, change needle to appropriate gauge and length according to route of medication administration.	Inserting needle through a rubber stopper dulls beveled tip. New needle is sharper and, because no fluid is along shaft, does not track medication through tissues.
l. For multidose vial, make label that includes date of opening vial and your initials.	Ensures that nurses will prepare future doses correctly. You discard some drugs after certain number of days after opening a vial.
5. ***Prepare vial containing a powder (reconstituting medications).***	
a. Remove cap covering vial of powdered medication and cap covering vial of proper diluent. Firmly swab both caps with alcohol swab and allow to dry.	Allowing alcohol to dry prevents it from coating needle and mixing with medication.
b. Draw up volume of desired diluent into syringe following Steps 4b through j.	Prepares diluents for injection into vial containing powdered medication.
c. Insert tip of needleless device or needle through center of rubber seal of vial of powdered medication. Inject diluents into vial. Remove needle.	Diluent begins to dissolve and reconstitute medication.
d. Mix medication thoroughly. Roll in palms. Do not shake.	Ensures proper dispersal of medication throughout solution.
e. Reconstituted medication in vial is ready for you to draw into new syringe. Read label carefully to determine dose after reconstitution.	Once you add diluent, concentration of medication (milligrams/milliliters) determines dose you give. Reading medication label carefully decreases administration errors.
f. Draw up reconstituted medication in syringe. Insert needleless device/needle into vial. Do not add additional air. Then follow Steps 4e to 4j.	Prepares medication for administration.

SAFETY ALERT Some agencies require that you verify dose of certain medications (e.g., insulin and heparin) for accuracy by another nurse. Check guidelines before administering medication.

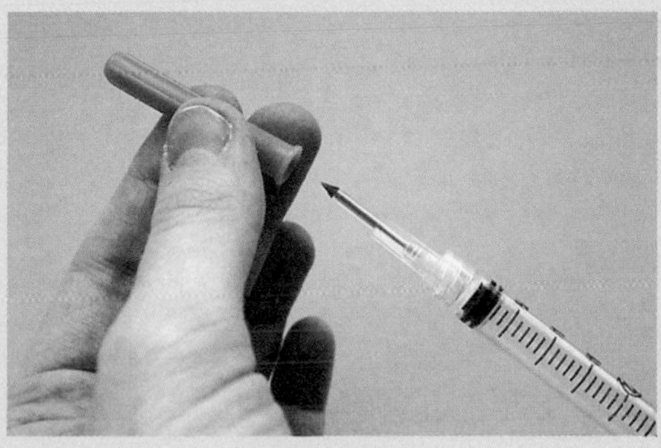

STEP 4b Syringe with needleless access device.

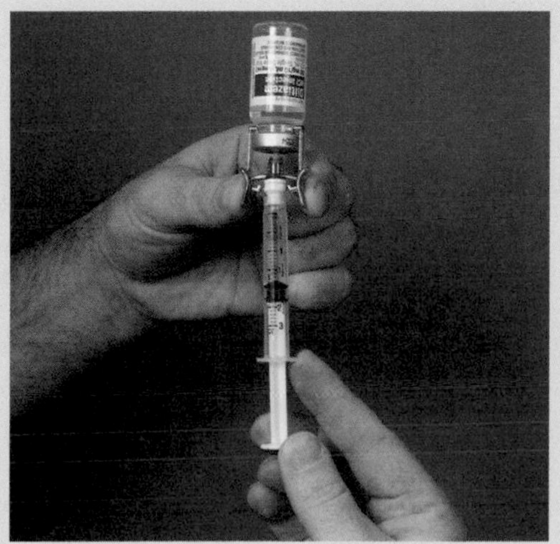

STEP 4g Withdraw fluid with vial inverted.

Continued

STEP	RATIONALE
6. Compare label of medication with MAR, computer screen, or computer printout.	*This is the second check for accuracy.*
7. See Completion Protocol (inside front cover).	
8. *The third check for accuracy occurs at patient's bedside.*	

EVALUATION

1. Compare dose in syringe with desired dose.

Unexpected Outcomes and Related Interventions

1. Air bubbles remain in syringe.
   a. Expel air from syringe and add medication to syringe until you prepare the correct dose.
2. You prepared incorrect dose.
   a. Discard prepared dose and prepare corrected new dose.

PROCEDURAL GUIDELINE 23.1
Mixing Medications in One Syringe

Some medications need to be mixed from two vials or from a vial and an ampule. Mixing compatible medications avoids the need to give a patient more than one injection. Most nursing units have medication compatibility charts, which are in drug reference guides or are posted within patient care areas. If you are uncertain about medication compatibilities, consult a pharmacist. When mixing medications, you must correctly aspirate fluid from each type of container. When using multidose vials, do not contaminate the contents of the vial with medication from another vial or ampule.

When you mix medications from a vial and an ampule, you prepare medications from the vial first. Then you withdraw medication from the ampule using the same syringe and a filter needle. When mixing medications from two vials, do not contaminate one medication with another, ensure that the final dose is accurate, and maintain aseptic technique.

Give special consideration to the proper preparation of insulin, which comes in vials. Insulin is the hormone used to treat diabetes mellitus. Insulin is classified by rate of action, including short acting, intermediate, and long acting. Often patients with diabetes mellitus receive a combination of different types of insulin to control their blood glucose levels. Before preparing insulin, gently roll all cloudy insulin preparations (Humulin-N) between palms of the hands to resuspend the insulin (Aschenbrenner and Venable, 2009). Do not shake insulin vials. Shaking causes bubbles that take up space in a syringe and alter the dose.

If more than one type of insulin is required to manage the patient's diabetes, you can mix them in one syringe if they are compatible. Always prepare the short- or rapid-acting insulin first to prevent it from becoming contaminated with the longer-acting insulin (Aschenbrenner and Venable, 2009). In some settings insulin is not mixed. Box 23-2 lists recommendations for mixing insulins.

BOX 23-2 RECOMMENDATIONS FOR MIXING INSULINS

Use the following principles when mixing insulins (ADA, 2004; Novo Nordisk, 2008):

- Patients who are well controlled on a particular mixed-insulin regimen should maintain their standard procedure for preparing their insulin doses.
- No other medication or diluent should be mixed with any insulin product unless approved by the prescribing physician.
- Do not mix insulin glargine with other forms of insulin because of the low pH of its diluent.
- Use commercially available premixed insulins only if the insulin ratio is appropriate to the patient's insulin requirements.
- When currently available NPH and short-acting insulin formulations are mixed, they may be used immediately or stored for future use.
- Rapid-acting insulin can be mixed with NPH, Lente, and Ultralente.
- When rapid-acting insulin is mixed with either an intermediate- or a long-acting insulin, the mixture should be injected within 15 minutes before a meal.
- Mixing short-acting and Lente insulins is not recommended except for patients already adequately controlled on such a mixture. If short-acting and Lente mixtures are to be used, the patient should standardize the interval between mixing and injection.
- Phosphate-buffered insulins (e.g., NPH) should not be mixed with Lente insulins.
- Insulin formulations may change; consult the manufacturer in cases in which its recommendations appear to conflict with the American Diabetes Association guidelines.

PROCEDURAL GUIDELINE 23.1
Mixing Medications in One Syringe—cont'd

Delegation and Collaboration

The skill of mixing medications in one syringe cannot be delegated to nursing assistive personnel (NAP).

Equipment

- Single-dose or multidose vials and ampules containing medication
- Syringe and two needles
- Needles:
  - Needleless blunt-tip vial-access cannula or needle for drawing up medication
  - Filter needle if indicated
  - SESIP needle for injection
- Alcohol swab
- Puncture-proof container for disposing of syringes, needles, and glass
- Medication administration record (MAR) or computer printout
- Medication in vial or ampule

Procedural Steps

1. **See Standard Protocol (inside front cover).**
2. Check accuracy and completeness of the MAR or computer printout with prescriber's written medication order. Check patient's name, medication name and dosage, route of administration, and time of administration. Recopy or reprint any portion of MAR that is difficult to read.
3. Review pertinent information related to medication including action, purpose, side effects, and nursing implications.
4. Assess patient's muscle size and weight if giving subcutaneous or intramuscular injections.
5. Consider compatibility of medications to be mixed and type of injection.
6. Check medication's expiration date printed on vial or ampule.
7. Perform hand hygiene.
8. Prepare medication for one patient at a time following the six rights of medication administration (see Chapter 21). Select an ampule or a vial from the unit-dose drawer or automated dispensing system. Compare the label of the medication with the MAR or computer printout. *This is the first check for accuracy.*
9. ***Mixing medications from two vials:***
   a. Take syringe with needleless access device or filter needle and aspirate volume of air equivalent to first medication dose (vial A).
   b. Inject air into vial A, making sure that needleless device or needle does not touch solution (see illustration).
   c. Holding on to plunger, withdraw needleless device or needle and syringe from vial A. Aspirate air equivalent to second medication dose (vial B) into syringe.
   d. Insert needleless device or needle into vial B, inject volume of air into vial B, and withdraw medication from vial B into syringe (see illustration).
   e. Withdraw needleless device or needle and syringe from vial B. Ensure that proper volume has been obtained.
   f. Determine on syringe scale what the combined volume of medications should measure.

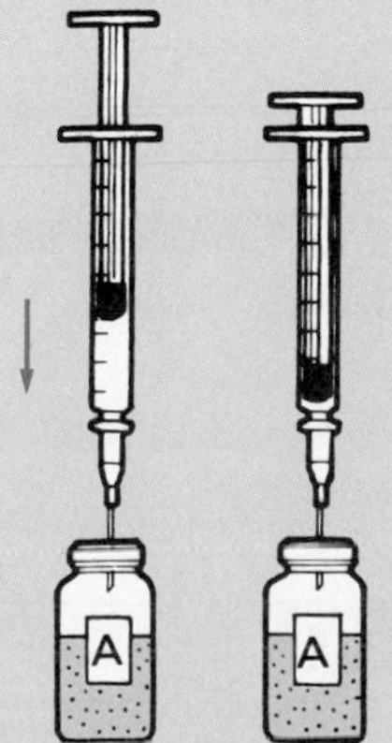

STEP 9b Injecting air into vial A.

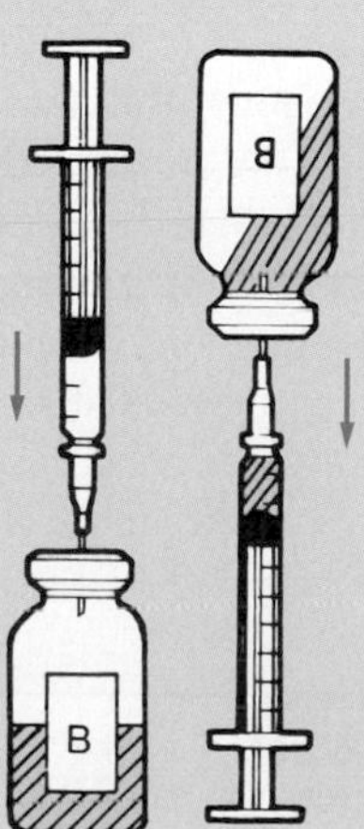

STEP 9d Injecting air into vial B and withdrawing dose.

Continued

PROCEDURAL GUIDELINE 23.1
Mixing Medications in One Syringe—cont'd

g. Insert needleless device or needle into vial A, being careful not to push plunger and expel medication within syringe into vial. Invert vial and carefully withdraw the desired amount of medication from vial A into syringe (see illustration).

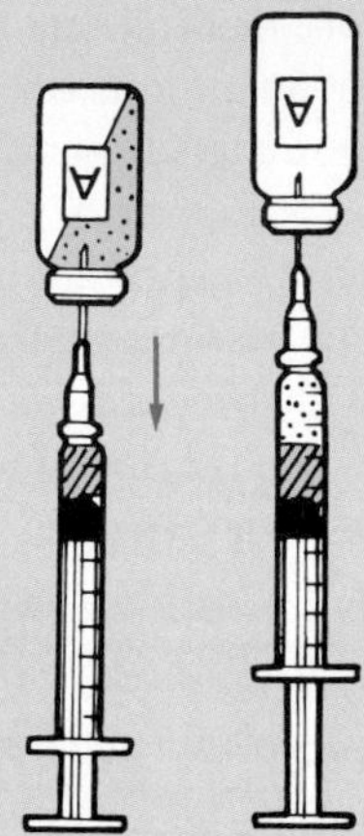

STEP 9g Withdrawing medication from vial A.

h. Withdraw needleless device or needle and expel any excess air from syringe. Check fluid level in syringe. Medications are now mixed.

> **SAFETY ALERT** If too much medication is withdrawn from second vial, discard syringe and start over. Do not push medication back into either vial.

i. Change needleless device or filter needle for appropriate-size needle if medication is being injected. Keep new needleless device or needle capped until administration time.

10. *Mixing insulin:*
   a. If patient takes insulin that is cloudy, roll the bottle of insulin gently between the hands to resuspend the insulin preparation.
   b. Wipe off tops of both insulin vials with alcohol swab.
   c. Verify insulin dose against MAR.
   d. If mixing rapid- or short-acting insulin with intermediate- or long-acting insulin, take insulin syringe and aspirate volume of air equivalent to dose to be withdrawn from intermediate- or long-acting insulin first. If two intermediate- or long-acting insulins are mixed, it makes no difference which vial is prepared first.

> **SAFETY ALERT** If long-acting insulin glargine (Lantus) is ordered, note this is a clear insulin that should not be mixed with another insulin.

   e. Insert needle and inject air into vial of intermediate- or long-acting insulin. Do not let the tip of the needle touch solution.
   f. Remove syringe from vial of insulin without aspirating medication.
   g. With the same syringe, inject air equal to the dose of rapid- or short-acting insulin into the vial and withdraw the correct dose into the syringe.
   h. Remove the syringe from the rapid- or short-acting insulin and remove any air bubbles to ensure accurate dose.

> **SAFETY ALERT** Some institutions require the dose of clear insulin verified before proceeding with mixing of insulin. Then have dose verified a second time after the medications are mixed.

   i. *Verify* insulin doses with MAR, show insulin prepared in syringe to another nurse to verify that correct dose of insulin was prepared. Then determine which point on syringe scale the combined units of insulin should measure by adding the number of units of both insulin together (e.g., 4 units regular + 10 units NPH = 14 units total).
   j. Place the needle of the syringe back into the vial of intermediate- or long-acting insulin. Be careful not to push plunger and inject insulin in syringe into the vial.
   k. Invert the vial and carefully withdraw the desired amount of insulin into syringe.
   l. Withdraw needle and check fluid level in syringe. Keep needle of prepared syringe sheathed or capped until ready to administer medication.

> **SAFETY ALERT** Administer mixture of insulin within 5 minutes of preparation. Rapid- or short-acting insulin can bind with intermediate- or long-acting insulin, thus reducing the action of the more rapid-acting insulin (ADA, 2007).

11. *Mixing medications from a vial and an ampule:*
   a. Prepare medication from vial first, following Skill 23.1, Step 4.
   b. Determine on syringe scale what the combined volume of medications should measure.

> **SAFETY ALERT** If needleless access device was used in preparing medication from vial, change needleless system to filter needle.

PROCEDURAL GUIDELINE 23.1
Mixing Medications in One Syringe—cont'd

c. Next, using same syringe, prepare medication from ampule following Step 3 in Skill 23.1.
d. Withdraw filter needle from ampule and verify fluid level in syringe. Change filter needle to appropriate SESIP needle. Keep device or needle sheathed or capped until administering medication.
e. Check syringe carefully for total combined dose of medications.

12. Compare MAR, computer printout, or screen with prepared medication and labels on vials/ampules. *This is the second check for accuracy.*
13. **See Completion Protocol (inside front cover).**
14. Check syringe again carefully for total combined dose of medication.
15. *The third check for accuracy occurs at patient's bedside.*

SKILL 23.2 ADMINISTERING SUBCUTANEOUS INJECTIONS

- **Nursing Skills Online: Injections Module, Lesson 3**
- *Video Clips*

Subcutaneous injections involve depositing medication into the loose connective tissue underlying the dermis. Because subcutaneous tissue does not contain as many blood vessels as muscles, medications are absorbed more slowly than IM injections. Physical exercise or application of hot or cold compresses influences the rate of drug absorption by altering local blood flow to tissues. Any condition that impairs blood flow is a contraindication for subcutaneous injections.

You give subcutaneous medications in small doses of 0.5 to 1 mL that are isotonic, nonirritating, nonviscous, and water soluble. Examples of subcutaneous medications include epinephrine, insulin, allergy medications, opioids, and heparin. Because subcutaneous tissue contains pain receptors, the patient often experiences some discomfort.

The best subcutaneous injection sites include the outer aspect of the upper arms, the abdomen from below the costal margins to the iliac crests, and the anterior aspects of the thighs (Fig. 23-8). These areas are easily accessible and are large enough to rotate multiple injections within each anatomical location.

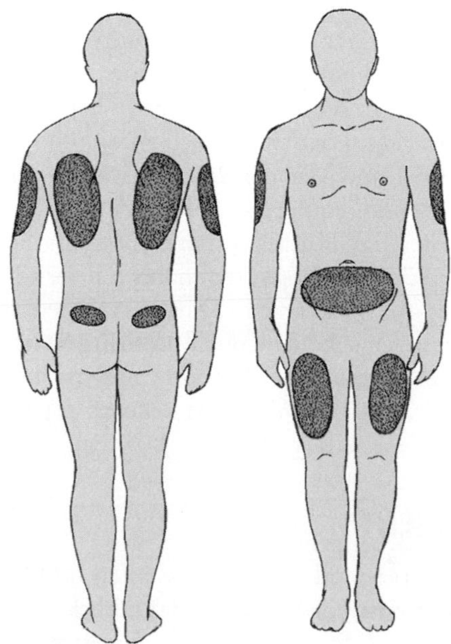

FIG 23-8 Sites recommended for subcutaneous injections.

Choose an injection site that is free of skin lesions, bony prominences, and large underlying muscles or nerves. Site rotation prevents the formation of lipohypertrophy or lipoatrophy in the skin. The patient's body weight and amount of adipose tissue indicate the depth of the subcutaneous layer. Therefore base the needle length and angle of needle insertion on the patient's weight and an estimate of subcutaneous tissue. Generally a 25-gauge ⅝-inch needle inserted at a 45- to 90-degree angle (Fig. 23-9) or a ½-inch needle inserted at a 90-degree angle deposits medications into the subcutaneous tissue of a normal-size patient. A child usually requires a 26- to 30-gauge ½-inch needle inserted at a 90-degree angle (Hockenberry and Wilson, 2009). Hunter (2008b) suggests that, to ensure that a medication reaches subcutaneous tissue, insert the needle at a 90-degree angle. If the patient is obese, pinch the tissue and use a needle long enough to insert through the fatty tissue at the base of the skin fold. Thin patients sometimes have insufficient tissue for subcutaneous injections. Therefore the upper abdomen is the best injection site for patients with little peripheral subcutaneous tissue. Special consideration needs to be given to obese or cachectic patients. Aspiration after a subcutaneous injection, including

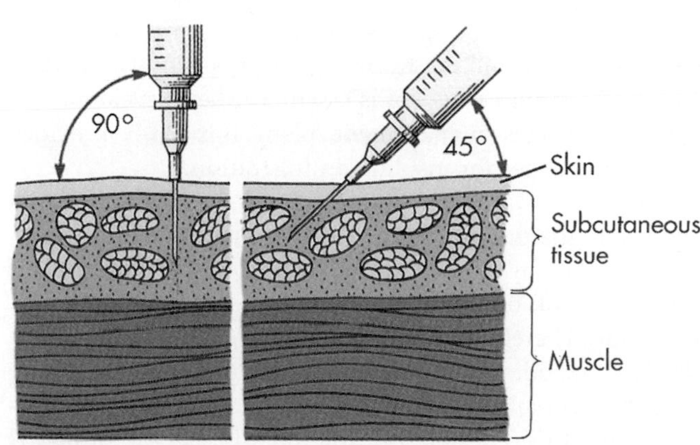

FIG 23-9 Subcutaneous injection. Angle and needle length depend on thickness of skin fold.

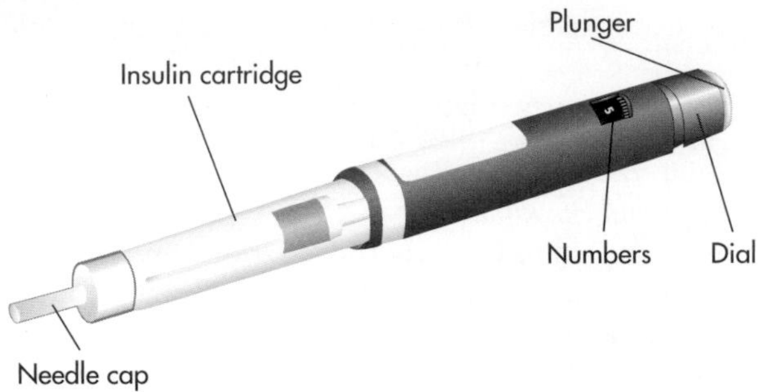

FIG 23-10 Insulin injection pen.

heparin and insulin, is not necessary. Piercing a blood vessel and causing a hematoma formation are rare (ADA, 2007; Hunter, 2008b).

Injection pens are a new technology that patients can use to self-administer medications (e.g., epinephrine, insulin, interferon) subcutaneously (Fig. 23-10). They offer a convenient delivery method using prefilled, disposable cartridges. The patient pinches his or her skin, inserts the needle, releases the skin, and injects a predetermined medication dose. Teaching is essential to ensure that patients use the correct injection technique and deliver the correct dose of medication. The disadvantages to this technology include increased risk of needlestick injury, lack of knowledge and skill concerning administration technique, and inappropriate storage of device (Aschenbrenner, 2009; Shih-Wen, 2007).

Special Considerations for Administration of Insulin

Most patients manage type I diabetes mellitus with injections. Anatomical injection site rotation is no longer necessary because newer human insulins carry a lower risk for hypertrophy. Patients choose one anatomical area (e.g., the abdomen) and systematically rotate sites within that region, which maintains consistent insulin absorption from day to day. Absorption rates of insulin vary based on the injection site. Insulin is most quickly absorbed in the abdomen, followed by the arms, thighs, and buttocks (Aschenbrenner, 2009).

The timing of injections is critical to correct insulin administration. When health care providers plan insulin injection times, blood glucose levels are used to determine when the patient will eat. Knowing the peak action and duration of the insulin protocol is essential when developing an effective diabetes management plan. Box 23-3 provides general guidelines for insulin administration.

Special Considerations for Administration of Heparin

Heparin therapy provides therapeutic anticoagulation to reduce the risk of thrombus formation by suppressing clot formation. Therefore patients receiving heparin are at risk for bleeding, including bleeding gums, hematemesis, hematuria, or melena. Results from coagulation blood tests (e.g., activated partial thromboplastin time [aPTT], partial thromboplastin time [PTT]) allow you to monitor the desired therapeutic range for heparin therapy.

BOX 23-3 GENERAL GUIDELINES FOR INSULIN ADMINISTRATION

- Store vials in the refrigerator. Keep vials currently being used at room temperature. Do not inject cold insulin.
- Inspect vials before each use for changes in appearance (e.g., clumping, frosting, precipitation, change in clarity or color), indicating lack of potency.
- The usual recommended interval between injection of short-acting insulin and a meal is 30 minutes.
- Have patient self-administer insulin whenever possible. Generally children begin self-administration by adolescence.
- Patients who take insulin need to self-monitor their blood glucose.
- All patients who take insulin should carry at least 15 g of carbohydrate (e.g., 4 ounces of fruit juice, 4 ounces of regular soft drink, 8 ounces of skim milk, 6 to 10 hard candies) in the event of a hypoglycemic reaction.

Adapted from American Diabetes Association: *American Diabetes Care 27*: 5106-5109, 2004.

Before administering heparin, know the preexisting conditions that contraindicate its use, including cerebral or aortic aneurysm, cerebrovascular hemorrhage, severe hypertension, and blood dyscrasias. In addition, assess for conditions in which increased risk of hemorrhage is present: recent childbirth, severe diabetes and renal disease, liver disease, severe trauma, and active ulcers or lesions of the gastrointestinal (GI), genitourinary (GU), or respiratory tract. Assess the patient's current medication regimen, including use of over-the-counter (OTC) and herbal medications (e.g., garlic, ginger, ginkgo, horse chestnut, or feverfew), for possible interaction with heparin. Other medications that interact with heparin include aspirin, nonsteroidal antiinflammatory drugs (NSAIDs), cephalosporins, antithyroid agents, probenecid, and thrombolytics.

You administer heparin subcutaneously or intravenously. Low-molecular-weight (LMW) heparins (e.g., enoxaparin [Lovenox]) are more effective than heparin in some patients. The anticoagulant effects are more predictable (Aschenbrenner and Venable, 2009). LMW heparins have a longer half-life and require less laboratory monitoring but are expensive. These medications often come from the manufacturer in a prepared syringe (see manufacturer's guidelines). To minimize the pain and bruising associated with LMW heparin, it is given subcutaneously on the right or left side of the abdomen at least 5 cm (2 inches) away from the umbilicus; this area is commonly referred to as a patient's "love handles."

ASSESSMENT

1. Check accuracy and completeness of each MAR with prescriber's original medication order. Check patient's name, drug name and dosage, route of administration, and time for administration. Recopy or reprint any portion of

printed MAR that is difficult to read. *Rationale: The prescriber's order is the most reliable source and only legal record of drugs patient is to receive. Ensures that patient receives the right medications. Handwritten MARs are a source of medication errors (Eisenhauer and others, 2007; Furukawa and others, 2008).*

2. Assess patient's medical and medication history. *Rationale: Identifies need for medication.*
3. Review medication reference information for medication action, purpose, side effects, normal dose, rate of administration, time of peak onset, and nursing implications. *Rationale: Knowledge allows you to give medication safely and monitor patient's response to therapy.*
4. Assess patient's history of allergies; known type of allergens, and normal allergic reaction. *Rationale: Certain substances have similar compositions; it may harm patients to give a medication if there is a known allergy.*
5. Observe patient's previous verbal and nonverbal responses toward injection. *Rationale: Anticipating patient's anxiety allows you to use distraction to reduce pain awareness.*
6. Assess for contraindication to subcutaneous injections, such as circulatory shock or reduced local tissue perfusion. *Rationale: Reduced tissue perfusion interferes with drug absorption and distribution.*
7. Assess patient's symptoms before initiating medication therapy. *Rationale: Provides information to evaluate desired effect of the medication.*
8. Assess adequacy of patient's adipose tissue. *Rationale: The amount of adipose tissue influences methods for administering injections.*
9. Assess patient's knowledge of medication.

PLANNING

Expected Outcomes focus on safe administration of subcutaneous injections.

1. Patient experiences no pain or mild burning at injection site.
2. Patient achieves desired effect of medication with no signs of allergies or undesired effects.
3. Patient explains purpose, dosage, and effects of medication.

Delegation and Collaboration

The skill of administering subcutaneous injections cannot be delegated to nursing assistive personnel (NAP). Instruct the NAP about the following:

- Potential medication side effects and reporting their occurrence to the nurse
- Reporting any change in the patient's condition to the nurse

Equipment

- Proper-size syringe and SESIP needle:
  - Subcutaneous: syringe (1 to 3 mL) and needle (25 to 27 gauge, $\frac{3}{8}$ to $\frac{5}{8}$ inch)
  - Subcutaneous U-100 insulin: insulin syringe (1 mL) with preattached needle (28 to 31 gauge, $\frac{5}{16}$ to $\frac{1}{2}$ inch)
  - Subcutaneous U-500 insulin: 1 mL TB syringe with needle (25 to 27 gauge, $\frac{1}{2}$ to $\frac{5}{8}$ inch)
- Small gauze pad (optional)
- Alcohol swab
- Medication vial or ampule
- Clean gloves
- Medication administration record (MAR) or computer printout
- Puncture-proof container

IMPLEMENTATION *for* ADMINISTERING SUBCUTANEOUS INJECTIONS

STEP	RATIONALE
1. Perform hand hygiene and prepare medication using aseptic technique (see Skill 23.1). Check label of medication carefully with MAR two times while preparing medication.	Ensures that medication is sterile. *First and second checks for accuracy* ensure that the correct medication is administered.
2. Take medications to patient at correct time, within 30 minutes before or after prescribed time (see agency policy). Give stat and single-order medications at the exact time ordered.	Ensures intended therapeutic effect. Giving stat medications immediately or single-order medications at time ordered decreases transfer of microorganisms.
3. **See Standard Protocol (inside front cover).**	
4. Identify patient using two identifiers (e.g., name and birthday or name and account number, according to facility policy). Compare identifiers with information on patient's MAR or medical record.	Ensures correct patient. Complies with The Joint Commission standards and improves patient safety (TJC, 2010).
5. At the bedside again compare the MAR or computer printout with the names of medications on the medication labels. Ask patient if he or she has allergies.	*This is the third check for accuracy* and ensures that patient receives correct medication. Confirms patient's allergy history.

Continued

STEP	RATIONALE
6. Discuss the purpose of each medication, action, and possible adverse effects. Allow patient to ask any questions. Tell patient that injection will cause a slight burning or sting.	Patient has the right to be informed, and patient's understanding of each medication improves adherence with drug therapy. Helps minimize patient's anxiety.
7. Keep sheet or gown draped over body parts not requiring exposure.	Respects dignity of patient while exposing injection area.
8. Select appropriate injection site. Inspect skin surface over sites for bruises, inflammation, or edema. Do not use an area that is bruised or has signs associated with infection.	Injection sites are free of abnormalities that interfere with drug absorption. Sites used repeatedly become hardened from lipohypertrophy (increased growth in fatty tissue).
9. Palpate sites and avoid those with masses or tenderness. Rotate insulin sites within an anatomic area (e.g., the abdomen) and systematically rotate sites within that area. Be sure that needle is correct size by grasping skin fold at site with thumb and forefinger. Measure fold from top to bottom. Make sure that needle is one-half length of fold.	You can mistakenly give subcutaneous injections in the muscle, especially in the abdomen and thigh sites. Appropriate size of needle ensures that you inject the medication in the subcutaneous tissue (Hunter, 2008b). Rotating injection sites within the same anatomical area maintains consistency in day-to-day insulin absorption (Aschenbrenner and Venable, 2009).
a. When administering insulin or heparin, use abdominal, arm, or thigh injection sites.	Risk for bruising is not affected by site (Aschenbrenner and Venable, 2009).
b. When administering LMW heparin subcutaneously, choose a site on the right or left side of the abdomen at least 5 cm (2 inches) away from the umbilicus.	Injecting LMW heparin on the side of the abdomen helps decrease pain and bruising at the injection site (Sanofi-Aventis, 2010).
10. Assist patient into comfortable position. Have patient relax arm, leg, or abdomen, depending on site selection.	Relaxation of site minimizes discomfort.
11. Relocate site using anatomical landmarks.	Injection into correct anatomical site prevents injury to nerves, bone, and blood vessels.
12. Cleanse site with antiseptic swab. Apply swab at center of site and rotate outward in circular direction for about 5 cm (2 inches) (see illustration).	Removes secretions containing microorganisms.
13. Hold swab or gauze between third and fourth fingers of nondominant hand.	
14. Remove needle cap or protective sheath by pulling it straight off.	Preventing needle from touching sides of cap prevents contamination.
15. Hold syringe between thumb and forefinger of dominant hand; hold as dart, palm down (see illustration).	Quick, smooth injection requires proper manipulation of syringe parts.

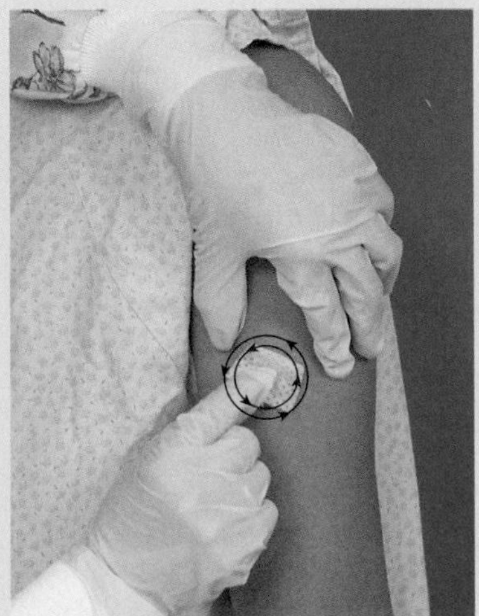
STEP 12 Cleansing site with circular motion.

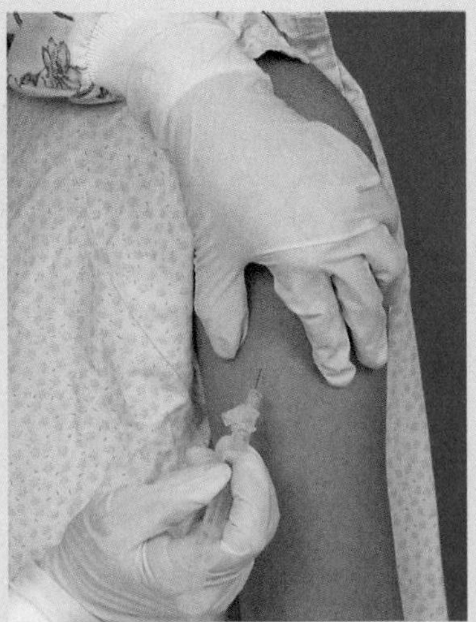
STEP 15 Holding syringe as if grasping a dart.

STEP	RATIONALE
16. Administer injection:	
a. For average-size patient, hold skin across injection site or pinch skin with nondominant hand.	Needle penetrates tight skin more easily than loose skin. Pinching skin elevates subcutaneous tissue and desensitizes area.
b. Inject needle quickly and firmly at 45- to 90-degree angle. Release skin if pinched. *Option:* When using injection pen or giving heparin, continue to pinch skin while injecting medication.	Quick, firm insertion minimizes discomfort. (Injecting medication into compressed tissue irritates nerve fibers.) Correct angle prevents accidental injection into muscle.
c. For obese patient pinch skin at site and inject needle at 90-degree angle below tissue fold.	Obese patients have fatty layer of tissue above subcutaneous layer (Zaybak and others, 2007).
d. After needle enters site, grasp lower end of syringe barrel with nondominant hand to stabilize it. Move dominant hand to end of plunger and slowly inject medication over several seconds (Hunter, 2008b). Avoid moving syringe.	Movement of syringe may displace needle and cause discomfort. Slow injection of medication minimizes discomfort.

SAFETY ALERT Aspiration after injecting a subcutaneous medication is **not necessary.** Piercing a blood vessel in subcutaneous tissue is very rare (Hunter, 2008b). Aspiration after injecting heparin is not recommended (Aschenbrenner and Venable, 2009).

STEP	RATIONALE
e. Withdraw needle quickly while placing antiseptic swab or gauze gently over site.	Supporting tissues around injection site reduces discomfort. Dry gauze may minimize patient discomfort associated with alcohol on nonintact skin.
17. Apply gentle pressure to site. Do not massage site. (If heparin is given, hold alcohol swab or gauze to site for 30 to 60 seconds.)	Aids absorption. Massage can damage underlying tissue. Time interval prevents bleeding at site.
18. Discard uncapped needle or needle enclosed in safety shield (see Fig. 23-1, *B*) and attached syringe into a puncture- and leak-proof receptacle.	Prevents injury to patients and health care personnel. Recapping needles increases risk for a needlestick injury (OSHA, 2009).
19. See Completion Protocol (inside front cover).	
20. Stay with patient for several minutes and observe for any allergic reactions.	Dyspnea, wheezing, and circulatory collapse are signs of severe anaphylactic reaction.

EVALUATION

1. Return to room in 15 to 30 minutes and ask if patient feels any acute pain, burning, numbness, or tingling at injection site.
2. Inspect site, noting bruising or induration.
3. Observe patient's response to medication at times that correlate with onset, peak, and duration of medication.
4. Ask patient to explain purpose and effects of medication.

Unexpected Outcomes and Related Interventions

1. Patient complains of localized pain, numbness, tingling, or burning at injection site.
   a. Assess injection site; may indicate potential injury to nerve or tissues.
   b. Notify patient's health care provider.
   c. Do not reuse site.
2. Patient displays adverse reaction with signs of urticaria, eczema, pruritus, wheezing, and dyspnea.
   a. Monitor patient's heart rate, respirations, blood pressure, and temperature.
   b. Follow agency policy for appropriate response to allergic reactions, (e.g., administration of antihistamine or epinephrine) and notify patient's health care provider immediately.
   c. Add allergy information to patient's record.
3. Hypertrophy of skin develops from repeated subcutaneous injection.
   a. Do not use site for future injections.
   b. Instruct patient not to use site for 6 months.

Recording and Reporting

- Record drug, dose, route, site, time, and date given on MAR immediately after administration, not before. Include initials or signature.
- Record patient teaching, validation of understanding, and patient's response to medication in nurses' notes.
- Report any undesirable effects from medication to patient's health care provider and document adverse effects in record.

Sample Documentation

0730 Patient's blood glucose 320 mg/dL; 8 units Humalog insulin administered subcutaneously in RLQ of abdomen.

0800 Patient complaining of dizziness and sweating; physician notified.

Special Considerations

Pediatric

- Administer only amounts up to 0.5 mL subcutaneously to small children (Hockenberry and Wilson, 2009).
- Children can be anxious or afraid of needles. Assistance with properly positioning and holding the child is sometimes necessary. Distraction such as blowing bubbles and pressure at the injection site before giving the injection helps reduce the child's anxiety (Schechter and others, 2007).

Geriatric

- Aging patients have less elastic skin and reduced subcutaneous skin fold thickness. The upper abdominal site is the best site to use when patient has little subcutaneous tissue.

Home Care

- Improper disposal of used needles and sharps in the home setting poses a health risk to the public and waste workers. Several options for safe sharps disposal at home exist, including, allowing patients to transport their own sharps containers from home to collection sites (e.g., doctor's office, a hospital, or a pharmacy); mailing their used syringes to a collection site (mail-back programs); syringe exchange programs; or special devices that destroy the needle on the syringe, rendering it safe for disposal. If the patient cannot implement any of these options, have him or her dispose of needles and other sharps in a hard plastic or metal container with a tightly sealed lid (e.g., empty detergent bottle or coffee can). Pamphlets for safe home disposal of sharps are on the Environmental Protection Agency (EPA) website (2004).
- Most insulin preparations have bacteriostatic properties that inhibit bacterial growth on the skin. Therefore patients with diabetes may reuse their syringes at home if they can safely recap their needles. Syringes should be discarded when the needles become dull or bent or contact any surface other than the skin. Wiping the needle off with alcohol is not recommended because the silicon coating on the needle is removed, making injections more painful. Patients with poor personal hygiene, acute illness, or open hand wounds or immunocompromised patients should not reuse syringes (ADA, 2007).
- Teach injection techniques to patient and family caregiver that minimize patient discomfort.

SKILL 23.3 ADMINISTERING INTRAMUSCULAR INJECTIONS

- **Nursing Skills Online: Injections Module, Lesson 5**

Video Clips

The IM injection route deposits medication into deep muscle tissue, which has a rich blood supply, allowing medication to absorb faster than the subcutaneous route. However, there is an increased risk of injecting drugs directly into blood vessels. Any factor that interferes with local tissue blood flow affects the rate and extent of drug absorption.

An IM injection requires a longer and larger-gauge needle to penetrate deep muscle tissue. The viscosity of a medication, injection site, patient's weight, and amount of adipose tissue influence needle size selection. Determine needle gauge by the medication to be administered. For example, give immunizations and parenteral medications in aqueous solutions with a 20- to 25-gauge needle. Give a viscous or oil-based solution with an 18- to 21-gauge needle. For children, a small-gauge needle (22- to 25-gauge) is used unless the medication is viscous. An obese patient requires a needle over 1.5 inches, whereas a thinner patient only requires a ½- to 1-inch needle (Zaybak and others, 2007). Recommendations for needle length in children include use of a 1-inch needle for infants, 1- to 1¼-inch in toddlers, and 1½- to 2-inch in older children (Hockenberry and Wilson, 2009). Length varies by injection site.

Muscle is less sensitive to irritating and viscous medication. A normal, well-developed adult can safely tolerate 2 to 5 mL of medication in larger muscles such as the ventrogluteal (Hunter, 2008a). However, clinically it is unusual to administer over 3 mL of medication in a single injection because the body does not absorb it well. Older adults and thin patients often tolerate only 2 mL in a single injection. The muscles of older infants and small children can tolerate 1 mL of medication in a single site. Larger muscles are often able to tolerate a maximum volume of 2 mL of medication (Hockenberry and Wilson, 2009).

Give IM injections so the needle is perpendicular to the patient's body and as close to a 90-degree angle as possible. Rotate IM injection sites to decrease the risk of hypertrophy. Emaciated or atrophied muscles absorb medication poorly; avoid their use when possible. The Z-track method, a technique for pulling the skin during an injection, is recommended for IM injections. The Z-track technique prevents leakage of medication into subcutaneous tissue, seals medication in the muscle, and minimizes irritation. This zigzag path seals the needle track wherever tissue planes slide across each other (Fig. 23-11, *A* and *B*). The medication is sealed in the muscle tissue.

Injection Sites

When selecting an IM site, determine that the site is free of pain, infection, necrosis, bruising, and abrasions. Also consider the location of underlying bones, nerves, and blood vessels and the volume of medication you will give. Because of the sciatic nerve location, the dorsogluteal muscle is not recommended as an injection site. If a needle hits the sciatic nerve, the patient may experience partial or permanent paralysis of the leg (Hunter, 2008a; Ramtahal and others, 2006).

Ventrogluteal muscle

The ventrogluteal muscle involves the gluteus medius and minimus and is the preferred site for adults and children of all ages (Hockenberry and Wilson, 2009). Research has shown that nerve and tissue injury and pain are associated with inappropriate site selection (Hunter, 2008a). To locate the ventrogluteal muscle, place the heel of the hand over the greater trochanter of the patient's hip with the wrist almost perpendicular to the femur. Use the right hand for the left hip and the left hand for the right hip. Point the thumb toward the patient's groin, point the index finger to the anterior superior iliac spine, and extend the middle finger back along the iliac crest toward the buttock. The index finger, the middle finger, and the iliac crest form a V-shaped triangle. The injection site is the center of the triangle (Fig. 23-12, *A* and *B*). To relax this muscle, patients lie on their side or back, flexing the knee and hip.

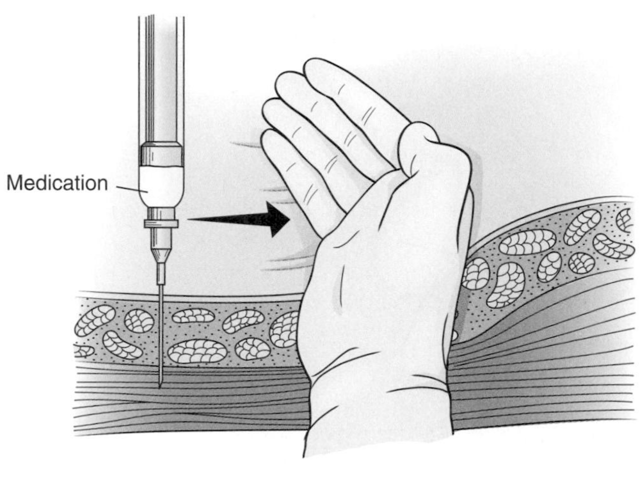

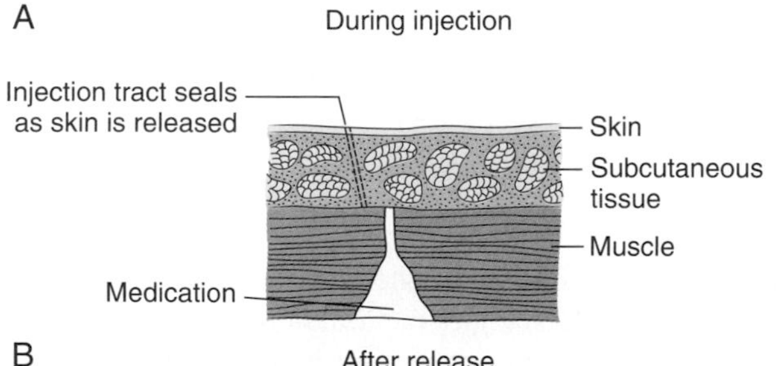

FIG 23-11 A, Pulling on overlying skin with dorsum of hand during IM injection moves tissue to prevent later tracking. **B,** The Z-track left after injection prevents the deposit of medication through sensitive tissue.

Vastus lateralis muscle

The vastus lateralis muscle is another injection site used in adults and is the preferred site for administration of biologicals (e.g., immunizations) to infants (Hockenberry and Wilson, 2009). The muscle is thick and well developed and is located on the anterior lateral aspect of the thigh. It extends in an adult from a handbreadth above the knee to a handbreadth below the greater trochanter of the femur (Fig. 23-13, *A* and *B*). Use the middle third of the muscle for injection. The width of the muscle usually extends from the midline of the thigh to the midline of the outer side of the thigh. With young children or cachectic patients it helps to grasp the body of the muscle during injection to be sure that the medication is deposited in muscle tissue. To help relax the muscle, ask the patient to lie flat with the knee slightly flexed and foot externally rotated or assume a sitting position.

Deltoid muscle

Although the deltoid site is easily accessible, the muscle is not well developed in many adults. There is potential for injury because the axillary, radial, brachial, and ulnar nerves and the brachial artery lie within the upper arm under the triceps and along the humerus (Fig. 23-14). Use this site for small medication volumes (0.5 to 1 mL); administration of routine immunizations in toddlers, older children, and adults; or when other sites are inaccessible because of dressings or casts.

Locate the deltoid muscle by fully exposing the patient's upper arm and shoulder and asking him or her to relax the arm at the side or by supporting the patient's arm and flexing the elbow. Do not roll up any tight-fitting sleeve. Allow the patient to sit, stand, or lie down. Palpate the lower edge of the acromion process, which forms the base of a triangle in line with the midpoint of the lateral aspect of the upper arm. The injection site is in the center of the triangle, about 2.5 to 5 cm (1 to 2 inches) below the acromion process (see Fig. 23-14, *B*). Locate the apex of the triangle by placing four fingers

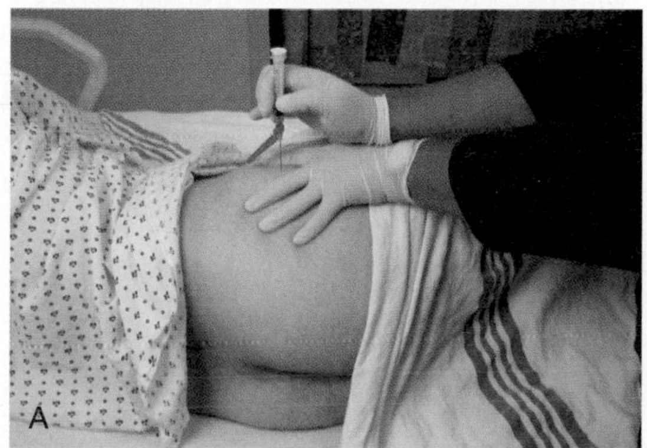

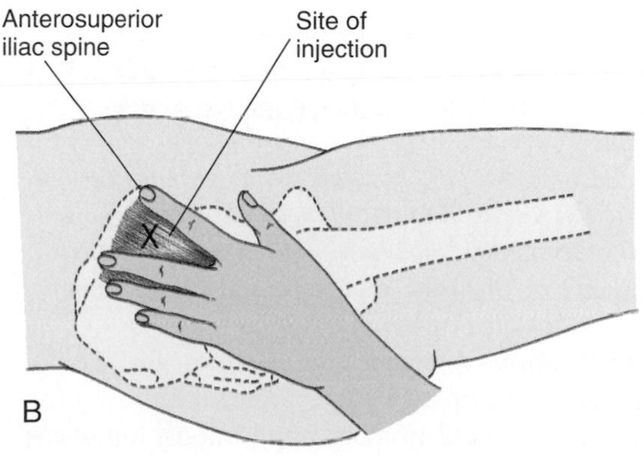

FIG 23-12 A, Injection into the ventrogluteal site avoids major nerves and blood vessels. **B,** Anatomical view of ventrogluteal site.

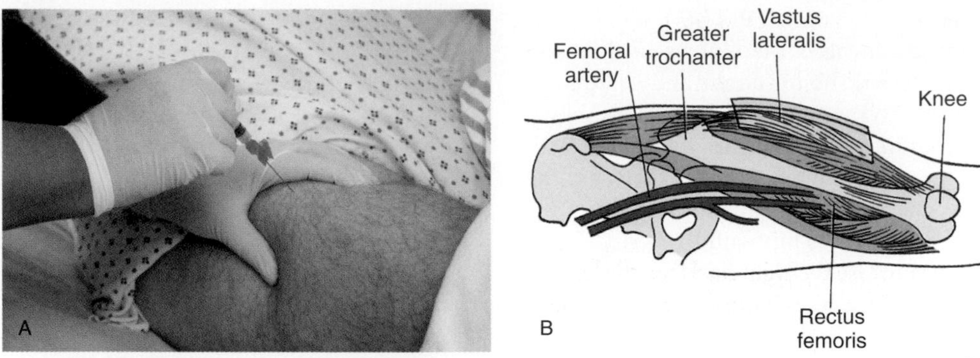

FIG 23-13 **A,** Injection into the vastus lateralis muscle. **B,** Landmarks of vastus lateralis site.

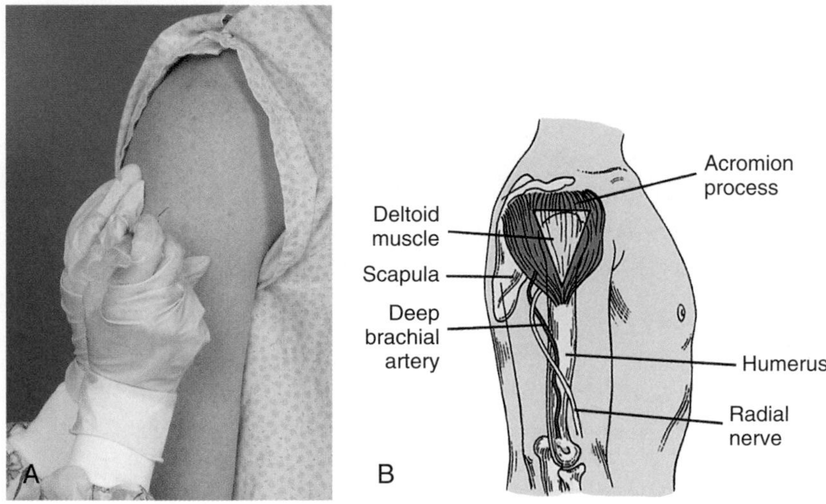

FIG 23-14 **A,** Administering IM injection in deltoid site. **B,** Anatomical view of the deltoid muscle.

across the deltoid muscle, with the top finger along the acromion process. The injection site is three fingerwidths below the acromion process.

ASSESSMENT

1. Check accuracy and completeness of each medication administration record (MAR) with prescriber's original medication order. Check patient's name, drug name and dosage, route of administration, and time for administration. Recopy or reprint any portion of printed MAR that is difficult to read. *Rationale: The prescriber's order is the most reliable source and only legal record of drugs patient is to receive. Ensures that patient receives the right medications. Handwritten MARs are a source of medication errors (Eisenhauer and others, 2007; Furukawa and others, 2008).*
2. Assess patient's medical and medication history. *Rationale: Identifies need for medication.*
3. Review medication reference information for action, purpose, side effects, normal dose, rate of administration, time of peak onset, and nursing implications. *Rationale: Knowledge of medication allows you to give medication safely and monitor patient's response to therapy.*
4. Assess patient's history of allergies, known type of allergens, and normal allergic reaction. *Rationale: Certain substances have similar compositions; it may harm patients to give a medication if there is a known allergy.*
5. Observe patient's previous verbal and nonverbal responses toward injection. *Rationale: Injections are sometimes painful. Anticipating patient's anxiety allows you to use distraction to reduce pain awareness.*
6. Assess for contraindication to IM injections, such as muscle atrophy, reduced blood flow, or circulatory shock. *Rationale: Atrophied muscle absorbs medication poorly. Factors interfering with blood flow to muscles impair drug absorption.*
7. Assess patient's symptoms before initiating medication therapy. *Rationale: Provides information to evaluate desired effect of medication.*
8. Assess patient's knowledge of medication.

PLANNING

Expected Outcomes focus on safe administration of intramuscular injection.

1. Patient experiences no pain or mild burning at injection site.
2. Patient achieves desired effect of medication with no signs of allergies or undesired effects.
3. Patient explains purpose, dosage, and effects of medication.

Delegation and Collaboration

The skill of administering IM injections cannot be delegated to nursing assistive personnel (NAP). Instruct the NAP about the following:

- Potential medication side effects and reporting their occurrence to the nurse
- Reporting any change in the patient's condition to the nurse

Equipment

- Syringe: 2 to 3 mL for adult, 0.5 to 1 mL for infants and small children
- Needle: length corresponds to site of injection and age and size of patient
- Needle gauge often depends on length of needle. Administer most biologicals and medications in aqueous solutions with 20- to 25-gauge needle
- Alcohol swab
- Small gauze pad
- Vial or ampule of medication
- Clean gloves
- MAR or computer printout
- Puncture-proof container

IMPLEMENTATION *for* ADMINISTERING INTRAMUSCULAR INJECTIONS

STEP	RATIONALE
1. Prepare medication from ampule or vial using aseptic technique (see Skill 23.1). Check label of medication carefully with the MAR two times while preparing medication.	Ensures that medication is sterile. *First and second checks for accuracy* ensure that the correct medication is administered.
2. Take medications to patient at correct time, within 30 minutes before or after prescribed time (see agency policy). Give stat and single-order medications at the exact time ordered.	Ensures intended therapeutic effect.
3. **See Standard Protocol (inside front cover).**	
4. Identify patient using two identifiers (e.g., name and birthday or name and account number, according to facility policy). Compare identifiers with information on patient's MAR or medical record.	Ensures correct patient. Complies with The Joint Commission standards and improves patient safety (TJC, 2010).
5. At the bedside again compare the MAR or computer printout with the names of medications on the medication labels. Ask patient if he or she has allergies.	*This is the third check for accuracy* and ensures that patient receives correct medication. Confirms patient's allergy history.
6. Discuss the purpose of each medication, action, and possible adverse effects. Allow patient to ask any questions. Tell patient that injection will cause a slight burning or sting.	Patient has the right to be informed, and patient's understanding of each medication improves adherence with drug therapy. Helps minimize patient's anxiety.
7. Keep sheet or gown draped over body parts not requiring exposure.	Respects dignity of patient while exposing injection area.
8. Select appropriate site. Note integrity and size of muscle. Palpate for tenderness or hardness. Avoid these areas. If you give injections frequently, rotate sites. Use ventrogluteal site if possible.	The ventrogluteal or deltoid site is the preferred injection site for adults. This ventrogluteal site is also preferred for children of all ages (Hockenberry and Wilson, 2009).
9. Assist patient to comfortable position. Position patient depending on chosen site (e.g., sit, lie flat, on side, or prone).	Reduces strain on muscle and minimizes injection discomfort.

SAFETY ALERT Ensure that medical condition (e.g., circulatory shock) does not contraindicate patient's position for injection.

STEP	RATIONALE
10. Relocate site using anatomical landmarks.	Injection into correct anatomical site prevents injury to nerves, bone, and blood vessels.

Continued

STEP	RATIONALE
11. Cleanse site with antiseptic swab. Apply swab at center of site and rotate outward in circular direction for about 5 cm (2 inches).	Removes secretions containing microorganisms.
Option: Apply EMLA cream on injection site at least 1 hour before IM injection or use a vapocoolant spray (e.g., ethyl chloride) just before injection.	Decreases pain at injection site.
12. Hold swab or gauze between third and fourth fingers of nondominant hand.	
13. Remove needle cap or sheath by pulling it straight off.	Preventing needle from touching sides of cap prevents contamination.
14. Hold syringe between thumb and forefinger of dominant hand; hold as dart, palm down.	Quick, smooth injection requires proper manipulation of syringe parts.
15. Administer injection.	
a. Position ulnar side of nondominant hand just below site and pull skin laterally approximately 2.5 to 3.5 cm (1 to 1½ inches). Hold position until medication is injected. With dominant hand, inject needle quickly at 90-degree angle into muscle (see Fig. 23-11, *A*).	Z-track creates zigzag path through tissues that seals the needle track to avoid tracking medication. A quick, dartlike injection reduces discomfort (Hunter, 2008a).
b. *Option:* If patient's muscle mass is small, grasp body of muscle between thumb and forefingers.	Ensures that the medication reaches the muscle mass (Hockenberry and Wilson, 2009; Hunter, 2008a).
c. After needle pierces skin, still pulling on skin with nondominant hand, grasp lower end of syringe barrel with fingers of nondominant hand to stabilize it. Move dominant hand to end of plunger. Avoid moving syringe.	Smooth manipulation of syringe reduces discomfort from needle movement. Skin remains pulled until after medication is injected to ensure Z-track administration.
d. Pull back on plunger 5 to 10 seconds. If no blood appears, inject medication slowly at a rate of 1 mL/10 sec.	Aspiration of blood into syringe indicates possible placement into a vein. Slow injection reduces pain and tissue trauma.

SAFETY ALERT If blood appears in syringe, remove needle, dispose of medication and syringe properly, and prepare another dose of medication for injection.

STEP	RATIONALE
e. Wait 10 seconds and smoothly and steadily withdraw needle, release skin, and apply alcohol swab or gauze gently over site.	Allows time for medication to absorb into muscle before syringe is removed and skin is released. Dry gauze minimizes discomfort associated with alcohol on nonintact skin.
16. Apply gentle pressure to site. Do not massage site. Apply bandage if needed.	Massage damages underlying tissue.
17. Discard uncapped needle or needle enclosed in safety shield and attached syringe into a puncture- and leak-proof receptacle.	Prevents injury to patients and health care personnel. Recapping needles increases risk for a needlestick injury (OSHA, 2009).
18. See Completion Protocol (inside front cover).	
19. Stay with patient for several minutes and observe for any allergic reactions.	

EVALUATION

1. Return to room in 15 to 30 minutes and ask if patient feels any acute pain, burning, numbness, or tingling at injection site.
2. Inspect site; note any bruising or induration.
3. Observe patient's response to medication at times that correlate with the onset, peak, and duration of medication.
4. Ask patient to explain purpose and effects of medication.

Unexpected Outcomes and Related Interventions

1. Patient complains of localized pain or continued burning at injection site, indicating potential injury to nerve or vessels.
   a. Assess injection site.
   b. Notify patient's health care provider.
2. During injection blood is aspirated.
   a. Immediately stop injection and remove needle.
   b. Prepare new syringe of medication for administration.

3. Patient displays adverse reaction with signs of urticaria, eczema, pruritus, wheezing, and dyspnea.
   a. Follow agency policy for appropriate response to adverse drug reactions (e.g., administration of antihistamine such as diphenhydramine [Benadryl] or epinephrine).
   b. Notify patient's health care provider immediately.
   c. Add allergy information to patient's record.

Recording and Reporting

- Record drug, dose, route, site, time, and date given on MAR immediately after administration, not before. Include initials or signature.
- Record patient teaching, validation of understanding, and patient's response to medication in nurses' notes.
- Report any undesirable effects from medication to patient's health care provider and document adverse effects in record.

Sample Documentation

0800 Patient diagnosed with vitamin B_{12} deficiency. Administered 100 mcg cyanocobalamin IM in right ventral gluteal muscle. Patient reports some burning during and following administration.

Special Considerations

Pediatric

- Children can be anxious or afraid of needles. Assistance with proper positioning and holding the child is sometimes necessary. Distraction such as blowing bubbles and pressure at the injection site before giving the injection can help alleviate the child's anxiety (Schechter and others, 2007).
- If possible, apply EMLA cream on injection site at least 1 hour before IM injection or use a vapocoolant spray (e.g., ethyl chloride) just before injection to decrease pain (Hockenberry and Wilson, 2009).

Geriatric

- Older patients may have decreased muscle mass, which reduces drug absorption from IM injections. In addition, older adults may have loss of muscle tone and strength that impairs mobility, placing them at high risk for falls from guarding an injection site.

Home Care

- Self-administration of an IM injection is difficult, especially in the vastus lateralis. Teach a family caregiver to identify and administer injections in this site.
- Instruct adult patients who require frequent injections to apply EMLA cream to the injection site 1 hour before administration.
- Patients will need instruction about safe disposal of syringes and needles (see Skill 23.2, Home Care Considerations).
- See Chapter 32 for information about modifying safety risks in the home.

SKILL 23.4 ADMINISTERING INTRADERMAL INJECTIONS

- **Nursing Skills Online: Injections, Lesson 4**

Video Clips

You typically give ID injections for skin testing (e.g., in TB screening and allergy tests). Because such medications are potent, you inject them into the dermis, where blood supply is reduced and drug absorption occurs slowly. A patient may have an anaphylactic reaction if the medications enter his or her circulation too rapidly. For patients with a history of numerous allergies, the physician may perform skin testing. Skin testing often requires the nurse to visually inspect the test site; therefore make sure that ID sites are free of lesions and injuries and are relatively hairless. The inner forearm and upper back are ideal locations.

To administer an ID injection, use a TB or small syringe with a short ($\frac{3}{8}$ to $\frac{5}{8}$ inch), fine-gauge (25 to 27) needle. The angle of insertion for an ID injection is 5 to 15 degrees (Fig. 23-15). Inject only small amounts of medication (0.01 to 0.1 mL) intradermally. Only administer amounts up to 0.1 mL to children (Hockenberry and Wilson, 2009). If a bleb does not appear or if the site bleeds after needle withdrawal, the medication may have entered subcutaneous tissues. In this situation skin test results will not be valid.

ASSESSMENT

1. Check accuracy and completeness of each medication administration record (MAR) with prescriber's original medication order. Check patient's name, drug name and dosage, route of administration, and time for administration. Recopy or reprint any portion of printed MAR that is difficult to read. *Rationale: The prescriber's order is the most reliable source and only legal record of drugs patient is to receive. Ensures that patient receives the right medications. Handwritten MARs are a source of medication errors (Eisenhauer and others, 2007; Furukawa and others, 2008).*
2. Assess patient's medical and medication history. *Rationale: Identifies need for medication.*

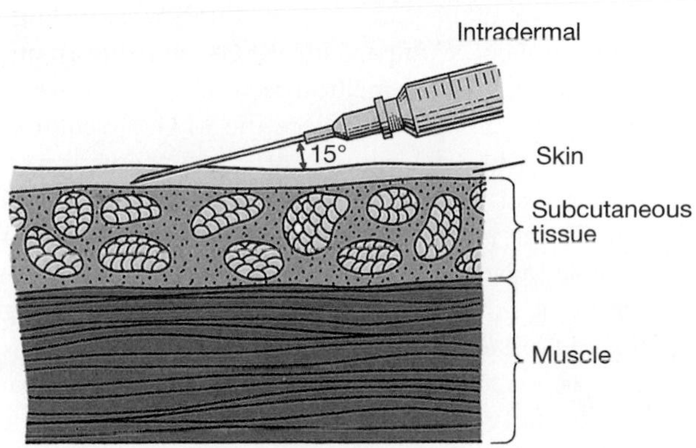

FIG 23-15 Intradermal needle tip inserted into dermis.

3. Review medication reference information for action, purpose, side effects, normal dose, rate of administration, time of peak onset, and nursing implications. *Rationale: Knowledge of medication allows you to give medication safely and monitor patient's response to therapy.*
4. Assess patient's history of allergies, known type of allergens, and normal allergic reaction. *Rationale: Certain substances have similar compositions; it may harm patients to give a medication if there is a known allergy.*
5. Observe patient's previous verbal and nonverbal responses toward injection. *Rationale: Injections are sometimes painful. Anticipating patient's anxiety allows you to use distraction to reduce pain awareness.*
6. Assess for contraindication to ID injections. Assess for history of severe adverse reactions or necrosis that happened after previous ID injection. *Rationale: Medications are potent and can cause severe anaphylaxis.*
7. Assess patient's symptoms before initiating medication therapy. *Rationale: Provides information to evaluate desired effect of medication.*
8. Assess patient's knowledge of purpose and response to skin testing. *Rationale: Patients need to know when to come back for follow-up reading of skin test and when and how to report any reaction.*

PLANNING

Expected Outcomes focus on safe ID injection.

1. Patient experiences no pain or mild burning at injection site.
2. Patient achieves desired effect of medication with no signs of allergies or undesired effects.
3. Patient explains purpose, dose, and effects of medication.

Delegation and Collaboration

The skill of administering ID injections cannot be delegated to nursing assistive personnel (NAP). Instruct the NAP about the following:

- Potential medication side effects and reporting their occurrence to the nurse
- Reporting any change in the patient's condition to the nurse

Equipment

- Syringe: 1-mL TB syringe
- Needle: 25 to 27 gauge, $\frac{3}{8}$ to $\frac{5}{8}$ inch
- Alcohol swab
- Small gauze pad
- Vial or ampule of medication
- Clean gloves
- MAR or computer printout
- Puncture-proof container

IMPLEMENTATION *for* ADMINISTERING INTRADERMAL INJECTIONS

STEP	RATIONALE
1. Prepare medication using aseptic technique (see Skill 23.1). Check label of medication carefully with the MAR two times while preparing medication.	Ensures that medication is sterile; preparation techniques differ for ampule and vial. *First and second checks for accuracy* ensure that the correct medication is administered.
2. Take medications to patient at correct time, within 30 minutes before or after prescribed time (see agency policy). Give stat and single-order medications at the exact time ordered.	Ensures intended therapeutic effect. Give stat medications immediately or single-order medications at the time ordered.
3. **See Standard Protocol (inside front cover).**	
4. Identify patient using two identifiers (e.g., name and birthday or name and account number, according to facility policy). Compare identifiers with information on patient's MAR or medical record.	Ensures correct patient. Complies with The Joint Commission standards and improves patient safety (TJC, 2010).
5. At the bedside again compare the MAR or computer printout with the names of medications on the medication labels. Ask patient if he or she has allergies.	*This is the third check for accuracy* and ensures that patient receives correct medication. Confirms patient's allergy history.
6. Discuss the purpose of each medication, action, and possible adverse effects. Allow patient to ask any questions. Tell patient that injection will cause a slight burning or sting.	Patient has the right to be informed, and patient's understanding of each medication improves adherence with drug therapy. Helps minimize patient's anxiety.
7. Keep sheet or gown draped over body parts not requiring exposure.	Respects dignity of patient while exposing injection area.

STEP	RATIONALE
8. Select appropriate site. Note lesions or discolorations of skin. If possible, select site three to four fingerwidths below antecubital space and one handwidth above wrist. If you cannot use the forearm, inspect the upper back. If necessary, use sites appropriate for subcutaneous injections.	An ID injection site is free of discolorations or hair so you can see the results of skin test and interpret them correctly (CDC, 2009).
9. Assist patient to comfortable position. Have patient extend elbow and support it and forearm on flat surface.	Stabilizes injection site for easiest accessibility.
10. Relocate site using anatomical landmarks.	Injection into correct anatomical site prevents injury to nerves, bone, and blood vessels.
11. Cleanse site with antiseptic swab. Apply swab at center of site and rotate outward in circular direction for about 5 cm (2 inches).	Mechanical action of swab removes secretions containing microorganisms.
Option: Use a vapocoolant spray (e.g., ethyl chloride) just before injection.	Decreases pain at injection site.
12. Hold swab or gauze between third and fourth fingers of nondominant hand.	Swab or gauze remains readily accessible when withdrawing needle.
13. Remove needle cap or sheath by pulling it straight off.	Preventing needle from touching sides of cap prevents contamination.
14. Hold syringe between thumb and forefinger of dominant hand. Hold bevel of needle pointing up.	With bevel up you are less likely to deposit medication into tissues below dermis.
15. Administer injection.	
a. With nondominant hand stretch skin over site with forefinger or thumb.	Needle pierces tight skin more easily.
b. With needle almost against patient's skin, insert it slowly at a 5- to 15-degree angle until resistance is felt. Advance needle through epidermis to approximately 3 mm (⅛ inch) below skin surface. You will see bulge of needle tip through skin.	Ensures that needle tip is in dermis. You will obtain inaccurate results if you do not inject needle at correct angle and depth (CDC, 2009).
c. Inject medication slowly. Normally you feel resistance. If not, needle is too deep; remove and begin again.	Slow injection minimizes discomfort at site. Dermal layer is tight and does not expand easily when you inject solution.
(1) While injecting medication, note that small bleb (approximately 6 mm [¼ inch]) resembling mosquito bite appears on skin surface (see illustration).	Bleb indicates that you deposited medication in dermis.

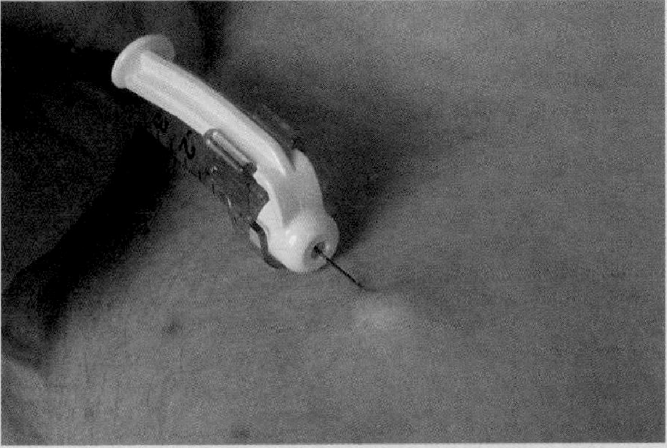

STEP 15c(1) Injection creates a small bleb.

STEP	RATIONALE
(2) After withdrawing needle, apply alcohol swab or gauze over site.	Do not massage site. Apply bandage if needed.

Continued

STEP	RATIONALE
16. Discard uncapped needle or needle enclosed in safety shield and attached syringe into a puncture- and leak-proof receptacle.	Prevents injury to patients and health care personnel. Recapping needles increases risk for a needlestick injury (OSHA, 2009).
17. See Completion Protocol (inside front cover).	
18. Stay with patient for several minutes and observe for any allergic reactions.	Dyspnea, wheezing, and circulatory collapse are signs of severe anaphylactic reaction.

EVALUATION

1. Return to room in 15 to 30 minutes and ask if patient feels any acute pain, burning, numbness, or tingling at injection site.
2. Inspect site; note any bruising or induration.
3. Observe patient's response to medication at times that correlate with the onset, peak, and duration of the medication.
4. Ask patient to explain purpose and effects of medication.
5. For ID injections use skin pencil and draw circle around perimeter of injection site. Read site within appropriate amount of time, designated by type of medication or skin test you give.

SAFETY ALERT Read TB test at 48 to 72 hours. Induration (hard, dense, raised area) of skin around injection site indicates positive TB reaction of:
- 15 mm or more in patients with no known risk factors for TB.
- 10 mm or more in patients who are recent immigrants; injection drug users; residents and employees of high-risk settings; patients with certain chronic illnesses; children less than 4 years of age; and infants, children, and adolescents exposed to high-risk adults.
- 5 mm or more in patients who are human immunodeficiency virus (HIV) positive, immunocompromised patients, or patients recently exposed to TB (CDC, 2009).

Unexpected Outcomes and Related Interventions

1. Patient complains of localized pain or continued burning at injection site, indicating potential injury to nerve or vessels.
   a. Assess injection site.
   b. Notify patient's health care provider.
2. Raised, reddened, or hard zone (induration) forms around ID test site.
   a. Notify health care provider
   b. Document sensitivity to injected allergen or positive test if TB skin testing was completed.
3. Patient has adverse reaction with signs of urticaria, eczema, pruritus, wheezing, and dyspnea.
   a. Follow agency policy for appropriate response to adverse drug reactions (e.g., administration of antihistamine or epinephrine).
   b. Notify patient's health care provider immediately.
   c. Add allergy information to patient's record.

Recording and Reporting

- Record drug, dose, route, site, time, and date administered on MAR immediately after administration, not before. Include initials or signature.
- Record patient teaching, validation of understanding, and patient's response to medication.
- Report any undesirable effects from medication to patient's health care provider and document adverse effects in record.

Sample Documentation

0900 Patient's ID site, right forearm noted 10 mm raised, reddened zone. Health care provider notified, and patient sent for chest radiograph at 1000.

Special Considerations

Pediatric

- Children who are exposed to persons with confirmed or suspected infectious TB should be tested for TB immediately following exposure (Hockenberry and Wilson, 2009).
- Children who are exposed to high-risk individuals (e.g., HIV-infected, homeless, incarcerated) should be tested for TB every 2 to 3 years.

Geriatric

- The older adult has skin that is less elastic and must be held taut to ensure that ID injection is administered correctly.

SKILL 23.5 ADMINISTERING MEDICATIONS BY INTRAVENOUS BOLUS

- **Nursing Skills Online: Intravenous Medication Administration, Lessons 1 and 3**

An IV bolus involves introducing a concentrated dose of a medication directly into a vein by way of an existing intravenous access (see Chapter 28). An IV bolus or "push" usually requires a small volume of fluid, which is an advantage for patients at risk for fluid overload. Administering medications by IV bolus is common in emergencies when you need to deliver a fast-acting medication quickly. Because these medications act quickly, it is essential that you monitor patients closely for adverse reactions. Institutions have policies and procedures that identify the medications that nurses are allowed to administer by IV push and other IV routes. These policies are based on the medication, capability and availability of staff, and type of monitoring equipment available.

The IV bolus is a dangerous method to administer medications because it allows no time to correct errors. Administering an IV push medication too quickly can cause death. Therefore be very careful in calculating the correct amount of the medication to give. In addition, a bolus may cause direct irritation to the lining of blood vessels; thus always confirm placement of the IV catheter or needle. Never give an IV bolus if the insertion site appears puffy, edematous, or reddened or if the IV fluids do not flow at the ordered rate. Accidental injection of some medications into tissues surrounding a vein can cause pain, sloughing of tissues, and abscesses.

Verify the rate of administration of IV push medication using institutional guidelines or a medication reference manual. Review the amount of medication the patient will receive each minute, the recommended concentration, and rate of administration. For example, if a patient is to receive 6 mL of a medication over 3 minutes, give 2 mL of the IV bolus medication every minute. Understand the purpose of the medication and any potential adverse reactions related to the rate and route of administration.

You give an IV push medication through either an existing continuous IV infusion or an intermittent venous access (commonly called a saline lock). A saline lock is an IV catheter with a small "well" or chamber covered by a rubber cap. An IV catheter can be converted into a lock by inserting a special rubber-seal injection cap into the end of the catheter (see Chapter 28). Use of a lock saves time by eliminating constant monitoring of an IV line. It also offers better mobility, safety, and comfort for patients by eliminating the need for a continuous IV line. After you administer an IV bolus through an intermittent venous access, flush with a normal saline solution to keep it patent.

ASSESSMENT

1. Check accuracy and completeness of each medication administration record (MAR) with prescriber's original medication order. Check patient's name, drug name and dosage, route of administration, and time for administration. Recopy or reprint any portion of printed MAR that is difficult to read. *Rationale: The prescriber's order is the most reliable source and only legal record of drugs patient is to receive. Ensures that patient receives the right medications. Handwritten MARs are a source of medication errors (Eisenhauer and others, 2007; Furukawa and others, 2008).*

> **SAFETY ALERT** Some IV medications can be pushed safely only when the patient is continuously monitored for dysrhythmias, blood pressure changes, or other adverse effects. Therefore you can push some medications only in specific areas within a health care agency. Confirm agency guidelines about requirements for special monitoring.

2. Assess patient's medical and medication history. *Rationale: Identifies need for medication.*
3. Collect drug reference information necessary to administer drug safely, including action, purpose, side effects, normal dose, time of peak onset, how slowly to give the medication, and nursing implications such as the need to dilute the medication or administer it through a filter. *Rationale: Knowledge of medication allows you to give it safely and monitor patient's response to therapy.*
4. If you give medication through an existing IV line, determine compatibility of medication with IV fluids and any additives within IV solution. *Rationale: IV medication is sometimes not compatible with IV solution and/or additives.*
5. Assess condition of IV needle insertion site for signs of infiltration or phlebitis. *Rationale: Do not administer medication if site is edematous or inflamed.*
6. Assess patient's history of medication allergies, known type of allergens, and normal allergic reaction. *Rationale: IV medications may cause rapid response. Allergic response is immediate.*
7. Assess patient's symptoms before administering medication. *Rationale: Provides information to evaluate desired effect of medication.*
8. Assess patient's understanding of purpose of medication therapy.

PLANNING

Expected Outcomes focus on safe administration of an IV bolus medication.

1. Desired effect of medication achieved with no signs of adverse reactions.
2. IV site remains intact without signs of swelling or inflammation or symptoms of tenderness at site.
3. Patient explains purpose and side effects of medication.

Delegation and Collaboration

The skill of administering medications by IV bolus cannot be delegated to nursing assistive personnel (NAP). Instruct the NAP about the following:

- Potential medication actions and side effects of the medications and reporting their occurrence to the nurse
- Reporting any change in the patient's condition to the nurse
- Reporting any patient complaints of moisture or discomfort around IV insertion site

Equipment

- Watch with secondhand
- MAR or computer printout
- Clean gloves
- Antiseptic swab
- Medication in vial or ampule
- Safety syringes for medication and saline flush preparation

- Needleless (SESIP) device or sterile needle (21 to 25 gauge)
- Intravenous lock: vial of normal saline flush solution (saline recommended [Infusion Nurses Society, 2006]; but, if agency continues to use heparin flush, the most common concentration is 10 units/mL; check agency policy)
- Puncture-proof container

IMPLEMENTATION *for* ADMINISTERING MEDICATIONS BY INTRAVENOUS BOLUS

STEP	RATIONALE
1. Prepare medication from ampule or vial using aseptic technique (see Skill 23.1). Check label of medication carefully with MAR two times while preparing medication.	Ensures that medication is sterile. *First and second checks for accuracy* ensure that the correct medication is administered.

SAFETY ALERT Some IV medications require dilution before administration. Verify with agency policy or pharmacist. If a small amount of medication is given (e.g., less than 1 mL), dilute medication in small amount (e.g., 5 mL) of normal saline or sterile water so the medication does not collect in the "dead spaces" (e.g., Y-site injection port, IV cap) of the IV delivery system.

STEP	RATIONALE
2. Take medication to patient at correct time, within 30 minutes before or after prescribed time. Give stat and single-order medications at the exact time ordered.	Ensures intended therapeutic effect. Give stat medications immediately or single-order medications at the time ordered.
3. See Standard Protocol (inside front cover).	
4. Identify patient using two identifiers (e.g., name and birthday or name and account number, according to facility policy). Compare identifiers with information on patient's MAR or medical record.	Ensures correct patient. Complies with The Joint Commission standards and improves patient safety (TJC, 2010).
5. Compare the names of medications on the medication label with the MAR one more time at patient's bedside.	*The third check for accuracy* ensures that the correct medication is administered.
6. Discuss the purpose of each medication, action, and possible adverse effects with patient. Allow patient to ask any questions about drugs. Explain procedure to patient. Encourage patient to report symptoms of discomfort at IV site.	Patient has the right to be informed, and patient's understanding of each medication improves adherence with drug therapy. Helps identify possible infiltration early.
7. ***Intravenous push (existing line):***	
a. Select injection port of IV tubing closest to patient. Whenever possible, use needleless injection port.	Follows provisions of the Needle Safety and Prevention Act of 2001 (OSHA, 2009).

SAFETY ALERT Never administer IV medications through tubing that is infusing blood, blood products, or parenteral nutrition solutions.

STEP	RATIONALE
b. Clean injection port with antiseptic swab. Allow to dry.	Prevents transfer of microorganisms during needle or blunt cannula insertion.
c. *Connect syringe to IV line:* Insert needleless tip of syringe (see illustration) or small-gauge needle containing medication through center of port.	Prevents introduction of microorganisms. Prevents damage to port diaphragm and possible leakage from site.
d. Occlude IV line by pinching tubing just above injection port (see illustration). Pull back gently on plunger of syringe to aspirate for blood return.	Final check ensures that medication is delivered into bloodstream.

SAFETY ALERT In the case of smaller-gauge IV needles, blood return sometimes is not aspirated, even if IV line is patent. If IV site shows no signs of infiltration and IV fluid is infusing without difficulty, give IV push.

STEP	RATIONALE
e. Release tubing and inject medication within amount of time recommended by agency policy, pharmacist, or medication reference manual. Use a watch to time administrations. You can pinch the IV line while pushing medication and release it when not pushing medication. Allow IV fluids to infuse when not pushing medication.	Ensures safe medication infusion. Rapid injection of IV drug can be fatal. Allowing IV fluids to infuse while pushing IV drug enables medication to be delivered to patient at prescribed rate.

SAFETY ALERT If IV medication is incompatible with IV fluids, stop the IV fluids, clamp the IV line, and flush with 10 mL of normal saline or sterile water. Then give the IV bolus over the appropriate amount of time and flush with another 10 mL of normal saline or sterile water at the same rate as the medication was administered. Restart the IV fluids at the prescribed rate. This allows you to give the medication through the existing line without creating potential risks associated with IV incompatibilities. If the IV line that is currently hanging is a medication, disconnect IV line and administer IV push medication as outlined in Step 7 to avoid giving a sudden bolus of the medication in the existing IV line to patient. Verify agency policy regarding stopping IV fluids or continuous IV medications. If unable to stop IV infusion, start a new IV site (see Chapter 28) and administer medication using the IV push (IV lock) method.

STEP	RATIONALE
f. After injecting medication, withdraw syringe and recheck fluid infusion rate.	Injection of bolus often alters rate of fluid infusion. Rapid fluid infusion causes circulatory fluid overload.
8. ***Intravenous push (intravenous lock):***	
a. Prepare flush solution according to policy.	
(1) *Saline flush method (preferred method)*: Prepare two syringes filled with 2 to 3 mL of normal saline (0.9%). *Heparin flush (not recommended, refer to agency policy)*	Normal saline is effective in keeping peripheral IV locks patent and is compatible with a wide range of medications.
b. Administer medication:	
(1) Clean injection port of lock with antiseptic swab.	Prevents transfer of microorganisms during needle insertion.

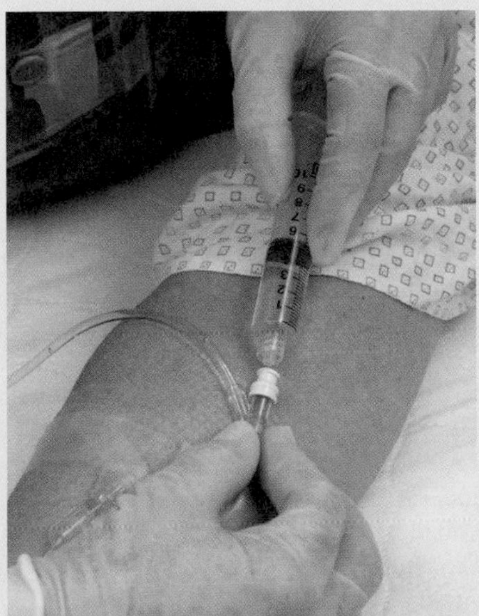

STEP 7c Connecting syringe to IV line with needleless blunt cannula tip.

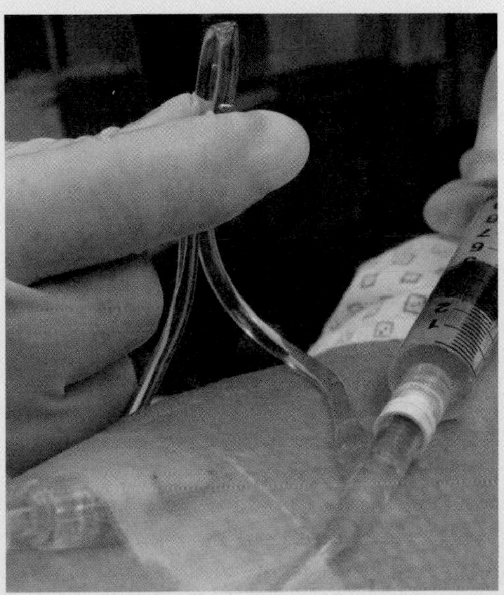

STEP 7d Occluding IV tubing above injection port.

Continued

STEP	RATIONALE
(2) Insert syringe with normal saline 0.9% through injection port of IV lock.	
(3) Pull back gently on syringe plunger and check for blood return.	Indicates if needle or catheter is in vein.
SAFETY ALERT In some cases, especially with a smaller-gauge IV needle, blood return is usually not aspirated, even if IV is patent. If IV site does not show signs of infiltration and IV flushes without difficulty, proceed with IV push.	
(4) Flush IV site with normal saline by pushing slowly on plunger.	Cleans needle and reservoir of blood. Flushing without difficulty indicates patent IV line.
(a) Carefully observe the area of skin above the IV catheter. Note any puffiness or swelling as you flush the IV line.	Swelling indicates infiltration into the vein and requires removal of catheter.
(5) Remove saline-filled syringe.	
(6) Clean injection port of lock with antiseptic swab.	
(7) Insert syringe containing prepared medication through injection port of IV lock.	Allows administration of medication.
(8) Inject medication within amount of time recommended by agency policy, pharmacist, or medication reference manual. Use a watch to time administration.	Many medication errors are associated with IV pushes being administered too quickly. Following guidelines for IV push rates promotes patient safety.
(9) After administering bolus, withdraw syringe.	
(10) Clean injection site of lock with antiseptic swab.	
(11) Flush injection port. Attach syringe with normal saline and inject flush at the same rate the medication was delivered.	Flushing IV line with saline prevents occlusion of IV access device and ensures that all medication is delivered. Flushing IV site at same rate as medication ensures that any medication remaining within IV needle is delivered at the correct rate.
9. Dispose of uncapped needles and syringes in puncture- and leak-proof container.	Prevents accidental needlestick injuries and follows CDC guidelines for disposal of sharps (OSHA, 2009).
10. See Completion Protocol (inside front cover).	
11. Stay with patient for several minutes and observe for any allergic reactions.	Dyspnea, wheezing, and circulatory collapse are signs of severe anaphylactic reaction.

EVALUATION

1. Observe patient closely for adverse reactions during administration and for several minutes thereafter.
2. Observe IV site during injection and for 48 hours after IV push for sudden swelling.
3. Assess patient's status after giving medication to evaluate the effectiveness of the medication.
4. Ask patient to explain the purpose and side effects of medication.

Unexpected Outcomes and Related Interventions

1. Patient develops adverse reaction to medication.
   a. Stop delivering medication immediately and follow agency policy for appropriate response (e.g., administration of antihistamine or epinephrine) and reporting of adverse drug reactions.
   b. Add allergy information to patient's medical record per agency policy.
2. Intravenous site shows symptoms of infiltration or phlebitis (see Chapter 28).
   a. Stop infusion immediately or discontinue access device and restart in another site.
   b. Determine how much damage the IV medication can produce in subcutaneous tissue.
   c. Provide IV extravasation care (e.g., injecting phentolamine [Regitine] around the IV infiltration site) as indicated by agency policy, use a medication reference, or consult pharmacist to determine appropriate follow-up care.
3. Patient is unable to explain medication information.
   a. Patient requires reinstruction or is unable to learn at this time.

Recording and Reporting

- Record drug, dose, route, time instilled, and date and time administered on MAR immediately after administration, not before. Include initials or signature.
- Record patient teaching and validation of understanding and ability to self-administer medication in nurses' notes.
- Record patient's response to medication in nurses' notes.
- Report any adverse reactions to patient's health care provider. Patient's response may indicate need for additional medical therapy.

Sample Documentation

1400 Lasix (furosemide) 20 mg IVP administered over 2 minutes via IV in right forearm. Site free from redness and edema. Patient denies any pain at IV insertion site.

Special Considerations

Pediatric

- The therapeutic dose of IV push medications for infants and children is often small and difficult to accurately prepare, even with a TB syringe. Infuse these medications slowly and in small volumes because of the risk for fluid volume overload (Hockenberry and Wilson, 2009). For child safety, use syringe pumps with pharmacy-preprinted medication labels when administering medications via IV bolus (Wesolowski, 2009).

Geriatric

- The renal and metabolic systems do not function as efficiently because of the aging process. To reduce the risk of adverse effects of IV push medications, have good drug knowledge about adverse effects and drug interactions (Aschenbrenner and Venable, 2009). Older patients may tolerate IV push medications if they are given over longer periods of time.

Home Care

- IV push medications are frequently given in the home. Nurses, pharmacists, and physicians need to collaborate closely in the care of these patients. Patients and families who are independently responsible for managing IV medications need to understand all aspects of administration safety. Adequate eyesight and manual dexterity are necessary to manipulate the syringe. Patients need to understand their venous access device, rate to give medications, and how to flush their access device. Patients need to safely store their medications, dispose of their IV supplies, and whom to contact in case of an emergency.

SKILL 23.6 ADMINISTERING INTRAVENOUS MEDICATIONS BY PIGGYBACK, INTERMITTENT INFUSION, AND MINI-INFUSION PUMPS

- **Nursing Skills Online: Intravenous Medication Administration Module, Lesson 4**

Another method of administering IV medications uses small volumes (25 to 250 mL) of compatible IV fluids infused over a desired period of time. This method reduces the risk of rapid dose infusion and provides independence for the patient. Patients must have an established IV line that is kept patent by either a continuous infusion or intermittent flushes of normal saline. You can administer intermittent infusion of medication with any of the following methods.

Piggyback

A piggyback is a small (25 to 250 mL) IV bag or bottle connected to a short tubing line that connects to the *upper* Y-port of a primary infusion line or to an intermittent venous access such as a saline lock. The IV container that holds the medication is labeled following the IV piggyback medication format of the ISMP (2008). The piggyback tubing is a microdrip or macrodrip system. The set is called a piggyback because the small bag or bottle is set higher than the primary infusion bag or bottle. In the piggyback setup the main line does not infuse when the piggybacked medication is infusing. The port of the primary IV line contains a back-check valve that automatically stops flow of the primary infusion once the piggyback infusion flows. After a piggyback solution infuses and the solution within the tubing falls below the level of the primary infusion drip chamber, the back-check valve opens, and the primary infusion begins to flow again.

Volume-Control Administration

Volume-control administration sets (e.g., Volutrol, Buretrol, Pediatrol) are small (50 to 150 mL) containers that attach just below a primary infusion bag or bottle. The set is attached and filled in a manner similar to that used with a regular IV infusion. However, the priming of the set is different, depending on the type of filter (floating valve or membrane) within the set. Follow package directions for priming sets.

Mini-Infusion Pump

The mini-infusion pump is battery operated and delivers medications in very small amounts of fluid (5 to 60 mL) within controlled infusion times (Fig. 23-16). It uses standard syringes.

ASSESSMENT

1. Check accuracy and completeness of each medication administration record (MAR) with prescriber's original medication order. Check patient's name, drug name and dosage, route of administration, and time for administration. Recopy or reprint any portion of printed MAR that

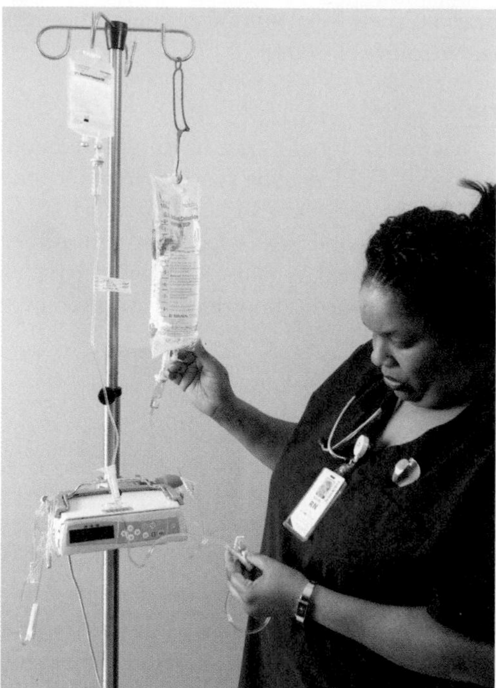

FIG 23-16 Mini-infusion pump.

is difficult to read. *Rationale: The prescriber's order is the most reliable source and only legal record of drugs patient is to receive. Ensures that patient receives the right medications. Handwritten MARs are a source of medication errors (Eisenhauer and others, 2007; Furukawa and others, 2008).*

2. Assess patient's medical and medication history. *Rationale: Identifies need for medication.*
3. Collect drug reference information necessary to administer drug safely, including action, purpose, side effects, normal dose, time of peak onset, how slowly to give the medication, and nursing implications such as the need to dilute the medication or administer it through a filter. *Rationale: Knowledge of medication allows you to give medication safely and monitor patient's response to therapy.*
4. If you give medication through existing IV line, determine compatibility of medication with IV fluids and any additives within IV solution. *Rationale: IV medication is sometimes not compatible with IV solution and/or additives.*

SAFETY ALERT Never administer IV medications through tubing that is infusing blood, blood products, or parenteral nutrition solutions.

5. Assess patency of patient's existing IV infusion line (see Chapter 28). *Rationale: Do not administer medication if site is edematous or inflamed.*
6. Assess patient's history of medication allergies, known type of allergens, and normal allergic reaction. *Rationale: IV administration of medications may cause rapid response. Allergic response is immediate.*
7. Assess patient's symptoms before initiating medication therapy. *Rationale: Provides information to evaluate desired effect of medication.*
8. Assess patient's knowledge of medication.

PLANNING

Expected Outcomes focus on safe administration of an IV bolus medication.

1. Medication is administered safely with desired therapeutic effect achieved.
2. Medication infuses within desired time frame.
3. IV site remains intact without signs of swelling, inflammation, symptoms of tenderness at site.
4. Patient explains the purpose and the side effects of medication.

Delegation and Collaboration

The skill of administering IV medications by piggyback, intermittent infusion sets, and mini-infusion pumps cannot be delegated to nursing assistive personnel (NAP). Instruct the NAP about the following:

- Potential medication actions and side effects and reporting their occurrence to the nurse
- Reporting any change in the patient's condition to the nurse
- Reporting any patient complaints of moisture or discomfort around IV insertion site

Equipment

- Adhesive tape (optional)
- Antiseptic swab
- IV pole
- MAR (electronic or in print)
- Puncture-proof container

Piggyback or mini-infusion pump

- Medication prepared in 5- to 250-mL labeled infusion bag or syringe
- Syringe prepared with vial of normal saline flush solution (for saline lock only)
- Short microdrip, macrodrip, or mini-infusion IV tubing set, preferably with needleless system attachment
- Needleless device or stopcocks preferred if available
- Needles (21 or 23 gauge, **only** if stopcocks or other needleless methods are not available)
- Mini-infusion pump if indicated

Volume-control administration set

- Volutrol or Buretrol
- Infusion tubing (may have needleless system attachment)
- Syringe (1 to 20 mL)
- Vial or ampule of ordered medication

IMPLEMENTATION *for* ADMINISTERING INTRAVENOUS MEDICATIONS BY PIGGYBACK, INTERMITTENT INFUSION, AND MINI-INFUSION PUMPS

STEP	RATIONALE
1. Prepare medication using aseptic technique (see Skill 23.1). Check the label of medication with the MAR two times while preparing medication.	Ensures medication is sterile. *First and second checks for accuracy* ensure that the correct medication is administered.
2. Take medication to patient at correct time, within 30 minutes before or after prescribed time (see agency policy). Give stat and single-order medications at the exact time ordered.	Ensures intended therapeutic effect.
3. See Standard Protocol (inside front cover).	
4. Identify patient using two identifiers (e.g., name and birthday or name and account number, according to facility policy). Compare identifiers with information on patient's MAR or medical record.	Ensures correct patient. Complies with The Joint Commission standards and improves patient safety (TJC, 2010).
5. At the bedside again compare the MAR or computer printout with the names of medications on the medication labels. Ask patient if he or she has allergies.	*This is the third check for accuracy* and ensures that patient receives correct medication. Confirms patient's allergy history.
6. Discuss the purpose of each medication, action, and possible adverse effects. Allow patient to ask any questions. Explain that you will give medication through existing IV line. Encourage patient to report symptoms of discomfort at site.	Keeps patient informed of planned therapies, minimizing anxiety. Patients who verbalize pain at the IV site help detect IV infiltrations early, lessening damage to surrounding tissues.
7. Administer infusion.	
a. Piggyback infusion:	
(1) Connect infusion tubing to medication bag (see Chapter 28). Fill tubing by opening regulator flow clamp. Once tubing is full, close clamp and cap end of tubing.	Filling infusion tubing with solution and freeing air bubbles prevent air embolus.
(2) Hang piggyback medication bag above level of primary fluid bag (see illustration). (Use hook to lower main bag.)	Height of fluid bag affects rate of flow to patient.

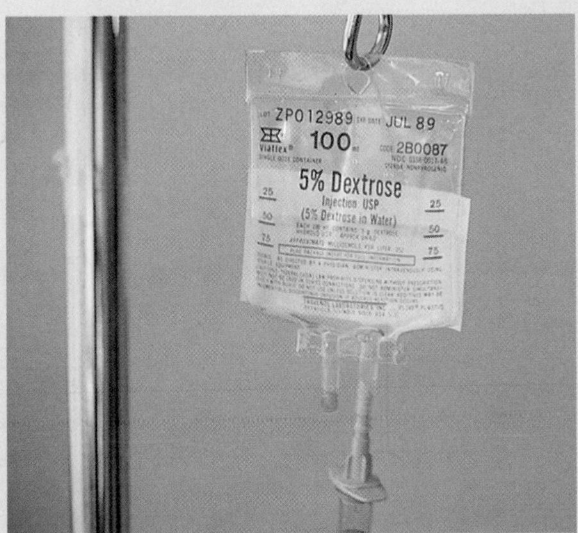

STEP 7a(2) Small-volume minibag for piggyback infusion.

STEP	RATIONALE
(3) Connect tubing of piggyback infusion to appropriate connector on upper Y-port of primary infusion line.	Connection allows IV medication to enter main IV line.

Continued

STEP	RATIONALE
(a) *Needleless system:* Wipe off needleless port of main IV with alcohol swab, allow to dry, and insert tip of piggyback infusion tubing (see illustrations).	Use needleless connections to prevent accidental needlestick injuries (OSHA, 2009).

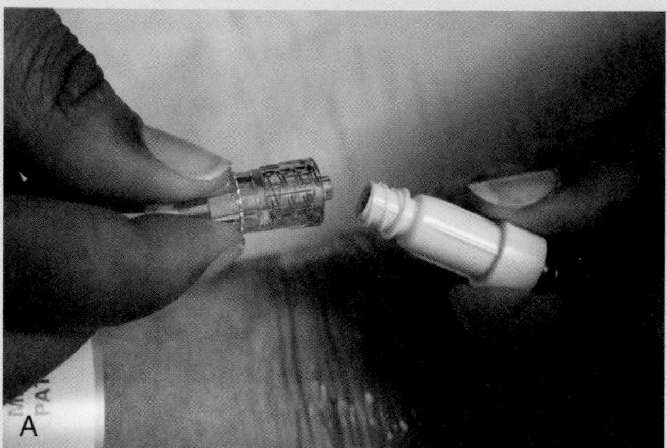

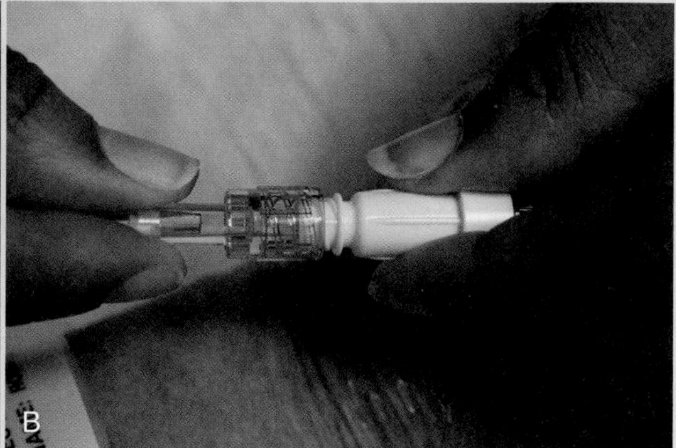

STEP 7a(3)(a) A and **B,** Needleless lock cannula system.

STEP	RATIONALE
(b) *Stopcock:* Wipe off stopcock port with alcohol swab, allow to dry, and connect tubing. Turn stopcock to open position.	Stopcock eliminates need for needle.
(c) *Tubing port:* Connect sterile needle to end of piggyback infusion tubing. Remove needle cap, cleanse injection port on main IV line with alcohol swab, allow to dry, and insert needle through center of port. Secure by taping connection.	Only use this method if needleless system is unavailable. Prevents introduction of microorganisms during needle insertion.
(4) *Option*: Saline lock: Follow Steps 8a(1) through 8b(6) in Skill 23.5 to flush and prepare lock. Wipe off port with alcohol swab, let dry, and insert tip of piggyback infusion tubing via needleless access.	Flushing of lock ensures patency.
(5) Regulate flow rate of medication solution by adjusting regulator clamp or IV pump infusion rate (see Chapter 28). Infusion times vary. Refer to medication reference or agency policy for safe flow rate.	Provides slow, safe infusion of medication and maintains therapeutic blood levels.
(6) Once medication has infused:	
(a) *Continuous infusion:* Check flow rate on primary infusion. The primary infusion automatically begins to flow after the piggyback solution is empty. If stopcock is used, turn stopcock to off position.	Back-check valve on piggyback stops flow of the primary infusion until medication infuses. Checking flow rate ensures proper administration of IV fluids.
(b) *Normal saline lock:* Disconnect tubing, cleanse port with alcohol, and flush IV line with 2 to 3 mL of sterile 0.9% sodium chloride. Maintain sterility of IV tubing between intermittent infusions.	
(7) Regulate continuous main infusion line to ordered rate.	Infusion of piggyback sometimes interferes with main line infusion rate.
(8) Leave IV piggyback bag and tubing in place for future drug administration (see agency policy) or discard in appropriate containers.	Establishing secondary line produces route for microorganisms to enter main line. Repeated changes in tubing increase risk of infection transmission (check agency policy).

STEP	RATIONALE
b. Volume-control administration set (e.g., Volutrol):	
(1) Fill Volutrol with desired amount of fluid (50 to 100 mL) by opening clamp between Volutrol and main IV bag (see illustration).	Small volume of fluid dilutes IV medication and reduces risk of fluid infusing too rapidly.
(2) Close clamp and check to be sure that clamp on air vent of Volutrol chamber is open.	Prevents additional leakage of fluid into Volutrol. Air vent allows fluid to exit at regulated rate.
(3) Clean injection port on top of Volutrol with antiseptic swab.	Prevents introduction of microorganisms during needle insertion.
(4) Remove needle cap or sheath and insert needleless syringe or syringe needle through port and inject medication (see illustration). Gently rotate Volutrol between hands.	Rotating mixes medication with solution to ensure equal distribution in Volutrol.
(5) Regulate IV infusion rate to allow medication to infuse in time recommended by agency policy, a pharmacist, or a medication reference manual.	For optimal therapeutic effect, drug needs to infuse in prescribed time interval.
(6) Label Volutrol with name of drug, dosage, total volume including diluent, and time of administration following ISMP (2008) safe IV medication label format.	Alerts nurses to medication being infused. Prevents other medications from being added to Volutrol.
(7) If patient is receiving a continuous IV infusion, check continuous infusion after Volutrol infusion is complete to ensure appropriate rate of IV fluid administration.	Ensures appropriate fluid balance.
(8) Dispose of uncapped needle or needle enclosed in safety shield and syringe in proper container.	Prevents accidental needlesticks.
c. Mini-infusion administration:	
(1) Connect prefilled syringe to mini-infusion tubing.	Special tubing designed to fit syringe delivers medication to main IV line.
(2) Carefully apply pressure to syringe plunger, allowing tubing to fill with medication.	Ensures that tubing is free of air bubbles to prevent air embolus.

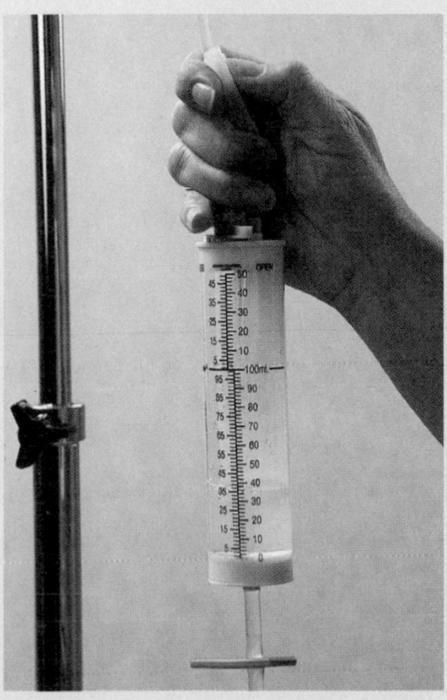

STEP 7b(1) Filling volume control device.

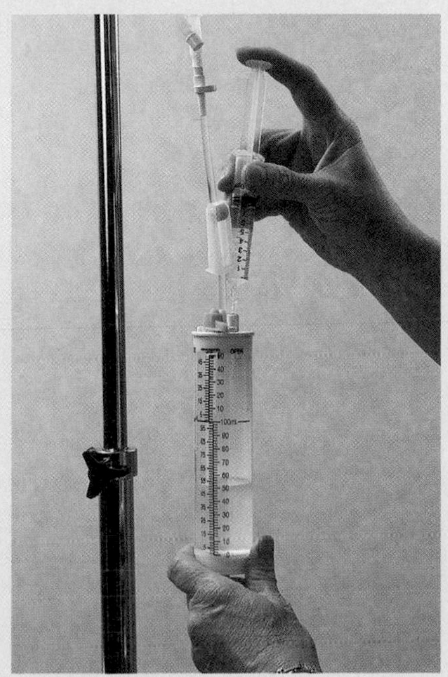

STEP 7b(4) Injecting medication into Volutrol.

Continued

STEP	RATIONALE
(3) Place syringe into mini-infusion pump (follow product directions) and hang on IV pole. Be sure that syringe is secured (see illustration).	Correct placement is necessary for proper infusion.

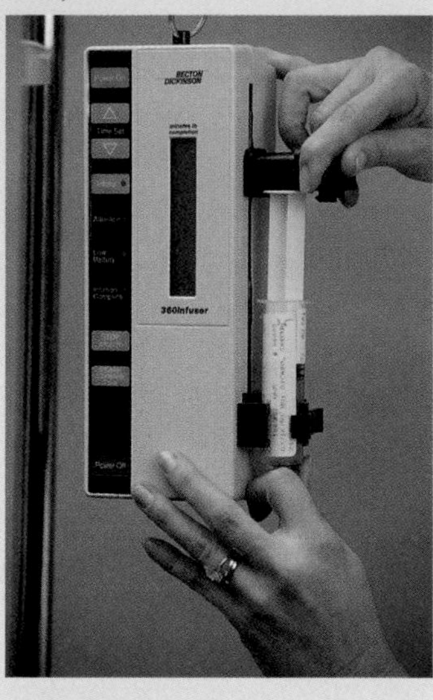

STEP 7c(3) Ensure that syringe is secure after placing it into mini-infusion pump.

STEP	RATIONALE
(4) Connect end of mini-infusion tubing to main IV line or saline lock.	
(a) *Needleless system:* Wipe off needleless port of IV tubing with alcohol swab, let dry, and insert tip of the mini-infusion tubing through center of port.	OSHA recommends needleless system to reduce risk of needlestick injuries (2007).
(b) *Stopcock:* Wipe off stopcock port on continuous infusion tubing with alcohol swab, let dry, and connect tubing. Turn stopcock to open position.	Stopcock reduces risk of needlestick injuries.
(c) *Needle system:* Connect sterile needle to mini-infusion tubing, remove cap, cleanse injection port on main IV line with alcohol swab, let dry, and insert needle through center of port. Consider placing tape where IV tubing enters port to keep connection secured.	Use this method only if needleless system is not available.
(d) *Saline lock:* Follow Steps 8a(1) through 8b(6) in Skill 23.5 to flush and prepare lock. Wipe off port with alcohol swab, allow to dry, and insert tip of mini-infusion tubing.	
(5) Set pump to deliver medication within time recommended by agency policy, a pharmacist, or a medication reference manual. Press button on pump to begin infusion.	Pump automatically delivers medication at safe, constant rate based on volume in syringe.
(6) Once medication has infused:	
Main IV infusion: Check flow rate. The infusion automatically begins to flow once the pump stops. Regulate infusion to desired rate as needed. (NOTE: If using a stopcock, turn off mini-infusion line and restart continuous infusion.)	Maintains patency of primary IV line.
Normal saline lock: Disconnect the tubing, cleanse the port with alcohol, and flush the IV line with 2 to 3 mL of sterile 0.9% sodium chloride.	

STEP	RATIONALE
(7) Dispose of supplies in puncture- and leak-proof container.	Prevents accidental needlesticks (OSHA, 2009).
8. See Completion Protocol (inside front cover).	
9. Stay with patient for several minutes and observe for any allergic reactions.	Dyspnea, wheezing, and circulatory collapse are signs of severe anaphylactic reaction.

EVALUATION

1. Assess patient's status after giving medication.
2. Observe patient for signs of adverse reactions.
3. During infusion periodically check infusion rate and condition of IV site.
4. Ask patient to explain purpose and side effects of medication.

Unexpected Outcomes and Related Interventions

1. Patient develops adverse drug reaction.
   a. Stop medication infusion immediately.
   b. Follow agency policy for appropriate response and reporting of adverse drug reactions.
   c. Add allergy information to patient's medical record.
2. Medication does not infuse over desired period.
   a. Determine reason (e.g., improper calculation of flow rate, poor positioning of IV needle at insertion site, infiltration).
   b. Take corrective action as indicated.
3. Intravenous site shows symptoms of infiltration or phlebitis (see Chapter 28).
   a. Stop infusion immediately and discontinue access device.
   b. Treat IV site as indicated by agency policy.
   c. For infiltration determine how harmful the IV medication is to subcutaneous tissue. Provide IV extravasation care (e.g., injecting phentolamine [Regitine] around the IV infiltration site) as indicated by agency policy or consult pharmacist to determine appropriate follow-up care.

Recording and Reporting

- Record drug, dose, route, infusion rate, and date and time administered on MAR immediately after administration, not before. Include initials or signature.
- Record volume of fluid in medication bag or Volutrol as fluid intake.
- Report any adverse reactions to patient's health care provider.

Sample Documentation

1600 Lasix (furosemide) 10 mg IV via mini-infusion started. IV insertion site left forearm free from redness, pain, or edema. Primary IV $D_5\frac{1}{2}$ normal saline infusing at 100 mL/hr without difficulty.

Special Considerations

Pediatric

- Infants and young children are more vulnerable to alterations in fluid balance and do not adjust quickly to changes in fluid balance. Monitor intake and output carefully when infusing intravenous medications (Hockenberry and Wilson, 2009).

Geriatric

- Altered pharmacokinetics of medications and the effects of polypharmacy place older adults at risk for medication toxicity. Carefully monitor the response of older adults to IV medication therapy (Aschenbrenner and Venable, 2009).
- Older adults are at risk for developing fluid volume overload and require careful assessment for signs of overload and heart failure.

Home Care

- Patients or family caregivers who administer IV medications at home require education about the steps of medication administration. The patient or family caregiver needs to perform several return demonstrations of IV medication administration before performing this skill independently. In addition, patients and family caregivers need to know signs of IV medication administration complications such as phlebitis and infiltration and what to do for any problems.

SKILL 23.7 ADMINISTERING CONTINUOUS SUBCUTANEOUS MEDICATIONS

The continuous subcutaneous infusion (CSQI or CSCI) route of medication administration is used for selected medications (e.g., opioids, insulin). The route is also effective with medications to stop preterm labor (e.g., terbutaline [Brethine]) and to treat pulmonary hypertension (e.g., treprostinil sodium [Remodulin]). One factor that determines the infusion rate of CSQI is the rate of medication absorption. Most patients can absorb 3 to 5 mL/hr of medication (Justad, 2009).

With CSQI patients are able to manage their illness and/or pain without the risks and expenses involved with IV medication administration. This route is relatively easy for patients and families to learn and understand in the home setting. CSQI improves oncologic and postoperative pain control in

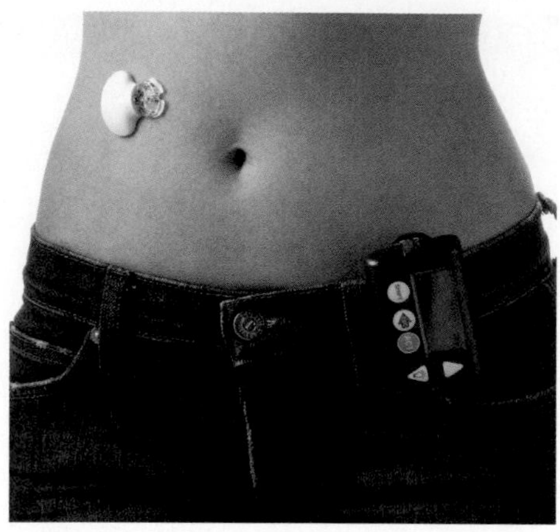

FIG 23-17 MiniMed Paradigm REAL-Time Insulin CSQI Pump and Continuous Glucose Monitoring System. (Courtesy Medtronic MiniMed, Northridge, Calif.)

different patients, including infants, children, and adults (Cope and others, 2008; Justad, 2009; Morton, 2007).

Patients with diabetes using CSQI for management of blood glucose levels receive intense diabetes self-management education from qualified diabetic educators and insulin pump trainers. The newest system integrates an insulin pump with real-time continuous glucose monitoring (Fig. 23-17) (Medtronic MiniMed, 2009). Patients with diabetes using insulin pumps generally require less insulin because insulin is absorbed and used more efficiently (Jakisch and others, 2008).

The procedure to initiate and discontinue CSQI therapy is similar, regardless of the type of medication being delivered. However, nursing assessment and interventions vary, depending on the type of medication administered. For example, if the medication is for diabetes glucose management, you evaluate the patient's blood glucose levels and episodes of hypoglycemia or hyperglycemia (Weissberg-Benchell and others, 2007).

Use a small-gauge (25 to 27) winged butterfly IV needle or special commercially prepared Teflon cannula to deliver medications. Although Teflon cannulas are generally more expensive, they tend to be more comfortable and have lower rates of complications than winged IV needles. They are associated with fewer needlestick injuries. Base the choice of needle type on institutional guidelines or patient preference. Use the needle with the shortest length and the smallest gauge needed to start and maintain the infusion.

Use the same anatomical sites as for subcutaneous injections and the upper chest (see Skill 23.2). Site selection depends on the patient's activity level and the type of medication. For example, pain medications given to ambulatory patients are best delivered in the upper chest, which allows the patient to move freely. Insulin is absorbed most consistently in the abdomen; thus choose a site in the abdomen away from the waistline. Always avoid sites where the tubing of the pump could be disturbed. Rotate sites at least every 72 hours or whenever complications such as leaking occur (INS, 2006; Medtronic MiniMed, 2009).

The CSQI route requires a computerized pump with safety features, including lockout intervals and warning alarms. Ideally medication pumps are individualized based on the medication being delivered and the patient's needs. You also need to consider the availability and cost of the pump and its supplies. When possible, have patients select the pump that fits their individual and home needs and is easiest to use.

ASSESSMENT

1. Check accuracy and completeness of each medication administration record (MAR) with prescriber's original medication order. Check patient's name, drug name and dosage, route of administration, and time for administration. Recopy or reprint any portion of printed MAR that is difficult to read. *Rationale: The prescriber's order is the most reliable source and only legal record of drugs patient is to receive. Ensures that patient receives the right medications. Handwritten MARs are a source of medication errors (Eisenhauer and others, 2007; Furukawa and others, 2008).*
2. Assess patient's medical and medication history. *Rationale: Identifies need for medication.*
3. Collect drug reference information necessary to administer drug safely, including action, purpose, side effects, normal dose, time of peak onset, how slowly to give the medication, and nursing implications. *Rationale: Knowledge of medication allows you to give medication safely and monitor patient's response to therapy.*
4. Assess for contraindications to CSQI (e.g., thrombocytopenia or reduced local tissue perfusion). *Rationale: Reduced tissue perfusion interferes with medication absorption and distribution.*
5. Assess adequacy of patient's adipose tissue to determine appropriate site. *Rationale: Physiological changes of aging or effect of illness on subcutaneous tissue affects choice of catheter insertion site.*
6. Assess patient's history of medication allergies, known type of allergens, and normal allergic reaction. *Rationale: CSQI administration of medications may cause rapid response. Allergic response is immediate.*
7. Assess patient's symptoms before initiating medication therapy. Determine severity of pain (if using analgesia) or measure blood glucose level (if using insulin). *Rationale: Provides information to evaluate desired effect of medication.*
8. Assess patient's knowledge of medication and medication delivered CSQI. *Rationale: Provides information about patient's understanding of medication and delivery device.*

PLANNING

Expected Outcomes focus on safe administration of CSQI.

1. Needle insertion site remains free from infection.
2. Patient achieves desired effect of medication with no signs of adverse reactions.

3. Patient explains purpose, dosage, and effects of medication and verbalizes understanding of CSQI therapy.

Delegation and Collaboration

The skill of administering CSQI medications cannot be delegated to nursing assistive personnel (NAP). Instruct the NAP about the following:

- Potential medication side effects or reactions and reporting their occurrence to the nurse
- Reporting complications (e.g., leaking, redness, discomfort) at the CSQI needle insertion site to the nurse
- Obtaining any required vital signs and reporting them to the nurse

Equipment

Initiation of CSQI

- Clean gloves
- Alcohol swab
- Antibacterial skin preparation such as chlorhexidine
- Small (25 to 27)–gauge winged IV catheter with attached tubing or CSQI-designed catheter (e.g., Sof-set)
- Infusion pump
- Occlusive, transparent dressing
- Tape
- Medication in appropriate syringe or container

Discontinuing CSQI

- Clean gloves
- Small, sterile gauze dressing
- Tape or adhesive bandage
- Alcohol swab and chlorhexidine (optional)
- Puncture-proof container

IMPLEMENTATION *for* ADMINISTERING CONTINUOUS SUBCUTANEOUS MEDICATIONS

STEP	RATIONALE
1. Review manufacturer's directions for pump.	Ensures proper use of equipment.
2. Prepare medication using aseptic technique (see Skill 23.1) or check dose on prefilled syringe. Connect syringe and prime tubing with medication being careful not to lose any medication. Compare label of the medication with the MAR.	Ensures that medication is sterile. Checking the label of the medication with transcribed order reduces error. *First check for accuracy* ensures that the correct medication is administered.
3. Obtain and program medication administration pump. Place syringe in pump.	Ensures that medication dose administered is accurate.
4. Read label on prefilled syringe and compare with MAR.	*This is the second check for accuracy.*
5. Take medications to patient at correct time, within 30 minutes before or after prescribed time (see agency policy). Give stat and single-order medications at the exact time ordered.	Ensures that patient will experience medication effects at right time.
6. See Standard Protocol (inside front cover).	
7. Identify patient using two identifiers (e.g., name and birthday or name and account number, according to facility policy). Compare identifiers with information on patient's MAR or medical record.	Ensures correct patient. Complies with The Joint Commission standards and improves patient safety (TJC, 2010).
8. At the bedside again compare the MAR or computer printout with the names of medications on the medication labels. Ask patient if he or she has allergies.	*This is the third check for accuracy* and ensures that patient receives correct medication. Confirms patient's allergy history.
9. Discuss the purpose of each medication, action, and possible adverse effects. Allow patient to ask any questions. Tell patient that needle insertion will cause slight burning or stinging.	Patient has the right to be informed, and patient's understanding of each medication improves adherence with drug therapy.
10. Initiate CSQI.	
a. Assist patient to comfortable position.	Eases pain associated with insertion of needle.
b. Select appropriate insertion site free of irritation and away from bony prominences and waistline. Most common sites are subclavicular and abdomen.	Ensures proper medication absorption.
c. Cleanse injection site with alcohol using a circular motion, followed by antiseptic, using straight cleansing strokes. Allow both agents to dry.	Reduces risk of infection at insertion site.

Continued

STEP	RATIONALE
d. Hold needle in dominant hand and remove needle guard.	Prepares needle for insertion.
e. Gently pinch or lift up skin with nondominant hand.	Ensures that needle will enter subcutaneous tissue.
f. Gently and firmly insert needle at a 45- to 90-degree angle (see illustration). Some shorter prepackaged needles (e.g., Sof-Set, Subcutaneous-Set) are inserted at a 90-degree angle. Refer to manufacturer's directions.	Decreases pain related to insertion of needle.
g. Release skin fold and apply tape over "wings" of needle.	Secures needle.

SAFETY ALERT Some cannulas have a sharp needle covered with a plastic catheter. In this case remove the needle and leave the plastic catheter in the skin.

STEP	RATIONALE
h. Place occlusive, transparent dressing over insertion site (see illustration).	Protects site from infection and allows you to assess site during medication infusion.
i. Attach tubing from needle to tubing from infusion pump and turn on pump.	Allows you to administer medication.
j. Dispose of any sharps in appropriate leak- and puncture-proof container.	Prevents accidental needlestick injuries and follows CDC guidelines for disposal of sharps (OSHA, 2009).
k. Assess site before leaving patient and instruct patient to inform you if site becomes red or begins to leak.	Initiate a new site with a new needle whenever erythema or leaking occurs. If the site is free from complications, rotate the needle every 3 to 5 days (INS, 2006).
11. Stay with patient for several minutes and observe for any allergic reactions.	Dyspnea, wheezing, and circulatory collapse are signs of severe anaphylactic reaction.
12. Discontinue CSQI.	
a. Verify order and establish alternative method for medication administration if applicable.	If medication will be required after discontinuing CSQI, a different medication and/or route is often necessary to continue to manage patient's illness or pain.
b. Stop infusion pump.	Prevents medication from spilling.
c. Perform hand hygiene.	Follows CDC recommendations to prevent accidental exposure to blood and body fluids (OSHA, 2009).
d. Remove dressing without dislodging or removing the needle.	Exposes needle.

SAFETY ALERT If site is infected or if included in institutional guidelines, cleanse site with alcohol and antiseptic. Apply triple antibiotic cream to site if it is excoriated (abraded).

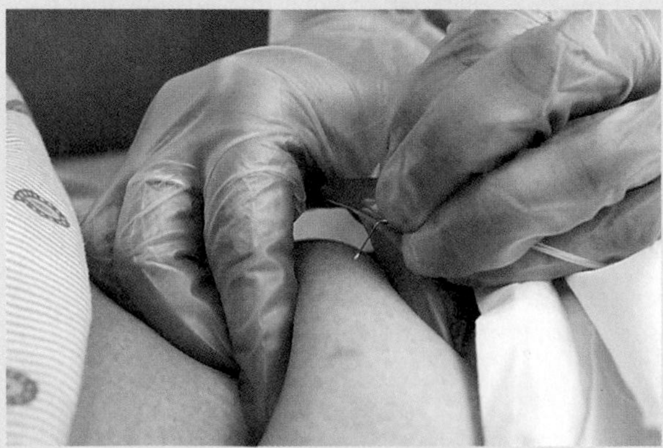

STEP 10f Insertion of needle into subcutaneous tissue of abdomen.

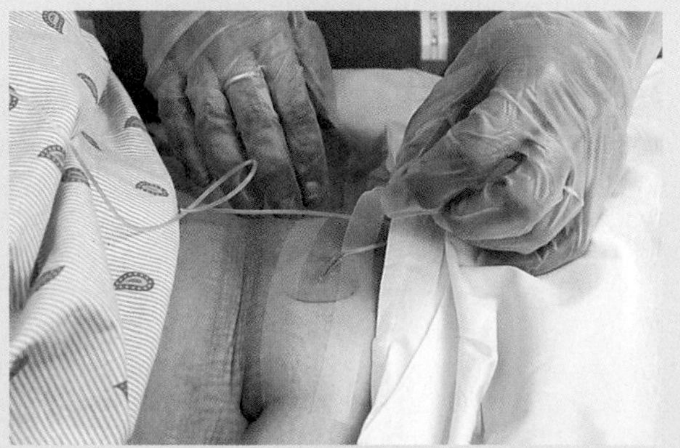

STEP 10h Securing injection site.

STEP	RATIONALE
e. Remove tape from the wings of needle and pull needle out at the same angle it was inserted.	Minimizes patient discomfort.
f. Apply gentle pressure at site until no fluid leaks out of skin.	Dressing adheres to site if skin remains dry.
g. Apply small sterile gauze dressing or adhesive bandage to site.	Prevents bacterial entry into puncture site.
13. Dispose of uncapped needles and syringe in puncture- and leak-proof container.	Prevents accidental needlestick injuries and follows CDC guidelines for disposal of sharps (OSHA, 2009).
14. See Completion Protocol (inside front cover).	

EVALUATION

1. Evaluate patient's response to medication.
2. Assess site at least every 4 hours for redness, pain, drainage, or swelling.
3. Ask patient to verbalize understanding of medication and CSQI therapy.

Unexpected Outcomes and Related Interventions

1. Patient complains of localized pain or burning at insertion site of needle or site appears red or swollen or is leaking, indicating potential infection or needle dislodgement.
   a. Remove needle and place new needle in a different site.
   b. Continue to monitor original site for signs of infection and notify health care provider if you suspect infection.
2. Patient displays signs of allergic reaction to medication.
   a. Stop delivering medication immediately and follow agency policy for appropriate response (e.g., administration of antihistamine or epinephrine) and reporting of adverse drug reactions.
   b. Notify patient's health care provider of adverse effects immediately.
   c. Add allergy information to patient's medical record per agency policy.
3. CSQI becomes dislodged.
   a. Stop the infusion, apply pressure at the site until no fluid leaks out of skin, cover site with a gauze dressing or adhesive bandage, and initiate a new site.
   b. Assess patient to determine effects of not receiving medication (e.g., assess patient's pain level using age-appropriate pain scale, obtain blood glucose level).

Recording and Reporting

- After initiating CSQI, immediately chart medication, dose, route, site, time, date, and type of medication pump in patient's medical record. Use initials or signature.
- If medication is an opioid, follow agency policy to document waste.
- Record patient's response to medication and appearance of site every 4 hours or according to agency policy in nurses' notes.
- Report any adverse effects from medication or infection at insertion site to patient's health care provider and document according to agency policy. Patient's condition often indicates need for additional medical therapy.

Sample Documentation

1400 CSQI initiated with 25-gauge Teflon catheter in RLQ of abdomen. Infusing morphine sulfate at 0.05 mg per hour. Site free from redness and edema.

Special Considerations

Pediatric

- CSQI improves glycemic control in children and adolescents. There is a decreased rate of severe hypoglycemia, catheter-site infection, and weight gain (Cope and others, 2008). Parents experience higher levels of confidence and independence in diabetes management with appropriate education and guidance (Weissberg-Benchell and others, 2007).
- Insulin pumps offer flexibility for adolescents, placing the responsibility of diabetes management on the child. Extensive child and family education is needed in using CSQI (Hockenberry and Wilson, 2009).

Home Care

- Patients in the home using CSQI need a responsible family caregiver if available. Educate the patient or family caregiver about the desired effect of the medication, side effects and adverse effects of the medication, operation of the pump, how to evaluate the effectiveness of the medication, when and how to assess and rotate insertion sites, and when to call a health care provider for problems. Patients need to know where and how to obtain and dispose of all required supplies.
- Patients managing CSQI at home may use an antibacterial soap (e.g., Hibiclens, PhisoHex) instead of alcohol and chlorhexidine to cleanse insertion site.

REVIEW QUESTIONS

1. The nurse is preparing to care for a patient with a newly diagnosed thrombophlebitis who is scheduled to receive heparin 5000 units subcutaneously now and every 8 hours. The heparin comes from the pharmacy as a multidose vial. What does the nurse need to know about the medication and vial before administering?
2. The nurse finds that, in addition to heparin, her patient is also receiving morphine sulfate 1 mg IV push every 8 hours as needed for pain. The patient has no allergies, and the nurse has reviewed medication references and the health care provider's order. What additional factors does the nurse need to assess before administering the morphine?
3. The nurse is mixing two medications in one syringe. One medication is in a vial, and the other is in an ampule. Which is the initial correct step to prepare the medication?
   1. Check the volume of medication in syringe.
   2. Draw up medication from the ampule first.
   3. Shake the medication in the vial to ensure that there is no cloudiness.
   4. Draw up the medication from the vial first.
4. Which of the following assessment findings indicates a positive TB reaction in a patient with no known risk factors for TB?
   1. A large area of redness and swelling at the injection site
   2. An induration of 18 mm
   3. Frequent, productive cough accompanied by a fever
   4. Sudden onset of shortness of breath and wheezing
5. Which of the following symptoms may indicate that a patient has sustained an injury to a nerve after an IM injection?
   1. Pain, numbness, and tingling at the injection site 2 hours after the injection
   2. Pain experienced during the injection
   3. Urticaria, eczema, wheezing, and dyspnea
   4. Nausea, vomiting, and diarrhea
6. Match the best needle size to use when administering an injection in each situation listed.
   1. 25-gauge, ⅝- to 1-inch ______
   2. 22-gauge, 1½-inch _______
   3. 27-gauge, ⅜ inch ______

   a. Intradermal Mantoux test
   b. Children older than 1 year
   c. Average size 30-year-old female
7. A patient is to receive a subcutaneous injection of heparin. The patient is 5 feet, 2 inches tall and weighs 135 pounds. The nurse plans to administer the injection in the abdomen. The most appropriate needle size to use for this injection is:
   1. 18 gauge, 1¼ inch
   2. 20 gauge, 1 inch
   3. 22 gauge, 1½ inch
   4. 25 gauge, ½ inch
8. The nurse needs to reconstitute a medication for a subcutaneous injection. Which action would indicate the procedure is completed correctly?
   1. She shakes the vial after the fluid is injected into the vial to mix it completely.
   2. She determines the amount of prepared medication and concentration before adding the appropriate diluent.
   3. The powder is injected into the vial of diluent.
   4. She evaluates the concentration after the diluent and powder are mixed.
9. When you assess your patient's intravenous site, before giving an IV push medication, you note that it is cool, pale and swollen. What should you do?
   1. Stop the IV infusion and change it to another site.
   2. Slow the rate of the IV infusion.
   3. Flush the IV line with a normal saline flush.
   4. Take off the IV dressing and place a new one on that is not as tight.
10. What is the most important action for the nurse to implement before giving an IV push medication?
    1. Assess the IV insertion site.
    2. Stop the primary (maintenance) fluid infusion.
    3. Dilute the medication to minimize vein irritation.
    4. Ensure that the correct filter needle is used to withdraw the medication from the vial.

REFERENCES

American Diabetes Association (ADA): Standards of medical care in diabetes-2007, *Diabetes Care* 30(suppl 1):S4, 2007.

American Diabetes Association (ADA): Insulin administration: position statement, *Diabetes Care* 27(suppl 1):S106, 2004.

Alexander M and others: *Infusion nursing: an evidence-based approach*, ed 3, St Louis, 2009, Elsevier.

American Nurses Association (ANA): *2008 study of nurses' views on workplace safety and needlestick injuries*, Washington, DC, 2009, ANA, http://www.nursingworld.org/MainMenuCategories/OccupationalandEnvironmental/occupationalhealth/SafeNeedles/2008InviroStudy.aspx.

Aschenbrenner D: Unsafe injection practices put patients at risk, *Am J Nurs* 109(7):45, 2009.

Aschenbrenner D, Venable S: *Drug therapy in nursing*, ed 3, Philadelphia, 2009, Lippincott, Williams & Wilkins.

Centers for Disease Control and Prevention (CDC): TB treatment guidelines, 2009, http://www.cdc.gov/tb/, accessed August 2009.

Cocoman A, Murray J: Intramuscular injection: a review of best practices for mental health nurses, *J Psychiatric Mental Health Nurs* 15(5):424, 2008.

Cope J and others: Adolescent use of insulin and patient-controlled analgesia pump technology: a 10-year food and drug administration retrospective study of adverse events, *Pediatrics* 121(5):1133, 2008.

Environmental Protection Agency (EPA): New information about disposing of medical sharps, October 2004, http://www.epa.gov/osw/nonhaz/industrial/medical/med-govt.pdf, accessed August 2009.

Eisenhauer LA and others: Nurses' reported thinking during medication administration, *J Nurs Sch* 39(1):82, 2007.

Furukawa MF and others: Adoption of health information technology for medication safety in U.S. hospitals, 2006, *Health Affairs* 27(3):865, 2008.

Hockenberry MJ, Wilson D: *Wong's essentials of pediatric nursing*, ed 8, St Louis, 2009, Mosby.

Hunter J: Intramuscular injection technique, *Nurs Stand* 22(24):35, 2008a.

Hunter J: Subcutaneous injection technique, *Nurs Stand* 22(21):41, 2008b.

Infusion Nurses Society: Infusion nursing standards of practice, *J Infus Nurs* 29(1 Suppl):S1, 2006.

Institute of Safe Medication Practices (ISMP): Principles of designing a medication label for intravenous piggyback medication for patient specific, inpatient use, 2008, http://www.ismp.org/tools/guidelines/labelFormats/IVPB.asp, accessed September 14, 2010.

Jakisch B and others: Comparison of continuous subcutaneous insulin (CSII) and multiple daily injections (MDI) in pediatric type I diabetes: a multicentre matched-pair cohort analysis over 3 years, *Diabetic Med* 25(1):80, 2008.

Justad M: Continuous subcutaneous infusion: an efficacious, cost-effective analgesia alternative at the end of life, *Home Healthcare Nurse* 27(3):140, 2009.

LePorte L and others: Effect of a distraction-free environment n medication errors, *Am J Health-System Pharmacy* 66(9):795, 2009.

Medtronic MiniMed: MiniMed Paradigm REAL-Time Insulin Pump and Continuous Glucose Monitoring System, 2009, http://www.minimed.com/products/insulinpumps, accessed August 2009.

Morton N: Management of postoperative pain in children, *Arch Dis Childh* 92:14, 2007.

Ng C and others: *Ethno-psychopharmacology: advances in current practice*, New York, 2008, Cambridge University Press.

Novo Nordisk: Levimir, 2008, http://www.levemir-us.com, accessed August, 2009.

Occupational Safety and Health Administration (OSHA): *Bloodborne pathogens and needlestick injuries*, 2009, http://www.osha.gov/SLTC/bloodbornepathogens/index.html, accessed August 2009.

Ramtahal J and others: Sciatic nerve injury following intramuscular injection: a care report and review of the literature, *J Neurosci Nurs* 38(4):238, 2006.

Sanofi-Aventis: Dosing and administration of Lovenox, March 2010, http://www.lovenox.com/hcp/dosingAdministration/default.aspx, accessed September 14, 2010.

Schechter NL and others: Pain reduction during pediatric immunizations: evidence-based review and recommendations, *Pediatrics* 119(5):1184, 2007.

Schim S: Culturally congruent care, *J Transcultural Nursing* 18(2):103, 2007.

Shih-Wen H: Evaluating the results of teaching epinephrine auto-injector use in an allergy clinic, *Pediatr Asthma Allergy Immunol* 20(1):19, 2007.

The Joint Commission: *2010 National Patient Safety Goals*, Oakbrook Terrace, Ill, 2010, The Commission, http://www.jointcommission.org/PatientSafety/NationalPatientSafetyGoals/.

Weissberg-Benchell J and others: The use of continuous subcutaneous insulin infusion (CSII): Parental and professional perceptions of self-care master and autonomy in children and adolescents, *J Pediatr Psychol* 32(7):1, 2007.

Wesolowski C: Preventing medication errors in hospitalized children, *Am J Health-System Pharmacy* 66(3):287, 2009.

Wolf Z: Pursuing safe medication use and the promise of technology, *MedSurg Nurs* 16(2):92, 2007.

Zaybak A and others: Does obesity prevent the needle from reaching muscle in intramuscular injections, *J Adv Nurs* 58(6):552, 2007.

CHAPTER

24

Wound Care and Irrigation

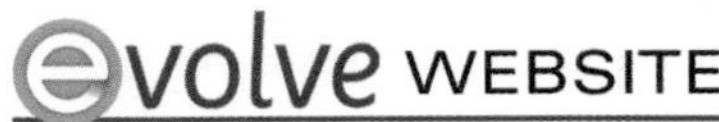

http://evolve.elsevier.com/Perry/nursinginterventions
Video Clips
Nursing Skills Online

Proper wound care promotes wound healing that results in an intact skin layer (Fig. 24-1). Nurses play a vital role in the management of a patient with a wound. Wound healing is extremely complex, involving a series of physiological processes among cells and tissues. The location, severity, and extent of the injury and the tissue layer(s) involved all affect the wound healing process (Doughty and Sparks-Defriese, 2007). Likewise, the rate of healing depends on numerous internal and external factors (Box 24-1). Effective wound management requires you to understand the processes of wound healing and the factors that may interfere with healing, as well as to know how to perform a comprehensive wound assessment. Assessment of a wound provides you with information needed to recognize changes in a wound so that you can institute appropriate wound care measures. The wound assessment is the foundation for the wound plan of care and helps to determine wound healing progress or deterioration.

A partial-thickness wound (loss of tissue to the epidermis and partial dermis) heals by regeneration. However, a full-thickness wound (total loss of skin layers as well as some deeper tissues) heals by scar formation. In a full-thickness wound, healing occurs in four phases (Box 24-2). Collagen deposition begins during inflammation and peaks during proliferation. It is important for nurses to assess for the buildup of this new tissue. This "healing ridge" is composed of newly formed collagen, and you can usually feel it along a healing wound (Doughty and Sparks-Defriese, 2007). Types of healing are primary, secondary, and tertiary intention (Fig. 24-2). Healing by primary intention occurs when the wound edges of a clean surgical incision remain close together. Wounds left open and allowed to heal by scar formation are classified as healing by secondary intention. Healing by tertiary intention is often called delayed primary intention. It occurs when surgical wounds are not closed immediately but left open for 3 to 5 days to allow edema or infection to diminish. Then the wound edges are stapled or sutured close. The type of wound and the manner in which it heals dictate the types of treatment and wound support required.

PATIENT-CENTERED CARE

Wound assessment is the first essential step in planning wound care. Discuss with your patient and family the importance of a thorough and periodic wound assessment so they understand the need for this procedure. It is important for them to understand that wounds heal in an organized fashion and that the ongoing assessments aid in determining wound progress and treatments. Determine what effect the wound may have from the patient's cultural perspective; for example, some cultures believe that the use of herbs or other folk remedies helps to support wound healing. It is important to be culturally sensitive to the patient's and family's beliefs; for example, some skin substitutes (used in severe wounds) are pork based and may not be acceptable to the Muslim or Jewish patient.

As in all clinical situations, approach wound assessment through the "patient's eyes," especially in the case of chronic wounds. Patients with chronic wounds have often seen multiple care providers and have used various therapies to manage their wounds. Become familiar with what they have used in the past, determine whether the therapies that they use are safe, and if the therapies are not safe, explain why. Always value and apply any expertise patients may have in managing their wound.

SAFETY

When you perform a wound assessment, wound irrigation, emptying of a wound collection device, or removal of staples

BOX 24-1 FACTORS THAT INFLUENCE WOUND HEALING

- With increasing age, the reproductive function of epidermal cells diminishes, replacement is slowed, and the dermis atrophies, which slows wound contraction and increases risk of wound dehiscence (Baranoski and others, 2008a).
- Inadequate nutrition, including proteins, carbohydrates, lipids, vitamins, and minerals, delays tissue repair and increases risk for infection (Posthauer and Thomas, 2008).
- The obese patient is at risk for wound infection and dehiscence or evisceration. Fat tissue has less vascularization, which decreases transport of nutrients and cellular elements required for healing (Colwell and Fichera, 2005).
- A hematocrit value below 20% and a hemoglobin value below 10 g/100 mL negatively influence tissue repair because of decreased oxygen delivery. Oxygen release to tissue is reduced in smokers.
- Impaired wound healing in patients with diabetes results from reduced collagen synthesis and deposition, decreased wound strength, and impaired leukocyte (white blood cell [WBC]) function.
- Wound infection prolongs the inflammatory response, and the micro-organisms use nutrients and oxygen that are intended for repair.
- Long-term steroid therapy and chemotherapy or the use of immunosuppressive medications may diminish the inflammatory response and reduce the healing potential.
- An open wound must be maintained in a moist environment, and a closed wound must be protected from microorganisms and stress.

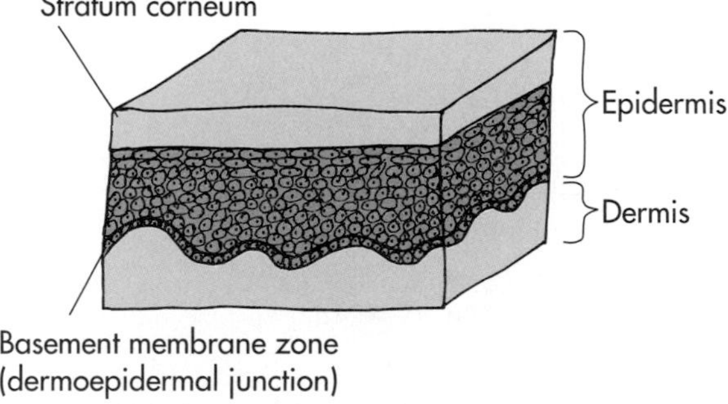

FIG 24-1 Layers of the integument.

or stitches, safety is a priority. One risk to a patient's safety is the risk for infection. When a wound is present, the patient no longer has the protection of intact skin. When you assess the wound or provide wound care, remember to use proper infection control practices to reduce the risk for a wound infection. Improper wound care can contaminate the wound bed with a microorganism, which delays wound healing. When measuring a wound using a wound measuring guide or cotton-tipped applicator, gently insert the guide around the perimeter of the wound so as not to cause any tissue injury, which also delays wound healing. Perform wound irrigation by gently introducing the ordered fluid into the wound to prevent tissue injury. When removing staples or stitches, use the correct instruments to prevent trauma to the newly healed incision.

BOX 24-2 PHASES OF WOUND HEALING (FULL-THICKNESS WOUNDS)

Hemostasis
Blood vessels constrict: clotting factors activate coagulation to stop bleeding. Clot formation seals disrupted vessels so blood loss is controlled and acts as a temporary bacterial barrier. Growth factors are released, which attract cells needed to begin tissue repair.

Inflammation
Vasodilation occurs, allowing plasma and blood cells to leak into a wound, noted as edema, erythema, and exudate. Leukocytes arrive in the wound to begin cleanup. Macrophages appear and regulate the wound repair. The result of inflammation is a clean wound bed in a patient with a noncomplicated wound.

Proliferation
Epithelization (the construction of new epidermis) begins. At the same time new granulation tissue is formed. New capillaries are created, restoring the delivery of oxygen and nutrients to the wound bed. Collagen is synthesized and begins to provide strength and structural integrity to a wound. Contraction reduces the size of a wound.

Remodeling
Collagen is remodeled to become stronger and provide tensile strength to a wound. Outer appearance in an uncomplicated wound will be that of a well-healed scar.

Data from Doughty DB, Sparks-Defriese B: Wound healing physiology. In Bryant RA, Nix DP, editors: *Acute and chronic wounds: current management concepts,* ed 3, St Louis, 2007, Mosby.

EVIDENCE-BASED PRACTICE TRENDS

Fernandez R and others: Water for wound cleansing, *Cochrane Database Syst Rev* 2008(2):CD003861, DOI: 10.1002/14651858.CD003861.pub2.

Romanelli M and others: Outcomes research: measuring wound outcomes, *Wounds* 19(11):1, 2007, http://www.woundsresearch.com/article/7986, accessed September 11, 2009.

Wound assessment is essential in wound management. The assessment of the following factors: location, dimensions, undermining, drainage, tissue type, exudate, wound edges, and pain, plays an important role in correct diagnosis and proper treatment of wounds and hard-to-heal pressure ulcers. A uniform approach to wound assessment that uses measurements can identify the appropriate treatment plan and appropriately evaluate progress to healing. In reports involving multiple assessment parameters, the percent reduction in wound surface area (the dimensions of the wound) during the first 2 weeks of care has been identified as the most reliable indicator for complete healing (Romanelli and others,

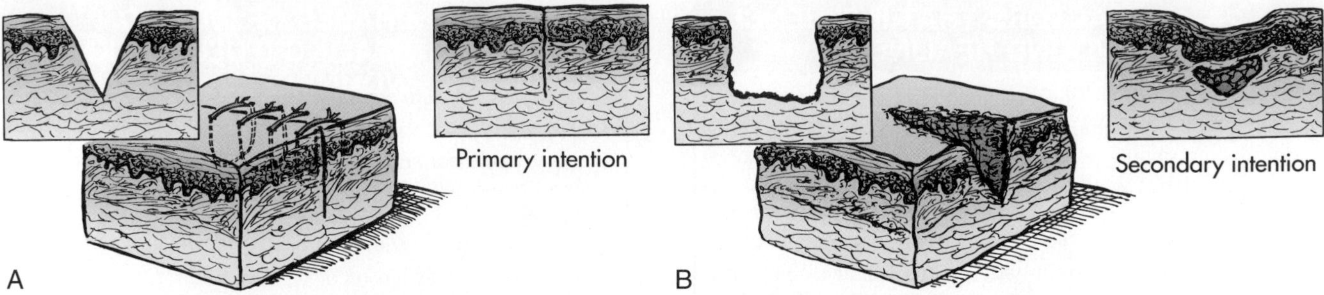

FIG 24-2 A, Wound healing by primary intention, such as with a surgical incision. Wound healing edges are pulled together and approximated with sutures, staples, or adhesive, and healing occurs by connective tissue deposition. **B,** Wound healing by secondary intention. Wound edges are not approximated, and healing occurs by granulation tissue formation and contraction of the wound edges. (Used with permission from Bryant RA, editor: *Acute and chronic wounds: nursing management,* ed 2, St Louis, 2000, Mosby.)

2007). Thus this finding reinforces the need for wound assessment and in particular obtaining and documenting wound dimensions. If wounds fail to show the expected progress toward healing, consider a change in the wound care plan.

When considering the type of solution to clean a wound, a recent review of clinical trials by the Cochrane Group noted that using tap water to cleanse acute wounds in adults does not increase the infection rate and may be as good as other methods such as saline. Although more research is needed to determine the best method to cleanse a wound, wound assessment and stage of wound healing helps to individualize the type of wound cleansing solution for an individual patient (Fernandez and others, 2008).

PROCEDURAL GUIDELINE 24.1
Performing a Wound Assessment

- **Nursing Skills Online:** Wound Care Module, Lesson 1

Wound assessment is the collection of data that characterizes the status of a wound and the periwound skin to determine the phase of healing (Nix, 2007). This information is used to continue the plan of care or alter the type of intervention (e.g., the type and frequency of dressing; use of adjunct wound therapies such as appropriate nutrition and antibiotics; or interventions such as debridement, a pressure relief device, or a surgical referral). The frequency of wound assessment depends on the condition of the wound as well as the standards of practice within the patient's health care setting. Acute care settings generally require assessment daily or with each dressing change, whereas long-term care facilities may require an initial admission assessment and generally a weekly assessment for a chronic wound; home care assessments depend on the frequency of visits. The type of wound assessment tool used by staff will depend on the facility. Regardless of the setting, determine the frequency of the wound assessment by the wound characteristics observed at the previous dressing change, facility protocols, and the provider's orders. The effectiveness of interventions cannot be determined unless baseline assessment data are compared to follow-up data (Baranoski and others, 2008a).

Delegation and Collaboration

The assessment of a wound cannot be delegated to nursing assistive personnel (NAP). Instruct the NAP about the following:

- Immediately reporting any drainage outside of the wound dressing to the nurse for further assessment
- Reporting any dressing that is no longer adherent

Equipment

- Clean gloves
- Measuring guide
- Cotton-tipped applicator
- Agency tool to document assessment
- Dressing supplies (as ordered)
- Disposable trash bag

Procedural Steps

1. **See Standard Protocol (inside front cover).**
2. Examine the medical record for the last wound assessment to use as a comparison for this wound assessment. Also, review the record to determine the etiology of the wound.
3. Remove soiled dressings, examine for quality of drainage (color, consistency), presence of odor, and quantity of drainage (the approximate amount of drainage in the removed dressing). Discard dressings in disposable trash bag; remove and discard gloves. Perform hand hygiene.
4. Inspect the wound and determine the type of wound healing (e.g., primary or secondary intention).

PROCEDURAL GUIDELINE 24.1
Performing a Wound Assessment—cont'd

5. Use the facility-approved assessment tool and assess the following:
   a. Wound healing by primary intention (surgical wound)
      (1) Assess the anatomical location of the wound on the body.
      (2) Note if the incisional wound margins are approximated or closed together. The wound edges should be together with no gaps.
      (3) Observe for the presence of drainage. A closed incision should not have any drainage.
      (4) Look for evidence of infection (presence of erythema, odor, or wound drainage).
      (5) Lightly palpate along the incision to feel a healing ridge. The ridge will appear as an accumulation of new tissue presenting as induration beneath the skin extending to about 1 cm (½ inch) on each side of the wound between 5 and 9 days after wounding. This is an expected positive sign (Whitney, 2007).
      (6) Assess for pain at the wound site, using an analog scale of 0 to 10.
   b. Wound healing by secondary intention (e.g., pressure ulcer or contaminated surgical or traumatic wound)
      (1) Assess the anatomic location of the wound.
      (2) Assess wound dimensions: Measure the size of the wound, including length, width, and depth, using a centimeter measuring guide. Measure length by placing a ruler on the wound at the point of greatest length (or head to foot). Measure width from side to side (Nix, 2007) (see illustration). Measure depth by inserting a cotton-tipped applicator in the area of greatest depth and placing a mark on the applicator at skin level. Discard the measuring guide and the cotton-tipped applicator in a trash bag.
      (3) Assess for undermining: Use a cotton-tipped applicator to gently probe the wound edges. Measure the depth and note the location using the face of the clock as a guide. The 12 o'clock position (top of the wound) would be the head of the patient, and the 6 o'clock position would be the bottom of the wound toward the patient's feet (see illustration). Document the number of centimeters the area of damage extends from the wound edge (e.g., underneath intact skin).

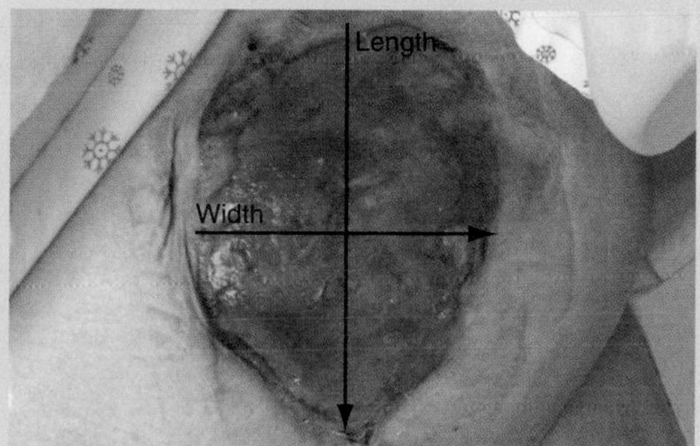

STEP 5b(2) Measuring wound depth and width.

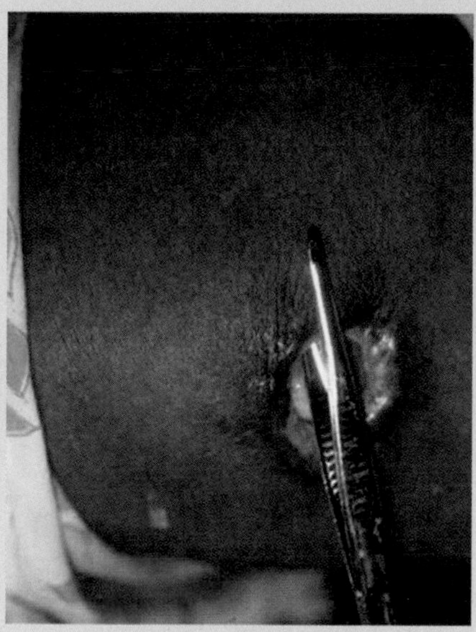

STEP 5b(3) Measuring undermining; note undermining at 6 o'clock.

      (4) Assess the extent of tissue loss: If the wound is a pressure ulcer, determine the deepest viable tissue layer in the wound bed. If necrotic tissue does not allow visualization of the base of the wound, the stage cannot be determined.
      (5) Notice the tissue type including percentage of tissue intact and the presence of granulation, slough, and necrotic tissue.
      (6) Note the presence of exudate: amount, color, consistency, and odor. Indicate amount of exudate by using part of dressing saturated or in terms of quantity (e.g., scant, moderate, or copious).
      (7) Note if wound edges are rounded toward the wound bed, this may be an indication of delayed wound healing. Describe the presence of epithelialization at wound edges (if present) because this indicates healing.
      (8) Inspect the periwound skin: Include color, texture, temperature, and a description of integrity (e.g., open macerated areas).
      (9) Assess for pain at the wound site, using an analog scale of 0 to 10.
6. Reapply dressing per order. Place time, date, and initials on the new dressing.
7. Record wound assessment findings and compare assessment with previous wound assessments to monitor wound healing.
8. **See Completion Protocol (see inside front cover).**

SKILL 24.1 WOUND IRRIGATION

Video Clips

Wound irrigation cleanses and irrigates surgical wounds or chronic wounds such as pressure ulcers. The cleansing solution is introduced directly into the wound with a syringe, a syringe and catheter, or a pulsed lavage device. When using a syringe, the tip remains 2.5 cm above the wound. If the patient has a deep wound with a narrow opening, attach a soft catheter to the syringe to permit the fluid to enter the wound. Irrigation should not cause tissue injury or discomfort. Avoid fluid retention in the wound by positioning the patient on the side to encourage the flow of the irrigant away from the wound. It is often helpful to use a 3-mL syringe with a 19-gauge needle to facilitate optimal pressure for cleansing with minimal risk for tissue injury (Rolstad and Ovington, 2007). Pulsatile high pressure lavage is an alternative to using the 35-mL syringe and the 19-gauge Angio catheter. It is the use of a machine to deliver intermittent high-pressure irrigation combined with suction to remove the irrigant and wound debris (Gardner and Frantz, 2008). This procedure provides force to remove wound debris without damaging healthy tissue.

Wound irrigation promotes wound healing through removing debris from a wound surface, decreasing bacterial counts, and loosening and removing necrotic tissue (Ramundo, 2007). Solutions used for irrigations include normal saline, warm water, and commercially available wound cleansers. Typically you use sterile technique for cleansing and irrigating surgical wounds and clean technique for certain chronic wounds.

ASSESSMENT

1. Review health care provider's order for wound irrigation, noting the type and amount of fluid and irrigation device. *Rationale: Open wound irrigation requires medical order, including the type of solution(s) to use.*
2. Perform wound assessment (see Procedural Guideline 24.1) and examine recent documented assessment of patient's open wound. *Rationale: Provides basis for comparing assessment findings with baseline to determine progress with healing.*
3. Assess patient for history of allergies to antiseptics, medications, tapes, or dressing materials. *Rationale: Known allergies suggest application of a sample of prescribed wound treatment as skin test before flushing wound with large volume of solution.*

PLANNING

Expected Outcomes focus on promoting wound healing.

1. Patient states acceptable level of comfort on pain scale of 0 to 10 after wound irrigation.
2. Wound begins to demonstrate signs of wound healing: wound is free of excessive drainage, exudate, and inflammation.
3. Skin integrity is maintained; no redness, edema, or inflammation is noted in surrounding tissue.

Delegation and Collaboration

The skill of sterile wound irrigation cannot be delegated to nursing assistive personnel (NAP). However, the cleansing of chronic wounds using clean technique can be delegated. It is the nurse's responsibility to assess and document wound characteristics. Instruct the NAP about the following:

- What to report when a wound is cleansed (e.g., wound color, presence of bleeding, drainage)
- Reporting patient pain

Equipment

- Sterile gloves (Steps 6 and 7)
- Clean gloves (Step 8)
- Irrigation/cleansing solution per order
- Irrigation delivery system per order: sterile irrigation 3-mL syringe with sterile soft Angio catheter with 19-gauge needle or handheld shower head.
- Protective equipment: gown, and goggles if splash/spray risk exists
- Waterproof underpad if needed
- Dressing supplies
- Disposable trash bag

IMPLEMENTATION *for* WOUND IRRIGATION

STEPS	RATIONALE
1. **See Standard Protocol (inside front cover).**	
2. Identify patient using two identifiers (e.g., name and birthday or name and account number, according to facility policy).	Ensures correct patient. Complies with The Joint Commission standards and improves patient safety (TJC, 2010).

STEPS	RATIONALE
3. Close room door or bed curtains, perform hand hygiene, and position patient. **a.** Position comfortably to permit gravitational flow of irrigating solution over wound and into collection receptacle. **b.** Position patient so wound is vertical to collection basin.	Maintains privacy; frequent hand hygiene reduces microorganisms. Directing solution from top to bottom of wound and from clean to contaminated area prevents further infection.
4. Place underpad under area where irrigation will take place.	Prevents bed linen from becoming wet.
5. Apply gown and goggles. Then apply sterile gloves for Steps 6 and 7 and use sterile precautions.	Protects from splashes or sprays of body fluids.
6. Irrigate wound with wide opening: **a.** Fill 35-mL syringe with irrigation solution.	
b. Attach 19-gauge Angio catheter or 19-gauge needle.	Catheter lumen delivers ideal pressure for cleansing and removal of debris (Ramundo, 2007).
c. Hold catheter needle tip 2.5 cm (1 inch) above upper end of wound and over area to be cleansed.	Prevents syringe contamination. Careful placement of syringe prevents unsafe pressure of flowing solution.
d. Using continuous pressure, flush wound; repeat Steps 6a to 6c until prescribed solution is used.	Clear solution indicates removal of all debris.
7. Irrigate deep wound with a very small opening: **a.** Attach soft catheter to filled irrigating syringe.	Catheter permits direct flow of irrigant into wound. Expect wound to take longer to empty when opening is small.
b. Gently insert tip of catheter into opening of wound, about 1.3 cm (0.5 inch).	Prevents tip from touching fragile inner wall of wound.

SAFETY ALERT Do not force catheter into the wound because this will cause tissue damage.

STEPS	RATIONALE
c. Using slow, continuous pressure, flush wound.	Use of slow mechanical force of a stream of solution loosens particulate matter on the wound surface and promotes healing (Ramundo, 2007).

SAFETY ALERT Pulsatile high-pressure lavage is often the irrigation of choice for necrotic wounds. Pressure settings should be set per provider order, usually between 4 and 15 psi, and should not be used on skin grafts, exposed blood vessels, muscle, tendon, or bone. Use with caution if patient has coagulation disorder or is on anticoagulants (Ramundo, 2007).

STEPS	RATIONALE
d. Pinch off catheter just below syringe while keeping catheter in place.	Prevents aspiration of solution into syringe and contamination of sterile solution.
e. Remove and refill syringe. Reconnect to catheter and repeat until prescribed solution is used.	
8. Cleanse wound with a handheld shower:	Helps patients shower with assistance or independently. May be accomplished at home.
a. With patient seated comfortably in shower chair, adjust spray to gentle flow; make sure that water is warm.	
b. Shower for 5 to 10 minutes with shower head 30 cm (12 inches) away from wound.	Ensure that wound is cleansed thoroughly.
9. Dry wound edges with gauze; dry patient after shower.	Prevents maceration of surrounding tissue from excess moisture.
10. Apply appropriate dressing and label with date, time, and nurse's initials.	Maintains protective barrier and healing environment for wound. Indicates time of most recent dressing change.
11. Assist patient to comfortable position.	
12. See Completion Protocol (see inside front cover).	

EVALUATION

1. Have patient rate level of comfort on a scale of 0 to 10.
2. Monitor type of tissue in wound bed and presence of drainage and inflammation. This assessment can identify where the wound is in the wound healing trajectory and helps determine the best dressing.

Unexpected Outcomes and Related Interventions

1. Bleeding or serosanguineous drainage appears.
   a. Flush wound during next irrigation using less pressure.
   b. Notify health care professional of bleeding.
2. Patient reports increased pain or discomfort during irrigation.
   a. Decrease force of pressure during wound irrigation.
   b. Assess patient for need for additional analgesia before wound care.

Recording and Reporting

- Record wound assessment before and after irrigation, amount and type of solution used, irrigation device used, patient tolerance of the procedure, and type of dressing applied after irrigation.
- Immediately report to attending health care professional any evidence of fresh bleeding, sharp increase in pain, retention of irrigant, or signs of shock.

Sample Documentation

0900 Patient rates abdominal wound pain as a 3 on a scale of 0 to 10. Abdominal wound 2 × 6 inches open with granulation tissue, minimal serous drainage in wound. Wound irrigated with 150 mL of NS, using irrigating syringe. Irrigant clear at end of procedure. Wound packed with moist sterile gauze and covered with one abdominal dressing. Patient had no complaints; rates abdominal wound pain as a 3 postprocedure.

Special Considerations

Pediatric

- Some pediatric patients may become frightened and may either verbally or physically attempt to prevent the wound irrigation. Describing the wound irrigation using a doll may help to alleviate the fear. When possible, include parents in procedure.
- Neonatal skin is immature and easily damaged from pressure irrigation. Check that products are approved for this patient population.

Geriatric

- Wound irrigation can be frightening for older adults with cognitive impairment and in some cases very painful. Assess patient's cooperation before irrigating the wound.
- With aging comes a 20% loss in dermal thickness. The skin is less resilient, and wound irrigation can easily result in skin tears and other trauma (Baranoski and others, 2008b).

Home Care

- Assess patient's home environment to determine adequacy of facilities for performing wound care: check especially for adequate lighting, running water, and storage of supplies.
- Provide support for patient and caregiver during the wound healing process. Chronic wounds do not heal properly and do not close in a timely manner (Doughty and Sparks-Defriese, 2007).

SKILL 24.2 MANAGING WOUND DRAINAGE EVACUATION

When wound drainage accumulates in a wound bed, it will interfere with wound healing. This is managed by the surgeon inserting a drain directly through the suture line into the wound or through a small stab wound near the surgical site. Jackson-Pratt and Hemovac drains are portable drainage devices that are self-contained suction units that connect to a drainage tube within the wound and provide constant low-pressure suction to remove and collect drainage. A Jackson-Pratt drain (Fig. 24-3) is used for small amounts of drainage (100 to 200 mL per 24 hours). A Hemovac or ConstaVac drainage system is used for larger amounts of drainage (as much as 500 mL per 24 hours). When a drainage device is more than half full, it should be emptied and reset to apply suction. If the patient has more than one drain, the drains must be numbered to accurately report drainage amount.

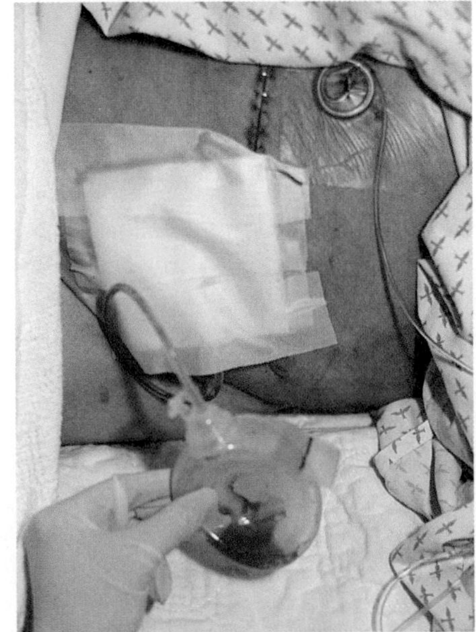

FIG 24-3 Jackson-Pratt drainage tube and reservoir.

ASSESSMENT

1. Perform wound assessment (see Procedural Guideline 24.1). *Rationale: Provides baseline to determine progress of wound healing.*

2. Identify the number and type of drainage systems when patient returns from surgery or from interventional radiology. *Rationale: Awareness of drain placement is needed to plan skin care and identify type and quantity of dressing supplies required.*
3. Inspect drainage tube for patency by observing drainage movement through tubing in direction of the reservoir and look for intact connection sites. Be sure that there is no pulling on the tubing. *Rationale: Properly functioning system maintains suction until reservoir is filled or drainage is no longer being produced or accumulated. Tension on drainage tubing causes injury to underlying tissue or skin.*

PLANNING

Expected Outcomes focus on promoting wound healing and comfort and preventing infection.

1. Quantity and appearance of wound drainage remain within expected guidelines based on type of surgery or involved area.
2. Vacuum is reestablished.
3. Patient reports less pain than initially assessed (scale of 0 to 10).

Delegation and Collaboration

Assessment of wound drains and the drainage systems may not be delegated to nursing assistive personnel (NAP). However, the skill of emptying a closed drainage container, measuring the amount of drainage, and reporting the amount on the patient's intake and output (I&O) record may be delegated. Instruct the NAP about the following:

- What to observe and report back to the nurse (e.g., appearance of drain contents and amount, patient's report of discomfort at wound site)
- Modification of the skill such as increased frequency of emptying the drain other than once a shift

Equipment

- Measuring container
- Alcohol wipes
- Gauze sponges
- Dressings
- Clean gloves
- Safety pin(s)
- Goggles, mask, and protective gown if risk of spray from drain is present
- Disposable drape or barrier

IMPLEMENTATION *for* MANAGING WOUND DRAINAGE EVACUATION

STEPS	RATIONALE
1. **See Standard Protocol (inside front cover).**	
2. 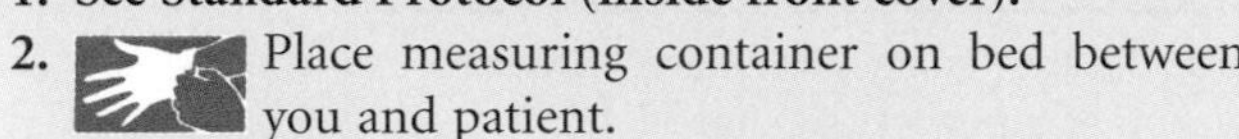 Place measuring container on bed between you and patient.	
3. ***Empty Hemovac or ConstaVac.***	
a. Maintain asepsis while opening plug on port indicated for emptying drainage reservoir. Tilt evacuator in direction of plug. Slowly squeeze the two flat surfaces together, tilting container toward measuring container.	Vacuum is broken, and reservoir pulls air in until chamber is fully expanded. Squeezing empties reservoir of drainage.
b. Drain contents into measuring container (see illustration).	Contents counted as fluid output.
c. Hold uncovered alcohol swab in dominant hand; place evacuator on a flat surface and press downward until bottom and top are in contact (see illustration).	Compression of surface of Hemovac recreates vacuum.

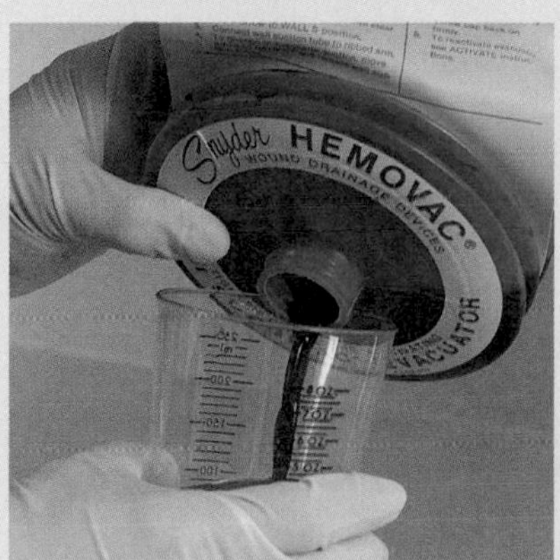

STEP 3b Emptying Hemovac contents into measuring container.

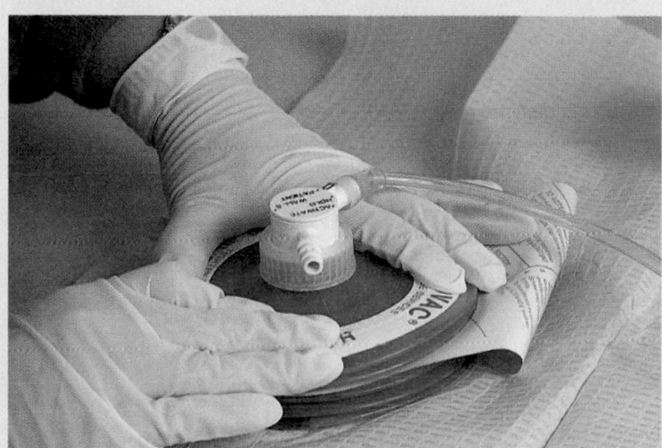

STEP 3c Hemovac suction.

Continued

STEPS	RATIONALE
d. Holding surfaces together with one hand, use other hand to cleanse port and tip of plug with alcohol wipe; immediately replace plug.	Cleansing plug reduces transmission of microorganisms.
e. Check evacuator for reestablishment of vacuum, patency of drainage tubing, and absence of tension on tubing.	Facilitates wound drainage and prevents pressure and trauma to tissues.
4. ***Empty Hemovac with wall suction.***	
a. Turn off suction.	
b. Disconnect suction tubing from Hemovac port.	
c. Empty Hemovac as described in Step 3.	Empties drainage and reestablishes suction to wound bed.
d. Cleanse port opening and end of suction tubing with alcohol wipe; reconnect suction tubing to open port of Hemovac.	Cleansing plug reduces transmission of microorganisms.
e. Set suction level as prescribed or on low if physician does not specify suction level.	
5. ***Empty Jackson-Pratt drain.***	
a. Open port on the end of bulb-shaped reservoir (see illustration).	Breaks vacuum.
b. Tilt bulb toward direction of port and drain toward opening to empty drainage into measuring container (see illustration). Cleanse end of emptying port and plug with alcohol wipe.	Reduces transmission of microorganisms into drainage evacuator
c. Compress bulb over drainage container. While compressing bulb, replace plug immediately.	Establishes vacuum.
6. Place and secure drainage system below exit site with safety pin to patient's gown.	Pinning system to patient's gown prevents tension or pulling on tubing and insertion site.

SAFETY ALERT Be sure that there is slack in the tubing from the reservoir to the wound, allowing patient movement and no tension at the insertion site.

STEPS	RATIONALE
7. Note characteristics of drainage; measure volume and discard by flushing in commode.	Contents counted as fluid output.
8. Proceed with inspection of skin and dressing change using drain sponges.	Drainage is irritating to skin and increases risk of skin breakdown.
9. Remind patient to keep drain lower than insertion site when ambulating, sitting, and lying.	Facilitates drainage.
10. See Completion Protocol (inside front cover).	

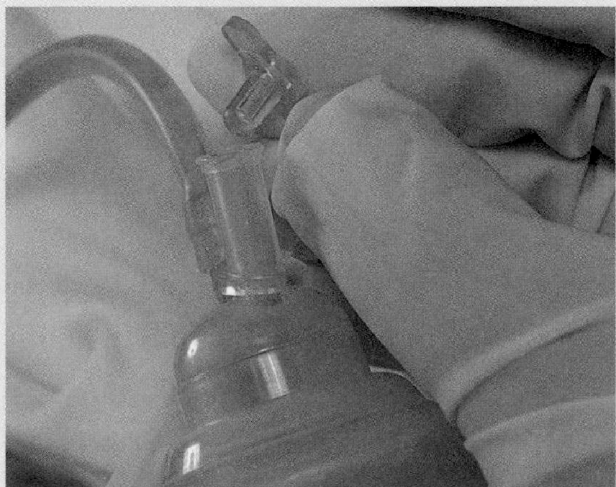

STEP 5a Opening port of Jackson-Pratt drain.

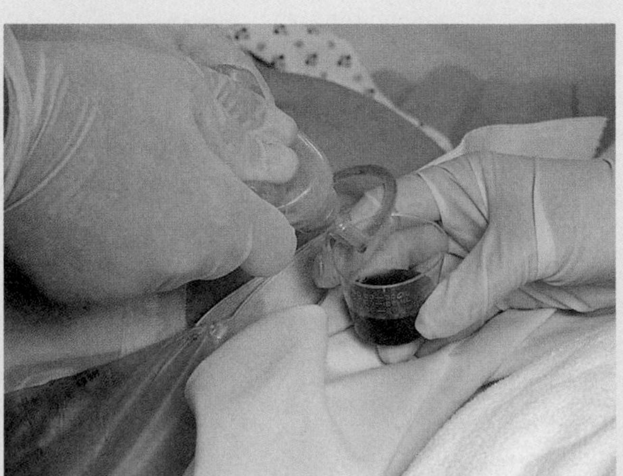

STEP 5b Emptying contents from Jackson-Pratt drainage device.

EVALUATION

1. Compare amount and characteristics of drainage with what is expected to determine patency of tubing and functioning of drainage evacuator.
2. Inspect for drainage around the tubing, which may indicate lack of vacuum or obstruction of drainage system.
3. Ask patient to describe level of comfort in relation to drain site.

Unexpected Outcomes and Related Interventions

1. Drainage is not accumulating in drainage system.
   a. Position tubing to enhance gravity flow and eliminate kinks or pressure on tubing.
   b. Gently "milk" tubing to release any clots that may block it.
   c. Check for loss of suction.
2. Excessive amount of bright bloody drainage accumulates over a short time (e.g., 4 hours). Drainage that is bright red in large amounts may indicate hemorrhage.
   a. Report excessive bright red drainage to surgeon.
   b. Confirm with surgeon and keep patient on nothing-by-mouth (NPO) status because it may be necessary for patient to return to surgery for suturing of a bleeding vessel.

Recording and Reporting

- Record results from emptying wound drainage system and dressing change in progress notes and I&O record. Note characteristics of insertion site and drainage; note volume. Record patient's level of comfort.
- Report presence of functioning drainage system and emptying frequency at end-of-shift report to oncoming nurse.

Sample Documentation

1800 Skin around drainage site is pink. Drain is secure with one suture. 200 mL of dark red drainage emptied from Hemovac. 4 × 4 drain dressing applied around drainage site. No reports of pain or discomfort with procedure.

Special Considerations

Pediatric

- Advise family members to keep drainage container less than one-third full to prevent tugging of drainage collector.
- Because children are very active, be sure to secure drainage device to avoid accidental removal.

Geriatric

- Be aware that patients with large amounts of drainage need additional fluid intake to prevent dehydration.
- Measures may need to be taken to prevent a confused patient from pulling out drain.

Home Care

- Instruct how to change dressings around drainage tube. Ask patient or caregiver to record the amount of drainage and bring the record to the health care professional at the next outpatient visit.

SKILL 24.3 REMOVING SUTURES AND STAPLES

Sutures are used to close a surgical incision both within tissue layers in deep wounds and for the outer skin layer. The patient's history of wound healing, site of incision, tissues involved, and purpose of the sutures determine the closure material selected. Deep sutures are a material that is absorbed or an inert wire that remains indefinitely. Nonabsorbable sutures (those that require removal) are available in silk, cotton, Prolene, wire, nylon, and Dacron. Removable skin sutures are interrupted or continuous. Interrupted sutures are separate stitches, each with its own knot (Fig. 24-4, *A*). A continuous suture is one long "thread" that spirals along the entire suture line at evenly spaced intervals. The surface appearance is very similar to a line of interrupted sutures, except that each section crossing the incision line does not have a knot (see Fig. 24-4, *B*). Another type of continuous stitch is a blanket continuous suture. This spirals along the incision with each turn pulled over to one side. The suture is looped around the thread of the previous stitch before making the next turn in spiral (see Fig. 24-4, *C*). When appearance and minimal scarring are important, very fine Dacron or subcutaneous sutures beneath the skin are used. An obese patient with abdominal surgery may have retention sutures covered with rubber tubing to provide greater strength (see Fig. 24-4, *D*).

Staples are made of stainless steel, are quick to use, and provide ample strength. They are used for skin closure of abdominal incisions and orthopedic surgery when appearance of the incision is not critical (Fig. 24-5). The time of

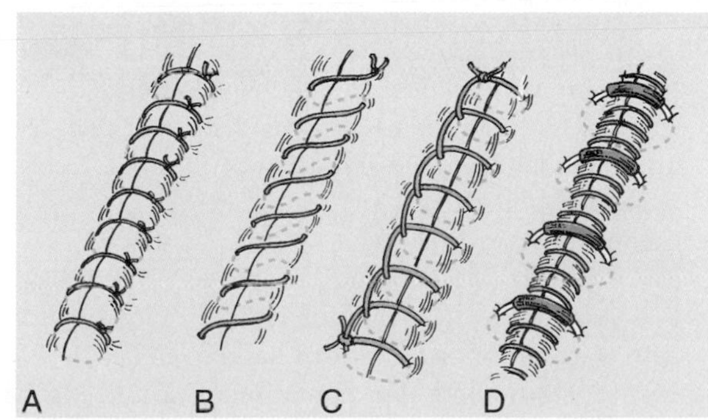

FIG 24-4 Sutures. **A,** Interrupted. **B,** Continuous. **C,** Blanket continuous. **D,** Retention.

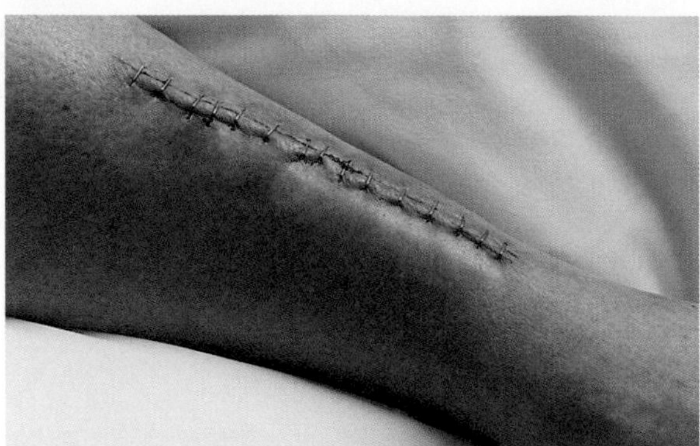

FIG 24-5 Suture line secured with staples.

removal is based on the stage of incisional healing and extent of surgery.

Institutional policy determines which health care providers may remove sutures and staples. Sutures and staples generally are removed within 7 to 10 days after surgery if healing is adequate. Retention sutures are left in place longer (14 days or more). Timing the removal of sutures and staples is important. They must remain in place long enough to ensure initial wound closure with enough strength to support internal organs and tissues. If any sign of suture line separation is evident during the removal process, the remaining sutures are left in place, and a description is documented and reported to the health care professional. In some cases these sutures are removed several days to a week later. Once sutures are removed, the nurse applies Steri-Strips over the incision to provide support. The strips loosen over time (5 to 7 days) and can be removed when half of the strip is no longer attached to the skin.

ASSESSMENT

1. Review health care professional's orders for specific directions related to suture or staple removal, including which sutures are to be removed (e.g., every other). *Rationale: Order is required due to the risk of premature or improper suture removal leading to wound damage.*
2. Assess patient's level of comfort on a scale of 0 to 10. If patient is uncomfortable, offer an analgesic at least 30 minutes before removal. *Rationale: Provides baseline to determine tolerance to procedure.*
3. Inspect surgical incision for healing ridge and skin integrity of suture line for uniform closure of wound edges, normal color, and absence of drainage and inflammation. *Rationale: Adequate healing needs to take place before sutures or staples are removed.*

PLANNING

Expected Outcomes focus on maintaining skin integrity, preventing infection, and promoting comfort.

1. Patient's incision is intact with edges well approximated after suture/staple removal.
2. Patient reports less pain than initially assessed (scale of 0 to 10) during suture removal.
3. Patient is able to perform incisional self-care by discharge.

Delegation and Collaboration

The skill of suture removal may not be delegated to nursing assistive personnel (NAP). Instruct the NAP about the following:

- Specific wound hygiene measures
- Expected drainage and what to observe and report back to the nurse
- Reporting any patient complaints of discomfort, pressure, or wound drainage

Equipment

- Disposable waterproof bag
- Sterile suture removal set (forceps and scissors) or sterile staple remover
- Sterile antiseptic applicators or swabs
- Gauze pads
- Steri-Strips
- Clean gloves

IMPLEMENTATION *for* REMOVING SUTURES AND STAPLES

STEPS	RATIONALE
1. **See Standard Protocol (inside front cover).**	
2. Identify the patient using two identifiers (e.g., name and birthday or name and account number, according to facility policy).	Ensures correct patient. Complies with The Joint Commission standards and improves patient safety (TJC, 2010).
3. Ensure there is direct lighting on suture line.	Aids visibility.
4. Remove dressing (if present) and discard; remove gloves and dispose of them directly into waterproof bag. Perform hand hygiene.	Reduces transmission of microorganisms.
5. Inspect incision for approximation of wound edges and absence of drainage and inflammation (redness, warmth, and swelling).	Presence of these findings may indicate need for delay of suture/staple removal.

STEPS	RATIONALE
6. Cleanse sutures or staples and healed incision with antiseptic swabs. Wipe across the sutures using a clean swab for each swipe.	Removes surface bacteria from incision and sutures or staples.
7. Remove staples.	
a. Place lower tip of staple extractor under first staple. As you close handles, upper tip of extractor depresses center of staple, causing both ends of staple to be bent upward and exit their insertion sites in the dermal layer simultaneously (see illustration).	Avoids excess pressure to suture line and secures smooth removal of each staple.
b. Carefully control staple extractor.	Avoids suture line pressure and pain.
c. As soon as both ends of staple are visible, move it away from skin surface (see illustration).	Prevents scratching tender skin surface with sharp pointed ends of staple for comfort and infection control.
d. Release handles of staple remover over disposable waterproof bag, allowing staple to drop into bag.	Avoids contamination of sterile field with used staples.
e. Repeat Steps 7a to 7d for removal of remaining staples as ordered.	Minimizes risk of separation of wound edges.
8. ***Remove interrupted sutures.***	
a. Place gauze a few inches from suture line. Hold scissors in dominant hand and forceps (clamp) in nondominant hand.	Gauze serves as a receptacle for removed sutures. Placement of scissors and forceps allows for efficient suture removal.
b. Grasp knot of suture with forceps and gently pull up knot while slipping tip of scissors under suture near skin (see illustration).	

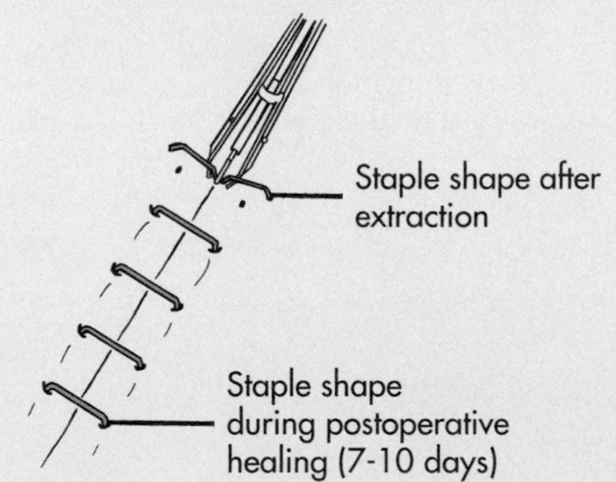

STEP 7a Staple extractor placed under staple.

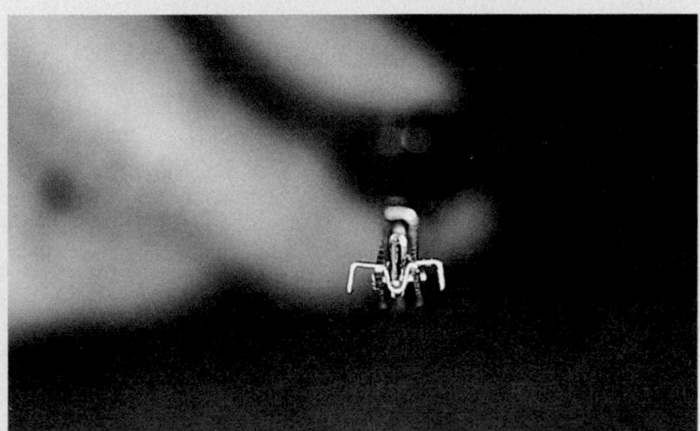

STEP 7c Metal staple removed by extractor.

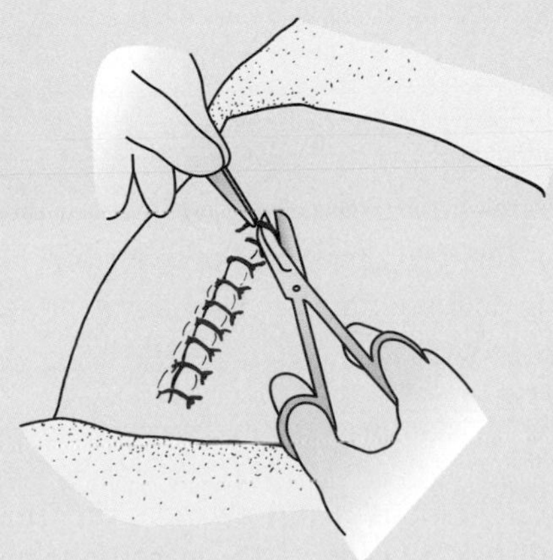

STEP 8b Removal of interrupted suture. Nurse cuts suture as close to skin as possible, away from the knot.

Continued

STEPS	RATIONALE
c. Snip suture as close to skin as possible at end distal to knot. With knot grasped with forceps, use one continuous smooth action to pull suture through from the other side. Place removed suture on gauze.	Smoothly removes suture without additional tension to suture line.

> **SAFETY ALERT** Never snip both ends of a suture. There will be no way to remove the part of the suture situated below the skin surface. Never pull exposed surface of any suture into tissue below dermis. The exposed surface of any suture is considered contaminated.

STEPS	RATIONALE
d. Repeat Steps 8a to 8c until every other suture has been removed.	
9. ***Remove continuous and blanket stitch sutures.***	
a. Place sterile gauze a few inches from suture line. Grasp scissors in dominant hand and forceps in nondominant hand.	Gauze serves as a receptacle for removed sutures. Placement of scissors and forceps allows for efficient suture removal.
b. Snip first suture close to skin surface at end distal to knot.	Releases suture. Prevents pulling contaminated portion of suture through skin.
c. Snip second "suture" on same side.	
d. Grasp knotted end and gently pull with continuous smooth action, removing suture from beneath the skin. Place suture on gauze.	Smoothly removes sutures without additional tension to suture line.
e. Repeat Steps 9a to 9d until entire line is removed.	
10. Inspect incision site to make sure that all sutures are removed and identify any trouble areas. Gently wipe suture line with antiseptic swabs to remove debris and cleanse wound. Cleanse in a direction out and away from incision.	Reduces risk of incision separation. Prevents contamination of incision.
11. Apply Steri-Strips according to facility policy or surgeon's preference.	Supports the wound by distributing tension across it.
a. Cut Steri-Strips to allow strips to extend 4 to 5 cm (1½ to 2 inches) on each side of the incision.	
b. Remove backing and apply across incision (see illustration).	

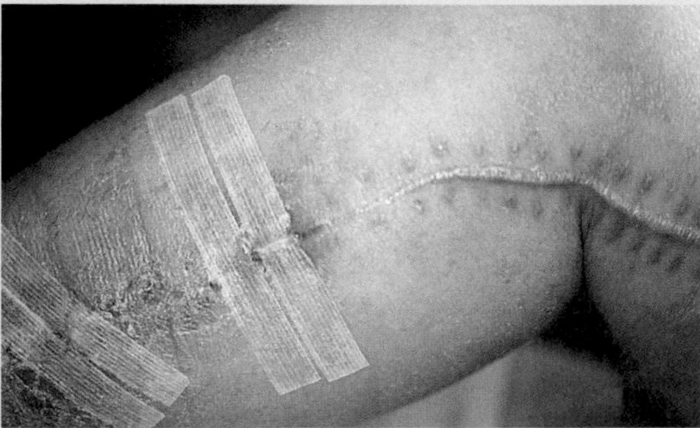

STEP 11b Steri-Strips over incision.

STEPS	RATIONALE
c. Inform patient to take showers rather than soak in the bathtub according to surgeon's preference.	Steri-Strips are not removed and are allowed to fall off gradually.
12. Apply light dressing if drainage is apparent, if clothing may rub and irritate suture line, or if the incision may be left open to air.	
13. Instruct patient about local and systemic indications of infection and tell patient to notify health care professional if these occur after discharge.	Provides information to patient for reporting wound infection to health care professional.
14. **See Completion Protocol (inside front cover).**	

EVALUATION

1. Inspect incision for approximation of wound edges.
2. Ask patient to rate pain using a scale of 0 to 10.
3. Ask patient to explain self-care guidelines before discharge.

Unexpected Outcomes and Related Interventions

1. Patient exhibits wound separation/dehiscence (surgical wound breaks, separates, and opens to the fascial level) and reports something "gave way."
   a. Notify surgeon.
   b. Keep any remaining sutures or staples in place.
2. Evisceration develops, involving protrusion of visceral organs through wound opening. This is a serious emergency because blood supply to tissues may be compromised when organs protrude.
   a. Keep organs moist by applying sterile towels that have been saturated in warm sterile saline solution.
   b. Immediately notify surgeon so surgical intervention can be arranged.

Recording and Reporting

- Record patient's response to suture removal in patient's progress note. Indicate that the entire suture was removed if appropriate.
- Notify health care professional immediately of any of the following findings: suture line separation, evisceration, bleeding, or new purulent drainage.

Sample Documentation

1300 Wound edges well approximated. Healing ridge palpated on abdominal wound. No redness, swelling, or wound drainage. All sutures removed from abdominal incision. Steri-Strips applied and left open to air. Patient instructed to shower, avoid tension on incision, and avoid heavy lifting. Patient instructed to return to his doctor in 1 week, and appointment slip given to wife.

Special Considerations

Pediatric

- Young patients need reassurance before suture removal. Involve parent; demonstrate removal technique before the actual removal.
- Talk to patient while removing sutures; reassure patient to remain inactive and calm.

Geriatric

- Older adults may need reassurance about the suture removal procedure. Assess mental status for comprehension of the procedure.
- Older skin may be at higher risk for dehiscence after sutures are removed because of delayed healing.
- Skin tears related to use of adhesives may occur in the patient with aged skin.

SKILL 24.4 NEGATIVE-PRESSURE WOUND THERAPY

Negative-pressure wound therapy (NPWT) is a mechanical wound care treatment that uses localized negative pressure (suction) to assist and accelerate wound healing (Frantz and others, 2007) (Figs. 24-6 and 24-7). NPWT assists and accelerates wound healing by removing wound fluids, stimulating granulation tissue, reducing the bacterial burden in the

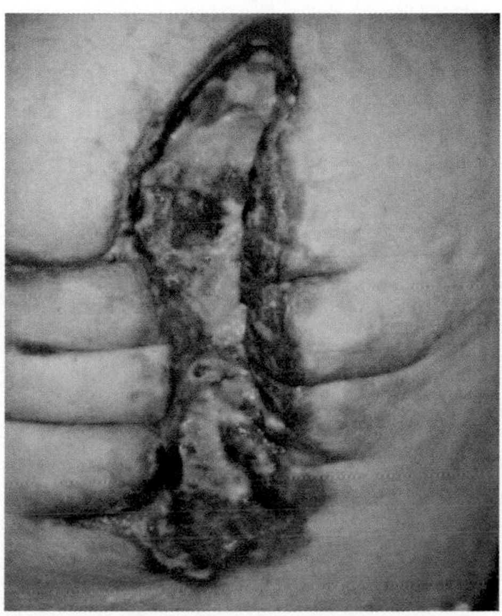

FIG 24-6 Dehisced wound before NPWT.

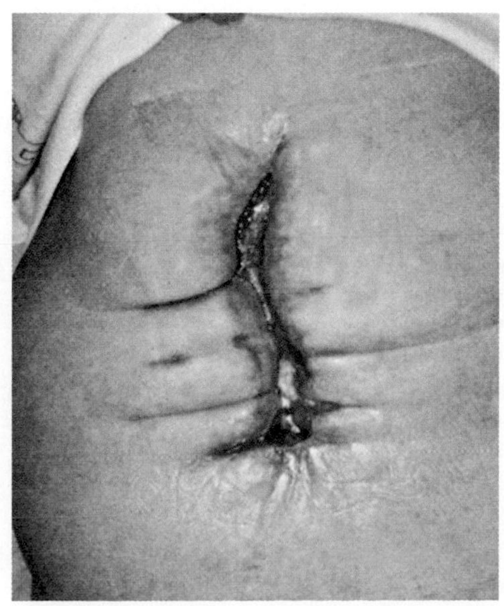

FIG 24-7 Dehisced wound after NPWT.

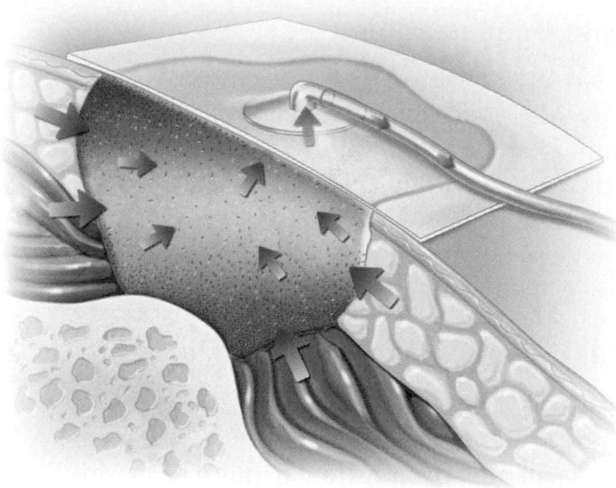

FIG 24-8 Wound NPWT in place. This is a wound vacuum-assisted closure (V.A.C.) system using negative pressure to remove fluid from area surrounding the wound, reducing edema, and improving circulation to the area. (Courtesy KCL, San Antonio, Tex.)

wound, and providing a moist wound environment. NPWT is available in several different forms and uses a dressing that is placed into the wound, a semiocclusive adhesive dressing or drape, and the application of suction via a tubing system that is connected and controlled by a computerized pump (Fig. 24-8).

Wounds managed by NPWT include acute (surgical) and traumatic wounds, surgical dehiscence, pressure ulcers, wounds caused by diabetes, arterial and venous ulcers, fresh flaps, and any compromised flap. Once the NPWT is selected for wound treatment, it is applied and changed every 48 hours for most wounds. The dressing is applied to the wound; the clear adhesive drape is placed over the dressing and secured to the periwound skin. Depending on the type of device used, evacuation tubing is placed over or into the dressing and attached to a suction source. The amount of suction or negative pressure varies from 75 mm Hg to 125 mm Hg, depending on the device and the characteristics of the wound. An airtight seal is necessary to maintain a negative-pressure environment. A snug and tight application of the dressing must be applied to ensure a good seal.

ASSESSMENT

1. Assess patient's knowledge of purpose of dressing change. *Rationale: Determines level of support and explanation required.*
2. Assess patient's comfort level using a scale of 0 to 10. *Rationale: Data determine effectiveness of comfort control interventions before, during, and after dressing change.*
3. Assess location, appearance, and size of wound (see Procedural Guideline 24.1). *Rationale: Provides information regarding status of wound healing, presence of complications, and the proper type of supplies and assistance needed.*

PLANNING

Expected Outcomes focus on promoting comfort and wound healing and preventing infection.

1. Patient's wound shows evidence of healing by smaller dimensions and less drainage or edema.
2. Dressing remains intact with airtight seal and prescribed negative pressure.
3. Patient reports less pain during and after dressing change.

Delegation and Collaboration

The skill of removal and application of NPWT may not be delegated to nursing assistive personnel (NAP). Instruct the NAP about the following:

- Reporting any change in the dressing shape or if the dressing is not flat to the wound
- Reporting any wound fluid leakage around the edges of the adhesive drape

Equipment

- NPWT unit (requires provider order)
- NPWT dressing (gauze or foam, depending on manufacturer's recommendations; adhesive drape)
- NPWT suction device
- Tubing for connection between NPWT unit and NPWT dressing
- Gloves, clean and sterile
- Scissors
- Skin preparation/skin barrier
- Waterproof, disposable trash bag

IMPLEMENTATION *for* NEGATIVE-PRESSURE WOUND THERAPY

STEPS	RATIONALE
1. **See Standard Protocol (inside front cover).**	Decreases patient anxiety.
2. Identify the patient using two identifiers (e.g., name and birthday or name and account number) according to facility policy.	Ensures correct patient. Complies with The Joint Commission standards and improves patient safety (TJC, 2010).

STEPS	RATIONALE
3. Determine if patient will require pain medication before removal; discuss previous NPWT changes with patient to determine pain tolerance with procedure. Medicate at least 30 minutes before dressing change.	Pain has been reported with NPWT removal and application; pain medication prior to dressing change can reduce procedural pain (Frantz and others, 2007).
4. Position patient comfortably and drape to expose only wound site. Instruct patient not to touch wound or sterile supplies. Place a disposable waterproof bag within reach of work area.	Maintaining patient comfort assists in completing skill smoothly. Draping provides access to wound while minimizing unnecessary exposure.
5. Follow manufacturer's directions for removal and replacement because each unit varies slightly with regard to removal and application.	
6. *Turn off NPWT unit by pushing therapy on/off button:*	Deactivates therapy and allows for proper drainage of fluid in drainage tube.
a. Raise tubing above unit and clamp and engage clamp on dressing tubing.	Prevents backflow of any drainage in tubing.
b. Engage clamp on dressing tubing.	
c. Allow drainage to flow from tubing into drainage collector.	Prevents drainage from exiting tubing when removed.
d. Gently stretch drape horizontally and remove slowly from dressing and skin.	Protects periwound skin.
e. Remove old dressing and discard.	
f. Perform wound assessment (see Procedural Guideline 24.1).	Provides baseline for change or maintenance of wound therapy plan.
7. Remove gloves; perform hand hygiene.	
8. Cleanse wound per facility policy. Oftentimes wound irrigation is performed (see Skill 24.1). Gently blot periwound with gauze to dry.	Irrigation removes wound debris.
9. Treat periwound skin with skin protectant product to prevent skin tears on removal and enhance adherence of adhesive drape.	Prevents skin blistering and excoriation when removing the adhesive drape (Baranoski and others, 2008c).
10. Application of NPWT (there are several manufacturers of NPWT; follow manufacturers' directions):	
a. Prepare NPWT foam.	
(1) If needed, measure wound and select appropriate foam dressing.	Establishes baseline for wound dimensions. Black polyurethane foam has larger pores and is most effective in stimulating granulation tissue and wound contraction. It is hydrophobic and does not absorb fluid but stays moist and promotes exudate removal (Jerome, 2007). Polyvinyl alcohol soft foam is denser with smaller pores and is used when the growth of granulation tissue needs to be restricted (Frantz and others, 2007).
(2) Using sterile scissors, cut foam to exact wound size, making sure to fit the size and shape of the wound, including tunnel and undermined areas.	Proper size of foam dressing is necessary to maintain negative pressure to the entire wound.
b. Place foam in the wound following manufacturer's instructions. Count the number of foam or gauze dressings and document in chart.	Edges of foam must be in direct contact with patient's skin. A foam count provides the nurse who removes the dressing with the number that should be removed.
c. If the NPWT system requires you to place a drain before the adhesive drape, place drain per manufacturer's recommendations.	With some wounds with large amounts of exudate, a drain facilitates wound healing.

Continued

STEPS	RATIONALE
d. Apply NPWT transparent dressing over the wound dressing (and suction drain if in wound). Trim dressing to cover wound dressing and extend onto periwound skin approximately 2.5 to 5 cm (1 to 2 inches) (see illustration).	Ensure that wound is properly covered and a negative pressure seal is achieved (Box 24-3).
(1) If using NPWT that has drain tubing that is applied after transparent dressing, cut hole in dressing large enough to accommodate tubing. Place into dressing and seal with adhesive drape.	Dressing should be airtight with no tunnels or gaps; this will ensure a good seal once the suction is activated.
11. After the wound is completely covered, connect tubing from the dressing to the tubing from the NPWT unit and set at ordered suction level. Examine the system to be sure that the seal is intact and the therapy is working; this is different for each type of NPWT unit. For example, on some units the display screen will show "Therapy On." Check facility policy and procedure for specific information.	Optimal negative pressure levels should be between –75 and –125 mm Hg (NPUAP, 2009).
12. Record initials and new date on new dressing.	
13. See Completion Protocol (inside front cover).	

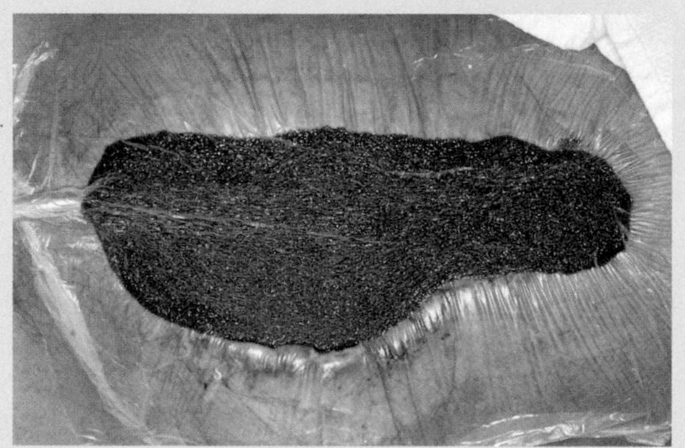

STEP 10d Foam dressing, transparent dressing over existing wound.

BOX 24-3 MAINTAINING AN AIRTIGHT SEAL

To avoid loss of suction (negative pressure), the wound and dressing must stay sealed once therapy is initiated. Problem seal areas include wounds around joints; near skin creases and folds; and near moisture such as diaphoresis, wound drainage, and urine or stool. The following points may assist in maintaining an airtight seal:

- Shave hair on skin around wound.
- Make sure that skin surface is dry.
- Cut adhesive drape to extend 2.5 to 5 cm (1 to 2 inches) beyond wound parameter.
- Avoid wrinkles when applying adhesive drape.
- Patch leaks with small pieces of adhesive drape.
- Avoid adhesive remover because it leaves a residue that hinders film adherence.

EVALUATION

1. **Perform wound inspection;** compare appearance of wound with previous assessment.
2. Ask patient to rate pain using a scale of 0 to 10.
3. Verify airtight dressing seal and proper negative pressure.

Unexpected Outcomes and Related Interventions

1. Wound appears inflamed and tender, drainage has increased, and an odor is present.
   a. Notify health care provider.
   b. Obtain wound culture.
2. Patient reports increase in pain.
   a. Patient may need more analgesic support.
   b. Negative pressure may need to be reduced.
3. Negative pressure seal has broken.
   a. Take preventive measures (see Box 24-3).
   b. Shave surrounding skin.

Recording and Reporting

- Record appearance of wound (characteristics of and amount of drainage), placement of NPWT, negative pressure setting, and patient's response.
- Report brisk, bright bleeding, evidence of poor wound healing, and possible wound infection to health care provider.

Sample Documentation

1100 Home visit. Wound on lower abdomen is pink, moist, and without edema in periwound region. Wound size is improving, currently 2 × 2.2 cm. Patient reports decrease in frequency and intensity of pain in wound area. Medicated with 600 mg Ibuprofen 30 minutes prior to dressing change. Dressing changed every 48 hours. Observed wife correctly change dressing and activated NPWT to –120 mm Hg. Family has sufficient NPWT supplies for the next week. Reviewed dressing care plan with wife and patient; dressing changes continue every 48 hours.

Special Considerations

Pediatric

- This wound application is not appropriate for fragile neonatal skin.

Geriatric

- Use skin care practices to protect periwound tissue. The adhesive film may be irritating to fragile skin. Skin protectant is one method to reduce the risk of tissue injury.
- Visual impairment may prevent self-care and require home care services.

Home Care

- When NPWT is used in the home, the patient and caregiver may benefit from initial visits with home care agency to monitor initial treatments.
- Provide information to family and caregiver regarding proper disposal of contaminated product.

REVIEW QUESTIONS

Case Study for Questions 1 to 3

Mr. Garcia underwent an emergency appendectomy 3 days ago. His abdominal wound was left open because of intraabdominal contamination at the time of surgery. The dressing to his abdominal wound is changed every 8 hours using a moist saline gauze dressing. Today when the nurse removes the dressing, she notes beige drainage on the gauze. As she examines the base of the wound, she notices yellow loose tissue adhering to the base and a foul odor. The edges of the wound are red and warm.

1. The nurse is assessing the wound and wound drainage. What should be included in the assessment? Select all that apply.
   1. Color, amount, and odor of drainage
   2. Tissue moist and adherent to the wound base
   3. Results of normal saline moist dressing application
   4. Color and temperature of wound edges
2. The nurse has consulted with the wound care nurse specialist about the best treatment for Mr. Garcia's wound. The wound care nurse has ordered a wound irrigation using 250 mL of normal saline. Which of the following steps would be included in the wound irrigation? Select all that apply.
   1. Leave the gauze dressing in place and irrigate into the gauze.
   2. Use a 19-gauge Angio catheter and a 35-mL syringe.
   3. Saturate several gauze pads with the normal saline and drizzle the solution into the wound.
   4. Direct the solution to the area of the slough tissue.
   5. Pour the solution into the wound directly from the container.
   6. Wear a protective gown and eye protection.
   7. Position patient to allow the wound irrigant to flow out of the wound into a collection device.
3. Mr. Garcia's wound is healing by what method?
   1. Primary intention
   2. Secondary intention
   3. Tertiary intention
4. Which of the following should be included in an assessment of a wound healing by secondary intention? Select all that apply.
   1. Wound location
   2. Estimated time to healing
   3. Wound dimensions
   4. Wound tissue type
   5. Dimensions of healing ridge
5. When the nurse attempts to empty the Jackson-Pratt bulb drainage collector from her patient with an intraabdominal abscess, she notes no drainage in the collector. Based on the report she received from the outgoing nurse at the beginning of her shift, she knows that he had 100 mL in the drainage collector 8 hours ago. What should her immediate actions be? Select all that apply.
   1. Call the surgeon to report her findings.
   2. Gently milk the tubing to see if there is a clot in the tubing preventing drainage.
   3. Assess the dressing around the tube for drainage.
   4. Observe the tube and the area for 8 hours.
   5. Gently irrigate the tube with 50 mL of normal saline.
6. Which of the follow care measures should be provided to a patient with a Jackson-Pratt drain?
   1. Empty the bulb only when it is filled to the top of the container.
   2. When the patient is ambulating, place a knot in the tubing to prevent excess drainage.
   3. Pin the bulb below the insertion site to facilitate drainage.
   4. Lubricate the insertion site to prevent crusting.
7. What is the correct sequence for staple removal from a healing surgical incision?
   a. Using staple removal, gently place under staple and press the extractor down.
   b. Put on clean gloves.
   c. Place Steri-Strips horizontally over the incision.
   d. Palpate and verify the presence of the healing ridge.
   e. Explain procedure to patient.
   1. c, d, e, b, a
   2. e, b, d, a, c
   3. e, c, b, a, d
   4. e, d, b, a, c
8. What is the recommended amount of pressure for a patient who has NPWT to facilitate wound healing?
   1. Up to –250 mm Hg
   2. –75 to –125 mm Hg
   3. –50 to –100 mm Hg
   4. –90 to –190 mm Hg

9. Which of the following interventions fix or prevent a break in the seal on an NPWT adhesive drape? Select all that apply.
   1. Use pieces of the adhesive drape over the areas where air is leaking.
   2. Stuff small pieces of gauze into the areas that appear to have the leak.
   3. Shave the skin before application.
   4. Do not use adhesive remover on the skin.
   5. Soap the skin around the wound and allow to air dry.

10. What is the purpose of using Steri-Strips across an incision after staple or suture removal?
    1. To keep the incision dry in the areas where the staples or stitches were removed
    2. To support the wound by distributing tension across it
    3. To keep a 2-cm (about 1 inch) separation together to facilitate healing
    4. To conceal the incision from the patient, reducing anxiety

REFERENCES

Baranoski S and others: Skin: an essential organ. In Baranoski S, Ayello EA, editors: *Wound care essentials: practice principles*, ed 2, Philadelphia, 2008a, Lippincott Williams & Wilkins.

Baranoski S and others: Wound assessment. In Baranoski S, Ayello EA, editors: *Wound care essentials: practice principles*, ed 2, Philadelphia, 2008b, Lippincott Williams & Wilkins.

Baranoski S and others: Wound treatment options. In Baranoski S, Ayello EA, editors: *Wound care essentials: practice principles*, ed 2, Philadelphia, 2008c, Lippincott Williams & Wilkins.

Colwell JC, Fichera A: Care of the obese patient with an ostomy, *J Wound Ostomy Continence Nurs* 32(6):378, 2005.

Doughty DB, Sparks-Defriese B: Wound healing physiology. In Bryant RA, Nix DP, editors: *Acute and chronic wounds: current management concepts*, ed 3, St Louis, 2007, Mosby.

Fernandez R and others: Water for wound cleansing, *Cochrane Database Syst Rev* 2008(2):CD003861, DOI: 10.1002/14651858.CD003861.pub2.

Frantz RA and others: Devices and technology in wound care. In Bryant RA, Nix DP: *Acute and chronic wounds: current management concepts*, St Louis, 2007, Mosby.

Gardner SE, Frantz RA: Wound bioburden. In Baranoski S, Ayello EA, editors: *Wound care essentials: practice principles*, ed 2, Philadelphia, 2008, Lippincott Williams & Wilkins.

Jerome D: Advances in negative pressure wound therapy: the VAC instill, *J Wound Ostomy Continence Nurs* 34(2):191, 2007.

National Pressure Ulcer Advisory Panel (NPUAP)/European Pressure Ulcer Advisory Panel, Pressure Ulcer Treatment Clinical Practice Guidelines, 2009, The Association.

Nix DP: Patient assessment and evaluation of healing. In Bryant RA, Nix DP: *Acute and chronic wounds: current management concepts*, ed 4, St Louis, 2007, Mosby.

Posthauer ME, Thomas DR: Nutrition and wound care. In Baranoski S, Ayello EA, editors: *Wound care essentials: practice principles*, ed 2, Philadelphia, 2008, Lippincott Williams & Wilkins.

Ramundo J: Wound debridement. In Bryant RA, Nix DP: *Acute and chronic wounds: current management concepts*, ed 4, St Louis, 2007, Mosby.

Rolstad BS, Ovington LG: Principles of wound management. In Bryant RA, Nix DP: *Acute and chronic wounds: current management concepts*, ed 4, St Louis, 2007, Mosby.

Romanelli M and others: Outcomes research; measuring wound outcomes, *Wounds* 19(11):1, 2007, http://www.woundsresearch.com/article/7986, accessed September 11, 2009.

The Joint Commission (TJC): *2010 National Patient Safety Goals*, Oakbrook Terrace, Ill, 2010, The Commission, http://www.jointcommission.org/PatientSafety/NationalPatientSafetyGoals.

Whitney JD: Acute surgical and traumatic wounds. In Bryant RA, Nix DP: *Acute and chronic wounds: current management concepts*, ed 4, St Louis, 2007, Mosby.

CHAPTER

25

Pressure Ulcers

evolve WEBSITE

http://evolve.elsevier.com/Perry/nursinginterventions

Video Clips

Nursing Skills Online

Pressure ulcers are localized areas of tissue destruction caused by the compression of soft tissue over a bony prominence and an external surface for a prolonged period of time (WOCN, 2010). The term *bedsore* is inaccurate because it is known that such ulcers result from positions other than lying. Pressure ulcers can occur when patients are sitting and/or when an external source such as a cast edge applies unrelieved pressure to skin. Fig. 25-1 shows pressure points over bony prominences where pressure ulcers can develop in sitting and lying positions. Common sites for the development of pressure ulcers include the sacrum, heels, elbows, lateral malleoli, trochanters, and ischial tuberosities (Ayello and others, 2008). Three pressure-related forces lead to the development of a pressure ulcer: (1) intensity of pressure (how much pressure is applied), (2) duration of pressure (how long the pressure is applied), and (3) tissue tolerance (the ability of skin and its supporting structures to endure pressure without adverse effects). The intensity of the pressure must exceed capillary closure pressure, thus compressing the blood flow to the skin. Both low pressure over a prolonged period of time and high pressure over a short time period can create a pressure ulcer. The greater the pressure and the longer pressure is applied, the greater the likelihood that a pressure ulcer will develop. Special mattresses and support surfaces help reduce this pressure (see Procedural Guideline 25.1). The third factor, tissue tolerance, refers to the ability of the tissue to react to the pressure.

Three external factors (i.e., shear, friction, and moisture) make the tissues less tolerant to pressure (Pieper, 2007). Shear is a parallel force that stretches tissue and blood vessels such as when a patient is in a semi-Fowler's position and slides toward the foot of the bed (Fig. 25-2). The skin over the sacrum sticks to the bed sheets, but the bony structure slides down, occluding the blood vessels, causing deep tissue destruction. Friction, the rubbing of the tissue against a surface, abrades the top layer of skin (epidermis), which makes tissue susceptible to pressure injury. Skin moisture (most often from fecal and urinary incontinence) softens skin, creating the risk for skin breakdown. Other factors related to pressure ulcer development include poor nutrition; advanced age; medical conditions causing poor tissue perfusion (low blood pressure, smoking, elevated temperature, anemia); and psychosocial status, in particular stress-induced cortisol secretion (WOCN, 2010).

Wound Healing

Skin, the largest organ in the body, protects the body from chemical and mechanical insults and bacterial and viral entry and regulates fluid loss and electrolytes. When wounded, the skin and supporting tissue go through a complex repair process. Nurses have an important role in wound healing, supporting the patient by providing the appropriate wound-healing environment. A comprehensive wound assessment provides information needed for planning wound care for a patient. To provide appropriate wound care, you must understand the process of wound healing. The physiology of wound healing occurs via two mechanisms: (1) regeneration (i.e., replacement of damaged or lost tissue with more of the same as occurs in partial-thickness wounds); or (2) connective tissue repair in wounds with tissue loss where scar formation replaces lost tissue such as in full-thickness wounds (Doughty and Sparks-Defriese, 2007). See Chapter 24 for a full discussion of wound healing.

Many factors influence wound healing and patient care. Nutrition is critical to healing because with injury more calories and substrates are needed for healing (Stotts, 2007).

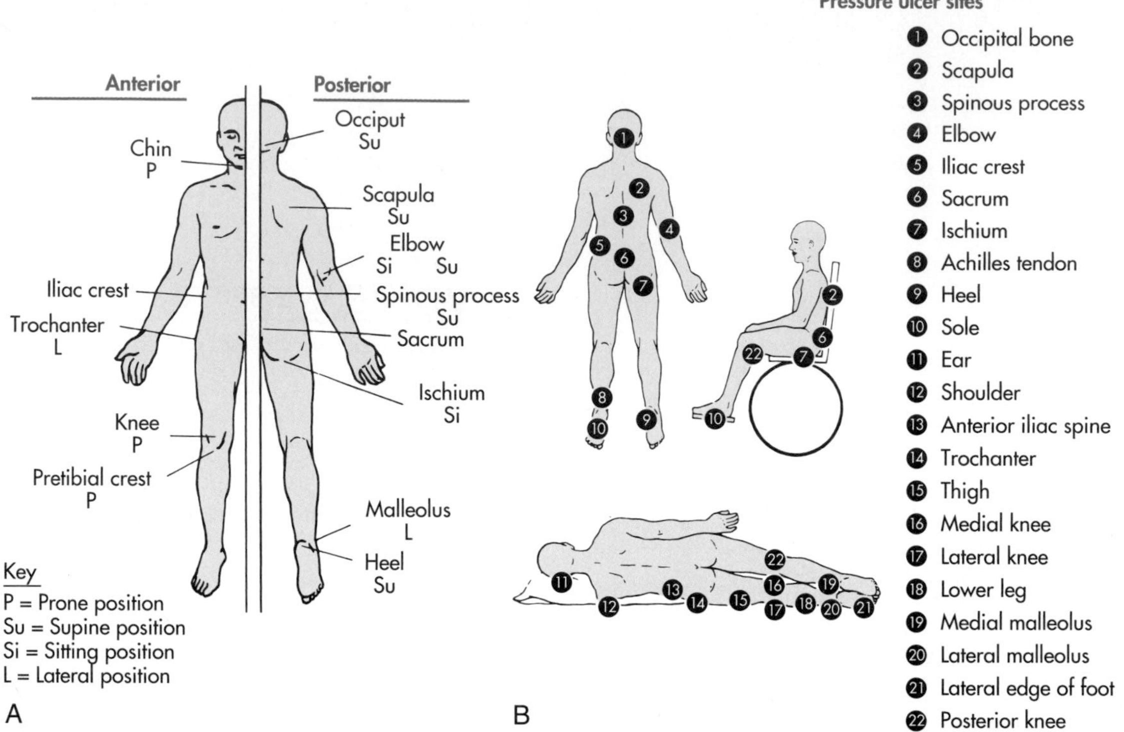

FIG 25-1 **A,** Bony prominences most frequently underlying pressure ulcers, **B,** Pressure ulcer sites. (From Trelease CC: Developing standards for wound care, *Ostomy Wound Manage* 26:50, 1988.)

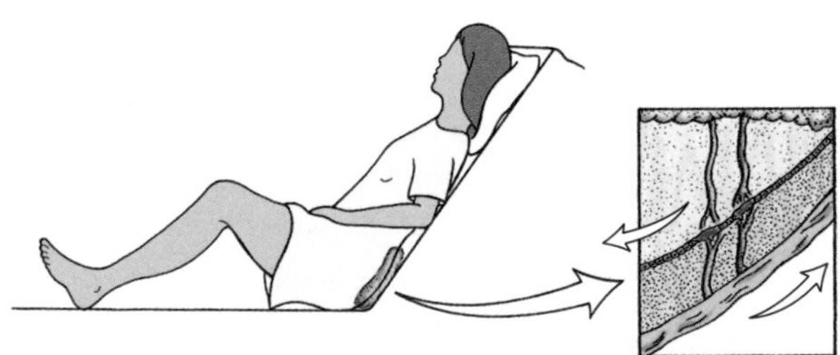

FIG 25-2 Shear exerted in the sacral area.

Infection prolongs the inflammatory phase, which prevents epithelialization. Medications such as steroids slow the inflammatory process, making wounds more prone to infection and delayed healing (Table 25-1). High levels of stress increase cortisol levels, which reduces the number of lymphocytes and decreases the inflammatory response.

PATIENT-CENTERED CARE

When assessing a patient for pressure ulcer risk, describe to the patient and family members the importance of determining possible risk factors. Informing them of the need to identify risk factors educates them on the increased risk for pressure ulcer development. Explaining that, once risk factors are identified, the appropriate interventions can be put into place helps them understand how to lessen the risk of pressure ulcer development. Describe to the patient and family members what interventions will be instituted for prevention and treatment. Be mindful that dark skin may need a close examination for color changes. Also let patients and family members help identify skin color changes (as appropriate). A patient is familiar with bodily changes and is an important resource in your assessment. In some instances the change in tissue may only be noted by touching the skin to note temperature changes.

When providing pressure ulcer care, a patient centered approach attends to the patient's comfort and emotional support. Describe what you are doing when you gently palpate areas of the skin and or apply treatments to wounds. Gather all supplies at the bedside just prior to a procedure so patients will not be left alone with their wounds uncovered.

SAFETY

Preventing pressure ulcers and skin breakdown is essential for safe patient care. Preventing injuries to the patient's skin and underlying muscle tissue not only saves health care resources but also protects the patient's overall level of health, independence, and optimal functioning. When performing a skin assessment, provide privacy for the patient and assist him or her as necessary in position changes, while keeping areas not under examination covered. Position the patient in bed to adequately assess the skin; and, when turning the patient onto the side, be sure that the side rail is up on the side of the bed to which the patient is turned to prevent falls.

TABLE 25-1 FACTORS THAT DELAY WOUND HEALING

FACTOR	RATIONALE
Older adult	Aging affects all phases of wound healing. The most significant change includes a diminished inflammatory response.
Obesity	Fatty subcutaneous tissue is less vascular.
Diabetes	Vascular changes reduce blood flow to peripheral tissues; leukocyte malfunction results from hyperglycemia, resulting in high risk for infection.
Compromised circulation	Vascular changes decrease the delivery of oxygen and nutrients.
Malnutrition	Inadequate nutrition slows healing because of lack of nutrients needed for wound healing (Doughty and Sparks-Defriese, 2007).
Immunosuppressive therapy	Immunosuppression decreases inflammatory response and collagen synthesis.
Chemotherapy	Chemotherapy interferes with leukocyte (white blood cell [WBC] count) production and immune response.
High levels of stress	Increased cortisol levels reduce number of lymphocytes and decrease inflammatory response.

EVIDENCE-BASED PRACTICE TRENDS

Bergstrom N and others: The National Pressure Ulcer Long-Term Care Study: outcomes of pressure ulcer treatments in long-term care, *J Am Geriatr Soc* 53(10):1721, 2005.

Comfort EH: Reducing pressure ulcer incidence thru Braden Scale risk assessment and support surface use, *Adv Skin Wound Care* 31:7, 300, 2007.

A review of the literature examined hospitals (nine) that implemented a pressure ulcer risk assessment policy for all admitted patients (Comfort, 2007). The policy included use of the Braden Scale to identify at-risk patients. Pressure redistribution surfaces were provided to those found to be at risk. All hospitals demonstrated a reduction in the occurrence of pressure ulcer formation. This study supports the practice of routinely using a risk assessment and implementing the appropriate intervention to help reduce the numbers of hospitalized patients that acquire a pressure ulcer.

A study by Bergstrom and others (2005) identified treatment characteristics associated with pressure ulcer healing in a long-term care setting. Patients studied had at least one pressure ulcer stage II or greater. Moist and dry dressings were used for treatment; patients using the moist dressings had a greater reduction in wound surface area. The other predictor for pressure ulcer healing in this population was adequate nutritional support; the patients with stage III and stage IV pressure ulcers were noted to have greater reduction in size of their ulcers. This study supports the use of moist wound healing and providing adequate nutrition in patients with pressure ulcers.

PROCEDURAL GUIDELINE 25.1
Selection of a Pressure-Reducing Support Surface

Pressure ulcers can occur in any setting. Patients in the operating room are also at risk for injury to the skin and underlying tissue. This injury occurs from a combination of factors such as surgical positioning and the effects of anesthetic agents. Because the damage resulting from intraoperative pressure develops in the muscle and subcutaneous tissues and progresses outward, damage is sometimes not visible for several days (Courtney and others, 2006). Use support surfaces in the operating room for patients at high risk for pressure ulcer development. The use of intraoperative pressure redistribution devices is associated with a decreased incidence of postoperative pressure ulcers (McInnes and others, 2008). When you care for postoperative patients, observe the skin for signs of injury or breakdown, even when a patient is ambulatory in the postoperative setting. In addition, instruct patients having surgery in ambulatory care settings how to observe for signs of skin breakdown once they return home.

Specialized support surfaces are foam, air, or gel mattresses, beds, and cushions (Table 25-2). Pressure-redistribution surfaces are classified as nonpowered (formerly called *static*) or powered (formerly called *dynamic*) support surfaces (NPUAP, 2007b). Nonpowered support surfaces include mattresses or mattress overlays filled with air, water, gel foam or a combination of any of these. Powered support surfaces change the pressure beneath the patient, reducing the duration of any applied pressure (Nix, 2007b). Mattresses or beds with a slick surface help decrease friction and shear. Surfaces with porous covers allow airflow, which reduces moisture, resulting in decreased risk for skin maceration.

Delegation and Collaboration

The selection of a pressure-reducing support device cannot be delegated to nursing assistive personnel (NAP).

Continued

TABLE 25-2 SUPPORT SURFACES

CATEGORY AND MECHANISM OF ACTION	INDICATIONS FOR USE	ADVANTAGES	DISADVANTAGES
Support Surfaces and Overlays			
Foam Overlays (Available As an Overlay or in a Full Mattress)			
Reduce pressure; the cover (top) reduces friction and shear; base height of 7.5 to 10 cm (3 to 4 inches); see manufacturer's guidelines regarding the amount of body weight supported	Use for moderate- to high-risk patients.	One-time charge No setup fee Cannot be punctured Available in various sizes (e.g., bed, chair, operating room table) Little maintenance Does not need electricity	Elevated patient body temperature Hot and may trap moisture Limited life span Plastic protective sheet needed for incontinent patients or patients with draining wounds
Water Overlays (Available As an Overlay or in a Full Mattress)			
Reduce pressure and pressure points because these surfaces provide flotation with pressure reduction by evenly redistributing patient's weight over the entire support surface	Use for high-risk patients.	Readily available Some control over motion sensations Easy to clean	Easily punctured Heavy Fluid motion may make procedures (e.g., dressing changes, cardiopulmonary resuscitation [CPR]) difficult Maintenance needed to prevent microorganism growth Patient transfers out of bed difficult Difficult to raise and lower head of bed
Gel Overlays			
Reduce pressure and pressure points because these surfaces provide flotation by evenly redistributing patient's weight over the entire support surface	Use for moderate- to high-risk patients. Use for patients who are wheelchair dependent.	Low maintenance Easy to clean Multiple-patient use Impermeable to needle punctures	Heavy Expensive Lack airflow for moisture control Variable friction control
Nonpowered Air-Filled Overlays			
Reduce pressure by lowering the mean interface pressure between patient's tissue and mattress	Use for moderate- to high-risk patients. Use for patients who can reposition themselves.	Easy to clean; multiple-patient use Low maintenance Potential repair of some air-filled products Durable	Damaged by punctures from needles and sharps Require routine monitoring to determine adequate inflation pressure Patient transfers out of bed difficult
Low-Air-Loss Overlays (Available in a Full Bed or Overlay)			
Maintain constant and slight air movement against skin to prevent buildup of moisture and skin maceration	Use for moderate- to high-risk patients.	Easy to clean Maintain constant inflation Deflate to facilitate transfer and CPR Control moisture Air permeable, bacteria impermeable, and waterproof fabric covering overlay Reduce shear and friction Setup provided by manufacturer	Damaged by needles and sharps Noisy Require electricity

TABLE 25-2 SUPPORT SURFACES—cont'd

CATEGORY AND MECHANISM OF ACTION	INDICATIONS FOR USE	ADVANTAGES	DISADVANTAGES
Specialty Beds			
Air-Fluidized Beds			
Bed frame contains silicone-coated beads and incorporates both air and fluid support. The silicone-coated beads become fluidized when air is pumped through the beads.	Use for high-risk patients. Use for patients with stage III or IV pressure ulcers or burns.	Less frequent turning or repositioning Improved patient comfort Quickly become firm for CPR or other treatments when device is turned off Reduce shear, friction, and edema to site May facilitate management of copious wound drainage or incontinence Setup provided by manufacturer	Patient risk for dehydration, especially in those with severe burns, possibly increased by continuous circulation of warm, dry air Possible increase in room temperature Possible patient disorientation Patient transfer difficult Heavy Expensive May not be wide enough for use for obese patients or patients with contractures
Low-Air-Loss Beds			
Bed frame with a series of connected air-filled pillows; amount of pressure in each pillow controlled and can be calibrated to patient need	Use is indicated in patients who need pressure relief, those who cannot be repositioned frequently, or those who have skin breakdown on more than one surface. They are contraindicated in patients with unstable spinal column.	Can raise and lower head and foot of bed Easy transfer in and out of bed Less frequent turning schedule Can transfer pillows to stretcher with patient Setup provided by the manufacturer	Requires a portable motor that is noisy Bed surface material slippery; patients can easily slide down mattress or out of bed when being transferred
Kinetic Therapy			
Provides continuous passive motion to promote mobilization of pulmonary secretions and provides low air loss, which provides pressure relief	Primarily indicated for patients needing spinal stabilization Should not be used when patient is hemodynamically unstable	Reduces pulmonary complications associated with restricted mobility Reduces risk of urinary stasis and urinary tract infections Reduces venous stasis	Does not reduce shear or moisture Cannot be used with cervical or skeletal traction Possible motion sickness initially Possible sensations of claustrophobia

Data from Bryant RA: *Acute and chronic wounds: nursing management,* ed 3, St Louis, 2007, Mosby; Morrison MJ: *The prevention and treatment of pressure ulcers,* St Louis, 2001, Mosby; Wound, Ostomy and Continence Nurses Society: *Guideline for prevention and management of pressure ulcers,* Glenview, Ill, 2003, WOCN.

PROCEDURAL GUIDELINE 25.1
Selection of a Pressure-Reducing Support Surface—cont'd

Equipment

- Agency pressure ulcer risk assessment tool (see Chapter 25)
- Body chart, tape measure, and/or camera to document existing areas of impaired skin integrity
- Documentation record
- Skin care products

Procedural Steps

1. Assess patient's risk for skin breakdown using a risk assessment tool (e.g., Braden Scale).
2. Assess patient's existing pressure ulcers, including areas of blistering, abnormal reactive hyperemia, and abrasion.
3. Assess patient's level of comfort using a pain scale of 0 to 10.
4. Identify patient using two identifiers (i.e., name and birthday or name and account number, according to facility policy).
5. Place "at-risk" patients on a pressure-reduction surface (Nix, 2007b; Gray, 2009).
6. Identify patient factors when selecting an appropriate surface.
   a. Does patient need pressure redistribution (e.g., you cannot reposition the patient or there is an existing pressure ulcer)?
   b. Is the surface needed for short- or long-term care? A short-term surface is usually needed for acute illness and hospitalization. A long-term surface is usually needed for extended or home care.
   c. What is the potential comfort level achieved by the surface? If patient is sensitive to noise, a device with a loud motor will increase his or her discomfort.
   d. Are patient, family, and caregivers adherent to repositioning? In addition, are they aware that a support surface should never replace repositioning? In a home setting a support surface is often necessary when the family, caregiver, or patient is unable to independently reposition or assist with repositioning.
   e. Does the support surface have a potential to interfere with patient's independent functioning? The height of the overlay and its soft edge may affect patient's ability to transfer, and a high-air-loss bed is not appropriate for a patient who needs to get in and out of bed frequently.
   f. What are the patient's financial limitations?
   g. If patient is using the device in the home, what are the environmental limitations? Will the home and existing electrical service accommodate the surface selected? Can the caregivers and family in the home manage the surface?
   h. What is the durability of the product? Is the surface easily subjected to puncture? What is the ease of cleaning the surface?
7. Determine the specific device (see Table 25-2).
   a. Pressure-redistribution devices redistribute pressure over bony prominences. Surfaces providing pressure redistribution include therapeutic mattress replacements, nonpowered and powered (i.e., moving) surfaces, low-air-loss beds and mattresses, and air-fluidized beds (Gray, 2009). Pressure-redistribution surfaces are also used in the operating room for individuals who are at high risk or for lengthy procedures.
   b. Use a nonpowered support surface if the patient can assume a variety of positions without bearing weight on a pressure ulcer without bottoming out. Bottoming out makes the support surface ineffective. To assess for bottoming out, place a hand (palm up) under the mattress or cushion below the area of risk for pressure areas (e.g., patient's pressure points when lying or sitting on surface). If less than 2.5 cm (1 inch) of support material is felt, patient has bottomed out (WOCN, 2010).
   c. Select a powered support surface when patient cannot assume a variety of positions without bearing weight on a pressure ulcer, if patient fully compresses the static support surface, or if the pressure ulcer does not show evidence of healing. Alternating or powered mattresses are associated with lower incidence of pressure ulcers than standard mattresses (Gray, 2009).
   d. High-specification foam is effective in decreasing the incidence of pressure ulcers in fairly high-risk patients, including older adults and patients with fractures of the neck of the femur (McInnes and others, 2008).
   e. Patients with stage III or IV pressure ulcers on multiple turning surfaces often benefit from an air-fluidized bed (Nix, 2007b; WOCN, 2010).
   f. There is limited evidence that low-air-loss beds reduce the incidence of pressure ulcers in intensive care (WOCN, 2010).
   g. When excess moisture is a potential risk, a support surface that provides airflow is important in drying the skin and reducing the incidence of pressure ulcers (NPUAP, 2007b).
8. Check agency policy regarding implementing support surface.
   a. Obtain a health care provider's order. This is usually required for a patient to obtain third-party reimbursement.
   b. Consult with agency case manager or social worker to assist with patient's financial eligibility and terms

PROCEDURAL GUIDELINE 25.1
Selection of a Pressure-Reducing Support Surface—cont'd

and length of third-party reimbursement for the surface.

c. Consult with agency home care or discharge planning if the device is anticipated for long-term use. Specific procedures and evaluations are needed for continuity of surface when patient is transferred to extended care or discharged home.

9. Inspect condition of skin regularly according to agency policy to evaluate changes in skin and effectiveness of therapy.
10. Observe existing pressure ulcers for evidence of healing.
11. Observe for side effects associated with specific pressure-reducing surface (e.g., nausea, dizziness, changes in fluid and electrolyte status).
12. Document pressure ulcer risk assessment and skin assessment in the patient's record.
13. Document the support surface selected and patient response to the surface (see specific skills for recording and reporting details).

SKILL 25.1 PRESSURE ULCER RISK ASSESSMENT AND PREVENTION STRATEGIES

- **Nursing Skills Online: Wound Care Module, Lesson 4**

A comprehensive program to prevent pressure ulcers includes the use of a risk assessment tool to identify factors that place the patient at risk for skin breakdown. Risk assessment allows a nurse to plan interventions to reduce or prevent skin breakdown. In addition to the risk assessment tool, a daily skin inspection, including an examination of pressure points, is essential. The Braden Scale for Predicting Pressure Sore Risk (Table 25-3) has six subscales that measure degrees of sensory perception, moisture, activity, mobility, nutrition, friction, and shear (Braden and Bergstrom, 1989). Each subscale is given a score, resulting in a total score indicative of the patient's risk for pressure ulcer development. The scale is used on admission to a health care facility and at periodic intervals.

Systematically inspect the skin of all patients at risk at least once a day, paying particular attention to bony prominences (Bergstrom and others, 1992). Inspect a patient's skin during routine care and always document your findings.

ASSESSMENT

1. Assess patient's risk for pressure ulcer formation, using agency pressure ulcer risk assessment tool. Determine the risk assessment score and compare patient's score with established score ranges that indicate high risk for skin breakdown. *Rationale: A validated risk assessment tool is recommended by the Wound, Ostomy and Continence Nurses Society (WOCN, 2010). Identifies individuals at risk early so risk factors can be reduced through interventions (WOCN, 2010).*
2. Assess patient for presence of potential pressure areas other than bony prominences, for example, nares (nasogastric [NG] tubes, oxygen cannula), tongue, and lips (oral airway, endotracheal [ET] tube); and skin next to drainage tubes or beneath orthopedic devices (braces, casts). *Rationale: Patients may have sites in addition to bony prominences that are at risk for pressure necrosis.*
3. Observe patient for preferred positions when in bed or chair. *Rationale: Weight of body is placed on certain bony prominences, and patient may resist repositioning of these areas.*
4. Observe patient's ability to initiate and assist with position changes. *Rationale: Prolonged lying or sitting in one position can cause capillary compression and tissue loss.*
5. Assess patient's and support person's understanding of risks for the development of pressure ulcers and knowledge of preventive measures. *Rationale: Patient and family are integral to prevention and management of pressure ulcers (WOCN, 2010).*

PLANNING

Expected Outcomes focus on identifying patient's risk for skin breakdown and preventing it.

1. Risk factors are identified.
2. Patient experiences no change from baseline skin assessment.
3. Patient experiences no new areas of erythema or signs of skin loss.
4. Patient has an acceptable comfort level (4 on a pain scale of 0 to 10) in pressure redistribution positions.

Delegation and Collaboration

The skill of pressure ulcer risk assessment may not be delegated to nursing assistive personnel (NAP). Instruct the NAP about the following:

- Explaining frequency of position changes and specific positions individualized for the patient
- Reviewing need to report to the nurse any redness or break in patient's skin or any abrasion from tubes or assistive devices

Equipment

- Risk assessment tool
- Positioning aids
- Clean gloves

TABLE 25-3	BRADEN SCALE FOR PREDICTING PRESSURE SORE RISK			
Sensory Perception Ability to respond meaningfully to pressure-related discomfort	1. Completely Limited Unresponsive (does not moan, flinch, or grasp) to painful stimuli because of diminished level of consciousness or sedation *Or* Limited ability to feel pain over most of body surface	2. Very Limited Responds only to painful stimuli; cannot communicate discomfort except by moaning or restlessness *Or* Has a sensory impairment that limits the ability to feel pain or discomfort over ½ of body	3. Slightly Limited Responds to verbal commands but cannot always communicate discomfort or need to be turned *Or* Has some sensory impairment that limits ability to feel pain or discomfort in one or two extremities	4. No Impairment Responds to verbal commands; has no sensory deficit that would limit ability to feel or voice pain or discomfort
Moisture Degree to which skin is exposed to moisture	1. Constantly Moist Skin kept moist almost constantly by perspiration, urine; dampness detected every time patient is moved or turned	2. Very Moist Skin often but not always moist; must change linens at least once a shift	3. Occasionally Moist Skin occasionally moist, requiring an extra linen change approximately once a day	4. Rarely Moist Skin usually dry; must change linens only at routine intervals
Activity Degree of physical activity	1. Bedfast Confined to bed.	2. Chairfast Ability to walk severely limited or nonexistent; cannot bear own weight and/or must be assisted into chair or wheelchair	3. Walks Occasionally Walks occasionally during day but for very short distances, with or without assistance; spends majority of each shift in bed or chair	4. Walks Frequently Walks outside room at least twice a day and inside room at least once every 2 hours during waking hours
Mobility Ability to change and control body position	1. Completely Immobile Does not make even slight changes in body or extremity position without assistance	2. Very Limited Makes occasional slight changes in body or extremity position but unable to make frequent or significant changes independently	3. Slightly Limited Makes frequent although slight changes in body or extremity position independently	4. No Limitation Makes major and frequent changes in position without assistance
Nutrition Usual food intake pattern	1. Very Poor Never eats a complete meal; rarely eats more than ⅓ of any food offered; eats 2 servings or less of protein (meat or dairy products) per day; takes fluids poorly; does not take a liquid dietary supplement *Or* Is NPO and/or maintained on clear liquids or intravenous (IV) fluids for more than 5 days	2. Probably Inadequate Rarely eats a complete meal and generally eats only about ½ of any food offered; protein intake includes only 3 servings of meat or dairy products per day; occasionally takes a dietary supplement *Or* Receives less than optimum amount of liquid diet or tube feeding	3. Adequate Eats over half of most meals; eats a total of 4 servings of protein (meat, dairy products) each day; occasionally refuses a meal but usually takes a supplement if offered *Or* Is on a tube feeding or TPN regimen that probably meets most nutritional needs	4. Excellent Eats most of every meal; never refuses a meal; usually eats a total of 4 or more servings of meat and dairy products; occasionally eats between meals; does not require supplementation

TABLE 25-3 BRADEN SCALE FOR PREDICTING PRESSURE SORE RISK—cont'd

Friction and Shear	1. Problem Requires moderate-to-maximum assistance in moving; complete lifting without sliding against sheets impossible; frequently slides down in bed or chair, requiring frequent repositioning with maximum assistance; spasticity, contractures, or agitation leads to almost constant friction	2. Potential Problem Moves feebly or requires minimum assistance; during a move skin probably slides to some extent against sheets, chair, restraints, or other devices; maintains relatively good position in chair or bed most of the time but occasionally slides down	3. No Apparent Problem Moves in bed and chair independently and has sufficient muscle strength to lift up completely during move; maintains good position in bed or chair
Total Score	____	____	____

Scoring: Very high risk, <9; high risk, 10-12; moderate risk, 13-14; at risk, 15-18; low risk, 19-22; no risk, >23. © 2001 Barbara Braden.

IMPLEMENTATION *for* PRESSURE ULCER RISK ASSESSMENT AND PREVENTION STRATEGIES

STEPS	RATIONALE
1. **See Standard Protocol (inside front cover).**	
2. Explain procedure to patient and family members.	Helps patient and family understand the importance of the risk assessment.
3. Gloves are needed when open draining wounds are present.	Reduces transmission of microorganisms.
4. Inspect skin at least once a day.	
a. Observe patient's skin; pay particular attention to bony prominences. If you find a reddened area, gently press the area with a gloved finger to check for blanching. If the area does not blanch, suspect tissue injury and recheck in 1 hour. Any discoloration may vary from pink to a deep red.	Routine skin inspection is fundamental to risk assessment and in designing interventions to reduce risk (WOCN, 2010). Persistent redness in lightly pigmented skin when pressed can indicate tissue injury (Ayello and others, 2008). If an area of redness blanches (lightens in color), this indicates that skin is not at risk for breakdown.
b. If patient has darkly pigmented skin, look for color changes that differ from patient's normal skin color such as red, blue, or purple tones.	Darkly pigmented skin may not have blanching. Although the skin may not show direct changes in color, the color may differ from the surrounding area (NPUAP, 2007a) (Box 25-1).
5. Check all treatment and assistive devices (catheters, feeding tubes, casts, braces) for potential pressure points. Remove gloves.	Pressure from these devices increases risk on bony prominences as well as other areas.
6. Review patient's pressure ulcer risk score.	Risk score aids in identifying interventions needed to lessen or eliminate the present risk factors (Braden and Maklebust, 2005).

SAFETY ALERT Do not massage reddened areas because this may cause additional tissue trauma. Reddened areas indicate blood vessel damage; massaging can further damage the vessels.

7. If immobility, inactivity, or poor sensory perception is a risk factor(s) for patient, consider one of the following interventions:	Immobility and inactivity reduce the patient's ability or desire to independently change position. Poor sensory perception decreases the patient's ability to feel the sensation of pressure or discomfort.

Continued

STEPS	RATIONALE
a. Reposition patient at least every 2 hours; use a written schedule (WOCN, 2010).	Reduces the duration and intensity of pressure. Some patients may require repositioning more often.
b. When patient is in the side-lying position in bed, use the 30-degree lateral position (see illustration).	Reduces direct contact of the trochanter with the support surface.
c. When needed, use pillow bridging (see illustration).	Use of pillows prevents direct contact between bony prominences.

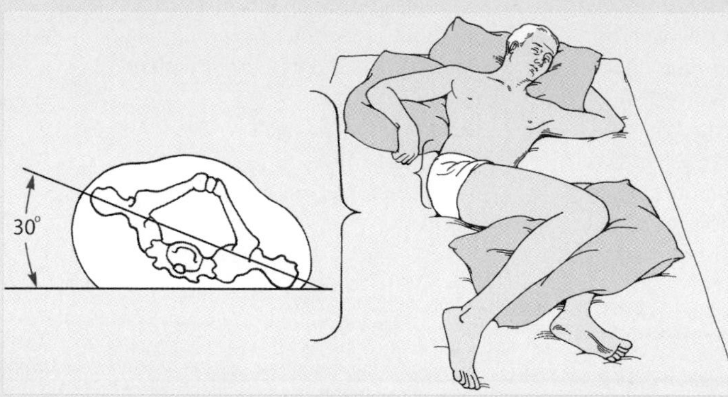

STEP 7b Thirty-degree lateral position with pillow placement.

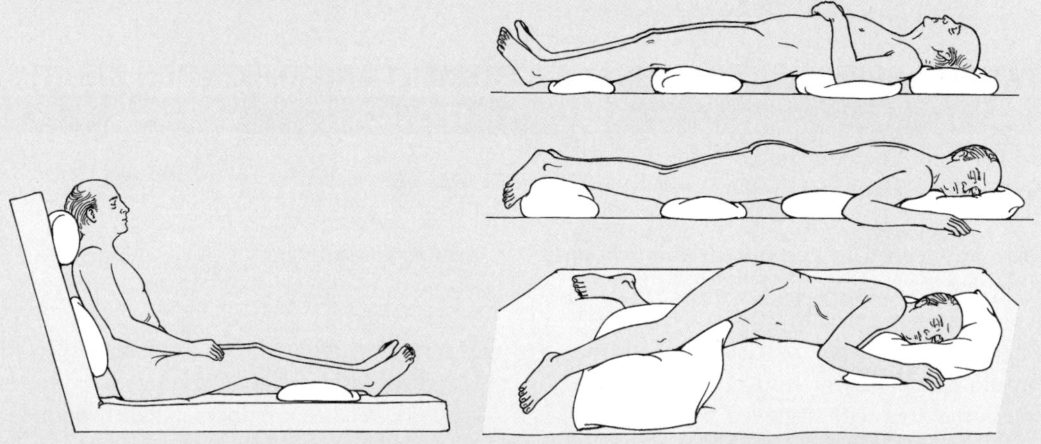

STEP 7c Pillow bridging.

BOX 25-1 CULTURAL CONSIDERATIONS FOR SKIN ASSESSMENT FOR PRESSURE ULCERS: THE PATIENT WITH INTACT, DARKLY PIGMENTED SKIN

Patients with darkly pigmented skin cannot be assessed for pressure ulcer risk by examining only skin color. Follow these recommended guidelines:

1. Assess localized skin color changes. Any of the following may appear:
   - Skin color changes are different from usual skin tone.
   - Darkly pigmented skin may not have visible blanching; its color may differ from the surrounding area.
   - Color is darker than the surrounding skin (purplish, bluish, eggplant).
2. Importance of lighting for skin assessment:
   - Use natural or halogen light.
   - Avoid fluorescent lamps, which can give the skin a bluish tone.
   - Avoid wearing tinted lenses when assessing skin color.
3. Tissue consistency:
   - Skin is taut, shiny, or indurated; edema occurs with induration of more than 15 mm in diameter.
   - Assess for edema, swelling.
   - Assess for firm or boggy feel.
4. Sensation:
   - Assess for pain or changes in skin sensation such as burning or itching.
5. Skin temperature:
   - Initially skin in the area of pressure may feel warmer than surrounding skin.
   - Subsequently skin may feel cooler than surrounding skin.
   - Feel areas of skin that are not involved in or around a pressure point to serve as a point of temperature reference.

Modified from Bennett MA: Report of the task force on the implications for darkly pigmented intact skin in the prediction and prevention of pressure ulcers, *Adv Wound Care* 8(6):34, 1995; and National Pressure Ulcer Advisory Panel (NPUAP): *Pressure ulcer stages revised by NPUAP,* February 2007, http://www.npuap.org/pr2.htm, accessed September 27, 2010.

STEPS	RATIONALE
d. Place patient (when lying in bed) on a pressure redistribution surface (see Procedural Guideline 25.1).	Reduces the amount of pressure exerted against the tissues.
e. Place patient (when in a chair) on a pressure redistribution device and shift the points under pressure at least every hour.	Reduces the amount of pressure on the sacral and ischial areas.
8. If friction and shear are identified as risk factors, consider the following interventions:	Friction and shear damage underlying skin.
a. Use two nurses and a pull sheet to reposition patient. Use a slide board (see Chapter 15) to transfer patient from bed to stretcher.	Proper repositioning of patient prevents dragging along the sheets. Slide board provides slippery surface to reduce friction.
b. Ensure that heels are free from the surface of the bed by using a pillow under the calves to elevate the heels.	"Floating" the heels from the bed surface eliminates shear and friction.
c. Maintain the head of the bed at 30 degrees.	Decreases potential for patient to slide toward foot of bed and incur a shear injury.
9. If patient receives a low score on a moisture subscale, consider one or more of the following interventions:	Continual exposure of body fluids to the patient's skin increases the risk for skin breakdown and pressure ulcer development.
a. Apply a moisture barrier ointment to perineum and surrounding skin after each incontinent episode.	Protects intact skin from fecal or urinary incontinence.
b. If skin is denuded, use a protective barrier paste after each incontinent episode.	Provides a barrier between the skin and the stool/urine, allowing for healing.
c. If incontinence is ongoing, consider a collection device: fecal incontinence collector, bowel management system, or indwelling urinary catheter.	Collection of the irritating substance may be appropriate if the cause of the incontinence cannot be controlled.
d. If source of moisture is from wound drainage, consider frequent dressing changes, skin protection with protective barriers, or collection devices.	Removes the frequent exposure of wound drainage from the skin.
10. If patient scores low on the nutrition subscale of the risk assessment, consider the following interventions:	There is a strong relationship between nutrition and pressure ulcer development.
a. Assess patient's nutritional status, including fluid intake. Determine if patient has been NPO recently.	Dehydration can affect albumin levels and tissue integrity.
b. Perform a nutritional screening in patient identified to be at risk on the nutrition subscale. Consider a referral to a registered dietitian per facility policy.	Malnutrition is a risk factor for pressure ulcer development.
c. Offer support with eating (see Chapter 12).	Encourages intake.
d. Institute oral supplements (tube feedings, dietary supplements) per physician order if patient is undernourished.	Oral supplements increase patient's protein intake and calorie count and supply essential vitamins and minerals.
11. Educate patient/family caregiver regarding pressure ulcer risk and prevention (Baharestani, 2008; WOCN, 2010).	Assists in adhering to interventions to reduce pressure ulcer risk.
12. See Completion Protocol (inside front cover).	

EVALUATION

1. Observe patient's skin for areas at risk for tissue damage, noting change in color, appearance, or texture.
2. Observe tolerance of patient for position change by measuring level of comfort on pain scale.
3. Compare subsequent risk assessment scores and skin assessments.

Unexpected Outcomes and Related Interventions

1. Skin becomes mottled, reddened, purplish, or bluish.
   a. Document and communicate interval for reevaluation of risk assessment score.
   b. Obtain health care provider's order (when needed) for identified consultations such as wound, ostomy, and continence nurse; dietitian; clinical nurse specialist

(CNS); and/or physical therapist (PT). Revise position change schedule as needed.

Recording and Reporting

- Record patient's risk and skin assessments, turning intervals, pressure redistribution support surface, and moisture protection interventions.
- Report need for additional consultations (if indicated) for the high-risk patient.

Sample Documentation

1500 Braden risk assessment scale completed on admission. Risk assessment score is 12 (high risk). Skin is intact over all surfaces; pressure ulcer prevention protocol implemented.

Special Considerations

Pediatric

- Immature skin in young patient is susceptible to skin tears.
- Moist skin covered with a diaper may soften, causing skin breakdown.

Geriatric

- In the older adult the epidermal-dermal junction becomes flatter, putting the patient at increased risk for epidermal damage.

Home Care

- Evaluate the home environment for the use of a pressure redistribution support surface (including a wheel chair).
- Evaluate the seating surface for an appropriate pressure redistribution support surface.

SKILL 25.2 TREATMENT OF PRESSURE ULCERS AND WOUND MANAGEMENT

- **Nursing Skills Online: Wound Care Module, Lesson 4**

Video Clips

Treatment for a patient with a pressure ulcer includes systematic support of the patient, reduction or elimination of the cause of the skin breakdown, and wound management that provides an environment conducive to healing. Wound healing does not occur or occurs slowly in the malnourished patient or the patient with a poor cardiovascular status; thus measures are needed to systemically support the patient. Other factors that impede wound healing include immunosuppressive therapy and uncontrolled diabetes mellitus.

The cause(s) of a wound must be assessed before wound therapy is instituted. If the contributing causes of a pressure ulcer (pressure, shear, friction, and/or moisture) are not addressed, the tissue damage continues, and healing does not take place. A wound environment conducive to healing is achieved by using topical wound therapy with the following objectives: prevent and manage infection, cleanse the wound, remove nonviable tissue, maintain appropriate level of moisture, eliminate dead space, control odor, eliminate or minimize pain, and protect the wound (Rolstad and Ovington, 2007). The choice of topical treatment (dressings and solutions) is dictated by these objectives. Ongoing monitoring evaluates the effectiveness of wound care.

ASSESSMENT

1. Assess patient's level of comfort on a pain scale of 0 to 10. If patient is in pain, determine if a prn medication has been ordered and administer along with appropriate nonpharmacological strategies (see Chapter 13). *Rationale: Patient should be as comfortable as possible during the dressing change.*
2. Determine if patient is allergic to topical agents. *Rationale: Topical agents contain elements that may cause localized skin reactions.*
3. Identify reasons for the pressure ulcer and control or eliminate the cause. *Rationale: Failure to address causative factors results in a nonhealing wound (Rolstad and Ovington, 2007).*
4. Review medical order for topical agent(s) and/or dressings. *Rationale: Ensures that right patient receives proper medication and treatment.*
5. Assess patient's wounds using the following wound parameters and continue ongoing wound assessment per agency protocol. Note: This may be done during procedure after dressing removal. *Rationale: Determines effectiveness of wound care and drives the treatment plan of care (WOCN, 2010).*
   a. *Wound location:* Describe the body site where the wound is located.
   b. *Stage of wound:* Describe the extent of tissue destruction (Table 25-4).
   c. *Wound size:* Length, width, and depth of the wound are measured per facility protocol. Use a disposable measuring guide for length and width. Use a cotton-tipped applicator to assess depth (Fig. 25-3).

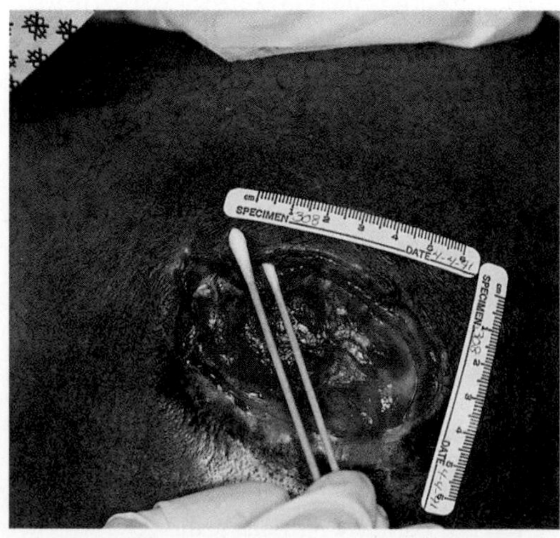

FIG 25-3 Measuring length, width, and depth of a pressure ulcer.

TABLE 25-4 STAGING OF PRESSURE ULCERS

Suspected Deep Tissue Injury

Purple or maroon localized area of discolored intact skin or blood-filled blister caused by damage of underlying soft tissue from pressure and/or shear. The area may be preceded by tissue that is painful, firm, mushy, boggy, warmer, or cooler compared to adjacent tissue.

Stage I

Skin is intact with nonblanchable redness of a localized area usually over a bony prominence. Darkly pigmented skin may not have visible blanching; its color may differ from the surrounding area.

Further description: The area may be painful, firm, soft, warmer, or cooler compared to adjacent tissue. Stage I may be difficult to detect in individuals with dark skin tones. May indicate at-risk persons (a heralding sign of risk).

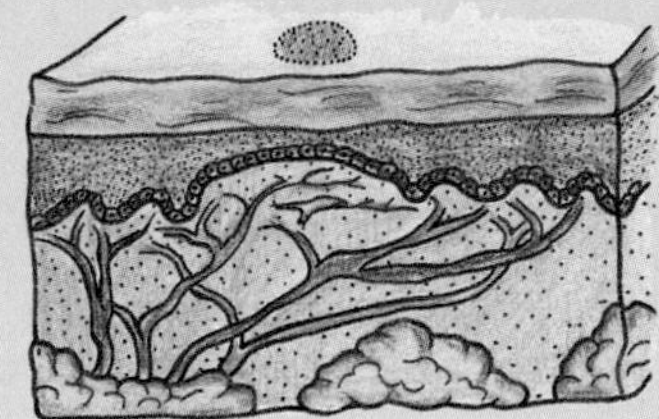

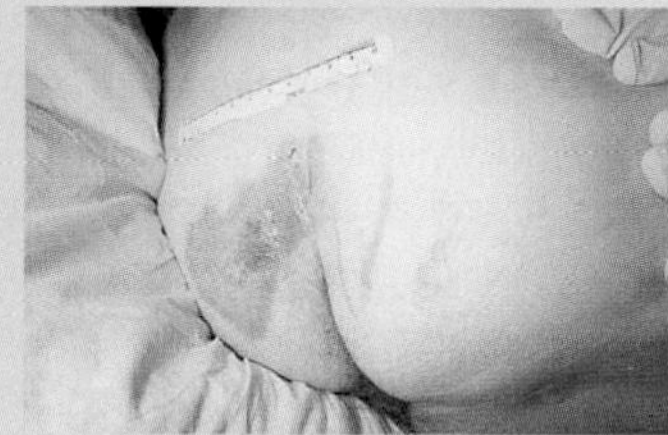

Stage II

Partial-thickness loss of dermis presents as a shallow open ulcer with a red pink wound bed without slough. This stage may also present as an intact or open/ruptured serum-filled blister.

Further description: This stage presents as a shiny or dry shallow ulcer without slough or bruising.* It should not be used to describe skin tears, tape burns, perineal dermatitis, maceration, or denudement.

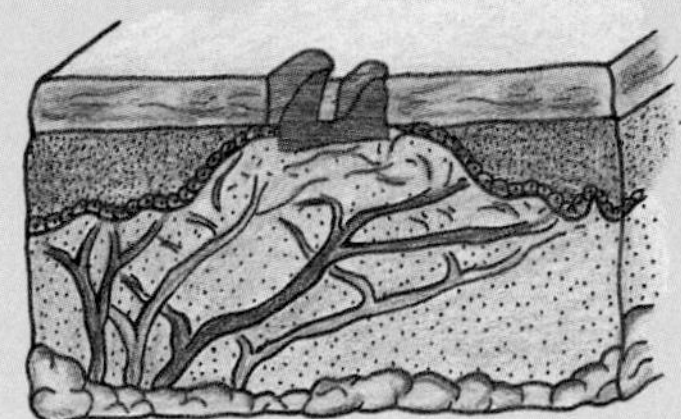

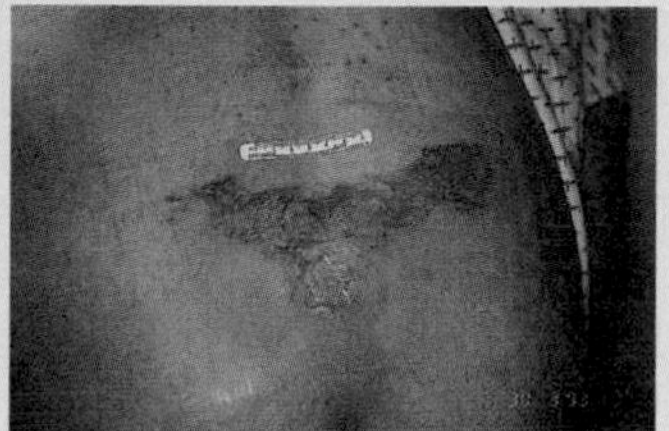

Stage III

Stage III is full-thickness tissue loss. Subcutaneous fat may be visible; but bone, tendon, or muscle *is not* exposed. Slough may be present but does not obscure the depth of tissue loss. It *may* include undermining and tunneling.

Further description: The depth of a stage III ulcer varies by anatomical location. The bridge of nose, ear, occiput, and malleolus do not have subcutaneous tissue; and stage III ulcers can be shallow. In contrast, areas of significant adipose tissue can develop extremely deep stage III ulcers. Bone or tendon is not visible or directly palpable.

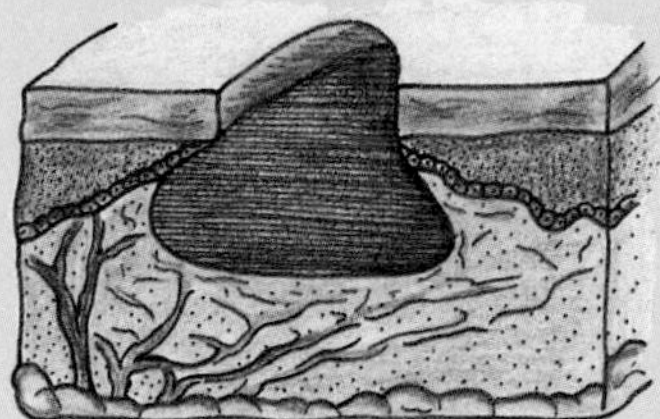

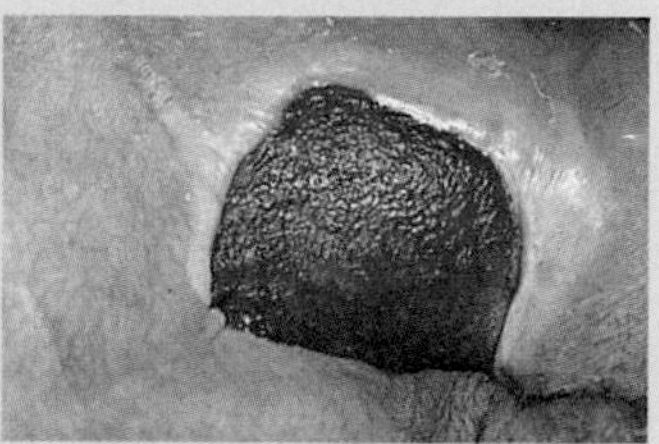

Stage IV

Stage IV is full-thickness tissue loss with exposed bone, tendon, or muscle. Slough or eschar may be present on some parts of the wound bed. It *often* includes undermining and tunneling.

Further description: The depth of a stage IV pressure ulcer varies by anatomical location. The bridge of the nose, ear, occiput, and malleolus do not have subcutaneous tissue; and these ulcers can be shallow. Stage IV ulcers can extend into muscle and/or supporting structures (e.g., fascia, tendon, or joint capsule), making osteomyelitis possible. Exposed bone/tendon is visible or directly palpable.

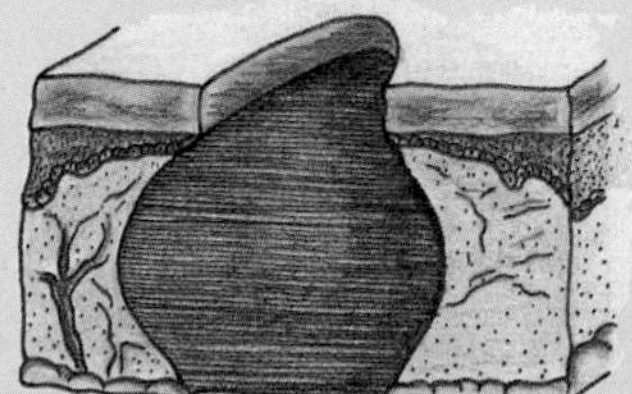

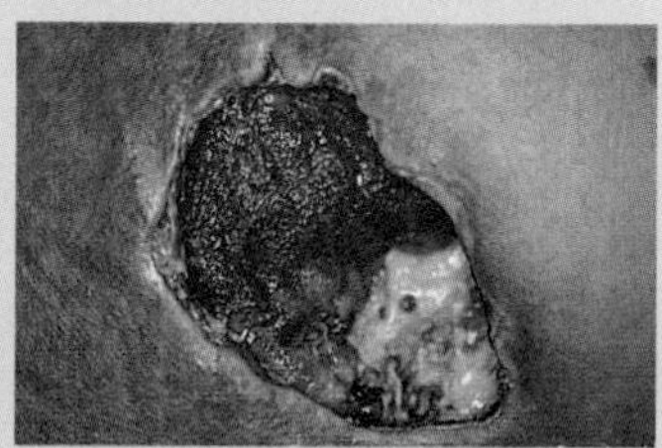

Unstageable

Full-thickness tissue loss in which the base of the ulcer is covered by slough (yellow, tan, gray, green, or brown) and/or eschar (tan, brown, or black) in wound bed.

Further description: Until enough slough and/or eschar is removed to expose the base of the wound, the true depth, and therefore stage, cannot be determined. Stable (dry, adherent, intact without erythema or fluctuance) eschar on the heels serves as "the body's natural (biological) cover" and should not be removed.

Data from National Pressure Ulcer Advisory Panel (NPUAP): *Pressure ulcer stages revised by NPUAP,* February 2007, http://www.npuap.org/pr2.htm, accessed September 27, 2010. Photos courtesy Laurel Wiersma, RN, MSN, CNS, Barnes-Jewish Hospital, St Louis, MO.

*Bruising indicates suspected deep tissue injury.

d. *Presence of undermining, sinus tracts, or tunnels:* Use a sterile cotton-tipped applicator to measure depth and, if needed, a gloved finger to examine the wound edges.
e. *Condition of the wound bed:* Describe the type and percentage of tissue in the wound bed.
f. *Volume of exudate:* Describe the amount, characteristics, odor, and color.
g. *Condition of periwound skin:* Examine the skin for breaks; dryness; and the presence of a rash, swelling, redness, or warmth.
h. *Wound edges:* Gives information regarding epithelialization, chronicity, and etiology (Nix, 2007a).
i. *Presence of pain:* Note pain at or around the wounded area; have patient rate pain on scale of 0 to 10.

6. Observe for factors affecting wound healing: poor perfusion, immunosuppression, or preexisting infection.
7. Assess patient's nutritional status. Clinically significant malnutrition is present if (1) serum albumin level is less than 3.5 g/dL, (2) lymphocyte count is less than 1800/mm^3, or (3) body weight decreases more than 15% (WOCN, 2010). *Rationale: Delayed wound healing occurs in poorly nourished patients.*
8. Assess patient's and family caregiver's understanding of pressure ulcer characteristics and purpose of treatment. *Rationale: Explanations relieve anxiety and promote cooperation during procedure.*

PLANNING

Expected Outcomes focus on healing ulcer and preventing further skin breakdown.

1. Ulcer drainage decreases.
2. Granulation tissue is present in wound base.
3. Nutrition is adequate to support wound repair.
4. Patient's skin is protected from further breakdown.

Delegation and Collaboration

The skill of treatment of pressure ulcers and wound management may not be delegated to nursing assistive personnel (NAP). Instruct the NAP about the following:

- Any patient-specific position changes
- Observing and reporting back to nurse any redness or break in patient's skin

Equipment

- Clean gloves
- Sterile gloves (optional)
- Goggles and cover gown (if splash is a risk)
- Plastic bag for dressing disposal
- Wound measuring device
- Cotton-tipped applicators
- Normal saline or cleansing agent (as ordered)
- Topical agent or solution (as ordered)
- Dressings
- Hypoallergenic tape if needed

IMPLEMENTATION *for* TREATMENT OF PRESSURE ULCERS AND WOUND MANAGEMENT

STEPS	RATIONALE
1. **See Standard Protocol (inside front cover).**	
2. Identify patient using two identifiers (e.g., name and birthday or name and account number, according to facility policy).	Ensures correct patient. Complies with The Joint Commission standards and improves patient safety (TJC, 2010).
3. Explain procedure to patient and family members.	
4. Select pressure ulcer management based on objectives of local wound care:	
a. Prevent and manage infection.	Infected wounds do not heal.
b. Cleanse wound.	Removes surface bacteria.
c. Remove nonviable tissue that promotes infection.	Many dressings support the softening and eventual loosening of nonviable tissue.
d. Maintain appropriate level of moisture.	A moist environment supports wound healing.
e. Eliminate dead space.	Prevents exudate buildup.
f. Control odor.	
g. Eliminate or minimize pain.	
h. Protect wound.	Prevents further injury.
5. Consult with physician or wound care specialist in selecting appropriate dressing (Table 25-5) based on pressure ulcer assessment, principles of wound management, and patient care setting. Dressing options include:	The dressing provides an appropriate wound-healing environment (WOCN, 2010).

STEPS	RATIONALE
a. Gauze pads	Used for wicking, maintaining a moist environment, packing, and delivering solutions to a wound.
b. Transparent film dressings	Used on partial-thickness wounds with minimal wound exudate.
c. Hydrogel (available in a sheet or in a tube)	Maintains moist environment to facilitate wound healing.
d. Hydrocolloid	Maintains moist environment to facilitate wound healing while protecting wound base.
e. Alginate dressings	Highly absorbent of wound exudate in heavily draining wounds.
f. Foam dressings	Protective and prevents wound dehydration; also absorbs small-to-moderate amounts of drainage. Maintains a moist environment.
g. Silver impregnated dressings/gels	Controls bacterial burden in wound.
h. Enzymatic debriding agents	Promotes removal of devitalized tissue.
i. Wound fillers	Fills shallow wounds, hydrates, and absorbs.
j. Antimicrobials	Control or decreases bioburden. Includes antibacterials and antiseptics.
6. Open packages and topical solution containers.	Prepares supplies for easy application so you can use supplies without contaminating them.
7. Position patient to expose ulcer, keeping rest of body covered with bed linen.	Prevents unnecessary exposure of body parts.

TABLE 25-5 DRESSING SELECTION BASED ON WOUND ASSESSMENT

WOUND DESCRIPTION	REQUIREMENTS	RATIONALE	DRESSING OPTIONS
Necrotic tissue	Debridement	Removal of dead tissue decreases risk of bacterial overgrowth and facilitates healing (healing will not take place in the presence of devitalized tissue).	Consider a dressing that traps the moisture from the wound (e.g., hydrogel, impregnated gauze, hydrocolloid) over the necrotic tissue, allowing the tissue to soften and be removed (autolysis). Consider use of enzyme preparations for chemical debridement.
Granulation tissue	Protection	Support granulation tissue with a moist environment to facilitate healing.	Consider the use of hydrocolloid, hydrogel, or foam dressing to maintain moisture.
Dry wound base	Hydration	A moist wound base facilitates healing by providing a surface for new cells to migrate.	Consider use of a hydrogel to bring moisture to the wound. *or* Consider use of gauze with saline to provide moisture to the wound.
Moderate-to-heavy exudate	Absorption	Excess wound drainage overhydrates cells, delaying healing and macerating the periwound skin.	Consider the use of a hydrocolloid, foam, alginate, or hydrofiber dressing, all of which absorb various amounts of drainage.
Significant depth	Packing	Packing prevents wound drainage from accumulating in the dead space of the deep wound.	Consider the use of gauze, alginate, or wound filler; pack lightly into the defect to fill the wound.
Erythema, warmth, edema, tenderness	Infection management	Wound infection prolongs the inflammatory response, delaying wound healing.	Antimicrobial dressings or solutions decrease bacterial overload.
Periwound skin maceration	Protection	Maceration can cause further skin breakdown and discomfort.	Skin sealant or barrier ointment provides protection.

Continued

STEPS	RATIONALE
8. Remove old dressings and discard in plastic bag. Discard gloves; perform hand hygiene per agency protocol.	
9. Cleanse wound with prescribed solution, cleansing from least contaminated to most contaminated area. Rinse with solution; gently wipe wound base and surrounding skin with moistened gauze. Use fresh piece of moistened gauze to clean skin surface; dry with fresh dry gauze.	Reduces surface bacteria; removes wound exudate and/or dressing residue.
10. Apply topical agents to wound using cotton-tipped applicators or gauze as ordered.	
a. *Antibacterials:* Examples include bacitracin, metronidazole, and silver sulfadiazine.	Destroy or stop bacterial growth.
b. *Antiseptics:* Examples include acetic acid and hypochlorite (Dakin's solution).	Reduce bacteria on the wound surface. Use is limited because of cell toxicity.
c. *Enzyme debriding agents:* Cover wound with debriding agent and apply a moist gauze dressing over wound.	Removes dead tissue. Moisture must be present for the enzyme preparation to work.
11. Apply prescribed wound dressing:	
a. ***Moist-to-dry dressing***	
(1) Apply saline to gauze; wring out excess.	Dampens gauze, allowing the gauze to "wick" drainage.
(2) Unfold gauze and, if wound has depth, loosely pack it with the dressing; if shallow, lay gauze over wound.	Unfolded gauze allows for wicking of the drainage.
(3) Cover with secondary dry dressing; tape dressing over wound.	
b. ***Transparent film dressings (see Chapter 26)***	Applied over superficial wounds only.
c. ***Hydrogel***	Hydrogel maintains a moist environment to facilitate wound healing.
(1) Cover wound base with a thick layer of the amorphous hydrogel or cut a sheet to fit wound base.	
(2) Cover with secondary dressing; tape.	
(3) If using impregnated gauze, pack loosely into wound; cover with secondary gauze dressing, and tape.	A loosely packed dressing delivers the gel to the wound base and allows any wound debris to be trapped in the gauze.
d. ***Hydrocolloid (see Chapter 26)***	Hydrocolloid forms a gel over the wounded area; the outer edge creates the seal.
e. ***Alginate***	
(1) Cut to size of wound and loosely pack into wound.	The dressing swells and increases in size; tight packing can compromise blood flow to the tissues.
(2) Cover with a secondary gauze dressing; apply tape.	
f. ***Foam dressings (see Chapter 26)***	Protective; prevents wound dehydration; absorbs small-to-moderate amount of drainage.
12. Reposition patient comfortably off wound.	
13. **See Completion Protocol (inside front cover).**	

EVALUATION

1. Observe skin surrounding wound for inflammation, edema, and tenderness.
2. Inspect dressings and exposed wounds; observe for drainage, foul odor, and tissue necrosis. Monitor patient for signs and symptoms of infection, including fever and elevated WBC count.
3. Compare subsequent wound measurements with each dressing change.
4. Ask patient to rate pain on a scale of 0 to 10 during and following pressure ulcer care.

Unexpected Outcomes and Related Interventions

1. Skin surrounding ulcer becomes macerated.
   a. Reduce exposure of surrounding skin to topical agents and moisture.
   b. Consider use of a liquid skin barrier on periwound skin.
2. Ulcer becomes deeper with increased drainage and/or development of necrotic tissue.
   a. Notify health care provider for possible change in pressure ulcer status.
   b. Additional consultations (e.g., wound care nurse specialist) may be indicated.
   c. Obtain necessary wound cultures.

Recording and Reporting

- Record assessment of ulcer, type of topical agent and or dressing used, and patient's response in medical record.
- Report any deterioration in ulcer appearance.

Sample Documentation

0900 Sacral pressure ulcer, stage II, 2 × 3 cm irregular shape. Base of wound covered 100% by granulation tissue; no drainage or odor present. Surrounding skin intact. Wound cleansed with NS and hydrocolloid dressing applied. On a low–air loss overlay, repositioned q2 hr as condition allowed. Nutritional supplements taken as offered. Patient and sister instructed in care and prevention of skin breakdown have correctly participated in repositioning.

Special Considerations

Pediatric

- Reinforce wound dressings in the diaper zone with a water-resistant tape. Carefully remove this tape to avoid skin stripping.

Geriatric

- Skin in older adults has a slower and less intense inflammatory reaction; therefore closely monitor older patients.

Home Care

- The bed at home should have the appropriate type of support surface.
- Be sure that patient and family caregiver know how to use the wound products chosen.
- Choose a dressing that does not require multiple dressing changes in a 24-hour period. This decreases the amount of time that the family will need to pay to the wound management program, increases compliance, and makes good use of home care resources.

REVIEW QUESTIONS

Case Study for Questions 1 and 2

Mr. Bass is admitted to a surgical unit following a small bowel resection. He is currently NPO and has had frequent loose stools and several incontinence episodes. He is alert and oriented but notes that he has abdominal discomfort when he moves. He has been wheelchair bound for several months following complications from hip surgery. His wife also has health issues and has been unable to provide direct care to her husband at home.

1. The nurse is assessing Mr. Bass for pressure ulcer risk using the Braden Scale. Under the moisture subscale she has determined that her patient's skin moisture is related to fecal incontinence. What are two interventions that the nurse can consider as she develops her plan of care to reduce the effects of skin moisture?
   1. Application of talcum powder in areas where stool is in contact with the skin
   2. Use of a moisture barrier ointment after each bowel movement
   3. A fecal incontinence collector
   4. Placing several towels under patient's buttocks
2. During Mr. Bass's skin assessment the nurse notes an ulcer at the sacral area. The base of the wound is covered with dark necrotic tissue, and, when she presses on the tissue, it feels soft. What stage is this ulcer?
   1. Stage II
   2. Stage III
   3. Stage IV
   4. Not stageable
3. Which of the following patients are likely to have factors that negatively affect wound healing? Select all that apply.
   1. A patient whose surgical wound is producing yellowish drainage and whose WBC count is elevated
   2. A cancer patient receiving the antiinflammatory drug cortisol
   3. An older adult who has been advised to add more sources of vitamin C to her diet
   4. A trauma patient who has an open wound that is being treated with a moist dressing
4. Mrs. Gibbs is a 71-year-old patient who has been in the intensive care unit for 48 hours. She has an endotracheal tube inserted through the mouth to maintain ventilation. She has an intravenous (IV) line infusing at 125 mL/hr. Her abdominal wound over the right lower quadrant is dry and intact. The nurses have placed pillows under both ankles. Turning the patient is difficult because she weighs 320 pounds. She is most likely to be at risk for pressure ulcers in which of the following locations? Select all that apply.
   1. Heels
   2. Posterior bony prominences
   3. Nose
   4. Mouth
   5. IV site
5. When using gauze moistened in normal saline for a wound dressing, why is the gauze pad wrung out before application?
   1. To prevent excessive delivery of the solution to the wound

2. To keep the healing wound moist and wick any excessive drainage
3. To prevent moistening the secondary dressing and causing maceration
4. To allow the wound to become slightly dry to facilitate healing

6. What is the primary mechanism of action of a hydrocolloid dressing?
   1. It covers the wound, preventing staff or patient from viewing the affected area.
   2. It forms a gel over the wound to facilitate moist wound healing.
   3. It forms a temporary membrane over the wound, allowing oxygen transport directly to the wound.
   4. It delivers epithelial growth factors to the wound base.
7. The dressing ordered for a patient's sacral pressure ulcer is a hydrocolloid dressing. Place the following steps in appropriate order for the dressing application:
   a. Cleanse wound with ordered solution.
   b. Remove paper backing from dressing.
   c. Explain to patient the purpose of the dressing change.
   d. Position patient to gain access to the pressure ulcer.
   e. Measure wound to determine correct size of dressing.
   f. Place dressing over wound; apply light pressure for 30 to 60 seconds.

   1. a, c, e, f, b, d
   2. c, d, a, e, b, f
   3. c, d, a, e, b, f
   4. e, a, c, d, b, f
8. Which of the following patients is most at risk for developing a pressure ulcer?
   1. An 80-year-old adult with Alzheimer's who has poor oral intake
   2. A 45-year-old male who is confined to a wheelchair as a result of paraplegia
   3. A 50-year-old male with type I diabetes who underwent major heart surgery 24 hours ago and has diaphoresis
   4. A 60-year-old female who underwent bladder surgery and now has urinary incontinence
9. A patient is admitted to the intensive care unit with pneumonia and renal failure. He is receiving IV fluids of $D_5\frac{1}{2}$NS and is NPO. He has been diaphoretic and febrile and requires linen changes each shift. He is able to turn in bed but requires reminding. He is confined to bed. He is able to respond verbally and describe sources of discomfort. Which category on the Braden Scale is not included in this assessment?
   1. Nutrition
   2. Activity
   3. Frictional shear
   4. Moisture

REFERENCES

Ayello EA and others: Pressure ulcers. In Baranoski S, Ayello EA, editors: *Wound care essentials: practice principles*, ed 2, Philadelphia, 2008, Lippincott Williams & Wilkins.

Baharestani MM: Quality of life and ethical issues. In Baranoski S, Ayello EA, editors: *Wound care essentials: practice principles*, ed 2, Philadelphia, 2008, Lippincott Williams & Wilkins.

Bergstrom N and others: *Pressure ulcers in adults: prediction and prevention*, Clinical Practice Guideline No 3, AHCPR Pub No 92-0047, Rockville, Md, May 1992, Agency for Health Care Policy and Research, Public Health Service, US Department of Health and Human Services.

Bergstrom N and others: The National Pressure Ulcer Long-Term Care Study: outcomes of pressure ulcer treatments in long-term care, *J Am Geriatr Soc* 53(10):1721, 2005.

Braden BJ, Bergstrom N: Clinical utility of the Braden Scale for predicting pressure sore risk, *Decubitus* 2(3):441, 1989.

Braden BJ, Maklebust J: Preventing pressure ulcers with the Braden Scale: an update on this easy-to-use tool that assesses a patient's risk, *Am J Nurs* 105(8):16, 2005.

Comfort EH: Reducing pressure ulcer incidence thru Braden Scale risk assessment and support surface use, *Adv Skin Wound Care* 31:7, 300, 2007.

Courtney BA and others: Save our skin: initiative cuts pressure ulcer incidence in half, *Nurs Manage* 37(4):35, 2006.

Doughty D, Sparks-Defriese B: Wound-healing physiology. In Bryant RA, Nix DP, editors: *Acute and chronic wounds current management concepts*, St Louis, 2007, Mosby.

Gray M: Context for WOC practice: assessment, prevention, and intervention in wound, ostomy, and continence care, *J Wound Ostomy Continence Care* 36(1):11, 2009.

McInnes E and others: Support surfaces for pressure ulcer prevention, *Cochrane Database of Systematic Reviews* 4, 2009.

National Pressure Ulcer Advisory Panel (NPUAP): Pressure ulcer stages revised by NPUAP, February 2007a, http://www.npuap.org/pr2.htm, accessed September 27, 2010.

National Pressure Ulcer Advisory Panel (NPUAP): Support surface standards initiatives: terms and definitions related to support surfaces, 2007b, http://www.npuap.org/NPUAP_S31_TD.pdf, accessed July 2009.

Nix, D. Patient assessment and evaluation of healing. In Bryant RA, Nix DP, editors: *Acute and chronic wounds current management concepts*, St Louis, 2007a, Mosby.

Nix D: Support surfaces. In Bryant RA, Nix DP, editors: *Acute and chronic wounds: current management concepts*, St Louis, 2007b, Mosby.

Pieper B. Mechanical forces: pressure, shear and friction. In Bryant RA, Nix DP, editors: *Acute and chronic wounds current management concepts*, St Louis, 2007, Mosby.

Rolstad BS, Ovington LG. Principles of wound management. In Bryant RA, Nix DP, editors: *Acute and chronic wounds current management concepts*, St Louis, 2007, Mosby.

Stotts NA: Nutritional assessment and support. In Bryant RA, Nix DP, editors: *Acute and chronic wounds current management concepts*, St Louis, 2007, Mosby.

The Joint Commission: *2010 National Patient Safety Goals*, Oakbrook Terrace, Ill, 2010, The Commission, http://www.jointcommission.org/PatientSafety/NationalPatientSafetyGoals/, accessed February 14, 2010.

Wound, Ostomy and Continence Nurses Society: *Guideline for prevention and management of pressure ulcers*, WOCN Clinical Practice Guidelines Series, Mount Laurel, NJ, 2010, WOCN.

CHAPTER

26

Dressings, Bandages, and Binders

evolve WEBSITE

http://evolve.elsevier.com/Perry/nursinginterventions

Wound healing is a complex physiological process. Dressings are an important part of this process because of their ability to control moisture, debride dead tissue, and protect a wound. Numerous dressings and products are available for the management of acute and chronic wounds (Table 26-1). Primary dressings are in direct contact with the wound bed. Secondary dressings cover or secure the primary dressing in place. It is important to match the wound characteristics, goals of wound management, and properties of the "ideal" dressing (Box 26-1).

Wounds heal best in a moist environment that allows epithelial cells to move more rapidly over a wound surface. Dressings are essential to maintaining the optimal level of moisture by absorbing exudate or hydrating cells to prevent the drying of a wound (Brett, 2006b). When a patient has a draining wound, the dressing must be highly absorbent. A patient with an excessively dry wound needs a dressing with moisturizing capability. This chapter reviews principles of wound care, current wound care products, and the proper techniques for the application of dressings.

The removal of necrotic tissue or slough is a component of wound healing because it allows for the growth of new tissue. Certain dressings have debriding properties. The traditional tissue debriding method is the moist-to-dry dressing (see Skill 26.1). Although effective, this method potentially causes trauma to new, healthy granulation tissue (Kirshen and others, 2006). Recent advances in wound care therapies have led to the development of a number of debriding products for use along with moist gauze for debriding necrotic wounds. Autolytic debriding products allow enzymes to self-digest dead tissue. Enzymatic debriding agents act by breaking down dead tissue. Enzymatic products are used in combination with moist-to-dry gauze but may also come as packaged dressings that do not require additional gauze packing (see Skill 26.3).

Dressings protect wounds, guarding them against contamination, heat loss, further tissue injury, and spread of microorganisms. Some dressings are impregnated with antimicrobial elements such as silver for use in wounds suspected to be infected (Baranoski, 2008). Dressings also control bleeding and drainage (see Skill 26.2). They promote hemostasis by direct pressure and absorption of drainage. They may also serve to support or immobilize a body part (see Procedural Guideline 26.3).

PATIENT-CENTERED CARE

Both acute and chronic wounds present any number of challenges to patients and their families. Wounds frequently are the cause of great distress to patients. Whether it is the pain of dressing changes, the emotional impact of deformity or viewing a wound, or the financial burdens associated with illness, it is important to consider the unique needs of patients, particularly those from specialized socioeconomic populations (Pieper, 2009).

Many patients and their families ultimately become the primary caretakers of their wounds. Wound care and pain management are frequently cited by surgical patients as the areas of greatest concern at discharge (Pieper and others, 2006). It is incumbent on nurses to instruct patients and family caregivers about wound care techniques. Successful wound care teaching results in faster healing and fewer post-discharge complications. Teaching should be initiated as soon as possible and should include patient participation.

TABLE 26-1 COMPARISON OF WOUND CARE PRODUCTS

PRODUCT CATEGORY	INDICATIONS FOR USE	CONTRAINDICATIONS	ADVANTAGES	DISADVANTAGES	FREQUENCY OF CHANGE (PER MANUFACTURER'S RECOMMENDATIONS)
Gauze Dressings					
Cotton or synthetic material; woven or nonwoven construction	Protection of surgical incisions Mechanical debridement (moist to dry) Secondary dressing for other wound products Packing wounds	Overgranulating wounds as primary treatment	Available in many sizes and forms Sterile and nonsterile	May adhere to healthy tissue, causing injury when removed Lint fibers may be left on wound May interfere with wound healing if gauze dries out in a moist-to-dry dressing	2 to 3 times per day as needed.
Transparent Films					
Adhesive membrane dressings; waterproof, impermeable to fluids and bacteria; allow oxygen and moisture vapor exchange	Shallow wounds with minimal exudate Skin protection from friction and shear Promote autolytic debridement Stage I or II pressure ulcers	Infected wounds; wounds that tunnel, undermine, or are full thickness; wounds with moderate-to-heavy exudate; burns	Easy to apply and remove without damage to underlying tissue Able to see the wound Waterproof Create a moist environment that softens thin slough and eschar Serve as a barrier to external fluids and bacteria	May cause skin maceration May not adhere to moist areas May cause skin stripping if improperly removed	Every 24-72 hours If using to facilitate autolytic debridement, every 24 hours
Hydrocolloids					
Adhesive dressings made of elastomeric, adhesive, and gelling agents; considered semiocclusive dressings	Minimal-to-moderate exudating wounds Stage I-IV pressure ulcers Can be used in combination with absorbent powder or alginate	Third-degree burns, infected wounds; arterial or diabetic ulcers Wounds with dry eschar	Available in many sizes Facilitates autolytic debridement Impermeable to fluids/bacteria Thermal insulator Easy to apply and remove	Potential for periwound maceration if dressing left in place too long Drainage often mistaken for pus/infection Adhesive possibly too aggressive for fragile skin	Every 3-5 days
Hydrogel					
Glycerin- or water-based dressings designed to hydrate a wound; may also absorb a small amount of exudate	Dry-to–minimally invasive wound with or without a clean granular wound base Shallow or deep wounds Wounds with undermining Necrotic wounds	Third-degree burns Wounds with heavy exudate	Facilitates autolysis Conforms to wound	Potential for maceration or candidiasis of periwound area	Daily if adhesive sheets or wound fillers are not used Up to 3 times per week for sheets with adhesive covers
Alginates					
Highly absorbent nonwoven material that forms a gel when exposed to wound drainage; fibrous product derived from brown seaweed	Moderate-to–heavily exudating wounds with or without depth Full-thickness, tunneling wounds Partial- and full-thickness wounds Leg ulcers, donor sites, traumatic wounds	Third-degree burns Nondraining wounds Dry, necrotic wounds	Nonadhering Nonocclusive May be packed into tunneled areas Promote autolytic debridement in exudating wounds Highly absorbent	More expensive than gauze or gauze packing strips Not practical for large wounds Gelled material possibly mistaken for purulence	Every 24 hours Loosely pack wound. Layer dressings in a deep wound
Foam Dressings					
Absorbent, nonadherent polyurethane pad used to protect wounds and maintain moist healing environment	Moderate or heavily exudating wounds Partial- and full-thickness wounds Stage II-IV pressure ulcers	Third-degree burns, wounds that tunnel, wounds with sinus tracts, nondraining wounds, caution with infected wounds	Highly absorbent while maintaining moist wound environment May be used with other dressings (films, absorbers) Nonadherent to wound bed	Nonadhesive foams require a secondary dressing Possible maceration of periwound if dressing left on too long	Up to 3 times per week Once per day when using foam wound fillers

Modified from Rolstad BS, Ovington LG: Principles of wound management. In Bryant RA, Nix DP: *Acute and chronic wounds: nursing management*, ed 3, St Louis, 2007, Mosby; Nelson D, Dilloway MA: Principles, products, and practical aspects of wound care, *Crit Care Nurs Q* 25(1):33, 2002.

BOX 26-1 PROPERTIES OF THE IDEAL DRESSING

- Able to absorb exudate without desiccating wound bed
- Serves as barrier against bacteria
- Allows for removal without trauma or dressing fragments left in wound
- Is permeable to moisture vapors and prevents overhydration and maceration of surrounding skin (Brett, 2006a)

SAFETY

Many wounds are colonized or contaminated with low levels of bacteria. Unlike bacterial infections, colonization is a chronic state in which low levels of bacteria exist in the wound but do not interfere with wound healing. Colonized wounds may not require active treatment but do need to be monitored for signs of bacterial overgrowth that may progress to infection. Wound infections interfere with healing and need to be addressed quickly. Signs of bacterial infection include a sudden deterioration of the wound along with changes in the amount, consistency, color, and odor of the drainage (Brett, 2006b).

Bacteria are often spread from patient to patient by health care workers. During any dressing change, follow precautions to protect a patient from the introduction or spread of bacteria. Appropriate personal protective equipment (PPE) (see Chapter 5) should be worn to protect you and your patients. Some agencies choose to isolate patients who are colonized or infected with certain organisms.

EVIDENCE-BASED PRACTICE TRENDS

Jones K: Identifying best practices for pressure ulcer management, *JCOM* 16(8), 375, 2009.

Best practices for chronic wounds require a moist environment to promote healing. Choice of dressing requires decisions based on wound location, infection risk, frequency of dressing change, who will change the dressing, what product is available, and product cost. New practice guidelines and wound care algorithms suggest that new products such as transparent film, hydrogel, or hydrocolloid dressings are preferred over traditional gauze dressings. Recent studies have shown that hydrocolloid dressings are more effective than saline-soaked gauze or paraffin gauze dressings for wound healing. However, studies have not shown that any one of the new products was the most ideal, but they were better than more traditional dressings.

SKILL 26.1 APPLYING A GAUZE DRESSING (DRY AND MOIST-TO-DRY)

Dry dressings are for wounds healing by primary intention with little drainage (Fig. 26-1). The dressing protects the wound from injury, prevents the introduction and spread of bacteria, reduces discomfort, and speeds healing. Dry woven gauze dressings do not interact with wound tissues and cause little wound irritation. They are commonly used for abrasions and nondraining postoperative incisions. Telfa gauze dressings contain a shiny, nonadherent surface on one side that does not stick to the wound. Drainage passes through the nonadherent surface to the outer gauze dressing (Table 26-2). Dry dressings are not appropriate for debriding wounds. On occasion a dry dressing may adhere to the wound (when there has been drainage). In that case moistening the dressing with sterile normal saline or sterile water before removing the gauze minimizes trauma to the wound.

FIG 26-1 Types of gauze dressings: 4 × 4, split, roll, and ABD.

Moist-to-dry dressings are gauze moistened with an appropriate solution. They are also called *wet-to-dry* or *damp-to-dry* dressings. The primary purpose is to mechanically debride wounds, specifically full-thickness wounds healing by secondary intention and wounds with necrotic tissue. A moist-to-dry dressing has a moist contact dressing layer that touches the wound surface. The moistened gauze increases the absorptive ability of the dressing to collect exudate and wound debris. This layer dries and adheres to dead cells, thus debriding the wound when removed. Isotonic solutions such as normal saline or lactated Ringer's are best to use to moisten this type of dressing. The outer absorbent layer of a moist-to-dry dressing is a dry dressing that protects the wound from invasive microorganisms.

Most dressings are secured with tape, which may be paper, plastic, woven, or elastic material with adhesive. Frequent removal of tape for dressing changes irritates the skin and causes skin tears. Several techniques are available to reduce tape-related injury. Montgomery straps are wide strips of tape with holes and laces that secure dressings when placed on opposite wound edges and tied. Strips of a stomadhesive or hydrocolloid dressing are used to create a window around the wound. Then tape is applied over the strips, thereby reducing contact with the periwound skin.

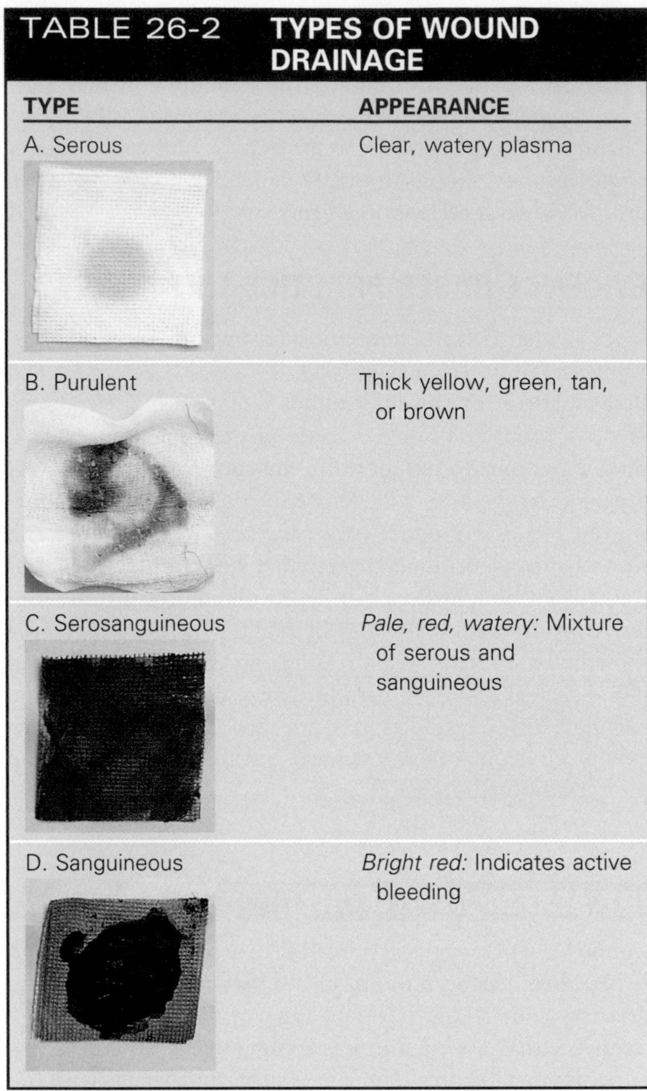

TABLE 26-2 TYPES OF WOUND DRAINAGE

TYPE	APPEARANCE
A. Serous	Clear, watery plasma
B. Purulent	Thick yellow, green, tan, or brown
C. Serosanguineous	*Pale, red, watery:* Mixture of serous and sanguineous
D. Sanguineous	*Bright red:* Indicates active bleeding

Delegation and Collaboration

The skill of applying dry and moist-to-dry dressings may sometimes be delegated to nursing assistive personnel (NAP) if the wound is chronic (see agency policy). However, all wound assessment, care of acute new wounds, and wound care that requires sterile technique should not be delegated. Instruct the NAP by:

- Explaining how to adapt the skill for a specific patient.
- Reviewing what to observe and report back to the nurse.

Equipment

- Clean gloves
- Sterile gloves
- Sterile dressing set (scissors and forceps)
- Sterile drape (optional)
- Necessary dressings: fine-mesh gauze, 4 × 4–inch gauze, and/or abdominal pads (ABDs) (see Fig. 26-1)
- Sterile basin (optional)
- Antiseptic ointment as prescribed
- Sterile Q-tips
- Cleansing solution as prescribed
- Sterile normal saline (or prescribed solution)
- Tape or ties as needed, including nonallergenic tape if necessary
- Measuring guide
- Adhesive remover (optional)
- Waterproof bag
- Debriding gel as ordered
- Protective gown, goggles, and mask (used when spray from wound is a risk)

ASSESSMENT

1. Determine the presence of allergies to antiseptics, tape, or latex. *Rationale: Patients may have localized or systemic allergic reactions to these supplies.*
2. During the dressing removal inspect and assess the condition of the wound (see Implementation, Step 8). *Rationale: Assists in planning choice of dressing materials to use. Provides baseline for condition of wound.*
3. Ask patient to rate wound pain using a scale of 0 to 10. *Rationale: Patient may require pain medication before dressing change to allow for peak effect of drug during procedure.*
4. Assess patient's knowledge of purpose of dressing change. *Rationale: Determines level of support and explanation required.*
5. Determine the need for patient or family member to participate in dressing wound. *Rationale: Prepares patient or family member if dressing will be changed at home.*

PLANNING

Expected Outcomes focus on preventing infection, promoting healing, controlling pain, and patient and family learning.

1. Patient's wound shows evidence of healing by smaller size and less drainage, redness, or swelling.
2. Patient reports pain less than previously assessed level (scale of 0 to 10) during and after dressing change.
3. Dressing remains clean, dry, and intact.
4. Patient or family demonstrates correct method of dressing changes.

IMPLEMENTATION *for* APPLYING A GAUZE DRESSING (DRY AND MOIST-TO-DRY)

STEPS	RATIONALE
1. **See Standard Protocol (inside front cover).**	
2. Identify patient using two identifiers (e.g., name and birthday or name and account number, according to facility policy).	Ensures correct patient. Complies with The Joint Commission standards and improves patient safety (TJC, 2010).

STEPS	RATIONALE
3. Premedicate patient with ordered analgesic 30 minutes before dressing change. Position patient comfortably and drape to expose only wound site. Instruct patient not to touch wound or sterile supplies.	Reduces discomfort during dressing change. Maintaining patient comfort assists in completing skill smoothly. Draping provides access to wound while minimizing unnecessary exposure.
4. Place disposable waterproof bag within reach of work area with top folded to make a cuff.	Facilitates safe disposal of soiled dressings.
5. Apply gown and mask/goggles if risk of splashing (see agency policy).	
6. Gently remove tape by using your nondominant hand to support the dressing and, with your dominant hand, pulling the tape parallel to the skin toward the dressing. If over hairy areas, remove in the direction of hair growth. Secure patient permission to clip or shave area (check agency policy).	Pulling tape toward dressing reduces stress on suture line or wound edges and reduces irritation and discomfort.
7. Remove dressing one layer at a time, observing appearance and drainage on dressing. Use caution to avoid tension on any drains that are present.	Determines dressings needed for replacement. Avoids accidental removal of an underlying drain because it may or may not be sutured in place.
a. If a moist-to-dry dressing sticks, gently free dressing and alert patient of discomfort.	Moist-to-dry dressing should debride a wound (Ramundo, 2007).
b. If a dry dressing sticks, moisten it with normal saline and remove.	Prevents injury to wound edges.
8. Inspect wound for appearance, color, size, depth, drainage, edema, drains, approximation (wound edges are together), granulation tissue, or odor. Use a measuring guide to measure size of wound (see Chapter 24).	Provides baseline assessment for drainage and wound integrity. Monitors status of wound healing.
9. Fold dressings with drainage turned inward and remove gloves inside out. With small dressings, remove gloves inside out over dressing (see illustrations). Dispose of gloves and soiled dressings according to agency policy. Cover wound lightly with a sterile gauze pad and perform hand hygiene.	Provides containment of soiled dressings, prevents contact of nurse's hands with drainage, and reduces transmission of cross-contamination microorganisms.

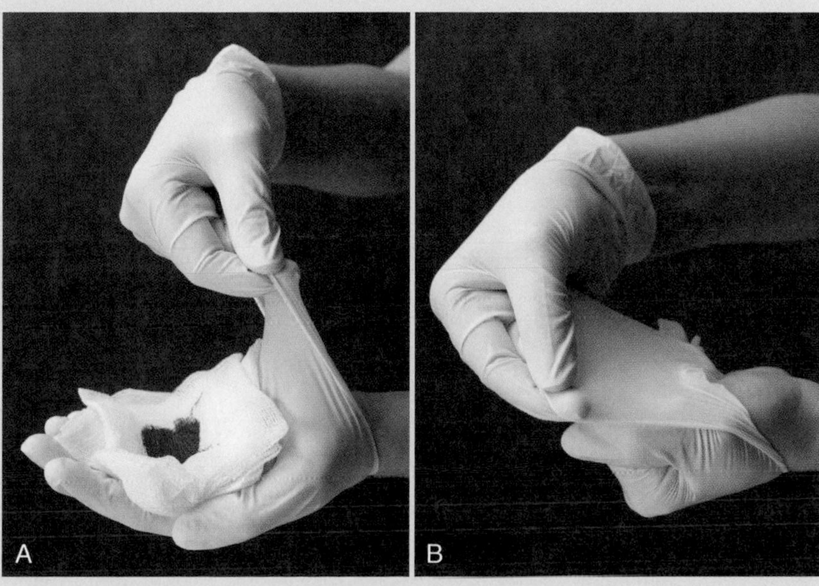

STEP 9 A and **B,** Dispose of soiled dressing and gloves.

Continued

STEPS	RATIONALE
10. Create a sterile field with a sterile dressing tray or individually wrapped sterile supplies on over-bed table (see Chapter 5). Pour prescribed solution into sterile basin.	Sterile dressings remain sterile while on or within sterile area.
11. Remove gauze cover over wound.	
12. Cleanse wound.	
a. Use an antiseptic swab for each cleansing stroke or spray wound surface.	Prevents transfer of organisms from previously cleaned area.
b. Clean from least contaminated to most contaminated area (see illustration).	Prevents spreading germs across cleaner incisional area.
c. Cleanse around drain (if present), using a circular stroke starting near the drain and moving outward away from insertion site (see illustration).	
13. Use sterile dry gauze to blot dry the wound, using same technique as Step 12.	Drying reduces excess moisture, which could harbor microorganisms.
14. Apply antiseptic ointment (if ordered) with sterile Q-tip or gauze, using same technique as Step 12. Dispose of clean gloves.	
15. Apply dressing. Apply sterile gloves (see agency policy).	Prevents transmission of organisms to wound site.
a. ***Dry sterile dressing:***	
(1) Apply loose woven gauze as contact layer.	Promotes proper absorption of drainage.
(2) If drain is present, apply precut, split 4 × 4–inch gauze around drain (see Fig. 26-1).	Secures drain and promotes drainage absorption at site.
(3) Apply additional layers of gauze as needed.	Ensures proper coverage and optimal absorption.
(4) Apply thicker woven pad (e.g., ABD, Surgipad) (see Fig. 26-1).	Dressing is used as an outer layer on postoperative wounds when there is excessive drainage.
b. ***Moist-to-dry dressing:***	
(1) Place fine-mesh or loose 4 × 4–inch gauze in container of prescribed sterile solution. Wring out excess solution.	Moist gauze absorbs drainage and removes tissue when dried (Kirshen and others, 2006).
(2) Apply moist fine-mesh or open-weave gauze as a single layer directly onto wound surface. If wound is deep, gently pack gauze into wound with forceps until all wound surfaces are in contact with moist gauze. Be sure that gauze does not touch surrounding skin (see illustrations).	Inner gauze should be moist, not dripping wet, to absorb drainage and adhere to debris. Wound should be packed loosely to facilitate wicking of drainage into absorbent outer layer of dressing. Moisture that escapes the dressing may cause maceration of the periwound skin (Gray and Weir, 2007).

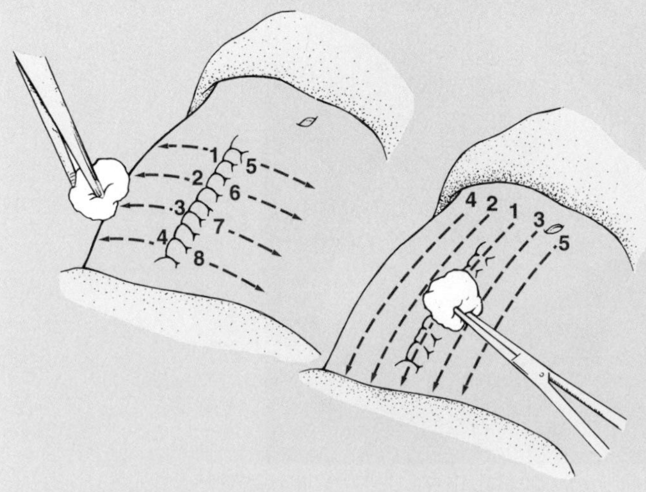

STEP 12b Methods for cleansing a wound.

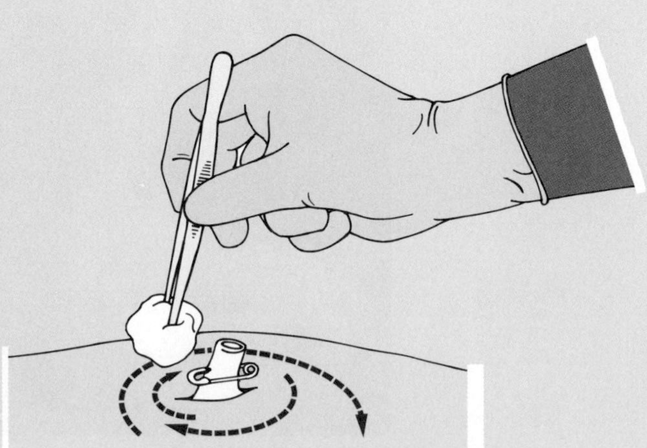
STEP 12c Cleansing a drain site.

STEPS	RATIONALE
(3) Observe packing to ensure that any dead space from sinus tracts, undermining, or tunneling is loosely packed with gauze.	Do not overpack the wound because it can lead to increased pressure within the wound bed, causing tissue damage and delayed healing.
(4) Apply dry, sterile 4 × 4–inch gauze over moist gauze.	Pulls moisture from wound.
(5) Cover with ABD pad, Surgipad, or gauze (see Fig. 26-1).	Protects wound from entrance of microorganisms.
16. Secure dressing.	
a. *Tape:* Apply tape to secure dressing. When necessary, use nonallergenic tape.	
b. *Montgomery ties (see illustrations):*	
(1) Be sure that skin is clean. Application of a skin barrier is recommended.	Skin barrier (stomadhesive) protects intact skin from stretch and tension of adhesive tape.
(2) Expose adhesive surface of tape ends.	

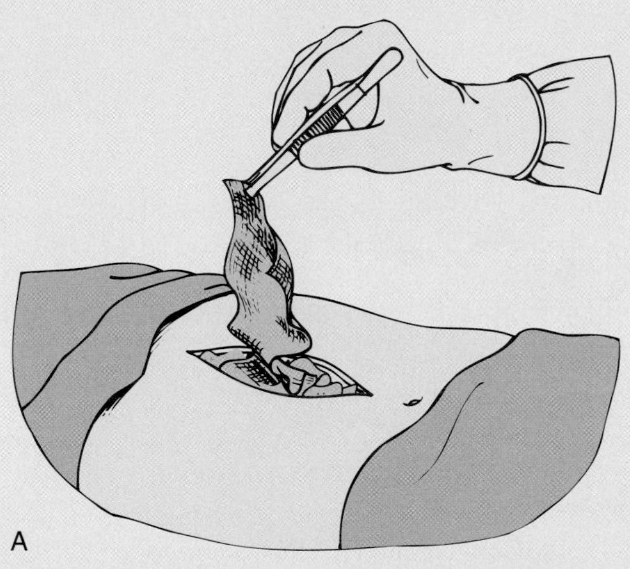

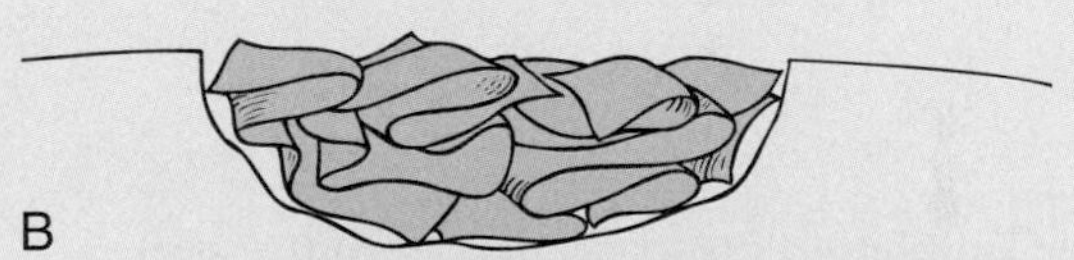

STEP 15b(2) A, Packing a wound with fine-mesh gauze. **B,** Cross-section of wound packed loosely.

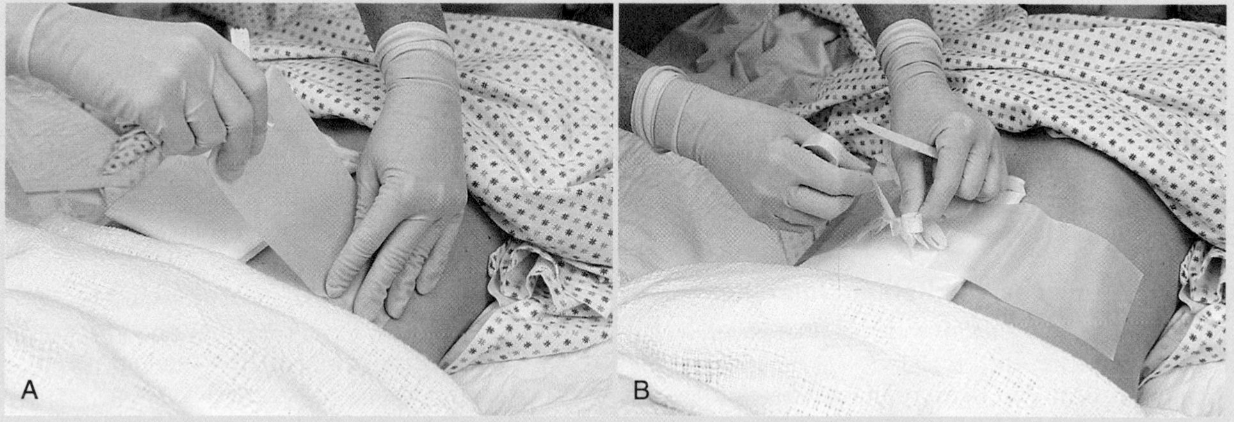

STEP 16b Montgomery ties. **A,** Each tie is placed at side of dressing. **B,** Securing ties encloses dressing.

Continued

STEPS	RATIONALE
(3) Place ties on opposite sides of dressing over skin or skin barrier.	
(4) Secure dressing by lacing ties across dressing snugly enough to hold dressing secure but without pressure on the skin.	
c. *Stomadhesive/hydrocolloid window:*	An alternative to Montgomery ties for smaller wounds. Creates a window with strips of stomadhesive or hydrocolloid dressings around the wound.
(1) Cut strips of the stomadhesive or hydrocolloid pad into 1 cm (½-inch) strips.	
(2) Use skin barrier to wipe areas where adhesive will be applied.	
(3) Apply adhesive strips to two or four sides of the wound, framing the wound.	
(4) Apply dressing, securing tape to the adhesive pads.	Tape is placed on window strips to reduce skin irritation.
d. For dressing on an extremity, dressing is secured with roller gauze (see illustration) or Surgiflex elastic net.	

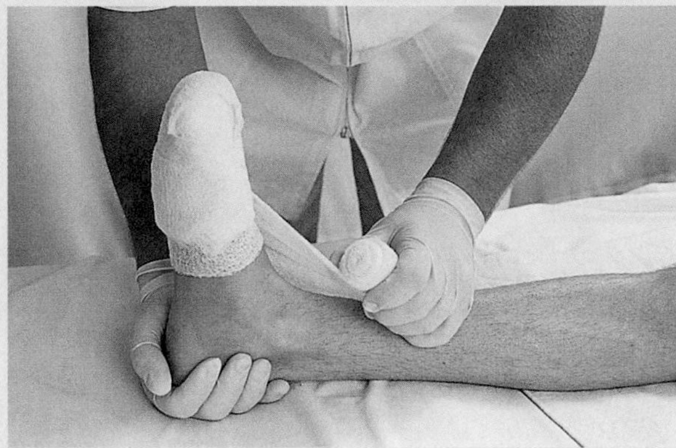

STEP 16d Wrap roller gauze around extremity.

STEPS	RATIONALE
17. See Completion Protocol (inside front cover).	Reduces transmission of microorganisms.
18. Label tape over the dressing with your initials and the date dressing is changed.	

EVALUATION

1. Observe appearance of wound for healing: measure size of wound, observe amount, color and type of drainage, and periwound erythema or swelling.
2. Ask patient to rate pain using a scale of 0 to 10.
3. Inspect status of dressing at least every shift or as ordered.
4. Observe patient's or family caregiver's ability to perform dressing change.

Unexpected Outcomes and Related Interventions

1. Wound appears inflamed and tender, drainage is evident, and/or an odor is present.
   a. Monitor patient for signs of infection (e.g., fever, increased white blood cell [WBC] count).
   b. Notify health care provider.
   c. Obtain wound cultures as ordered.
2. Wound bleeds during dressing change.
   a. Observe color and amount of drainage. If excessive, may need to apply direct pressure.
   b. Inspect area along dressing and directly underneath to determine the amount of bleeding.
   c. Obtain vital signs as needed.
   d. Notify health care provider of findings.
3. Patient reports a sensation that "something has given way under the dressing."
   a. Observe wound for increased drainage or dehiscence (partial or total separation of wound layers) or evisceration (total separation of wound layers and protrusion of viscera through the wound opening).
   b. Protect wound by covering with sterile moist dressing.
   c. Instruct patient to lie still.
   d. Notify health care provider.

Recording and Reporting

- Record size and appearance of wound, characteristics of drainage, type of dressings applied, response to dressing change, and patient's level of comfort in nurses' notes.
- Report brisk, bright bleeding or evidence of wound dehiscence or evisceration to health care provider immediately.

Sample Documentation

1000 Midline abdominal wound dressing changed. Wound measures 6 × 2 cm with 1.5 cm depth. Wound bed with 90% pink granulation tissue and 10% yellow slough. Minimal amount of serosanguineous drainage, no odor. Surrounding skin intact. Wound bed cleansed with wound cleanser spray. Saline moistened gauze lightly packed into wound. Covered with an ABD. Skin protectant wipe applied to surrounding skin. ABD secured with hypoallergenic cotton tape. Reported 0 pain on a scale of 0 to 10 pre and post dressing change, 3/10 during change.

Special Considerations

Pediatric

- Pediatric patients may be fearful of dressing changes. Use age-specific interventions such as having personnel available to keep child from moving during procedure, diversion such as music for older children, or letting children observe dressings before procedure (Hockenberry and Wilson, 2007).

Geriatric

- Adhesive tape may be too irritating to older adults' skin and cause skin tears. Use paper tape, nonallergenic tape, or wraps or mesh without tape contacting patient's skin.
- Normal changes associated with aging may delay wound healing (Meiner and Lueckenotte, 2006).

Home Care

- Some wounds may be cleansed in the shower. Have patient verify this practice with health care provider before discharge.
- Clean dressings may be used in the home environment.
- Contaminated dressings should be disposed of in a manner consistent with local regulations.

SKILL 26.2 APPLYING A PRESSURE BANDAGE

Pressure bandages are a temporary treatment to control excessive bleeding. The bleeding is a sudden and often unanticipated event. A pressure dressing exerts pressure over an area to prevent the collection of fluid in the underlying tissues. A frequent routine use of pressure dressings is following an invasive procedure or surgery such as cardiac catheterization, arterial puncture, or organ biopsy punctures. They are also used in emergency situations such as postoperative hemorrhages or traumatic injuries. Pressure dressings are essential to stopping the flow of blood and promoting clotting at the site until definitive action can be taken to stop the source. The following skill describes the steps to take when dressing an acute injury or bleed. Given the emergent nature of an acute bleeding episode, the aseptic techniques considered essential in most other dressing applications are secondary to the goal of halting the bleeding. A pressure dressing applied in an emergency is usually temporary and can be cleansed and changed once the bleeding has been controlled.

Delegation and Collaboration

The skill of applying a pressure bandage in an emergency situation cannot be delegated to nursing assistive personnel (NAP). If application requires more than one person, the NAP can assist the nurse as directed.

Equipment

- Clean gloves
- Necessary dressings: fine-mesh gauze, dressings, roller gauze and/or ABDs
- Tape or ties as needed, including hypoallergenic tape if necessary
- Adhesive remover (optional)
- Protective gown, goggles, and mask (used when spray from wound is a risk)
- Equipment for vital signs

ASSESSMENT

1. Anticipate any patients at risk for unexpected bleeding, including traumatic injury, arterial puncture, or postoperative wound. *Rationale: Prepares you to rapidly respond and prioritize actions.*
2. Assess the location and circumstance of the area where hemorrhage is expected. *Rationale: Assists in planning for proper type and amount of supplies needed.*
3. Assess patient for presence of allergies to antiseptics, tape, or latex. If patient is not responsive and no history is available, use nonlatex or nonallergenic supplies. *Rationale: Patients may have localized or systemic reactions to these supplies and should be assessed for allergies before use.*
4. Assess patient's anxiety level and knowledge of the clinical situation and purpose of dressing application.

PLANNING

Expected Outcomes focus on minimizing blood loss and fluid collection, preventing infection, promoting healing, and patient and family education.

1. Patient shows complete cessation of bleeding and no evidence of hematoma formation.
2. Patient maintains hemodynamic stability following application of pressure bandage.
3. Distal circulation is maintained, and no further injury is sustained.
4. Patient maintains sufficient level of pain control.

IMPLEMENTATION *for* APPLYING A PRESSURE BANDAGE

STEPS	RATIONALE
1. See Standard Protocol (inside front cover).	Maintaining asepsis and privacy are considered only if time and severity of blood loss permit.
Phase I: Immediate action—First Nurse	
2. Locate external bleeding site.	Wounds to groin area can result in large amounts of blood loss, which is not always visible.
3. Apply immediate manual pressure to the site of bleeding with a gloved hand and dry gauze.	Maintains hemostasis until supplies are prepared.
4. Seek assistance.	
Phase II: Applying pressure bandage—Second Nurse	
5. Quickly observe location of bleeding.	Determines method and supplies to apply.
a. Arterial is bright red and gushes forth in waves, related to heart rate. If vessel is very deep, flow will be steady.	
b. Venous is dark red and flows smoothly.	
c. Capillary is oozing of dark red; self-sealing controls bleeding.	
6. Elevate the affected body part if possible (e.g., extremity).	Assists in slowing rate of hemorrhage.
7. First person continues direct pressure as second nurse unwraps roller bandage and places within easy reach. Next, second nurse quickly cuts three to five lengths of adhesive tape and places them within reach; do not cleanse wound.	Pressure dressing controls bleeding temporarily. Preparation allows nurses to secure pressure bandage quickly.
8. In simultaneous coordinated actions:	
a. Rapidly cover bleeding area with multiple thicknesses of gauze compresses. First nurse slips fingers out as other nurse exerts adequate pressure to continue controlling bleeding.	Gauze is absorbent. Layers provide bulk against which local pressure can be applied to bleeding site.
b. Place adhesive strips 7 to 10 cm (3 to 4 inches) beyond width of dressing with even pressure on both sides of the fingers as close as possible to central bleeding source (see illustrations). Secure tape on distal end, pull tape across dressing, and keep firm pressure as the proximate end of tape is secured.	Tape exerts downward pressure, promoting hemostasis. To ensure blood flow to distal tissues and prevent tourniquet effect, adhesive tape must not be continued around entire extremity.

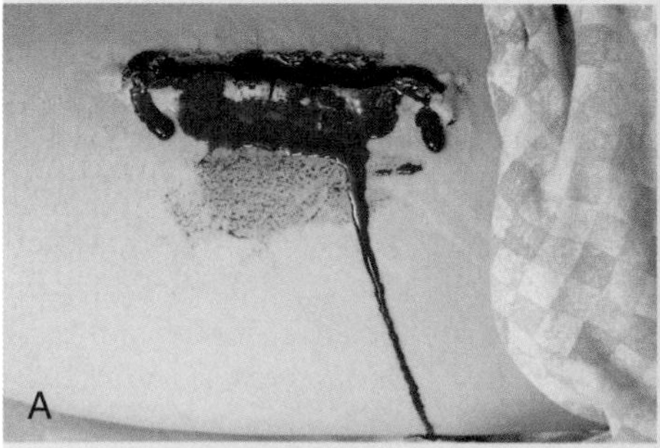

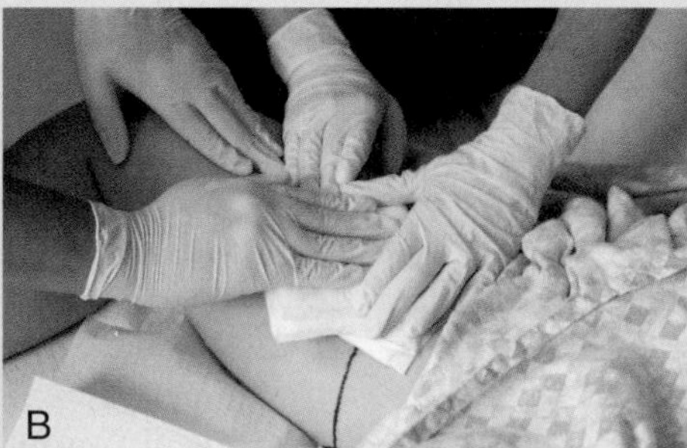

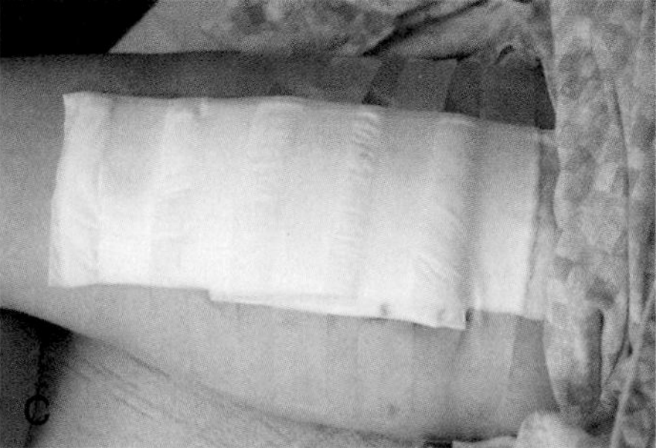

STEP 8b A, Bleeding wound. **B,** Nurses applying pressure dressing. **C**, Dressing applied

STEPS	RATIONALE
c. Remove fingers temporarily and quickly cover center of area with a third strip of tape.	Provides pressure to source of bleeding.
d. Continue reinforcing area with tape as each successive strip is overlapped on alternating sides of center strip. Keep applying pressure.	

STEPS	RATIONALE
e. When bandage is on lower extremity, apply roller gauze: apply two circular turns tautly on both sides of fingers that are pressing the gauze. Compress over bleeding site. Simultaneously remove finger pressure and apply roller gauze over center. Continue with figure-eight turns. Secure end with two circular turns and strip of adhesive.	Roller gauze acts as pressure bandage, exerting more even pressure over extremity
9. See Completion Protocol (inside front cover).	

EVALUATION

1. Observe dressing for control of bleeding.
2. Evaluate adequacy of circulation (distal pulse, skin character).
3. Measure vital signs.

Unexpected Outcomes and Related Interventions

1. There is continued bleeding and fluid and electrolyte imbalance, tissue hypoxia, confusion; hypovolemic shock and cardiac arrest develop.
   a. Notify health care provider.
   b. Reinforce or adjust pressure dressing.
   c. Initiate intravenous (IV) therapy per health care provider's order.
   d. Place patient in Trendelenburg's position; provide warmth.
   e. Monitor vital signs every 5 to 15 minutes (apical pulse, distal pulses, and blood pressure).
2. Pressure dressing is too tight and occludes circulation.
   a. Inspect areas distal to pressure dressing to ensure that circulation has not been occluded.
   b. Adjust dressing as needed.
   c. Notify health care provider of findings.

Recording and Reporting

- Report immediately to health care provider present status of patient's bleeding control, time bleeding was discovered, estimated blood loss (amount of initial dressings), nursing interventions (type and amount of bandages), vital signs, and patient's mental status and signs of restlessness.
- Record interventions taken and patient's response in progress notes and vital sign flow sheet.

Sample Documentation

2230 Patient noted to have excessive bleeding from left mastectomy site 2 hours post-op. Dressing saturated with frank red blood. Two ABDs applied over saturated dressing and held in place with pressure. Dressing then bound tightly with 5-cm (2-inch) surgical tape. No further blood noted on reinforced dressing applied at 2200. Health care provider notified. Vital signs are stable.

Special Considerations

Pediatric

- Child will calm down if care providers and family remain calm.

Geriatric

- Older adults have an increased risk for vascular and tissue changes distal to the pressure dressing. Assess skin and pulse distal to the pressure bandage frequently.

Home Care

- Prepare patient and family caregiver in how to respond if there is a risk of sudden hemorrhage (e.g., cancer patient with eroding tumor).
- Patient/family caregiver may use clean towels or linen to apply pressure.
- Have emergency 911 activated or called immediately.
- Position patient to promote elevation of affected body part and relaxation.

PROCEDURAL GUIDELINE 26.1
Applying a Transparent Dressing

A transparent dressing is a clear, adherent, nonabsorptive polyurethane moisture- and vapor-permeable dressing. These dressings are appropriate for superficial, minimally draining wounds and are often used following laparoscopic surgery, for protection over high-friction areas, and as a dressing over an IV catheter. The synthetic permeable membrane acts as a temporary second skin, adheres to undamaged skin to contain exudate, minimizes wound contamination, and allows the wound surface to "breathe." These occlusive or moisture-retentive dressings cover and encapsulate wounds. They may be used as a primary or a secondary dressing over a packed wound. They protect wounds and surrounding skin from maceration, dehydration, heat loss, and exposure to pathogens. With transparent

Continued

PROCEDURAL GUIDELINE 26.1 Applying a Transparent Dressing—cont'd

dressings a moist exudate forms over the wound surface, which prevents tissue dehydration and allows for rapid, effective healing (Rolstad and Ovington, 2007).

Delegation and Collaboration

The skill of applying transparent dressings in certain situations may be delegated to nursing assistive personnel (NAP) (see agency policy). The wound assessment and care of sterile or new acute wounds cannot be delegated. Instruct the NAP by:

- Explaining how to adapt the skill for a specific patient.
- Reviewing what to observe and report back to the nurse (e.g., loosening of dressing, appearance of drainage).

Equipment

- Clean and sterile gloves
- Dressing set (optional)
- Sterile saline or other cleansing agent
- Cotton swabs
- Waterproof bag
- Transparent dressing
- Sterile 4 × 4–inch gauze pads
- Skin preparation materials
- Moisture-proof gown, goggles, and mask (when splashing from wound is a risk)

Procedural Steps

1. **See Standard Protocol (inside front cover).**
2. Identify patient using two identifiers (i.e., name and birthday or name and account number, according to facility policy).
3. Assess for presence of allergies to cleansing agents or latex.
4. Review health care provider's orders for frequency and type of dressing change.
5. Assess patient's comfort level using a scale of 0 to 10. Medicate with pain medications as needed before dressing removal.
6. Assess patient's knowledge of purpose of dressing change.
7. Position patient comfortably to allow access to dressing site.
8. Assess location, appearance, and size of wound to be dressed. Determine size of transparent dressing needed.
9. Apply PPE (gown, mask, goggles as needed).
10. Cuff top of disposable waterproof bag and place within reach of work area.
11. Remove old dressing by placing nondominant hand gently over wound; use dominant hand to pick up ends and slowly pull back in a direction parallel to the wound rather than upward.
12. Remove any packing from wound.
13. Dispose of dressings in waterproof bag. Remove and discard gloves. Perform hand hygiene.
14. Prepare dressing supplies. Use sterile supplies for new wounds.
15. Apply sterile (or clean) gloves (check agency policy).
16. Pour saline or prescribed solution over sterile 4 × 4–inch gauze pads if needed for cleansing.
17. Cleanse area gently with moistened swab or gauze or spray with a wound cleanser (see agency policy or health care provider preference). Cleanse from least contaminated to most contaminated area (see Skill 26.1).
18. Dry skin around wound thoroughly using dry sterile gauze. Make sure that skin surface is dry.
19. Inspect wound for color, odor, and drainage; measure if indicated.
20. Apply transparent dressing according to manufacturer's directions. Do not stretch film during application and avoid wrinkles.
    a. Remove paper backing, taking care not to allow adhesive areas to touch each other.
    b. Place film smoothly over wound without stretching (see illustrations).

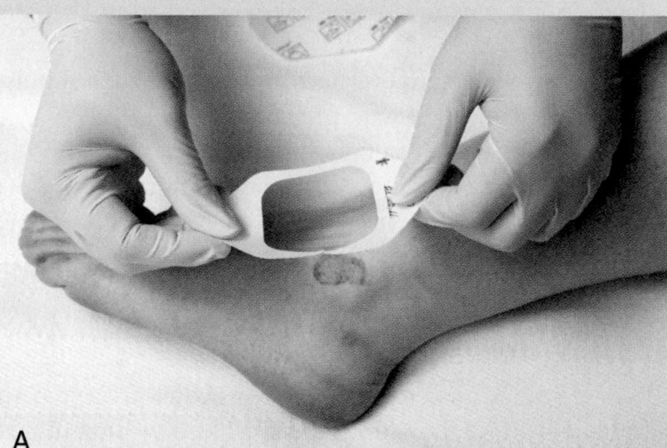

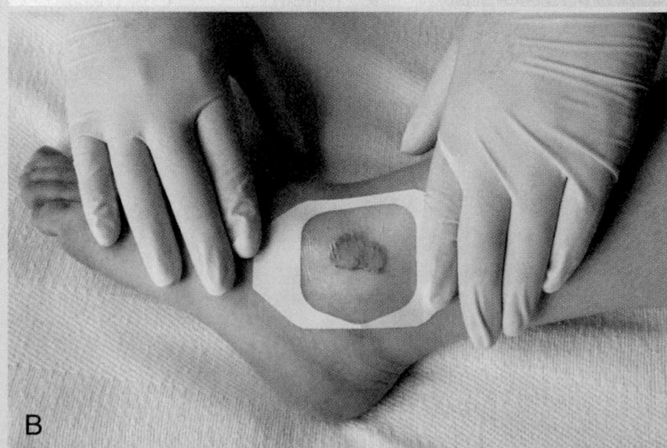

STEP 20b A, Transparent dressing placed over small wound on ankle. **B,** Place film smoothly without stretching.

PROCEDURAL GUIDELINE 26.1
Applying a Transparent Dressing—cont'd

c. Use your fingers to smooth and adhere the dressing. Label with date, initials, and time of dressing change on outer label of dressing (see illustration).

21. **See Completion Protocol (inside front cover).**
22. Record appearance of wound and presence of drainage or odor, dressing applied, and patient's response and level of comfort in nurses' notes.
23. Evaluate periwound area and the appearance of wound for changes.

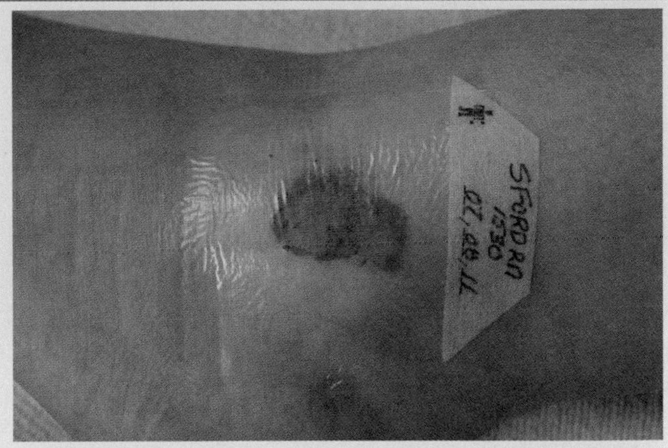

STEP 20c Transparent dressing correctly labeled.

SKILL 26.3 APPLYING HYDROCOLLOID, HYDROGEL, FOAM, OR ABSORPTION DRESSINGS

Wound care continues to advance. Today there are numerous classes of dressings whose properties can be carefully matched with the characteristics of a wound. Dressings can be divided into two classes: hydrating and absorbent.

Hydrocolloid dressings are composed of elastometric, adhesive, and gelling agents. They have absorptive, hydrating, and debriding properties. When in contact with wound drainage, the hydrocolloid forms a gel that promotes a moist environment and facilitates autolytic and enzymatic debridement. Hydrocolloid adhesive dressings help diminish pain because the cushioning effect of the dressing protects the wound and skin. This type of dressing conforms well to different body contours. Hydrocolloids come in the form of granules, paste, or wafer dressings. Wound exudate is absorbed into the dressing, forming a jellylike substance next to the wound surface. The dressing maintains a moist, insulated environment for rapid, effective healing.

Hydrogel dressings are glycerin- or water-based dressings designed to hydrate a wound (Rolstad and Ovington, 2007). They have some absorptive properties. These dressings are similar to hydrocolloids and come in the form of sheets, amorphous gels, and impregnated gauze. The gel dressings are nonadherent and less painful to remove and must be covered with a secondary dressing to hold them in place.

Two examples of absorbent dressings are foam and hydrofiber. A foam dressing absorbs moderate-to-heavy exudates in superficial or deep wounds, protects friable periwound skin, provides autolytic debridement, and pads high trauma areas. Foam dressings are used with infected wounds following appropriate intervention and close monitoring of wound healing. However, the dressing is not appropriate when there is tunneling of a wound. Application directions for the different brands of foam dressings vary. Some foam dressings are designed to fit around tubes such as a tracheostomy.

Hydrofiber dressings may come as a sheet or rope that can be packed into a wound that has moderate-to-heavy drainage. A hydrofiber dressing works by wicking exudate away from a wound (Dinah and Adhikari, 2006). It requires a secondary dressing.

Delegation and Collaboration

The skill of applying a hydrocolloid, hydrogel, foam, or absorption dressing cannot be delegated to nursing assistive personnel (NAP). Instruct the NAP about the following:

- The approach to assist in positioning patient during dressing change
- What to observe (e.g., leakage of drainage, slippage of dressing) and report back to the nurse

Equipment

- Clean gloves
- Sterile gloves (optional)
- Sterile dressing set (Fig. 26-2)
  - Sterile drape (optional)
  - Necessary primary dressings: gauze, hydrocolloid, hydrogel, or foam; and secondary dressings of choice
  - Sterile saline for cleansing or cleansing spray as prescribed
  - Skin barrier wipe
  - Tape (nonallergenic paper or adhesive) or ties as needed
  - Measuring guide (optional)
  - Adhesive remover (optional)
  - Waterproof bag
  - Debriding gel as ordered
- Protective gown, goggles, and mask (used when spray from wound is a risk)

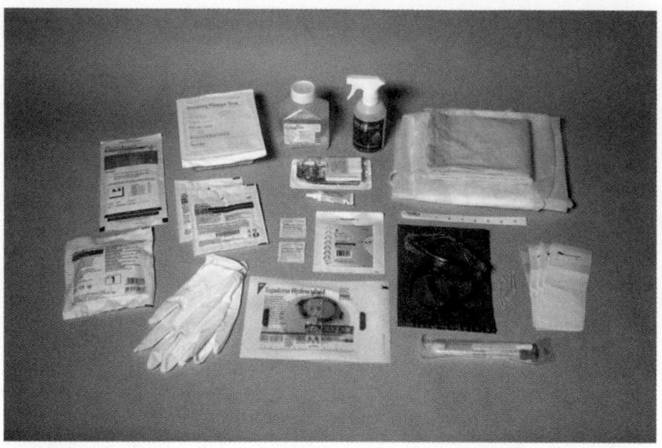

FIG 26-2 Dressing set with personal protective equipment and wound cleansers.

ASSESSMENT

1. Assess for presence of allergies to antiseptics, tape, or latex. *Rationale: Patients may have localized or systemic reactions to these supplies.*
2. During dressing removal, inspect and assess the condition of wound (see Implementation, Step 7). *Rationale: Assists in planning choice of materials to use. Provides baseline for condition of wound.*
3. Ask patient to rate pain using a scale of 0 to 10. *Rationale: Patient may require pain medication before dressing change to allow for peak effect of drug during procedure.*
4. Assess patient's knowledge of purpose of dressing change. *Rationale: Determines level of support and explanation required.*
5. Determine the need for patient or family member to participate in dressing wound. *Rationale: Prepares patient or family member if dressing will be changed at home.*

PLANNING

Expected Outcomes focus on preventing infection, promoting healing, pain control, and patient and family education.

1. Patient's wound shows evidence of healing by smaller size and less drainage, redness, or swelling.
2. Patient reports pain less than previously assessed level (scale of 0 to 10) during and after dressing change.
3. Dressing remains clean, dry, and intact.
4. Patient or family demonstrates correct method of dressing change.

IMPLEMENTATION *for* APPLYING HYDROCOLLOID, HYDROGEL, FOAM, OR ABSORPTION DRESSINGS

STEPS	RATIONALE
1. **See Standard Protocol (inside front cover).**	
2. Identify patient using two identifiers (e.g., name and birthday or name and account number, according to facility policy).	Ensures correct patient. Complies with The Joint Commission standards and improves patient safety (TJC, 2010).
3. Premedicate patient with ordered analgesic 30 minutes before dressing change. Position patient comfortably and drape to expose only wound site. Instruct patient not to touch wound or sterile supplies.	Reduces discomfort during dressing change. Maintaining patient comfort assists in completing skill smoothly. Draping provides access to wound while minimizing unnecessary exposure.
4. Place disposable waterproof bag within reach of work area with top folded to make a cuff.	Facilitates safe disposal of soiled dressings.
5. Apply moisture-proof gown, mask, and goggles if risk for splashing exists.	Reduces transmission of infectious microorganisms.
6. Remove old dressing one layer at a time, observing appearance and drainage on dressing. Use caution to avoid tension on any drains that are present.	Determines dressings needed for replacement. Avoids accidental removal of drain because it may or may not be sutured in place.

SAFETY ALERT Check removal directions for specific brand of dressing used. Some brands need to have old dressing soaked or moistened for removal. Others require use of adhesive remover, which should not directly come in contact with a wound.

STEPS	RATIONALE
7. Inspect and measure wound for appearance, drainage, edema, drains, approximation (wound edges are together), granulation tissue, odor, size, and depth.	Provides assessment data for drainage and wound integrity. Monitors status of wound healing.
8. Fold old dressings with drainage contained inside and dispose in paper bag. Remove gloves and dispose. Cover wound lightly with a sterile gauze pad and perform hand hygiene.	Provides containment of soiled dressings, prevents contact of nurse's hands with drainage, and reduces transmission of cross-contaminating microorganisms.

STEPS	RATIONALE
9. Create a sterile field with a sterile dressing kit or individually wrapped sterile supplies on over-bed table (see Chapter 5).	Sterile dressings remain sterile while on or within sterile area.
10. Pour saline or prescribed solution over 4 × 4–inch sterile gauze pads or prepare spray wound cleanser.	
11. Remove gauze cover. Apply sterile gloves or use no-touch technique with sterile forceps, which maintains sterility of all items in direct contact with the wound.	Sterile gloves may be used for more complex situations with extensive drainage.
12. Cleanse wound.	
a. Cleanse area gently with moist 4 × 4–inch gauze pads, swabbing exudates away from wound; or spray with wound cleanser; or irrigate (see Chapter 24) with commercial wound cleanser or saline.	Technique removes exudate without spreading organisms onto wound site.
b. Cleanse around any drain, using a circular stroke starting near the drain and moving outward away from insertion site (see Skill 26.1).	Cleans in direction from least contaminated to most contaminated area.
13. Use sterile dry gauze to blot dry any excess saline or cleanser.	Drying reduces excess moisture, which could harbor microorganisms.
14. Apply dressing.	
a. Hydrocolloid dressing:	
(1) Select proper size, allowing at least 2.5 cm (1 inch) to extend beyond wound edges.	
(2) Remove paper backing from adhesive side and place over wound.	
(3) In the case of a deep wound, apply hydrocolloid granules or paste before applying wafer. Do not stretch dressing and avoid wrinkles or tenting. Mold wafer to the affected body part. Secure edges of dressing with nonallergenic paper tape.	Granules/paste helps to absorb drainage to increase wearing time of dressing (Rolstad and Ovington, 2007). Tape prevents edge of dressing from rolling or adhering to sheets and clothing.
(4) Hold the dressing in place for 30 to 60 seconds after application.	Hydrocolloid dressings are most effective at body temperature. Holding dressing facilitates dressing action (Rolstad and Ovington, 2007).
(5) Apply a secondary dressing such as an ABD pad if needed. Use nonallergenic tape to secure.	Secondary dressing may be used instead of tape to hold hydrocolloid dressing in place.
b. Hydrogel:	
(1) Apply skin barrier wipe to surrounding skin that will come in contact with adhesive.	Protects periwound skin.
(2) Apply gel or impregnated gauze directly into the wound, spreading evenly over the wound bed. Fill wound cavity with gel about ½ to ⅔ full or pack the gauze loosely into wound bed and any undermined areas. Cover with a moisture-retentive dressing (moist-to-dry [see Skill 26.1] or hydrocolloid wafer).	Hydrogels hydrate and debride (autolyze) wounds. Filling wound cavity partially full allows for expansion with absorption of exudate.
(3) Prepare a hydrogel sheet so it extends 2.5 cm (1 inch) onto intact periwound skin. Cover with a moisture-retentive secondary dressing.	Protects skin around wound.
(4) Secure hydrogel dressing with nonallergenic tape if secondary dressing is not self-adhering.	
c. Foam:	
(1) Know the removal and application characteristics of specific brand of foam dressing.	Various forms are available.
(2) Apply skin barrier wipe to surrounding skin that will come in contact with adhesive.	Protects periwound skin.

Continued

STEPS	RATIONALE
(3) Cut foam sheet to extend 2.5 cm (1 inch) onto intact periwound skin. Make sure that you know which side of foam dressing should be placed toward wound bed and which side should face away from wound bed (check product instructions).	Ensures proper absorption and keeps wound exudates away from wound bed (Rolstad and Ovington, 2007).
(4) Some foam dressings need slight tension on the dressing during application. Others need to be covered with a secondary dressing (Rolstad and Ovington, 2007).	
(5) Cut foam to fit around a drain or tube if present.	
(6) Place foam gel or gauze into a deep wound bed or into wound cavity. Cover with a secondary dressing.	Provides for adequate absorption of exudate in deep wound.
15. See Completion Protocol (inside front cover).	
16. Initial and date the dressing.	

EVALUATION

1. Observe appearance of wound for healing, including size of wound, amount, color and type of drainage, and periwound erythema or swelling.
2. Ask patient to rate pain using a scale of 0 to 10.
3. Inspect status of dressing at least every shift or as ordered.
4. Observe patient's or caregiver's ability to perform dressing change.

Unexpected Outcomes and Related Interventions

1. Wound develops more necrotic tissue and increases in size.
   a. In rare cases some wounds do not tolerate hypoxia induced by hydrocolloid dressings. Discontinue use and notify health care provider.
   b. Evaluate appropriateness of wound care protocol.
   c. Assess for other factors interfering with wound healing.
2. Dressing does not stay in place.
   a. Evaluate size of dressing used for adequate margin (2.5 to 3.75 cm [1 to 1½ inches]) or dry the skin more thoroughly before application.
   b. Consider custom shapes for difficult body parts.
   c. Dressing may be secured with roll gauze, tape, or dressing sheet.
3. Periwound skin appears macerated or shows signs of breakdown.
   a. Assess skin for maceration. If present, assess moisture-control property of dressing or application technique. May need to consider a new dressing type.
   b. Inspect areas in contact with tape or adhesive because allergies may be the cause of breakdown.
   c. Consider alternatives for securing dressing.

Recording and Reporting

- Record appearance of wound, color, size, characteristics of drainage, response to dressing change, condition of periwound skin, and patient's level of comfort in nurses' notes.
- Report signs of infection or deteriorating wound status to health care provider immediately.

Sample Documentation

0930 Stage II ulcer on R medial malleolus measuring 4 × 2 cm, 0.5 cm in depth. Wound bed with 50% pink granulation tissue and 50% yellow slough tissue. Minimal serous drainage noted. No odor. Surrounding skin intact. Wound cleansed with saline. Hydrogel applied to wound bed. Skin protectant applied to periwound skin. Covered with a 4 × 4 hydrocolloid dressing. Patient reported 4/10 pain with removal of old dressing. 0/10 pain at present.

Special Considerations

Geriatric

- Avoid early and frequent removal of a hydrocolloid dressing to reduce injury to surrounding intact skin.

PROCEDURAL GUIDELINE 26.2
Applying Gauze and Elastic Bandages

Gauze and elastic bandages secure or wrap hard-to-cover areas of the body. For example, they can be used to secure dressings on extremities, amputation stumps, and the hand. Bandages are a secondary dressing, providing protection, pressure, immobilization, and anchoring of underlying dressings or splints. There are numerous types of and applications for bandages. Bandages are available in rolls of various widths and materials, including gauze, elastic

PROCEDURAL GUIDELINE 26.2
Applying Gauze and Elastic Bandages—cont'd

webbing, elasticized knit, flannel, and muslin. Gauze bandages are lightweight and inexpensive, mold easily around body contours, and permit air circulation to prevent skin maceration. Elastic bandages conform well to body parts but can also be used to exert pressure over a body part. Flannel and muslin bandages are thicker than gauze and thus stronger for supporting or applying pressure.

When applying a bandage, select a type of bandage turn and width, depending on the size and shape of the body part to be bandaged (Table 26-3). For example, 7.5 cm (3-inch) bandages are most commonly used for the adult leg. A smaller 2-inch bandage is normally used for the wrist.

Delegation and Collaboration

The skill of applying an elastic bandage for compression cannot be delegated to nursing assistive personnel (NAP). A nurse assesses the condition of any wound or dressing before applying a bandage. The skill of applying bandages to secure nonsterile dressings can be delegated. Instruct the NAP by:

- Explaining how to adapt the skill for a specific patient.
- Reviewing what to observe and report back to the nurse (e.g., patient's complaint of pain, numbness or tingling after application, or changes in patient's skin color or temperature).

Equipment

- Clean gloves (if drainage present)
- Correct width and number of gauze or elastic bandages
- Clips or adhesive tape

TABLE 26-3 TYPES OF BANDAGE TURNS

TYPE	DESCRIPTION	PURPOSE OR USE
Circular Circular turns	Bandage turn overlapping previous turn completely	Anchors bandage at the first and final turn; covers small part (finger, toe)
Spiral Spiral turns	Bandage ascending body part with each turn overlapping previous one by one-half or two-thirds width of bandage	Covers cylindrical body parts such as wrist or upper arm
Spiral-reverse Spiral-reverse turns	Turn requiring twist (reversal) of bandage halfway through each turn	Covers cone-shaped body parts such as the forearm, thigh, or calf; useful with nonstretching bandages such as gauze or flannel
Figure eight Figure-eight turns	Oblique overlapping turns alternately ascending and descending over bandaged part, each turn crossing previous one to form figure eight	Covers joints; applies low-grade pressure for venous return; snug fit provides excellent immobilization
Recurrent Recurrent turns	Bandage first secured with two circular turns around proximal end of body part; half turn made perpendicular up from bandage edge; body of bandage brought over distal end of body part to be covered with each turn folded back over on itself	Covers uneven body parts such as head or stump

Continued

PROCEDURAL GUIDELINE 26.2
Applying Gauze and Elastic Bandages—cont'd

Procedural Steps

1. **See Standard Protocol (inside front cover).**
2. Review patient's medical record for specific orders related to application of gauze or elastic bandage. Note area to be covered, type of bandage required, and frequency of change.
3. Identify patient using two identifiers (i.e., name and birthday or name and account number, according to facility policy).
4. Inspect the condition of any wound.
5. Observe adequacy of circulation by noting temperature of skin, skin color, pulses (distal to area to be bandaged), presence of edema, sensation, and movement.
6. Assess patient's level of comfort (pain scale of 0 to 10).
7. Assess for size of bandage.
8. Position patient comfortably in bed in supine position.
9. Apply gloves if drainage is present.
10. *Gauze or elastic bandage to secure dressing:*
    a. With patient in bed, elevation of dependent extremities for 15 minutes before elastic bandage application enhances venous return.
    b. Make sure that primary dressing is in place.
    c. Hold roll of bandage in dominant hand and use other hand to lightly hold beginning layer of bandage at distal body part.
    d. While rolling bandage around body part in two circular turns, continue transferring roll to dominant hand as you wrap the bandage (see illustration).

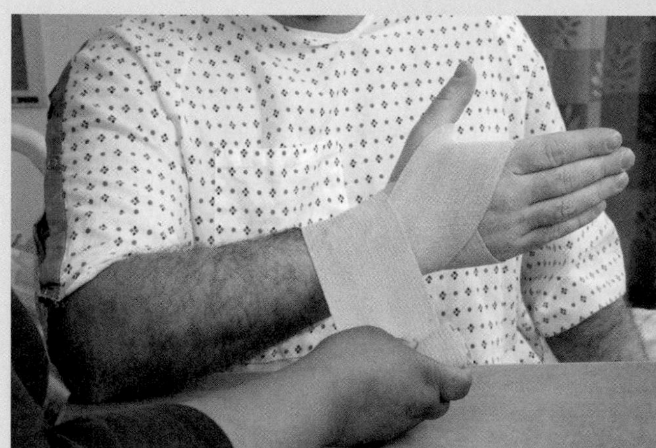

STEP 10d Hold bandage in dominant hand and apply using circular turns.

    e. Apply bandage from distal point toward proximal boundary (see illustration) using turns appropriate to cover various shapes of body parts. Roll gauze overlapping each layer by one half to two thirds the width of the bandage.

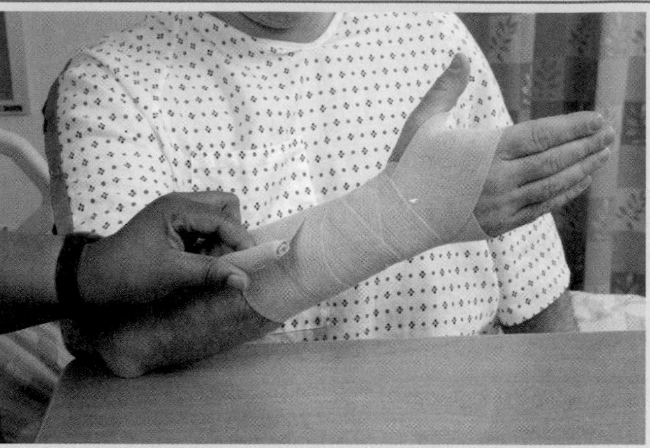

STEP 10e Apply bandage from distal to proximal.

    f. Alternate ascending and descending turns (figure-eight pattern) when wrapping a joint.
    g. Ensure that bandage is snug but not tight and that the primary dressing or splint is positioned correctly.
    h. While unrolling elastic bandage, stretch bandage slightly. Explain to patient that smooth, even pressure will be applied to improve circulation, reduce swelling, immobilize body part, and provide pressure.
    i. Secure end of gauze or elastic bandage to outside layer of bandage, not skin, with tape or clips (see illustration).

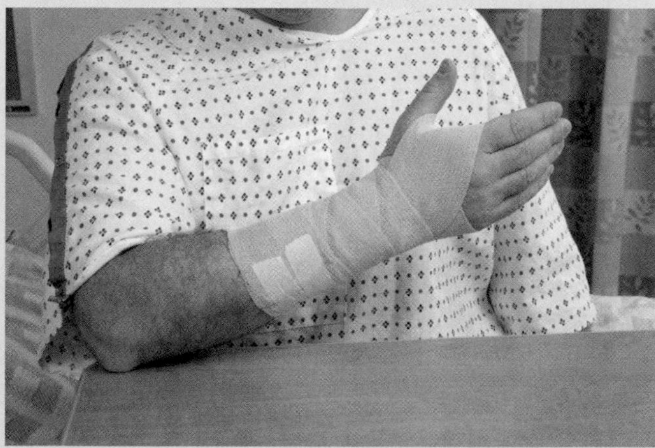

STEP 10i Secure with tape or closure device.

11. *Elastic bandage over stump:*
    a. Elevate stump by using a pillow or supporting with the assistance of another person.
    b. Secure bandage by wrapping it twice around proximal end of stump or person's waist (depending on size of stump) (see illustration).
    c. Make a half turn with bandage perpendicular to its edge.

PROCEDURAL GUIDELINE 26.2
Applying Gauze and Elastic Bandages—cont'd

- **d.** Bring body of bandage over distal end of stump.
- **e.** Continue to fold bandage over stump, wrapping from distal to proximal points.
- **f.** Secure with metal clips, Velcro if provided, or tape.

12. Assess degree of tightness of bandage.

13. Evaluate distal circulation when bandage application is complete, at least twice during the next 8 hours, and then at least every shift.

- **a.** Observe skin color for pallor or cyanosis.
- **b.** Palpate skin for warmth.
- **c.** Palpate distal pulses and compare bilaterally.
- **d.** Ask patient to rate any pain on scale of 0 to 10 and to describe any numbness, tingling, or other discomfort.

14. Evaluate bandage for wrinkles, looseness. and presence of drainage.

15. Have patient or family caregiver demonstrate bandage application.

16. Record patient's baseline and postbandage application level of comfort, dressing status, integrity of wound and periwound skin, appearance of extremity, and patient's tolerance in nurses' notes.

17. See Completion Protocol (inside front cover).

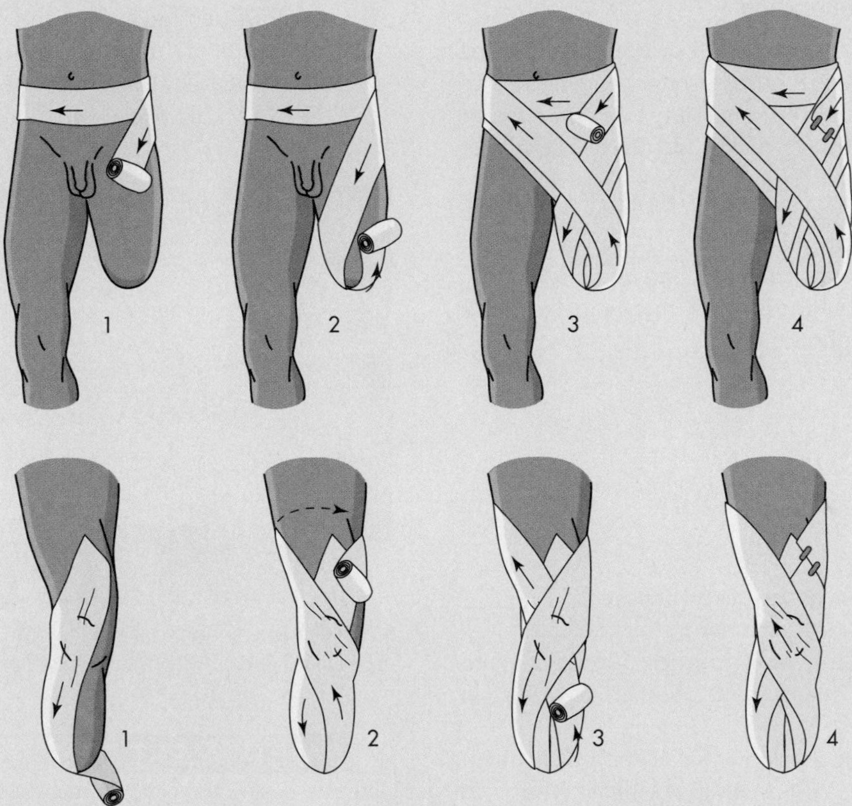

STEP 11b-f *Top,* Correct method for bandaging midthigh amputation stump. Note that bandage must be anchored around patient's waist. *Bottom,* Correct method for bandaging midcalf amputation stump. Note that bandage need not be anchored around the waist. (From Monahan F and others: *Phipps' medical-surgical nursing: health and illness perspectives,* ed 8, St Louis, 2006, Mosby).

PROCEDURE GUIDELINE 26.3
Applying Abdominal and Breast Binders

Binders are bandages made of large pieces of material specially designed to fit a specific body part. Most binders are made of elastic or cotton. The most common types of binders are the breast binder and the abdominal binder. An abdominal binder supports large abdominal incisions that are vulnerable to tension or stress as a person moves or coughs. If not fitted correctly, there is a risk of an abdominal binder impairing ventilation. In a recent study by Larson and others (2009), the researchers found that abdominal binders in patients who underwent midline abdominal incisions had no significant effect on postoperative pulmonary function but seemed to help with pain control.

A breast binder looks like a tight-fitting sleeveless vest. It conforms to the shape of the chest wall and is available in

Continued

PROCEDURE GUIDELINE 26.3
Applying Abdominal and Breast Binders—cont'd

various sizes. Breast binders are common after breast surgery.

Binders are applied over or around dressings. The therapeutic benefits of a binder include supporting a wound, reducing or preventing edema, protecting surrounding skin, and decreasing pain, thereby promoting physical activity and respiratory function. It is important that a binder be applied correctly and monitored for movement. Misplaced binders have the potential to injure the wound and the underlying skin, cause discomfort to the patient, and interfere with respirations and mobility.

Delegation and Collaboration

The skill of applying binders can be delegated to nursing assistive personnel (NAP). A nurse assesses the condition of any incision; the skin; and patient's ability to breathe deeply, cough effectively, and move independently before binder application. Instruct the NAP by:

- Explaining how to adapt the skill for a specific patient.
- Reviewing what to observe and report back to the nurse (e.g., patient's complaint of numbness, pain, tingling, difficulty breathing, or change in skin color below area of application).

Equipment

- Clean gloves (if drainage present)
- Correct type and size of binder
- Velcro closure or fastening device

Procedural Steps

1. **See Standard Protocol (inside front cover).**
2. Review medical record for order for binder.
3. Identify patient using two identifiers (i.e., name and birthday or name and account number, according to facility policy).
4. Inspect skin for actual or potential alterations in integrity. Observe for irritation, abrasions, and skin surfaces that rub together.
5. Observe patient's ability to breathe deeply, cough effectively, and turn or move independently.
6. Cover any exposed area of an incision or wound with a dressing.
7. Apply binder.
   a. *Abdominal binder:*
      (1) Position patient in supine position with head slightly elevated and knees slightly flexed.
      (2) Assist patient to roll on side away from you toward raised side rail while firmly supporting abdominal incision and dressing with hands.
      (3) Fanfold far side of binder toward midline of binder.
      (4) Place fanfolded ends of binder under patient.
      (5) Instruct or assist patient in rolling over folded binder. For overweight patients have a colleague assist.
      (6) Unfold and stretch ends of binder out smoothly on far side of bed. Then stretch out ends on near side of bed.
      (7) Instruct patient to roll back into supine position.
      (8) Adjust binder so supine patient is centered over binder using symphysis pubis and costal margins as lower and upper landmarks.
      (9) If patient is very thin, pad the bony prominences with gauze bandages.
      (10) Close binder. Pull one end of binder over center of patient's abdomen. While maintaining tension on that end of binder, pull opposite end of binder over center and secure with Velcro closure tabs, metal fasteners, or horizontally placed safety pins (see illustration).

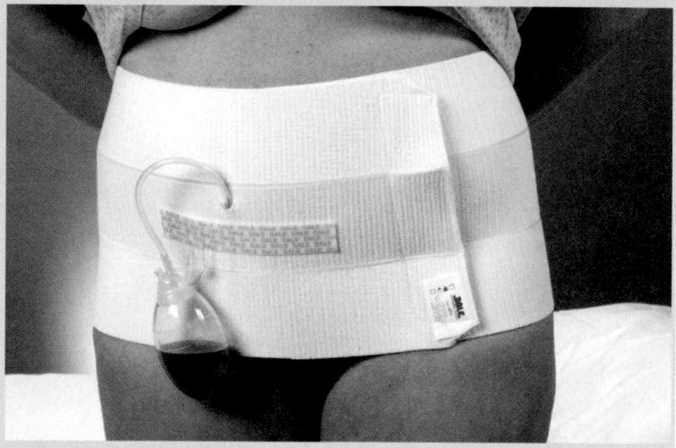

STEP 7a(10) Abdominal binder with Velcro closures. (Courtesy Dale Medical Products, Inc, Plainsville, Mass.)

> **SAFETY ALERT** Recheck patient's ability to breathe deeply and cough effectively. Shallow respirations continuing after a tight binder has been loosened may indicate beginning signs of serious respiratory problems.

   b. *Breast binder:*
      (1) Assist patient to sit up and place arms through binder's armholes.
      (2) Assist patient to supine position if needed.
      (3) Pad area under breasts if necessary.
      (4) Using Velcro closure tabs, secure binder at nipple level first. Continue closure process above and then below nipple line until entire binder is closed.
      (5) Make appropriate adjustments, including individualizing fit of shoulder straps and pinning waistline darts to reduce binder size.
      (6) Assess patient's comfort level and adjust binder as needed.

PROCEDURE GUIDELINE 26.3
Applying Abdominal and Breast Binders—cont'd

8. **See Completion Protocol (inside front cover).**
9. Ask patient to rate pain on a scale of 0 to 10.
10. Remove binder and any underlying dressing to evaluate skin and wound characteristics at least every 8 hours.
11. Evaluate patient's ability to breathe deeply and cough without discomfort every 4 hours.
12. Record type and application of binder, condition of skin, circulation, ease of breathing and coughing, level of comfort, dressing status, integrity of wound and periwound skin, and tolerance of binder.
13. After loosening binder, report any continued changes in ventilation to health care provider.

REVIEW QUESTIONS

Case Study for Questions 1 and 2

Mr. Alberts is a 73-year-old male who is 2 weeks postoperative for an open right colectomy. His surgical course was complicated by a wound dehiscence and subsequent infection. He has an open abdominal wound that measures 4 × 3 cm with a depth of 1.5 cm and 2 cm with undermining at 12:00. The wound has a moderate amount of serosanguineous drainage. The periwound skin is intact. His wound care regimen consists of daily packing with a hydrogel gauze.

1. Mr. Alberts has been premedicated and is ready for his dressing change. The nurse has removed the old dressing and inspected the wound bed and drainage. Place the following steps for applying Mr. Alberts' new dressing in the correct order:
   a. Cleanse wound.
   b. Moisten 4 × 4–inch gauze in sterile saline.
   c. Perform hand hygiene.
   d. Cover gel gauze with a moisture-retentive dressing.
   e. Blot dry any remaining saline on skin with gauze.
   f. Gently cover the wound bed with hydrogel gauze.
   g. Apply sterile gloves or use no-touch technique with sterile forceps.
2. Mr. Alberts' packing strips are impregnated with hydrogel gauze. What are the benefits of using this type of dressing for his wound? Select all that apply.
   1. Impregnated dressings have antimicrobial properties.
   2. Dressings are less painful to remove.
   3. Dressing has absorptive properties.
   4. Gauze strips can be used to pack wound bed and undermined area.
3. A transparent film dressing is indicated for all but which of the following types of applications?
   1. A 2-cm deep wound with copious amounts of serous drainage
   2. A newborn with a skin tear
   3. A laparoscopic cholecystectomy wound 1 day after surgery
   4. A protective cover for an intravenous catheter
4. Which of the following is not characteristic of an ideal dressing?
   1. Maintains a core temperature of 37° C
   2. Is impermeable to microorganisms
   3. Removes exudate and allows the wound to dry
   4. Is cost effective
5. One hour ago an NAP applied an abdominal binder after the nurse observed the patient's condition. Which of the following observations pertain to the patient's tolerance to the binder?
   1. The length of time the binder has been applied
   2. The patient's ability to cough
   3. The condition of the wound under the binder
   4. The patient's heart rate
6. Which of the following statements about bacterial wound colonization is correct?
   1. Signs of bacterial colonization include a sudden deterioration of the wound along with changes in the amount, color, and odor of the drainage.
   2. Most chronic wounds are colonized or contaminated with low levels of bacteria.
   3. Bacterial colonization is an urgent issue that requires an aggressive response to preserve wound healing.
   4. Bacterial infection and colonization present with similar symptoms and require similar interventions.
7. Which of the following signs indicate that an abdominal binder has been applied too tightly? Select all that apply.
   1. The patient reports a pulling sensation while ambulating.
   2. A new skin abrasion is noted under the binder, just proximal to the intact dressing.
   3. The patient is able to perform cough and deep-breathing exercises.
   4. The patient reports new pain with deep inspiration.
8. Which of the following dressings are appropriate for a wound that requires debriding? Select all that apply.
   1. Transparent dressing
   2. Moist-to-dry dressing
   3. Hydrocolloid gel
   4. Dry dressing
9. Which of the following wound characteristics would be appropriately treated by a foam dressing?
   1. A dry venous stasis ulcer
   2. A heavily exudating stage III sacral ulcer
   3. A small, open abdominal wound with tunneling and copious drainage
   4. A skin abrasion with minimal drainage.

10. A nurse who is changing a dry gauze dressing over a patient's postoperative incision notices that the dressing is soiled with old sanguineous drainage. The gauze is sticking to dried drainage from the incision line. What should the nurse do to remove the dressing without causing injury to the incision?
1. Pull it off and alert the patient to possible discomfort.
2. Moisten the dressing with normal saline and then remove it.
3. Remove all layers of gauze at the same time, lifting off the incision.
4. Irrigate the wound before applying the dry dressing.

REFERENCES

Baranoski S: Choosing a wound dressing, part I, *Nursing 2008* 38(1):60, 2008.

Brett D: A review of moisture control dressings in wound care, *J Wound Ostomy Continence Nurs* 33(6S):S3, 2006a.

Brett D: Impact on exudate management, maintenance of a moist wound environment, and prevention of infection, *J Wound Ostomy Continence Nurs* 33(6S):S9, 2006b.

Dinah F, Adhikari A: Gauze packing of open surgical wounds: empirical or evidence-based practice? *Ann R Coll Surg Engl* 88:33, 2006.

Gray N, Weir D: Prevention and treatment of moisture-associated skin damage (maceration) in the periwound skin, *J Wound Ostomy Continence Nurs* 34(2):153, 2007.

Hockenberry MJ, Wilson D: *Wong's nursing care of infants and children*, ed 8, St Louis, 2007, Mosby.

Jones K: Identifying best practices for pressure ulcer management, *JCOM* 16(8):375, 2009.

Kirshen C and others: Debridement: a vital component of wound bed preparation, *Adv Skin Wound Care* 19(12):506, 2006.

Larson C and others: The effect of abdominal binders on postoperative pulmonary function, *Am Surg* 75(1):169, 2009.

Meiner SE, Lueckenotte AG: *Gerontologic nursing*, ed 3, St Louis, 2006, Mosby.

Pieper B: Vulnerable populations: considerations for wound care, *Ostomy Wound Manage* 55(5):24, 2009.

Pieper B and others: Discharge information needs of patients after surgery, *J Wound Ostomy Continence Nurs* 33(3):281, 2006.

Ramundo J: Wound debridement. In Bryant R, Nix D: *Acute and chronic wounds: current management and concepts*, ed 3, St Louis, 2007, Mosby.

Rolstad BS, Ovington LG: Principles of wound management. In Bryant RA, Nix DP: *Acute and chronic wounds: nursing management*, ed 3, St Louis, 2007, Mosby.

The Joint Commission: *2010 National Patient Safety Goals*, Oakbrook Terrace, Ill, 2010, The Commission, http://www.jointcommission.org/PatientSafety/NationalPatientSafetyGoals/, accessed February 14, 2010.

CHAPTER

27

Therapeutic Use of Heat and Cold

evolve WEBSITE

http://evolve.elsevier.com/Perry/nursinginterventions

Local application of moderate heat and cold to a body part provides comfort and pain relief, reduces muscle spasm, improves mobility, and promotes healing. The therapeutic effects of heat and cold applications result from changes in blood vessel size and subsequent blood flow to an area.

Local heat application produces vasodilation. You apply moist heat to the body using a moist compress or sitz bath and dry heat through an aquathermia or heating pad. Heat relieves pain, improves circulation and metabolism to an affected area, increases edema and inflammation, and promotes consolidation of exudate in a wound. Cold applications, such as compresses, promote vasoconstriction. Cold therapies reduce recovery time as part of the rehabilitation program for the treatment for acute and chronic injuries. They physiologically create pain relief, reduce muscle spasm, and reduce edema and inflammation secondary to vasoconstriction. In addition, cold decreases the metabolism of the area of application, thus reducing tissue injury.

PATIENT-CENTERED CARE

Patient comfort and privacy are of the utmost importance in the application of heat and cold therapy. During heat or cold therapy the patient or patient's extremities may be exposed. Maximize comfort and privacy by providing warm blankets, adequate attire, and the use of privacy curtains and doors during treatment. Educating the patient to report excessive heat, cold, tingling, numbness, or any discomfort requiring the termination of treatment assists in providing safe and effective care. Introducing caregivers to the strategies of applying heat and cold is an opportunity for the nurse to prepare the patient for discharge to home or an extended-care facility.

SAFETY

Normally, stimulation of heat or cold receptors sends sensory impulses that travel via sensory afferent fibers to the hypothalamus and cerebral cortex. The cerebral cortex makes a person aware of temperature sensation. The body also reacts protectively through a reflex response, causing a person to withdraw from a stimulus. However, sensory adaptation to local temperature extremes can occur quickly within the body. As a nurse you must know the normal physiologic changes due to heat and cold and anticipate the risk of injury to a patient.

Exposure to heat or cold causes both systemic and local responses. Local cold application produces vasoconstriction, increasing the risk of chilling, ischemia, and frostbite. The application of cold therapy may decrease circulation to the affected area and, if allowed to remain in place, can lead to excessive tissue ischemia. When ischemia is present, there is insufficient blood flow to tissues, causing cellular death. Excessive cold exposure triggers a sensation of numbness before the patient senses pain. In contrast, excessive heat application triggers a burning sensation. In the presence of edema the application of heat may increase the risk for injury. The risks of injury associated with local application of cold and heat therapies increase in patients with decreased sensation, decreased voluntary movement, confusion, or dementia. These patients do not perceive or process sensations associated with excessive heat or cold or are unable to move away from the heat or cold exposure.

Close attention to the duration of therapy and assessment of the patient's tolerance to therapy are essential to patient safety. An order from a health care provider is needed for the application of heat or cold. The order includes the duration

TABLE 27-1 TEMPERATURE RANGES FOR HOT AND COLD APPLICATIONS

TEMPERATURE	CELSIUS RANGE	FAHRENHEIT RANGE
Hot	37° to 41°	99° to 106°
Warm	34° to 37°	93° to 98°
Tepid	26° to 34°	80° to 92°
Cool	18° to 26°	65° to 79°
Cold	10° to 18°	50° to 64°

of therapy and the desired temperature when temperature settings can be controlled (Table 27-1). Adherence to these guidelines is critical for maximum benefit of either heat or cold therapy. Checking the temperature and the patient's tolerance of the treatment frequently aids in preventing injury.

EVIDENCE-BASED PRACTICE TRENDS

Janwantanakul P: Different rate of cooling time and magnitude of cooling temperature during ice bag treatment with and without damp towel wrap, *Phys Ther Sport* 5:156, 2004.

Pescasio M and others: Clinical management of muscle strains and tears, *J Musculoskelet Med* 25(11):526, 2008.

The application of ice or cryotherapy is a mainstay in the management of acute musculoskeletal injury (Pescasio and others, 2008). Cold also reduces recovery time as part of the rehabilitation program for the treatment of both acute and chronic injuries and therefore is recommended for the care of patients with musculoskeletal injuries in the immediate postoperative period (Janwantanakul, 2004). Because of the reduction of temperature in the affected area, positive physiological effects such as pain relief, reduction of muscle spasm, decrease of nerve conduction velocity, and decrease in inflammation edema can be achieved.

SKILL 27.1 MOIST HEAT

Warm compresses and commercial moist heat packs are examples of moist heat applications used for a variety of conditions (Table 27-2). A warm compress is a section of sterile or clean gauze moistened with a prescribed heated solution and applied directly to an affected area. Compresses can be warmed and replaced intermittently or, in the case of a gauze compress, heated continuously with a temperature-controlled aquathermia pad (Fig. 27-1) placed over the compress. Moist heat application also includes use of warm baths and sitz baths. A bath or soak involves immersion of a body part into a warmed solution. Sitz baths are disposable and especially easy to use in the home. Patients who have painful hemorrhoids, have had an episiotomy, or have undergone perineal or rectal surgery benefit from a sitz bath because the therapy promotes circulation and debrides wounds. Moist heat penetrates quickly and deeply and effectively increases the temperature of subcutaneous tissue. Table 27-3 outlines advantages and disadvantages of moist versus dry heat. Use caution when applying any form of moist heat because prolonged exposure increases the risk for a burn.

TABLE 27-2 CHARACTERISTICS OF HOT AND COLD APPLICATION

	EXAMPLES OF CONDITIONS TREATED	PRECAUTIONS	ADVERSE TREATMENT EFFECTS
Cold applications	Immediately after direct trauma such as sprains, strains, fractures, muscle spasms; after superficial lacerations or puncture wounds; after minor burns; chronic pain of arthritis, joint trauma; delayed-onset muscle soreness; inflammation	Circulatory insufficiency Cold allergy Advanced diabetes	Cardiovascular effects (bradycardia) Raynaud's phenomenon Cold urticaria Nerve and tissue damage Slowed wound healing Frostbite
Hot applications	Inflamed or edematous body part; new surgical wound; infected wound; arthritis; degenerative joint disease; localized joint pain, muscle strains; low back pain; menstrual cramping; hemorrhoidal, perianal, and vaginal inflammation; local abscess	Pregnancy Laminectomy sites Spinal cord Malignancy Vascular insufficiency Eyes, testes, heart	Burns Infections Increased pain Increased inflammation

Data from Nadler S and others: The physiologic basis and clinical applications of cryotherapy and thermotherapy for the pain practitioner, *Pain Physician* 7(3):395, 2004.

TABLE 27-3 WARM APPLICATIONS: MOIST VERSUS DRY

TYPE	ADVANTAGES	DISADVANTAGES
Moist application	Reduces drying of skin and softens wound exudates Moistened material conforms well to body area being treated Penetrates deep into tissue layers Lessens sweating and insensible fluid loss	Can cause maceration of the skin with prolonged exposure Cools rapidly because of moisture evaporation Creates greater risk for burns to skin because moisture conducts heat
Dry application	Less likely to burn skin Does not cause skin maceration Retains temperature longer because it is not influenced by evaporation	Increases body fluid loss through sweating Does not penetrate deep into tissue Causes increased drying of skin

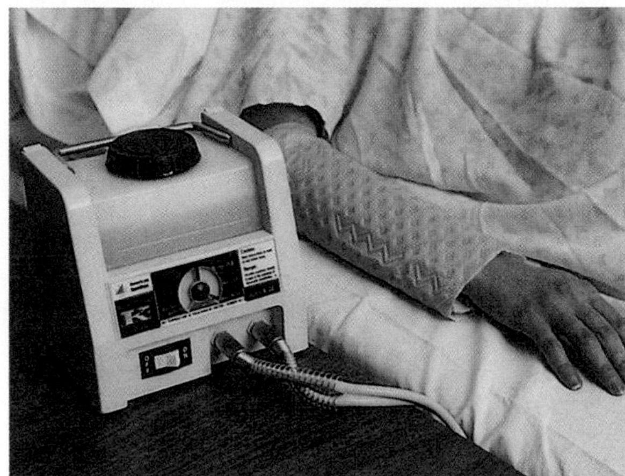

FIG 27-1 Aquathermia pad.

ASSESSMENT

1. Refer to health care provider's order for type of heat application, location and duration of application, and desired temperature. *Rationale: Ensures safe and correct application.*
2. Assess skin around area to be treated. Perform neurovascular check for sensitivity to temperature and pain by measuring light touch, pin prick, and temperature sensation (see Chapter 7). *Rationale: Certain conditions alter conduction of sensory impulses that transmit temperature and pain. Patients insensitive to heat or cold sensations must be monitored closely during treatment.*
3. Inspect wound for size, color, drainage volume and character, presence of pain (rate on a scale of 0 to 10), and odor. *Rationale: Provides a baseline to determine changes in wound after heat application.*
4. Assess patient's level of comfort on a scale of 0 to 10. *Rationale: Provides baseline measure.*
5. Measure joint range of motion (ROM) of any affected joint. *Rationale: Provides baseline to determine changes in joint mobility.*
6. Refer to patient's medical record for any contraindications to moist heat application. *Rationale: Patients with certain cardiovascular conditions and who exhibit side effects of certain medications may be at risk for sudden changes in blood pressure and blood flow caused by vasodilation. Patients insensitive to heat sensation must be monitored closely during treatment.*
7. Assess blood pressure and heart rate for patient using moist heat. *Rationale: Patient may become hypotensive during procedures; establishes a baseline for comparison.*
8. Determine patient's or family members' knowledge of procedure and related safety factors. *Rationale: Warm compresses are frequently used in homes; assessment determines patient's health teaching needs.*

PLANNING

Expected Outcomes focus on promoting wound healing, increasing mobility, decreasing pain, and preventing burns.

1. After multiple applications, healing is demonstrated by wound showing tissue granulation and reduced edema, inflammation, and drainage.
2. Affected area is pink and warm to touch immediately after heat application.
3. Patient denies any burning sensation at the conclusion of treatment.
4. Patient reports a decrease in pain.
5. Patient's blood pressure and pulse are within his or her range.
6. Patient's joint mobility improves.

Delegation and Collaboration

Assessment of patient's condition may not be delegated. However, the skill of applying moist heat may be delegated to nursing assistive personnel (NAP). Instruct the NAP about the following:

- Proper temperature of the application
- Skin changes to immediately report to the nurse (e.g., burning, excessive skin redness)
- Informing the nurse if patient complains of dizziness or light-headedness
- Reporting when treatment is complete so that an evaluation of patient's response can be made.

Equipment

All moist heat

- Bath blanket
- Warmed prescribed solution (i.e., normal saline)

- Dry bath towel
- Biohazard waste bag

All compresses
- Waterproof pad
- Ties or cloth tape
- Aquathermia pad

Clean compress
- Clean basin
- Clean gauze or towel

Sterile compress
- Sterile basin
- Clean gloves
- Sterile gloves

Soak or sitz bath
- Clean or sterile basin or sitz bath

IMPLEMENTATION *for* MOIST HEAT

STEPS	RATIONALE
1. See Standard Protocol (inside front cover).	
2. Identify patient using two identifiers (e.g., name and birthday or name and account number, according to facility policy).	Ensures correct patient. Complies with The Joint Commission standards and improves patient safety (TJC, 2010).
3. Explain to patient the sensations he or she will feel, such as decreasing warmth and wetness. Explain precautions to prevent burning.	Minimizes anxiety and promotes cooperation.
4. Place waterproof pad under patient (except for sitz bath).	Protects bed linen from moisture and soiling.
5. ***Apply moist sterile compress.***	
a. Position patient carefully, keeping affected body part in proper alignment. Expose body part to be covered with compress and drape patient with bath blanket.	Limited mobility in an uncomfortable position causes muscular stress. Draping prevents unnecessary cooling.
b. Heat prescribed solution to desired temperature by immersing closed bottle in basin of very warm water.	Prevents burns by ensuring proper temperature.
c. Prepare aquathermia pad if needed. Temperature is usually preset by biomedical personnel.	
d. Remove existing dressing (if present), and dispose of old dressing and gloves in biohazard bag.	
e. Inspect condition of wound and surrounding skin. Inflamed wound appears reddened, but surrounding skin is less red in color.	Provides baseline or ongoing data to measure wound healing against existing baseline information.
f. Perform hand hygiene. Prepare sterile supplies. Pour the warmed solution into sterile container. If using commercially prepared compress, follow manufacturer's directions.	Sterile compress is needed for an open wound.
g. Use sterile technique (see Chapter 5) to add sterile gauze to warmed sterile solution to immerse gauze.	Maintains sterility of compress.
h. Apply sterile gloves if dressing change is sterile; otherwise use clean gloves.	Sterile glove allows for manipulation of gauze without contamination.
i. Pick up one layer of immersed gauze, wring out any excess solution, and apply gauze lightly to open wound; avoid surrounding skin.	Excess moisture macerates skin and increases risk of burns and infection. Skin is sensitive to sudden change in temperature.
j. After a few seconds, lift edge of gauze to assess for redness.	Increased redness indicates burn.
k. If patient tolerates compress, pack gauze snugly against wound. Be sure to cover all wound surfaces with warm compress.	Packing compress prevents rapid cooling from underlying air currents.
l. Cover moist compress with dry sterile dressing and bath towel. If necessary, pin or tie in place. Remove gloves.	Dry sterile dressing prevents transfer of microorganisms to wound via capillary action caused by moist compress. Towel insulates compress to reduce heat loss.
m. Apply aquathermia or waterproof heating pad over towel (optional) (see Skill 27.2). Keep in place for duration of application.	Maintains constant temperature to compress.

STEPS	RATIONALE
SAFETY ALERT Local application of heat longer than 20 to 30 minutes without interruption may result in changes to the microcirculation such as reflex vasoconstriction (Stitik and Nadler, 1999). Thus prolonged exposure can reduce circulation to treated area.	
n. If an aquathermia pad is not used, change warm compress using sterile technique every 5 to 10 minutes or as ordered for duration of treatment.	Prevents cooling and maintains therapeutic benefit of compress.
o. After prescribed time, remove pad, towel and compress. Evaluate wound and condition of skin and replace the type of dressing ordered for patient.	Continued exposure to moisture will macerate skin. Prevents entrance of microorganisms into wound site.
6. ***Provide sitz bath or warm soak.***	
a. Remove any existing dressing covering wound. Dispose of gloves and dressings in proper receptacle. Perform hand hygiene.	Reduces transmission of microorganisms.
b. Inspect condition of wound and surrounding skin. Pay particular attention to suture line.	Provides baseline or ongoing data to measure wound healing against existing baseline information.
c. When exudate is present, cleanse intact skin around open area with clean cloth and soap and water or sterile gauze (sterile gloves needed) and sterile water or saline. Dispose of gloves. Perform hand hygiene.	Cleansing area prevents transfer of microorganisms.
d. Fill sitz bath or bath tub in bathroom with warmed solution. Check temperature (see agency policy for guidance on solution temperature).	Ensures proper temperature and prevents transfer of microorganisms from solution to wound.
e. Assist patient to immerse body part in sitz bath, tub, or basin. Cover patient with bath blanket or towel as needed. Assess heart rate and ask if patient feels light-headed or dizzy or if the water feels too warm. Have call light within reach.	Assisting patient prevents falls. Covering patient prevents heat loss through evaporation and assists in maintaining a constant temperature. Heart rate provides baseline to determine response to therapy. If water is too warm, remove patient from bath.
f. Maintain constant temperature throughout 15- to 20-minute soak. After 10 minutes, remove body part from soak, check skin for burning, empty cooled solution, add newly heated solution, and reimmerse body part.	Avoids chilling and enhances ability of patient to relax. Constant temperature ensures therapeutic effect.
g. After prescribed time, remove patient from soak or tub; dry body parts thoroughly. NOTE: Wear clean gloves if drainage is present.	
h. Drain solution from basin or tub. Clean bath according to agency policy.	Reduces transmission of microorganisms.
7. See Completion Protocol (inside front cover).	

EVALUATION

1. Inspect wound for size and evidence of healing; observe skin color, temperature, edema, and sensitivity to touch.
2. Ask patient to describe level of comfort on a scale of 0 to 10. Ask about any sensation of burning at the conclusion of treatment.
3. Measure blood pressure and compare to baseline.
4. Measure affected joint ROM (if appropriate).
5. Observe patient demonstrate application of therapy.

Unexpected Outcomes and Related Interventions

1. Patient's skin is reddened and sensitive to touch (either during treatment or as long as 30 minutes after treatment).
   a. Stop treatment.
   b. Ensure proper temperatures or check equipment for proper functioning.
   c. Notify health care provider.

2. Patient complains of burning and/or increased discomfort.
   a. Inspect underlying skin.
   b. Reduce temperature.
   c. Notify health care provider.

Recording and Reporting

- Record and report procedure, noting solution and type, location, and duration of application. Include condition of body part, wound, and skin before and after treatment and patient's response to therapy.
- Record instructions given to patient and patient's ability to explain and perform procedure.

Sample Documentation

0930 Warm moist compress applied for pain at discontinued IV site, L forearm (patient reports pain at 5 on a scale of 0 to 10). Area red, edematous, 6 cm long, 3 cm wide, slightly raised, tender to touch, and warm. States pain has been worsening since IV discontinued early AM.

Special Considerations

Pediatric

- The skin of infants and children is thin and fragile and therefore easily damaged. Use special caution in this population (Hockenberry and Wilson, 2007). Remain with children during procedure for safety and effectiveness.
- Incorporate play into the time the child is required to soak. Placing items in the basin to keep the child occupied may be helpful. Continuous adult supervision is necessary.
- Perform frequent neurovascular evaluations to ensure adequate blood flow before and after treatment.

Geriatric

- Older patients, especially those undergoing long-term steroid therapy, may have thinner, more fragile skin.
- Older patients may have impaired circulation or diminished subcutaneous fat, leading to alterations in thermoregulation (Meiner and Lueckenotte, 2006).
- In some cases, such as with patients who have cardiac conditions, it may be necessary to monitor vital signs throughout the procedure.

Home Care

- When necessary, assess availability of family caregiver to assist patient in application of moist heat. Assess caregiver's understanding of purpose of procedure and willingness to comply with procedure and not leave patient.
- Assess physical environment to determine adequacy of facilities for use by patient. Contact medical equipment companies for assistance in determining best products for patient.
- Warn patient and family caregiver never to warm a gauze compress in a microwave because the temperature will be very hot or uneven and potentially very injurious to the skin.

SKILL 27.2 DRY HEAT

You can apply dry heat directly to the skin with an aquathermia pad, electric heating pad, or commercial heat pack. The aquathermia pad used in health care settings consists of a waterproof rubber or plastic pad connected by two hoses to an electrical control heating unit. Dry heat treatments penetrate superficially but maintain temperature changes longer than moist heat treatments (see Table 27-3). This superficial heating is not effective in penetrating deep joints such as the knee or hip. You must control the temperature and duration of these treatments carefully. It is important to protect the patient from burns, skin dryness, and loss of body fluids through diaphoresis. Because of the constant temperature control, aquathermia pads tend to be safer than electric heating pads. A conventional heating pad is used in the home care setting and can be used only when a patient or family caregiver is able to correctly adjust the temperature and monitor the condition of the patient's skin.

ASSESSMENT

1. Refer to physician's order for location of application and duration of therapy. *Rationale: Order required to ensure patient safety.*
2. Assess patient's skin over area to be treated for integrity, color, temperature, sensitivity to touch, blistering, and excessive dryness. *Rationale: Establishes baseline for condition of skin.*
3. Ask patient to report pain on scale of 0 to 10. *Rationale: Provides baseline to determine if pain relief is achieved.*
4. Assess ROM of body part. *Rationale: Provides baseline to determine changes in joint mobility.*
5. Refer to patient's medical record for any contraindications to dry heat application. *Rationale: May require more frequent monitoring or necessitate different form of therapy.*
6. Check electrical plugs and cords for obvious fraying or cracking. *Rationale: Prevents injury from accidental electrical shock.*
7. Determine patient's or family caregiver's knowledge of procedure and related safety factors. *Rationale: Heating pads are frequently used in homes; assessment determines patient's and family's health teaching needs.*

PLANNING

Expected Outcomes focus on decreasing pain and improving mobility while preventing burns and dehydration.

1. Patient reports decreased level of pain.

2. Patient's ROM increases.
3. Patient's skin remains intact, pink, warm, and sensitive to touch, with no excessive dryness and no blisters. Immediately after treatment, skin may be pink to red and warm.
4. Patient correctly applies pad.

Delegation Considerations

Assessment of the patient's condition may not be delegated; however, the skill of applying dry heat may be delegated to nursing assistive personnel (NAP). Instruct the NAP about the following:

- Specific positioning and time requirements for the patient
- What to observe and report immediately, such as excessive redness of skin and patient's report of pain
- Reporting when treatment is complete so that an evaluation of patient's response can be made

Equipment

- Aquathermia pad, electric heating pad, or commercial chemical heat pack
- Electrical control unit
- Distilled water (for aquathermia pad)
- Bath towel or pillow case
- Ties or tape

IMPLEMENTATION *for* DRY HEAT

STEPS	RATIONALE
1. **See Standard Protocol (inside front cover).**	
2. Identify patient using two identifiers (e.g., name and birthday or name and account number, according to facility policy).	Ensures correct patient. Complies with The Joint Commission standards and improves patient safety (TJC, 2010).
3. Position patient to expose area to be treated.	
4. Apply aquathermia or heating pad; cover or wrap affected area with bath towel or enclose pad in pillowcase.	Prevents heated surface from touching patient's skin directly and increasing risk for injury to patient's skin.
a. Place pad over affected area (see Fig. 27-1) and secure with tape or ties as needed.	

> **SAFETY ALERT** Never position patient so he or she is lying directly on pad. Lying directly on pad prevents dissipation of heat and increases risk of burns.

STEPS	RATIONALE
b. Turn heating pad on low or medium setting. Turn on aquathermia unit and check temperature. Most units are preset to 105° F or 40.5° C to 43° C.	To determine correct function of equipment and check for proper temperature. Prevents exposure of patient to temperature extremes.
5. Apply commercially prepared heat pack; break pouch inside larger packet (follow manufacturer's instructions for use).	Activates chemicals within pack to warm outer surface.

> **SAFETY ALERT** Do not puncture outer pack. Do not allow chemicals to come in contact with skin or eyes.

STEPS	RATIONALE
6. Monitor condition of skin over site every 5 minutes and ask patient about sensation of burning.	Determines if heat exposure is resulting in burn.
7. Remove treatment after 20 to 30 minutes (or time ordered by health care provider).	Local application of heat longer than 20 minutes without interruption may result in burn or changes to the microcirculation such as vasoconstriction (Stitik and Nadler, 1999).
8. **See Completion Protocol (inside front cover).**	

EVALUATION

1. Inspect patient's skin for integrity, color, temperature, dryness, and blistering. Evaluate again 30 minutes after procedure.
2. Ask patient to rate pain level on scale of 0 to 10.
3. Measure patient's ROM.
4. Observe patient or family caregiver apply pad.

Unexpected Outcomes and Related Interventions

1. See Unexpected Outcomes, Skill 27.1.
2. Body part is painful to move.
   a. Discontinue treatment.
   b. Assess for edema or increased swelling.
   c. Notify health care provider.

Recording and Reporting

- Record pain level; ROM of body part; skin integrity, color, temperature, sensitivity to touch, dryness, and blistering; type of application; temperature and duration of treatment; and patient response to treatment.
- Report any unusual findings such as blistering, decreased ROM, or increased pain.

Sample Documentation

1000 Family caregiver (sister) applied heating pad on low setting to right bicep for pain with motion. Pain severity 6 on a scale of 0 to 10. Flexion 140 degrees and extension 20 degrees. Skin intact, pink, and warm; skin turgor is elastic.

1020 Heating pad removed. Right bicep pink to red and warm. No blisters; skin turgor is elastic. Patient states feels light touch to affected area and rates pain a 2 on a scale of 0 to 10. Flexion 145 degrees, extension 20 degrees.

Special Considerations

Pediatric

- Because of risk of injury from heating pads, aquathermia pads are used infrequently in children. If prescribed, remain with patient to ensure safety and effectiveness.

Geriatric

- Older patients have thinner, more fragile skin that is more susceptible to burns. Use extreme caution with electric heating pads in older patients.
- Older patients have an increased risk of burns because of diminished heat sensation.

Home Care

- Assess patient's use of alternative treatments at home (e.g., use of rice socks or herb packs). Evaluate for proper use of such treatments.
- Assess the home environment for facilities to adhere to implementation of the procedure.

SKILL 27.3 COLD APPLICATIONS

Cooling can be applied in many different ways such as ice bags, moist cold compresses, commercial cold packs or compresses, and electromechanical devices. Cold exerts a profound physiological effect on the body, reducing inflammation, pain, and swelling caused by injuries to the soft tissues of the musculoskeletal system (Kullenberg and others, 2006). Because reduction of inflammation is the primary goal, application of cold (cryotherapy) is the treatment of choice for the first 24 to 48 hours after a soft tissue injury.

Cold applications cause vasoconstriction and reduce blood flow to the injured part; as a result, fluid accumulation, bleeding, and hematoma formation associated with trauma are decreased. The lower temperature also reduces muscle spasm and produces a local anesthetic response (McGuire and Hendricks, 2006).

There are electrically controlled cooling devices that work much like aquathermia pads. The cooling pads deliver a constant cool temperature. Woolf and others (2008) found that cold devices that simultaneously provide compression are effective in treating acute musculoskeletal injury with soft tissue swelling. Whether using one of these devices or a cold compress, use the acronym *RICE: R*est, *I*ce, *C*ompression bandages (such as snug elastic wraps), and *E*levation of the injured area to effectively manage musculoskeletal injuries (Hume and others, 2006).

ASSESSMENT

1. Refer to physician's order for type, location, and duration of application. Temperature of an electronic device will be ordered. *Rationale: Order is required for all cold applications.*
2. Inspect condition of affected area or injury; palpate for edema. *Rationale: Provides baseline to determine changes in soft tissue after treatment.*
3. Perform neurovascular check. Assess surrounding skin for integrity, adequacy of circulation (presence of pulses), color, temperature, and sensitivity to touch. *Rationale: Provides baseline for determining change in condition of injured tissues.*
4. Determine time of injury. *Rationale: Cold reduces edema and soft tissue injury. Cold applications are most effective within the first 24 to 48 hours after injury (Airaksinen and others, 2003).*
5. Refer to patient's medical record for any contraindications to cold application. *Rationale: Patient with a preexisting condition that impairs circulation would be at greater risk for injury.*
6. Assess patient's pain on a scale of 0 to 10. *Rationale: Provides baseline to determine pain relief.*
7. Assess patient's understanding of procedure. *Rationale: Determines need for health teaching.*

PLANNING

Expected Outcomes focus on decreasing pain, edema, bleeding (in tissues), and bruising while preventing ischemia.

1. Patient reports decreased pain and uses fewer analgesics.
2. There is decreased edema and/or bleeding in tissues at site of injury.

3. Surrounding skin is slightly pale and cool to touch.
4. Patient or family caregiver correctly states how to apply cold.

Delegation Considerations

Assessment of patient's condition may not be delegated; however, the skill of applying cold applications may be delegated to nursing assistive personnel (NAP). Instruct the NAP about the following:

- Any mobility restrictions caused by the injury
- What to observe (e.g., expected mobility, pain, wound status) and report back to nurse
- Reporting when treatment is complete so that an evaluation of patient's response can be made

Equipment

All compresses, bags, and packs

- Soft cloth covering, stockinette, towel, or pillowcase
- Cloth tapes or ties
- Bath towel
- Bath blanket for warmth
- Waterproof pad

Cold compress

- Towel or gauze
- Prescribed solution, ice
- Basin

Ice bag or gel pack

- Ice bag
- Ice chips and water
- Reusable commercial gel pack (cold pack)
- Disposable commercial chemical cold pack

Electrically controlled cooling device

- Gauze roll or elastic wrap
- Cool-water flow pad or cooling pad and electrical pump

IMPLEMENTATION *for* COLD APPLICATIONS

STEPS	RATIONALE
1. **See Standard Protocol (inside front cover).**	
2. Identify patient using two identifiers (e.g., name and birthday or name and account number, according to facility policy).	Ensures correct patient. Complies with The Joint Commission standards and improves patient safety (TJC, 2010).
3. Provide warm covering for patient.	To prevent chilling.
4. Position patient comfortably, keeping affected body part in proper alignment. Expose only the area to be treated and drape patient with bath blanket.	Prevents further injury to area. Avoids unnecessary exposure of body parts, maintaining patient's warmth, comfort, and privacy.
SAFETY ALERT In cases of strains, sprains, or fractures, align extremity or body part following physician's recommendation to prevent further injury.	
5. Place towel or absorbent pad under area to be treated.	
6. ***Apply cold compress.***	
a. Place ice and water into basin and test temperature.	Extreme temperature can cause tissue injury.
b. Place gauze into basin and wring out excess moisture.	Dripping gauze is uncomfortable to patient.
c. Apply compress, molding it gently over site. Remove, remoisten, and reapply to maintain temperature as needed.	Ensures that cold is directed over site of injury.
7. ***Apply ice pack or bag.***	
a. Fill bag with water, secure cap, and invert.	Prevents skin maceration by testing bag for leaks.
b. Empty water. Then, fill bag two-thirds full with small ice chips and water.	Bag is easier to mold over body part when it is not full.
c. Express air from bag, secure closure, and wipe bag dry.	Allows ice bag to conform to area and promotes maximum contact.
d. Squeeze or knead a commercial ice pack.	Releases alcohol-based solution to create cold temperature.

Continued

STEPS	RATIONALE
e. Wrap pack or bag with towel, stockinette, or pillowcase (see illustration). Wrap prepared ice pack directly over area.	Prevents direct exposure of cold against patient's skin. Cold is applied directly over site of injury and assists in reducing inflammation and swelling.
f. Secure with elastic wrap bandage, gauze roll, or ties.	Secures therapeutic cold to area of injury.

SAFETY ALERT Sterile supplies must be used with open wounds.

STEPS	RATIONALE
8. ***Apply commercial gel pack.***	
a. Remove pack from freezer.	
b. Wrap pack in towel, stockinette, or pillowcase or cover patient's skin with towel.	Prevents direct exposure of cold application to skin, reducing risk of tissue injury.
c. Place gel pack on affected area (see illustration).	
d. Secure with gauze roll, cloth tape, or ties as needed.	Secures therapeutic cold to area of injury.
9. ***Apply electrically controlled cooling device (see illustration).***	
a. Make sure that all connections are intact and temperature (if adjustable) is set. (See agency policy and manufacturer's directions.)	Ensures safe temperature for application.
b. Wrap cool-water flow pad in pillow case or towel. Then wrap pad around body part.	Ensures even temperature during cold application.
c. Turn device on and set or check correct temperature.	
d. Secure with elastic wrap bandage, gauze roll, or ties.	Secures therapeutic cold to area of injury.
10. Check condition of skin every 5 minutes for duration of any cold application.	Determines presence of adverse reactions to cold, including mottling, redness, burning, blistering, and numbness (Nadler and others, 2004).
a. If area is edematous, sensation may be reduced; use extra caution during cold therapy and assess the site more often.	Reduced sensation does not allow patient to perceive numbness or tingling in the area; as a result the site is at greater risk for injury.
b. Numbness and tingling are common sensations with cold applications and indicate adverse reactions only when severe and coupled with other symptoms. Stop when patient complains of burning sensation or skin feels numb.	Initially cold is sensed followed by pain relief. As treatment progresses, patient may report burning sensation, pain in the skin, and finally numbness (Nadler and others, 2004).

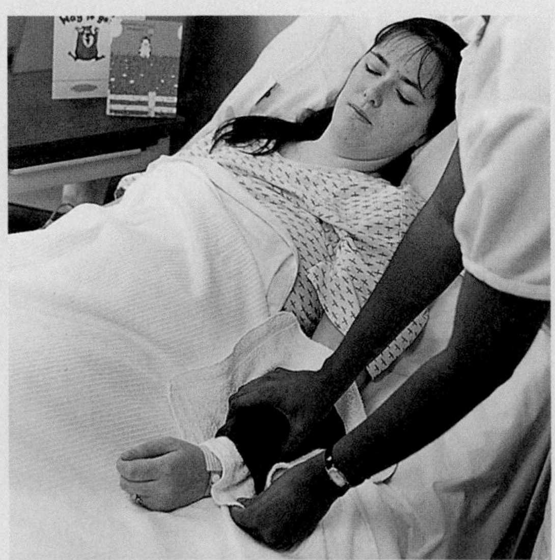
STEP 7e Protecting patient's skin.

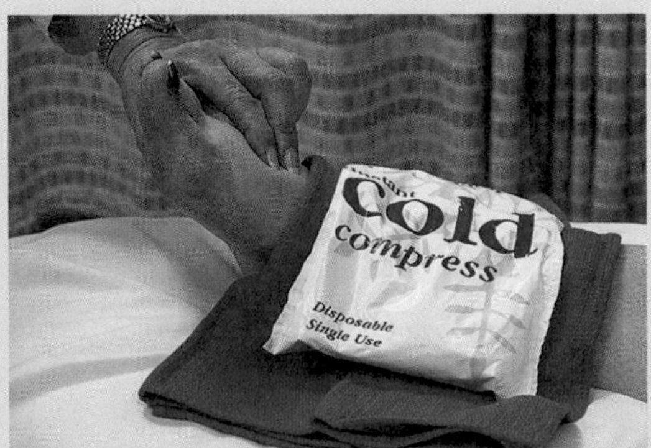

STEP 8c Cold compress application.

STEPS	RATIONALE
11. After 15 to 20 minutes (or as ordered by health care provider), remove compress or pad and gently dry off any moisture.	Drying prevents maceration of the skin.

SAFETY ALERT Areas with little body fat such as knees and ankles do not tolerate cold as well as fatty areas such as thighs and buttocks. For bony areas reduce time of cold application.

12. See Completion Protocol (inside front cover).

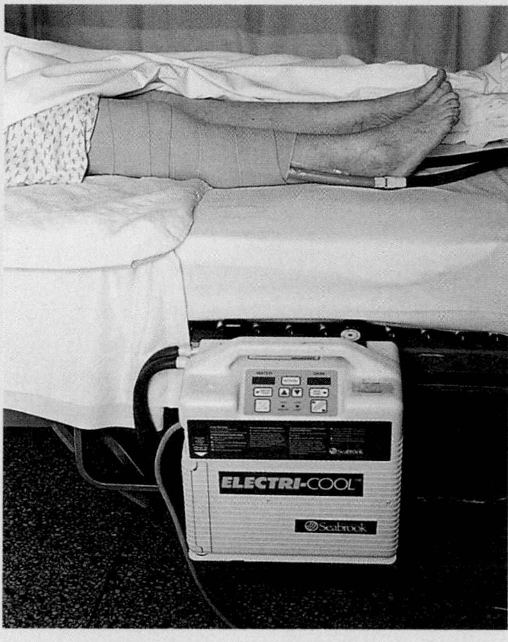

STEP 9 Electric cooling device.

EVALUATION

1. Inspect surrounding tissues for integrity, color, and temperature; ask patient to describe sensitivity to touch. Reevaluate 30 minutes after procedure.
2. Palpate tissue or wound for edema, bruising, and bleeding.
3. Ask patient to report pain level on a scale of 0 to 10.
4. Monitor patient's use of analgesics.
5. Observe patient apply cold application and discuss risks of treatment.

Unexpected Outcomes and Related Interventions

1. Skin appears mottled, reddened, or bluish purple.
   a. Stop treatment; symptoms indicate prolonged exposure.
   b. Report to health care provider if symptoms persist for more than 30 minutes.
2. Patient complains of burning-type pain and numbness.
   a. Stop treatment; symptoms indicate possible ischemia.
   b. Report to health care provider if symptoms persist for more than 30 minutes.

Recording and Reporting

- Record pain level; presence of bleeding, bruising, and edema in area of injury; skin integrity, color, temperature, and sensitivity to touch; and type of application, temperature and duration of treatment, and patient's response.
- Report any sensations of burning, numbness, or unrelieved changes in skin color.

Sample Documentation

0930 Left ankle edematous and tender to touch after twisting injury. Ankle measures 32 cm at medial malleolus and 31 cm across metatarsal region of foot. Pain at 7 on a scale of 0 to 10. Ecchymosis present, extending 8 cm on medial aspect with surrounding skin warm and pink. Dorsalis pedis and posterior tibialis pulses present and strong. Left extremity elevated with ice pack applied to ankle.

0950 Ice pack removed from ankle. Ankle measures 32 cm. Pain at 2 on a scale of 0 to 10. Ecchymosis unchanged. Skin pink and cool; patient reports numbness on palpation.

Special Considerations

Pediatric

- A greater metabolic rate and larger trunk in relation to the rest of the body make children more prone to hypothermia. Exercise caution with young patients.
- Infants have an unstable temperature-control mechanism; thus mottling of extremities is common and may not indicate an adverse reaction if this symptom is seen alone.
- Further assessment in children with frequent soft tissue or musculoskeletal injuries may be necessary.

Geriatric

- Older patients are more at risk for tissue damage because of loss of temperature sensation (Nicoll, 2002). Check site frequently during all treatments.
- Anticipate shortening duration of treatment.
- Older patients may require more covering for warmth.

Home Care

- A bag of frozen vegetables conforms nicely to an affected area and is effective for brief periods of treatment. Place a thin towel between the bag and skin or place bag inside a pillowcase.

REVIEW QUESTIONS

Case Study for Questions 1 to 4

A 73-year-old patient arrives in the nursing unit following a total knee arthroplasty procedure. The nurse notes swelling and redness of the affected extremity, and the patient complains of pain of 7 on a scale of 0 to 10. The patient has an order for an ice bag to the region.

1. Which of the following is most appropriate for the nurse to do to correctly prepare ice for application to the wound?
   1. Fill the bag with ice; add air to increase surface area.
   2. Water test the bag to be sure that it has no leaks.
   3. Expose the skin in the affected area to ready it for ice application.
   4. Assess the area for numbness and tingling before application.
2. The patient is 5 minutes into having the ice pack applied. The patient reports that pain is still 7 on a scale of 0 to 10 and slight numbness to the area that is iced. The patient also reports feeling chilled and uncomfortable. Which of the following actions would be most appropriate for the nurse to take at this time?
   1. Add fresh ice to the treatment to ensure that continuous cold is applied.
   2. Discontinue the cold therapy and document that patient was chilled.
   3. Administer prescribed pain medication to reduce pain to the affected area.
   4. Inform patient that chilling is normal and continue the treatment for an additional 10 minutes.
3. Which of the following would indicate a successful treatment plan using cold therapy? Select all that apply.
   1. Patient reports a reduction of pain from 5 to 2 on a scale of 0 to 10.
   2. Edema has been reduced over a 12-hour shift.
   3. The skin has become mottled.
   4. The patient has decreased his need for oral analgesics.
4. Which of the following assessment findings is a contraindication for use of cold therapy?
   1. A patient with acute inflammation
   2. A patient with impaired circulation
   3. A patient with severe pain
   4. A patient suffering trauma within the past 24 hours
5. What is a major concern with the prolonged application of moist heat?
   1. Maceration
   2. Cramping
   3. Erythema
   4. Dermatitis
6. Performing which of the following actions would be inappropriate when applying moist heat therapy to a patient?
   1. Performing a neurovascular assessment before heat application
   2. Using a low setting on the microwave to heat the compress
   3. Checking affected joint ROM after application
   4. Removing compress before 20 minutes has passed
7. The application of ______________________ would achieve the most effective deep penetrating heat. Fill in the blank.
8. Assessment findings of ______________ skin would be an indication of prolonged exposure to cold from a cold gel pack. Fill in the blank.
9. A patient has an order for heat application following a muscle strain to the back. Which nursing intervention would be the priority for the prevention of injury in this situation?
   1. Frequently assessing the setting on the heat delivery system
   2. Placing a plastic wrap over the compress for better penetration
   3. Frequently assessing the area where the heat is being applied
   4. Encouraging the patient to increase his oral fluid intake

REFERENCES

Airaksinen OV and others: Efficacy of cold gel for soft tissue injuries: a prospective randomized double-blinded trial, *Am J Sports Med* 31(5):680, 2003.

Hockenberry MJ, Wilson D: *Wong's nursing care of infants and children*, ed 8, St Louis, 2007, Mosby.

Hume PH and others: Epicondylar injury in sport; epidemiology, type, mechanisms, assessment, management, and prevention, *Sports Med* 36(2):151, 2006.

Janwantanakul P: Different rate of cooling time and magnitude of cooling temperature during ice bag treatment with and without damp towel wrap, *Phys Ther Sport* 5:156, 2004.

Kullenberg B and others: Postoperative cryotherapy after total knee surgery: a prospective study of 86 patients, *J Arthroplasty* 21(8):1175, 2006.

McGuire DA, Hendricks SD: Incidences of frostbite in arthroscopic knee surgery postoperative cryotherapy rehabilitation, *Arthroscopy* 22(10):1141, 2006.

Meiner SE, Lueckenotte AG: *Gerontologic nursing*, ed 3, St Louis, 2006, Mosby.

Nadler S and others: The physiologic basis and clinical applications of cryotherapy and thermotherapy for the pain practitioner, *Pain Physician* 7(3):395, 2004.

Nicoll L: Heat in motion: evaluating and managing temperature, *Nursing* 32(5):S1, 2002.

Pescasio M and others: Clinical management of muscle strains and tears, *J Musculoskelet Med* 25(11):526, 2008.

Stitik T, Nadler S: Sports injuries: when and how to apply heat, *Consultant* 39(1):144, 1999.

The Joint Commission: *2010 National Patient Safety Goals*, Oakbrook Terrace, Ill, 2010, The Commission, http://www.jointcommission.org/PatientSafety/NationalPatientSafetyGoals/, accessed February 14, 2010.

Woolf S and others: Comparison of a continuous temperature-controlled cryotherapy device to a simple icing regimen following outpatient knee arthroscopy, *J Knee Surg* 21:15, 2008.

CHAPTER

28

Intravenous Therapy

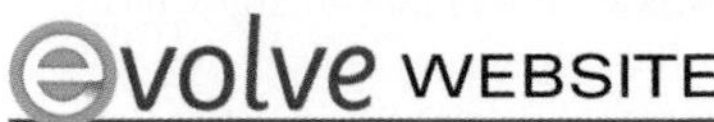

http://evolve.elsevier.com/Perry/nursinginterventions

Video Clips

Nursing Skills Online

Placement of an intravenous (IV) device is one of the most invasive procedures a nurse can perform, putting a patient at risk for complications associated with infusion therapy. Critical thinking is required before initiation of infusion therapy and during the course of treatment. Assessment of a patient's anatomy and physiology of the circulatory system, fluid and electrolyte balance, disease pathophysiology, type and duration of prescribed therapy, allergies, and the patient's response to illness play a key role in decision making to ensure safe delivery of infusion solutions or medications. The goal of IV therapy is to maintain and prevent fluid and electrolyte imbalances, administer continuous or intermittent medications, replenish blood volume, and assist in pain management. For all the skills in this chapter, follow the six rights of medication administration and IV administration: *R*ight drug/solution, *R*ight dose/concentration, *R*ight patient, *R*ight route, *R*ight date/time, and *R*ight documentation and *R*ight indication when providing IV therapy (Alexander and others, 2010).

The Infusion Nurses Society standards of practice include evidence-based practice (EBP) and are integrated throughout the skills in this chapter (INS, 2006). Additional guidelines published by The Joint Commission (TJC, 2007), the Centers for Disease Control and Prevention (CDC, 2002), and the Occupational Safety and Health Administration (OSHA, 2006) are incorporated to support safe, efficient, and quality care when providing infusion therapy. Know and follow these standards, your employer's policy and procedures, and your state or government practice guidelines and standards when providing IV care.

PATIENT-CENTERED CARE

The approach you take can directly affect a patient's response to infusion therapy. Preparing the patient before placing a peripheral IV device may help to alleviate fears associated with infusion therapy. Psychological factors also need to be considered because your patient's previous experience with infusion therapy will affect both your placement of the IV device and the patient's ability to understand the therapy prescribed (Alexander and others, 2010). You can make the experience less traumatic if you appear confident, speak directly to the patient, ensure his or her privacy, and answer questions as directly and honestly as possible. Depending on the age of the patient or factors that may affect his or her ability to comprehend, you need to establish a rapport with a significant person associated with the patient's care. Using various communication and diversional techniques will help to lessen anxiety. Such techniques would include having the patient breathe in and out slowly, avoid looking at the catheter during insertion, and focus on a pleasant image or past experience (Alexander and others, 2010). As a nurse you must be aware of the diversity found within health care, including age, gender, race, ethnicity, sexual orientation, and religious beliefs (Alexander and others, 2010). Such diversity means that you must provide culturally competent care. It is impossible to be aware of all the various cultures you may encounter, but a careful assessment of a patient's beliefs and the meaning behind those beliefs helps you to know your patient and be better able to meet his or her physical, psychosocial, spiritual, and cultural needs (Alexander and others, 2010).

SAFETY

During the insertion of a peripheral-short IV device and when managing infusion therapy, the potential for you to incur a needlestick injury or be exposed to a bloodborne pathogen is a significant safety concern. Bloodborne pathogens such as human immunodeficiency virus (HIV), hepatitis B, and hepatitis C affect approximately 100,000 health care workers annually, and the incidence of sharps injuries is about 30 per 100 hospital beds per year (Gabriel, 2008). The Needlestick Safety and Prevention Act (OSHA, 2006) requires health care employers to identify and make use of effective and safer medical devices. In addition, the INS standards state that all devices should have engineered sharps injury protection mechanisms that should be activated before disposal (INS, 2006). Most devices have either a self-sheathing mechanism that covers the needle tip once the catheter is placed or a spring action mechanism in which the needle is retracted into a protective housing after the catheter is inserted.

It would be impossible to eliminate the need to use short-peripheral IV devices; however devices with built-in sharps injury protection features can reduce the risk of an accidental needlestick injury. The use of rigid sharps disposal containers is an additional method for sharps injury prevention, and all sharps material should be disposed of in the appropriate container (CDC, 2002; Gabriel, 2008; INS, 2006). You will become familiar with your agency-specific safety devices and the correct method to activate the safety mechanism. The skills in this chapter outline how to use the safety features of peripheral-short IV devices. Further safety issues related to placing and removing the peripheral-short IV device and initiating and completing the setup of the infusion equipment are covered in each skills section.

EVIDENCE-BASED PRACTICE TRENDS

Ahlqvist M and others: Handling of peripheral intravenous cannula: effects of evidence-based clinical guidelines, *J Clin Nurs* 15(11):1354, 2006.

Alexander M and others: *Infusion nursing: an evidence-based approach,* ed 3, St Louis, 2010, Elsevier.

Eggimann P: Prevention of intravascular catheter infection, *Curr Opin Infect Disease* 20(4):360, 2007.

Richardson D: Vascular access nursing-standards of care and strategies in the prevention of infection: a primer on central venous catheters, *J Assoc Vasc Access* 12(19):21, 2007.

Adhering to evidence-based practice (EBP) in the placement of an IV device while administering infusion solutions and medications can significantly reduce the risk of infusion-related complications. Infusion-related complications can be either local or systemic. The CDC has demonstrated that the increased risk of infusion-related complications can be directly linked to poor infection control practices. These include poor hand hygiene, inadequate site preparation, and inadequate nursing judgment when assessing for the appropriate insertion site and catheter selection. According to the CDC, "serious infectious complications produce considerable annual morbidity because of the frequency with which such catheters [peripheral] are used" (Ahlqvist and others, 2006; Alexander and others, 2010; CDC, 2002; Eggimann, 2007; Richardson, 2007).

SKILL 28.1 INSERTION OF A PERIPHERAL-SHORT INTRAVENOUS DEVICE

- **Nursing Skills Online: Intravenous Fluid Administration Module, Lessons 1 and 2** *Video Clips*

To maintain or correct fluid and electrolyte balance, isotonic, hypotonic, or hypertonic fluids are delivered through a variety of devices using continuous or intermittent infusion. Infusion therapy provides access to the venous system to deliver various medications in emergent and non-emergent situations and to infuse blood or blood products. Reliable venous access for infusion therapy administration is essential.

Successful IV therapy depends on patient preparation, site selection, catheter selection, and catheter insertion. Several vascular access devices are available for use in peripheral veins (Table 28-1). The Infusion Nurses Society (INS) standards of practice recommend using the smallest device and smallest gauge possible to give the prescribed therapy (INS, 2006). Because potential exposure to bloodborne pathogens is high during insertion and care of IV devices, adherence to asepsis

TABLE 28-1 INTRAVENOUS ACCESS DEVICE OPTIONS

TYPE	USE	TYPES OF INFUSIONS
Winged infusion butterfly needle	One-time infusion, IV push administration	Solutions or medications with a pH between 5.0 and 9.0 Osmolarity less than 600 mOsm/L (INS, 2006)
Short, over-the-needle catheter (7.5 cm [less than 3 inches])	Continuous infusion, intermittent infusion, short-term duration (rotate site every 72 hours) (INS, 2006)	Solutions or medications with a pH between 5.0 and 9.0 Osmolarity less than 600 mOsm/L (INS, 2006)
Midline peripheral catheters (7.5 to 20 cm [3- to 8-inches])	Continuous and intermittent infusion (1 to 4 weeks) (INS, 2006)	Solutions or medications with a pH between 5.0 and 9.0 Osmolarity less than 600 mOsm/L (INS, 2006)

and standard precautions is required (see Chapter 5). In addition, to minimize the complications of IV therapy it is important to change peripheral IV access every 72 hours (INS, 2006), per health care provider's orders, or more frequently if complications such as phlebitis occur.

Steel-winged infusion devices (butterfly needles) should be limited to short-term or single-dose IV administration. They are easier to insert but may easily infiltrate. Commonly used over-the-needle catheters include (1) a metal stylet to pierce the skin, and (2) a catheter made of silicone, polyurethane, PVC, or Teflon, which threads into a vein and remains there for the infusion of fluid. These flexible catheters do not dislodge from the vein as easily as stainless steel needles. Improved product design provides many choices, all of which should be radiopaque in the event of catheter shearing.

ASSESSMENT

1. Verify prescriber's order, including patient name and correct solution type, volume, rate, frequency, dosage, and route. Medications and additives must be checked for the correct dosage, frequency, rate, and their compatibility with primary and secondary solutions. *Rationale: Ensures safe and correct administration of IV therapy by verifying order. Assists in selection of an appropriate access device and early placement of longer-term infusion devices and minimizes multiple venipunctures.*
2. Assess patient's previous experience and understanding of IV therapy. *Rationale: Determines level of emotional support and instruction necessary.*
3. Determine if patient is to undergo any planned surgeries or procedures. *Rationale: Allows nurse to place an appropriate-size catheter and avoids placement in an area that will interfere with surgeries or procedures.*
4. Assess patient's hand/arm dominance. *Rationale: Ensures that placement does not impair therapy or interfere with activities of daily living (ADLs) or mobility and that it improves patient's comfort.*
5. Assess for risk factors: child or older adult, presence of heart failure or renal failure, skin lesions, infection, low platelet count; or anticoagulant use. *Rationale: Conditions pose a risk for fluid overload, affect IV site selection, and determine the patient's risk for bleeding.*
6. Assess condition of both arms, including palpation of veins. *Rationale: Allows for appropriate selection of vein to accommodate device and therapy. Avoids veins that are sclerosed or damaged from previous IV therapy or contraindicated for an IV start such as mastectomy or dialysis shunt.*
7. Assess for clinical conditions such as dehydration, peripheral edema, body weight, dry mucous membranes, altered vital signs, and lung sounds that will be affected by IV fluid administration. *Rationale: Provides baseline for monitoring reactions and response to therapy.*
8. Assess laboratory data and patient's history of allergies. *Rationale: May reveal information that affects insertion of devices such as fluid and electrolyte imbalances or coagulation problems. Prepping agents, gloves, and certain catheter materials may create a serious problem for patients with allergies to iodine, adhesive, or latex or previous allergies to medications such as antibiotics.*
9. Assess patient's medical history for chronic illnesses and all prescribed and over-the-counter medications. *Rationale: Provides background information that might result in adverse effects on patient (e.g., heart failure may require slower infusion rate) or conflict with the prescribed therapy such as drug-drug interactions.*

PLANNING

Expected Outcomes focus on avoiding complications related to IV therapy, minimizing patient discomfort, and establishing a patent route for delivery of therapies.

1. Fluid and electrolyte balance returns to normal, and/or blood volume is replenished.
2. Vital signs are stable, and laboratory values return to within normal limits for patient.
3. Intake and output (I&O) are within normal limits for patient's condition.
4. No signs or symptoms of IV-related complications are observed.
5. IV access is patent, and infusion is delivered at prescribed rate and volume.

Delegation and Collaboration

Infusion therapy should only be performed by nurses who meet the established educational experience and technical clinical criteria set forth by the nurse practice act of their state and agency policies and procedures (INS, 2006). The skills of inserting, maintaining, and discontinuing an IV device and initiating and monitoring infusion solutions and medications cannot be delegated to nursing assistive personnel (NAP). Instruct the NAP about the following:

- What to observe such as complaints of pain, bleeding, or swelling at IV site and when this information is to be reported back to the nurse
- When to inform the nurse (e.g., when the volume of fluid is low in the IV bag or the electronic infusion device [EID] is sounding its alarm)

Equipment

- IV start kit, which contains tourniquet, tape, clear occlusive dressing, cleansing agent(s) (2% chlorhexidine or povidone-iodine, and 70% alcohol), and 2 × 2–inch gauze pads
- Appropriate IV catheter (see Table 28-1). In adult, 22-gauge cannula is appropriate for fluid maintenance.
- Clean gloves (latex-free for patient with latex allergy)
- Extension set with needleless connection device
- Prefilled 5-mL syringe with flush agent (preservative-free normal saline [NS])
- Alcohol pads
- IV tubing appropriate for electronic infusion device (EID)
- Prescribed IV solution or medications
- EID and IV pole

IMPLEMENTATION *for* INSERTION OF A PERIPHERAL-SHORT INTRAVENOUS DEVICE

STEPS	RATIONALE
1. See Standard Protocol (inside front cover).	
2. Identify patient using two identifiers (e.g., name and birthday or name and account number, according to facility policy). Compare identifiers with information on patient's medication administration record (MAR) or medical record.	Ensures correct patient before insertion of IV device and initiation of solution or medications. Complies with The Joint Commission standards and improves patient safety (TJC, 2010).
3. Select appropriate-size catheter and prepare sterile packages.	The catheter selected uses the smallest size and shortest length to accommodate prescribed therapy (INS, 2006).
4. Prepare IV infusion tubing and solution for continuous infusion using sterile technique.	Maintaining the sterility of a closed IV system decreases the risk of bacterial contamination (CDC, 2002).
a. Check IV solution using the six rights of medication administration. Check solution for leaks, color, clarity, and expiration date.	IV solutions are medications and need to be carefully checked to reduce the risk for error.
b. Open infusion set, maintaining the sterility of both tubing ends. Many EID pumps have special administration sets.	Prevents touch contamination, which prevents micro-organisms from entering infusion equipment and bloodstream.
c. Place roller clamp 2 to 5 cm (1 to 2 inches) below drip chamber, and move roller clamp to "off" position (see illustration).	Close proximity of clamp to drip chamber allows more accurate regulation of flow rate. Off position prevents leakage during priming.
d. Remove protective sheath from IV tubing port on plastic IV solution bag (see illustration) or top of bottle. Insert infusion set into fluid bag or bottle by removing protector cap from insertion spike (not touching the spike) and inserting it into opening of IV container (see illustration). Cleanse rubber stopper on glass-bottled solution with single-use antiseptic, and insert spike into black rubber stopper of IV bottle. Bottle needs vented tubing.	Provides access for insertion of infusion tubing into the solution using sterile technique. Flat surface on top of a bottled solution may contain contaminants, whereas the port on the plastic bag is recessed.

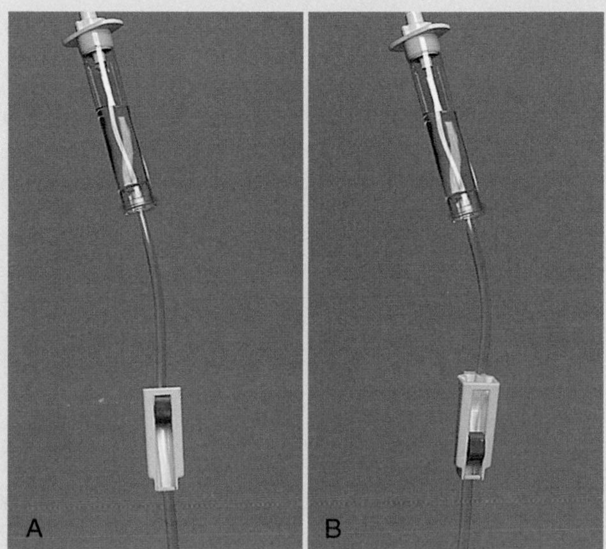

STEP 4c A, Roller clamp in open position. **B,** Roller clamp in off or closed position.

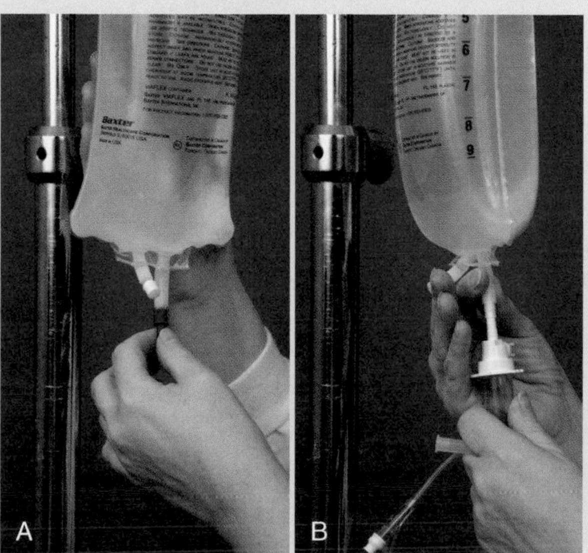

STEP 4d A, Remove protective covering from IV solution tubing port, **B,** Insert tubing spike into IV container,

Continued

STEPS	RATIONALE
e. Prime infusion tubing by filling with IV solution: Compress drip chamber and release, allow it to fill one-third to one-half full (see illustration).	Ensures tubing is cleared of air and filled with saline before connection with IV catheter.

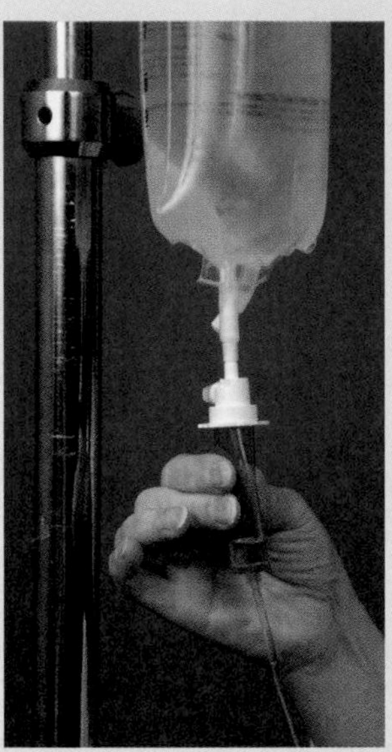

STEP 4e Squeeze drip chamber to fill with fluid.

STEPS	RATIONALE
f. Remove protector cap on end of tubing (you can prime some tubing without removal) and slowly open roller clamp to allow fluid to travel from drip chamber through tubing to needle adapter. Invert Y-connector sites to displace air. Close roller clamp. Be certain tubing is clear of air and air bubbles. Remove small air bubbles by firmly tapping IV tubing where bubbles are located. Check entire length of tubing to ensure that all air bubbles are removed. Replace cap protector on end of infusion tubing.	
5. Prepare an extension set, which can be used as an extender for standard tubing or as a saline lock (capped catheter).	Extension set used when continuous infusions are not needed.
a. For a saline lock, swab injection cap with antiseptic swab. Insert syringe with sterile saline flush and inject through the cap into the loop or short extension tubing. Keep syringe attached.	Removes air from tubing and prevents air from being introduced into vein. Sterile syringe will be used later once IV line is established.
6. Perform hand hygiene. NOTE: Gloves may be left off to locate the vein but must be applied before preparing the site. Apply tourniquet around arm above antecubital fossa or 10 to 15 cm (4 to 6 inches) above proposed insertion site. Do not apply too tightly to cause injury or bruising to skin. Verify presence of a radial pulse.	Tourniquet should be tight enough to impede venous return but not occlude arterial flow. Use of blood pressure cuff reduces trauma to underlying skin.
7. Select the vein for device insertion.	
a. Use most distal site in patient's nondominant arm if possible. Clip arm hair with scissors if necessary. Do not shave IV site area because shaving causes microabrasions and increases risk of infection.	Venipuncture should be performed distal to proximal, which increases availability of other sites for future IV therapy. Hair impedes venipuncture and adherence of dressing (INS, 2006).

STEPS	RATIONALE
b. Avoid areas that have already been compromised from previous IV insertions (e.g., areas that are painful, bruised, or inflamed or have a rash).	It would be difficult to assess for any signs or symptoms of complications if an IV device were inserted in an area already compromised.
c. Select a well-dilated vein large enough for device placement (see illustration).	Prevents interruption of venous flow while allowing adequate blood flow around catheter.
d. Choose a site that does not interfere with patient's ADLs or planned surgery or procedures.	Maintains patient's mobility as much as possible.
e. With the index finger palpate the vein by pressing downward and noting a resilient, soft, bouncy feeling as the pressure is released (see illustration). Avoid veins that feel hard.	Use of the same finger causes a development of sensitivity to better assess the vein condition. Hard veins are those that are sclerosed and have been damaged from previous IV insertions.
f. If needed, place patient's arm in a dependent position to select the well-dilated vein.	Promotes venous distention.
g. Methods to improve venous distention include:	
(1) Stroking extremity from distal to proximal below the proposed venipuncture site.	Promotes venous filling.

SAFETY ALERT Vigorous friction and multiple taping of veins, especially in older adults, causes hematoma and/or venous constriction.

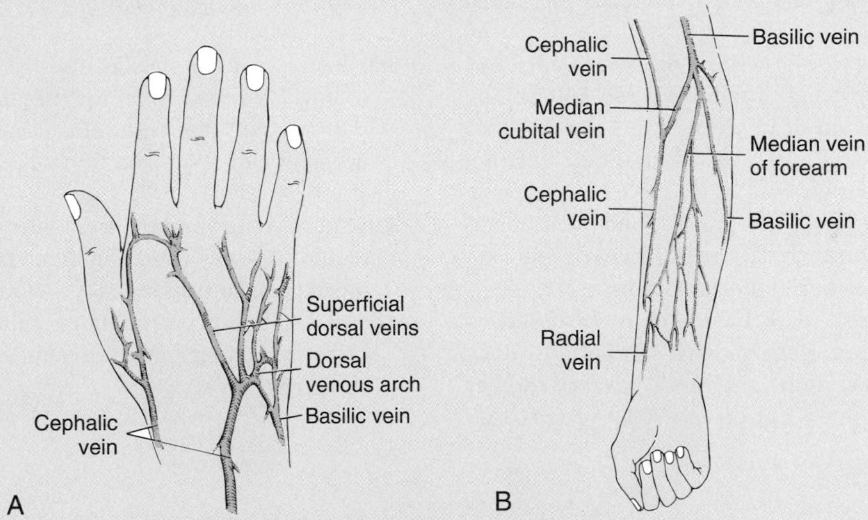

STEP 7c Common intravenous sites. **A,** Dorsal surface of hand. **B,** Inner arm.

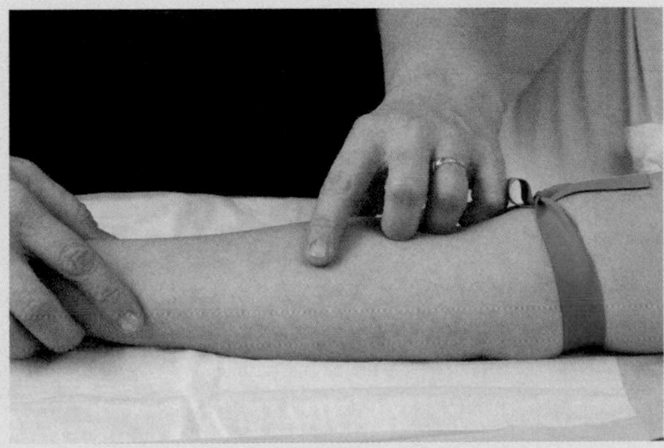

STEP 7e Palpate vein for resilience.

Continued

STEPS	RATIONALE
(2) Applying warmth to extremity for several minutes (e.g., use a warm washcloth).	Heat increases blood supply through vasodilation.
h. Avoid sites distal to a previous venipuncture site, veins in the antecubital fossa or inner wrist, sclerosed or hardened cordlike veins, an infiltrated site or phlebotic vessels, bruised areas, and areas of venous valves or bifurcation.	Such sites increase risk of IV-related complications. Veins in antecubital fossa are used for blood draws, placement of midlines or peripherally inserted central catheter (PICC) lines. Placement here limits mobility (INS, 2006).
i. Avoid fragile dorsal veins in older adults and vessels in an extremity with compromised circulation (e.g., in cases of mastectomy, dialysis graft, or paralysis).	Venous alterations can increase risk of complications (e.g., infiltration, decreased catheter dwell time).
8. Release tourniquet temporarily and carefully. Option: You may apply a local anesthetic to site at least 30 minutes before IV start.	Prevents damage to skin and restores blood flow while preparing for venipuncture. Local anesthetic is effective in reducing discomfort of venipuncture.
9. Apply gloves if not done in Step 6. Place adapter end of filled infusion tubing or extension set nearby, keeping it inside the sterile packing in which it came. Cleanse insertion site using friction for a minimum of 30 seconds (see illustration). Use antiseptic preparation as a single agent or in combination. Allow to dry between agents if agents are used in combination.	Mechanical friction allows penetration of antiseptic into epidermal layer of skin. Drying prevents chemical reactions between agents and allows time for maximum microbicidal activity of agents. Chlorhexidine (2%) has recently been shown to be an effective agent (INS, 2006). Touching cleansed area would introduce organisms from nurse's hand to site (Hadaway, 2006a).
10. Reapply tourniquet and verify presence of radial pulse.	Promotes vein engorgement.
11. Perform venipuncture. Anchor vein below proposed insertion site by placing thumb over vein and pulling skin against direction of insertion 4 to 5 cm (1½ to 2 inches) distal to the site (see illustration). Instruct patient to relax hand.	Stabilizing vein for needle insertion prevents vein from rolling. Provides ease for needle insertion for skin puncture and then into vein. Skin becomes taut, thereby decreasing drag on insertion of IV device.
12. Warn patient of a sharp, quick stick. Puncture skin and vein, holding catheter at a 10- to 30-degree angle with bevel in the up position (see illustration).	Superficial veins require a smaller angle. Deeper veins require a greater angle. Depth of vein is related to amount of subcutaneous tissue.
13. Observe for a brisk, dark blood return in flashback chamber of catheter, lower catheter until almost flush with skin (see illustration), and slowly advance another 0.6 cm (¼ inch) into vein. Loosen stylet of over-the-needle catheter.	Allows for full penetration of vein wall, placement of catheter in inner lumen of vein, and easy advancement of catheter off stylet.

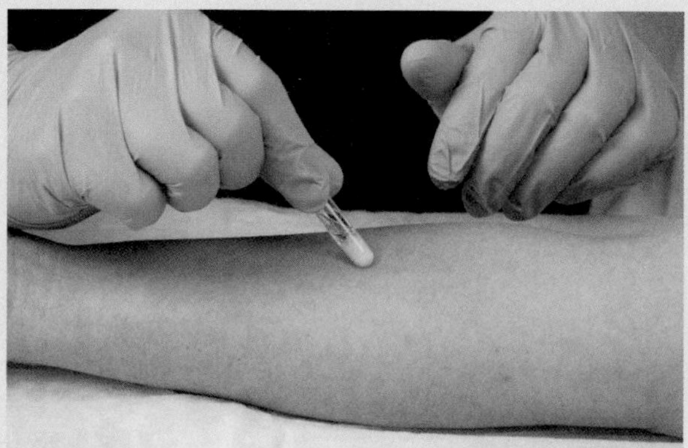

STEP 9 Cleanse site with chlorhexidine.

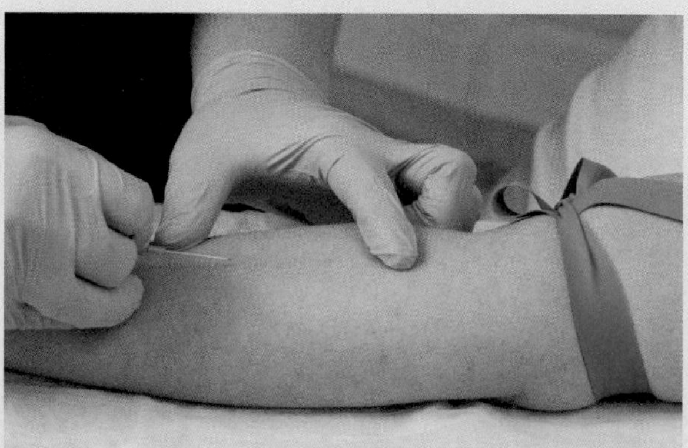

STEP 11 Stabilize vein below insertion site.

STEPS	RATIONALE
14. If no blood return is observed or catheter does not advance, venipuncture was unsuccessful; device should be removed, with firm direct pressure applied to insertion site until bleeding stops. Obtain a new catheter and attempt a second time in another location proximal to the previous attempt.	If venipuncture is unsuccessful, always obtain a new catheter before a second attempt. Never reinsert the stylet (needle) into the catheter because this may damage the catheter and cause catheter embolism. When the catheter is partially withdrawn through the stylet and/or reinserted, the damage can range from a small nick in the catheter to complete severing of the distal tip (INS, 2006). After a second unsuccessful attempt, ask another practitioner to perform venipuncture.
15. Advance catheter off stylet to thread catheter into vein. Continue until catheter hub rests at venipuncture site (see illustration). *Do not reinsert the stylet once it is loosened.* Continue to hold skin taut.	Reduces risk of introduction of infectious microorganisms along catheter length.
16. Stabilize catheter with one hand and release tourniquet with the other.	Restores blood flow to arm.
17. Apply gentle but firm pressure with index finger of nondominant hand 3 cm (1¼ inches) above insertion site. For the safety device, glide the catheter off the stylet while gliding the protective guard over the stylet. A click indicates that the device is locked over the stylet. (Techniques vary with each IV device.) Remove the stylet.	Obstructs venous flow, minimizing blood loss. Use of safety devices prevents inadvertent needlestick injury.
18. Hold catheter firmly with dominant hand and quickly connect Luer-Lok end of the continuous infusion tubing set (see illustration). Do not touch point of entry of connection. Secure connection.	Stabilizing cannula prevents accidental withdrawal or dislodgment (INS, 2006). Prompt connection of infusion set maintains patency of vein.
Option. Quickly connect end of primed extension set tubing (saline lock), and flush with remaining fluid in the sterile prefilled syringe containing flush solution. Flush extension set slowly with flush solution (see illustration).	Positive-pressure flushing allows fluid to displace removed needle, creates positive pressure in catheter, and prevents reflux of blood into catheter lumen.

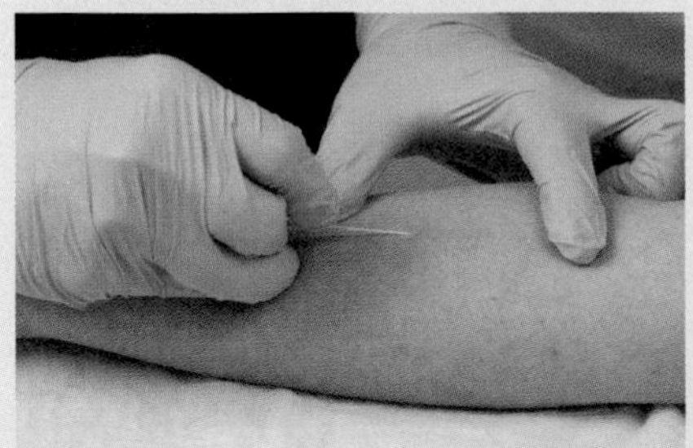

STEP 12 Puncture vein with catheter held at a 10- to 30-degree angle. Catheter enters vein.

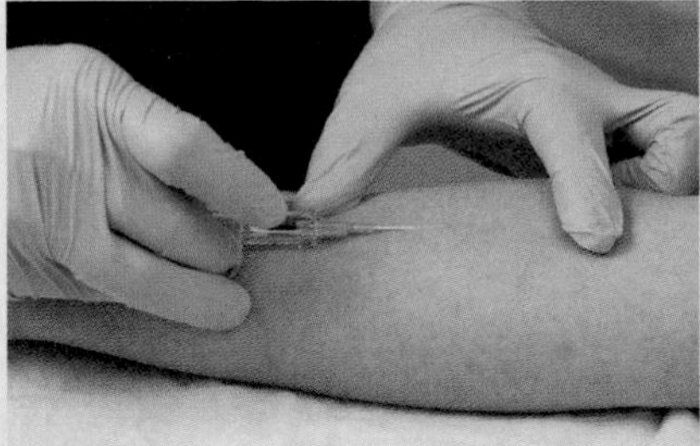

STEP 13 Observe for blood return in flashback chamber.

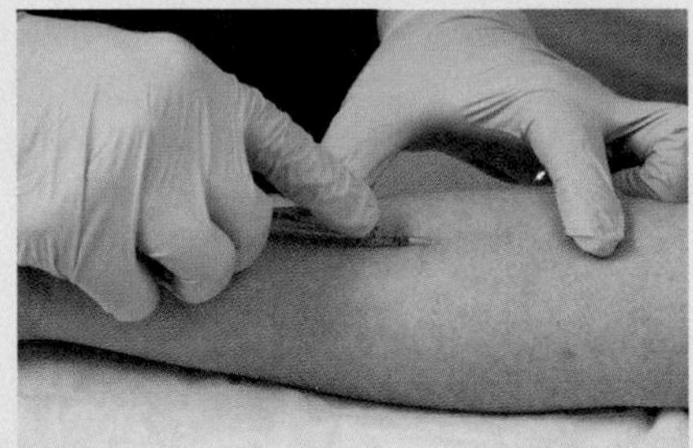

STEP 15 Advance catheter into vein until hub is near insertion site.

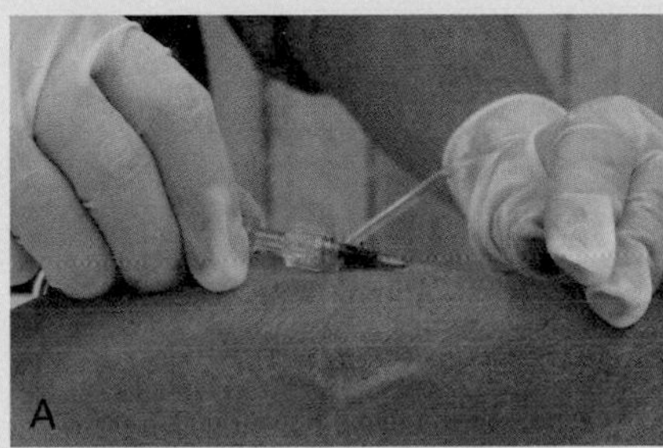

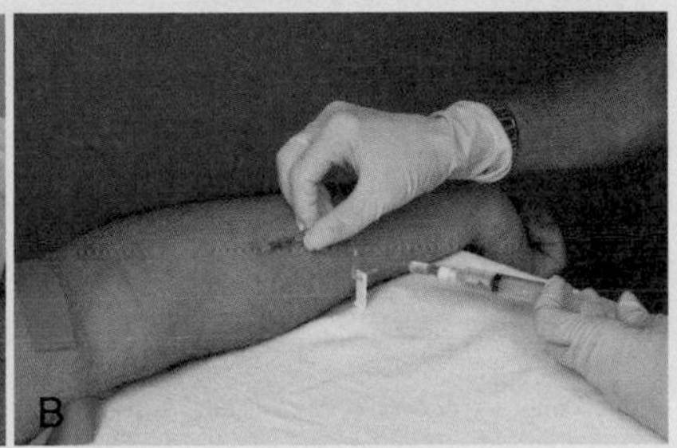

STEP 18 **A,** Connect end of continuous infusion tubing. **B,** Flush extension set slowly.

Continued

STEPS	RATIONALE
19. Secure IV catheter.	
a. Sterile transparent dressing Secure catheter with nondominant hand while preparing to apply dressing.	Prevents accidental catheter dislodgement.
b. Manufactured catheter stabilization device Wipe selected area with single-use skin protectant and allow to dry. Slide device under catheter hub, and center hub over device. Holding catheter in place, peel off half of liner, press to adhere to skin. Repeat on the other side. Holding catheter in place, pull tab out from center of device to create opening, insert catheter into slit. This frames the IV site. Cover insertion site with a transparent dressing (see Step 20a) (see illustration).	The stabilization device is a sterile adhesive pad that holds the catheter in place, reduces the risk for infection and needle-stick injuries, and improves patient outcomes (INS, 2006).
c. Sterile gauze dressing Place a narrow, 1.25-cm (½-inch) piece of sterile tape, about 10 cm (4 inches) long over catheter hub. Place tape only on the catheter hub, not over the insertion site (see illustration).	Use sterile tape under a sterile dressing to prevent site contamination. Regular adhesive tape is a potential source of pathogenic bacteria (INS, 2006). Prevents back-and-forth motion of catheter.
20. Apply sterile dressing over IV site.	
a. Transparent dressing.	
(1) Carefully remove adherent backing. Apply one edge of dressing over IV site and gently smooth remaining dressing. Leave connection between IV tubing and catheter hub uncovered (see illustration). Remove outer covering and smooth dressing gently over site.	Transparent dressing allows continuous inspection of site and surrounding tissue and is more comfortable. Transparent dressings are occlusive to moisture and microorganisms (INS, 2006). Prevents accidental dislodgement of catheter.
(2) Take a 1-inch piece of tape and place it over the end of tubing just behind connection point with catheter, but not over transparent dressing.	
b. Sterile gauze dressing	
(1) Place 2 × 2–inch gauze pad over venipuncture site and catheter hub (see illustration). Secure all edges with tape. Do not cover the connection between the IV tubing and catheter hub with the dressing.	Optional method of securing IV device if patient is allergic to transparent dressing. However, it is not the preferred method to cover and secure IV device because gauze prevents visualization of the insertion site (INS, 2006).
21. Loop the continuous infusion or extension set tubing along the outside of the arm and secure with a strip of tape (see illustration). Begin continuous infusion by slowly opening the slide clamp, adjusting roller clamp of IV tubing, or turning on already programmed electronic infusion pump.	Initiates flow of fluid through IV catheter, preventing clotting and initiating therapy.

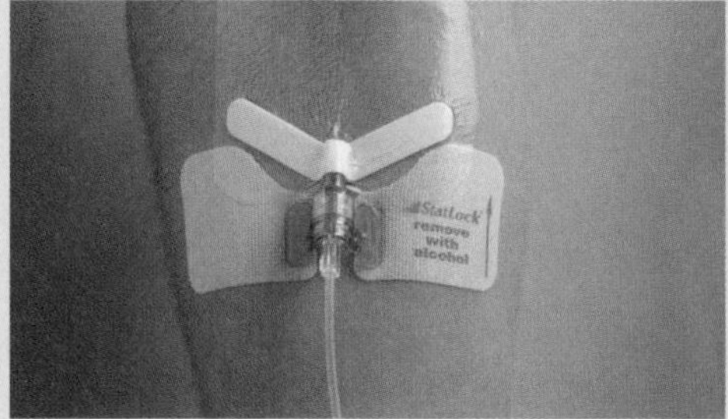

STEP 19b Catheter stabilization device in place. (Courtesy CR Bard Inc.)

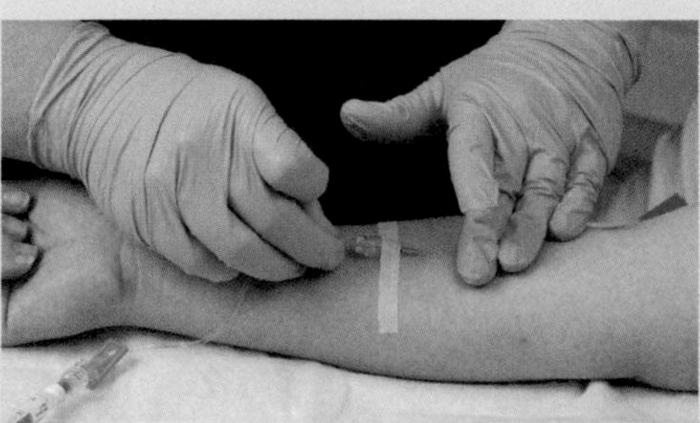

STEP 19c Apply tape over catheter hub.

STEPS	RATIONALE
22. Remove and dispose of gloves.	
23. Label IV dressing, including date, time, catheter gauge size and length, and nurse's initials (see illustration).	Allows for easy recognition of type of device and time interval for site rotation. INS standard for site rotation of peripheral IV access devices is every 72 hours (INS, 2006). CDC (2002) allows for replacement every 96 hours (observe agency policy).
24. Show patient how to avoid placing pressure on venipuncture site and/or catheter dislodgement when attempting to reposition in bed or getting out of bed. Discuss signs and symptoms of possible infiltration or phlebitis to report (e.g., pain, swelling, burning, redness, or moisture on dressing).	
25. Dispose of sheathed stylet and any uncapped sharps(s) in appropriate sharps container as soon as device is secured. Dispose of remaining trash.	Prevents accidental needlestick injury, and transmission of microorganisms is reduced (OSHA, 2006).
26. **See Completion Protocol (inside front cover).**	

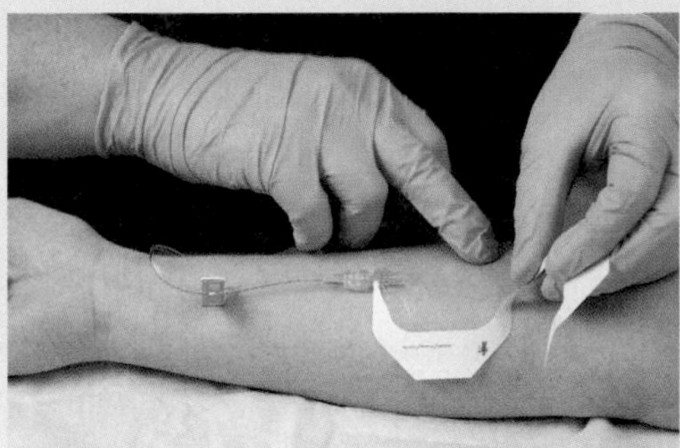

STEP 20a(1) Apply transparent dressing.

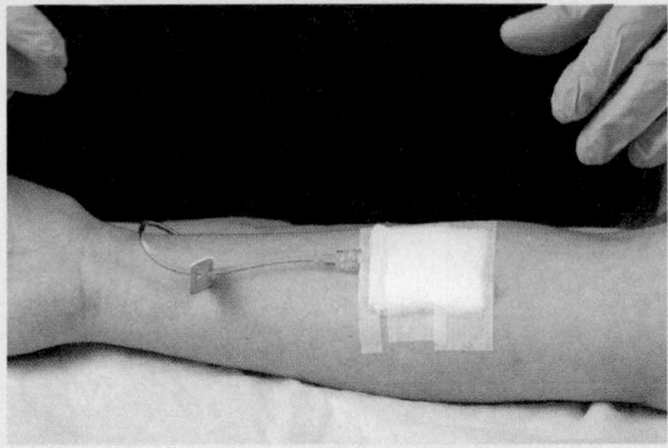

STEP 20b(1) Place 2 × 2–inch gauze over insertion site and catheter hub.

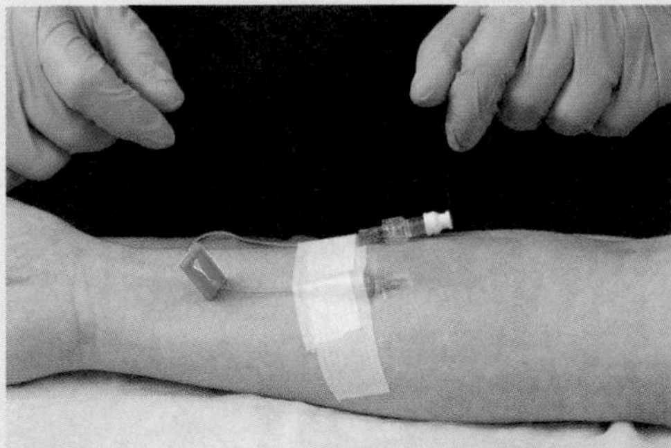

STEP 21 Loop and secure extension set tubing.

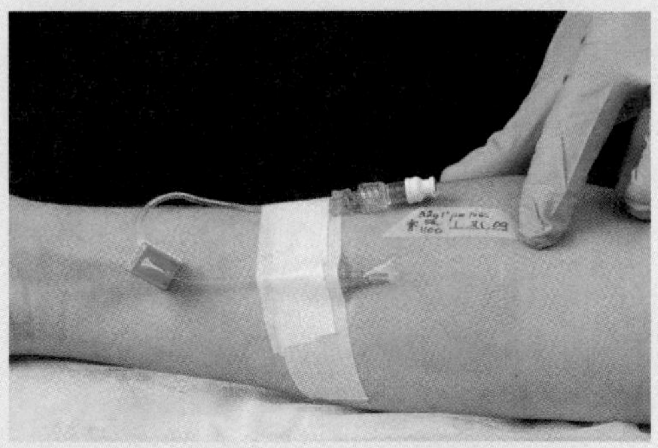

STEP 23 Label IV dressing.

EVALUATION

1. Observe patient every hour and check for:
   a. Patency of IV cannula.
   b. Correct type/amount of IV solution that has infused by comparing time tape or EID record.
   c. The infusion drip rate (if gravity drip) or the rate/volume on the infusion pump.
2. Monitor patient's I&O, daily weights as indicated, and evidence that prescribed therapy is working: return of normal fluid volume, resolution of infection, laboratory values in appropriate range.
3. Inspect patient's IV site and extremity every 1 to 2 hours for signs and symptoms of IV-related complications such as pain, swelling, heat, or redness during the infusion (see Tables 28-2 and 28-3).
4. On completion of IV insertion and during IV infusion, ask if patient is comfortable.

TABLE 28-2 PHLEBITIS SCALE

SCORE	CLINICAL SIGNS
0	No symptoms
1	Erythema at access site with or without pain
2	Pain at access site with erythema and/or edema
3	Pain at access site with erythema and/or edema Streak formation Palpable venous cord
4	Pain at access site with erythema and/or edema Streak formation Palpable venous cord >2.5 cm (1 inch) in length Purulent drainage

From Intravenous Nurses Society: 2006 Infusion nursing standards of practice, *J Infus Nurs* 29(suppl 1):S1, 2006.

TABLE 28-3 INFILTRATION SCALE

GRADE	CLINICAL CRITERIA
0	No symptoms
1	Skin blanched Edema <2.5 cm (1 inch) in any direction Cool to touch With or without pain
2	Skin blanched Edema 2.5 to 15 cm (1 to 6 inches) on skin surface in any direction Cool to touch With or without pain
3	Skin blanched, translucent Gross edema >2.5 to 15 cm (6 inches) in any direction Cool to touch Mild-to-moderate pain Possible numbness
4	Skin blanched, translucent Skin tight, leaking Skin discolored, bruised, swollen Gross edema >15 cm (6 inches) in any direction Deep pitting tissue edema Circulatory impairment Moderate-to-severe pain Infiltration of any amount of blood product, irritant, or vesicant

From Intravenous Nurses Society: 2006 Infusion nursing standards of practice, *J Infus Nurs* 29(suppl 1):S1, 2006.

Unexpected Outcomes and Related Interventions

1. *Phlebitis:* Patient complains of pain and tenderness at IV site with erythema at site or along path of vein. Insertion site is warm to touch, and rate of infusion may stop.
   a. Stop the infusion and discontinue IV. Reinsert new IV if continued therapy is required, Restart in opposite extremity or proximal to previous site.
   b. Apply moist warm compress over area of phlebitis. Monitor site according to agency policy.
   c. Document degree of phlebitis and nursing interventions per agency policy and procedure (Table 28-2).
2. *Infiltration:* Patient's rate of infusion slows; insertion site is swollen, cool to touch, pale, and painful.
   a. Stop infusion and discontinue the IV. Reinsert new IV if continued therapy is necessary, preferably in opposite extremity.
   b. Elevate affected extremity.
   c. Monitor previous insertion site per agency protocol until resolution of swelling.
   d. Document degree of infiltration and nursing intervention (Table 28-3).
3. Infusion is completed before or after appropriate time frame.
   a. Evaluate access device for position and patency; regulate remainder of infusion over prescribed time; assess need for EID.
   b. Assess IV site for need to restart IV infusion at another site.
   c. Continue to monitor hourly for proper rate of infusion.
   d. Monitor and document patient with too-rapid infusion for fluid overload. Obtain vital signs, respiratory status, and I&O.
   e. Notify health care provider.
4. IV site infections
   a. Assess insertion site for signs and symptoms of infection, which include redness, edema, induration, temperature changes, and drainage.
   b. Notify health care provider for appropriate interventions.
   c. Document the presence and severity of the infection.

Recording and Reporting

- Record number of attempts for insertion; type of solution or medication infusing, rate and method of infusion (e.g., gravity or name of EID), purpose of infusion; insertion site by location and vessel; brand, length and gauge of IV device; patient's response to insertion (e.g., what he or she reports); and when infusion was started. Use agency infusion therapy flow sheet. Always complete entry with full signature and credentials.
- Report any significant information, such as any signs or symptoms of IV-related complications (e.g., infiltration, phlebitis, change in flow rate, infection).

Sample Documentation

1400 IV started in left midcephalic vein with 22-gauge 1-inch Insyte catheter × 1 attempt. Infusion of 1 g Rocephin initiated via Baxter Flo Guard Pump at 100 mL/hr for UTI. No signs or symptoms of IV-related complications observed. Patient stated, "I hardly felt that at all."

Special Considerations

Pediatric

- In addition to usual venipuncture sites, the four scalp veins and the dorsum of the foot are used in infants. Needle selection is based on age: 26 to 24 gauge for neonates; 24 to 22 gauge for children (Alexander and others, 2010; Earhart and others, 2007; INS, 2006).

- Apply latex-free tubing or rubber band or use a blood pressure cuff inflated to just below the patient's diastolic blood pressure. In accessing scalp veins aim the catheter downward, toward the heart, so the flow of infusion can follow venous return (INS, 2006).
- Maintain skin integrity, especially in neonates. Use adhesives such as tape sparingly and remove tape gently.
- Stabilization is essential, especially in young children who cannot comprehend the importance of not "playing" with IV device.

Geriatric

- Older adults have loss of subcutaneous tissue, making veins more prominent. Loss of elasticity makes skin more fragile and prone to skin tears. Anchor catheters carefully to prevent damage to skin. Attempt to insert catheter without the use of a tourniquet if veins are visible and skin is fragile to prevent any damage. Place tourniquet over clothing to prevent bruising or skin tears. Use of smaller-gauge devices is recommended; ideal size is 22 or 24 gauge (INS, 2006).

Home Care

- Ensure the patient's/family caregiver's ability and willingness to administer and monitor IV therapy in the home. Determine if patient or caregiver has the manual dexterity and cognitive ability to manage the infusion and/or seek assistance in an emergency.
- Ensure that all sharps and equipment contaminated by blood are disposed in leak-proof, puncture-resistant containers with lids.
- Ensure availability of 24-hour assistance with provider of home infusion therapy pharmaceuticals and equipment.

SKILL 28.2 REGULATING INTRAVENOUS INFUSION FLOW RATES

- **Nursing Skills Online: Intravenous Fluid Therapy Management Module, Lesson 2** *Video Clips*

Accurate infusion rates in IV therapy are essential to deliver infusion solutions and medications safely. Complications associated with IV therapy (e.g., infiltration, phlebitis, clotting of device, or circulatory overload) are reduced or eliminated with a properly regulated IV infusion. Various factors interfere with infusion rates (Table 28-4). Hourly observation of the flow rate and IV system assist in achieving the therapeutic outcome and reducing complications.

Recent advances in infusion technology have resulted in a variety of devices available for use to ensure accurate hourly infusion of IV therapy (Alexander and others, 2010). Fluids that run by gravity are adjusted through use of a flow control/regulator clamp. A rate controller used on gravity infusions regulates the infusion but, unlike an electronic pump, it can be affected by many mechanical and patient factors. Fluids infused by an EID or rate controller are regulated by a mechanical pump set at the prescribed rate. Health care providers usually order the volume of fluid a patient is to receive within a specific time frame. For example, "1 L of D_5NS over 8 hours." You must be able to calculate hourly flow rates to ensure that the prescribed amount of fluid to be infused over the prescribed hours is correct. Regardless of whether gravity infusion or infusion via an electronic device is used, you must assess infusion rates hourly. Infusion pumps are necessary for patients who require low hourly volumes, are at risk for volume overload, have impaired renal clearance, or are receiving medications or fluids that require a specific hourly volume. EIDs deliver fluids using positive pressure. An electronic sensor with an alarm signals if the pressure in the system changes or if the desired flow rate alters. The minimal rate used to keep a vein patent is about 10 to 15 mL/hr in an adult and as low as 5 mL/hr in neonatal or pediatric patients. The use of an EID does not absolve the nurse from checking to ensure that the pump is functioning and infusing at the prescribed rate.

Many EIDs have operating and programming capabilities that allow for single- and multiple-solution infusions at different rates. A variety of detectors and alarms respond to air in IV lines, completion of infusion, high and low pressure, low battery power, occlusion, and the inability to deliver at a preset rate. An antifree-flow safeguard (preventing bolus infusion in the event of machine malfunction) is an

TABLE 28-4 FACTORS THAT ALTER INTRAVENOUS FLOW RATES

PATIENT FACTORS	MECHANICAL FACTORS
Change in patient position	Height of parenteral container (should be higher than 90 cm [36 inches] above heart)
Flexion of involved extremity	Positional access device
Partial or complete occlusion of IV device	Viscosity or temperature of IV solution; occluded air vent
Venous spasm	Occluded in-line filter
Vein trauma (phlebitis)	Improperly placed IV devices
Manipulated by patient or visitor	Crimped administration set tubing; tubing dangling below bed; low battery of an electronic device

From Intravenous Nurses Society: 2006 Infusion nursing standards of practice, *J Infus Nurs 29*(suppl 1):S1, 2006.

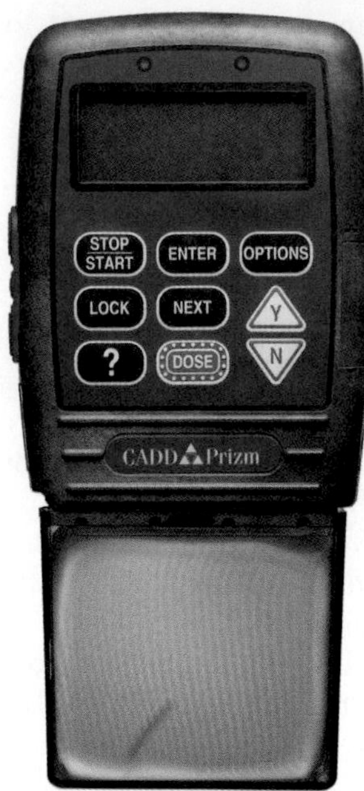

FIG 28-1 Patient-controlled ambulatory infusion pump. (Courtesy Smiths Medical ASD, Inc., St Paul, Minn.)

important element of an electronic infusion pump. Know and follow the agency and manufacturer's recommendations for selecting infusion pump controls: infusion volume, rate, alarm settings, and/or pump malfunction (Alexander and others, 2010; Cohen, 2007; TJC, 2007).

Patients in alternative care settings achieve infusion accuracy with ambulatory infusion pumps. Most pumps weigh less than 6 pounds and range from palm to backpack size. They function on battery power, allowing the patient freedom to return to normal life. Programming capabilities include automatic rate adjustments, remote site adjustments via a telephone modem, and therapy-specific settings such as patient-controlled analgesia (Fig. 28-1). Follow the manufacturer's recommendations for specific device features.

ASSESSMENT

1. Verify provider's order in patient's medical record for patient's name and correct IV solution: type, volume, additives, rate, and duration of IV fluid order. Apply the six rights of medication administration. *Rationale: Ensures that correct IV fluid is administered (INS, 2006).*
2. Assess patient's experience with having an IV, including knowledge about how positioning of IV site affects flow rate. *Rationale: Determines level of patient instruction or reinforcement needed.*
3. Inspect existing IV site, verify patency, and verify with patient how the site feels (e.g., determine if there is pain, burning, or tenderness at site). *Rationale: Pain or burning may be early indicators of phlebitis and the need to change IV site.*
4. Identify patient's risk for fluid imbalance (e.g., child; older adult; history of heart, renal, or respiratory disease; electrolyte imbalance). *Rationale: Strict infusion volume control is required.*

PLANNING

Expected Outcomes focus on infusion of prescribed solutions or medications without any adverse effects.

1. Patient receives prescribed volume of solutions/medication over desired time interval.
2. Response to prescribed therapy is achieved (e.g., return to normal fluid and electrolytes, laboratory values within normal limits for patient).

Delegation Considerations

The skill of regulating IV flow rates cannot be delegated to nursing assistive personnel (NAP). Instruct the NAP about the following:

- Reporting delayed or sudden emptying of IV bag
- Reporting sounding of the alarm on the infusion pump
- Reporting patient complaints of burning, bleeding, or swelling at IV site

Equipment

- Watch with a second hand
- Calculator, paper, and pencil
- Tape
- Label
- IV regulating device: EID (optional); volume control device (optional)

IMPLEMENTATION *for* REGULATING INTRAVENOUS INFUSION FLOW RATES

STEPS	RATIONALE
1. **See Standard Protocol (inside front cover).**	
2. Identify the patient using two identifiers (e.g., name and birthday or name and account number, according to facility policy).	Ensures correct patient before initiation of solution or medications. Complies with The Joint Commission standards and improves patient safety (TJC, 2010).

STEPS	RATIONALE
3. Obtain IV solution or medication and appropriate tubing and know calibration (drop factor) in drops per milliliter (gtts/mL) of infusion set used by agency:	Use of correct tubing ensures more accurate infusion delivery.
a. *Macrodrip:* Used to deliver rate *greater than* 100 mL/hr. (Drip factor is 10 to 20 gtts/mL, depending on equipment used. Drop factor is printed on box.) For example: • Travenol Laboratories: 10 gtts/mL • Abbott Laboratories: 15 gtts/mL • McGraw Laboratories: 15 gtts/mL	Macrodrip tubing allows for higher infusion volumes.
b. *Microdrip:* Used to deliver rates *less than* 100 mL/hr. Microdrip: 60 gtts/mL.	Microdrip tubing is used for slow delivery and smaller volumes.
4. Calculate desired flow rate (hourly volume) of prescribed infusion by dividing volume hours: **a.** $\text{Flow rate (mL/hr)} = \frac{\text{Total infusion (mL)}}{\text{Hours of infusion}}$ *Example*: 1000 mL/8 hr = 125 mL/hr	
5. Calculate the drop rate based on drops per minute and the drop factor of infusion set. **a.** Drop factor × mL/min = Drops/min or **b.** mL/hr × drop factor/60 min = Drops/min *Example:* Infuse 125 mL/hr via 10 gtts/mL drop factor: $\frac{125}{60} \times \frac{10}{1} = 21 \text{ gtts/min}$ Via 15 gtts/mL: $\frac{125}{60} \times \frac{15}{1} = 31 \text{ gtts/min}$ Via 20 gtts/mL: $\frac{125}{60} \times \frac{20}{1} = 41 \text{ gtts/min}$ Via 60 gtts/mL (microgtts): $\frac{125}{60} \times \frac{60}{1} = 125 \text{ gtts/min}$	
6. Time-tape the IV bag by securing marked adhesive tape or fluid indicator tape alongside of fluid container. Document each IV fluid bag sequentially and note type of fluid, patient's name, infusion span, and beginning and expected end of infusion.	Gives a visual scale to assess progress of infusion hourly. Avoid use of felt-tip pens or permanent markers on plastic bag; these can contaminate IV solutions.
7. Prepare IV tubing and infusion bag and prime tubing (see Skill 28.1).	Removes air from tubing.
8. ***Gravity infusion*** With IV fluid bag hung on pole at a minimum of 90 cm (36 inches) above IV insertion site, adjust rate-controlling clamp to deliver drops per minute. Using a watch, count drops in drip chamber for 1 minute. Then adjust roller clamp to increase or decrease rate of infusion.	Fluid container heights of 95 to 120 cm (36 to 48 inches) usually are sufficient to overcome venous pressure and other resistance from tubing and catheter (INS, 2006).

Continued

STEPS	RATIONALE
9. ***Electronic infusion device (EID).*** (Follow manufacturer's guidelines)	
a. Insert IV tubing into chamber of control mechanism (see illustration). (Consult manufacturer's instructions for use of pump.)	Pump chamber moves fluid through IV tubing.
b. Secure portion of IV tubing through "air in line" alarm system.	Allows for detection of air in tubing, which can enter vascular system, causing an embolus.
c. Close door to control chamber. Turn on pump and select rate per hour and total volume to be infused.	Follow pump instructions. Ensures that correct volume will be administered.
d. Open rate-controlling clamp on tubing if closed and press start button.	Rate control clamp should be open completely while infusion controller or pump is in use to ensure accurate volume of infusion.
e. Monitor infusion on a scheduled frequency to assess patency of system when in alarm mode and monitor for proper infusion rate and infiltration.	Ensures patient receives proper volume of fluid and ensures any complications are identified early.
10. ***Smart pump***	
a. Place pump module into the computer. Insert the IV tubing into the pump module and close the door.	
b. Follow manufacturer's instructions for use of pump. Smart pump instructions vary by manufacturer.	The pump checks programming against medication database to ensure accuracy.
11. ***Volume control device***	
a. Place volume control device between IV bag and infusion set using sterile technique.	Delivers small volume but must be refilled as it empties.
b. Fill volume control device with fluid by opening regulator clamp (see illustration). Place 2 hours of fluid allotment in chamber device. Regulate flow rate, counting for a full minute.	This prevents infusion from running dry if 60 minutes elapse before nurse returns. Should infusion rate accidentally increase, only 2 hours of fluid will infuse.
12. Instruct patient about the following:	
a. To avoid raising hand or arm to a position that will affect flow rate	Instruction informs patient about how to protect IV site and importance of not altering rate control.
b. To avoid manipulation of rate control clamp	
c. Purpose and significance of alarms	
13. See Completion Protocol (inside front cover).	

STEP 9a Insert IV tubing into chamber of control mechanism.

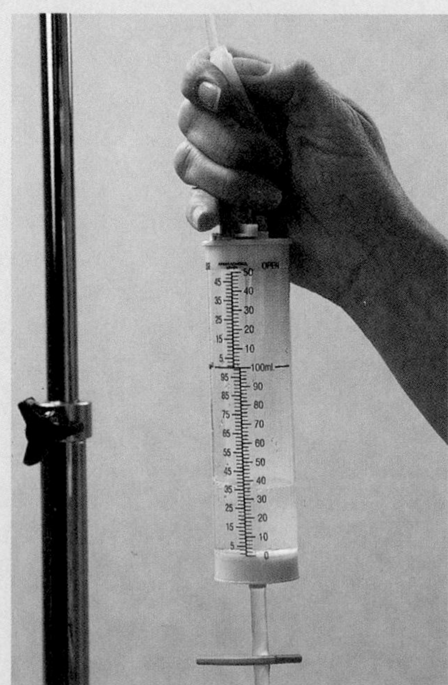

STEP 11b Open regulator clamp to fill volume control device.

EVALUATION

1. Monitor IV infusion at least every 1 to 2 hours, noting volume of IV fluid infused and rate.
2. Observe patient and monitor his or her response to therapy. Evaluate laboratory values, fluid, and electrolytes.
3. Observe for signs and symptoms of IV-related complications such as infiltration, phlebitis, clot in catheter, kink or knot in infusion tubing, and/or infusion pump malfunction.

Unexpected Outcomes and Related Interventions

1. Sudden infusion of large fluid volume of solution occurs with patient having symptoms of dyspnea, crackles in lung, and increased urine output, indicating fluid overload.
   a. Temporarily slow infusion rate to 10 gtts/min and notify health care provider.
   b. Place patient in high-Fowler's position; patient may require diuretic medications.
   c. New IV orders are required from health care provider.
2. IV infusion is slower than prescribed.
   a. Assess patient for positional change that might affect rate such as IV catheter or tubing obstruction.
   b. If volume is deficient, consult with health care provider for new prescribed order to provide required volume.

Recording and Reporting

- Record type of solution and/or medication being infused, rate of infusion, drops per minute, and milliliters per hour in patient's medical record; any ordered change in fluid rates; and use of any EID or controlling device.
- At change of shift or break time, report rate of infusion to nurse in charge or next nurse assigned to care for patient.

Sample Documentation

1400 Complaining of SOB. HOB elevated. Lungs auscultated with inspiratory crackles bilaterally. Physician notified. Order noted to decrease IV fluids of D_5NS to 25 mL/hr. IV site left midcephalic without signs or symptoms of IV-related complications observed. IV infusion converted to IMED Gemini infusion pump at 25 mL/hr. Purpose of fluid restriction and symptoms of pulmonary edema reviewed with patient and wife, who verbalized understanding. O_2 at 4 L/min per nasal cannula applied.

Special Considerations

Pediatric

- Containers exceeding 150 mL should not be used in children younger than 2 years of age; no more than 250 mL for children younger than 5 years; and no more than 500 mL for children younger than 10 years. *Always* use tamper-resistant volume-controlled infusion pumps to ensure accurate fluid delivery (Hockenberry and Wilson, 2007; INS, 2006).

Geriatric

- Use an EID with microdrip tubing. Carefully monitor patient's clinical status, laboratory results, vital signs, weight gain or loss, and I&O (INS, 2006).
- Infusing dextrose too rapidly may cause cerebral edema more readily in older patients. NS given to an older patient with impaired renal function can cause hypernatremia (INS, 2006).

Home Care

- Ensure that patient/family caregiver is able and willing to operate the ambulatory infusion pump. Assess any physical or visual limitations with ability to connect/disconnect infusion therapy and problem-solve pump malfunction (INS, 2006).
- The nurse should be in the home during initiation of IV therapy to ensure correct pump settings regarding solution, rate, time, and alarms.
- Provide telephone numbers for 24-hour service and emergencies with written instructions regarding infusion procedure and pump use.

SKILL 28.3 MAINTENANCE OF INTRAVENOUS SITE

- **Nursing Skills Online: IV Fluid Therapy Management Module, Lessons 3 and 4**
- **Nursing Skills Online: IV Fluid Administration Module, Lesson 3**

Peripheral-short IV catheters and infusion therapy are frequently associated with complications, which can be either local or systemic. Appropriate ongoing management of IV sites prevents or minimizes these complications (INS, 2006).

The skin insertion site is the most common source of infection for vascular catheters (Eggimann, 2007); therefore catheter dressings must be applied securely and changed when loose, wet, or soiled. A transparent dressing or sterile gauze secured with tape is used to cover the site (INS, 2006; Smith, 2007). A transparent dressing is changed with each catheter site rotation and immediately if integrity of dressing is compromised (INS, 2006). Gauze dressings are changed every 48 hours and immediately if integrity is compromised. When gauze is used in conjunction with a transparent dressing, it is considered a gauze dressing and changed every 48 hours (CDC, 2002; INS, 2006).

Solution and medication containers include plastic bags, plastic bottles, and glass bottles. These containers are changed frequently, depending on the rate of infusion, volume in the container, and stability of the solution or medication (INS, 2006). The CDC (2002) does not make a recommendation for the hang time of IV solutions or medications, but the INS recommends that each container be changed within 24 hours after the administration set is added (INS, 2006). Solution and medication containers on ambulatory infusion devices may remain longer than 24 hours if aseptic technique is used, the system remains closed without injection ports or add-on tubing, and the medication is stable for the anticipated infusion time (Depledge, 2006; INS, 2006).

It is more efficient to change infusion tubing when hanging a new fluid container. The CDC (2002) recommends changing continuous tubing no more frequently than every 96 hours, but the INS (2006) recommends 72- to 96-hour intervals for continuous tubing changes. Check your agency policy. The INS also recommends changing tubing used for intermittent infusion through an injection/access port every 24 hours because both ends of this tubing are manipulated more frequently than tubing used for continuous infusion.

A short extension tubing or loop may be placed between the catheter hub and injection cap, which allows manipulation of the injection cap without moving the catheter. This extension tubing remains attached to the peripheral-short catheter and is changed when the catheter is changed. The caps of midline and central venous catheters should be changed at least every 7 days (INS, 2006). The fluid pathway and capped ends on all infusion tubing, stopcocks, extension tubing, and injection caps are sterile. Use caution to prevent contamination of these surfaces during changes (INS, 2006).

You may need to assist patients with many aspects of hygiene (e.g., gown changes, bathing) while patients are receiving IV therapy. Infusion tubing is *never* disconnected to change a gown or any article of clothing. Coordinate care so bathing or hygiene activities are done after discontinuing an IV site and before another venipuncture is performed.

ASSESSMENT

1. Determine patient understanding of the need for continued IV infusion. *Rationale: Determines level of instruction or reinforcement needed.*
2. Changing a peripheral short IV dressing:
   a. Determine when the dressing was last changed by checking the dressing label. *Rationale: This labeling provides instant identification for determining status of the site (INS, 2006).*
   b. Observe present dressing for moisture and occlusiveness. Determine if moisture is caused by leaking from a puncture site or an external source. *Rationale: A soiled or wet dressing should be changed immediately.*
   c. Observe IV system for proper functioning (tubing or catheter kinks). Note if fluid is infusing at proper rate. *Rationale: Unexplained decrease in flow rate may indicate problems with catheter placement or patency.*
   d. Inspect exposed catheter site or palpate covered site for signs and symptoms of IV-related complications such as tenderness, swelling, redness, drainage, or blanching. *Rationale: Signs indicate phlebitis or infiltration.*
   e. Monitor body temperature. *Rationale: Rise in body temperature could be sign of infection at IV site.*
3. Changing infusion tubing:
   a. Determine when new infusion set is needed (e.g., according to agency policy, after contamination, or after puncture of infusion tubing). *Rationale: Changing of continuous infusion tubing and intermittent infusion tubing at recommended times reduces bloodstream infection.*
   b. Observe for occlusions in tubing such as kinking, drug or mineral precipitate, and blood. *Rationale: Infusion of incompatible medications can lead to precipitate formation. Blood may flow retrograde from vein and adhere to tubing. Infusion of viscous blood components may cause adherence to walls of tubing and decrease size of lumen.*
4. Changing infusion solution:
   a. Verify prescriber's original order. Check patient's name; IV solution or medication name and any medication additives; and dose, rate, route, and time of administration. *Rationale: The original order is the more reliable source of infusion and medication information. Ensures safe and correct administration of IV therapy by verifying order. A specific rate must be ordered; KVO is not an appropriate order (INS, 2006).*
   b. Determine the compatibility of all IV fluids and additives by consulting appropriate literature or the pharmacy. *Rationale: Patency of inside of catheter depends on prevention of chemical interactions. Precipitation can occur because of concentration of drugs in solution. When pH changes by contact between solutions or medications, a precipitate can occur (INS, 2006).*
   c. Verify patency of current IV access site. Carefully adjust roller clamp to regulated ordered rate or place tubing into EID and reset rate. Lowering IV container below level of IV site for blood return is an unreliable indicator. *Rationale: If patency is not verified, a new IV access site may be needed.*
   d. Palpate site for swelling, coolness, or tenderness around IV site. *Rationale: These symptoms are consistent with infiltration, indicating need to discontinue IV site.*

PLANNING

Expected Outcomes focus on reducing risk of IV-related complications, minimizing patient discomfort, reducing risk of overhydration, providing appropriate therapy, and maintaining a patent IV catheter.

1. IV site remains free of signs and symptoms of IV-related complications, including but not limited to infection, redness, swelling, pain, or drainage.
2. Patient's IV catheter and tubing are patent.
3. IV solution and medication infuse at proper rate.

Delegation Considerations

The skills of maintaining an IV site cannot be delegated to nursing assistive personnel (NAP). Instruct the NAP by:

- Explaining appropriate position for patient to maintain to avoid injury at insertion site

- Reviewing what to observe (e.g., changes in patient's temperature; signs and symptoms of IV-related complications such as pain, tenderness; and drainage at IV site) and reporting back to the nurse

Equipment

Changing a peripheral-short IV dressing

- Antiseptic swabs (2% chlorhexidine, or 70% alcohol, povidone-iodine)
- Skin protectant solution
- Adhesive remover (optional)
- Clean gloves
- Strips of sterile, precut tape (or 36-inch roll of tape)
- Transparent dressing or sterile 2 × 2–inch gauze pads and tape
- Commercially available IV site protector (*optional*) (Fig. 28-2)

Changing infusion tubing

- Clean gloves
- Sterile 2 × 2–inch gauze pads (*optional*)
- Microdrip or macrodrip infusion tubing or appropriate EID tubing. (Check manufacturer's requirements)
- 0.22-mcg filter and extension tubing if necessary
- Tubing label
- 5-mL syringe filled with preservative-free NS (observe agency policy)
- Antiseptic swabs

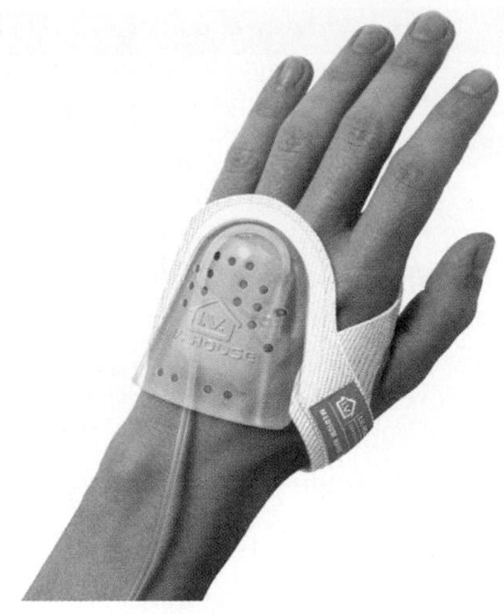

FIG 28-2 Commercially available intravenous site protector. (Courtesy I.V. House.)

Changing infusion container

- Bottle/bag of IV solution with medications as ordered by physician or appropriate prescriber
- Time tape
- Pen

IMPLEMENTATION *for* MAINTENANCE OF INTRAVENOUS SITE

STEPS	RATIONALE
1. **See Standard Protocol (inside front cover).**	
2. Identify the patient using two identifiers (e.g., name and birthday or name and account number, according to agency policy). If changing IV solution containing medication, compare identifiers with information on the patient's medication administration record (MAR) or medical record.	Ensures correct patient. Complies with The Joint Commission standards and improves patient safety (TJC, 2010).
3. ***Changing peripheral-short IV dressing***	
a. Remove transparent membrane dressing by picking up one corner and pulling the side laterally while holding catheter hub and tubing with non-dominant hand. Repeat for other side (see illustration). Discard dressing in trash container.	Technique minimizes discomfort during removal. Use alcohol swab on transparent dressing next to patient's skin to loosen dressing.

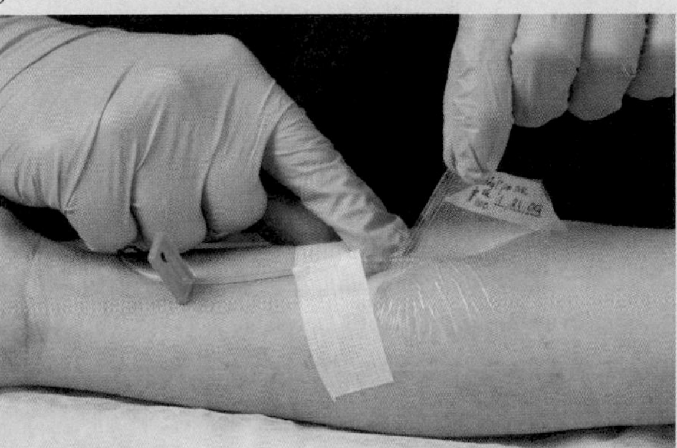

STEP 3a Remove transparent dressing by pulling side laterally.

Continued

STEPS	RATIONALE
Or	
b. Remove gauze dressing and tape from old dressing one layer at a time by pulling away from insertion site while holding catheter hub and tubing (follow agency policy). Be cautious if IV tubing becomes tangled between two layers of dressing.	Prevents accidental catheter displacement.
c. Observe insertion site for signs and symptoms of IV-related complications per Step 2d under Assessment above. If present, discontinue infusion (see Procedural Guideline 28.1).	Catheter moved during dressing change could accidentally dislodge and puncture blood vessel.
d. If IV solution is infusing properly, gently remove any tape securing catheter. Stabilize hub of catheter with one finger.	Exposes venipuncture site and prevents accidental displacement of cannula. Adhesive residue decreases ability of new tape to adhere securely to the skin.
e. Cleanse insertion site with antiseptic using friction, moving from insertion site outward. Allow antiseptic solution to dry completely.	Friction penetrates antiseptic into epidermal layer of skin. Antimicrobial solutions should be allowed to air dry completely to effectively reduce microbial counts (INS, 2006).
f. Secure catheter with nondominant hand.	Prevents accidental catheter dislodgment.
g. Apply sterile dressing over site.	
(1) Transparent dressing: See Skill 28.1, Step 20a.	Transparent dressing allows for inspection of IV site.
(2) Gauze dressing: See Skill 28.1, Step 20b.	Gauze dressings must be occlusive to prevent air flow (Alexander and others, 2010).
h. Curl a loop of the infusion tubing along the outside of the arm, and place a piece of tape directly over tubing.	Securing loop of tubing reduces risk of dislodging catheter from accidental pull.
i. Anchor IV tubing with additional pieces of tape if needed. When using transparent dressing, avoid placing tape over dressing.	
j. Label dressing with date and time of insertion, date and time of dressing change, gauge and length of catheter, and identification of nurse.	Allows easy recognition of type of device and time interval for site rotation.
4. *Changing infusion tubing*	
a. Open new infusion set and connect add-on pieces such as filters or extension tubing. Keep protective covering over spike and distal adapter. Secure all connections.	Separation of infusion tubing increases risk of air emboli, hemorrhage, and infection. Protective covers reduce entrance of microorganisms.
b. Expose catheter hub or end of extension set on existing IV. Avoid removing tape or transparent dressing securing catheter to skin.	Movement of catheter may cause it to dislodge. IV solutions and medications can be administered either by connecting directly to the IV device or through an end cap or extension set.
c. For continuous IV solutions:	
(1) Move roller clamp to "off" position of new tubing.	
(2) Slow rate of infusion to existing IV by regulating roller clamp on old tubing.	
(3) Compress and fill drip chamber of old tubing.	Ensures that fluid chamber remains full until new tubing is changed.
(4) Remove old tubing from IV container. Continue to hold it upright until you are ready to connect new tubing.	Fluid in drip chamber runs slowly to keep catheter patent.
(5) Place insertion spike of new tubing into old fluid container opening. Hang container on IV pole, compress and release drip chamber on new tubing, and fill drip chamber one-third to one-half full.	Permits drip chamber to fill and promotes rapid, smooth flow of solution through tubing.

STEPS	RATIONALE
(6) Slowly open roller clamp, remove protective cap from adapter (if necessary), and prime new tubing with solution. Stop infusion and replace cap. Place end of adapter near patient's IV site.	Removes air from tubing and replaces it with fluid. Position equipment for quick, smooth connection of new tubing.
(7) Turn roller clamp on old tubing to "off" position.	Prevents leakage of fluid.
d. Prepare tubing with extension set or saline lock:	IV tubing is attached to extension set without disconnecting from the hub of the catheter.
(1) If a loop or short extension tubing is needed, use sterile technique to connect the new injection cap to the new loop or tubing.	Prepares extension set for connecting with IV.
(2) Swab injection cap with antiseptic swab. Insert syringe with saline solution and inject through the injection cap into the loop of the extension tubing.	Prevents introduction of microorganisms.
e. Re-establish infusion	
(1) Gently disconnect old tubing or old extension set from IV catheter. Quickly insert adapter of new tubing or new extension set/saline lock into hub of IV catheter (see illustration).	Allows smooth transition from old to new tubing, minimizing time system is open.

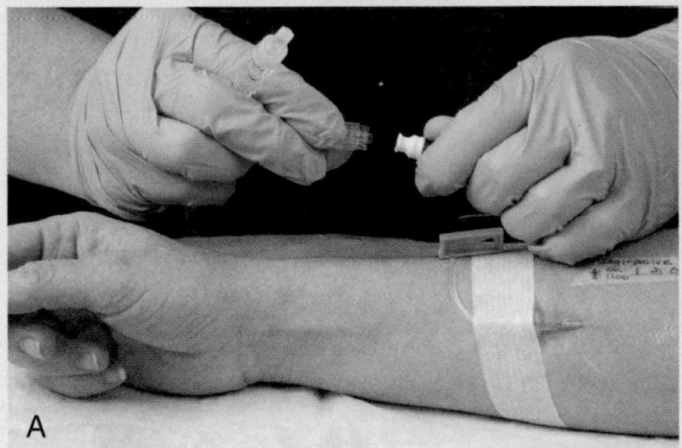
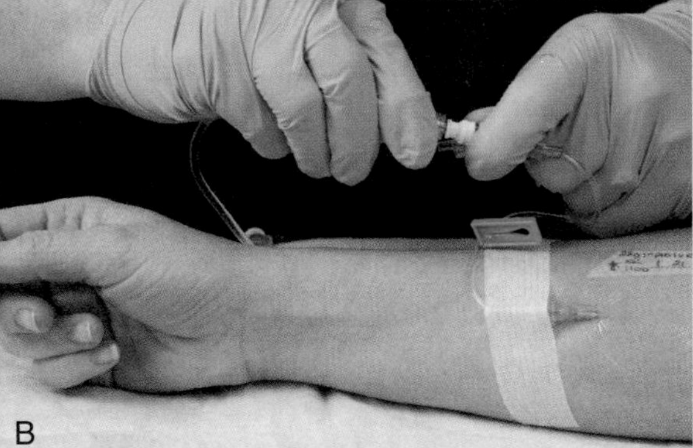

STEP 4e(1) A, Disconnect old intravenous tubing. **B,** Luer-Lok adaptor of new intravenous tubing.

STEPS	RATIONALE
(2) For continuous infusion, open roller clamp on new tubing, allowing solution to run rapidly for 30 to 60 seconds, and then regulate IV drip to ordered rate.	Ensures catheter patency and prevents occlusion.
(3) See agency policy. When re-establishing extension set, you will irrigate tubing and catheter with sterile saline flush.	
f. Attach a piece of tape or a preprinted label with date and time of tubing change onto tubing below the drip chamber.	Provides reference to determine next time for tubing change.
g. Form a loop of tubing and secure it to patient's arm with a strip of tape.	
h. If it was necessary to remove old dressing in order to access tubing, apply new dressing (see Step 3).	Avoids accidental pulling against site and catheter movement.
5. ***Changing IV solution***	
a. Prepare next solution at least 1 hour before needed. Ensure that the solution is correct and properly labeled. Follow six rights of drug administration. Verify solution expiration date. Observe for precipitate and discoloration.	Ensures no disruption in fluid therapy to patient.

Continued

STEPS	RATIONALE
b. Change solution when fluid remains only in neck of container or when new type of solution has been ordered.	Prevents waste of solution.
c. Move roller clamp to stop flow rate and remove old IV fluid container from IV pole.	
d. Quickly remove spike from old container and, without touching tip, insert spike into new container.	Maintains sterility of solution and reduces risk of solution in drip chamber running dry. If spike is contaminated, a new IV tubing set is required.
e. Hang new bag or bottle of solution on IV pole.	
f. Check for air in infusion tubing. If bubbles form, they can be removed by closing the roller clamp, stretching the tubing downward, and tapping the tubing with the finger (the bubbles rise in the tubing to the drip chamber).	Infusion of air in tubing can result in air embolus, which can be fatal to patient.
g. Make sure that drip chamber is one-third to one-half full. If drip chamber is too full, pinch off tubing below it, invert the container, squeeze the drip chamber, hang the container, and release the tubing (see illustration).	If chamber is completely filled, nurse cannot observe drip rate.
h. Regulate flow to prescribed rate or set up EID per manufacturer's instructions.	
i. Place time label on side of container and label with time hung, time of completion, and appropriate interval. If using plastic bags, mark only on the label and not the container.	
6. ***Discontinuing IV solutions or medications***	
a. Move roller clamp on infusion tubing to the "off" position.	Prevents spillage of fluid.
b. Remove any clasping devices and disconnect medication delivery tubing from injection port or end cap of main IV.	If the tubing spike, connector end, fluid pathway, or solution container is contaminated, a new tubing set or solution container is required.

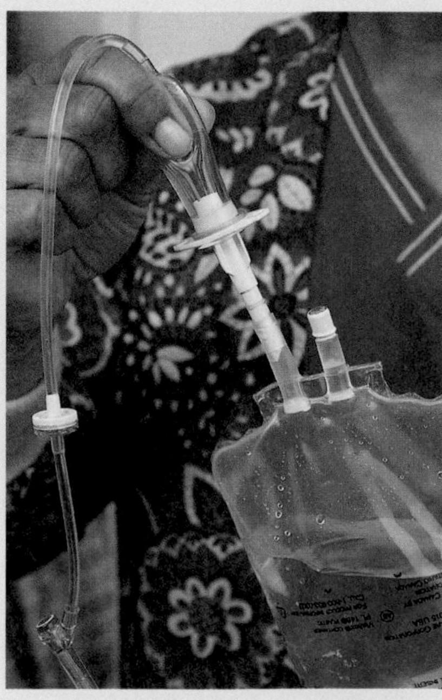

STEP 5g Remove excess fluid from the drip chamber.

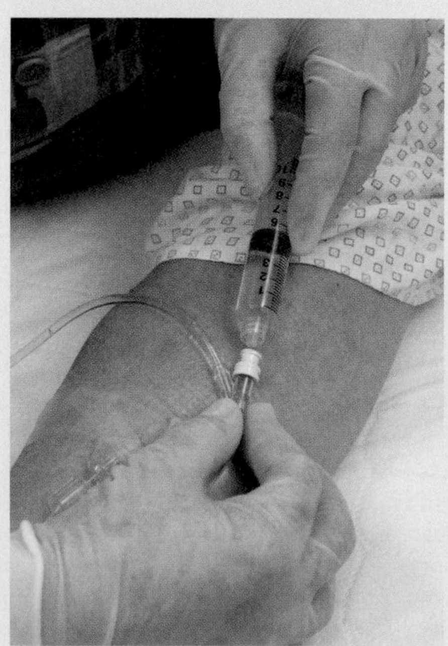

STEP 6e Flush injection port slowly.

STEPS	RATIONALE
c. Cover end of IV medication tubing with a sterile cap or cover as required.	Infusion tubing can be reused with next ordered medication.
d. Swab injection port or end cap on main IV tubing with antiseptic swab.	Ensures sterility of injection port or end cap.
e. For intermittent medication piggybacked into a continuous infusion, attach 5-mL saline-filled syringe to injection port and flush the line gently (see illustration). Regulate fluid flow of the continuous infusion as ordered.	Saline flush prevents incompatible medications from coming into contact in the infusion tubing. There is no way to know how much pressure is exerted inside catheter lumen. A 5-mL or 10-mL syringe generates less pressure than a 3-mL syringe. Do not force irrigation if resistance is felt.
f. For intermittent medications through an end cap or extension set, attach saline-filled 5-mL needleless syringe to injection port and flush catheter gently or attach heparin flush solution-filled needleless syringe to injection port and flush gently if necessary per agency policy. Do not force flushing of solution.	Flushing with saline instills any remaining medication in tubing. Volume of flush depends on lumen size, catheter length, and medication infused (Hadaway, 2006a). Size of syringe used for flushing should be in accordance with manufacturer's guidelines. The smaller the syringe, the higher the pressure exerted (INS, 2006). If resistance is met, assess for mechanical causes such as closed clamps or kinked tubing. Forcing the flush may cause catheter to fracture within the vein.
7. See Completion Protocol (inside front cover).	

EVALUATION

1. Observe functioning, intactness, and patency of IV system and flow rate after changing dressing and tubing and after administering IV medications.
2. Inspect condition of IV site for signs and symptoms of IV-related complications. Palpate for skin temperature, edema, and tenderness.
3. Monitor patient's body temperature.
4. Observe patient for signs of fluid volume excess or deficit to determine response to new IV solution.
5. Monitor laboratory values and I&O.

Unexpected Outcomes and Related Interventions

Changing Peripheral IV Dressing

1. IV catheter is infiltrated; phlebitis is present; or site is red, edematous, painful, and/or has presence of exudate.
   a. Stop the infusion and discontinue IV (see Procedural Guideline 28.1).
   b. Notify health care provider to evaluate patient for source of infection; antibiotic therapy may be prescribed.
   c. Culture of cannula may be ordered; confirm before removal of IV device.
   d. Restart new IV infusion in other extremity if continued therapy is required. Follow agency policy for complication management.

Changing Infusion Tubing

1. Decreased or absent flow of IV fluid indicated by a slowed or obstructed flow.
   a. Open roller clamp, slide clamps, and recalibrate drip rate. Check for kinks in tubing.
   b. Evaluate any pain or discomfort at the site for infiltration or temporary venous spasm.

Changing Fluid Container

1. Flow rate is incorrect; patient receives too little or too much fluid.
   a. Regulate to the correct rate.
   b. Determine and correct the cause of the incorrect flow rate (e.g., change in patient position, change in catheter position, kinked tubing).
   c. Use EID when accurate flow rate is critical.
   d. Notify health care provider if patient's anticipated infusion is less than or greater than 100 to 200 mL as expected (follow agency policy).

Discontinuing IV Medications

1. Solution in tubing below piggyback site turns cloudy because of precipitate formation, indicating medication incompatibility.
   a. Stop all infusions.
   b. Change tubing on continuous infusion.
   c. Assess need to restart IV infusion because precipitate may have formed within catheter lumen.

Recording and Reporting

- Record time peripheral-short dressing was changed, reason for dressing change, type of dressing material used, patency of system, and observation of venipuncture site.
- Record tubing change, infusion solution type, volume, and rate of infusion on patient's record. A special IV flow sheet may be used for IV solutions or medications.
- Record time of discontinuing medication; tubing/catheter flush with type, volume, and concentration of flush solution; and the IV site condition.

- Report to charge nurse or oncoming nurse dressing change, any significant information about the IV site or system, and time the medication or IV was discontinued.

Sample Documentation

0700 IV dressing became wet during shower; new transparent dressing applied; insertion site without signs or symptoms of phlebitis or infiltration. D_5NS infusing at 125 mL/hr via gravity. Patient states, "It does not hurt at all."

1125 Rocephin infusion complete; line flushed with 5 mL NS. D_5W continues infusing at 125 mL/hr via gravity. IV site without signs and symptoms of complications observed. Patient states, "When will this be over?"

Special Considerations

Pediatric

- Use commercially available IV site protectors to cover and protect the IV site in young active children. Ensure that ID band is visible and nonrestricting.

Geriatric

- Infiltration in older adults may go unnoticed because of the decreased elasticity of the skin and loose skin folds. Because of decreased tactile sensation, a large amount of fluid may infiltrate before patient experiences pain (Alexander and others, 2010).
- In older adults, because of decreased skin elasticity, skin turgor may not be a good indicator of fluid balance; the best assessment sites are the forehead and sternum.
- Phlebitis may develop without pain but with significant inflammation resulting from the decreased sensitivity of the nerve endings of the skin.

Home Care

- Have family caregiver demonstrate hand hygiene and aseptic technique for changing IV site dressing. If the catheter comes out, instruct caregiver to apply gauze pressure dressing and notify home care agency nurse.
- Teach patient to keep site dry during bath (preferred) or shower by wrapping in plastic bag and taping occlusively. Ensure EID or ambulatory infusion pump safety during hygiene activity.
- Discuss the signs and symptoms of possible IV-related complications such as infiltration or phlebitis swelling, pain, redness, or moisture at dressing site.

PROCEDURAL GUIDELINE 28.1
Discontinuing Peripheral-Short Intravenous Access

You discontinue a peripheral-short IV line when the prescribed length of therapy is completed or a complication occurs (e.g., phlebitis, infiltration, or catheter occlusion). The technique for discontinuing a peripheral IV line follows infection control guidelines.

Delegation and Collaboration

The skill of discontinuing a peripheral-short IV line cannot be delegated to nursing assistive personnel (NAP). Instruct the NAP about the following:

- Reporting to the nurse any bleeding at the site after the catheter has been removed

Equipment

- Clean gloves
- Sterile 2 × 2–inch or 4 × 4–inch gauze sponge
- Antiseptic swab
- Tape

Procedural Steps

1. **See Standard Protocol (inside front cover).**
2. Observe existing site for signs and symptoms of infection, infiltration, or phlebitis.
3. Review health care provider's order for discontinuation of IV therapy.
4. Identify the patient using two identifiers (e.g., name and birthday or name and account number, according to facility policy).
5. Explain procedure to patient, describing sensation (burning) the patient will feel and the need to hold affected extremity still.
6. Turn IV tubing roller clamp to "off" position or turn EID off and turn roller clamp to "off" position.
7. Remove IV site dressing or stabilizing IV device. Remove tape securing catheter.
8. With dry gauze held above site, apply light pressure and withdraw the catheter, using a slow, steady movement, keeping the hub parallel to the skin (see illustration).

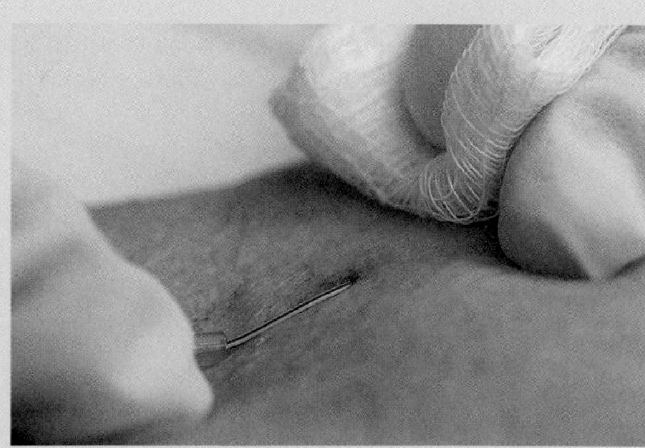

STEP 8 IV catheter is removed slowly, keeping catheter parallel to vein.

PROCEDURAL GUIDELINE 28.1
Discontinuing Peripheral-Short Intravenous Access—cont'd

9. Apply pressure to the site for 2 to 3 minutes until the bleeding stops, using a dry, sterile gauze pad. Secure with tape. NOTE: Apply pressure for 5 to 10 minutes if patient is on anticoagulants.
10. Inspect catheter for intactness, noting tip integrity and length.
11. Apply clean folded gauze dressing over insertion site and secure with tape.
12. Instruct patient to report any redness, pain, drainage, or swelling that may occur after catheter removal.
13. **See Completion Protocol (inside front cover).**

SKILL 28.4 ADMINISTRATION OF PARENTERAL NUTRITION

Video Clips

Parenteral nutrition (PN) is a specialized form of nutritional supplement in which nutrients are given intravenously (IV). PN is composed of a base IV solution with the addition of various electrolytes, minerals, and trace elements, along with amino acids and a fat emulsion as a means to provide complete or partial nutritional supplementation (Alexander and others, 2010). The base solution of PN is a dextrose solution ranging from 5% to as high as 70% dextrose with the addition of amino acids and fat emulsion. In some situations the fat emulsion is added directly to the solution rather than being administered separately. When the fat emulsion is added to the PN solution, it is referred to as a 3:1 solution. If the patient has fluid restrictions such as with heart failure (HF), this method allows for the appropriate nutritional support without the addition of fluid. Because of the high osmolarity of total PN (TPN) (more than 600 mOsm/L), this solution would be administered through a CVAD and not peripherally because of the increased risk of complications such as phlebitis (INS, 2006). With the lower dextrose and amino acid concentration of partial PN (PPN) (less than 600 mOsm/L), the solution is given through a peripheral IV device but may also be administered via CVAD.

PN regimens are individually designed for patients with the formulas prescribed by the physician and are reviewed daily, with special consideration given to each patient's fluid, electrolyte, and nitrogen balance. Nurses collaborate with the health care providers, which include the nutritional support team, in administering PN and monitoring the patient's nutritional status, blood glucose levels, and signs or symptoms of catheter-related complications. Indications for short-term PN is seen in patients requiring preoperative bowel rest and in patients whose gastrointestinal (GI) tracts are unusable for more than 4 to 5 days. Long-term indications include but are not limited to a nonfunctional GI tract seen with massive bowel resection/GI surgery/massive GI bleed or trauma to abdomen, head, or neck. The skill of infusing PN requires you to know the composition and indications thoroughly and follow the policy and procedure of your agency or institution.

ASSESSMENT

1. Assess indications of and risks for protein/calorie malnutrition: weight loss from baseline or ideal body weight, muscle atrophy/weakness, failure to wean from a ventilator, edema, lethargy, chronic illness, and nothing by mouth (NPO) for more than 6 days. Confer with nutritional support team. *Rationale: Indications for use of PN (ASPEN, 2002).*
2. Inspect venous access device to ensure that correct device is in place based on final formula concentration (peripheral versus central access). *Rationale: Final concentration of formula with osmolarity greater than 600 mOsm/L requires CVAD to prevent complications such as phlebitis (INS, 2006).*
3. Assess status of vascular access device for presence of tenderness, inflammation, edema, and drainage or inability to flush or aspirate blood return. *Rationale: Identifies early signs of catheter-related complications, which contraindicate infusion of PN and may indicate need to establish a new IV site.*
4. Consult with physician and nutritional support team on calculation of calorie, protein, and fluid requirements for patient. *Rationale: Provides multidisciplinary plan for patient's nutritional support and goals for therapy.*
5. Assess baseline vital signs, auscultate lung sounds, and measure weight. *Rationale: Provides baseline for monitoring patient's response to infusion of PN.*
6. Assess levels of serum albumin, total protein, transferrin, prealbumin, and blood glucose. *Rationale: Provides baseline for measuring patient's nutritional status and tolerance to PN.*
7. Verify physician's order for nutrients, vitamins, minerals, trace elements, electrolytes, and added medication and flow rate. Check for compatibility of added medications. *Rationale: Physician must order PN daily, usually after reviewing laboratory values. Ensures safe and accurate PN administration.*

PLANNING

Expected Outcomes focus on adequacy of nutrition, adequacy of fluid volume, and prevention of complications related to PN therapy.

1. Patient's ideal weight gain is usually between 1 and 3 pounds (0.5 to 1.5 kg) per week.
2. Serum glucose levels are less than 150 mg/dL or maintained between 80 and 110 mg/dL. Check physician's order for desired glucose level.

3. Venous access device is patent and free of signs or symptoms of IV-related complications.

Delegation and Collaboration

Administration of PN cannot be delegated to nursing assistive personnel (NAP). Instruct the NAP about the following:

- Immediately reporting to the nurse when the infusion pump is alarming
- Reporting to the nurse patient's complaints of shortness of breath, headache, weakness, feeling shaky
- Monitoring patient's urinary output and reporting to the nurse
- Reporting complaints of pain, bleeding, or swelling at IV site back to the nurse
- Performing blood glucose monitoring and reporting the results

Equipment

- PN solution (IV)
- EID
- Luer-Lok IV tubing with appropriate filter (0.22 μm for dextrose/amino acids; 1.2 μm for 3 : 1 solution)
- 5- to 10-mL syringe with sterile saline flush
- Bedside blood glucose monitoring kit
- Adhesive tape
- Alcohol swabs
- Clean gloves

IMPLEMENTATION *for* ADMINISTRATION OF PARENTERAL NUTRITION

STEPS	RATIONALE
1. See Standard Protocol (inside front cover).	
2. Prepare solution at least 1 hour before needed by removing from refrigerator. Review transcriber's order. Ensure that solution is correct and properly labeled. Follow six rights of drug administration. Verify solution expiration date.	Ensures no disruption in fluid therapy to patient. *This is the first check for accuracy.*
3. Compare label of PN with medication administration record (MAR) or computer printout; check for correct additives.	Ensures that patient receives correct PN and prevents medication errors. *This is the second check for accuracy.*
4. Inspect PN solution for particulate matter (if fat emulsion is contained in solution 3 : 1). Inspect emulsion for a cream layer or separation of fat into a layer.	Presence of particulate matter or fat emulsion separation requires that solution be discarded.
5. Identify the patient using two identifiers (e.g., name and birthday or name and account number, according to facility policy). Compare identifiers with information on the patient's MAR or medical record.	Ensures correct patient. Complies with The Joint Commission standards and improves patient safety (TJC, 2010). *This is the third check for accuracy.*
6. Obtain appropriate IV tubing with filter (0.22 μm for dextrose/amino acids; 1.2 μm for 3 : 1 solutions).	Filters allow for various particles to be removed before infusion, which prevents catheter-related complications such as infection.
7. Attach appropriate IV filter to IV tubing. Prime tubing with PN solution, making sure that no air bubbles remain; turn off the flow with the roller clamp (see Skill 28.1).	Maintains sterility of solution. Air introduced into central circulation can result in air embolus, a fatal IV complication.
8. Wipe end port of IV device with alcohol, allow to air dry, and attach syringe of 0.9% saline solution to CVAD; aspirate for blood return, then flush with saline per agency policy.	Determines patency of IV device before infusing PN.
9. Remove syringe. Connect Luer-Lok end of parenteral nutrition IV tubing to end cap of the IV device; for multilumen lines, label lumen used for PN.	Ensures that tubing is securely connected to IV line. Dedicated line should be used for multilumen devices.
10. Place IV tubing into EID. Open roller clamp and regulate flow rate on pump as ordered (see illustration). Flow rate can be continuous or cycled.	Flow rates are ordered to meet patient's metabolic and electrolyte needs. Maintaining rates prevents electrolyte imbalances.
a. *Continuous infusion (optional):* Flow rate is immediately set at ordered rate and given over a 24-hour period.	Ensures that blood glucose levels are maintained to prevent hypoglycemia/hyperglycemia (Alexander and others, 2010; ASPEN, 2002).

STEPS	RATIONALE
b. *Cycle infusion (optional):* Flow rate is initiated at about 40 to 60 mL/hr, and the rate is gradually increased until patient's nutritional needs are met. Before the completion of the infusion, the rate is decreased at about the same amount of milliliters per hour until PN has completed. This infusion is generally given over a shorter time frame (12 to 18 hours).	Infusion rates are gradually increased and decreased to prevent hypoglycemia/hyperglycemia (Alexander and others, 2010; ASPEN, 2002).
11. Infuse all IV medications or blood through an alternative IV site or line (multilumen devices). Do not obtain blood samples through same lumen or port used for PN.	Prevents drug incompatibility and IV device occlusion.
12. Do not interrupt a PN infusion (e.g., during showers, transport, blood transfusion). Change IV administration set for standard PN solution every 72 hours, for 3:1 solution every 24 hours. PN bags should be discarded in 24 hours even if there is solution left in the bag.	Prevents development of catheter-related bacteremia (INS, 2006).
13. See Completion Protocol (inside front cover).	

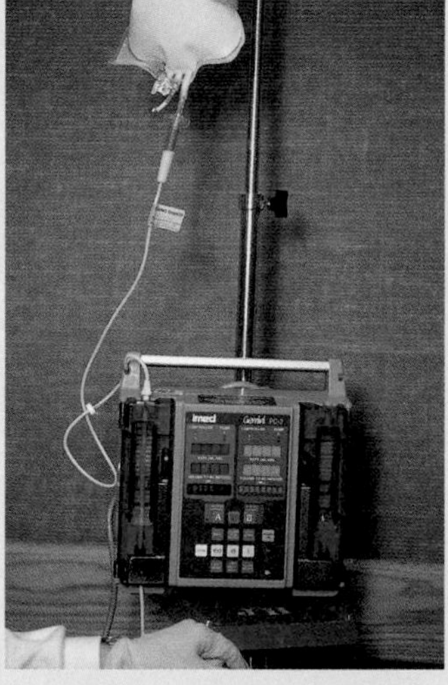

STEP 10 Place parenteral nutrition intravenous tubing into EID.

EVALUATION

1. Monitor flow rate according to agency policy and procedure. If infusion is not running on time (behind or ahead of prescribed order), do not attempt to catch up because this could cause hypoglycemic/hyperglycemic reaction and fluid overload.
2. Inspect IV site routinely for swelling, inflammation, drainage, warmth, tenderness, or edema.
3. Measure glucose levels every 6 hours or as ordered, and check other laboratory values as ordered by physician or nutrition support team.
4. Measure weights daily or as ordered.
5. Monitor I&O and assess for signs of fluid retention: palpate skin of extremities and auscultate lung sounds, which could indicate fluid retention.
6. Monitor for signs of systemic infection such as fever, elevated white blood cell count (WBC), or malaise.

Unexpected Outcomes and Related Interventions

1. Patient develops signs and symptoms of hypoglycemia/hyperglycemia or has blood glucose level lower or greater than target set by health care provider.
   a. Gradually adjust concentration of glucose in PN solution per orders.
   b. Insulin may be ordered to maintain proper blood glucose levels.
2. Infusion stops flowing or flows at rate slower than ordered
   a. Check patency of IV device and attempt to flush.
   b. Infusion of thrombolytic agent may be necessary (see agency policy).
   c. If line remains occluded, prepare for removal.

3. Patient experiences weight gain greater than 1 pound (½ kg) per day, taut skin turgor is present, and crackles are auscultated over lung fields.
   a. Notify health care provider and obtain orders to reduce infusion rate.
   b. Anticipate need to administer diuretics.
4. Development of fever, chills, malaise, and elevated WBC, indicating systemic infection.
   a. Notify health care provider and discuss possibility of obtaining cultures from insertion site and peripheral blood cultures.
   b. Systemic antibiotic therapy may be initiated, and/or IV device removed.
5. Solution is unavailable or unable to be infused because of particulate matter, leakage of bag, or separation of fat emulsion.
   a. Obtain and infuse 10% dextrose in water solution at same flow rate that PN was infusing to prevent sudden drop in blood glucose level.
   b. Evaluate for signs and symptoms of hypoglycemia (e.g., weakness, confusion) and report to health care provider.
   c. Monitor blood glucose levels and report to health care provider.

Recording and Reporting

- Report to health care provider deviation from baseline assessment or laboratory parameters and signs or symptoms of dehydration or fluid overload.
- Document assessment of physical condition, bedside blood glucose values, condition of IV site, and IV solution infusing on applicable flow sheet.
- Document I&O and weights on graphic sheets per agency policy and procedure.
- Report any signs or symptoms of local or systemic IV-related complications.

Sample Documentation

0800 TPN solution initiated through proximal lumen of nontunneled triple lumen subclavian IV device. Daily infusion to continue with 2000 mL/day as ordered of 3:1 solution. Rate at 150 mL/hr via Smart pump. Laboratory results reported to Dr. Laurie with no new changes to formula. Complete chemistry panel to be obtained in AM. Current weight maintained at 58 kg for last week. IV site without signs or symptoms of related complications observed. Patient states, "I don't feel as tired as I did last week."

Special Considerations

Pediatric

- Consider children's developmental needs when they are on long-term PN.
- Perform regular assessments of development to determine child's progress (Hockenberry and Wilson, 2007).

Geriatric

- Some older adults have impaired ability to manage higher fluid volumes or are at risk for an increased incidence of hypoglycemia.

Home Care

- Patients requiring long-term PN benefit from referral to a home nutrition therapy team.
- Patient and family members need to learn to perform catheter site care, dressing changes, and techniques for adding and removing PN solutions.
- Some patients receive PN at night during sleep (cycle therapy) to allow freedom to leave home or work during the day.
- Teach patient and primary caregiver to monitor patient's weights, calorie count, I&O, and serum glucose levels.

SKILL 28.5 TRANSFUSION OF BLOOD PRODUCTS

The transfusion of blood and blood components is a major factor in restoring and maintaining quality of life for the patient with hematological disorders, cancer, injury, or surgical intervention. Caring for the patient receiving blood or blood components is a nursing responsibility. However, the nurse should never view the transfusion of blood products as routine; overlooking a minor detail is dangerous and life threatening to a patient (Alexander and others, 2010; Knippen, 2006; Scarlet, 2006).

Transfusion of blood and blood products is closely regulated and monitored. Standards of operations for all blood bank centers are set by the American Association of Blood Banks (AABB, 2005), OSHA, the U.S. Food and Drug Administration (FDA), and the American Red Cross. These standards include the collection of donor blood, distribution of the product, and standards for transfusion. Always verify specific agency policy regarding specific procedural requirements before any transfusion.

Blood and blood component therapies treat and restore hemodynamic homeostasis or provide treatment for diseases related to coagulation deficiencies. A written health care provider's order to transfuse should always include which component to transfuse and the duration of the transfusion. A single unit of whole blood or blood components should be infused within a 4-hour period (INS, 2006). If more than one blood product is to be given, the sequence or order of transfusion should be specified. Any additional medications such as an antihistamine (given when the history shows previous allergic response), antipyretics (given when the history shows previous febrile nonhemolytic response), diuretics (given when the history shows potential for HF), or other special treatment of the components should also be included in the written order for the transfusion.

Three blood typing systems, ABO, Rh, and most recently HLA typing (such as single donor), are used to ensure that transfusion products match the recipient's blood as closely as

TABLE 28-5 ABO SYSTEM

PATIENT'S BLOOD TYPE	RED BLOOD CELLS ANTIGEN	TRANSFUSION WITH TYPE A	TRANSFUSION WITH TYPE B	TRANSFUSION WITH TYPE AB	TRANSFUSION WITH TYPE O	TRANSFUSION OPTIONS
A(+)	A	Yes	No	No	Yes	A+, A– O+, O–
A(–)	A	Yes	No	No	Yes	A–, O–
B(+)	B	No	Yes	No	Yes	B+, B– O+, O–
B(–)	B	No	Yes	No	Yes	B–, O–
AB(+)	AB	Yes	Yes	Yes	Yes	A+, A– B+, B– O+, O– Universal recipient
AB(–)	AB	Yes	Yes	Yes	Yes	A–, B–, O–
O(+)	None	No	No	No	Yes	O+, O–
O(–)	None	No	No	No	Yes	O–, universal donor

possible (Table 28-5). Before transfusion in nonemergent situations, the patient's blood type and Rh factor must always be verified to be compatible with the donor transfusion.

There is increasing public awareness of the possible transmission of infectious diseases through transfusion of blood products. Because of improved testing of donor blood, the risk of the blood recipient developing an infectious disease is lower than ever before. However, viral, bacterial, and parasitic diseases can still be transmitted through blood. Screening of blood donors is one of the most important steps to identify persons with a medical history, behavior, or events that put them at risk of transmissible disease (Katz, 2009). Nurses must be prepared to inform patients thoroughly about the options, benefits, and risks of transfusion and reassure them that every effort is taken to ensure a safe blood supply and transfusion. Patients should know that there is never a completely risk-free transfusion.

One avenue for preventing the transmission of infectious diseases during blood transfusion is the use of autologous blood (e.g., the patient's own blood). This can be done in several ways; however, the most frequent method is preoperative collection from the patient. AABB standards establish the process for determining patient eligibility, collecting, testing, and labeling the blood product unit. Before transfusion, ABO and Rh typing of the patient are performed. Autologous units must be used before units from the general blood supply. Identification and verifying processes and methods of administration for autologous units are the same as those used for other units of blood (Murphy and others, 2007). This method is still not without risk because human error still exists in collection and storing of the blood.

The skill of transfusing blood or blood products requires you to know agency policy and procedure thoroughly and to follow it completely. To ensure the safe administration of the product, closely monitor your patient before, during, and after the transfusion.

ASSESSMENT

1. Verify health care provider's order for specific blood or blood product with appropriate date, time to begin transfusion, duration, and any pretransfusion or posttransfusion medications to be given. *Rationale: Correct identification of ordered blood product is the first step to ensure safe administration.*
2. Obtain patient's transfusion history, including known allergies and previous transfusion reaction. Verify that type and crossmatch have been completed within 72 hours of transfusion and that patient consent for transfusion is provided. *Rationale: Identifies patient's prior response to blood/blood product transfusion. If patient has experienced a reaction in the past, anticipate a similar reaction and be prepared to rapidly intervene. Most agencies require patients to sign a consent form before receiving blood component therapy due to inherent risks.*
3. Verify that IV catheter is patent and site is without signs or symptoms of IV-related complications such as infiltration or phlebitis. In emergency situations that require rapid transfusions, a 16- or 18-gauge cannula is preferred. However, transfusions for therapeutic indications may be infused with cannulas ranging from 20 to 24 gauge. *Rationale: Catheters used for blood transfusion must be patent and large enough to accommodate the appropriate flow rate but not large enough to damage the vein. The major concern is completing the transfusion within the recommended 4-hour time frame. If a smaller-gauge catheter is used, consider requesting split blood units to ensure timely administration.*
4. Know the indications or reasons for a transfusion (e.g., low hematocrit secondary to postoperative bleeding). *Rationale: Allows nurse to anticipate patient's response to therapy.*
5. Obtain and record pretransfusion baseline vital signs (blood pressure, pulse, respiration, temperature). If patient

is febrile (temperature greater than 100° F [37.8° C]), notify physician or licensed independent practitioner before initiating transfusion (follow agency policy). *Rationale: This provides comparison to detect change in patient's condition during transfusion.*

6. Assess patient's level of comfort and understanding of the procedure and rationale. *Rationale: Clarifying patient's need for and associated benefits of therapy may alleviate some of the anxiety patient may have.*

PLANNING

Expected Outcomes focus on safe, complication-free transfusion therapy, including restoration of normal hemodynamics and improvement in clinical condition.

1. Patient's systolic blood pressure improves, urine output is 0.5 to 1 mL/kg/hr, and cardiac output returns to baseline.
2. Patient's laboratory values reflect improvement in targeted areas (hematocrit and hemoglobin values; factor levels within therapeutic range for patient; improved coagulation function).
3. Mucous membranes are pink, and patient has brisk capillary refill.
4. Patient verbalizes understanding of rational for therapy.

Delegation Considerations

Skills of initiating blood therapy cannot be delegated to nursing assistive personnel (NAP). Instruct the NAP about the following:

- Reporting complaints of shortness of breath, hives, and/or chills back to the nurse
- Reporting when volume of blood is low in the blood bag
- Reporting signs or symptoms of IV site complications such as swelling, pain, or redness

Equipment

- Blood administration set with standard filter. (NOTE: Depending on blood product, special tubing and filters may be necessary.)
- Prescribed blood product
- IV 250-mL bag 0.9% NaCl (NS) IV solution
- Clean gloves
- Tape
- Antiseptic wipes/swabs
- Vital sign equipment: thermometer, blood pressure cuff, stethoscope, and pulse oximeter
- Signed transfusion consent

Optional equipment

- Infusion pump (Verify that infusion pump can be used to deliver blood or blood products.)
- Use prescribed leukocyte-depleting filter. (Institution may irradiate blood products within its blood bank facility.)
- Blood warmer (used mainly when large volume or rapid transfusion is needed) (Ackley and others, 2008).
- Pressure bag (used for rapid infusion in acute blood loss)

IMPLEMENTATION *for* TRANSFUSION OF BLOOD PRODUCTS

STEPS	RATIONALE
1. **See Standard Protocol (inside front cover).**	
2. Obtain blood bag from laboratory following agency protocol. Blood transfusions must be initiated within 30 minutes after release from laboratory, blood bank, or controlled environment (INS, 2006) (see illustration).	Agencies differ as to personnel who can release a blood bag from a blood bank, but they always require two witnesses and some form of patient identification. Usually only one unit is released at a time.

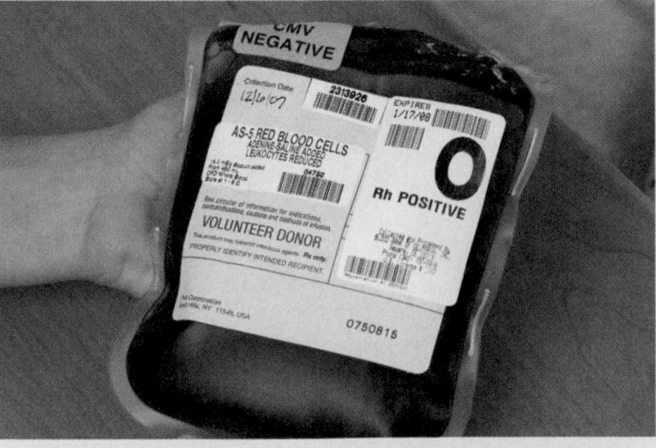

STEP 2 Blood bag with label.

STEPS	RATIONALE
3. Check appearance of blood product for leaks, bubbles, clots, or purplish color.	Determines integrity of bag. Air bubbles, clots or discoloration indicate bacterial contamination or inadequate anticoagulation of components and are contraindications for transfusion.
4. Verify that component received from blood bank matches blood or blood product ordered by physician or health care provider.	Ensures that patient receives correct blood or blood product (Davis and others, 2006; Dzik, 2007).
a. Identify patient using two identifiers (e.g., name and birthday or name and account number, according to facility policy). Compare identifiers with information on patient's medication administration record (MAR) or medical record. When a discrepancy is noted during verification process, do not administer blood or blood product. Notify blood bank and appropriate personnel per agency policy.	Ensures that correct patient receives transfusion. Complies with The Joint Commission standards and improves patient safety (TJC, 2010).
b. Correctly verify blood product and identify patient with a person considered qualified by your agency (e.g., RN, licensed practical nurse [LPN]; follow agency policy) (see illustrations).	Strict adherence to verification procedures before administration of blood or blood components reduces the risk of administering the wrong blood to patient. Most hemolytic transfusion reactions are caused by clerical errors (Gray and others, 2007; Katz, 2009).

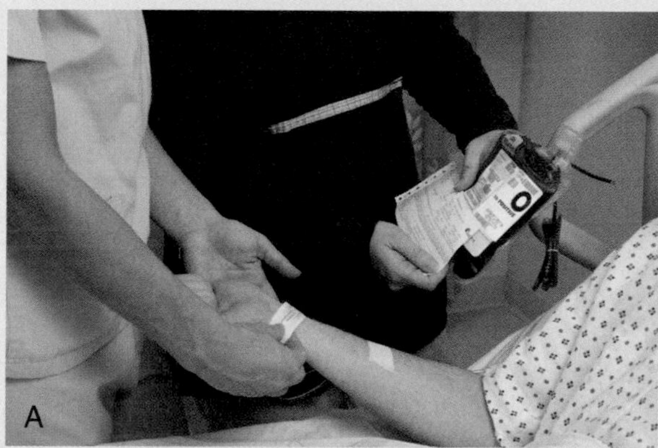

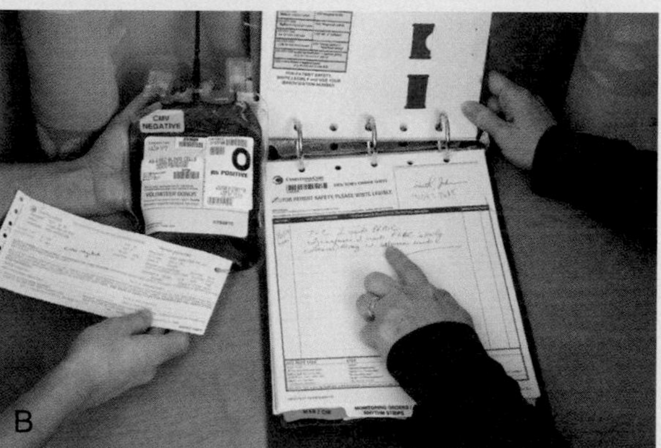

STEP 4b A, Checking patient identification, comparing information with arm band. **B,** Two clinicians verifying identification of patient and blood product.

STEPS	RATIONALE
c. Check that patient's blood type and Rh type are compatible with donor blood type and Rh type.	Verifies accurate donor blood and Rh type.
d. Check that unit number on unit of blood and form from blood bank match.	Further verification prevents accidental administration of wrong blood component.
e. Check expiration date and time on unit of blood.	Expired blood should never be used because the cell components deteriorate and may contain excess citrate ions.
f. Record verification process as directed by agency policy.	Documents process on legal medical record.
5. Have patient void or empty urinary drainage collection container.	If transfusion reaction occurs, urine specimen obtained must be recent and preferably taken after transfusion is initiated to assess for presence of red blood cells from a hemolytic reaction.
6. Review with patient the purpose of the transfusion. Ask patient to report immediately any signs and symptoms (during or after transfusion), including chills, low back pain, shortness of breath, nausea, excessive perspiration, rash, itching, or even a vague sense of uneasiness (Scarlet, 2006).	Once transfusion reaction occurs, staff must respond immediately with treatment.

Continued

STEPS	RATIONALE
7. Perform hand hygiene. Reinspect blood product for signs of leakage or unusual appearance. Gently invert bag 2 to 3 times.	Verifies quality of blood product. If signs of contamination are present, return blood product to laboratory. Inversion equally distributes cells throughout preservative solution.
8. Open blood administration set and spike bag of 0.9% NS with one of Y-tubing spikes. Hang bag on pole and prime tubing, completely filling filter with saline. Maintain sterility of system and close lower clamp. Maintain clamp on blood product side of Y-tubing in the "off" position.	Eliminates air in tubing. If filter is not completely primed with NS, transfusion will slow because of collection of debris in partially primed filter. NS wets the filter and dilutes RBCs to reduce their viscosity if necessary.
9. Remove protective covering from access port on blood bag. Spike blood component bag with other Y-tubing located next to NS 0.9% tubing (see illustration). Close NS clamp above filter and open clamp above filter to blood product; prime Y-tubing with blood. Blood will flow into drip chamber.	Prevents blood product from entering NS bag.

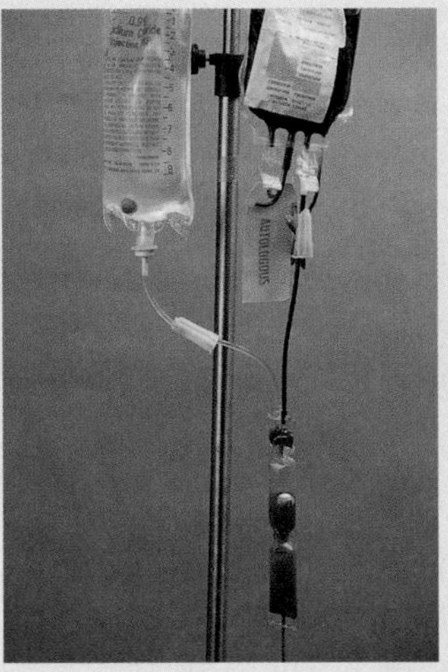

STEP 9 Unit of blood connected to Y-tubing setup.

STEPS	RATIONALE
10. Turn off any existing IV infusion and flush line with NS solution. Disconnect and cap tubing. Quickly connect NS-primed blood administration tubing directly to patient's IV site or insert IV tubing to newly placed IV catheter.	Ensures aseptic technique. Once blood or blood product begins to infuse, no other IV medications will be administered through the same IV line or device. The only IV fluids appropriate would be 0.9% NS.
11. Open lower clamp and regulate blood infusion to allow only 2 mL/min to infuse in the initial 15 minutes. Remain with patient for the first 5 to 15 minutes of the transfusion. Remove and discard gloves. Perform hand hygiene.	Most transfusion reactions occur within the first 5 to 15 minutes. Infusing a small amount of blood component initially minimizes the amount of incompatible blood to which patient is exposed, thereby minimizing the severity of a reaction.
12. Obtain vital signs (temperature, pulse, respiration, blood pressure) 5 minutes after initiation of transfusion and per agency policy after that.	Change from baseline vital signs may indicate transfusion reaction.
13. If there is no transfusion reaction, regulate rate according to physician's orders and infuse the remaining volume of blood as ordered. Packed red blood cells (PRBCs) are usually infused over 2 hours, and whole blood over 3 to 4 hours. Drop factor for blood tubing is 10 gtts/mL; check blood tubing package. For other blood products such as IV immunoglobulin (IVIG) or factor replacement, follow agency recommendations.	Careful regulation prevents adverse response. Patient's condition and health care provider's orders dictate rate of blood infusion. Blood must be transfused within 4 hours of initiation. Even if infusion is not completed, blood must be discontinued. This reduces the potential for exposure to bacterial infection from the blood. If patient is at risk for fluid overload, blood bank can split units.

STEPS	RATIONALE
14. After blood has infused, close roller clamp above filter to blood, open NS, and infuse until blood administration tubing is completely clear. Restart primary IV fluids as ordered only after assessing IV site for patency and signs and symptoms of IV-related complications. Discard blood bag according to agency policy.	NS infusion clears IV catheter of blood product. If transfusing more than one unit of blood or blood products, maintain 0.9% NS via blood administration set at prescribed rate until second unit is started. Because of risk of bacterial growth, blood administration sets and add-on filters should be changed after each unit or at the end of 4 hours, whichever comes first (INS, 2006).
15. See Completion Protocol (inside front cover).	

EVALUATION

1. Observe for any changes in vital signs and any sign of transfusion reaction such as chills, flushing, itching, hives, dyspnea, or tachycardia during transfusion.
2. Monitor I&O and laboratory values (hemoglobin, hematocrit, prothrombin time, partial thromboplastin time, and platelet count) after transfusion. (In the hematologically stable adult, one unit of PRBCs should increase the hemoglobin by 1 g/100 mL and the hematocrit by 3%. A unit of platelet concentrate prepared from a single unit of whole blood should increase the patient's platelet count by 5000 to 10,000/mL) (INS, 2006).
3. Monitor IV site for signs and symptoms of IV-related complications each time vital signs are taken.

Unexpected Outcomes and Related Interventions

1. Patient displays signs and symptoms of transfusion reaction.
   a. Stop the transfusion. Stay with patient and *notify* the physician or health care provider.
   b. A new NS infusion solution should be connected to the IV access site to prevent any subsequent blood from infusing from original blood tubing. Keep vein open with slow infusion at 10 to 12 gtts/min to ensure patency and maintain venous access for medication and/or to resume transfusion.
   c. Monitor vital signs.
   d. Send entire blood setup back to blood bank (per agency policy).
2. Rate of infusion slows in the absence of infiltration.
   a. Verify patency of IV catheter and that all clamps and stopcocks are open.
   b. Ensure that blood bag is elevated to proper height and filter is completely primed.
   c. Gently flush IV line with NS or use a pressure bag or EID that permits blood transfusion.
3. Patient experiences pain, swelling, or discoloration at IV site.
   a. Stop the transfusion and discontinue the IV infusion and catheter.
   b. Reinsert a new IV catheter in another site.
4. Fluid overload occurs, and/or patient exhibits difficulty breathing or has crackles on auscultation.
   a. Slow or stop the transfusion, elevate the head of the bed, and notify physician or health care provider.
   b. Administer prescribed diuretics, analgesics, and/or oxygen as prescribed.
   c. Continue frequent assessments and closely monitor vital signs and I&O.

Recording and Reporting

- Record pretransfusion medications, vital signs, and location and condition of the IV site.
- Record the type/volume of blood component, blood unit/donor/recipient identification, compatibility, and expiration date according to agency policy.
- Record volume of NS and blood component infused.
- Record vital signs obtained before, during, and after transfusion.
- Report signs and symptoms of a transfusion reaction immediately.

Sample Documentation

0900 Early AM CBC noted. Physician aware of Hct 22. Type and crossmatch drawn with two witnesses per phlebotomy.

1330 Voided 320 mL clear, amber urine. 20 g 1 inch Insyte inserted into L midcephalic × 1 attempt. Patient stated, "Only hurt a little." NS 0.9% initiated at 25 mL/hr. 1 unit PRBCs started at 40 mL/hr; vital signs: Temp 98.9°, Pulse 80, Resp 20 BP 140/78. Patient verbalized understanding of transfusion and to report any feeling of SOB, back pain, headache, or chills. Transfusion assessment and vital sign record initiated per policy.

Special Considerations

Pediatric

- Blood and blood products may be administered via 27-, 26-, or 24- gauge peripheral-short IV access in the neonate and via 24- or 22-gauge peripheral-short access in older children.
- Pediatric blood units are prepared in special units (Pedi-packs) and usually equal half the volume of a conventional adult unit.
- Initiate the transfusion slowly (5 mL/min for initial 15 minutes). Remain with child during this period of time and monitor vital signs and the infusion process (Hockenberry and Wilson, 2007).

Geriatric

- Older adults may have compromised cardiac, renal, and respiratory systems. Adjust flow rate if patient cannot tolerate prescribed flow rate. Flow rate should be 1 mL/kg/hr in patient at risk for circulatory overload.
- Vigilance in monitoring an access site during transfusion is vital in an older adult who may be less sensitive to the symptoms of infiltration and the generalized symptoms of a transfusion reaction.

Home Care

- Patients who have had prior transfusion reactions, acute angina, or CHF are not considered good candidates for home transfusion.
- Nursing personnel must be present for the entire transfusion process and for 30 to 60 minutes after transfusion.
- Whole blood must not be administered in the home.
- Blood and blood products must be transported in a container with appropriate coolant. Verify and record the temperature at the time of delivery.
- Posttransfusion instructions must be given in writing, and the patient/caregiver must be provided with names/phone numbers of individuals available to be called in the event of a delayed problem (e.g., unexplained fever, malaise, jaundice). Complications may occur days to weeks after transfusion.
- The container, empty bags, and tubing should be returned to the home care agency on completion of the transfusion.

REVIEW QUESTIONS

Case Study for Questions 1 to 3

Mrs. Jones, a 62-year-old, white female, is 3 days post-op following a left total knee replacement. She has been receiving IV fluids of $D_5\frac{1}{2}$NS solution at 83 mL/hr via an EID. Mrs. Jones has a 20-g 1-inch Insyte IV device in her L midcephalic. When getting report, the nurse finds out she has been c/o nausea and is unable to eat. Her blood work reveals she is mildly dehydrated, but her VS are stable. After calling her surgeon, Mrs. Jones is to continue her IV fluids for 2 more days. Her IV site is without signs/symptoms of IV-related complications and had been restarted yesterday.

1. Mrs. Jones is due for her next bag of IV fluids. Place in order the steps to change the IV bag.
   a. Remove spike from old IV bag.
   b. Label new IV bag with date, time, and time of completion.
   c. Close roller clamp on old IV tubing.
   d. Check for air in tubing.
   e. Regulate flow rate.
   f. Insert spike into new IV bag.
   g. Remove new IV bag from refrigerator at least 1 hour before hang time.
2. Thirty minutes after hanging her new 1 L bag of IV fluids, Mrs. Jones rings her call bell. On entering her room the nurse notices that her IV bag is $\frac{3}{4}$ empty and she is complaining of shortness of breath and is dyspneic. The nurse's assessment reveals bilateral crackles in lung bases, tachycardia, and increased urinary output. What should she suspect is happening?
   1. Fluid volume deficit
   2. Fluid volume overload
   3. Obstructed IV catheter
   4. Air emboli
3. Nursing interventions for Mrs. Jones's condition would include which of the following? Select all that apply.
   1. Slow infusion.
   2. Check for kinks in IV tubing.
   3. Place her in high-Fowler's position.
   4. Remove IV device.
4. Which of the following symptoms are indicative of phlebitis?
   1. Tenderness, pitting edema, dyspnea, cough
   2. Chest pain, cyanosis, hypotension, weak pulse
   3. Headache, nausea, diarrhea, chills
   4. Pain, erythema, induration, swelling
5. A patient is receiving a blood transfusion of PRBC following a total hip replacement. The nurse checks the vital signs 30 minutes after beginning the transfusion and finds an oral temperature of 101° F, pulse 100 bpm, and a respiratory rate of 20. What is the nurse's first priority?
   1. Notify the physician.
   2. Stop the transfusion and begin the NSS infusion.
   3. Notify the Blood Bank immediately.
   4. Wait 30 minutes and repeat the vital signs.
   5. Administer acetaminophen (Tylenol) 650 mg by mouth.
6. Considerations for selecting an IV catheter for a patient include which of the following?
   1. Selecting the longest catheter with a larger gauge
   2. Selecting the longest catheter with the smallest gauge
   3. Selecting the shortest catheter with a larger gauge
   4. Selecting the shortest catheter with the smallest gauge
7. Which is the correct anatomical tip location for a PICC line?
   1. Inferior vena cava
   2. Midaxillary
   3. Antecubital fossa
   4. Superior vena cava
8. A patient returning from surgery has an order for 1000 mL D_5NS to infuse at 100 mL/hr. The drop factor on the patient's infusion tubing is 10 gtts/mL. What would be the correct infusion rate?
   1. 34 gtts/min
   2. 10 gtts/min
   3. 60 gtts/min
   4. 17 gtts/min
9. Partial PN can only be administered through a CVAD.
   1. True
   2. False

REFERENCES

Ackley BJ and others: *Evidence-based nursing care guidelines: medical-surgical interventions*, St Louis, 2008, Mosby.

Ahlqvist M and others: Handling of peripheral intravenous cannula: effects of evidence-based clinical guidelines, *J Clin Nurs* 15(11):1354, 2006.

Alexander M and others: *Infusion nursing: an evidence based approach*, ed 3, St Louis, 2010, Elsevier.

American Association of Blood Banks (AABB): *Technical manual*, ed 15, Bethesda, Md, 2005, The Association.

American Society for Parenteral and Enteral Nutrition (ASPEN): Guidelines for the use of parenteral and enteral nutrition in the adult and pediatric patient, *JPEN J Parenteral Enteral Nutr* 26(suppl 1):1SA, 2002.

Centers for Disease Control and Prevention: Guidelines for the prevention of intravascular catheter-related infections, *MMWR* 52:RR-10, 2002.

Cohen M: Only as smart as the user, *Nursing* 37(7):12, 2007.

Davis K and others: Transfusing safely: a 2006 guide for nurses, *Aust Nurs J* 13(6):38, 2006.

Depledge J and others: Developing a strategic approach for IV therapy in the community, *Br J Community Nurs* 11(11):462, 2006.

Dzik WH: New technology for transfusion safety, *Br J Haematol* 136(2):181, 2007.

Earhart A and others: Assessing pediatric patients for vascular access and sedation, *J Infus Nurs* 30(4):226, 2007.

Eggimann P: Prevention of intravascular catheter infection, *Curr Opin Infect Dis* 20(4):360, 2007.

Eisen LA and others: Mechanical complications of central venous access catheters, *J Intensive Care Med* 21(1):40, 2006.

Gabriel J: Infusion therapy part two: prevention and management of complications, *Nurs Stand* 22(32):41, 2008.

Gray A and others: Safe transfusion of blood and blood components, *Nurs Stand* 21(51):40, 2007.

Hadaway LC: Heparin locking for central venous catheters, *J Assoc Vasc Access* 11(4):224, 2006a.

Hadaway LC: Practical considerations in administering intravenous medications, *J Neurosci Nurs* 38(2):119, 2006b.

Hamilton H: Complications associated with venous access devices: Part 1, *Nurs Stand* 20(26):43, 2006.

Hockenberry MJ, Wilson D: *Wong's nursing care of infants and children*, ed 8, St Louis, 2007, Mosby.

Infusion Nurses Society (INS): 2006 Infusion nursing standards of practice, *J Infus Nurs* 29(suppl 1):S1, 2006.

Katz E: Blood transfusion, *AACN Adv Crit Care* 20(2):155, 2009.

Knippen MA: Transfusion-related acute lung injury intervention can save lives, *Am J Nurs* 106(6):61, 2006.

Miller PA: Central venous access devices, *Radiol Technol* 77(4):297, 2006.

Murphy MF and others: Prevention of bedside errors in transfusion medicine (PROBE-TM) study: a cluster randomized, matched-paired clinical areas trial of a simple intervention to reduce errors in the pretransfusion bedside check, *Transfusion* 47(5):763, 2007.

Occupational Safety and Health Administration: Occupational exposure to blood borne pathogens, needlestick, and other sharps injuries: final rule, CFR 29, part 1910 (Fed Regist 66:5317, Jan 18, 2001), updated April 2006, http://www.osha.gov/SLTC/bloodbornepathogens/index.html accessed September 27, 2010.

Richardson D: Vascular access nursing-standards of care and strategies in the prevention of infection: a primer on central venous catheters, *J Assoc Vasc Access* 12(19):21, 2007.

Scarlet C: Anaphylaxis, *J Infus Nurs* 29(1):39, 2006.

Smith B: New standards for improving peripheral IV catheter securement, *Nursing* 37(3):72, 2007.

The Joint Commission: Maximizing the benefits of smart pump technology: addressing potential error proactively, *Joint Commission Perspect Patient Safety* 7(6):7, 2007.

The Joint Commission: *2010 National Patient Safety Goals*, Oakbrook Terrace, Ill, 2010, The Commission, http://www.jointcommission.org/PatientSafety/NationalPatientSafetyGoals/, accessed September 29, 2010.

CHAPTER

29

Preoperative and Postoperative Care

evolve WEBSITE

http://evolve.elsevier.com/Perry/nursinginterventions

Video Clips

Surgery is both psychologically and physiologically stressful for the patient. The patient has little control over the situation or the outcome, resulting in feelings of anxiety, fear, and powerlessness. Preoperative care reduces stress and places the patient in the best condition possible to undergo surgery. The nurse thoroughly assesses the patient's condition, teaches the patient and family what to expect, and prepares the patient physically and psychologically for surgery.

The care of postoperative patients is divided into three phases: immediate postanesthesia recovery, early recovery, and the convalescent phase. The immediate postanesthesia phase extends from the time the patient leaves the operating room (OR) to the time of transfer from the postanesthesia care unit (PACU) to the nursing unit. This phase requires 2 or more hours and frequent assessments for complications. Patients having surgery in ambulatory outpatient surgery centers have the same recovery needs as patients having surgery in a hospital. The early recovery phase includes several days after surgery followed by a convalescent recovery phase of several additional days or weeks at home for the continued healing process. Patients with chronic medical conditions such as chronic respiratory disease or diabetes mellitus may require a longer convalescent phase.

PATIENT-CENTERED CARE

Often the patient is unsure of what to expect and has concerns about the amount of pain, possible disfigurement, and length of recovery after surgery. Many patients return home the same day, and family members may be unsure about their role in the patient's care and recovery. Before the patient undergoes surgery and throughout the recovery stay, teach the patient and family what to expect and what they can do to assist in the recovery process. In addition, educate patients and their families, as needed, on surgical site infection (SSI) prevention (The Joint Commission, 2010).

Newer technologies such as laser and laparoscopy are less invasive and decrease the need for inpatient admission. More ambulatory outpatient surgeries and shorter hospitalizations lower costs and decrease the risk for the development of a health care–associated infection (HAI).

Patients must be asked about their cultural practices and religious beliefs that may alter their or their family's acceptance of necessary education and procedures. You also need to communicate information pertaining to these practices and beliefs to all members of the health care team so the patient receives comprehensive and holistic care. Before and after surgery it is helpful to assess patient preference for pain medication. Certain groups such as Buddhists and Hindus prefer to endure pain without medication (Andrews and others, 2007).

SAFETY

Physically preparing the patient to undergo surgery and anesthesia involves important skills, including a thorough preoperative assessment. Regardless of the setting, the preoperative assessment forms the basis for a plan of care for the patient during and after surgery. Safety measures such as verifying correct patient, correct procedure and surgical site, signed consent, and relevant documentation (e.g., history and physical, nursing assessment, and pre-anesthesia assessment) and ensuring the availability of required blood products, implants, devices and/or special equipment for the procedure are critical preparation steps. The timing and duration of antibiotic administration and proper surgical site preparation are critical in preventing SSIs. Other physical preparation procedures focus on minimizing the risks involved with surgery and anesthesia while optimizing the patient's condition. The surgical site must be marked before surgery to allow staff to clearly identify the intended site for the procedure, and a "Time-Out" must be performed immediately before starting the procedure (The Joint Commission, 2010). Glycemic control and normothermia restoration in the immediate postoperative period are also important care goals in specific surgical populations that help reduce the risk of SSIs (MedQIC, 2009).

Patient assessment in the immediate postoperative recovery phase emphasizes the ABCs: *A,* airway; *B,* breathing; and *C,* circulation. Postoperative patients are still under sedation and can easily become hypoxic. Nurses routinely monitor oxygen saturation levels and provide supplemental oxygen for as long as needed. Assess the wound size, location, and depth, all of which influence the type and amount of drainage. It is important to know what type of drainage to expect from the dressing, tubes, and catheters. You must implement prophylactic venous thromboembolism (VTE) measures. Patients who are overweight or obese have increased risk of postoperative complications such as obstructive sleep apnea (OSA). Patients with OSA have a greater incidence of airway management problems in the PACU and postoperative pulmonary complications. Longer lengths of stay and unanticipated postoperative admission to the intensive care unit are common.

EVIDENCE-BASED PRACTICE TRENDS

Hedrick TL and others: Prevention of surgical site infections, *Expert Rev Anti Infect Ther* 4(2):223, 2006.

Institute for Healthcare Improvement (IHI): *5 million lives campaign; getting started kit: prevent surgical site infections how-to-guide,* 2007.

MedQIC: *Surgical Care Improvement Project (SCIP). SCIP Project Information,* http://qualitynet.org/dcs/ContentServer?c=MQParents&pagename=Medqic%2FContent%2FParentShellTemplate&cid=1122904930422&parentName=Topic, accessed September 1, 2009.

The Surgical Care Improvement Project (SCIP), a national quality partnership of organizations interested in improving surgical care by significantly reducing surgical complications, developed a list of evidence-based interventions that have proven effective in reducing certain surgical complications such as infection, blood clots, and pneumonia. The Joint Commission (TJC), Centers for Medicare and Medicaid Services (CMS), Centers for Disease Control and Prevention (CDC), Association of periOperative Registered Nurses (AORN), and others have endorsed these evidenced-based initiatives, which focus on the prevention of adverse cardiac events, SSIs, postoperative pneumonia, and venous thrombosis.

SCIP literature indicates that adverse cardiac events are complications of surgery, occurring in 2% to 5% of patients undergoing noncardiac surgery and nearly 34% of patients undergoing cardiac surgery. Recent studies have suggested that beta blockers, when administered appropriately, reduce perioperative ischemia, especially in patients considered to be at risk. As a result of this information, the SCIP guidelines state that surgery patients on a beta blocker before arrival should receive a beta blocker during the perioperative period (MedQIC, 2009).

Postoperative SSIs are the most common HAIs in surgical patients (Hedrick and others, 2006). They contribute to increased medical costs, morbidity, and mortality. The Institute for Healthcare Improvement (IHI) estimates that 40% to 60% of SSIs are preventable (IHI, 2007). SCIP guidelines to reduce SSIs include:

- Do not remove hair unless it will interfere with the operation and remove it using only electric clippers if possible.
- Administer prophylactic antibiotics within 1 hour before surgical incision (2 hours when administering vancomycin and fluoroquinolones), redosed for longer surgeries, and discontinued within 24 hours after surgery end time (48 hours for cardiac patients).
- Maintain glucose control for major cardiac patients. (The IHI defines glucose control as serum glucose levels below 200 mg/dL, collected once on each of the first two postoperative days.)

Without prophylaxis, deep vein thrombosis (DVT) occurs in 25%, and PE occurs in 7% of all major surgical procedures. Despite the well-established efficacy and safety of preventive measures, studies show that prophylaxis is often underused or used inappropriately (MedQIC, 2009).

SKILL 29.1 PREOPERATIVE ASSESSMENT

To identify risks and plan for care during and after surgery, perform a thorough preoperative assessment of the patient's physiological and psychological condition. Many health care facilities have a designated department devoted to completing thorough preoperative screening and testing. Laboratory tests, electrocardiograms (ECGs), chest x-ray films, and other tests are often obtained in these facilities 1 to 2 weeks in advance of the scheduled surgical procedure. Perioperative staff performs a thorough assessment and review the test results to identify any potential abnormalities that may need further evaluation and treatment before surgery. The nurse assesses patients again 1 to 2 hours before the scheduled time of surgery to ensure that there are no changes to their medical condition. Advanced planning allows time for nurses to follow up on any unexpected outcomes. Before beginning this assessment, establish a trusting relationship with the patient.

It is not unusual for the patient to remember and report at this time facts that were not previously told to the physician. Provide the patient privacy and a location free of interruption to encourage open communication. A preprocedure checklist is initiated, beginning with the decision to perform a procedure, maintained with ongoing data collection and assessment, and verified immediately before moving the patient to the procedure room (TJC, 2010).

PLANNING

Expected Outcomes focus on obtaining accurate information and identifying risk factors related to the intended surgery.

- Patient provides the information required to establish a plan of care.
- Patient remains alert and appropriately responsive to nurse's assessment questions.

Delegation and Collaboration

The skills of preoperative assessment cannot be delegated to nursing assistive personnel (NAP). However, for stable patients instruct the NAP about the following:

- Obtaining vital signs and weight and height measurements
- Reporting any abnormal assessment findings to the nurse

Equipment

- Stethoscope
- Blood pressure cuff
- Pulse oximeter
- Thermometer
- Watch or clock with a second hand
- Scale
- Preprocedure checklist
- Preoperative assessment form

IMPLEMENTATION *for* PREOPERATIVE ASSESSMENT

STEPS	RATIONALE
1. See Standard Protocol (inside front cover).	
2. Identify patient using two identifiers (e.g., name and birthday or name and account number, according to facility policy).	Ensures correct patient. Complies with The Joint Commission standards and improves patient safety (TJC, 2010).
3. Determine if patient has any communication impairment (e.g., blindness, hearing loss), is able to read and understand English, and is mentally competent. For example, give patient an informational brochure and have him or her explain a portion of the contents.	Patient may not fully comprehend a diagnosis, understand proposed treatment, or effectively consider alternatives that are presented without effective communication (Sandberg and others, 2008).
4. Assess patient's understanding of the intended surgery and anesthesia. Ask patient to offer a description rather than asking a simple yes or no question (e.g., "Do you understand your surgery?"). Have patient describe in his or her own words. Ask about patient's and family members' expectations of surgery and care. Include questions concerning fears, cultural practices, and religious beliefs if applicable.	Patients may have misconceptions and incomplete knowledge (Sandberg and others, 2008). Asking about fears, cultural practices, and religious beliefs allows you to anticipate patient's/family's priorities and adapt plan so you can give appropriate instruction and support.
5. Ask if patient has an advance directive (see Chapter 31).	Advance directives protect patient's rights by communicating patient's treatment preferences if he or she is unable to communicate.
6. Collect nursing history and identify risk factors.	Allows for anticipation of possible complications and planning for interventions to reduce risks. Allergies, particularly to latex, can be life threatening.
a. Condition leading to surgery	Allows you to anticipate postoperative needs and complications.
b. Chronic illnesses and associated risks (e.g., hypertension: bleeding and stroke; OSA: postoperative respiratory depression and arrest; asthma: impaired ventilation; hiatal hernia: aspiration; diabetes mellitus: poor wound healing; methicillin-resistant *Staphylococcus aureus* (MRSA): impaired wound healing and sepsis)	Some chronic conditions increase the risk of complications from surgery and anesthesia.
c. Last menstrual period (for female patients in childbearing years)	Anesthetic agents and other medications could injure the fetus.

STEPS	RATIONALE
d. Previous hospitalizations	Determines if patient is familiar with hospital procedures.
e. Medication history, including prescription, over-the-counter (OTC), and herbal remedies and date/time of last doses	Patient may not report OTC medications and herbal remedies unless specifically asked. All may interact with anesthetic agents or other medications given during surgery. Patient may be instructed to take any routine blood pressure, cardiac, or seizure medications. Changes in dosages of oral diabetic agents or insulin may be ordered.
f. Previous experience with surgery and anesthesia (Have patient clarify if any undesirable outcomes occurred.)	Information assists in preventing recurrent problems with the planned surgery.
g. Family history of complications from surgery or anesthesia	A family history of reactions to anesthetic agents may indicate a familial condition such as malignant hyperthermia, which is life threatening.
h. Allergies to medications, food, or tape, including specific questions about natural rubber latex. Ask patients if they have had any problem with medication or anything placed on their skin.	Reactions to latex can be life threatening, and prevention in sensitized patients requires specific precautions. Often patients with latex allergies are scheduled as first case of the day. In addition, many patients do not understand that rubber and latex are the same. Using both words helps obtain accurate information.
i. Physical impairment	Physical impairments may cause limited mobility and situations that could lead to problems with positioning during surgery. Communicate this information to the OR nurse because these patients may need special positioning or considerations.
j. Prostheses and implants (e.g., implantable medication delivery pump, dentures, hearing aid, pacemaker, internal defibrillator, hip prosthesis)	These devices could become damaged or malfunction from electrical equipment used during surgery. Report this information to the OR nurse.
k. Smoking, alcohol, and drug use	Increases risk of intraoperative and postoperative complications.
l. Occupation	Anticipates how postoperative restrictions affect patient's return to work.
7. Obtain patient's weight, height, and vital signs (see Chapters 6 and 7).	Height and weight are used to calculate drug dosages. Vital signs provide a baseline for postoperative comparison.
8. Assess patient's respiratory status, including character and rate of respirations, oxygen saturation, ability to breathe lying flat, use of oxygen or continuous positive airway pressure (CPAP) at home, and chest x-ray film report.	Poor respiratory condition can affect patient's response to general anesthesia. Use of CPAP may indicate that patient has OSA, a condition that poses risks after surgery.
9. Evaluate patient's circulatory status, including apical pulse, ECG report, and peripheral pulses (see Chapter 7, Skill 7.4).	Circulation may be a factor in positioning patient on the OR table.
10. Determine patient's neurological status, including level of consciousness (LOC) (see Chapter 7, Skill 7.7).	Patient's neurological status affects attentiveness to instruction. Offers important baseline for postoperative evaluation.
11. Evaluate patient's musculoskeletal system, including range of motion (ROM) of joints (see Chapter 7, Skill 7.7).	If ROM is limited, extra care is needed to prevent injury related to positioning in surgery.
12. Examine patient's skin; identify any breaks in skin integrity and determine level of hydration (see Chapter 7, Skill 7.1). Pay particular attention to area of body on which patient will be positioned.	If skin is thin, broken, or bruised, extra padding is needed in surgery. Hydration may affect skin integrity.
13. Evaluate patient's emotional status, including level of anxiety, coping ability, and family support.	If patient has high level of anxiety or fear, consultation with a social worker, pastoral care, or advanced practice nurse (APN) might be useful.

Continued

STEPS	RATIONALE
14. Review the results of laboratory tests, including complete blood count (CBC), electrolytes, urinalysis, and other diagnostic tests.	Laboratory work provides an assessment of major body systems.
15. Identify the time of patient's last intake of food or drink.	With patient under general anesthesia, the esophageal sphincter relaxes, and the stomach contents can be aspirated.
16. See Completion Protocol (inside front cover).	

EVALUATION

1. Determine if patient information is complete so plan of care can be established. Validate unclear information with family.
2. Evaluate patient's ability to cooperate (e.g., makes eye contact, answers appropriately).

Unexpected Outcomes and Related Interventions

1. The patient does not understand English.
   a. Obtain a professional medical interpreter.
2. The patient is not mentally competent.
   a. Determine who is legally authorized to consent to surgery (see agency policy).
   b. Determine who can provide health history.
3. Patient does not understand what surgery will be performed.
   a. Notify the surgeon.
4. The patient reports a condition that is a risk factor for surgery or after surgery such as hiatal hernia, pregnancy, family history of complications with anesthesia, cold or upper respiratory infection, recent chest pain, or sleep apnea.
   a. Notify the surgeon and anesthesia provider.
5. Patient has been taking anticoagulants.
   a. Notify the surgeon.
6. Patient reports an allergy to latex.
   a. Remove all supplies containing latex from patient's room.
   b. Post a latex precautions sign on the door or stretcher.
   c. Notify surgeon, anesthesia provider, and OR nurse.
7. Appropriate laboratory tests were not ordered or completed.
   a. Notify surgeon and anesthesia provider and make arrangements for tests to be completed.
8. Chest x-ray film report, ECG, or laboratory tests show abnormal findings.
   a. Notify surgeon and anesthesia provider.
9. Patient has a blister, abrasion, or boil near the incision site.
   a. Notify surgeon.

Recording and Reporting

- Document findings on the preoperative portion of the nurses' detailed preoperative notes or other designated agency form.
- Report abnormal laboratory values or other concerns to the surgeon or anesthesiologist.

Sample Documentation

0830 Nursing history completed. Patient states that after knee surgery last year she "vomited for 6 hours." Anesthesiologist notified of patient history of vomiting after surgery.

Special Considerations

Pediatric

- Consider a child's developmental level when performing preoperative preparation (e.g., use films, books, tours, toys, and games to demonstrate preoperative procedures (Hockenberry and Wilson, 2009).
- Allow the parents to be present during induction if institution policy allows. If not, allow them to wait with the child until initial sedation begins to take effect. The child does not remember the parents leaving. Reunite parents with child after surgery as soon as the child is waking in recovery.

Geriatric

- Age-related changes may result in diminished short-term memory. Additional assessment and teaching may be necessary in this area.
- An older adult may have some limitation in ROM. If this limitation is significant, notify the OR nurse so surgical position can be modified.

SKILL 29.2 PREOPERATIVE TEACHING

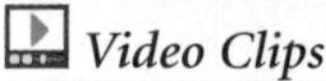
Video Clips

With shortened lengths of stay and growth in ambulatory surgical procedures, there is a greater demand for patient preparation and support. Patient education must go beyond simply providing information because patients and families must assume more preoperative and postoperative responsibilities (Johansson and others, 2006; Thomas and Sethares, 2008). Preoperative patient teaching involves assisting a patient to understand and mentally prepare for the surgical experience. Effective education leads to empowered patients who have sufficient knowledge that meets their needs, expectations, or preferences.

Preoperative teaching increases patient satisfaction, promotes psychological well-being, and may decrease complications leading to an increased length of stay (Lewis and others, 2007). Plan your teaching based on the preoperative assessment. Make every attempt to ensure the patient's privacy. Select the best learning method for the patient. In many settings videotape and written materials are available to assist you. Whenever possible, have the family members responsible for the patient's care after surgery present. Later they serve as coaches and assist the patient in performing exercises. Plan to have the patient demonstrate expected postoperative skills to allow for practice and facilitate understanding.

Patients and their families are often anxious about impending surgery, which impairs learning. Speak in a clear, slow voice to reduce the patient's anxiety and promote understanding. You may need extra time for teaching and reinforcement to ensure patient understanding. After surgery high anxiety can lead to negative psychological and physiological outcomes. Preoperative information about expected perioperative sensations decreases the distress associated with surgery. By teaching the patient before surgery, the nurse can make a significant contribution to its success and to the patient's postoperative recovery.

ASSESSMENT

1. Ask about patient's previous experiences with surgery and anesthesia. *Rationale: This allows you to individualize teaching and address specific patient concerns.*
2. Determine patient's and family's understanding of surgery. *Rationale: This information determines if correction of misunderstanding is necessary.*
3. Identify patient's cognitive level, language, and culture. *Rationale: These factors may alter patient's ability to understand the meaning of surgery and can affect the postoperative healing course if there are mixed messages or misunderstanding.*
4. Assess patient's anxiety related to surgery. *Rationale: Directs you to provide additional emotional support and indicates patient's readiness to learn.*
5. Assess patient's medical orders. *Rationale: Preoperative and postoperative orders often require adaptations in the way a patient performs exercises.*

PLANNING

Expected Outcomes focus on reducing the anxiety level of patient and family and having patient demonstrate understanding of key information and specific skills necessary to prevent complications.

- Patient demonstrates eye contact and asks and answers questions appropriately.
- Patient correctly performs splinting, turning and sitting, breathing exercises, and leg exercises.
- Family identifies the location of the waiting room.
- Family verbalizes the ability to care for patient at home.
- Family provides emotional support for patient before surgery.

Delegation and Collaboration

The skills of preoperative teaching cannot be delegated to nursing assistive personnel (NAP). NAP can reinforce and assist patients in performing postoperative exercises. Instruct the NAP about the following:

- Any precautions for turning a particular patient
- Informing the registered nurse (RN) if the patient is unable to perform the exercises correctly

Equipment

- Stretcher or bed
- Pillow
- Incentive spirometer
- Preoperative education flow sheet

IMPLEMENTATION *for* PREOPERATIVE TEACHING

STEPS	RATIONALE
1. **See Standard Protocol (inside front cover).**	
2. Inform patient and family of date, time, and location of surgery; anticipated length of surgery; additional time in the postanesthesia recovery area; and where to wait.	Accurate information helps reduce the stress associated with surgery.
3. Answer questions patient and family ask.	Responding to patient and family questions helps to decrease anxiety and demonstrates your concern for them.
4. Instruct patient on preoperative bowel or skin preparations as needed. Check institutional policy regarding number of preoperative showers and agent to be used for each shower (4% chlorhexidine gluconate [CHG] is used most often). Following each preoperative shower, the skin should be rinsed thoroughly and dried with a fresh, clean, dry towel; and patient should don clean clothing.	Proper skin preparation is a critical element in preventing SSIs. Rinsing the skin removes residual antiseptic preparation that may cause skin irritation. After use, towels contain microorganisms that can grow in the presence of moisture. Using a fresh towel after each shower and donning clean clothing minimizes the risk of reintroducing microorganisms to clean skin (AORN, 2009).

Continued

STEPS	RATIONALE
5. Instruct patient on extent and purpose of food and fluid restrictions for period specified before surgery (e.g., no oral intake for 2 hours before surgery; no meat or fried foods 8 hours before surgery, unless otherwise specified by surgeon or anesthesiologist).	During use of general anesthesia muscles relax, and gastric contents can reflux into esophagus, leading to aspiration. Anesthetic eliminates patient's ability to gag.
6. Describe perioperative routines (e.g., "Time Out," site marking, intravenous [IV] therapy, urinary catheterization, enema, hair clipping/removal, laboratory tests, transport to OR).	Allows patient to anticipate and recognize routine procedures, reducing anxiety.
7. Describe planned effect of preoperative medications.	Provides information about what to expect, thereby decreasing anxiety.
8. Review which routine medications patients need to discontinue before surgery.	Some medications are discontinued before surgery to minimize effects that can cause surgical risks. For example, anticoagulants may increase bleeding and are usually discontinued several days before surgery. Insulin dosages are usually adjusted because of the reduced intake of food before surgery.
9. Describe perioperative sensations (e.g., blood pressure cuff tightening, ECG leads, cool room, beep of monitor).	Misconceptions and concerns about anesthesia have been ranked high among preoperative patients.
10. Describe pain-control methods. Many patients have a patient-controlled analgesia (PCA) pump (see Chapter 13).	Patients are fearful of postoperative pain. Explaining pain-management techniques reduces this fear.
11. Describe what patient will experience after surgery (e.g., frequent vital signs, turning, catheters, drains, tubes, alternating pressure from sequential compression device [SCD]).	Provides a concrete description of what patient can expect after surgery so patient is prepared.
12. Teach turning.	
a. Instruct patient on turning and sitting up (especially suited for abdominal and thoracic surgery).	
(1) Turn onto right side: Instruct patient to flex knees while lying supine and move toward left side of bed.	Promotes circulation and ventilation.
(2) Have patient splint incision with right arm and pillow; keep right leg straight and flex left knee up; and grab right side rail with left hand, pull toward right, and roll onto right side. Reverse process to turn to left side.	Supports incision and decreases discomfort while turning.
(3) Instruct patient to turn every 2 hours from side to side while awake.	Reduces risk of vascular and pulmonary complications.
(4) Sit up on right side of bed: Elevate head of bed and have patient turn onto right side. While lying on right side, patient pushes on mattress with right arm and swings feet over edge of bed with nurse's assistance. To sit up on left side of bed, reverse this process.	Sitting position lowers diaphragm to permit fuller lung expansion.
13. Teach deep breathing and coughing:	Patient may be unable or reluctant to deep breathe because of weakness or pain, resulting in secretions remaining in the base of the lungs. Collection of secretions increases the risk of pulmonary atelectasis and pneumonia.
a. Assist patient to high-Fowler's position in bed with knees flexed or sitting on side of bed or chair in upright position.	Sitting position facilitates diaphragmatic expansion.
b. Instruct patient to lightly place palms of hands across from each other along the lower border of the rib cage or upper abdomen (see illustration).	This allows patient to feel the rise and fall of the abdomen during deep breathing (Lewis and others, 2007).

STEPS	RATIONALE
c. Have patient take slow, deep breaths, inhaling through nose. Explain that patient will feel normal downward movement of diaphragm during inspiration. Demonstrate as needed.	Helps to prevent hyperventilation or panting. Slow deep breath allows for more complete lung expansion.
d. Have patient avoid using chest and shoulder muscles while inhaling.	Increases unnecessary energy expenditure and does not promote full lung expansion.
e. Have patient take slow, deep breath, hold for count of 3 seconds, and slowly exhale through mouth as if blowing out a candle (pursed lips).	Resistance during exhalation helps to prevent alveolar collapse.
f. Have patient repeat breathing exercise 3 to 5 times.	Repetition reinforces learning.
g. Have patient take two slow, deep breaths, inhaling through nose and exhaling through pursed lips.	Deep breaths expand lungs fully so air moves behind mucus to facilitate coughing.
h. Have patient inhale deeply a third time and hold breath to count of 3. Cough fully for two to three consecutive coughs without inhaling between coughs.	Deep breathing moves up secretions in the respiratory tract to stimulate the cough reflex without voluntary effort on the part of patient (Lewis and others, 2007).
i. Caution patient against just clearing throat.	Clearing throat does not remove mucus from deeper airways.
j. Have patient practice several times. Instruct him or her to perform turning, coughing, and deep breathing every 2 hours.	Ensures mastery of technique. Frequent pulmonary exercises and movement decrease risk of postoperative pneumonia (Lewis and others, 2007).
14. Teach use of an incentive spirometer (see illustration).	Provides visual aid of respiratory effort. Encourages deep breathing to loosen secretions in lung bases.
a. Position in sitting or reclining position.	Facilitates diaphragm lowering and lung expansion.
b. Instruct patient to exhale completely and place mouthpiece so lips completely cover it and inhale slowly, maintaining constant flow through unit.	Promotes complete inflation of lungs and minimizes atelectasis.
c. After maximum inspiration, patient should hold breath for 2 to 3 seconds and exhale slowly.	Promotes alveolar inflation.
d. Set marker on spirometer at maximum inspiration point to establish postoperative target.	Establishes measure of normal maximum breath for patient. Provides outcome measure to determine postoperative return to preoperative volumes.
e. Instruct patient to breathe normally for a short period and repeat process for total of 10 times every hour while awake.	Prevents hyperventilation and fatigue.

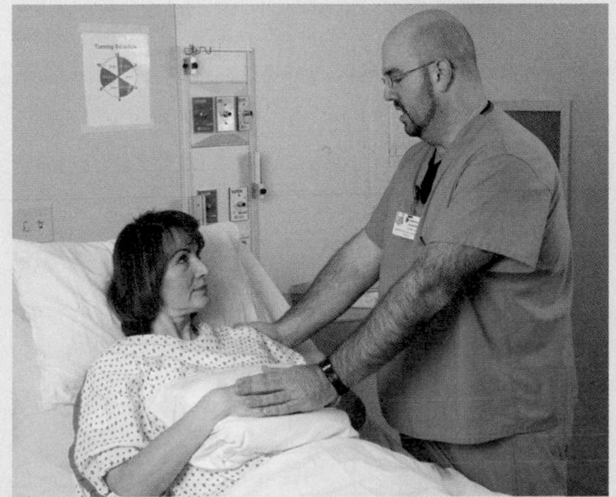

STEP 13b Deep-breathing exercise—placement of hands on upper abdomen during inhalation.

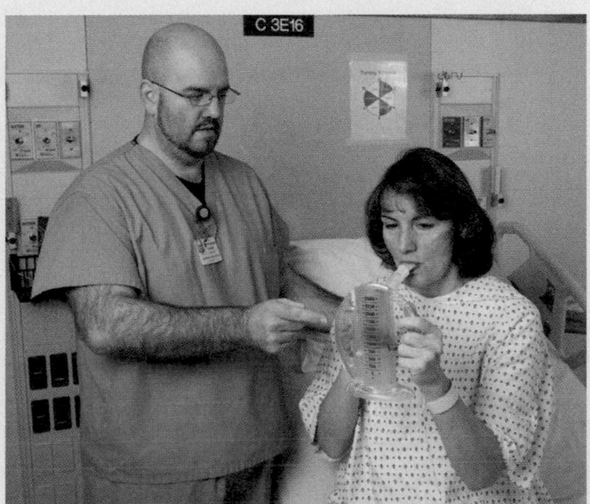

STEP 14 Patient demonstrates incentive spirometry.

Continued

STEPS	RATIONALE
15. Teach leg exercises:	
a. Instruct and encourage patient in leg exercises to be performed every 1 to 2 hours while awake: ankle rotation, dorsiflexion and plantar flexion, leg extension and flexion, straight leg raises.	Leg exercises facilitate venous return from the lower extremities and reduce the risk of circulatory complications such as a venous thrombus.
b. Position patient supine.	
c. Instruct patient to rotate each ankle in a complete circle and draw imaginary circles with the big toe 5 times (see illustration).	Promotes joint mobility.
d. Alternate dorsiflexion and plantar flexion while instructing patient to feel calf muscles tighten and relax. Repeat 5 times (see illustration).	Helps maintain joint mobility and promote venous return to prevent thrombus formation.
e. Instruct patient to alternate flexing and extending knees one leg at a time. Repeat 5 times (see illustration).	Maintains knee joint mobility and contracts muscles of upper leg.
f. Instruct patient to alternate raising legs straight up from bed surface. Leg should be kept straight. Repeat 5 times (see illustration).	Causes quadriceps muscle contraction and relaxation that helps promote venous return (Lewis and others, 2007).
g. Instruct patient to perform these four leg exercises 10 to 12 times every 1 to 2 hours while awake.	Leg exercises stimulate circulation, which prevents venous stasis to help prevent formation of DVT (Lewis and others, 2007).
16. Verify that patient's expectations of surgery are realistic. Correct expectations as needed.	Can prevent postoperative anxiety or anger.
17. Reinforce therapeutic coping strategies. If ineffective, encourage alternatives.	Therapeutic coping strategies promote postoperative compliance and recovery.
18. See Completion Protocol (inside front cover).	

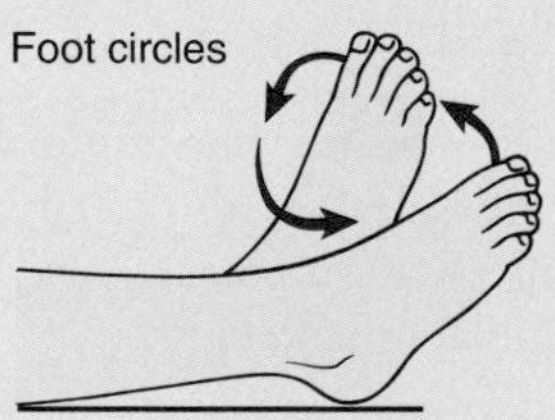

STEP 15c Foot circles. (From Lewis S and others: *Medical-surgical nursing: assessment and management of clinical problems,* ed 7, St Louis, 2007, Mosby.)

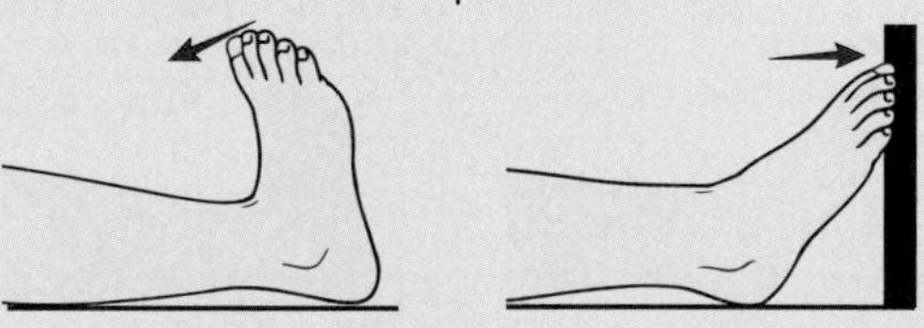

STEP 15d Alternate dorsiflexion and plantar flexion. (From Lewis S and others: *Medical-surgical nursing: assessment and management of clinical problems,* ed 7, St Louis, 2007, Mosby.)

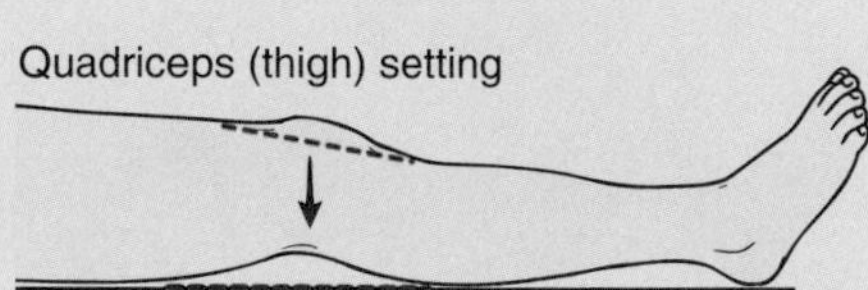

STEP 15e Hips and knee movements. (From Lewis S and others: *Medical-surgical nursing: assessment and management of clinical problems,* ed 7, St Louis, 2007, Mosby.)

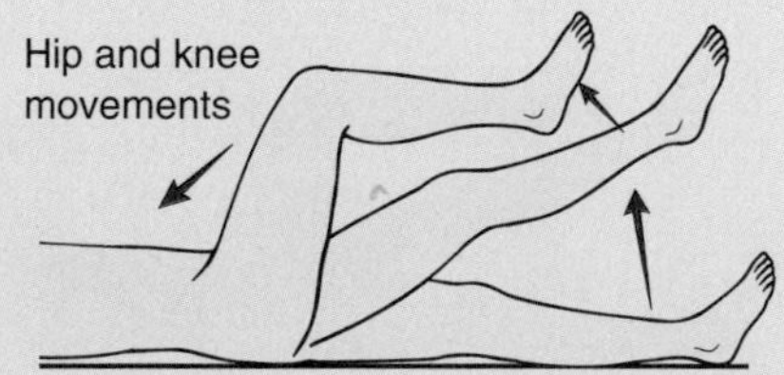

STEP 15f Quadriceps (thigh) setting. (From Lewis S and others: *Medical-surgical nursing: assessment and management of clinical problems,* ed 7, St Louis, 2007, Mosby.)

EVALUATION

1. Ask patient to repeat key information (e.g., rationale for withholding food and fluids).
2. Observe patient demonstrating splinting, turning and sitting, deep breathing, and leg exercises.
3. Ask family to identify location of the waiting room.
4. Ask family if they are able to care for patient at home after discharge.
5. Observe the level of emotional support family provides patient.
6. Observe patient and family coping strategies.

Unexpected Outcomes and Related Interventions

1. Patient identifies an incorrect procedure, site, date, or time of surgery.
   a. Provide the correct information verbally and in writing for patient and family.
2. Patient questions the importance of not drinking the morning of surgery.
   a. Explain that under anesthesia the fluid can come up from the stomach and go into the lungs.
3. Patient incorrectly performs breathing exercises.
   a. Explain and demonstrate the correct breathing technique.
   b. Explain the importance of postoperative breathing.
   c. Instruct patient to repeat the demonstration.
4. Family verbalizes anxiety about caring for patient at home.
   a. Explain that these feelings are normal.
   b. Provide written instructions and a telephone number for contact if there are further questions.
5. Family indicates that they are unable to care for patient at home.
   a. Contact health care provider and discuss the alternative of a home health care referral.

Recording and Reporting

- Record preoperative teaching on the preoperative education flow sheet or designated agency form.

Sample Documentation

0940 Preoperative teaching completed. Instructed on continued need to be NPO; routine events to expect in OR and recovery room; presence of oxygen; IV fluid; postoperative drains; and postoperative activities, including turn, cough, and deep breath (TCDB); use of IS; and leg exercises. Daughter expressed concern about her mother being able to care for herself at home after surgery. Home health nurse contacted to see patient before discharge.

Special Considerations

Pediatric

- Use an age-appropriate level of communication and provide simple explanations using familiar terms.
- The use of pictures, models, equipment, and play rather than verbal explanations increases preschool and school-age children's learning.

Geriatric

- Age-related changes in the central nervous system (CNS) may diminish short-term memory. Additional time and reinforcement may be necessary for older adults to learn and comprehend information (Spry, 2009). The greater the number of different exposures to new material, the higher the probability that the material will be learned.
- Reinforce teaching with verbal explanations, audiovisual resources, pamphlets, and demonstrations. Consider sight and hearing deficits when providing both written and verbal instructions (Spry, 2009).

Home Care

- Review coughing, deep breathing, abdominal splinting, relaxation, leg exercises, and ambulation before admission to hospital or surgical clinic and after discharge.

SKILL 29.3 PHYSICAL PREPARATION FOR SURGERY

Physical preparation of the patient for surgery involves providing nursing care immediately before surgery, verifying required procedures and tests, and documenting care in the patient's record. You follow specific steps to prepare every patient. These steps depend on the type of surgery being performed and the risks involved. For example, you use compression stockings, intermittent compression devices (ICDs), and the venous foot pump for adult patients undergoing surgery that will last several hours and require a long period of immobilization afterward. You provide a bowel preparation, administering an enema, laxative, or cathartic (this may be done at home by patients admitted the morning of surgery) for abdominal surgery on or near the intestine. You may need to clip hair near the incision site. Always check the physician's orders to determine what procedures are needed for the surgical patient. Regardless of the type of surgery, the goal of physical preparation is to place the patient in the best condition possible to minimize the risks of the planned surgery.

ASSESSMENT

1. The preoperative assessment forms the basis for physical preparation of the patient for surgery (see Skill 29.1).

PLANNING

Expected Outcomes focus on the proper physical preparation of the patient for surgery.

- Patient cooperates during preparatory measures (e.g., starting an IV line, undergoing an enema).
- Patient undergoes measures to reduce the risk of infection (e.g., preoperative antibiotic, skin preparation).

Delegation and Collaboration

The skill of coordinating the patient's preparation for surgery cannot be delegated to nursing assistive personnel (NAP). However, the NAP may administer an enema or a douche; obtain vital signs in stable patients; apply antiembolic stockings; and assist patients in removing clothing, jewelry, and prostheses. Instruct the NAP about the following:

- Using proper precautions when preparing a patient for surgery
- Observing and using precautions if the patient has an IV catheter in place

Equipment

NOTE: Equipment varies by procedure ordered.

- Hospital gown

- IV solution and equipment (see Chapter 28)
- Skin cleansing solution
- Compression (antiembolism) stockings
- Intermittent Compression Device (ICD)
- Venous foot pump
- Urinary catheterization kit (see Chapter 18)
- Preoperative checklist
- Medications (e.g., sedative)
- Enema set and prescribed solution (see Chapter 19)
- Douche set and prescribed solution

IMPLEMENTATION *for* PHYSICAL PREPARATION FOR SURGERY

STEPS	RATIONALE
1. See Standard Protocol (inside front cover).	
2. Identify patient using two identifiers (e.g., name and birthday or name and account number, according to facility policy). Ask patient to state name. Apply identification bracelet if all information is correct. Apply blood band if applicable and used by agency.	Ensures correct patient. Complies with The Joint Commission standards and improves patient safety (TJC, 2010). Application of blood band ensures that patient receives correct blood product.
3. Assist patient with putting on hospital gown and removing personal items. Patients are often anxious before surgery. Before any procedure, decrease anxiety by explaining how equipment or preparation will feel (e.g., cold, tight) before touching patient.	
4. Instruct patient to remove makeup, nail polish, hairpins, and jewelry.	During and after surgery, anesthesiologist and nurse must assess the skin and nails to determine tissue perfusion. (In some settings patients are allowed to have a ring taped and remove polish from only one nail.)
5. Ensure that money and valuables have been locked up or given to a family member.	Patient may not return to same location after surgery. Prevents valuables from being misplaced or lost.
6. Ensure that patient has followed appropriate fluid and food restrictions per surgeon or anesthesiologist order (see Skill 29.2).	Extent and type of restriction vary by institution and practitioner. Under general anesthesia the sphincters in the stomach relax, and contents can reflux into the esophagus and trachea.
7. Verify that patient has followed request for omission or ingestion of medications as instructed.	Missed or inaccurate dosage could precipitate complications.
8. Verify that a bowel preparation (e.g., laxative, cathartic, enema) is completed if ordered.	For patients admitted the morning of surgery, this may have been performed at home.
9. Ensure that a medical history and physical examination results are in patient's record.	Establishes database for future comparison.
10. Verify that surgical consent is complete. The name of procedure, name of surgeon, date, name of person authorized to obtain consent, and patient's signature should all be present.	Ensures patient's agreement to undergo intended procedure. In most settings the surgeon obtains the consent, and the RN verifies that it is complete and consistent with patient's understanding (refer to agency policy).
11. Ensure that necessary laboratory work, ECG, and chest x-ray film studies are completed and results are on the chart.	Diagnostic test results may indicate a medical problem and provide data for postoperative comparison.
12. Verify that blood type and crossmatch are completed if ordered by the physician and that blood transfusions are available as needed.	In many cases surgery cannot begin without availability of blood units.
13. Ask if patient has an advance directive. If so, place it in patient's record.	Document conveys patient's wishes if life support measures are necessary.
14. Assess and record patient's heart rate, blood pressure, respiratory rate, oxygen saturation, and temperature.	Provides a baseline for patient's preoperative status.
15. Administer cathartics or enemas if ordered (see Chapter 19, Skill 19.2).	Emptying the bowel is necessary for bowel surgery and the procedure to decrease the risk of postoperative ileus. Enemas are used when surgery is near the lower intestine.
16. Instruct patient to void.	Prevents risk of bladder distention or rupture during surgery.

STEPS	RATIONALE
17. Start an IV line; refer to unit standards or physician's orders (see Chapter 28).	IV provides access for fluids and medications administered in OR.
18. Administer preoperative medications as ordered.	Preoperative medications may be used for a variety of reasons and should be administered as ordered for maximum effectiveness.
19. Apply compression stockings (see Chapter 16, Procedural Guideline 16.2).	Compression stockings promote circulation during periods of immobilization, reducing the risk of an embolism.
20. Apply ICD if ordered (see illustrations) (see Procedural Guideline 16.2. NOTE: ICDs may or may not be used in combination with compression stockings. Verify order.	ICDs push blood from the superficial veins into the deep veins, thus decreasing venous stasis.

SAFETY ALERT ICDs do not provide effective DVT prophylaxis if the device is not applied correctly or if the patient does not wear the device continuously except during bathing, skin assessment, and ambulation. ICDs are *not* to be worn when a patient has an active DVT because of risk of pulmonary embolism (PE).

STEPS	RATIONALE
21. Apply venous plexus foot pump if ordered. Apply foot cover. Attach cover to device and verify correct settings (see illustration).	Venous plexus foot pumps promote circulation by mimicking the natural action of walking by intermittently compressing the sole of the foot and relaxing it so the venous plexus can fill with blood.

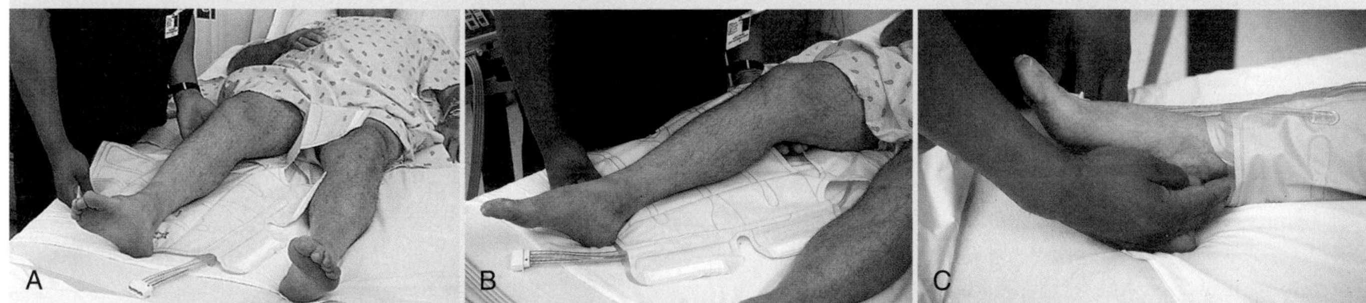

STEP 20 A, Correct leg position on inner lining. **B,** Position back of patient's knee with popliteal opening. **C,** Check fit of ICD sleeve.

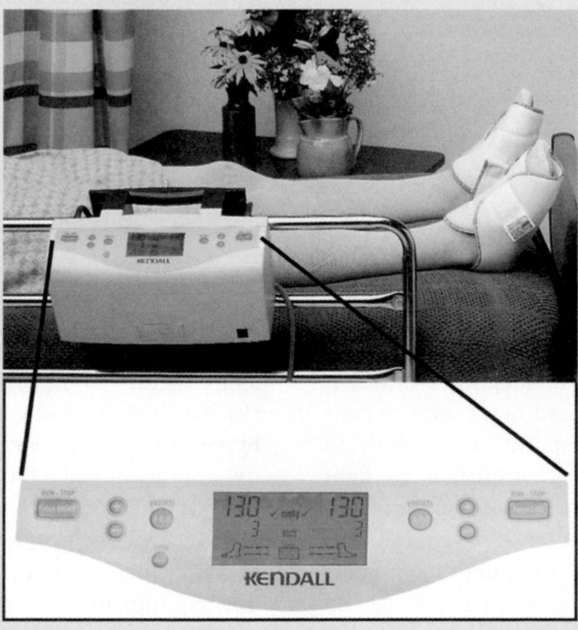

STEP 21 Venous plexus foot pump with bedside controls. (Courtesy Tyco Healthcare Group LP.)

Continued

STEPS	RATIONALE
22. Cleanse and prepare the surgical site if ordered.	Cleansing with an antimicrobial soap decreases bacterial flora on the skin.
23. Insert a urinary catheter if ordered (see Chapter 18). Maintains bladder decompression and provides for monitoring output during surgery.	
24. Allow the patient to wear eyeglasses, dentures, or hearing aid as long as possible before surgery. Remove contact lenses, eyeglasses, hairpieces, and dentures just before surgery.	These aids facilitate patient cooperation by ensuring that patient has clear vision and maximal auditory perception throughout the preoperative phase. In some settings dentures are left in place.
25. Place cap on patient's head.	The cap contains the hair and minimizes OR contamination during surgery. Plastic or reflective caps reduce heat loss during surgery.
26. Assist patient onto stretcher for transport to OR.	Some ambulatory surgery patients walk to OR.
27. See Completion Protocol (inside front cover).	

EVALUATION

1. Observe patient's level of cooperation during preparation.
2. Ask patient to assist with measures to reduce the risk of infection (preoperative antibiotics, skin preparation).

Unexpected Outcomes and Related Interventions

1. Patient reports having eaten breakfast or drinking fluids.
   a. Notify surgeon and anesthesia provider.
2. Patient refuses to go to surgery until contacting a family member.
   a. Notify surgeon.
   b. Assist patient with contacting family member.
3. Consent is incomplete or incorrect.
   a. Notify surgeon and anesthesia provider.
4. Patient did not follow instructions regarding medications.
   a. Notify surgeon.
5. Patient has a reaction to a preoperative medication.
   a. Discontinue the medication.
   b. Treat the reaction per institutional policy.
   c. Notify surgeon.

Recording and Reporting

- Document preoperative physical preparation on preoperative checklist

Sample Documentation

0850 Verified patient has been NPO since midnight. Dentures, yellow wedding band, and wallet given to patient's wife. Fleets enema given with results of large amount soft brown stool. Compression stockings applied. Patient stated he did not take his bedtime dose of 30 units of Lantus insulin. Bedside blood sugar 110. Surgeon notified. 20 units of Lantus insulin administered subcutaneously per order. IV of D_5 ½ Normal Saline started in right hand per order. Voided and taken to OR by stretcher per transporter.

Special Considerations

Pediatric

- Give the child as many choices related to procedures as possible.
- Keep parent-child separation to the minimum time possible. When a parent cannot be present, it is important to leave a favorite possession with the child.

Geriatric

- Because of cognitive, sensory, or physical impairments, it may take the older patient increased time to dress for surgery and complete needed physical preparation.

SKILL 29.4 MANAGING THE PATIENT RECEIVING MODERATE SEDATION

Moderate sedation is used during certain diagnostic or therapeutic procedures and is a drug-induced depression of consciousness during which patients respond purposefully to verbal commands, either alone or accompanied by light tactile stimulation. In addition, no interventions are required to maintain a patent airway, and spontaneous ventilation is adequate (ASA, 2004). (Patients most often undergo moderate sedation outside of the operative setting. See facility policy.) Benefits of moderate sedation are that it helps to improve the patient's cooperation with the procedure, allows a rapid return to the preprocedure status, and minimizes the risk for injury. Risks during moderate sedation include hypoventilation, airway compromise, hemodynamic instability, and/or altered LOCs that include an overly depressed LOC or agitation and combativeness. Emergency equipment appropriate for the patient's age and size and staff with skill in airway management, oxygen delivery, and use of resuscitation equipment are essential. Because of the risk of deep sedation, the use of moderate sedation is closely controlled and normally restricted to physicians and nurses who receive specialized training or credentialing (American Association of Nurse Anesthetists [AANA], 2004; Association of periOperative Registered Nurses [AORN], 2009). During and after the procedure patients need continuous monitoring of vital signs, oxygen saturation, heart rhythm, lung sounds, and LOC.

ASSESSMENT

1. Verify that a preprocedural history and physical examination was completed. *Rationale: Accrediting agencies such as The Joint Commission require a documented preprocedural history and physical examination before the administration of moderate sedation.*
2. Verify that informed consent was obtained. *Rationale: Federal regulations, many state laws, and accreditation agencies require informed consent for procedure.*
3. Assess patient's past history of adverse reaction to procedural sedation (e.g., hemodynamic instability nausea and vomiting, airway compromise, altered LOC). *Rationale: Patients with history of these reactions are at higher risk for procedural complications if procedural sedation is used.*
4. Verify patient's ASA Physical Status Classification (Box 29-1).

SAFETY ALERT An ASA classification of 3 or higher or a patient history of difficult intubation, sleep apnea, or complications related to sedation/anesthesia may necessitate anesthesiologist consultation (ASA, 2008). Check agency policy.

5. Assess patient's current or past history for substance abuse. *Rationale: A history of substance abuse usually requires dose adjustment of the sedative.*
6. Verify that the patient has not ingested food or fluids, except for oral medications, for at least 4 hours. Verify specific agency requirements. *Rationale: Because a risk of procedural sedation is loss of airway protection, an empty stomach reduces the risk for aspiration.*
7. Determine if patient is allergic to latex, antiseptic, or anesthetic solutions. *Rationale: Allergic reactions to latex range from mild skin reaction to anaphylaxis. Common allergic reactions to local anesthetic agents include CNS depression, respiratory difficulty, and hypotension.*
8. Assess patient's level of understanding of procedure, including any concerns. *Rationale: Determines extent of instruction or level of support required and decreases anxiety.*
9. Assess baseline heart rate, breath sounds, respiratory rate, blood pressure, LOC, pain level, and oxygen saturation. *Rationale: Establishes a baseline for comparison during the procedure.*
10. Determine patient's height and weight. *Rationale: Needed to calculate drug dosages.*
11. Assess and document patient's baseline status via agency designated scoring system. Many agencies use the "Aldrete score" (see Table 29-4). *Rationale: Establishes a baseline for comparison after the procedure.*

BOX 29-1 ASA PHYSICAL STATUS CLASSIFICATION

P1 = Normal healthy patient
P2 = Patient with mild systemic disease
P3 = Patient with severe systemic disease
P4 = Patient with severe systemic disease that is a constant threat to life
P5 = Moribund patient who is not expected to survive without the operation
P6 = Declared brain-dead patient whose organs are being removed for donor purposes

From American Society of Anesthesiologists: *Relative value guide,* 2008, The Society.

Delegation and Collaboration

The skill of assisting with moderate sedation cannot be delegated to nursing assistive personnel (NAP). In most agencies an RN, health care provider, or physician assesses and monitors the patient's level of sedation, airway patency, and LOC. Roles in monitoring depend on scope-of-practice guidelines as determined by state regulations and agency policy and practitioner credentialing. Check agency procedures regarding specific monitoring parameters and frequency required before, during, and after the procedure.

Equipment

- Protective equipment: gloves, mask, gown, goggles
- Sedation agent as prescribed: diazepam (Valium), midazolam (Versed), fentanyl (Sublimaze) and labels for each
- Emergency equipment: crash cart, defibrillator, and ET equipment in various sizes
- Equipment for insertion of a peripheral IV catheter (see Chapter 28)
- Oxygen and airway supplies: bag and mask device, oral/nasopharyngeal airways, suction equipment
- Sphygmomanometer or noninvasive blood pressure monitor
- Pulse oximeter
- ECG machine
- Appropriate reversal drugs (e.g., flumazenil [Romazicon] for reversal of benzodiazepines, naloxone [Narcan] for reversal of opiates), and labels for each
- Pain medication for procedures anticipated to cause discomfort

PLANNING

Expected Outcomes focus on safety and comfort during and after the procedure.

- Adhere to Universal Protocol (Box 29-2).
- Patient's airway remains patent.
- Patient's level of comfort is equivalent to a score of 4 or less on a pain scale of 1 to 10.

BOX 29-2 THE JOINT COMMISSION UNIVERSAL PROTOCOL

- Verification of correct person, correct site, and correct procedure occurs.
- When patient is in preprocedure area immediately before moving him or her to procedure room, a checklist (e.g., paper, electronic, or other medium such as a wall-mounted whiteboard) is used to review and verify that required items are available and accurately matched to the patient.
- Procedure site is marked before moving to procedure area.
- A "Time-Out" is performed immediately before starting procedures.

From The Joint Commission: *National Patient Safety Goals,* 2009, TJC, http://www.jointcommission.org/PatientSafety/NationalPatientSafetyGoals/npsg_facts.htm, accessed October 29, 2010.

IMPLEMENTATION *for* MANAGING THE PATIENT RECEIVING MODERATE SEDATION

STEPS	RATIONALE
1. **See Standard Protocol (inside front cover).**	
2. Identify the patient using two identifiers (e.g., name and birthday or name and account number, according to facility policy).	Ensures correct patient. Complies with The Joint Commission standards and improves patient safety (TJC, 2010).
3. Establish a peripheral IV access (see Chapter 28).	Provides for administration of sedation and any emergency changes (as needed).
4. Implement Universal Protocol in presence of appropriate health care team members (as applicable) and in accordance with agency policy (see Box 29-2).	Must ensure patient safety by correctly identifying correct patient to correct procedure.
5. During the diagnostic procedure, monitor heart rate and oxygen saturation (SpO_2) continuously via pulse oximetry equipment. Monitor airway patency, respiratory rate, blood pressure, and appropriate LOC and responsiveness every 5 to 15 minutes.	Vital signs provide a comparison with patient's baseline status.
6. Observe for verbal or nonverbal evidence of pain, facial grimacing, and eye opening.	Physical responses indicate level of sedation.
7. Monitor LOC/responsiveness to physical and/or verbal stimulation. Assess level of sedation using the Modified Ramsay sedation scale (Table 29-1) or other criteria adopted by the agency.	Determines patient's level of sedation. Use of a numeric rating scale ensures consistency in assessments and an accurate judgment of patient's changing status and verbal/physical stimulation.

SAFETY ALERT Report a Ramsay sedation score of 4 or higher to the physician.

8. **See Completion Protocol (inside front cover).**

TABLE 29-1 MODIFIED RAMSAY SEDATION SCALE

LEVEL	STATUS
Minimal sedation (anxiolysis)	1. Anxious and agitated or restless or both 2. Cooperative, oriented, and tranquil
Moderate sedation/analgesia	3. Responds to commands spoken in normal voice
Deep sedation/analgesia	4. Brisk response to a light forehead tap or loud auditory stimulus 5. Sluggish response to light forehead tap or loud auditory stimulus 6. No response to light forehead tap or loud auditory stimulus

From Sessler C and others: Evaluating and monitoring analgesia and sedation in the critical care unit, *Crit Care* 12(suppl 3):S2, 2008.

EVALUATION

1. Monitor patient throughout the procedure using the Ramsey Sedation Scale (or other criteria adopted by the agency).
2. *After procedure:* Use Aldrete score (see Table 29-4) and monitor airway patency, oxygen saturation, and pain score every 5 minutes for at least 30 minutes, then every 15 minutes for an hour, and then every 30 minutes until the patient meets discharge criteria on the agency designated scoring system.
3. Ask patient to repeat back what he or she understands regarding the procedure or any postprocedure patient instructions.
4. Have patient's "designated driver" explain any postprocedure education and sign appropriate documents. Patients who receive moderate sedation are restricted from driving for 24 to 48 hours, depending on the procedure, type of sedation, and postprocedure restrictions.

Unexpected Outcomes and Related Interventions

1. Oversedation, evidenced by:
   - Decreasing oxygen saturation; cyanosis; slow, shallow respirations with periods of apnea.
   - Tachycardia.
   - Sedation score of 4 or higher on the Modified Ramsay Sedation Scale, score less than 8 on Aldrete score.

   a. Support patient's breathing via positioning and manual bagging.
   b. Immediately notify physician or health care provider.
   c. Be prepared to administer reversal agents. Naloxone is for reversal of opioids and flumazenil is for reversal of benzodiazepines.
2. Patient develops cardiac instability evidenced by irregular heart rate, change in pulse rate, or change in blood pressure.
   a. Obtain ECG as ordered.
   b. Immediately notify physician or health care provider.

Recording and Reporting

- Document vital signs, oxygen saturation, and sedation level at baseline, then every 5 minutes during the procedure, and every 15 minutes for at least 30 minutes after the procedure according to agency policy.
- Record dosage, route, time of drugs administered during and after the procedure, including the use of reversal agents and significant patient reactions during the procedure. Include IV fluids and blood products if administered.
- Immediately report to patient's physician or health care provider any respiratory distress, cardiac compromise, or altered mental status.

Sample Documentation

1330 Patient tolerated procedure without complications. Patient received a total of Fentanyl, 40 mcg IVP and Versed 1 mg IVP. Patient awake and oriented X 3. Current VS BP 128/70, P 72, R 14, T 98.4; O_2 saturation 98% (on 2L per NP); Aldrete score 10. See Sedation Flowsheet for complete medication administration record, VS history, and Ramsay. Report called to R. Murke, RN. Pt transferred per stretcher to room 3456.

Special Considerations

Pediatric

- Sedation is used in pediatric patients to attain their cooperation with procedures. For this reason, deep sedation is used more often than moderate sedation in children under age 6 or those who did not progress as expected through their developmental stages (American Academy of Pediatrics, 2006).
- Children are more likely than adults to sustain a serious complication resulting from anesthesia. Such complications are often linked to either the cardiovascular or respiratory system. For this reason the American Academy of Pediatrics recommends that personnel who are able to manage a child's airway be present for the procedure (American Academy of Pediatrics, 2006).
- A preprocedure medical evaluation is required. To safely administer sedation to the pediatric patient, consider anatomical and physiological variations, preprocedure assessments, and pharmacological techniques (American Academy of Pediatrics, 2006).
- During the preprocedure assessment, answer the patient's questions in a relaxed and confident manner. When communicating with children, take into account the child's developmental stage.

Geriatric

- Closely monitor the effects of medication on patient's respiratory status and pulse. These drugs interfere with breathing or increase or decrease heart rate as a result of the reduced drug clearance through the kidneys or liver (Lewis and others, 2007).
- Physical limitations of the patient, including hearing and vision loss, contribute to frustration and confusion, compounding the sense of loss of control.

Home Care

- Instruct patient to avoid making any legally binding decisions until at least 24 hours after the procedure.
- Assess the need for a home health care referral.

SKILL 29.5 PROVIDING IMMEDIATE ANESTHESIA RECOVERY IN THE POSTANESTHESIA CARE UNIT (PACU)

The first phase of postoperative care takes place during the immediate recovery period. This phase extends from the time the patient leaves the OR to the time he or she is stabilized in the PACU, meets discharge criteria, and is transferred to the nursing unit. Table 29-2 provides an overview of expected monitoring following anesthesia.

The first 1 to 2 hours are the most critical for assessing the aftereffects of anesthesia, including airway clearance, cardiovascular complications, temperature control, and neurological function. The patient's condition can change rapidly; and assessments must be timely, knowledgeable, and accurate. You need to be aware of the common complications and problems associated with specific types of anesthesia (Table 29-3). Quick judgment regarding the most appropriate interventions is essential. The patient is usually ready for discharge to the general unit when specific standardized criteria are met. The Aldrete score is one of several scoring systems for assessment (Table 29-4). It uses parameters of

TABLE 29-2 POSTANESTHESIA MONITORING

CONDITION	INTERVENTIONS
Airway	
Mechanical obstruction: Decreased LOC and muscle relaxants, resulting in flaccid muscles and tongue blocking airway	Hyperextend neck; pull mandible forward; use nasal or oral airway; encourage deep breathing.
Retained thick secretions: Irritation from anesthesia; anticholinergic medications; history of smoking	Suction; encourage coughing.
Laryngospasm: Stridor from excessive secretions or airway irritation	Encourage to relax and breathe through the mouth. If extreme, it may require positive-pressure ventilation with oxygen, small dose of muscle relaxant (ordered by anesthesiologist), and intubation.
Laryngeal edema: Allergic reaction, irritation from endotracheal (ET) tube, fluid overload	Administer humidified oxygen, antihistamines, steroids, sedatives; and in some cases perform reintubation.
Bronchospasm: Preexisting asthma, anesthetic irritation (expiratory wheeze)	Administer bronchodilators as ordered.
Aspiration: Vomiting from hypotension, accumulated gastric secretions and delayed gastric emptying, pain, fear, position changes	Position on side; suction airway; administer antiemetic as ordered.
Breathing: Hypoventilation/Hypoxemia	
CNS depression: Anesthesia, analgesics, muscle relaxants (respiratory rate shallow)	Encourage to cough and deep breathe; use mechanical ventilator; administer narcotic antagonist, muscle relaxant reversal agent.
Mechanical restriction: Obesity, pain, tight cast or dressings, abdominal distention	Reposition; give analgesic; loosen cast or dressings; implement measures to reduce gastric distention (e.g., nasogastric [NG] intubation, NG suction).
Circulation	
Hypovolemia: Blood loss, dehydration	Administer IV fluids or blood replacement.
Hypotension: Anesthesia/drug effects, vasodilation (possibly from spinal anesthesia); narcotics	Elevate legs; give oxygen, IV fluids, or blood replacement; administer vasopressors; monitor intake and output (I&O), stimulation, hemoglobin, and hematocrit.
Cardiac failure: Preexisting cardiac disease; circulatory overload; excessive/too-rapid fluid replacement	Provide digitalization, diuretics; monitor ECG.
Cardiac arrhythmias: Hypoxemia; myocardial infarction (MI); hypothermia; imbalance of potassium, calcium, magnesium	Provide IV fluid replacement; monitor ECG, urine output; identify and treat cause.
Hypertension: Pain; distended bladder; preexisting hypertension; vasopressor drugs	Compare to preoperative baseline; identify and determine cause.
Compartment syndrome: Pressure from edema causing enough compression to obstruct arterial and venous circulation resulting in ischemia, permanent numbness, loss of function; forearm and lower leg most common sites	Elevate extremity no higher than heart level; remove or loosen bandage or cast to relieve compression; if left untreated, amputation may be required. Do not apply ice.

TABLE 29-3 FOCUSED ASSESSMENT OF PATIENT PROBLEMS RELATED TO ANESTHESIA TYPE

ANESTHESIA TYPE	FOCUSED ASSESSMENT
General	Hypotension; changes in heart rate or rhythm; lowered body temperature; respiratory depression; emergence delirium in the form of shivering, trembling, confusion, or hallucinations
Spinal	Headache, hypotension, decreased cardiac output, cyanosis, difficulty breathing
Local	Skin rash; allergic reaction with edema of the face, lips, mouth, or throat; restlessness; bradycardia; hypotension; ischemic necrosis at injection site
Conscious sedation	Respiratory depression, bradycardia, hypotension, nausea and vomiting
Epidural	Cyanosis, breathing difficulties, decreased heart rate, irregular heart rate, pale skin color, nausea and vomiting

Data from McKenry LM and others: *Mosby's pharmacology in nursing*, ed 22, St Louis, 2006, Mosby; and Rothrock JC: *Alexander's care of the patient in surgery*, ed 13, St Louis, 2007, Mosby.

TABLE 29-4 ALDRETE SCORE FOR POSTANESTHESIA MONITORING

		SCORE
Activity (moving voluntarily on command)	4 extremities	2
	2 extremities	1
	0 extremities	0
Respiration	Able to deep breathe and cough freely	2
	Dyspnea, shallow or limited breathing	1
	Apneic	0
Circulation	BP + 20 mm Hg of presedation level	2
	BP + 20-50 mm Hg of presedation level	1
	BP + 50 mm Hg of presedation level	0
Consciousness	Fully awake	2
	Arousable on having name called	1
	Not responding	0
Color	Normal	2
	Pale, dusky, blotchy, jaundiced or other change	1
	Cyanotic	0

From Aldrete JA: The post-anesthesia recovery score revisited, *J Clin Anesth* 7:89, 1995; Aldrete JA: Post-anesthetic recovery score, *J Am Coll Surg* 205(5):3, 2007.
BP, Blood pressure.

activity, respiration, circulation, consciousness, and oxygen saturation. A score of 8 or less requires additional monitoring. A score of 10 indicates a fully recovered patient.

Recovery from ambulatory surgery requires the same assessments. However, the depth of general anesthesia may be less because the surgery is less involved and of shorter duration. Some patients have only IV conscious sedation, for which intensive monitoring is required for a shorter time period. As soon as the patient is stable and alert, give instructions for home care to the patient and caregiver, including demonstrations and written instructions.

ASSESSMENT

1. Obtain report from circulating nurse and anesthesia provider and a review of patient's surgery course, physiological status, and baseline data. *Rationale: Information helps you assess for potential problems, identify changes in condition, and plan appropriate nursing interventions for patient in PACU.*
2. Review patient's preexisting conditions during operative procedure, including baseline and intraoperative vital signs; oxygen saturation; blood volume or fluid loss; fluid replacement; type of anesthesia; type of airway and size; and extent of surgical wound, including presence of surgical drains. *Rationale: Determines patient's general status and allows you to anticipate the need for special equipment, nursing care, and activities in PACU.*
3. Consider the effects of patient's type of surgery, anesthesia, and restrictions to movement. *Rationale: Information influences type of assessments you initiate, type of complications for which you observe, and specific nursing interventions.*

PLANNING

Expected Outcomes focus on early detection of complications from surgery or anesthesia and adequate pain control by the time of transfer (usually 1 to 2 hours).

- Patient's airway remains clear; and respirations are deep, regular, and within normal limits by the time of transfer. Oxygen saturation remains above 95%.
- Patient's blood pressure, pulse, and temperature remain within previous baseline or normal expected range by the time of transfer.
- Dressings are clean, dry, and intact by discharge from recovery.
- I&O is within expected parameters by discharge from recovery.
- Patient reports relief of discomfort after analgesia or other pain-relief measures by the time of transfer from the immediate recovery area (usually 1 to 2 hours).
- Patient's postoperative assessments are within expected normal postoperative parameters.

Delegation and Collaboration

The skill of initiating and managing postoperative care of the patient cannot be delegated to nursing assistive personnel (NAP). The NAP may obtain vital signs, apply nasal cannula or oxygen mask, and provide basic comfort and hygiene measures. Instruct the NAP by:

- Explaining how often to take vital signs
- Reviewing what to observe and report back to the RN
- Explaining the basic hygiene and comfort measures the patient needs

Equipment

- Stethoscope, sphygmomanometer, pulse oximeter, cardiac monitor, thermometer
- Oxygen equipment such as mask, oxygen regulator and tubing, and positive-pressure delivery system
- Suction equipment
- Dressing supplies
- Warmed blanket or active rewarming device
- Emergency equipment
- Emergency medications

IMPLEMENTATION *for* PROVIDING IMMEDIATE ANESTHESIA RECOVERY IN THE POSTANESTHESIA CARE UNIT (PACU)

STEPS	RATIONALE
1. See Standard Protocol (inside front cover).	
2. On patient's arrival in PACU, identify the patient using two identifiers (e.g., name and birthday or name and account number, according to facility policy).	A patient hand-off identification protocol ensures patient safety and continuity of care. Complies with The Joint Commission standards and improves patient safety (TJC, 2010).
3. As patient enters PACU on stretcher, immediately attach oxygen tubing to regulator and check IV flow rates.	Inhaled oxygen promotes tissue oxygenation during recovery from anesthesia. IV fluids maintain circulatory volume and provide route for emergency drugs.
4. Connect or secure drainage tubes to intermittent suction, depending on drain and order.	Drainage tubes must remain patent to prevent pressure within wound cavity.
5. Attach monitoring devices (e.g., blood pressure cuff, pulse oximeter, ECG, arterial lines).	Provides continual assessment and monitoring of physiological parameters.
6. Compare vital signs with patient's preoperative baseline. Continue assessing vital signs at least every 5 to 15 minutes until stable.	Vital signs may show respiratory depression, cardiac irregularity, hypotension, or hypothermia.
7. Maintain airway after general anesthesia.	
a. If patient is supine, elevate head of bed slightly, pull jaw forward, or turn head to side unless contraindicated. Initially patient may need to be reminded to breathe.	Maintains open airway by keeping tongue out of the way while patient has decreased LOC.

SAFETY ALERT Always stay with the sedated patient until respirations are well established. Patients with an artificial airway may gag and vomit, become restless, or stop breathing.

STEPS	RATIONALE
b. Suction artificial airway and oral cavity with Yankauer suction tip if secretions accumulate (see Chapter 14). Encourage patient to spit out oral airway as gag reflex returns.	Indicates that patient is able to maintain patent airway independently.
8. Call patient by name in normal tone of voice. If there is no response, attempt to arouse patient by touching or gently moving a body part. Explain that surgery is over and patient is in the recovery area.	Determines patient's LOC and ability to follow commands. Assists patient in being oriented to place.
9. Encourage patient to cough and deep breathe every 15 minutes (see Skill 29.2).	Promotes lung expansion, elimination of inhalation anesthetic, and expectoration of mucus secretions.
10. Inspect color of nail beds and skin. Palpate for skin temperature.	Indicators of peripheral tissue perfusion.
11. Assess closely for potential cardiovascular and pulmonary complications of general anesthesia (see Table 29-2).	Postoperative patients who are sedated often become hypoxic.
12. Monitor sensory, circulatory, and neurological responses after spinal or epidural anesthesia.	
a. Monitor for hypotension, bradycardia, and nausea and vomiting.	Blockage of sympathetic nervous system results in vasodilation of major vessels and systemic hypotension.
b. Maintain adequate IV infusion.	Maintains blood pressure by increasing fluid volume and fills temporarily expanded vascular space.
c. Keep patient supine or with head slightly elevated and maintain position.	Minimizes risk of postspinal anesthesia headache from leakage of spinal fluid at injection site, with increased pressures caused by elevation of upper body. Headache is more common with spinal than epidural anesthesia. Occurrence of headache is less with use of smaller-gauge spinal needles (Lewis and others, 2007).

STEPS	RATIONALE
d. Observe patients in PACU until they regain movement in extremities.	Patients fear permanent loss of function.
e. Assess respiratory status, level of spinal sensation, and mobility in lower extremities. Drowsiness will be apparent after IV sedation. The level of anesthesia depends on the location of sensation change. Have patient close eyes and use an alcohol wipe to test sensation along sensory dermatomes Have patient identify if warm or cold. *If patient had general anesthesia:* As patient arouses, introduce yourself and orient him or her to surroundings. *If patient had spinal anesthesia:* Remind him or her that loss of extremity sensation and movement is normal and will return in several hours.	Spinal block is set within 20 minutes of onset. However, if level of anesthesia moves above sixth thoracic vertebra (T6), respiratory muscles are affected. Patients often feel short of breath and, if severe, may require mechanical ventilation.
13. Monitor drainage.	
a. Observe dressing and drains for any evidence of bright red blood.	Dressing maintains hemostasis and absorbs drainage. First dressing changes usually occur 24 hours after surgery and are done by the surgeon unless otherwise ordered.
b. Inform physician of unexpected bloody drainage and reinforce dressing as indicated. Apply direct pressure. Also look underneath patient for any pooling of bloody drainage. Monitor for decreased blood pressure and increased pulse.	Hemorrhage from a surgical wound is most likely within first few hours, indicating inadequate hemostasis during surgery. As dressing becomes saturated, blood often oozes down patient's side and collects under him or her.
c. Inspect condition and contents of any drainage tubes and collecting devices. Note character and volume of drainage.	Determines patency of drainage tube and extent of wound drainage.
d. Observe amount, color, and appearance of urine from indwelling Foley catheter (if present).	Urine output of less than 30 mL/hr is a sign of decreased renal perfusion or altered renal function.
e. If NG tube is present, assess drainage. If not draining, check placement and irrigate if necessary with normal saline (see Chapter 19).	Maintains patency of tube to ensure gastric decompression. Expected drainage is dark or pale, yellow, or green and 100 to 200 mL/hr. Bloody drainage occurs after some surgeries.
f. Monitor IV fluid rates. Observe IV site for signs of infiltration (see Chapter 28).	Provides adequate hydration and circulatory function.
14. Promote comfort.	
a. Provide mouth care by placing moistened washcloth to lips, swabbing oral mucosa with dampened swab, or applying petrolatum to lips.	Mouth is dry from nothing-by-mouth (NPO) status and preoperative anticholinergics such as atropine.
b. Provide a warm blanket or active rewarming therapy to promote warmth and minimize shivering.	General anesthesia impairs thermoregulation, the OR environment is cold, and exposure of the body cavity results in internal heat loss. Shivering increases oxygen consumption predisposes patient to arrhythmias and hypertension, impairs platelet function, alters drug metabolism, impairs wound healing, and increases hospitalization costs because of cumulative adverse outcomes (ASPAN, 2008).
c. Assist with position changes and provide supportive pillows.	Improves ventilation and circulation.
15. Assess pain as patient awakens and until transfer to surgical unit or discharge, including quality, severity, and location. Do not assume that all postoperative pain is incisional pain.	Pain is often not directly related to the surgical procedure (e.g., chest pain [MI/PE] or muscle pain (trauma from positioning). Referred pain (in shoulder) often occurs after a laparoscopy. Systematic assessment of pain helps patients achieve functional status.
16. Provide pain medication as ordered and when vital signs have stabilized.	

Continued

STEPS	RATIONALE
17. Explain patient's condition to patient and inform of plans for transfer to nursing unit or discharge.	Decreases anxiety that can interfere with recovery process.
18. When patient's condition is stabilized (see Table 29-4), contact anesthesiologist to approve transfer to nursing unit or release to home.	A physician is responsible for authorizing transfer or discharge.
19. Before discharge to home from the ambulatory surgery unit, provide verbal and written instructions about: **a.** Signs and symptoms of possible complications. **b.** Not driving for 24 hours. **c.** Avoiding important legal decisions for 24 hours. **d.** Surgical site care. **e.** Activity restrictions. **f.** Pain control. **g.** Dietary modifications or restrictions. **h.** Medications as prescribed. **i.** Plan for follow-up visit. **j.** Reasons to call physician and number to call.	Patients and home care providers must be aware of potential complications and follow-up care.
20. See Completion Protocol (inside front cover).	

EVALUATION

1. Observe respirations: rate, depth, and rhythm. Auscultate breath sounds. Monitor pulse oximetry.
2. Compare all blood pressure, pulse, and temperature readings with patient's baseline and expected normal values.
3. Inspect dressings for drainage.
4. Measure I&O. Urine output should be at least 30 to 50 mL/hr.
5. Ask patient to rate pain on a scale of 0 to 10 and determine location and characteristics.
6. Conduct complete physical assessments with special attention to appropriate assessments according to patient's unique type of surgery (e.g., craniotomy: neurological assessment; neck surgery: airway status; vascular surgery: circulation and bleeding; orthopedic surgery: neurovascular status and immobility or positioning).

Unexpected Outcomes and Related Interventions

1. Patient exhibits respiratory depression (pulse oximetry less than 95%, respiratory rate less than 10 breaths per minute and/or shallow).
   a. Promptly report to physician.
   b. Administer oxygen as ordered by nasal cannula. Give patients with chronic obstructive pulmonary disease (COPD) 2 L/min or less of oxygen.
   c. Encourage deep breathing every 5 to 15 minutes.
   d. Position to promote chest expansion (on side or semi-Fowler's).
   e. Administer prescribed medications (e.g., epinephrine, muscle relaxant, or narcotic reversal agent).
2. Patient exhibits respiratory obstruction (e.g., abnormal lung sounds, snoring, stridor, or crowing sounds, wheezing).
   a. Reposition head/jaw to open airway.
   b. Administer oxygen at 6 to 10 L/min by mask as ordered.
   c. Encourage to cough and deep breathe.
   d. Suction if needed.
   e. Notify anesthesiologist if unresponsive to interventions; may need to be reintubated if severe.
3. Patient exhibits signs of hypovolemia related to internal or incisional hemorrhage.
   a. Elevate patient's legs enough to maintain a downward slope toward the trunk of the body. Do not lower the head past the flat position because this position increases respiratory effort and potentially decreases cerebral perfusion.
   b. Promptly report to physician patient's present status.
   c. Administer oxygen at 6 to 10 L/min by mask per order.
   d. Increase rate of IV fluid or administer blood products as ordered.
   e. Monitor blood pressure and pulse every 5 to 15 minutes.
   f. Apply pressure dressings as follows per order:
      (1) *Abdominal dressing:* Cover bleeding area with several thicknesses of gauze compresses and place tape 7 to 10 cm (3 to 4 inches) beyond width of dressing with firm, even pressure on both sides close to bleeding source. Maintain pressure as you tape entire dressing to maximize pressure at source of bleeding.
      (2) *Dressing on extremity:* Apply rolled gauze, pressing gauze compress over bleeding site. Do not continue tape around entire extremity.

(3) *Dressing in neck region:* Cover with several thicknesses of gauze and place tape 7 to 10 cm (3 to 4 inches) beyond width of dressing. Apply with pressure but do not occlude carotid artery or airway. Assess every 5 to 15 minutes for carotid pulse and evidence of airway obstruction.

g. Patient remains NPO because it is often necessary to return to surgery for control of bleeding.

4. Patient complains of severe incisional pain.
   a. The earliest symptom of compartment syndrome in an extremity is pain unrelieved by analgesics. Other symptoms include numbness, tingling, pallor, coolness, and absent peripheral pulses. The physician *must* be notified. Do not elevate extremity above the level of the heart because this raises venous pressure. Application of ice is contraindicated because vasoconstriction will occur (Lewis and others, 2007).
   b. Perform a pain assessment and administer analgesics before the pain is severe. It is not necessary to wait for patient to request pain medication.
   c. Pain sometimes lowers blood pressure; thus analgesia may restore vital signs to normal. Monitor vital signs carefully.
   d. For patients with PCA, be sure that patient is using device correctly. Warn family not to manipulate the PCA.
5. Patient has hypothermia (temperature less than 36° C [96.8° F]). Shivering increases oxygen consumption, predisposes patient to arrhythmias and hypertension, impairs platelet function and wound healing, and alters drug metabolism. This problem is seen more in infants and children because of immature thermoregulation centers.
   a. Use warm blankets, socks, head coverings, or active rewarming device.
   b. Monitor temperature and patient's thermal comfort level every 30 minutes until normal is reached.

Recording and Reporting

- Document in progress notes patient's arrival time at PACU; include vital signs, LOC, and assessment findings. Also include condition of the dressings and tubes, character of drainage, and all nursing measures initiated.
- Record vital signs and I&O on appropriate flow sheets.
- Report any abnormal assessment findings and signs of complications to physician.

Sample Documentation

1000 Received from OR via stretcher. Alert and oriented ×3. Oxygen administered at 3 L/min per nasal cannula. Abdominal dressing saturated with bright red blood, and pad under patient saturated, 12-cm to 20-cm area. Dressing reinforced with pressure dressing. IV in left forearm infusing with Lactated Ringer's at 150 mL/hr. Surgeon notified of excessive drainage and immediate interventions. Vital signs: BP 110/60, HR 98, R 22, SpO_2 96%. Remains NPO. Warm blanket applied.

Special Considerations

Pediatric

- Maintenance of body temperature in infants and children after surgery is a priority because of their immature temperature-control mechanisms.
- Infants and children normally have higher metabolic rates and differences in physiological makeup than adults, resulting in greater oxygen, fluid, and calorie needs.

Geriatric

- The ability of older adults to tolerate surgery depends on the extent of physiological changes that have occurred with aging, the presence of any chronic diseases, and the duration of the surgical procedure.
- When communicating with older adults, be aware of any auditory, visual, or cognitive impairment that may be present.

Home Care

- Teach patient and primary caregiver about any postoperative exercises, home modifications, or activity limitations.
- If patient is discharged with dressing changes, bedroom or bathroom is usually ideal for procedure. Have primary caregiver perform return demonstration of dressing change.
- Assess need for a home health care referral.

SKILL 29.6 PROVIDING EARLY POSTOPERATIVE AND CONVALESCENT PHASE RECOVERY

Careful monitoring and comfort measures are essential during the early postoperative recovery period, which extends from the time the patient is discharged from the PACU to the time he or she is discharged from the hospital. Patients who have outpatient surgery undergo convalescence at home. Individualize your nursing care depending on the type of surgery, preexisting medical conditions, the risk or development of complications, and the rate of recovery. Teaching promotes the patient's independence, educates the patient about any limitations, and provides resources needed for the patient to achieve an optimal state of wellness.

The convalescent phase lasts for several days or weeks after discharge. During this phase it is important to promote the patient's independence and active participation in care. The patient must have adequate nutrition and hydration to enhance healing. Make sure that his or her goals are realistic.

It is also important that the patient and caregiver have the required supplies and support services at home to promote healing. Some patients require a home health nurse.

ASSESSMENT

1. Obtain phone report from nurse in PACU. *Rationale: A preliminary report allows you to prepare hospital room with necessary supplies and equipment for patient's special needs.*
2. Next, assist with transfer and complete an initial assessment. Review chart to identify type of surgery, preoperative medical risks, and baseline vital signs. *Rationale: Provides baseline to detect any change in patient's condition.*
3. Review surgeon's postoperative orders.

PLANNING

Expected Outcomes focus on preventing complications, maintaining pain control adequate for recovery activities, and promoting patient's self-care postoperatively.

- Patient's breath sounds remain clear bilaterally.
- Patient's vital signs remain within normal limits consistent with preoperative baseline.
- Patient describes pain as less than 4 on a scale of 0 to 10 while engaged in moderate activity by discharge.
- Fluid balance is evident by I&O records.
- Normal bowel sounds are present after bowel surgery or general anesthesia within 48 to 72 hours after surgery.
- Incision wound edges are well approximated; no drainage is noted.
- Patient (or caregiver) describes plans for coping with stress of surgery.
- Patient (or caregiver) describes evidence of complications that should be reported to physician by discharge.
- Patient (or caregiver) describes or demonstrates incision care, dietary modifications, activity restriction, and plans for follow-up visit.

Delegation and Collaboration

The skill of providing early postoperative and convalescent phase recovery cannot be delegated to nursing assistive personnel (NAP). NAP may obtain vital signs, apply nasal cannula or oxygen mask, and provide hygiene or repositioning for comfort. Instruct the NAP by:

- Explaining how often to take vital signs.
- Reviewing what to observe and report back to the nurse.
- Explaining the basic hygiene and comfort measures that the patient needs.

Equipment

- Postoperative bed (recliner for day surgery recovery)
- Stethoscope, sphygmomanometer, thermometer
- IV fluid poles and infusion pumps as needed
- Emesis basin
- Washcloth and towel
- Waterproof pads
- Equipment for oral hygiene
- Pillows
- Facial tissue
- Oxygen equipment and mask
- Suction equipment (to suction airway)
- Dressing supplies
- Intermittent suction (to connect to NG or wound drainage tubes)
- Orthopedic appliances (if needed)
- Clean gloves

IMPLEMENTATION *for* PROVIDING EARLY POSTOPERATIVE AND CONVALESCENT PHASE RECOVERY

STEPS	RATIONALE
1. See Standard Protocol (inside front cover).	
Early Recovery Initial Postoperative Care	
2. If patient is being transported by stretcher, prepare for transfer with bed in high position (level with the stretcher), with sheet folded to side and room for a stretcher to be placed beside bed easily (see Chapter 15).	Arrangement of equipment facilitates safety and smooth transfer process.
3. Assist transport staff to move patient from stretcher to bed (see Chapter 15). Identify patient using two identifiers (e.g., name and birthday or name and account number, according to facility policy).	Ensures correct patient. Complies with The Joint Commission standards and improves patient safety (TJC, 2010).
4. Attach any existing oxygen tubing, position IV fluids, verify IV flow rate settings on infusion pump, and check drainage tubes (e.g., Foley catheter or wound drainage).	Maintains patency of IV and integrity of drainage tubing.
5. Maintain airway. If patient remains sleepy or lethargic, keep head extended and support in side-lying position (see Chapter 14, Skill 14.2).	Minimizes chances of aspiration and obstruction of airway with tongue.

STEPS	RATIONALE
6. Take vital signs and compare findings with vital signs in recovery area and patient's baseline values. Continue monitoring as ordered.	During transfer patient's status may change. Movement of patient and pain level influence stability of vital signs.
7. Encourage coughing and deep breathing (see Skill 29.2) to prevent atelectasis.	Anesthesia, medications, and intubation irritate airways, resulting in secretions and atelectasis. Coughing expands chest, aerates lungs, and mobilizes secretions.
8. If NG tube is present, check placement and irrigate (see Chapter 19, Skill 19.3). Connect to proper drainage device. Connect all other drainage tubes to appropriate suction or collection device. Secure to prevent tension on tubing.	Transfer and movement may dislodge tubes, which would interfere with drainage.
9. Assess patient's surgical dressing for appearance, presence, and character of drainage. Unless contraindicated by physician, outline drainage along the edges with a pen and reassess in 1 hour for change. If no dressing is present, inspect condition of wound (see Chapter 24).	Hemorrhage is most likely to occur on the day of surgery. Dressing should be clean, dry, and intact.
10. Palpate abdomen for bladder distention or use bladder ultrasound when available. If Foley catheter is present, check placement. Be sure that it is draining freely and properly secured. Patient may have continuous bladder irrigations or suprapubic catheter (see Chapter 18).	Anesthesia often contributes to urinary retention. Urinary stasis increases the risk for urinary tract infection (UTI).
11. If no urinary drainage system is present, explain that voiding within 8 hours after surgery is expected. Male patients may void successfully if allowed to stand.	After spinal or epidural anesthesia, risk for urinary retention is increased. Other risks for urinary retention include men, age older than 50 years, previous history of pelvic surgery or voiding problems, and concurrent neurologic diseases (Baldini and others, 2009). Patients may not feel the urge to void. If patient is unable to void and bladder is distended, catheterization is required.
12. Measure all sources of fluid I&O (including estimated blood loss during surgery).	Altered fluid and electrolyte balance is a potential complication of major surgery.
13. Describe the purpose of equipment and frequent observations to patient and significant others.	Unfamiliar sights (equipment, patient's appearance) are often anxiety provoking.
14. Position patient for comfort, maintaining correct body alignment. Avoid tension on surgical wound site.	Reduces stress on suture line. Helps patient relax and promotes comfort.
15. Place call light within reach and raise side rails (one of two or three of four). Instruct to call for assistance to get out of bed.	Promotes patient's safety as effects of anesthesia continue to diminish. A full set of raised side rails may be considered a physical restraint.
16. Assess patient's level of pain on an age-appropriate pain scale. Assess the last time analgesic was given. PCA may be used for pain control (see Chapter 13). Medicate patient as ordered either around-the-clock or prn as ordered during the first 24 to 48 hours.	Determines level of discomfort. Adequate pain control is needed to permit patient to participate with breathing exercises, coughing, and ambulation.
Continued Postoperative Care	
17. Assess vital signs at least every 4 hours or as ordered.	Temperature above 38° C (100.4° F) in the first 48 hours may indicate atelectasis, the normal inflammatory response, or dehydration. Elevation above 37.7° C on the third day or after often indicates wound infection, pneumonia, or phlebitis (Lewis and others, 2007). Altered blood pressure and/or pulse are associated with cardiovascular complications (see Table 29-2).
18. Provide oral care at least every 2 hours as needed. If permitted, offer ice chips.	Medication given before surgery such as an anticholinergic makes mouth dry. Oral care and ice chips promote comfort.

Continued

STEPS	RATIONALE
19. Encourage patient to turn, cough, and deep breathe at least every 2 hours.	Promotes adequate ventilation and minimizes hypoventilation and atelectasis. Especially necessary for patients with a history of smoking, pneumonia, or COPD or patients who are confined to bed rest.
20. Encourage use of incentive spirometer as ordered (see Skill 29.2).	Promotes adequate ventilation.
21. Promote ambulation and activity as ordered. Assess vital signs before and after activity to assess tolerance. Patients often are encouraged to be up in a chair the evening of surgery or the next morning and progress to walking in room or hallway.	Ambulation is the most significant nursing intervention to prevent postoperative complications. Mobility promotes circulation, lung expansion, and peristalsis. Postural hypotension is caused by sudden position changes.
22. Progress from clear liquids to regular diet as tolerated if nausea and vomiting do not occur.	Nausea and vomiting are associated with anesthesia and surgery. IV fluids are usually discontinued when oral intake is tolerated. Some patients must be NPO for several days until bowel sounds are heard.
23. Include patient and family in decision making; answer questions as they arise.	Promotes patient's sense of control and independence and improves self-esteem.
24. Provide opportunity for patients who must adjust to a change in body appearance or function to verbalize feelings.	Radical surgery, amputation, or inoperable cancer often results in anxiety and depression. The grief response to loss of a body organ is common and should be expected.
Convalescent Phase	
25. Assess patient's home environment for safety, cleanliness, and availability of assistance for patient.	Provides information about patient's need for home care.
26. Discuss discharge plans with patient and caregivers: dietary modifications or restrictions, wound care, medications, activity restrictions, and symptoms to report to physician. Clarify follow-up appointments and encourage quick access to emergency telephone numbers. Provide answers to individual patient questions or concerns.	Verifies patient's and caregiver's level of knowledge and any additional teaching needs for discharge. Assists in promoting uncomplicated discharge and patient's independence and participation in care.
27. Keep patient and family informed of progress made toward recovery. Explain the time expected to reach a level of maximal recovery. Provide answers to individual patient questions or concerns.	Decreases anxiety and helps patient know what to anticipate during the convalescent period.
28. See Completion Protocol (inside front cover).	

EVALUATION

1. Auscultate breath sounds bilaterally.
2. Obtain vital signs.
3. Ask patient to describe pain on a scale of 0 to 10 after moderate activity.
4. Evaluate I&O records. Assess time of patient's first post-operative urination.
5. Auscultate bowel sounds.
6. Inspect incision (wound edges well approximated, no drainage noted).
7. Ask patient to describe ability to cope with stress of surgery.
8. Ask patient (or caregiver) to indicate symptoms of complications that should be reported to the physician by discharge.
9. Have patient (or caregiver) describe incision care, dietary modifications or restrictions, activity restrictions, and plans for follow-up visit.

Unexpected Outcomes and Related Interventions

1. Vital signs are above or below patient's baseline or expected range. Initially this could be related to anesthesia efforts, pain, hypovolemic shock, airway obstruction, fluid and electrolyte imbalance, or hypothermia.
   a. Identify contributing factors.
   b. Notify physician.
2. Bowel sounds are absent or decreased. Patient experiences nausea and vomiting. Patient is unable to pass flatus, and abdomen is hard and distended. Paralytic ileus is a common complication after bowel surgery. Intestinal motility may return slowly.
   a. Report to physician.
   b. Insert NG tube as ordered (see Chapter 19).

Recording and Reporting

- Document patient's arrival at nursing unit; describe vital signs, assessment findings, and all nursing measures

initiated in progress note. Document every 4 hours or more frequently as patient's condition warrants.
- Record vital signs and I&O on appropriate flow sheet.
- Report any abnormal assessment findings and signs of complications to physician.

Sample Documentation

Third Postoperative Day After Abdominal Surgery

1800 Vomited 300 mL dark green mucus. Abdomen firm and distended. No bowel sounds heard. Not passing flatus. Rates pain at 7 (scale 0 to 10). Morphine sulfate 10 mg IV. Instructed not to eat or drink anything.

1910 Vomited 200 mL dark green material and C/O being "very nauseated." Abdominal pain now rated at 6 (scale 0 to 10). Dr. K notified. NG tube inserted and connected to low intermittent suction as ordered with return of 400 mL dark green material within 15 minutes. Phenergan 5 mg given intramuscularly for nausea.

1950 Resting comfortably. Denies nausea. Pain now rated at 4 (scale 0 to 10). NG draining 200 mL of dark green drainage.

Special Considerations

Pediatric

- Assessment of a child's perceptions of the surgical experience enforces positive experiences and clarifies misconceptions. Drawing and storytelling are effective methods that allow children to share their thoughts and feelings (Hockenberry and Wilson, 2009).
- Use appropriate pain assessment tools to determine child's pain level.

Geriatric

- Older adults often experience a longer and more difficult postoperative recovery. Assess carefully for the development of postoperative complications.
- Assess for postoperative delirium and changes in mental status along with potential causes.
- Postoperative pain tends to be undertreated in older adults. Some patients fear "becoming addicted" or minimize pain because they are stoic. Assess for pain and encourage use of nonpharmacological measures such as relaxation and imagery along with pain medications (Lewis and others, 2007).

Home Care and Long-Term Care

- Teach patient and primary caregiver about any postoperative exercises, home modifications, activity limitations, wound dressing care, medications, and nutritional needs.
- If patient is discharged with dressing changes, the bedroom or bathroom is usually ideal for procedure. Have patient and primary caregiver perform return demonstration of dressing change.
- Make referral to home health services if patient and caregiver will have difficulty providing the expected level of care needed.

REVIEW QUESTIONS

Case Study for Questions 1 to 3

Mr. Gates, a 39 year-old, arrived as a same-day-surgery admission to have arthroscopic surgery on his left knee. He is scheduled to have spinal anesthesia with light sedation. He is a runner, nonsmoker, drinks 1 to 2 beers daily, and has a negative health history.

1. At which points in his procedural planning and actual procedure should the Universal Protocol for preoperative verification of correct person, correct site, and correct procedure occur for Mr. Gates? Select all that apply.
   1. At the time the procedure was scheduled
   2. At the time of preadmission testing and assessment
   3. At the time of admission or entry into the agency for a procedure
   4. Before the patient leaves the preprocedure area or enters the procedure room
   5. Any time the responsibility of care of the patient is transferred to another member of the procedural care team
2. Which of the following elements are required on Mr. Gates' procedural checklist? Select all that apply.
   1. Assessment (physician, nursing, anesthesia)
   2. Signed consent form
   3. Family contact information
   4. Any required blood products, implants, and/or special equipment for the procedure
   5. Test results
3. Which of the following is true regarding when Mr. Gates' operative site should be marked?
   1. Immediately after he receives sedation and spinal anesthesia so he doesn't become fearful that the surgery team is unsure how to perform his surgery
   2. In the holding area outside of the OR, with Mr. Gates awake, alert and participating in the site-marking procedure
   3. In the OR by the circulating nurse while the surgeon is scrubbing
   4. It doesn't need to be marked since it is a minor surgical procedure.
4. A new admission has arrived, and the surgical unit is very busy. Which of the following activities is not delegated to the NAP?
   1. Vital sign collection
   2. Preoperative teaching
   3. Placement of antiembolic stockings
   4. Assisting patient with deep-breathing exercises

5. The nurse's role in informed consent includes which of the following?
   1. Informing the patient of the prognosis if patient refuses surgery
   2. Explaining the risks, benefits, and alternatives of the planned surgery
   3. Verifying the patient's understanding of the surgical procedure and being sure the patient's signature is complete on the consent form
   4. Asking the patient for consent for the planned surgery
6. A nurse is responsible for properly instructing patients on breathing exercises before surgery. Place the following steps for deep breathing and coughing in the correct order.
   - a. Have patient place palms of hands across from each other along the lower rib cage or upper abdomen.
   - b. Have patient take slow, deep breath; hold for count of 3 seconds; and exhale.
   - c. Have patient sit in high-Fowler's position with knees bent.
   - d. Have patient take slow, deep breaths, inhaling through nose.
   - e. Have patient repeat breathing exercise 3 to 5 times.
   1. a, c, b, d, e
   2. c, a, d, b, e
   3. b, c, a, d, e
   4. c, b, a, d, e
7. Which assessment findings in the patient in PACU need to be reported to the physician? Select all that apply.
   1. Respiratory rate <10 per minute with shallow breathing
   2. Bright red wound drainage saturating dressing
   3. Pain rating of 3 on a scale of 0 to 10
   4. Scattered crackles in posterior lung bases
8. The nurse is checking a patient into the room on the surgical unit after abdominal surgery. There is a 1.5-cm (½ in) diameter spot of serosanguineous drainage on the dressing. What action should the nurse take at this time?
   1. Notify the physician of bleeding from the wound.
   2. Note the amount of drainage on the dressing and continue to monitor.
   3. Remove the dressing to check for bleeding from the suture line.
   4. Apply gentle pressure to the site for 5 minutes.
9. Which position is used to minimize the chance of aspiration in a patient who is lethargic after general anesthesia?
   1. High-Fowler's
   2. Semi-Fowler's
   3. Side-lying
   4. Supine

REFERENCES

American Academy of Pediatrics: Guidelines and management of pediatric patients during and after sedation for diagnostic and therapeutic procedures: an update, *Pediatrics* 118:2387, 2006.

American Association of Nurse Anesthetists: AANA_ASA joint statement regarding propofol administration, 2004, accessed September 30, 2010.

American Society of Anesthesiologists (ASA): *Continuum of depth of sedation definition of general anesthesia and levels of sedation/analgesia,* 2004, http://www.asahq.org/publicationsAndServices/standards/20.pdf, September 30, 2010.

American Society of Anesthesiologists (ASA): *Relative value guide,* Park Ridge, Ill, 2008, The Society.

American Society of PeriAnesthesia Nurses (ASPAN): *2008-2010 Standards of perianesthesia nursing practice,* Cherry Hill, 2008, ASPAN.

Andrews M and others: *Transcultural concepts in nursing care,* ed 5, Philadelphia, 2007, Lippincott.

Association of Peri Operative Registered Nurses (AORN): *Perioperative standards and recommended practices,* Denver, 2009, AORN.

Baldini G and others: Postoperative urinary retention, *Anesthesiology* 110(5):1139, 2009.

Hedrick TL and others: Prevention of surgical site infections, *Expert Rev Anti Infect Ther* 4(2):223, 2006.

Hockenberry MJ, Wilson D: *Wong's essentials of pediatric nursing,* ed 8, St Louis, 2009, Mosby.

Institute for Healthcare Improvement (IHI): *5 million lives campaign; getting started kit: prevent surgical site infections how-to-guide,* 2007. http://www.ihi.org/IHI/Programs/Campaign/BoardsonBoard.htm; accessed October 29, 2010.

Lewis SM and others: *Medical-surgical nursing: assessment and management of clinical problems,* ed 7, St Louis, 2007, Mosby.

Johansson K and others: Empowering orthopedic patients through preadmission education: results from a clinical study, *Patient Educ Couns* 66:84, 2006.

MedQIC: *Surgical Care Improvement Project (SCIP). SCIP Project Information,* http://qualitynet.org/dcs/ContentServer?c=MQParents&pagename=Medqic%2FContent%2FParentShellTemplate&cid=1122904930422&parentName=Topic, accessed September 1, 2009.

Sandberg EH and others: Clinicians consistently exceed a typical person's short-term memory during preoperative teaching, *Anesth Analg* 107(3):972, 2008.

Spry C: *Essentials of perioperative nursing,* ed 4, Gaithersburg, Md, 2009, Aspen.

The Joint Commission: *2010 National Patient Safety Goals,* Oakbrook Terrace, Ill, 2010, The Commission, http://www.jointcommission.org/PatientSafety/NationalPatientSafetyGoals.

Thomas KH, Sethares KA: An investigation of the effects of preoperative interdisciplinary patient education on understanding postoperative expectations following a total joint arthroplasty, *Orthop Nurs* 27(6):374, 2008.

CHAPTER

30

Emergency Measures for Life Support in the Hospital Setting

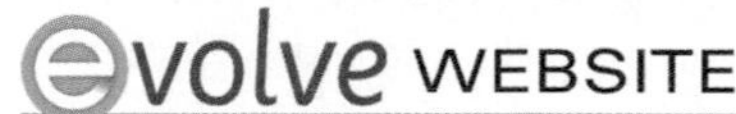

http://evolve.elsevier.com/Perry/nursinginterventions

Cardiac arrest is the cessation of circulating blood flow that eliminates oxygen transport and perfusion. Certain types of irregular heart rhythms or dysrhythmias increase the patient's risk for a cardiac arrest. Ventricular fibrillation or ventricular tachycardia without a pulse requires defibrillation, which is an externally applied electrical shock to attempt to restore a perfusing rhythm. Early defibrillation may return the heart quickly to a normal rhythm, and the patient may not progress to a respiratory arrest. Cardiopulmonary arrest involves the collapse of both the respiratory and cardiovascular systems. All patients receive cardiopulmonary resuscitation (CPR) in the event of an arrest unless otherwise indicated, such as a patient having an advance directive for final health care or a "do not resuscitate" status.

PATIENT-CENTERED CARE

Advance directives offer valuable information concerning a patient's resuscitation status and individual patient decisions regarding resuscitation efforts. Although advance directives are often addressed before or during the patient's hospital admission, you play an important role in encouraging patients to complete the document. Because of their unique relationship with patients and the associated high level of trust, nurses are the ideal facilitators for the initiation of advance directives. They have the opportunity to assist patients and their families in making informed decisions about end-of-life care. Patients want to discuss end-of-life care, and they expect providers to initiate these conversations. An advance directive can minimize disagreements among family members when the patient is physically or mentally unable to make decisions.

SAFETY

Perform emergency procedures quickly and efficiently to ensure the patient's best chance of survival. Some of these procedures involve the use of electrical energy, including defibrillation. Good skin contact between the paddle or pad and patient's chest is essential to avoid the release of live electricity into the environment. Clear communication to all other staff in the room is essential at the time of defibrillation so everyone is aware and does not touch the patient or the bed at time of the shock. Other safety issues include the appropriate hand position when performing chest compressions. Last, using a respiratory barrier between the patient and rescuers during artificial ventilation provides safety measures for both the staff performing mouth-to-mask ventilations and the patient.

EVIDENCE-BASED PRACTICE TRENDS

Ewy, G and Kern, K: Recent advances in cardiopulmonary resuscitation, *J Am Coll Cardiol* 53, 149, 2009.

Cardiocerebral resuscitation (CCR) presents new guidelines for the resuscitation of patients with cardiac arrest. It includes continuous chest compressions for bystanders, a new emergency medical services (EMS) algorithm, and aggressive postresuscitation care (Table 30-1). The CCR method has been shown to dramatically improve survival in a group of patients with witnessed arrest and shockable rhythm. The CCR method suggests the use of continuous chest compressions without mouth-to-mouth ventilations for witnessed cardiac arrest. For bystanders with access to automated external defibrillators (AED) and EMS personnel who arrive

TABLE 30-1 ADULT, CHILD, AND INFANT CPR TECHNIQUES (HEALTH CARE PROVIDER)

TECHNIQUE	ADULT	CHILD (1 TO 8 YEARS OLD)	INFANT (UNDER 1 YEAR) DOES NOT INCLUDE NEWBORNS
Chest compressions: Push hard and fast to allow complete recoil	Begin compressions if no pulse Lower half of sternum, between nipples Heel of one hand, other hand on top 1½ to 2 inches One or two rescuers: 30 compressions, 2 breaths (30:2). Continue until AED is available and ready to analyze rhythm	Begin compressions if no pulse or pulse <60/min Lower half of sternum, between nipples Heel of one hand or as for adults At. least ⅓ depth of chest One rescuer: 30 compressions, 2 breaths (30:2) Two rescuers: 15 compressions, 2 breaths (15:2)	Begin compressions if no pulse or pulse <60/min Just below nipple line (lower ½ of sternum) Two fingers, two thumb (encircling hands) At least ⅓ depth of chest One rescuer: 30 compressions, 2 breaths (30:2) Two rescuers: 15 compressions, 2 breaths (15:2)
Defibrillation using AED	Use adult pads. Provide 5 cycles of CPR before shock if response time is greater than 4 to 5 minutes and arrest was not witnessed. Otherwise AED should be applied as soon as available and shock as soon as advised. Resume compressions immediately after shock.	Use child pads whenever possible. If none, use adult pads but do not overlap them. Apply AED as soon as available and shock as soon as advised.	Use child pads whenever possible. If none, use adult pads but do not overlap them. Apply AED as soon as available and shock as soon as advised.
Airway	Head tilt–chin lift (HCP: Suspected trauma, use jaw thrust)	Head tilt–chin lift (HCP: Suspected trauma, use jaw thrust)	Head tilt–chin lift (HCP: Suspected trauma, use jaw thrust)
HCP: Rescue breathing with mouth-to-mask or bag-mask without chest compressions	10 to 12 breaths/min (approximate) 1 breath every 5-6 seconds	12 to 20 breaths/min (approximate) 1 breath every 3 seconds	12 to 20 breaths/min (approximate) 1 breath every 3 seconds
HCP: Rescue breaths for CPR with advanced airway (endotracheal tube/ tracheotomy)	8 to 10 breaths/min (approximate) 1 breath every 6-8 seconds	8 to 10 breaths/min (approximate) 1 breath every 6-8 seconds	8 to 10 breaths/min (approximate) 1 breath every 6-8 seconds
Foreign body airway obstruction	Abdominal thrusts	Abdominal thrusts	Back slaps and chest thrusts

Data from American Heart Association: Part 5 and 13. Adult and Pediatric Basic Life Support, *Circulation* 122 (Suppl 3): S685-S705 and S862-S875, 2010.
HCP, Health care provider.

during the first 4 or 5 minutes of the arrest, the delivery of a defibrillator shock is recommended. The updated CPR guidelines from the American Heart Association (AHA) also include a hands-only approach (continuous chest compressions) for the untrained lay rescuer. The sequence of actions has changed from A B C (airway, breathing, circulation) to C A B (circulation, airway, breathing) The AHA's "chain of survival" includes:

- Immediate recognition and activation of emergency medical response
- Early CPR that emphasizes chest compressions
- Rapid defibrillation if indicated
- Effective advanced cardiac life support
- Integrated post–cardiac arrest care

SKILL 30.1 INSERTING AN OROPHARYNGEAL AIRWAY

An oropharyngeal airway is a semicircular-shaped, minimally flexible, curved piece of hard plastic (Fig. 30-1). When inserted, it extends from just outside the lips, over the tongue, and to the pharynx (Fig. 30-2). Oral airways allow you to suction through a central core or along the side of the airway, facilitate resuscitation, and maintain airway patency in the unconscious patient.

The oral airway is sized for adults and children, varying in length and width (Table 30-2). Choose the size of an oral airway on the basis of the patient's age and the width and length of the patient's mouth. Size is correct if, when the flange is held parallel to the front teeth with the airway against the patient's cheek, the end of the curve reaches the angle of the jaw.

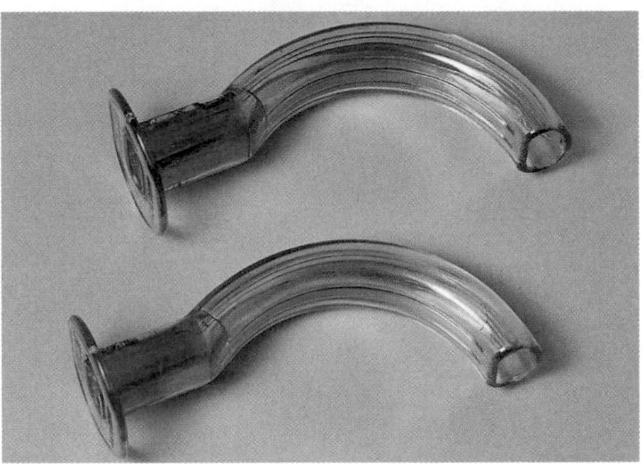

FIG 30-1 Oral airways.

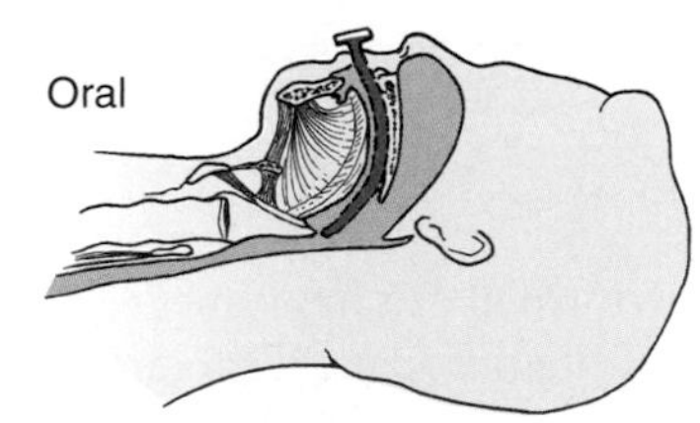

FIG 30-2 Placement of oral airway.

TABLE 30-2 ORAL AIRWAY GUIDELINES FOR SIZE BY AGE

SIZE	AGE
000	Premature neonates
00	Newborn
0	Newborn to 1 yr
1	1 to 2 yr
2	2 to 6 yr
3	6 to 18 yr
4 and larger	Older than 18 yr

ASSESSMENT

1. Observe for "gurgling" with respiratory cycle, absent cough or gag reflex, increased oral secretions or excretions, excessive drooling, grinding teeth, clenched teeth, biting of oral tracheal or gastric tubes, labored respirations, and increased respiratory rate. *Rationale: These conditions place patients at risk for obstruction of upper airway.*

> **SAFETY ALERT** An oral airway is only used for unresponsive patients without an active gag reflex. Placement of an oral airway may stimulate vomiting and possible aspiration or cause laryngospasm if inserted in a semiconscious patient.

> **SAFETY ALERT** Never insert an oropharyngeal airway in a patient with recent oral trauma, oral surgery, or loose teeth.

2. Determine factors that may be contributing to upper airway obstruction, such as presence of nasal and oral airway and drainage tubes (swallowing is more difficult with tubes in place). *Rationale: Allows you to accurately assess need for oral airway. Patients at greater risk for upper airway obstruction are adults with loss of consciousness, seizure disorders, neuromuscular diseases, increased oral secretions or excretions, or facial trauma.*
3. In postoperative patients awakening from anesthesia, assess for presence of cough or gag reflex; gently place tongue blade on back of patient's tongue. *Rationale: Provides guide as to when oral airway can be safely removed following general anesthesia.*

PLANNING

Expected Outcomes focus on the improvement in airway patency and respiratory status.

1. Patient's respiratory status improves, as evidenced by easier respirations with normal rate, easier removal of secretions, and lack of gurgling noise in throat with respirations.
2. Patient is not able to grind teeth or bite tubes.
3. Patient's tongue does not relax back into pharynx and obstruct airway.

Delegation and Collaboration

The skill of inserting an oropharyngeal airway cannot be delegated to nursing assistive personnel (NAP). Respiratory therapists have the training to insert an oral airway on delegation. Instruct the NAP to:

- Immediately report to the nurse any signs of airway distress, vomiting, or change in level of consciousness.

Equipment

- Appropriate-size oral airway
- Clean gloves
- Gown if needed
- Tissues or washcloths
- Suction equipment if indicated
- Tape
- Face shield if indicated
- Tongue blade
- Stethoscope

IMPLEMENTATION *for* INSERTING AN OROPHARYNGEAL AIRWAY

STEPS	RATIONALE
1. See Standard Protocol (inside front cover).	
2. Position unconscious patient; semi-Fowler's position is preferred.	Provides easy access to oral cavity.
3. Apply face shield (when possible).	Reduces transmission of microorganisms.
4. Whenever possible use padded tongue blade if you need to open patient's mouth.	Provides access to oral cavity.
5. Insert oral airway.	When inserting airway, take care not to push patient's tongue into pharynx.
a. Hold oral airway with curved end up and insert distal end until airway reaches back of throat; then turn airway over 180 degrees and follow natural curve of tongue. *Option:* Hold airway sideways and insert halfway; rotate airway 90 degrees while gliding it over natural curvature of tongue.	Provides patent airway and prevents displacement of patient's tongue into posterior oropharynx. Secure airway temporarily with tape on upper and lower flange. May need to insert an endotracheal (ET) airway as soon as possible.
6. Suction secretions as needed.	Removes secretions; maintains patent airway.
7. Reassess patient's respiratory status; auscultate lungs.	Verifies respiratory status and patent airway.
8. Clean patient's face with soft tissue or washcloth.	Promotes hygiene.
9. Administer frequent oral hygiene.	Increases patient comfort and removes debris. Provides moisture to oral mucosal tissues.
10. Oral airway needs to be removed, cleaned, and reinserted routinely in patients with a copious amount of oral mucus secretions (see agency policy).	Reduces risk of aspiration.
11. See Completion Protocol (inside front cover).	

EVALUATION

1. Observe patient's respiratory status and compare respiratory assessments before and after insertion of oral airway.
2. Assess that airway is patent, that patient does not occlude airway by biting tube, and that patient's tongue does not obstruct airway.

Unexpected Outcomes and Related Interventions

1. Patient pushes airway out of place or out of mouth.
   a. If patient regains consciousness and is gagging, place in lateral recumbent (rescue) position and suction.
   b. Determine patient's continued need for oral airway.
2. Airway obstruction is not relieved.
   a. Obtain immediate assistance.
   b. Reinsert airway.

Recording and Reporting

- Record and report assessment findings while inserting oral airway; size of oral airway; placement; any other procedures performed at same time, especially positioning, secretions obtained, patient's tolerance of procedure.

Sample Documentation

1000 Unresponsive, airway secretions increasing, upper airway gurgling auscultated. Gag reflex absent. Size 4 oropharyngeal airway inserted without trauma. Airway suctioned for yellow airway secretions. Bilateral lung sounds; no adventitious sounds.

Special Considerations

Pediatric

- Oral airways are seldom used in treatment of airway obstruction in children and infants. Because the child's airway is narrow, oral airways are often more occlusive than beneficial (Hockenberry and Wilson, 2007).
- For infants and small children sliding oral airway along side of mouth rather than with tip up is recommended because the soft palate is easily injured.

SKILL 30.2 USING AN AUTOMATED EXTERNAL DEFIBRILLATOR

The AED incorporates a rhythm analysis system. It eliminates the need for training in rhythm interpretation and makes early defibrillation practical and achievable. The device is attached to a patient by two adhesive pads and connecting cables. Most AEDs are stand-alone boxes with a very simple three-step function (Fig. 30-3) and verbal prompts to guide the responder. All AEDs offer automated rhythm analysis whereby the rhythm is compared to thousands of other rhythms stored in the computer software of the AED. On rhythm identification some AEDs automatically provide the electrical shock after a verbal warning (fully automated). Other AEDs recommend a shock, if needed, and prompt the responder to press the shock button.

Delegation and Collaboration

BLS certification provides hands-on training with an AED for laypersons, assistive personnel (AP), and licensed health care professionals. Most hospitals using AEDs have given the authority to use an AED to all CPR-certified personnel, including AP. Refer to specific hospital policies for use of the AED.

Equipment

- Automated external defibrillator
- Pair of AED adhesive pads

FIG 30-3 Automated external defibrillator device. (Courtesy Philips Medical Systems.)

ASSESSMENT

1. Establish patient's unresponsiveness and call for help. *Rationale: Assists the nurse in determining if the patient is unresponsive rather than asleep, intoxicated, hearing impaired, or post seizure (postictal).*
2. Establish absence of respirations and the lack of circulation within 10 seconds: no palpable pulse, no respirations, no movement. *Rationale: Indicates need for emergency measures, including AED.*

SAFETY ALERT An AED should only be applied to a patient who is unconscious, not breathing, and pulseless. For infants or children younger than 8 years old, AED pads designed for children should be used. If child pads are not available, use adult AED pads but do not allow the pads to overlap (Haskell and Atkins, 2010).

PLANNING

Expected Outcomes focus on improving cardiac rhythm and pulse rate and the return of respirations.

1. Patient's cardiac rhythm is converted back to a stable rhythm.
2. Patient regains pulse and respirations.

IMPLEMENTATION *for* USING AN AUTOMATED EXTERNAL DEFIBRILLATOR

STEPS	RATIONALE
1. Assess patient for unresponsiveness, no breathing and pulselessness within 10 seconds.	
2. Activate code team in accordance with hospital policy and procedure.	First available person to bring the resuscitation cart and AED.
3. Start chest compressions and continue until AED is attached and verbal prompt advises you, "do *not* touch the patient."	To minimize the interruption time of chest compressions, continue CPR while AED is being applied and turned on.
4. Place AED next to the patient near the chest or head.	

SAFETY ALERT If the AED is available immediately, attach it to patient as soon as possible. The faster defibrillation is delivered, the better the survival rate (Ewy and Kern, 2009).

Continued

STEPS	RATIONALE
5. Turn on the power (see illustration).	Turning on the power begins the verbal prompts to guide you through the next steps.

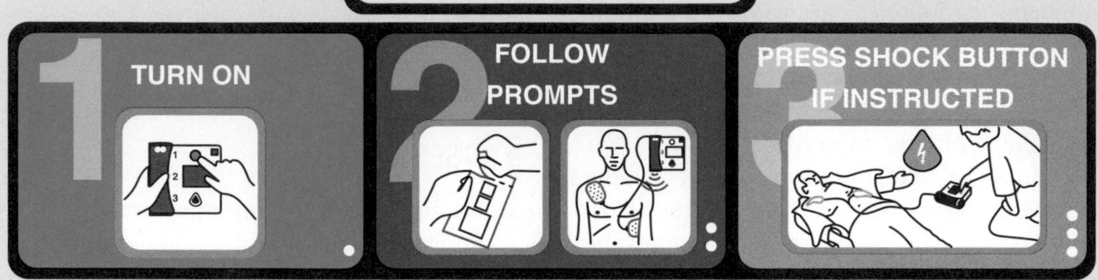

STEP 5 Power panel with automated external defibrillatory prompts. (Courtesy Philips Medical Systems.)

STEPS	RATIONALE
6. Attach the device. Place the first AED pad on the upper right sternal border directly below the clavicle. Place the second AED pad lateral to the left nipple with the top of the pad a few inches below the axilla (see illustration for Step 5). Ensure that the cables are connected to the AED. Do not attach pads to a wet surface, over a medication patch, or over a pacemaker or implanted defibrillator.	Alternative pad placement of AED pads is not recommended. The fastest application technique is the one mentioned. AEDs analyze most heart rhythms using lead II. If AED pads are placed as directed, patient's heart rhythm will be analyzed in lead II. Patients with large amounts of chest hair may require shaving to obtain adequate pad contact. Wet surfaces, implanted defibrillators, and medication patches reduce the effectiveness of the defibrillation attempt and result in complications.
7. Do *not* touch the patient when the AED prompts you. Direct rescuers and bystanders to avoid touching the patient by announcing "Clear!" Allow the AED to analyze the rhythm. Some devices require that an analysis button be pressed. The AED takes approximately 5 to 15 seconds to analyze the rhythm.	Each brand of AED is different; thus familiarity with the model is important. Not touching the patient when directed prevents artifact errors, avoids all movement during analysis, and prevents shock from being delivered to bystanders.
8. Before pressing the shock button, announce loudly to clear the victim and perform a visual check to ensure that no one is in contact with victim.	Clearing patient ensures safety for those involved in rescue efforts.
9. Immediately begin chest compression after the shock and continue for 2 minutes with a ratio of 30:2 (30 compressions and 2 breaths).	
10. After 2 minutes of CPR, AED prompts you not to touch patient and resume analysis of patient's rhythm. This cycle continues until patient regains a pulse or the physician determines death.	

EVALUATION

1. Inspect pad adhesion to chest wall. If pads are not in good contact with chest wall, remove them and apply a new set. Attach new set of pads to AED.
2. Monitor vital signs and continue resuscitative efforts until patient regains pulse or physician determines death.

Unexpected Outcomes and Related Interventions

1. Patient's heart rhythm does not convert into a stable rhythm with pulse after defibrillation.
   a. Observe pad contact with patient's chest wall.
   b. Do not touch patient during AED rhythm analysis.
2. Patient's skin has burns under AED pads.
   a. Observe that AED pad contacts with patient's chest wall.
   b. Ensure that patient's chest wall is dry before applying pads.

Recording and Reporting

- Immediately report arrest via hospital-wide communication system, indicating exact location of victim.
- Record in nurses' notes or on designated CPR worksheet: onset of arrest, time and number of AED shocks (you will not know the exact energy level used by the AED), time

and energy level of manual defibrillations, medications given, procedures performed, cardiac rhythm, use of CPR, and patient's response.

Sample Documentation

0900 Patient found unresponsive on floor of room; code team activated. No palpable pulse or observable respirations. CPR initiated at 0905.

0910 AED attached and pads placed on patient's chest, 1 shock applied, no palpable pulse. CPR resumed at 0912.

0915 Second shock applied; no palpable pulse and CPR continued. Code team arrived at 0918.

Special Considerations

Pediatric

- Many AEDs are equipped to deliver energy suitable for infants and children under 8 years of age using specific pads for children. Adult pads can be used if child pads are not available, but be sure not to overlap the pads. Manual defibrillation using lower energy settings (2 to 4 joules/kg) is preferred for infants (Haskell and Atkins, 2010).

Home Care

- AEDs are available for use in the community and home setting.
- Patient and family should keep emergency numbers taped to phone or consider programming them into speed dial function on both home and mobile phones. Stress the use of 911.

SKILL 30.3 CODE MANAGEMENT

This skill includes the initial response and management of cardiopulmonary arrest. All who respond to cardiopulmonary arrests should arrive well trained in a simple, easy-to-remember approach. The Advanced Cardiac Life Support (ACLS) Provider Course teaches the primary and secondary survey approach to arrest situations. With each step the responder performs an assessment and then, if the assessment so indicates, a management intervention. Initially a code is managed by the first responder performing the basic skills of CPR, which includes the primary survey of *C* (circulation), *A* (airway), *B* (breathing), *D* (early defibrillation). This survey continues until the code team arrives. The initial process also includes the notification of the hospital resuscitation team or code team. Most of the code team members have been trained in the ACLS guidelines and the performance of the secondary survey: *C* (rhythm analysis of cardiac rhythm), *A* (airway intubation), *B* (confirmation of airway and ventilation), and D (differential diagnosis of the cause). Both surveys must be reassessed continually and managed as appropriate throughout the code situation.

The hospital response team usually includes a physician; intensive care nurse; respiratory therapy personnel; anesthesia personnel; and possibly radiology, pharmacists, and laboratory technologists. A representative from pastoral care is often available to be with the family. If the patient is in a two-bed room, assist the roommate to leave. If the roommate cannot leave, have the chaplain or AP remain with the person. In addition, move excess furniture out of the way and bring resuscitation equipment into the room.

CPR is initiated and maintained by the discovering staff until the code team arrives. As soon as possible, determine the patient's cardiac rhythm and, if appropriate, defibrillate the patient with a manual defibrillator or an AED.

CPR certification is required of most nursing students or for entry into the nursing program. As a result, CPR is not covered in detail in this chapter. Table 30-1 details a few summary points about CPR. This skill focuses on code management of the patient with cardiac arrest.

ASSESSMENT

1. Determine if patient is unconscious by shaking patient and shouting, "Are you OK?" Assess patient's unresponsiveness. *Rationale: Confirms that patient is unconscious rather than asleep, intoxicated, or hearing impaired. Substance abuse, hypoglycemia, ketoacidosis, and shock can also cause unconsciousness.*

> **SAFETY ALERT** If an unconscious patient has adequate respirations and pulse, remain with him or her until further assistance is present. Place victim in a modified lateral recovery position (see illustration) if patient is not injured. Continue to determine presence of respirations and pulse throughout because a respiratory or cardiopulmonary arrest is still possible. Lateral recovery position helps to avoid airway blockage by the tongue and aspiration of oral fluids.

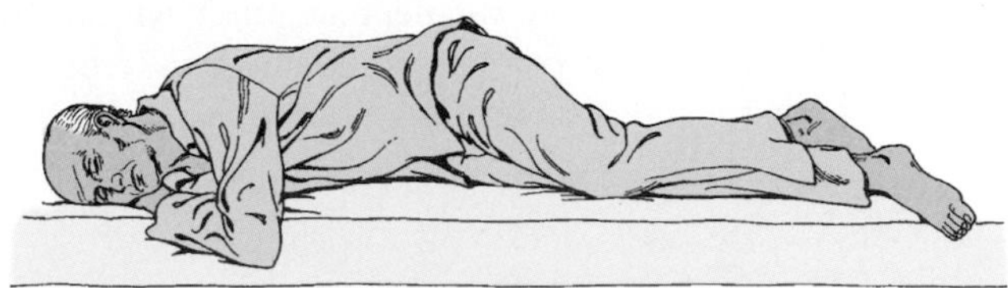

STEP 1 Recovery position.

2. Activate emergency medical service in accordance with hospital policy and procedure (e.g., call a code blue or 99) to ensure the timely delivery of the AED or manual defibrillator. *Rationale: Many adult victims are in ventricular fibrillation and need defibrillation and antidysrhythmic*

drugs as soon as possible. Early access to emergency cardiac care systems improves patient outcomes (Ewy and Kern, 2009).

PLANNING

Expected Outcomes focus on the restoration of cardiac and pulmonary function before irreversible organ damage occurs.

1. Patient regains pulse and respirations or is assisted with a ventilator as long as a pulse exists.
2. No complications occur from the resuscitation.
3. Physician may terminate CPR and pronounce death.

Delegation and Collaboration

The skill of code management cannot be delegated to nursing assistive personnel (NAP). However, NAP who are certified in BLS techniques can perform the basic skills of CPR. Most NAP are certified in BLS and may use an AED. However, manual defibrillation is usually reserved for licensed personnel who have ACLS certification. All other skills in the code situation are directed by the code team leader and performed by nurses, respiratory therapists, and other health care professionals.

Equipment

- Crash cart (Fig. 30-4): Most adult crash carts have the following equipment:
  - Clean and sterile gloves, gown, protective eyewear
  - Oxygen source
  - Bag mask
  - Oral airways
  - Laryngoscope, handle, and laryngoscope blades, straight and curved
  - ET tube, various sizes (6 to 8 Fr)
  - Carbon dioxide monitors (optional, see agency policy)
  - Tape
  - Backboard
  - AED and/or manual defibrillator
  - Intravascular needles (14- to 22-gauge)
  - Central vascular access kit
  - IV tubing, fluids (9% normal saline [NS], D_5W)
  - Syringes
  - Laboratory specimen tubes
  - Arterial blood gas kit
  - Emergency medications
  - ACLS guidelines or algorithms
  - Suction machine and suction equipment if not with crash cart

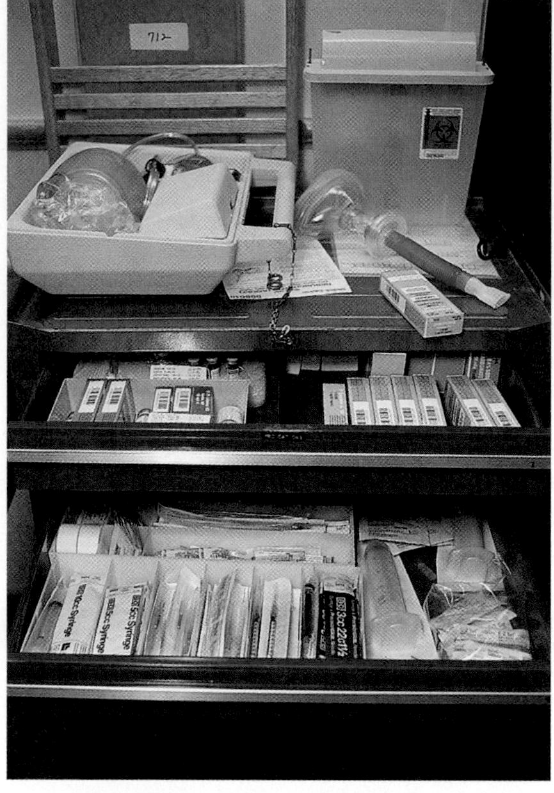

FIG 30-4 Emergency resuscitation cart.

IMPLEMENTATION *for* CODE MANAGEMENT

STEPS	RATIONALE
Primary Survey: C (Circulation)	
1. Check carotid pulse on adult or child; use brachial pulse on an infant. If no definite pulse within 10 seconds, begin chest compressions. Check if victim is unresponsive and not breathing or only gasping.	Carotid pulse is present when other peripheral pulses are not palpable. Because the neck of an infant is short, the carotid pulse is difficult to locate. Compressions are contraindicated when a pulse is present in adults. Compressions are to be started in children or infants who have no pulse or a pulse rate <60/min and are unresponsive and not breathing.
2. Place victim on a hard surface such as floor, ground, or backboard. Victim must be flat. If necessary, logroll victim to flat, supine position using spine precautions.	Facilitates external compression of heart. Heart is compressed between sternum and spinal vertebrae, which must be on a hard, flat surface.
Primary Survey: A (Airway)	
3. Open airway.	Determines if patient has spontaneous respirations.
a. Head tilt–chin lift (no trauma) (see illustration). *or*	

STEPS	RATIONALE
b. Jaw thrust (spinal cord trauma suspected) (see illustration).	Suspect a spinal cord injury with any type of trauma. Jaw thrust maneuver prevents head extension and neck movement and further paralysis or spinal cord injury.

SAFETY ALERT A cervical brace should be applied as soon as possible to maintain cervical-spine stability.

STEPS	RATIONALE
Primary Survey: B (Breathing)	
4. Attempt to ventilate patient with slow breaths, using one of these methods.	Slow breaths deliver air at a low pressure to reduce the risk of gastric distention.
a. Mouth-to-mouth using barrier device	Forms airtight seal and prevents air from escaping through nose.
b. Mouth-to-mask using a pocket mask (see illustration)	Provides secure seal and permits use of supplemental oxygen.
c. Bag-mask ventilation (see illustration)	Give breaths with enough force to make chest rise.
5. If readily available, insert oral airway (see Skill 30.1).	Maintains tone on anterior floor of mouth and prevents obstruction of posterior airway by tongue.
6. Suction secretions if necessary or turn victim's head to one side unless trauma is suspected.	Suctioning prevents airway obstruction. Turning patient's head to one side allows gravity to drain any secretions, decreasing risk of aspiration.
Primary Survey: D (Defibrillation)	
7. If pulse is absent and an AED is available, apply AED immediately as appropriate.	Most successful defibrillation rates occur when AED is applied and used within 5 minutes following collapse. Survival rates decline when defibrillation is delayed.
a. After one shock, resume CPR for 5 cycles and then begin rhythm analysis and shock sequence again.	One shock followed by chest compressions for 5 cycles provides sufficient blood movement and improved perfusion before another set of shocks is delivered.
8. If pulse is absent and an AED is unavailable, immediately initiate chest compressions:	

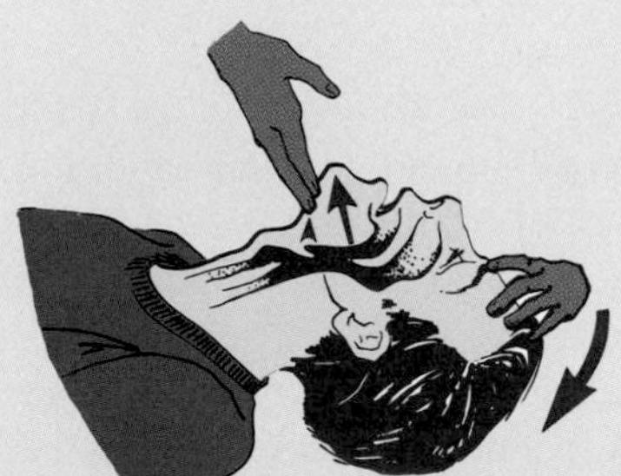

STEP 3a Head tilt–chin lift.

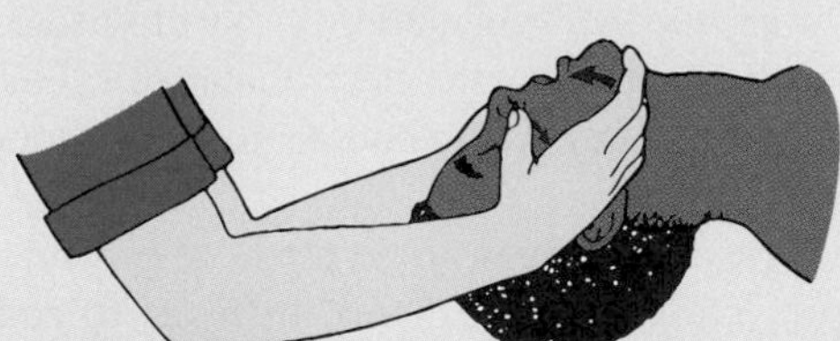

STEP 3b Jaw thrust without head tilt.

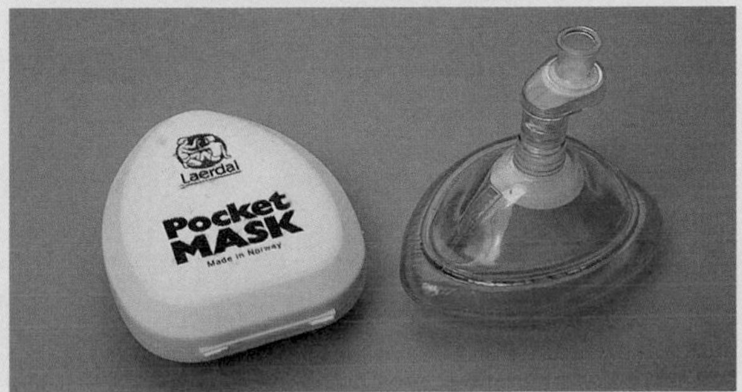

STEP 4b Pocket mask.

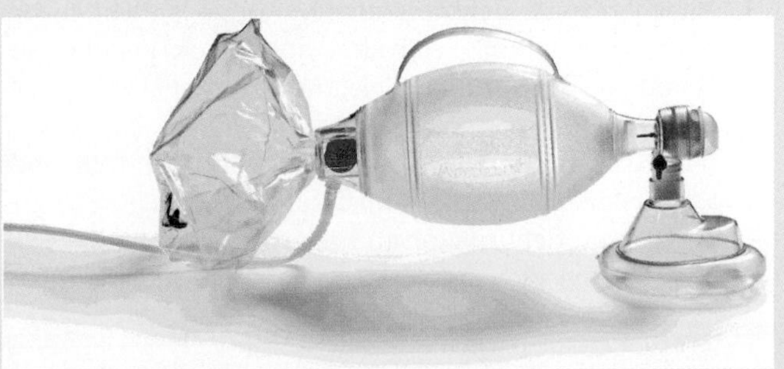

STEP 4c Bag-mask. (Courtesy AMBU, United States.)

Continued

STEPS	RATIONALE
a. Assume correct hand position and compression ratio for patient (see illustration).	Specific hand position, compression depth, and ratio are different for adult, child, and infant to avoid injury to heart, lung, or liver.

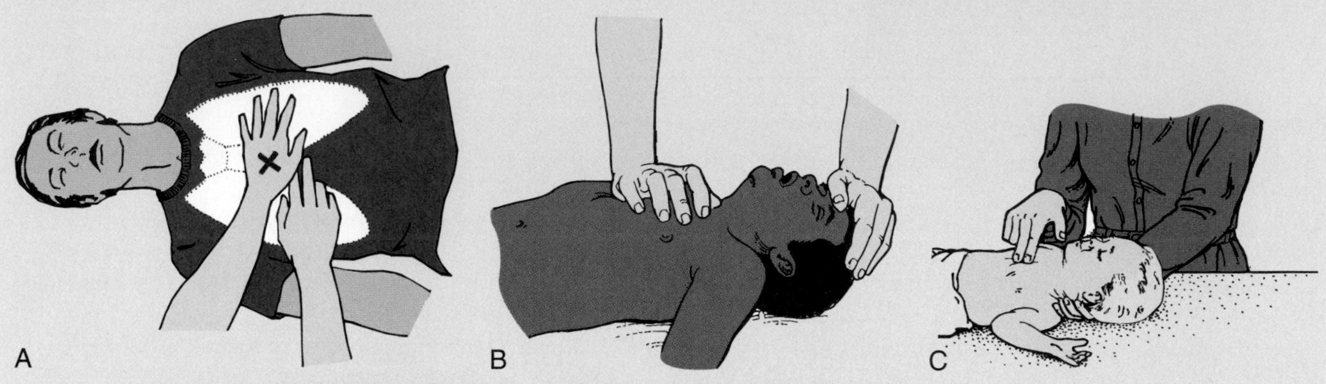

STEP 8a A, Proper hand position: adult. **B,** Proper hand position: child. **C,** Proper hand position: infant.

> **SAFETY ALERT** Ensure that fingers are off ribs and lowermost part of the xiphoid process. This reduces chance of rib fractures that could result in punctured lung or liver lacerations, which can further compromise cardiopulmonary status. Continue chest compressions, ventilation, and AED use.

STEPS	RATIONALE
Secondary Survey: Implementation	
1. Give code leader brief verbal report on events performed before code team's arrival (i.e., code, vital signs, medical diagnosis, and code intervention).	This information is critical in selection of appropriate treatment for patient.
2. On arrival of sufficient personnel, delegate tasks as appropriate.	Delegation of duties is essential to meet all needs of patient and his or her family in a timely manner.
a. Assist victim's roommate or visitors away from code scene. Assign pastoral care or other nurses to communicate with family.	
b. Delegate someone to remove excess furniture or equipment from room.	
c. Have someone bring patient's chart to bedside or be able to access patient's electronic medical record.	Clarifies patient's present medical condition, code status, and presence of any allergies.
d. Assign a nurse as recorder to record/document events of code.	Documents events of code and medications and treatments administered.
e. Assign another nurse to get medications and supplies from crash cart and hand them off to code team members. The bedside nurse is involved in tasks such as medication administration, vital signs, and assisting with procedures.	Provides code personnel with appropriate medication and equipment in a timely manner.
Secondary Survey: C (Analysis of Cardiac Rhythm)	
3. Attach manual defibrillator/monitor to patient using electrocardiogram electrodes, quick-look paddles, or "hands-off" defibrillation electrodes to visualize cardiac rhythm.	Cardiac rhythm monitor devices provide immediate rhythm display for analysis without disruption of rescue breathing and chest compression.
4. If cardiac rhythm is "shockable," continue CPR and assist code team with manual defibrillation.	Manual defibrillation is performed by ACLS-certified personnel.
a. Turn on defibrillator and select proper energy level following agency policy and equipment directions.	Energy is delivered in prescribed doses. Manual biphasic devices deliver shocks at a lower level (200 joules); monophasic waveforms use 360 joules.

STEPS	RATIONALE
b. Apply conductive gel or gel pads to patient's chest where defibrillator paddles will be placed. Some defibrillators use "hands-off pads" that are applied to patient's chest and directly connected to the manual defibrillator.	Decreases thoracic impedance and helps minimize burns to patient's skin (Craig, Hopkins-Pepe, 2006).
c. Paddles are placed on patient's chest wall.	Ensures appropriate discharge of current.
d. Verify that no one is in physical contact with patient, bed, or any item contacting patient during defibrillation. A warning must be called out before initiating the charge.	Prevents accidental delivery of shock or injury to personnel.
5. Establish IV access with large-bore needle (14- to 22-gauge) and begin infusion of 0.9% NS.	Provides a route for rapid drug administration and access for blood samples and fluid administration. Physiological saline is isotonic.
6. Assist with procedures as needed.	Much of the equipment needed for special procedures during a code is on the crash cart. Knowledge of crash cart contents and their location is essential to provide personnel with appropriate equipment without delay.
7. Continue CPR until relieved, until victim regains spontaneous pulse and respirations, until rescuer is exhausted and unable to perform CPR effectively, or until physician discontinues CPR.	Artificial cardiopulmonary function is maintained. Interruption of CPR is planned and organized. Interruptions occur seamlessly during changing of CPR personnel, defibrillation, and intubation. Interruptions must be kept to a minimum and not exceed 30 seconds.
Secondary Survey: A (Intubate Airway)	
8. If respirations are absent, assist code team with ET intubation.	Intubation provides patent airway and improves pulmonary ventilation. The use of laryngeal mask airway or esophageal-tracheal combitube can also be used to provide advanced airway support.
a. Have available laryngoscope blade, laryngoscope handle, curved and straight blades, and ET tubes. Ensure that light source on laryngoscope is functional.	Functional laryngeal light facilitates visualization of vocal cords and placement of ET tube into trachea.
Secondary Survey: B (Confirmation of Airway and Ventilation)	
9. Assist in confirmation of ET tube placement or advanced airway support by auscultating lungs for bilateral breath sounds. Carbon dioxide (CO_2) detector or esophageal detector devices are used as secondary methods to confirm correct airway placement.	Auscultation of lungs and exhaled CO_2 monitoring or esophageal detector device further verifies correct airway placement and adequacy of ventilation and gas exchange.
10. Ventilate using a bag upon intubation.	Bag provides ventilation through ET tube.
Secondary Survey: D (Differential Diagnosis)	
11. Assist physician in obtaining laboratory and diagnostic studies.	Helps in determining cause of the arrest.
12. See Completion Protocol (inside front cover).	

EVALUATION

1. Reassess primary and secondary survey ABCDs throughout code event.
2. Palpate carotid pulse at least every 5 minutes after first minute of CPR.
3. Observe for spontaneous return of pulse or respirations.
4. Observe that interruptions in CPR are minimized.

Unexpected Outcomes and Related Interventions

1. Patient experiences skeletal injury such as fractured ribs or sternum or internal organ injury such as lacerated lung or liver.
   a. Obtain appropriate diagnostic tests to document fractures.
   b. Assess patient's postarrest breathing or symmetry and pain.
   c. Observe for hemoptysis or gastrointestinal bleeding.
   d. Observe for distended abdomen.

2. Patient's CPR is unsuccessful.
   a. Contact chaplain services, social worker, or other family support systems.
   b. Provide privacy for patient's family to begin grieving process (see Chapter 31).
   c. Complete postmortem care on patient.

Recording and Reporting

- Record in nurses' notes or on designated CPR worksheet: onset of arrest, time, and number of AED shocks (you need to know the device-specific energy level delivered by the AED), time and energy level of manual defibrillations, medications given, procedures performed, cardiac rhythm, use of CPR, and patient's response. Most hospitals use a form designed specifically for in-hospital arrests.
- Immediately report arrest, indicating exact location of victim. In hospital setting follow agency policy for alerting the code team. In community setting activate emergency response system.

Sample Documentation

1030 Telemetry called with report of lethal arrhythmia. Immediately went to room to discover patient unconscious, not breathing, and pulseless. CPR started. AED applied. Advised shock, shock delivered × 1. Pulse returned. BP 76/50. Dopamine started. Patient intubated. Transferred to ICU with physician and ICU nurse.

Special Considerations

Pediatric

- Infants and children experience respiratory arrest more frequently than full cardiopulmonary arrest.

Geriatric

- Older adults, especially those with osteoporosis, are at greater risk for rib fractures.
- Whenever possible remove loose-fitting dentures to avoid airway obstruction during CPR and airway insertions. Properly fitting dentures should be left in place because they assist in ensuring a tight seal during artificial ventilation.

REVIEW QUESTIONS

Case Study for Questions 1 to 3

Mrs. Leibowitz is an 84-year-old female with a long history of heart failure and renal disease. She was admitted to the cardiology division with pulmonary edema. A telemetry monitor was attached to patient while diuretics were administered. Two hours after the last IV diuretic was administered, the nurse receives a call from centralized telemetry stating that Mrs. Leibowitz is in a lethal heart arrhythmia.

1. What is the first thing the nurse would do on receiving this phone call?
   1. Tell the nurse manager.
   2. Assess the patient and tell his or her co-workers to bring the AED.
   3. Hang up the phone and activate the hospital's code team.
   4. Prepare or draw laboratory specimens on Mrs. Leibowitz.
2. Place the following interventions in correct sequence on entrance into Mrs. Leibowitz's room.
   a. Check responsiveness.
   b. Begin 30 chest compressions.
   c. Provide 2 breaths.
   d. Attach the AED when available.
   e. Check for pulse.
   1. e, b, c, a, d
   2. a, e, d, b, c
   3. b, c, e, d, a
   4. a, e, b, c, d
3. After one shock of AED, the nurse should do which of the following first?
   1. Palpate the carotid pulse.
   2. Perform CPR for 5 cycles.
   3. Perform a rhythm analysis.
   4. Place patient in the recovery position.
4. Name the preferred technique to open the airway when there is no suspected trauma.
   1. Head tilt–chin lift
   2. Jaw thrust
   3. Lateral-lying position
   4. All of the above
5. _______________ minutes is the ideal time goal from victim discovery to first defibrillation for in-hospital patients.
   1. Three
   2. Five
   3. Seven
   4. Ten
6. Identify a possible unexpected outcome when performing chest compressions.
   1. Return of spontaneous pulse
   2. Possible skin burns from defibrillation
   3. Lacerated lung or liver
   4. Intubated airway

7. Which of the following is true about an oral airway?
   1. It eliminates the need to position the head of the unconscious patient.
   2. It eliminates the possibility of an upper airway obstruction.
   3. It is of no value once an ET tube is inserted.
   4. It may stimulate vomiting in the semiconscious patient.
8. During a cardiac arrest an advanced airway is inserted. How many breaths per minute should be delivered to the patient via the bag?
   1. 8 to 10
   2. 4 to 6
   3. 20 to 24
   4. 18 to 20
9. Which of the following is true regarding quality chest compressions?
   1. Adults required chest compression depth of 1.25 to 2.5 cm(½ to 1 inch).
   2. After each shock the pulse should be checked before beginning chest compressions.
   3. Chest compressions to ventilation rate should be 30:2.
   4. Adult CPR can be performed using one hand.

REFERENCES

American Heart Association: Part 5 and 13. Adult and Pediatric Basic Life Support, *Circulation* 122(Suppl 3):S685-S705 and S862-S875, 2010.

Craig KJ, Hopkins-Pepe L: Understanding the new AHA guidelines, Part II, *Nursing 2006* 36(5):52, 2006.

Ewy G, Kern K: Recent advances in cardiopulmonary resuscitation, *J Am Coll Cardiol* 53:149, 2009.

Haskell S, Atkins D: Defibrillation in children, *Journal of Emergencies, Trauma, and Shock*, 3(3):261, 2010.

Hockenberry MJ, Wilson D: *Wong's nursing care of infants and children*, ed 8, St Louis, 2007, Mosby.

CHAPTER

31

Palliative Care

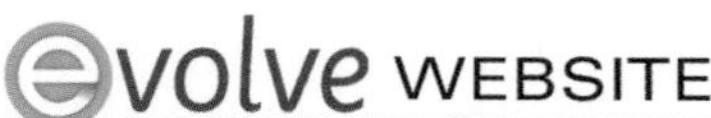

http://evolve.elsevier.com/Perry/nursinginterventions

Nurses play a vital role in helping patients with chronic, incurable illness maintain the best possible quality of life. They also help to ensure that patients at the end of life experience a peaceful death. Palliative care is a growing specialty in nursing. The World Health Organization (2002) defines it as an approach that improves the quality of life of individuals and their families facing life-threatening illness by preventing and relieving suffering through early identification and assessment and treatment of pain and other physical, psychological, and spiritual problems. As a patient's condition changes over time, the goals of care may shift to include more palliative care with a decreased emphasis on remission or cure. However, patients of all ages with any diagnosis receive palliative care, even as they seek treatment and cure for their illness. Patients who are in the process of dying will receive only palliative care if they are in a hospice program (Fig. 31-1).

You need to understand the similarities and differences between palliative and hospice care when helping patients and family members make important care decisions as their circumstances change (Box 31-1). Sometimes patients, family members, and health care professionals resist palliative care interventions, believing that palliative care is only for the dying (Kuebler and others, 2005). Because end-of-life care provides an excellent example of palliative care, the remainder of this chapter focuses on nursing care at the end of life.

PATIENT-CENTERED CARE

Patient-centered care lies at the heart of palliative and hospice care nursing. Each person will die in his or her own way, influenced by culture, religion, ethnicity, belief systems, support structures, and key relationships. As the plan of care shifts toward patient comfort and quality of life, less emphasis is placed on following medical regimens. Listen carefully to patient's and family members' descriptions of their needs and wishes through their eyes, and set your nursing care priorities accordingly. Think creatively about how to help patients live as well as possible as they approach the end of life. For example, you might extend visiting hours in the hospital setting to accommodate the needs of a family to be together as a loved one dies. Nurses giving palliative care should develop the ability to understand, acknowledge, and be present with people experiencing intense and changing emotional reactions to their situation. Compassion and attentiveness are conveyed in many ways, including the therapeutic use of touch (Fig. 31-2), active listening, or silently sitting with the patient.

Spiritual concerns often arise in situations of serious chronic illness and impending death. All patients, including those who do not practice a particular religion, have spiritual strengths, needs, and practices. The terms *spirituality* and *religion* are often used interchangeably and for many people are closely related. However, there are important differences in these terms. Religion refers to a person's specific beliefs and behaviors associated with a religious tradition. Spirituality refers to an innate human need for deeper meaning and purpose in life (Hermann, 2007). When exploring spirituality with your patient, think of four basic conceptual areas: meaning, hope, community, and a sense of the Holy Other (Vandecreek and Lucas, 2001) (Box 31-2).

Cultural sensitivity is crucial in providing patient-centered end-of-life care. The patient's culturally influenced health care beliefs and practices, communication patterns, and family structures affect the dying process (Crawley, 2005). To provide appropriate care, look beyond your own cultural assumptions and preconceived ideas and focus on the needs and cultural practices of those in your care. Be especially aware of religious diversity in end-of-life care (Box 31-3). Remember that people with the same religion have varying beliefs or practices or adhere more or less strictly to their beliefs.

Your ability to give patient-centered care is greatly aided when patients clearly communicate their preferences for end-of-life care. An advance directive helps patients make their values and wishes known and guides family members' and

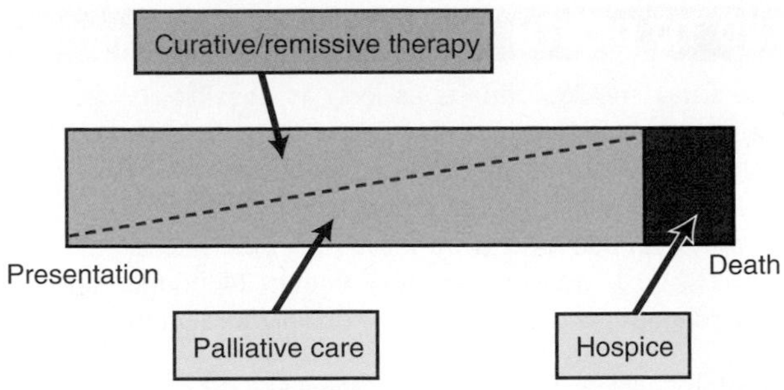

FIG 31-1 Palliative care and hospice. (Emanuel L and others: *The education in palliative and end of life care (EPEC) curriculum: The EPEC Project*, 2003, Northwestern University Feinberg School of Medicine.)

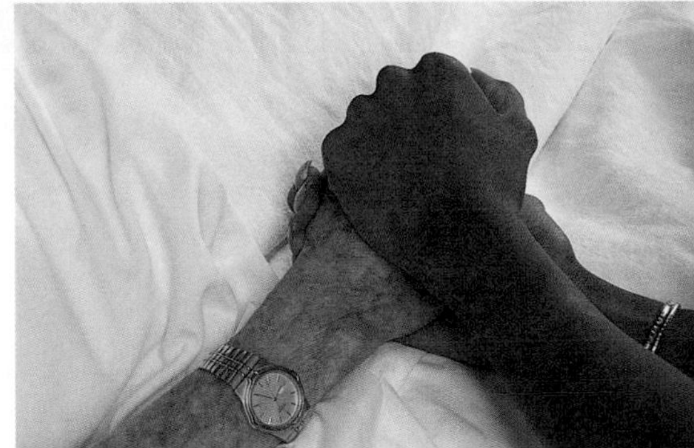

FIG 31-2 Touch can communicate caring and compassion.

BOX 31-1 SIMILARITIES AND DIFFERENCES BETWEEN PALLIATIVE AND HOSPICE CARE

Similarities

1. Prioritize for quality of life and relief from pain and other distressing symptoms, not curing
2. Integrate the physical, psychological, social, and spiritual dimensions into plan of care
3. Affirm life and regard dying as a normal process
4. Involve the patient and family as active participants in all decisions and care
5. Rely on skills of an interdisciplinary team for planning and implementing care
6. Appropriate for all patients, regardless of diagnosis or age

Differences

1. Palliative care is used in varying degrees at any time during an illness. Hospice care is designed exclusively for patients near the end of life.
2. Palliative care is often used in conjunction with curative interventions. To be eligible for hospice, patients can no longer be pursuing curative care.
3. Palliative care helps people living with chronic illness over an extended period of time rather than the shorter time frame (approximately 6 months) designated for hospice.

BOX 31-2 SPIRITUALITY CONCEPTS

Meaning

- What gives your life meaning and purpose in your current situation?
- What are your goals? What do you still want to achieve?
- What do you live for now?

Hope

- What do you hope for?
- How have your hopes changed?
- What gives you hope during difficult times?

Community

- Who are the people most important to you?
- Who gives you comfort in difficult times?
- Are you able to participate in community activities (i.e., church, family, friends, neighborhood)?

Sense of Holy Other or God

- What is God like for you? What is your concept of that which is larger than yourself?
- Is religion or God significant to you? If yes, can you describe how?
- Are certain religious practices or rituals meaningful to you?

caregivers' decisions when the patient can no longer participate (e.g., overwhelming illness, unconsciousness, or sedating drugs). Advance directives are written documents or are negotiated by a patient-appointed representative known as a durable power of attorney for health care. In an advance directive patients express their wishes concerning the use of extraordinary medical procedures, artificial nutrition and fluids, comfort measures, life support interventions, or other care preferences. Laws relating to advance directives vary from state to state; know those that apply in your state. Facilities usually have policies and sample forms for advance directives to help patients and families in their deliberations. Patients should give copies of completed advance directives to their physician and responsible family members and request that their advance directive be placed in their medical record. If a patient's wish to forego cardiopulmonary resuscitation (CPR) is expressed in an advance directive, a physician must also write a "do not resuscitate" (DNR) order in the medical chart. Because care decision discussions are very sensitive and emotional for patients and families, provide a quiet setting for conversation and participate when your involvement is appropriate. Recognize that cultural, ethnic, and religious values influence the likelihood of a patient using an advance directive and its content (Cox and others, 2006).

End-of-life care poses many challenging ethical questions, including patients' right to have assisted dying, use of artificial food and hydration, pain management, going against patient or family wishes, or the appropriate use of technology. To best ensure that you are providing patient-centered care

BOX 31-3 SOME RELIGIOUS PRACTICES RELATED TO DEATH AND DYING

Judaism
Persons dying in the Jewish faith may want to hear prayers and scripture at the time of death. After death there should be minimal handling of the body by non-Jews. A family member may stay with the body until burial. The eyes should be closed after death. It is customary to be buried within 24 hours, except on the Sabbath. Families participate in a mourning period during which grief is expressed openly and in keeping with ritual. Because life is valued as a gift of God, efforts to continue life are supported, especially in Orthodox Judaism. In some but not all types of Judaism, cremation, autopsy, and embalming are avoided.

Christianity
Christians believe in life after death and eternal life. Some may request rituals of confession, laying on of hands, anointing the sick, baptism, or Holy Communion. Prayer and reading from the Bible may be appropriate. There may be a period of viewing the body or a wake before burial. A funeral or memorial service is the norm. Cremation, autopsy, and embalming are usually allowed.

Islam
Muslims believe in eternal life and the will of God (Allah). Patients may wish to face Mecca (the East) as they are dying. Cleanliness and modesty are very important. Regular prayer 5 times a day should continue as long as possible. Loved ones usually remain with the dying person 24 hours a day. Non-Muslims should wear gloves when touching the body. Cover the body with a sheet until a person of the Muslim faith can give the ritual bath and wrap the body in a white cloth. Burial is usually in a Muslim cemetery within 24 hours. Autopsy, organ donation, and cremation are usually forbidden.

Hinduism
Hindus believe in one supreme deity and in lesser gods with power and interest in specific areas of life. Beliefs include reincarnation and karma (how one has lived in this world affects how one might return in the next one). Patients may want the presence of a Brahmin priest who may chant prayers. Only the family should touch the body after death, and they are responsible for washing and preparing it. Cremation is traditional.

Buddhism
In Buddhism the state of the mind at the time of death is relevant in the person's rebirth into a new life. The goal of life and death is to reach the eternal state of nirvana, or inner peace and happiness. The patient may want to remain conscious to be able to think right thoughts during the dying process. Notify a Buddhist priest at the time of death. Time from death to burial varies from 3 to 7 days. Mourners wear white to the funeral. Cremation and autopsy are usually allowed.

Adapted from: Matzo M: Peri-death nursing care. In Matzo M, Sherman D, editors: *Palliative care nursing: quality care to the end of life,* New York, 2006, Springer, p 443.

in ethical deliberations, listen carefully and nonjudgmentally to patient's and family members' concerns. To determine the best course of action, the patient, family, and members of the interdisciplinary team need to have meaningful conversations together.

SAFETY

Seriously ill patients experience decreased muscle strength and limited endurance. However, they may prefer to get out of bed for meals or walk to the bathroom as long as possible. Guard against falls by having patients use appropriate assistive devices for walking. Remain with the patient until he or she is safely seated or lying down. Patients at the end of life also lose the ability to chew and swallow safely (Cinocco, 2007). Place a patient who wants to eat or drink in an upright position and slowly offer small bites of food or sips of water to avoid aspiration.

In some facilities patients who do not want to be resuscitated (DNR) wear a wrist bracelet that alerts care providers that they should not start CPR when the patient's heart or breathing stops. Identify the patient with DNR status by using two identifiers (i.e., name and birthday or name and account number, according to facility policy). Compare identifiers with information on the patient's identification bracelet. Placing a DNR bracelet on the wrong patient may lead to unintentional death or the resuscitation of a patient against his or her wishes. Use the same patient identification methods before sending a body to the morgue. Improper identification of a body may lead to a serious miscommunication with family members.

NURSES' SELF-CARE

To nurture your capacity to remain empathically engaged with patients and family members, you must also care for yourself physically, spiritually, and emotionally. Nurses involved in palliative and hospice care are positively affected, touched, and changed by their intimate experiences with patients and families. They also share in the patient's grief and feelings of sadness, helplessness, and loss, which can lead to compassion fatigue. Compassion fatigue leaves nurses feeling tired, depressed, angry, "stressed out," and eventually apathetic (Bush, 2009). With each loss nurses may be reminded of their own personal losses, or they might struggle with moral distress. Talk about your feelings and experiences with a trusted friend or peer. Identify ways in which you can work with others to address workplace barriers to effective self-care. Sometimes a debriefing after a particularly long or difficult death helps nurses feel support and gain perspective. Regularly practice stress management techniques: physical exercise, nutritious eating patterns, humor, hobbies, and adequate sleep (Aycock and Boyle, 2009). Strengthen yourself spiritually with meditation, prayer, or consultation with a spiritual care provider. It may help to attend the funeral of a patient with whom you shared special bonds. You might also gain insight by reflecting on your own personal beliefs and feelings about death and loss.

EVIDENCE-BASED PRACTICE TRENDS

Phillips L, Reed P: Into the abyss of someone else's dying: the voice of the end of life caregiver, *Clin Nurs Res* 18(1):80, 2009.

Cox and others: Implications of cultural diversity in do not attempt resuscitation (DNAR) decision making, *J Multicult Nurs Health* 12 (1):20, 2006.

Interviews with family caregivers of older adults at the end of life revealed some common themes. Caregivers described attending a dying loved one as complex, unpredictable, frightening, and anguishing. In addition to the difficult aspects of end-of-life caregiving, those interviewed also described the experience as profoundly moving and affirming. The researchers noted that caregivers benefit when nurses give them practical information on the physical and emotional aspects of caregiving. Professional caregivers have similar experiences with the complexities of working with dying patients (Phillips and Reed, 2009).

Advance directives are generally accepted as a method by which people communicate their wishes for end-of-life care. Caregivers frequently urge patients and family members to complete an advance directive. In this study researchers found that, among black and minority ethnic groups, advance directives were not often used and held little or no relevance. The study reminds caregivers that a patient's cultural values and ethnicity play an important role in making health care decisions and that significant cultural differences exist regarding advance care planning (Cox and others, 2006).

SKILL 31.1 SUPPORTING PATIENTS AND FAMILIES IN GRIEF

During end-of-life situations, patients and family members experience intense feelings such as anxiety, sadness, regret, or relief. They ask questions of spiritual significance about the meaning of life, pain, suffering, and loss of personal power and control. In short, they experience grief, an intense emotional and behavioral response to perceived and actual losses. People express grief in physical, psychological, and spiritual ways. It is expressed as sadness, relief, denial, shock, guilt, or anger. Grief is a process that often begins before a patient dies. Survivors grieve as they anticipate a loss and continue to feel the grief after the patient dies. Most people gradually move through their grief and learn to adjust to life without their loved one. Nurses walk with patients and family members in their grief and provide emotional and spiritual support to help them move forward.

ASSESSMENT

1. Limit your initial grief assessment to concerns most important to patient and family. Expand the assessment through observation and explore concerns as they arise. *Rationale: Discussing emotional and spiritual concerns may arouse uncomfortable feelings, anxiety, or uncertainty. Refrain from probing issues before people are ready to talk about them.*
2. Discuss spiritual and emotional concerns at an appropriate time in a quiet place and in an unrushed manner. *Rationale: People participate when timing and location are right for them.*
3. Observe for physical symptoms and behaviors that might be related to grief. *Rational: Grief might cause insomnia, lack of interest in life, isolation, or frequent crying. In nonverbal patients, restlessness may indicate emotional distress.*
4. Listen for statements that might indicate spiritual distress such as, "I haven't accomplished what I wanted to in life," "I wasted so much of my life," or "Without him my life doesn't mean anything." *Rationale: Spiritual matters are often expressed in nonreligious language and should be recognized for their spiritual significance.*
5. Identify barriers to expression of feelings. *Rationale: Lack of privacy, pain, stress, distrust, or fatigue may create barriers to self-expression.*
6. Gather information about the person's coping style in previous losses, relationship to the deceased, and the nature of the loss. *Rationale: A person's usual coping patterns are of more use near the end of life than trying new strategies or those designed by others.*
7. Identify spiritual and religious needs, resources, and strengths. *Rationale: Acts of forgiveness, reconciliation, blessing, and community often help.*
8. Request services of a priest, rabbi, pastor, or the facility's spiritual care provider to obtain a full spiritual assessment. *Rationale: Patients and family members may benefit from the professional assessment skills of spiritual care experts.*

PLANNING

Expected Outcomes focus on providing emotional and spiritual support for patients and family members in a grief process.

1. Patient/family are able to share feelings and grief related to perceived and actual losses.
2. Patient/family verbalize sources of strength and hope.
3. Patient/family express satisfaction with emotional and spiritual aspects of palliative care.

Delegation and Collaboration

Psychosocial/spiritual care cannot be delegated to nursing assistive personnel (NAP). Instruct the NAP about the following:

- Specific changes in patient's affect or interaction with others that need to be reported to the nurse immediately
- How to maintain a respectful, quiet demeanor when interacting with grieving patient and family members

IMPLEMENTATION *for* SUPPORTING PATIENTS AND FAMILIES IN GRIEF

STEPS	RATIONALE
1. See Standard Protocol (inside front cover).	
2. Provide emotional support for grieving patients and family members.	
a. Use active listening, therapeutic communication skills, and quiet presence to help people feel and express their grief. Validate that grief feelings are normal.	Listening to patients and family members without interruption or trying to "fix" things validates their feelings.
b. Allow sufficient time for patients and family members to have conversations when they are ready.	Patients and family members may be in different phases of grief or have unresolved conflicts.
c. Respect individual differences in willingness to share. Remain alert for opportunities to have discussions when patient is ready.	Some people share feelings more than others. As a trusting relationship develops, people may share what they have been working on privately.
d. Explore realistic goals and offer practical help to address immediate problems. Do not focus on long-term problems that cannot be solved at the time.	Gives patients and family members sense of control and achievement even in limited circumstances (Clayton and others, 2005).
3. Promote emotional well-being.	A peaceful death is characterized by emotional comfort.
a. Talk with patient and family about fears, stressors, anxieties, and care options. Assure them that they will not be abandoned.	Patients feel valued and respected when included in discussions. Many patients fear being alone or abandoned (AACN and COH, 2008).
b. Consult interdisciplinary team for help with emotional, relational, and psychological issues.	Creative team approaches enhance care. Patient/family may benefit from professional counseling.
c. Administer prescribed anti-anxiety medication in cases of significant depression or anxiety.	Although sadness is normal with significant loss, severe anxiety or depression decreases quality of life (Block, 2006).
4. Promote spiritual well-being.	Grief experiences affect a person's sense of self, meaning, and relationships.
a. Facilitate spiritual activities (prayer, meditation, or reading patient's spiritual texts).	Spiritual activities sustain patients' hope and help them find sources of peace and reconciliation.
b. Consult with spiritual care team as appropriate.	A spiritual care professional can design individualized interventions.
c. Promote hope with your therapeutic presence and active listening. Provide information and answer questions in an honest, helpful manner.	Allowing patients to talk about their feelings and providing information and help promotes hope and sense of community (Chi, 2007).
d. Help patients and family members identify shifts in what they hope for (e.g., to live until an anniversary, eat at the family table, or have a peaceful death).	New sources of hope help people move forward.
e. Honor cultural and religious beliefs and rituals. People without a religious affiliation may have rituals for remembering and honoring their loved one.	Provides opportunity for closure, community support, and belief that the dying process conformed to one's own valued customs and behaviors (Kemp, 2005).
5. Assist patient and family members in advance planning and involve them in care decisions. Identify who will manage the patient's affairs and make funeral plans.	Minimizes fear and loss of control in decision making. Increases sense of having one's death supported and honored.
6. See Completion Protocol (inside front cover).	

EVALUATION

1. Evaluate degree of relief from grief and emotional and spiritual symptoms.
2. Monitor effectiveness of decision making related to important concerns.
3. Observe quality of interactions among patient, family members, and caregivers.
4. Evaluate patient and family satisfaction with emotional/spiritual support.

Unexpected Outcomes and Related Interventions

1. Emotional symptoms and spiritual distress are not managed well with current approaches.
   a. Collaborate with interdisciplinary team to develop new strategies. Make referrals as needed.
   b. Talk with patient/family about what actions they believe may be helpful.
2. Patient/family experience ethical conflicts or disagreements in decision making.

a. Clarify patient wishes or consult patient advance directives.
b. Use active listening to identify and clarify the issues impacting decision making.

Recording and Reporting

- Record in nurses' notes: interventions for psychological and spiritual grief responses, including patient response; patient/family preferences; family presence and involvement; and evidence of unresolved issues and concerns.
- Report when a patient or family member requests therapeutic intervention from social worker, counselor, or spiritual care provider.

Sample Documentation

1500 Patient stated that she wanted to talk more openly with family members about her impending death and wants to make decisions about her funeral and disposition of her possessions. Requested that a conversation with her pastor and family members be arranged for tomorrow afternoon. Patient states she knows this will be difficult but believes that decisions must be made.

Special Considerations

Pediatric

- Encourage parents to share information about their child's coping style and the openness with which death is addressed in the family.
- Decisions to end treatment can be more difficult when children are involved.
- Many children know they are dying and are able to have age-appropriate conversations about their feelings and fears.

Geriatric

- Older adults have experienced multiple losses in their lives, which may impact their reactions to subsequent losses and their grief response.
- Do not assume that older adults accept or have addressed their feelings about death.
- Older adults may have fewer relatives and friends available to offer support (Derby and O'Mahony, 2006).

Home Care

- Family members need support and role modeling for talking about emotional, relational, and spiritual issues.
- Family members may have ambivalent feelings about having a loved one die at home. Encourage them to express their concerns.
- Family members need respite care to meet caregiving demands and attend to their own grief and responses to loss (Osse and others, 2006).

SKILL 31.2 CARE OF THE DYING PATIENT

Providing palliative care at the end of life involves caring for the whole person—body, mind, and spirit. Skill 31.1 addresses the importance of emotional and spiritual care of patients and family members dealing with loss and grief. This skill provides information about symptom management to help maintain a patient's quality of life. Do not underestimate the importance of attending to the patient's physical needs. Patients and family members identify relief from pain and other troublesome physical symptoms as a high priority in end-of-life care. Their grief and response to loss are based in part on memories of their loved one's care and whether or not it was free from suffering (Lynch and Dahlin, 2007). You can begin to lessen the fear and uncertainty often associated with the dying process by helping patients and family members understand and anticipate the common physical changes associated with impending death (Table 31-1).

ASSESSMENT

1. Make assessments without imposing judgment on patient's reports of pain and discomfort. *Rationale: A symptom is what a patient says it is, not what the nurse says it is. Patients who have had persistent pain or other symptoms often exhibit behaviors different from those noted in patients with acute pain.*
2. Assess each symptom for onset, precipitating factors, quality, severity, and what has helped to relieve symptoms in the past. In nonverbal patients look for facial grimacing and restlessness as indicators of distress and validate with family members (Herr and others, 2006). *Rationale: Determines level of distress for planning patient-specific interventions.*
3. Perform thorough, frequent, ongoing assessments before and after an intervention. *Rationale: Good symptom management depends on early identification of a problem, prompt intervention to avoid symptom breakthrough, and reevaluation to assess for medication effectiveness and potential side effects.*
4. Involve family members in symptom assessment. *Rationale: Patients near the end of life may not be able to self-report. Family members who know patient behavior patterns provide valuable assessment information.*

PLANNING

Expected Outcomes focus on promoting comfort, autonomy, family involvement, and dignity throughout the dying experience.

1. Patient demonstrates relief from pain and other physical symptoms.

TABLE 31-1 PHYSICAL CHANGES COMMONLY ASSOCIATED WITH IMPENDING DEATH

SIGNS AND SYMPTOMS	INTERVENTIONS
Coolness and color changes in extremities	Use slippers or socks; cover person with light blankets, not tucked tightly over toes.
Increased periods of sleeping/unresponsiveness	Sit with patient, perhaps holding a hand and talking quietly; speak to patient even though there may be a lack of response.
Bowel or bladder incontinence	Change bedding as appropriate, use bed pads, and give frequent skin care. An indwelling urinary catheter may be indicated for patient fatigue or skin breakdown.
Congestion/increased secretions	Elevate head of bed, turn the head to drain secretions. Use prescribed medication to help decrease secretions. Avoid suctioning.
Restlessness or disorientation	Speak calmly, reduce lights. Gently massage hands or feet. Play soothing music.
Decreased intake of food or fluids	Do not force patient to eat or drink. Offer ice chips, popsicles, sips of fluid; apply lip balm; moisten mouth.
Decreased urine output	Consider advocating for the removal of indwelling urinary catheters. Change bed pads as needed.
Altered breathing patterns (apnea, labored, and irregular breathing)	Elevate the head, hold hand, and use quiet voice tones. Administer prescribed anxiolytics and/or opioids for pain and apprehension.

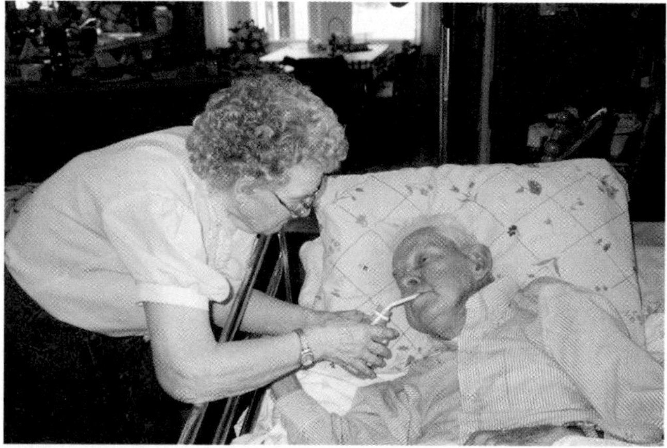

FIG 31-3 Encourage family involvement in care.

2. Patient/family participate in decisions regarding end-of-life care as desired.
3. Patient/family are involved in care based on their abilities and preferences (Fig. 31-3).
4. Patient/family express satisfaction with all aspects of palliative care.

Delegation and Collaboration

Physical care activities for dying patients may be delegated to nursing assistive personnel (NAP). When providing physical care, instruct the NAP about the following:

- Specific signs of patient discomfort to report for immediate nursing intervention
- How to use gentle touch and quiet tone of voice
- Specific patient care measures to promote comfort such as bathing or repositioning

Equipment

- Personal care items most preferred by patient
- Comfort and hygiene products
- Clean gloves

IMPLEMENTATION *for* CARE OF THE DYING PATIENT

STEPS	RATIONALE
1. See Standard Protocol (inside front cover).	
2. Promote pain relief (see Chapter 13).	
a. Administer prescribed analgesics around the clock (ATC); give extra doses for breakthrough pain.	ATC dosing is most effective method for maintaining adequate pain control. Using breakthrough doses minimizes pain episodes without overmedicating (Paice and Fine, 2006).
b. Collaborate with health care provider to consider use of adjuvant pain medications (e.g., antidepressants and anticonvulsants for neuropathic pain and antiinflammatory drugs for bone pain).	Adjuvant medications can enhance opioid effectiveness or treat pain not relieved by opioids (Paice and Fine, 2006).

STEPS	RATIONALE
c. Advocate for the most effective, least invasive route for analgesic administration.	Best route is based on patient's level of consciousness, gastrointestinal (GI) and circulatory status, type of medication, and ease of delivery.
d. Monitor effectiveness of medication regimen and adverse side effects at regular intervals.	Patients may need larger opioid doses to get relief as disease progresses, drug tolerance builds, and symptoms increase. Pain medication doses may have to be decreased when liver and kidney function declines. Treating symptoms before they worsen ensures more consistent pain relief (Paice and Fine, 2006).
e. Monitor for constipation, sedation (usually transitory), nausea, vomiting, or dry mouth.	These are side effects of opioids and sedatives. Excessive sedation may require decrease in opioid dose.
f. Use nonpharmacological methods of pain control (e.g., relaxation, repositioning, heat/cold, massage, diversion).	Nonpharmacological therapies enhance effectiveness of pain mediation and allow patients to participate in their symptom management (Matzo and Sherman, 2006).
3. Promote skin integrity and implement actions to prevent pressure ulcers (see Chapter 25).	Skin integrity is compromised by immobility, poor nutrition, and weight loss.
a. Reposition every 2 hours or more often for comfort and use pressure-reducing devices.	Immobility and prolonged pressure on an area cause pain, skin breakdown, and stiffness.
b. Apply alcohol-free lotion as needed and desired.	Lotion massage of hands, feet, or back may increase patient comfort.

SAFETY ALERT Do not massage any reddened area on patient's skin. Massaging causes breaks in the surface of the skin capillaries and increases risk of skin breakdown.

STEPS	RATIONALE
c.  Cleanse perineal area frequently if incontinent.	Promotes skin integrity and patient dignity and well-being.
4. Provide nutrition and hydration, accommodating changed patterns at end of life.	
a. Offer patient preferred food and liquids as tolerated, slowly, and in small amounts at patient-determined times.	Anorexia and difficulty swallowing are common at end of life. Patients are more likely to enjoy eating favorite foods.
b. Provide oral care q2h or as requested.	Reduces oral bacteria, mouth odor, and bad taste.
c. Avoid exposing patient to foods with strong odors.	Strong smells can intensify nausea.
d. Patients should determine what and when they eat or drink. Accept their refusal of food or liquids.	Gradual dehydration may be a natural way for the body to decrease distressing symptoms such as congestion, excess secretions, shortness of breath, vomiting, and edema (Plonk and Arnold, 2005).
e. Inform family members about normal decrease in appetite at end of life. Help family shift hope focus and find other ways to help.	Education can reduce family distress. Offering food and fluid symbolizes life, love, and nurturing. No longer sharing meals can be a difficult adjustment.
5. Assist with changing elimination patterns.	
a. Administer prescribed stool softeners and laxatives, especially with use of opioid analgesia.	Opioid analgesia, inactivity, and decreased fluid intake contribute to constipation.
b. Use bedside commode as long as possible.	Natural position for defecation promotes elimination and maintains patient autonomy.
6. Promote comfort with breathing patterns.	
a. Enhance patient respiratory effort by elevating head of the bed.	Diaphragm can move more easily in sitting position than when lying flat.
b. Increase air movement with fans or open windows.	Airflow stimulates trigeminal nerve in the cheek, which inhibits feelings of dyspnea. Use of oxygen is not routine at end of life unless for comfort (Kehl, 2008).
c. Use actions that conserve energy and balance rest and activity.	Reducing activity decreases patient oxygen use and minimizes shortness of breath.

Continued

STEPS	RATIONALE
d. Offer prescribed oral, intravenous (IV), or inhaled opioids for severe dyspnea and benzodiazepines for anxiety.	Medications decrease anxiety and may alter perception of breathlessness.
e. Decrease anxiety related to shortness of breath by massage therapy, relaxation therapy, and listening to music.	Air hunger is a very distressing, frightening symptom that may require use of multiple methods for symptom relief.
f. Decrease respiratory congestion ("death rattle") by elevating head of bed, side positioning, anticholinergic drugs. Educate family that patient cannot clear throat and is not choking.	Noise is caused by secretions at back of throat rattling with breath airflow and relaxed tongue. Anticholinergic drugs used before buildup of secretions dry secretions. Suctioning increases discomfort and does not help (Hipp and Letizia, 2009).
7. See Completion Protocol (inside front cover).	

EVALUATION

1. Evaluate patient's degree of symptom relief and effectiveness of each intervention.
2. Observe level of patient's and family members' participation and comfort in giving care.
3. Evaluate patient/family satisfaction with and knowledge of symptom management interventions.

Unexpected Outcomes and Related Interventions

1. Pain and/or other symptoms are not well managed with prescribed treatment plan.
   a. Collaborate with interdisciplinary team for alternative medications or adjuvant therapies.
   b. Talk with patient/family about what they believe may be helpful.
   c. Consider emotional or spiritual issues that may interfere with symptom management.
2. Family members are not present or participating in care.
   a. Determine cause of nonparticipation. Provide information to increase family members' comfort with care interventions.
   b. Maintain a nonjudgmental attitude and support patient/family coping styles and relationships.

Recording and Reporting

- Record in nurses' notes: interventions for pain and symptom management, including patient response; changes in physical, mental, emotional, or spiritual status; patient/family preferences; family presence and involvement; evidence of unresolved issues and concerns with physical care or patient symptoms.
- Report when a previously alert patient becomes unresponsive.

Sample Documentation

1500 Patient less responsive to verbal stimuli with occasional periods of restlessness. No oral intake this shift. Mouth care given every 2 hours. Unable to rate pain. Hospital spiritual care provider and grandchildren visiting. Family members tearful and verbalize awareness that death is near. A family member wishes to remain with patient until the time of death.

Special Considerations

Pediatric

- Treat family and child as a unit. Encourage parents to stay with child and participate in care as much as desired or possible.
- Consider child's age and developmental level in care planning, symptom management, and sibling support (Hellsten and Kane, 2006).

Geriatric

- Older patients may have more than one disease process and multiple physical symptoms.
- Many older adults do not want invasive treatments at the end of life but want comfort measures. Preferences can change over time; thus revaluate periodically (Bolmsjo, 2008).
- Pain, respiratory distress, and confusion are common symptoms in older adults at end of life.

Home Care

- Family members assume primary care responsibility and need ongoing teaching and support.
- Educate family members about symptom management approaches and when to seek help.
- Volunteers may be needed to give family members' respite time.

SKILL 31.3 CARE OF THE BODY AFTER DEATH

After a patient dies, the designated health care provider, most often a physician or nurse practitioner, certifies the death and records the time and actions taken at the time of death in the medical record. The health care provider may request permission from the family for an autopsy or postmortem examination, although this is less likely with an anticipated death or when the cause of death is known. An autopsy may be performed to confirm or determine the cause of death, gather data regarding the nature and progress of a disease, study the effects of therapies on body tissues, and provide statistical data for epidemiology and research purposes. An autopsy consent form must be signed by the appropriate family member and the physician or designated requestor. Autopsies normally do not delay burial. The nurse is responsible for providing respectful, thorough care of the body after death. Some family members wish to view the body immediately after death, or they may wish to help with preparing the body. Give family members and significant others ample time to say good-bye before transferring the body to the morgue or funeral home.

ASSESSMENT

1. Assess for presence of family members or significant others and determine whether they have been informed of patient's death. Determine who is responsible for any legal matters after death. *Rationale: Assists in coordinating facility-based procedures for care after death.*
2. Assess family members' grief response. *Rationale: Determines level of support and guidance needed.*
3. Determine if patient is an organ/tissue donor. Federal law mandates that family members be given a chance to authorize organ/tissue donation (Ferrell and Coyle, 2006). Call organ/tissue request and procurement team (consult facility policy). *Rationale: Trained requestors usually approach families for donation and manage care of the body for successful organ retrieval. Successful recovery of organs/tissues depends on skillful and timely requests.*
4. Assess patient's religious preference and/or cultural heritage. *Rationale: Patient's religious or cultural practices for body preparation may require changes in routine procedures.*
5. Determine if autopsy will be done. *Rationale: If autopsy is planned or required, procedures such as removal of tubes and lines may be altered or prohibited. Consult facility guidelines.*
6. Assess the general condition of the body and note presence of dressing, tubes, and medical equipment. *Rationale: Validates tissue damage and type of postmortem care required.*

PLANNING

Expected Outcomes focus on preventing injury to the body and facilitating grieving of family and friends.

1. Survivors able to grieve in a manner consistent with religious, cultural, and personal values.
2. Patient's body is prepared in a respectful manner consistent with cultural and religious practices and with family involvement if desired.
3. Patient's body is free of new skin damage and optimally prepared for mortuary.

Delegation and Collaboration

Emotional and supportive care at time of death cannot be delegated to nursing assistive personnel (NAP). NAP can provide physical care. Instruct the NAP about the following:

- Any specific physical measures needed for postmortem care of the body
- Preparing room and area for family to view the body

Equipment

- Clean gloves, gown, and other protective clothing if needed
- Plastic bag for hazardous waste disposal
- Washbasin, washcloth, warm water, and bath towel
- Clean gown or disposable gown for body (consult facility policy)
- Absorbent pads
- Body bag or shroud kit (consult facility policy)
- Paper tape and gauze dressing
- Paper bag, plastic bag, or other suitable receptacle for patient's clothing, belongings, and other items to be returned to family
- Envelope for valuables
- Identification tags as specified by facility policy

IMPLEMENTATION FOR CARE OF THE BODY AFTER DEATH

STEPS	RATIONALE
1. **See Standard Protocol (inside front cover).**	
2. Place pillow under head or slightly elevate head of bed.	Helps decrease pooling of blood and discoloration of the face while you make other preparations (Sherman and others, 2005).
3. Discuss routine postmortem care with family members and ask if they wish to include their own cultural or religious practices. Offer support from spiritual care provider in facility.	Seeking family input provides culturally sensitive patient-centered care. Family members may welcome the presence of a spiritual care professional immediately after a death. Some facility policies include calling spiritual care department at time of death.
4. Ask family members if they wish to be involved in preparation of the body.	Facilitates grieving.
5. If tissue, body, or organ donation has been made, consult facility policy for specific guidelines.	Retrieval of tissues (e.g., corneas, skin) may require special body preparation.

Continued

STEPS	RATIONALE
6. Prepare body in private room or move roommate to another room during end-of-life care.	Provides staff and family with privacy for rituals, body preparation, and expressions of grief.
7. Don't rush. Proceed at pace that honors family's cultural, spiritual, and personal preferences and expectations.	A rushed pace may seem disrespectful and increases family distress. Allow time for reflection and saying good-bye.
8. Apply gown or protective barriers as needed.	Withdrawal of IV lines or tubes may cause oozing of blood or release of body fluids.
9. Identify body and leave identification (tag) in place as directed in facility policy.	Ensures proper identification of body in morgue, autopsy room, and funeral home.
10. Remove indwelling catheters, tubes, tape, and airways (check agency policy). Disconnect and cap off (no need to remove) intravenous lines. Leave all devices in place if autopsy is requested or required (coroner's case).	Creates a normal, nonmedical appearance for family at time of viewing the body.
11. Remove soiled dressings and replace with clean gauze dressings using paper tape. Cover puncture wounds with a small dressing.	Changing dressings helps to control odors caused by microorganisms and creates more acceptable appearance. Paper tape minimizes skin trauma.
12. If person wore dentures, insert them. If mouth fails to close, place a rolled-up towel under chin. If dentures do not stay securely in mouth, place in denture cup and transport with body to mortuary.	It is easiest to insert dentures immediately after death. Dentures maintain natural facial expression if body is to be viewed.
13. Close eyes by gently pulling eyelashes over eyes. Some cultures prefer eyes remain open.	Closed eyes present a more natural appearance.
14. Wash body parts soiled by blood, urine, feces, or other drainage. Place an absorbent pad under patient's buttocks.	Prepares body for viewing and reduces odors. Relaxation of sphincter muscles at death releases urine or feces.
15. Place clean gown on patient. Facility policy may require removal after viewing. Do not tie hands together on top of body (see agency policy).	Presents body in natural, modest, and dignified state for viewing.
16. Brush and comb patient's hair. Remove any clips, hairpins, or rubber bands.	Patient should appear well-groomed. Objects can damage or discolor face and scalp.
17. Remove all jewelry and give all personal belongings to designated family member. Exception: If family requests that wedding band be left in place, place a small strip of tape around patient's finger over the ring.	Prevents loss of patient's valuables.
18. Place a sheet or light blanket over body with only head and upper shoulders exposed. Remove medical equipment from room. Provide soft lighting and offer chairs. Determine if family prefers to be alone or have a nurse with them during viewing.	Maintains dignity and respect for patient and limits exposure of body. People viewing body are provided with pleasant, comfortable environment for this important phase of grief process (Marthaler, 2005).
19. After body has been viewed, remove all linen and patient's gown. Place body in body bag with extremities straight at side and cover with shroud in accordance with facility policy (see illustration).	Tying wrists together can cause discoloration and skin damage on a visible part of the body.

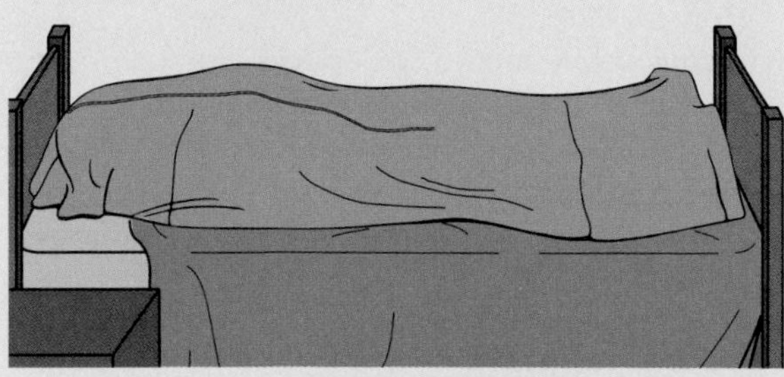
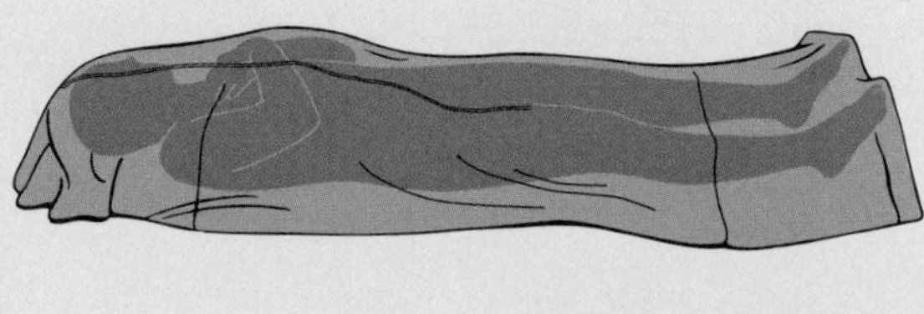

STEP 19 Body in body bag covered by shroud.

STEPS	RATIONALE
20. Before transport to the morgue, place identification on outside of body bag as directed by facility policy. Identify patient using two identifiers (i.e., name and birthday or name and account number, according to facility policy). Compare identifiers with information on patient's identification bracelet. Place isolation tag on body bag if applicable.	Ensures proper identification of body and alerts transporters and morgue personnel of potential infectious hazard.
21. Arrange transportation of body to morgue or mortuary.	Body should be kept in a cooled morgue to delay tissue decomposition.
22. Respond to family questions or concerns. Remind family members to notify others of the death. Confirm name of funeral home.	Following a death, grieving people may have difficulty remembering details and may need guidance.
23. See Completion Protocol (inside front cover).	

EVALUATION

1. Observe family/significant others' response to the loss.
2. Ask family members if they feel they have received emotional/spiritual support after the death.
3. Note appearance and condition of patient's skin during preparation of the body.

Unexpected Outcomes and Related Interventions

1. Grieving survivors become immobilized by grief and have difficulty functioning.
   a. Maintain a calm, unhurried atmosphere. Allow time for questions and expressions of grief.
   b. Offer spiritual or psychological consultation from interdisciplinary team.
2. Lacerations, bruises, or abrasions are noted on deceased's skin surfaces.
   a. Cleanse areas thoroughly before family viewing.
   b. Inform family of any notable bruises or lacerations that they may see.
   c. Document any new skin tears or breakdown.

Recording and Reporting

- Record in nurses' notes the date and time of death as determined by designated health care professional, the time professional notified, name of professional pronouncing death, completion of postmortem care, identification and disposition of body, information provided to significant others, and whether autopsy consent (if needed) was signed.
- Document any marks, bruises, or wounds on body before death or those observed during care of body.
- Document how valuables and personal belongings were handled and who received them. Secure signatures as required by facility policy.

Sample Documentation

0245 Pronounced dead by Dr. S. Williams. Wife and daughter present at time of death and assisted with preparation of the body. Spiritual care provider was present, offering support. Two bruises on left forearm, both approximately 1 cm in diameter. Allen and Sons Funeral Home notified of death. Glasses and clothes sent with body to morgue with transport personnel. White colored metal ring left in place at wife's request, taped to left hand ring finger.

Special Considerations

Pediatric

- Parents need opportunity to hold their deceased child and/or help with body preparation.
- In conjunction with parents, assess siblings' developmental level and readiness to view their brother's or sister's body.
- In cases of neonatal deaths or stillbirths, many parents appreciate having a picture or lock of hair from their child as a remembrance.

Geriatric

- Some geriatric patients have a limited support group. The nurse may be the person who stays with the patient in the final stages of life.
- For older adults who live in an extended-care facility, the residents and staff are often regarded as family members and should be notified of the patient's death.

Home Care

- More people are choosing to die at home with hospice care.
- Family members need ongoing education on end-of-life care, signs of impending death, who to call for help with symptom control, what to do and who to call at the time of death, and how to arrange for transportation of the body.

REVIEW QUESTIONS

Case Study for Questions 1 and 2

Mr. Robinson, a retired auto worker, has advanced incurable lung cancer and is now hospitalized for pneumonia. While in the hospital, he tells his wife that he is tired of fighting his illness and wants to go home to die. His wife becomes alarmed by what she perceives as giving up and urges him to stay in the hospital until he is strong enough to go home again. Mrs. Robinson asks the nurse to help convince him to keep fighting. Mr. Robinson has also told the nurse that he wants to go home.

1. Which of the following responses would be best at this time?
   1. "Your husband has talked to me about this too, and we always support the patient's decision."
   2. "You and your husband are facing some difficult decisions. It sounds like you both want to talk about what is happening."
   3. "I think we should ask the palliative care team to visit your husband."
   4. "I agree. How will he ever get better if he doesn't fight the pneumonia?"
2. Mrs. Robinson was confused about why a nurse from the palliative care team came in to visit with them. Which of the following statements accurately describe(s) palliative care? Select all that apply.
   1. Palliative care is only for people who are at the end of life.
   2. Palliative care focuses on managing patients' physical, emotional, and spiritual symptoms.
   3. Palliative care is only given in the home setting.
   4. Once you are in palliative care, you must stop all treatments to cure your disease.
   5. Members from the palliative care team will play a role in how to address symptoms.
3. A patient tells the nurse that she was given information about preparing an advance directive when she entered the hospital. She asks you to explain how advance directives work. Which of the following explanation(s) is/are accurate? Select all that apply.
   1. "Advance directives have to be written documents."
   2. "Be sure to store your advance directive in a safe deposit box."
   3. "Advance directives are the same across the country."
   4. "You can indicate in an advance directive what kind of care you want and do not want if you are unable to speak for yourself."
   5. "Advance directives help your family members know your wishes for care at the end of life."
4. Which of the following statements best describes the nurse's first response to a family member who states that he believes a decision in his father's end-of-life care is unethical?
   1. Tell the family member that she will call the ethics committee to provide him with good information.
   2. Advise the family member to discuss the matter with the health care provider who wrote the order.
   3. Inform the family member of how commonly that particular intervention is used.
   4. Seek further clarification of the family member's ethical viewpoint.
5. A woman exhibiting confusion has just entered home hospice care. Which of the following nurse activities help(s) to ensure that the patient will get patient-centered care? Select all that apply.
   1. Talk to her husband about her daily routine.
   2. Have her husband prepare an advance directive for her.
   3. Delete salty foods from her diet because she has heart disease.
   4. Observe the patient to determine which positions seem most comfortable for her.
6. The wife of a patient who is at home receiving hospice care says that she does not feel comfortable giving his medications and wonders if he can go to the hospital when he is close to death. Which of the following responses would be most therapeutic?
   1. "When a patient receives hospice care at home, a friend or family member must provide the care. If you can't do it, he will not be able to have hospice services."
   2. "Your husband really wants to die at home. This is the last gift you can give him."
   3. "Medications are really easy to give. He only gets his pain pill and laxative."
   4. "It sounds like you have a lot of questions about being the primary caregiver for your husband."
7. The nurse notices that a patient who has just been diagnosed with a recurrence of her breast cancer is becoming increasingly withdrawn and does not want to take her medications. In which of the following areas should the nurse assess to better understand what the patient is facing? Select all that apply.
   1. Medication regimen
   2. Spiritual and emotional needs and resources
   3. Activity level and last physical therapy session
   4. Usual support persons and when they last visited
   5. Treatment plan
8. A patient at the end of life reports unrelieved pain shortly after getting a pain medication. Which of the following considerations would help the nurse select the most appropriate intervention? Select all that apply.
   1. If patient's disease has progressed, she may need to receive higher doses of the same medication to get pain relief.
   2. The medication has worked all along; the patient must just want more medication.
   3. Spiritual or emotional issues may be complicating the patient's pain perception.

4. The nature of the pain may have changed, requiring the use of an adjuvant medication.
5. The patient's physical assessment and vital signs have not changed; thus the medication will likely work in a short time.

9. A patient receiving home hospice care wants to get out of bed for meals. What would be the nurse's best response to the patient's request?
1. "Let's try it. Your wife and I will help you to the wheelchair and pull you up to the table."
2. "You are so weak, Mr. Jones, that it's probably safer to keep you in bed."
3. "Your appetite has been so poor that it will take too much energy to get up."
4. "Why don't you let us bring our food into the bedroom to eat with you?"

10. The nurse begins to prepare the body of a deceased patient for family viewing and transport to the morgue. Place the following actions in proper sequence, beginning with what the nurse should do first.
a. Wash body parts soiled by blood, urine, feces or other drainage.
b. Elevate the head of the bed.
c. Place a clean gown on the patient.
d. Apply gloves, gown, or protective barriers as applicable.
e. Apply fresh dressings to open wounds.
f. Ask family members if they want to be involved in final preparation of the body.
1. d, f, a, e, c, b
2. b, f, d, e, a, c
3. d, a, f, e, b, c
4. f, a, d, e, c, b

REFERENCES

American Association of Colleges of Nursing (AACN) and City of Hope (COH): *ELNEC-CORE: End of life nursing education consortium (core)*, Duarte, Calif, 2008, AACN.

Aycock N, Boyle D: Interventions to manage compassion fatigue in oncology nursing, *Clin J Oncol Nurs* 13(2):183, 2009.

Block S: Psychological issues in end of life care, *J Palliat Med* 9(3):751, 2006.

Bolmsjo I: End of life care for old people: a review of the literature, *Am J Hosp Palliat Med* 25(4):328, 2008.

Bush N: Compassion fatigue: are you at risk? *Oncol Nurs Forum* 36(1):24, 2009.

Chi G: The role of hope in patients with cancer, *Oncol Nurs Forum* 34(2):415, 2007.

Cinocco D: The difficulties of swallowing at the end of life, *J Palliative Med* 10(2):506, 2007.

Clayton JM and others: Fostering coping and nurturing hope when discussing the future with terminally ill cancer patients and their caregivers, *Cancer* 103(9):1965, 2005.

Cox CL and others: Implications of cultural diversity in do not attempt resuscitation (DNAR) decision making, *J Multicult Nurs Health* 12(1):20, 2006.

Crawley L: Racial, cultural, and ethnic factors influencing end of life care, *J Palliat Med* 8(1):S58, 2005.

Derby S, O'Mahony S: Elderly patients. In Ferrell B, Coyle N, editors: *Textbook of palliative nursing*, New York, 2006, Oxford Press, p 635.

Ferrell B, Coyle N: *Textbook of palliative nursing*, ed 2, New York, 2006, Oxford University Press.

Hellsten M, Kane J: Symptom management in pediatric palliative care. In Ferrell B, Coyle N, editors: *Textbook of palliative nursing*, New York, 2006, Oxford Press, p 895.

Hermann C: The degree to which spiritual needs of patients near the end of life are met, *Oncol Nurs Forum* 34(1):70, 2007.

Herr K and others: Pain assessment in the nonverbal patient: position statement with clinical practice recommendations, *Pain Manage Nurs* 7(2):44, 2006.

Hipp B, Letizia M: Understanding and responding to the death rattle in dying patients, *Medsurg Nurs* 18(1):17, 2009.

Kehl K: Caring for the patient and family in the last hours of life, *Home Health Care Manag Pract* 20(5):408, 2008.

Kemp C: Cultural issues in palliative care, *Semin Oncol Nurs* 21(1):44, 2005.

Kuebler K and others: Perspectives in palliative care, *Semin Oncol Nurs* 21(1):2, 2005.

Lynch M, Dahlin C: The national consensus project and national quality forum preferred practices in the case of the imminently dying: implications for nursing, *J Hosp Palliat Nurs* 9(6):316, 2007.

Marthaler M: End of life care: practical tips, *Dimens Crit Care Nurs* 24(5):215, 2005.

Matzo M, Sherman D: *Palliative care nursing: quality care to the end of life*, New York, 2006, Springer.

Osse B and others: Problems experienced by the informal caregivers of cancer patients and their needs for support, *Cancer Nurs* 29(5):378, 2006.

Paice J, Fine P: Pain at the end of life. In Ferrell B, Coyle N, editors: *Textbook of palliative nursing*, New York, 2006, Oxford Press, p 131.

Plonk W, Arnold R: Terminal care: the last weeks of life, *J Palliat Med* 8(5):1042, 2005.

Phillips L, Reed P: Into the abyss of someone else's dying: the voice of the end of life caregiver, *Clin Nurs Res* 18(1):80, 2009.

Sherman and others: Preparation and care at the time of death, *J Nurses Staff Dev* 21(1):93, 2005.

Vandecreek L, Lucas A, editors: *The discipline for pastoral caregiving: Foundations for outcome-oriented chaplaincy*, Binghamton, NY, 2001, Haworth Press.

World Health Organization National Cancer Control Programs: *Policies and managerial guidelines*, ed 2, Geneva, 2002, World Health Organization.

CHAPTER

32

Home Care Safety

evolve WEBSITE

http://evolve.elsevier.com/Perry/nursinginterventions

The collaborative relationship between the nurse and recipient of care in the home requires the use of the term *client* rather than *patient* in these settings. Clients need instruction so they feel less anxious about self-care in the home and moving about in their environment. Home care instruction begins at the time of admission to a health care facility and includes multiple topics on health care promotion (e.g., prenatal care and exercise), coping with impaired function (e.g., speech therapy and making adaptive changes in the home), and restoration of health due to disease (e.g., learning how to take medicines and modify diet). It continues into the home and community settings, and it helps clients learn, assess available education programs, establish health education goals, and prioritize home care needs. During this instruction you encourage clients to provide feedback to ensure that the information provided is understood, appropriate, and useful. Document client education and achievement of outcomes in the client's medical record, according to agency policy.

CLIENT-CENTERED CARE

Home care clients include older adults, the chronically ill, disabled adults and children, and those who have experienced an acute illness or injury. The nurse focuses on the client, taking into account the client-family interaction, and provides education and interventions appropriate for all parties (Motyka and Nies, 2007). In addition, completion of a cultural assessment increases understanding of the client's beliefs, values, and practices to determine appropriate nursing interventions (Andrews, 2007). A home care nurse is sensitive to a client's surroundings and delivers care in a culturally sensitive manner, respectful of the client and support system.

Home care is part of the continuum of care. Nurses are instrumental in helping clients to achieve their maximum functional ability and adjust to changes once back in their home. Older adults can be at greater risk for environmental hazards and mistreatment as they age. The nurse works with clients in the home and encourages them to share the responsibility for maintaining a healthy lifestyle (Ebersole and others, 2008). An in-depth assessment gives nurses clues as to areas of needed education and intervention.

SAFETY

The Joint Commission (TJC, 2010) identified 16 goals related to client safety in home care. Included in these goals are improving the effectiveness of communication among caregivers, improving the safety of using medications, reducing the risk of injury from falls, and encouraging active involvement in one's care.

Home safety modifications affect all people living in the home. The nurse must include the client and family caregivers in all discussions. Be prepared to discuss concerns about the number of modifications required, costs of modifications, and change in home decor. Accident prevention begins with making timely and adequate home repairs; however, it may also be necessary to modify the home to make it more accessible for the client. The goal is to provide an environment in which the client and family caregiver can provide self-care safely and effectively.

EVIDENCE-BASED PRACTICE TRENDS

Drury LJ: DP and home care need improved communication, *J Contin Educ Nurs* 39(5):198, 2008.

Stolee P and others: Risk factors for hip fracture in older home care clients, *J Gerontol* 64A(3):403, 2009.

Drury (2008) explained that nurses need to take steps to transition their clients from the hospital to the home. Included in this transition is reconciling preadmission lifestyles (e.g., medications, diet, activity restrictions) with discharge lifestyles. The need for teaching clients and family caregivers before discharge to ensure their ability to perform procedures needed at home was emphasized.

Stolee and others (2009) examined the risk factors for hip fractures in home care of older adults. The researchers analyzed data from 40,279 home care clients 65 years of age and older. Males and females had different risk profiles; however, tobacco use and use of an ambulation aid were risk factors for both. Older females were at an increased risk; and those with osteoporosis, history of falls, unsteady gait, malnutrition, and cognitive impairment were also vulnerable. The researchers found that frail older adult home care clients needed fall and hip fracture prevention strategies and emphasized the importance of screening clients for risk factors and educating them on prevention.

SKILL 32.1 HOME HEALTH SAFETY AND ASSESSMENT

The home environment should be a place in which individuals feel healthy, comfortable, and safe. Older adults are at risk for threats to safety as a result of physiological changes that come with aging. Fall prevention is a critical component of home care safety. After a fall an older adult may experience greater functional decline in ADLs; prevention is imperative to help maintain independence and quality of life (Aykol, 2007).

Injury and violence prevention is a proposed objective identified by *Healthy People 2020* (US Department of Health and Human Services, [HHS], 2010). Knowledge of specific motor and cognitive developmental needs helps the nurse in the home setting to assess the potential for injury for each client. After areas of risk are identified, he or she designs interventions to eliminate or reduce threats to the client's safety.

ASSESSMENT

1. Determine client's actual or potential limitations resulting from sensory, motor, cognitive, or physical changes. *Rationale: These factors increase client's risk of injury.*
2. Assess client's physical and mental status and determine type of adaptations necessary in the home. *Rationale: The nature of physical and cognitive limitations determines the type of adjustments to be made in the home.*
3. Assess client's attitudes about returning home and following health care provider recommendations. Determine client's perceived benefit of action, perceived barrier to action, interpersonal influences such as family and peers, and commitment to a plan of action. *Rationale: These variables are major sources of motivation for changing behavior, and nursing interventions are targeted toward these variables (Pender and others, 2006).*
4. Consult other health care team members about client needs in the home. Make appropriate referrals. *Rationale: Members of all health care disciplines collaborate to determine client's needs and functional abilities.*
5. Assess developmental stage of client. *Rationale: Safety needs of clients vary based on their developmental age.*
6. Assess client's history of falls in the past. If client has fallen at home, use the mnemonic, SPLATT to assess the client. *Rationale: Previous falls often indicate an increased risk for falling or a client's fear of falling. Assessing prior falls helps identify factors that contribute to or prevent future falls.*
   Symptoms at time of fall
   Previous fall
   Location of fall
   Activity at time of fall
   Time of fall
   Trauma after fall (Meiner and Lueckenotte, 2006)

PLANNING

Expected Outcomes focus on identifying risk factors and providing a safe environment in the home.

1. Client/family identifies safety risks in the home.
2. Client/family identifies community resources available and how to initiate contact.
3. Client/family does not experience injury in the home.

Delegation and Collaboration

The skill of risk assessment and accident prevention cannot be delegated to nursing assistive personnel (NAP). However, the nurse may need to consult with a physical or an occupational therapist to conduct a thorough home safety assessment and determine appropriate adaptations needed based on client's physical and/or cognitive limitations.

Equipment

- Home safety checklist

IMPLEMENTATION *for* HOME HEALTH SAFETY AND ASSESSMENT

STEPS	RATIONALE
1. **See Standard Protocol (inside front cover).**	
2. Involve client and family as active participants in a home safety assessment using a checklist (Table 32-1).	Active participation enhances learning and empowers making decisions about care.
3. General safety in the home	

Continued

TABLE 32-1 HOME SAFETY CHECKLIST

CRITERIA FRONT AND BACK ENTRANCES	YES	NO
1. Walkways and steps are smooth and well lighted. Sturdy handrail is on both sides of stairs to entrance.	_____	_____
2. Nonskid strips/safety treads or bright paint is used on outdoor steps. All steps have the same depth and rise.	_____	_____
3. A shelf or bench is kept by front/back doors to place grocery bags or packages if needed.	_____	_____
4. Doormats are in good condition.	_____	_____
Kitchen		
1. Client wears clothes with short or close-fitting sleeves when cooking.	_____	_____
2. Stove control dials are easy to see and use, and stove top and oven are clean and grease free.	_____	_____
3. Items in kitchen cabinets and shelves are easy to reach.	_____	_____
4. Lighting over sink, stove, and work areas is bright.	_____	_____
5. Client stays in kitchen while cooking.	_____	_____
6. Fire extinguisher is available.	_____	_____
Floors		
1. All carpeting and mats are secure. Skid backing is present under area rugs, or throw rugs are removed.	_____	_____
2. Walkways are free of clutter.	_____	_____
Bathrooms		
1. Door lock can be unlocked from both sides.	_____	_____
2. Tub or shower has nonskid mats or abrasive strips.	_____	_____
3. Tub or shower has at least one grab bar kept free of towels or other items.	_____	_____
4. Shower has a stable stool or chair and handheld sprayer.	_____	_____
5. Cold and hot water faucets are clearly marked, and temperature on water heater is 120° F (49° C) or less.	_____	_____
6. A night-light is available.	_____	_____
Bedroom		
1. Client can turn on light without having to get out of bed in the dark.	_____	_____
2. Furniture is arranged to provide clear path from bed to bathroom.	_____	_____
3. Phone with emergency numbers is within easy reach of bed.	_____	_____
4. Alarm systems are available. There are listening devices for invalid clients.	_____	_____
Living Room/Family Room		
1. Light can be turned on without having to walk into dark room.	_____	_____
2. Lamp, extension, or phone cords are kept out of traffic ways.	_____	_____
3. Furniture is arranged so it can be walked around easily.	_____	_____
Fire Safety		
1. Sufficient numbers of working smoke detectors are in appropriate locations.	_____	_____
2. Emergency exit plans are in place in case of fire.	_____	_____
3. Family has determined a meeting place outside the house.	_____	_____
4. Portable space heaters are used and kept 3 feet away from flammable items.	_____	_____
5. Furnace area is free of things that can catch on fire.	_____	_____
6. Furnace and chimney are checked annually by a qualified professional.	_____	_____
7. Emergency numbers for police, fire, and poison control are posted near phone.	_____	_____
8. Fire extinguisher is available and easy to handle and use.	_____	_____
Electrical Safety		
1. Electrical cords are in good condition and not frayed, spliced, or cracked.	_____	_____
2. Electrical cords are kept away from water.	_____	_____
3. Extension cord/outlet extenders have built-in circuit breaker or fuse.	_____	_____
4. Wall outlets and switches have cover plates.	_____	_____
5. Light bulbs are of correct wattage for each fixture.	_____	_____
6. Fuse box is easily accessible and clearly labeled.	_____	_____
7. Lamp switches are easy to turn on to avoid burns from hot light bulbs.	_____	_____
Carbon Monoxide Prevention		
1. Furnace flues are checked regularly for patency.	_____	_____
2. Carbon monoxide detector is in home.	_____	_____

Modified from Meiner SE, Lueckenotte AG: *Gerontologic nursing,* ed 3, St Louis, 2006, Mosby.

STEPS	RATIONALE
a. With client and family identify ways to make home environment safe; post emergency phone numbers near all telephones.	A safe environment helps maintain or improve level of independence and function.
b. If client is an older adult who is alone frequently, suggest use of a home monitoring system (HMS) and set a schedule for client to "check in" with family, neighbors, or friends.	HMS technologies support and enable safe independent living (Mihailidis and others, 2008). Checking in with others at regular times communicates that client is safe at home (Meiner and Lueckenotte, 2006).
c. Reduce the number of different pain medications the client uses if possible (consult with physician).	Prevents oversedation and enhances ability of client to make safe decisions.
d. Offer client and family appropriate information about community health care resources.	The emphasis is to keep client in the home for as long as it is safe and desirable to do so. During decision-making period regarding need for care outside the home, the role of the nurse is to support client and family and provide information about available options (Hockenberry and others, 2008; Meiner and Lueckenotte, 2006).
4. Electrical safety	
a. Verify that major electrical appliances are grounded and that there are no overloaded plugs or sockets. Examine plugs, cords, and switch plates for signs of damage.	Reduces risk of electrical shock and fire (Electrical Safety Foundation International [ESFi], 2010).
b. If small children are in the house, cover unused outlets with safety plugs.	Prevents child from electrical shock.
c. Check fuse box accessibility and wattage of light bulbs.	Correct wattage lessens risk of fire.
5. Fire safety/burn prevention	
a. Instruct client to keep thermostat on hot water heater below 120° F (49° C).	Prevents scalding burns from hot water (Meiner and Lueckenotte, 2006).
b. Encourage client not to smoke. If he or she smokes, educate client him or her not to smoke while tired or in bed.	Smoking and secondhand smoke are health hazards; falling asleep while smoking is associated with preventable deaths and injuries (Meiner and Lueckenotte, 2006).
c. Instruct clients, especially those with small children in the home, about stove safety (e.g., turn pot handles inward, away from edge of stove; install stove knob protectors and a stove lock).	Safe stove use helps prevent burns.
d. Instruct client on safe usage of portable space heaters.	Prevents accidental fire.
e. Discuss emergency exit plan with client.	Assists in rapid evacuation of home.
6. Fall prevention	
a. Schedule diuretics early in the day and space antihypertensives and antiarrhythmics at different times to minimize side effects.	Appropriate diuretic schedule minimizes interruption in sleep and trips to the bathroom at night. Antihypertensives and antiarrhythmics often cause hypotension and dizziness, increasing risk of falls (Touhy and Jett, 2010).
b. Consider changing the physical environment to reduce predisposition to falls such as removing trip hazards on the floor and installing safety grab bars in the bathroom.	Modifying the home environment is effective in preventing falls (Meiner and Lueckenotte, 2006).
c. Inspect client's shoes. Teach him or her to wear shoes with thin, firm soles and moderate traction, especially if he or she has a shuffling gait.	Better stability and proprioception are provided by shoes that have a thin, firm sole with moderate traction. Footwear with thicker soles (e.g., sneakers) can result in tripping if the client has a shuffling gait.
d. Refer client to physical therapist for rehabilitative and/or therapeutic exercise if indicated.	Tailored exercise programs help decrease the risk of falls.
e. Teach client and family about risks for falling and plan for reducing falls in the home.	Clients who are educated about their fall risk and understand their illnesses are less fearful of falling.

Continued

STEPS	RATIONALE
f. Have client keep a fall diary if he or she falls or almost falls at home. Organize diary so client enters date and time of each fall, activity at time of fall, and any related symptoms or injury. If family caregiver witnesses fall, he or she should make an entry. Instruct client to share diary with physicians, nurses, and other health care providers.	Information in diary provides helpful information about what happened before and after the fall. Information can be used by health care providers to develop strategies for preventing falls (Meiner and Lueckenotte, 2006).
7. Firearm safety	
a. Teach client about dangers associated with keeping guns in the home.	The risk of suicide increases in homes with firearms (Edelman and Mandle, 2009).
b. If guns are in the home, teach client to install trigger locks on them and store them unloaded in a locked cabinet. Teach client to store ammunition in a secured area separate from the guns. Store keys in a place inaccessible to children.	Following gun safety standards decreases the risk of injury and death related to gun use (Hockenberry and others, 2008).
8. Ask client to verbalize information taught.	
9. See Completion Protocol (inside front cover).	

EVALUATION

1. Ask client to identify safety risks present in the home.
2. Have client describe plan that minimizes risk for injury and leads to safe health behavior choices.
3. Ask client and family to identify resources available for a particular problem and how to initiate contact with that resource.
4. Ask client and family if anyone has experienced an injury in the home.

Unexpected Outcomes and Related Interventions

1. Client is unable to identify safety risks.
   a. Reevaluate home environment with client and family.
   b. Reinforce information about preventing and removing potential hazards from home environment.
2. Client and family do not follow through with plan to reduce risks in home.
   a. Assess client's concerns or views about making changes.
   b. Assess client's finances.
   c. Establish a plan that includes changes that client will accept.
3. Client and family are unaware of community resources.
   a. Reinforce information about available resources.
   b. Provide informational brochures and contact information for resources.
4. Client/family reports that an injury has occurred in the home.
   a. Determine cause and extent of injury.
   b. Suggest further modifications that can be made in the home to prevent future injuries.

Recording and Reporting

- Retain copy of the home safety assessment in client's home health record.
- Record assessment of cognitive and mental status, recommended interventions, and client's and caregiver's response to the assessment.
- Record any instruction provided, client's response, and changes made to the environment.

Sample Documentation

0900 Safety checklist completed with client and family members. Spouse states will remove throw rugs and have hand rails installed in bathroom. Referred client to physical therapy for selection of ambulation assist device.

Special Considerations

Pediatric

- Ensuring the safety of children in the home is based on child's developmental level. Instruct families to use safety devices as applicable.
- Suggest that parents or caregivers get down on the floor to look at the environment from child's view to identify dangers present in the home (Hockenberry and others, 2008).
- Children imitate and copy what they see and hear. Instruct parents that practicing safety teaches safety (Hockenberry and others, 2008).
- Teach families car safety based on child's age, developmental level, and size. Children are placed in appropriate restraint system; if the car has airbags, children less than 12 years of age need to ride in the back seat or as defined by state law.

Geriatric

- Physiological and mental status changes (e.g., slower reaction time, reduced pain and temperature perception, and reduced visual acuity) place older adults at risk for injury in the home environment.
- Older adults are usually more aware of potential dangers when they are in a familiar setting.
- Frail older adults should not ride in the passenger side of the car if the car has airbags. Teach them to sit in the back seat or at least 10 inches away from the airbag.

Home Care

- Make changes in client's home environment to keep him or her as independent as possible.
- Before making any revisions to a client's home, know his or her financial resources and let him or her be the final decision maker in the types of changes to be made whenever possible. Consider client's physical strengths and remaining functional abilities, not just the disabilities.
- Educate caregivers about the importance of preserving client autonomy.

SKILL 32.2 ADAPTING THE HOME SETTING FOR CLIENTS WITH COGNITIVE DEFICITS

Clients with cognitive impairments and their families need assistance in making adaptations to preserve their ability to function safely within the home. To be safe, a person needs to be able to perform routine ADLs and make sound decisions. When there are cognitive limitations, a person's independence is threatened. Family members often do not understand changes in cognition and function and need help to determine whether a client is competent to remain at home safely.

It is a myth that all older adults experience cognitive dysfunctions; however, older adults are more likely to develop them. Accurate assessment includes mental and physical health, social and economic status, functional status, and the environment (Ebersole and others, 2008). Some mental processes may be intact (e.g., orientation to name, time, and place), whereas at the same time other processes are compromised (e.g., short-term memory of life events).

In addition to mental status and cognitive changes, it is important to recognize that many older adults suffer from depression (Meiner and Lueckenotte, 2006). Depression occurs alone or in combination with cognitive disorders such as dementia. Depression often results from social isolation (e.g., the older adult is homebound and has few visitors).

ASSESSMENT

1. Assess client over several short periods and be ready to adapt your assessment if client has sensory disabilities. *Rationale: Improves likelihood of gathering relevant data (Ebersole and others, 2008).*
2. Listen carefully to client in a quiet, well-lit space, without interruptions or distractions. Speak slowly, clearly, and in a normal tone of voice. *Rationale: Providing an optimal environment ensures accurate assessment of client's cognitive and mental status.*
3. Ask client to describe own level of health and ability to provide self-care skills. Ask family members to confirm description. Also assess for risky behaviors (e.g., unsupervised use of stove, handling of weapons). *Rationale: Question requires client to describe abilities and health challenges. Family members are able to provide helpful insight, especially about risky behaviors. Minimizing risky behaviors is essential in making the environment safe.*
4. Ask how client is doing with home management responsibilities and with managing medical care. *Rationale: Data gathered allow you to assess short-term memory, judgment, and problem solving.*
5. If you suspect that client is wandering or at risk for wandering, observe and assess for the following characteristics and behaviors. *Rationale: Clients who exhibit these behaviors or have these characteristics are more prone to wandering:*
   - Higher level of cognitive impairment
   - Difficulty sleeping
   - Active lifestyle before becoming cognitively impaired
   - Use of psychotropic medications
   - Pacing or walking that cannot be redirected easily
   - Getting lost in familiar places
   - Client explains he or she is searching for "missing" people or places
6. Determine if client has a family member or friend who helps with self-care or home management responsibilities. *Rationale: Determines availability of potential resources for client.*
7. Assess competency of family caregiver and caregiver's perception of ability to care for client safely in the home. *Rationale: Caring for caregiver and ensuring that caregiver can care for client competently are essential in providing a safe environment for client.*

PLANNING

Expected Outcomes focus on adaptation of the home environment and promoting client's ability to perform ADLs.

1. Client is able to complete as many home management responsibilities as possible within existing limitations.
2. Caregiver(s) use adaptations in the home that help client perform home management activities as needed.

Delegation and Collaboration

The skill of adapting the home setting for clients with cognitive deficits cannot be delegated to nursing assistive personnel (NAP). Instruct the NAP about the following:

- Observing for and reporting any changes in client mood, memory, and ability to maintain the home

Equipment

- Mini-Mental State Examination
- Calendar
- Paper for making lists
- Bulletin board or poster board (optional)
- Motion detector (optional)

IMPLEMENTATION *for* ADAPTING THE HOME SETTING *for* CLIENTS WITH COGNITIVE DEFICITS

STEPS	RATIONALE
1. See Standard Protocol (inside front cover).	
2. If client has difficulty remembering when to perform self-care routines, create a list or post reminder notes written in large print in a noticeable place. Suggest use of a wristwatch with an alarm to signal time of scheduled activity and use of a medication organization container to help with medication administration.	Memory function in older adults tends to be preserved for relevant, well-known material (Meiner and Lueckenotte, 2006). Lists and other reminders help client remember and complete required tasks. Large print is helpful when client has limited eyesight.
3. Schedule medications that cause confusion or drowsiness at bedtime.	Maintains mental status during the day at the maximum level possible.
4. Instruct family caregiver to focus on client's abilities rather than disabilities.	Retains client's autonomy and sense of self-worth.
5. When client has difficulty completing tasks with multiple steps, reduce number of steps or simplify task.	Prevents frustration and forgetting one or more steps that lead to not finishing task.
6. Help client and family develop a schedule for routine ADLs such as eating, bathing, and exercise.	Consistency creates a sense of security and helps keep client oriented to ADLs.
7. Have caregiver set up activities so client can complete them (e.g., lay out clothes to wear for the day, place food for meals out on the counter).	Helps client complete tasks even though unable to plan and perform all the steps.
8. Instruct caregiver to use simple and direct communication using calm and relaxed approach. Use eye contact and touch. Speak in simple words and short sentences.	Facilitates effective communication and reduces anxiety.
9. Place clocks, calendars, and personal mementos throughout rooms within the home.	Maintaining familiar surroundings maximizes cognitive function.
10. Enhance the environment with addition of tactile boards or three-dimensional art.	
11. If client wanders, consider the following interventions:	
a. Provide a safe place (e.g., large room in den free of obstacles) for client to wander.	Reduces risk of client leaving residence.
b. Provide clues (e.g., signs) to guide client to a desired location.	Reduces aimless wandering.
c. Recommend that caregiver install door locks or electronic guards.	Reduces chance of wandering.
d. Address the cause of wandering (e.g., provide food if hungry) and eliminate or lessen stressors (e.g., pain).	Reduces causes of wandering.
12. Have caregiver routinely remind client of who he or she is and what the next step will be.	Improves client's responses to activities and environment (Meiner and Lueckenotte, 2006).
13. Facilitate regular naps or rest periods.	Fatigue adds to mental status changes.
14. Encourage and support frequent visits by family and friends. Encourage use of humor and reminiscing about favorite stories.	Prevents boredom and reduces restlessness.
15. See Completion Protocol (inside front cover).	

EVALUATION

1. Ask client to review the home management activities completed that day and the previous day.
2. Ask family caregiver to describe approaches used to help client maintain independence.

Unexpected Outcomes and Related Interventions

1. Client is unable to complete daily activities as planned.
   a. Review what occurred and identify barriers.
   b. Identify strategies for maintaining adequate support and overcoming barriers.
2. Family caregiver is unable to carry out techniques that improve orientation and ability of client to complete activities.
   a. Offer reinstruction for caregiver.
   b. Reassess caregiver's ability to provide necessary support. Consider other living arrangements or support services if indicated.

Recording and Reporting

- Record cognitive abilities and mental status, recommended interventions, and client's and caregiver's responses.
- Report significant decline in cognitive or mental status to physician or health care provider.

Sample Documentation

2100 Oriented to person and place but not to time. States is "waiting for breakfast." Reoriented by having client look outside to see that it is dark and telling her that it will soon be bedtime. Sister reports that client has wandered less since offering more frequent meals and planning naps.

Special Considerations

Pediatric

- Children with cognitive impairments often are not aware of dangers normally present during play and daily activities. Adult supervision is critical.

Geriatric

- Many clients experience progressive loss of function, requiring continuous adaptations and adjustments. If client becomes unable to complete any ADLs or experiences major behavioral changes (e.g., excessive wandering), you may need to help family member determine need for a skilled nursing facility.
- The nurse can reduce caregiver stress by educating him or her about problematic behaviors and how to manage them (Meiner and Lueckenotte, 2006).

SKILL 32.3 MEDICATION AND MEDICAL DEVICE SAFETY

Older adults are prone to medication toxicities resulting from polypharmacy and physiological changes from advanced age (Zillich and others, 2008). Preventable adverse effects such as depression, constipation, falls, delirium, and confusion may occur (Zillich and others, 2008). Assess the client's use of prescribed medications, herbal remedies, and over-the-counter medications to ensure safety and prevent untoward effects.

The use of different medical devices in the home further complicates the ability of clients to care for themselves. Medical devices include syringes, blood glucose monitoring equipment, dressings, and intravenous devices. Clients need to understand medication administration, storage of medical devices and medications, proper waste disposal, and prevention of infection.

Clients who have special needs include those with acute sensory or neurological impairment, chronic illnesses such as diabetes or arthritis, and physical limitations that make manipulation of medical devices and handling medications difficult. In some cases a family member or other caregiver must learn to provide this care (Fig. 32-1).

ASSESSMENT

1. Assess client's visual, cognitive, musculoskeletal, and neurological function; level of consciousness or sedation; vision; hearing; literacy; and willingness to learn. *Rationale: Helps to identify approaches to use in instruction and appropriate assistive devices needed.*
2. Assess client's knowledge of medication regimen and compare with actual regimen. Also assess length of time client has been receiving each drug. *Rationale: Determines complexity of medication regimen and client's familiarity with each drug.*
3. Identify where medications are stored and the type of storage containers used. *Rationale: Determines safe use of medications.*
4. Assess resources for obtaining medications when needed. *Rationale: Lack of resources interferes with self-medication at home.*

PLANNING

Expected Outcomes focus on client's ability to manage medications and medical devices safely.

1. Client states purpose of each medication, common side effects, and when to notify health care provider about problems.
2. Client is able to read each label and explain when each drug is to be taken.

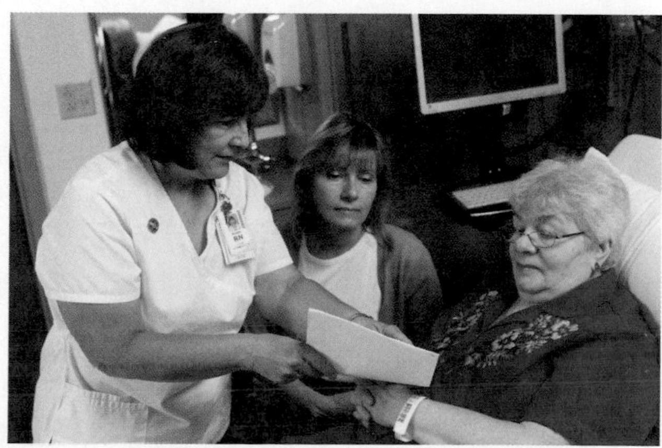

FIG 32-1 A family member or other caregiver often needs to learn about prescribed medications.

3. Client/caregiver prepares and administers prescribed medications independently.
4. Client/caregiver stores medications and medical devices properly and disposes of medical wastes safely.

Delegation and Collaboration

The skill of medication and medical device safety cannot be delegated to nursing assistive personnel (NAP). Instruct the NAP about the following:

- Observing for and reporting unsafe behaviors, improper disposal of sharps and contaminated supplies, and use of infection control practices

Equipment

- Written instructions or charts
- Medications
- Container for daily or weekly medication preparation
- Measuring devices (e.g., medicine cup, teaspoon, syringe) if needed
- Colored marking pens
- Labels
- Assistive device (e.g., syringe magnifier) or medical device (e.g., blood glucose monitor)
- Puncture-resistant sharps container or other hard plastic bottle (e.g., fabric softener bottle) with cap

IMPLEMENTATION *for* MEDICATION AND MEDICAL DEVICE SAFETY

STEPS	RATIONALE
1. See Standard Protocol (inside front cover).	
2. Educate client and caregiver about prescribed medications and over-the-counter medications that are scheduled and taken prn, including: a. Purpose of medications and their expected effects. b. How medications work. c. Dosage schedules and rationale. d. Common side effects and what to do to relieve side effects. e. What to do if dose is missed. f. When to call the physician or health care provider.	Education about medications enhances compliance with medication therapy and reduces errors in medication administration.
3. Suggest use of appropriate devices to help client take medications as scheduled: a. Make calendars for each week with plastic bags of medications to take at specific times. b. Divide egg cartons into color-coded sections with medications for the day, using color-coding for drug types (e.g., blue for sedative, red for pain pill). c. Use pillboxes that are set up daily or weekly to separate pills into slots for each day of the week and appropriate time of day (see illustration).	Helps client decrease medication administration errors.

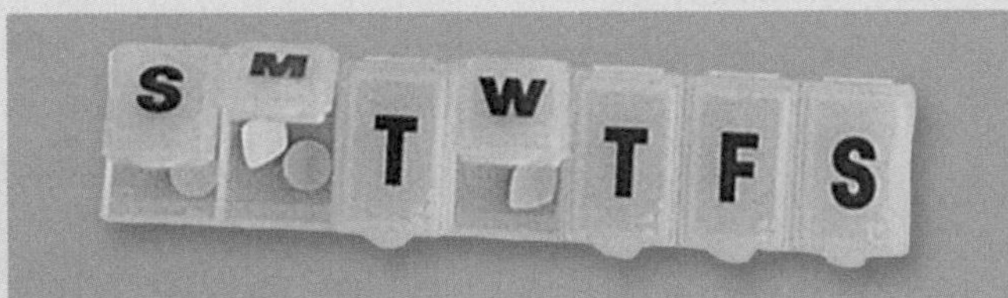

STEP 3c Pill organizer for each day of the week.

STEPS	RATIONALE
4. Educate client and caregiver about the principles of safe medication administration and the recommended modifications for safe administration.	Medication prescriptions specify frequency, dosage, and special instructions (e.g., take before meals).
a. Prescribed medication must be used only as prescribed and by person for whom it was prescribed.	It is unsafe for members of the household to take medications prescribed for another person.
b. Do not take expired medications.	Medication may be toxic or no longer effective.
c. Keep medications in original containers and make sure that label is clear and legible. Have pharmacy provide large print or Braille labels if needed.	Putting several different kinds of medications in the same container is unsafe because client can mix up dosages or schedules of administration. Large print makes label reading easier.

STEPS	RATIONALE
d. Finish prescribed medications and, if ordered, get refills before container is empty.	It is unsafe for client to keep some medication when symptoms are gone, planning to use it later. It is essential to order refills so there is no interruption in medication routine.
e. Have pharmacist put medications in a container that client can open easily if manual dexterity is limited.	Childproof containers may be difficult to open if client has limited mobility of fingers/hands.
SAFETY ALERT Help identify a safe place for storage of medication to reduce risk of accidental ingestion by children.	
f. Use color-coding system for prescribed medications by marking tops of medication containers with the same color when they are taken at the same time.	Often helps clients take medications at right time.
5. Instruct client or caregiver about safe use and disposal of medical devices and supplies.	Prevents injuries from contaminated supplies.
a. Instruct client or caregiver how to use medical device, using diagrams, written information, and other resources (e.g., Internet), and provide for return demonstration when possible.	Clear written information, diagrams, and other resources enhance client learning and allow reinforcement of information.
b. Instruct client or caregiver on proper storage and care of medical device.	Ensures that device will continue to work safely and accurately.
c. Instruct client to place needles, syringes, lancets, or other sharp objects in hard plastic or metal container such as a soda bottle or laundry detergent container with screw-on or tightly secured lid.	Reduces transmission of microorganisms and prevents exposure to body fluids (OSHA, 2001).
d. Instruct client to put soiled bandages, disposable sheets, and medical gloves in securely fastened plastic bag before being placed in garbage can.	Ensures safe disposal of medical supplies (OSHA, 2001).
6. See Completion Protocol (inside front cover).	

EVALUATION

1. Ask client to state purpose of each medication, common side effects, and when to notify health care provider about problems associated with medications.
2. Ask client to explain when each medication is to be taken.
3. Observe client/caregiver preparing and administering medications and using medical devices independently.
4. Complete a pill count at specific intervals.
5. Ask to see where client/caregiver stores items and observe disposal of medical supplies.

Unexpected Outcomes and Related Interventions

1. Client makes errors in preparing medications or is unable to recall information.
   a. Provide written instructions at client's/caregiver's level of understanding. Pictures are very helpful.
   b. Repeat and reinforce important information. Give positive feedback for accurate recall of information.
   c. Provide repeated supervised practice until client is able to self-administer medications safely.
2. Client's self-care deficits prevent safe self-medicating.
   a. Develop alternate plan, which may require family, friends, or home health agency.
   b. Consider need for alternative living arrangements.
3. Excess or insufficient pills are found in pill container during pill count.
   a. Reevaluate use of dosage reminders.
   b. Establish monitoring system until client is able to self-medicate accurately.
4. Medications and medical devices/supplies are not stored and/or disposed of in a secure or appropriate location.
   a. Identify barriers and appropriate alternatives.
   b. Explain risks posed when supplies/devices are not handled safely.

Recording and Reporting

- Document all instructions given, including details of medication administration, use of medical devices, and client's response to instruction.
- Describe system planned to ensure safe medication administration and use of medical devices.

Sample Documentation

0900 Instructed on self-administration of digoxin. Client states purpose of medication, common side effects, and when to notify physician about medication-related concerns. Able to read each label and state when drug is to be taken. Demonstrated how to take pulse correctly.

Special Considerations

Pediatric

- Keep all medications, medical supplies, and equipment safely out of reach of children.
- Tell family caregivers not to refer to medications as treats; this could add to risk of child overdosing by mistaking medicine for candy.

Geriatric

- Capacity for learning new information remains as adults age (in the absence of dementia). Additional time is needed to accomplish learning; allow adequate time and number of teaching sessions to support successful learning.
- The assistance of a home health nurse is often needed to fill weekly pillbox containers.

REVIEW QUESTIONS

Case Study for Questions 1 and 2

Mrs. Jones is the parent of a 4-year-old girl who was recently discharged from the hospital after an acute asthma attack. Mrs. Jones is a stay-at-home mother who exercises regularly and reports that she smokes a pack of cigarettes daily. The home health nurse visits Mrs. Jones to assess the 4-year-old child's respiratory function after discharge and becomes concerned that the home environment contains hazards that can affect the child.

1. The home care nurse instructs Mrs. Jones in ways to prevent burns. Her instructions include which of the following safety measures? Select all that apply.
   1. Turn pot handles to face inward when cooking on stovetop.
   2. Install a stove lock.
   3. Set hot water heater above 120° F (49° C).
   4. Offer smoking cessation classes.
2. The home care nurse observes that Mrs. Jones' elderly mother lives with her and uses a cane to walk. The nurse is concerned about risk for falls. Which of the following actions could the nurse take to prevent a fall?
   1. Discourage use of the cane.
   2. Encourage client to wear shoes with thick soles.
   3. Advise client to remove area rugs from home.
   4. Schedule diuretic medications in late evening.
3. When should discharge planning begin?
   1. When the client is able to participate fully
   2. On client's admission to a health care facility
   3. After client has been stabilized
   4. Only when client is going to a long-term care facility
4. Which of the following approaches does a nurse use when assessing a client with cognitive deficits?
   1. Assess client over a time period of at least 1 year.
   2. Only acknowledge the answers given by caregivers.
   3. Have client describe his or her own level of health.
   4. Meet with client in a public area.
5. A client who is at risk for wandering must be monitored carefully. The nurse educates caregivers of these clients in safety measures by encouraging caregivers to use which of the following tactics? Select all that apply.
   1. Provide signs in the home to guide the client.
   2. Remove locks from doors.
   3. Allow wandering in a safe place.
   4. Use restraints to discourage wandering.
6. The home care nurse visits an 83-year-old woman who has multiple health problems. The client takes eight different medicines. Which of the following measures would help prevent a medication administration error?
   1. Have client get a refill before a medicine container is empty.
   2. Have pharmacist place pills in an easy-to-open container.
   3. Dispense pills into a pill organizer for a full week.
   4. Do not take expired medications.
7. In helping an older adult self-administer his or her medications, the nurse performs which of the following actions? Select all that apply.
   1. Use color coding to identify drugs to take at the same time.
   2. Have client develop own unique way to store medications.
   3. Dispose of used needles in a plastic bag.
   4. Review safe storage techniques for medications.
   5. Have pharmacist put medication in container that client can open easily.
8. The home care nurse visits a client who has an ulcer on his lower leg. The client's wife performs the dressing change for the nurse. The nurse knows that the wife is able to dispose of medical supplies correctly by which of the following?
   1. Does not wear gloves because they would offend her husband
   2. Places sharp objects in a trash bag
   3. Uses a disposable sheet during dressing change
   4. Places the soiled bandages in a securely fastened plastic bag
9. The home care nurse visits a family with two children, ages 10 and 15 years. While visiting with the father of the children, the nurse observes that a gun is lying on a table in the living room. What is the best response the nurse can make to this observation?
   1. Engage the father in conversation about how he uses the gun.
   2. Encourage the father to move the gun to a nightstand in his bedroom.
   3. Advise the father to install trigger locks and store the gun in a locked cabinet.
   4. Suggest that he teach his children how to use the gun by practicing in their backyard.

REFERENCES

Andrews MM: Cultural diversity and community health nursing. In Nies MA, McEwen M, editors: *Community health nursing: promoting the health of populations*, ed 4, St Louis, 2007, Elsevier.

Aykol AD: Falls in the elderly: What can be done? *Int Nurs Rev* 54(2):191, 2007.

Drury LJ: DP and home care need improved communication, *J Contin Educ Nurs* 39(5):198, 2008.

Ebersole P and others: *Toward healthy aging: human needs and nursing response*, ed 7, St Louis, 2008, Mosby.

Edelman CL, Mandle CL: *Health promotion throughout the lifespan*, ed 6, St Louis, 2009, Mosby.

Electrical Safety Foundation International (ESFi): How to conduct a *basic home electrical safety check*, http://esfi.org/index.cfm?cd=FAP&cdid=11246&pid=10272, last accessed September 30, 2010.

Hockenberry MJ and others: *Wong's essentials of pediatric nursing*, ed 8, St Louis, 2008, Mosby.

Meiner SE, Lueckenotte AG: *Gerontologic nursing*, ed 3, St Louis, 2006, Mosby.

Mihailidis A and others: The acceptability of home monitoring technology among community-dwelling older adults and baby boomers, *Assist Technol* 20(1):1, 2008.

Motyka CL, Nies MA: Home health and hospice. In Nies MA, McEwen M, editors: *Community health nursing: promoting the health of populations*, ed 4, St Louis, 2007, Elsevier.

Occupational Safety and Health Administration (OSHA): Occupational exposure to bloodborne pathogens; needlestick and other sharp injuries; final rule, *Fed Reg* CFR 29, part 1910(66:5317), January 18, 2001, http://www.osha.gov/pls/oshaweb/owadisp.show_document?p_table=FEDERAL_REGISTER&p_id=16265, accessed September 30, 2010.

Pender NJ and others: *Health promotion in nursing practice*, ed 5, Upper Saddle River, 2006, Prentice Hall.

Stolee P and others: Risk factors for hip fracture in older home care clients, *J Gerontol* 64A(3):403, 2009.

The Joint Commission (TJC): *2010 National Patient Safety Goals*, Oakbrook Terrace, Ill, 2010, The Commission, http://www.jointcommission.org/PatientSafety/NationalPatientSafetyGoals/, accessed September 30, 2010.

Touhy TA, Jett KF: *Ebersole and Hess' Gerontological nursing health aging*, ed 3, St Louis, 2010, Mosby.

US Department of Health and Human Service (HHS): *Proposed Healthy People 2020 objectives: list for public comment*, last revised October 30, 2009, http://www.healthypeople.gov/hp2020/Objectives/TopicAreas.aspx, accessed September 30 2010.

Zillich AJ and others: Quality improvement toward decreasing high-risk medications for older veteran outpatients, *J Am Geriatr Soc* 56:1299, 2008.

APPENDIX

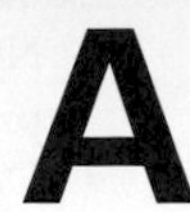

Answer Key to End-of-Chapter Exercises

CHAPTER 1

1. Does the use of an instructional DVD program (I) compared with a standard teaching booklet (C) improve cancer patient's (P) ability to manage the side effects of oral chemotherapy (O)?
2. An outcome would be the patient's ability to identify the side effects of oral chemotherapy, and the approach for measurement would be having patients complete a survey on knowledge of side effects.
3. Answer: 3, 5, 2, 4, 6, 1
4. 3; *Rationale:* Evidence review and critique determine if the evidence is strong enough to eventually apply in practice.
5. 3; *Rationale:* The nurses seek scientific information about local anesthesia as an opportunity to build knowledge about a new procedure.
6. 1 and 3; *Rationale:* Background questions are broad and less focused than a foreground or PICO question; thus they often lead to too many articles to read on diverse topics not relevant to your question.
7. 1; *Rationale:* A descriptive study describes phenomena, in this case perceptions of nurses. It usually involves analysis of surveys, interviews, or questionnaires.
8. 2, 3; *Rationale:* Randomized trials are experimental studies involving a control and experimental (intervention) group. Both the control and intervention groups are measured by the same outcomes to determine if the intervention was more effective than the control.
9. 1; *Rationale:* The literature review summarizes available literature on the researcher's topic of interest. A good review explains why the author decided to study or report on a topic, usually because of a gap in the literature.
10. *P:* Medical inpatients; *I:* Hourly rounds; *C:* Standard observations; *O:* Fall incidence or rate.

CHAPTER 2

1. 2; *Rationale:* This is an example of an ineffective/nontherapeutic communication technique and will likely result in increased agitation and frustration in the patient.
2. 3; *Rationale:* The correct order for structured communication hand-off is SBAR: Situation, Background, Assessment, and Recommendation.
3. 4; *Rationale:* Nonverbal communication is very powerful; however, the nurse must validate that the message perceived is the intended message.
4. 1; *Rationale:* Touch can be a therapeutic nonverbal communication technique, but it should not be used with suspicious patients. This may be perceived as an invasion of personal space and may heighten the level of suspiciousness.
5. 1, 2, 4, 6 are examples of therapeutic techniques.
6. 2; *Rationale:* Nurses should never give advice to patients, even if it is solicited by the patient. The nurse-patient relationship is patient centered; and patients should make decisions on their own, without such input from the nurse.
7. 3; *Rationale:* The nurse is brushing off the patient's concerns and minimizing them. The issue is a concern of the patient and should be addressed by the nurse.
8. 2, 4; *Rationale:* Asking why questions is nontherapeutic and sets up a feeling of defensiveness in the patient. Information may be obtained by asking questions using other words such as how, where, what, and when. It is not therapeutic to challenge patients, demanding proof from them.
9. 4; *Rationale:* Many factors may adversely affect patient outcomes; all of the factors listed have the potential to negatively affect patients.
10. 3; *Rationale:* Maintaining personal space, encouraging safe coping behaviors, and using silence are all therapeutic techniques. The use of touch is discouraged with angry patients because it may escalate the situation.

CHAPTER 3

1. 3; *Rationale:* Nurses should document only factual and objective information and not express opinions or assumptions in the medical record.
2. 4; *Rationale:* The nurse should quote what the patient states if it is relevant and appropriate to nursing care.
3. 2, 5; *Rationale:* Administration of any treatments should be documented as soon as possible after administration. The other activities should be included in routine charting either periodically during the shift or at end of shift.
4. 2 matches **S**: 'The pain increases every time I turn on my left side." *Rationale:* This is subjective data. 4 matches **O**: Left lower surgical incision sutures intact, no drainage noted. *Rationale:* This is objective data. 3 matches **A**: Acute pain related to surgical incision. *Rationale:* This is the assessment of the situation. 1 matches **P**: Repositioned patient on right side. This is the plan of care.

5. Examples:
   - Never share passwords and keep own password private.
   - Delete documentation mistakes from the record using agency protocol.
   - Do not leave patient information on the monitor where others can view.
6. 1, 2; *Rationale:* When completing an incident report, information specific to the individual involved in the incident and information from witnesses, if any, should be included. Data that are hearsay or the nurse's opinions about the incident should not be included.
7. False; *Rationale:* HIPAA provides patients with the right to review their medical records. Patients have to follow protocols established by the institution.
8. 3; *Rationale:* 0530 is equivalent to 5:30 AM; 1530 is equivalent to 3:30 PM; and 1630 is equivalent to 4:30 PM.
9. 1, 4; *Rationale:* Objective data are those that are observed. To say that the patient is demanding is neither objective nor subjective data, but the writer's opinion. When the patient reports feelings, it is subjective data.
10. 3; *Rationale:* When an incident report is completed, the nurse does not document in the chart that the incident report was completed.

CHAPTER 4

1. 3; *Rationale:* Because the goal is to maintain the least restrictive environment, restraint alternatives must be tried before deciding to restrain the patient. A restraint alternative does not require a physician's order. It must be something that the patient is cognitively and physically able to remove on her own.
2. 1, 2, 3, 5; *Rationale*: Evidence has shown that being on four or more medications, advancing age, patient care equipment, and altered cognition are independent factors that increase the risk for fall.
3. 3; *Rationale*: It is important to eliminate the electric current. Unplug the refrigerator without stepping in the water or touching your co-worker. Call the rapid response team after you have unplugged it or if you are unable to unplug it. Do not wipe up the water or take his vital signs until after the refrigerator is unplugged.
4. 3; *Rationale*: The nurse's first responsibility is to protect the patient from harm. Different interventions may be needed, depending on what is occurring, and may include putting up the side rails.
5. 2; *Rationale*: The purpose of a root cause analysis is to investigate the cause of an error without placing blame or relieving accountability. It is a systematic process with the goal of preventing future similar errors.
6. 4; *Rationale*: The registered nurse has a responsibility to listen to patient concerns. Many patients are very aware of their medications. Do not give the medication without verifying that he is indeed supposed to receive it.
7. 3; *Rationale*: Using the acronym *RACE*, the nurse would remove Mr. Macalister from the room. Although the steps are not necessarily always sequential, it is important to remove the patient from harm first.
8. 1, 2, 3, 4; *Rationale*: All of these interventions are important for the patient in restraints. Without ROM, the patient may rapidly decondition. Restraints can restrict circulation and lead to skin breakdown. Therefore these assessments must be made at least every 2 hours. Toileting and hydration are basic human needs that a restrained person cannot provide for himself. All of these interventions also show respect for the patient.
9. 1, 2, 3; *Rationale*: Planned activities such as walks or other activities can decrease wandering. Keeping a patient near the nurses' station where her activities can be watched more closely is also helpful.

CHAPTER 5

1. 2; *Rationale:* Small droplets cannot be transmitted when there is a barrier such as a hand or tissue in place. This reduces the risk of transmission of infection.
2. 3, 4, 2, 6, 5, 1, 7; *Rationale:* This sequence ensures that the risk of contaminating any other surfaces or health care personnel is reduced.
3. 2, 4, 5*; Rationale:* No. 1 has happened outside of the hospital, and No. 3 is not acquiring a problem but just testing for that problem. All other answers are acquired in a hospital setting.
4. 4; *Rationale:* Gloves protect health care personnel from contamination with body fluids, which is a method of blocking the portal of exit from the patient.
5. 1; *Rationale:* A dressing serves as a source of a reservoir for microorganisms. Changing dressings reduces the risk of bacterial growth.
6. 1: S, 2: S, 3: M, 4: M, 5: S, 6: M; *Rationale:* Nos. 1, 2 and 5 all require sterile technique because of the high risk of bacterial entrance into sterile body cavities through the urethra, trachea, or central nervous system.
7. 1; *Rationale:* The second glove was picked up incorrectly. The nurse should have picked up the second one under the cuff, not at the top of the cuff.
8. 2; *Rationale:* To maintain a sterile field, objects must be maintained and handled above the waist.
9. 2, 3, 4; *Rationale:* Reactions to latex-containing products such as gloves and food reactions such as peaches and kiwis place patients at high risk for developing latex reactions.
10. 1; *Rationale:* The first flap in a sterile field is opened away from, not toward, the nurse.

CHAPTER 6

1. 4; *Rationale***:** If patient is unable to keep the mouth closed, the nurse should select another site.
2. 2, 3, 5; *Rationale:* Insufficient information is available to notify the health care provider. The nurse cannot assume that Mrs. Kilty has not taken her medications. A complete vascular assessment is not indicated until blood

pressure measurements are verified. Lower-extremity blood pressure measurements are not needed in this situation. The correct blood pressure cuff should be used for the initial measurement. The measurements should be verified before taking any action and compared to baseline.

3. 2; *Rationale*: Pain increases heart rate and respiratory rate. Pain causes vasoconstriction, which increases blood pressure. There is no effect on temperature.
4. 2; *Rationale*: The IV line in the left arm may be influencing the blood pressure and needs to be reconfirmed. The perspiration suggests the patient may be febrile and should be reconfirmed. The pulse is acceptable and does not require an apical rate.
5. 3; *Rationale:* The blood pressure and heart rate are acceptable for a patient with a fever. The respiratory rate reflects complications of pneumonia, and interventions are needed.
6. 3; *Rationale:* The associated symptoms of hypertension (e.g., headache) support the blood pressure measurements, making repeating the blood pressure values unnecessary. Although the social worker should be contacted, the physician needs to be notified to treat the hypertension.
7. 3; *Rationale*: An irregular pulse rate should be verified by assessing the apical pulse. If there are still irregularities, a pulse deficit assessment is indicated.
8. 2; *Rationale:* Cheyne-Stokes is a pattern of apnea and hyperventilation. The respiratory rate of 12 was counted with the apneic phase.
9. 1; *Rationale*: Nos. 2 and 3 create a false low blood pressure. A blood pressure does not fluctuate with an asymptomatic patient. Flexing increases resistance to flow.
10. 4; *Rationale*: Decreased pulse strength on affected side may indicate vascular compromise.

CHAPTER 7

1. Focused assessments would include cardiovascular and peripheral neurovascular, respiratory, abdominal and perineal, I&O. Key elements of each system:
   a. Cardiovascular: Blood pressure; heart rate; inspection, palpation, and auscultation of the heart
   b. Peripheral neurovascular: Inspection and palpation of the extremities; checking peripheral pulses, edema, skin color and temperature, capillary refill; sensation and movement
   c. Respiratory: Checking rate and depth of respirations, chest excursion, and lung sounds
   d. Abdominal: Checking size and shape of abdomen, palpation of bladder, assessing bowel sounds, assessing dressing
   e. I&O: Intake, output (Foley, Jackson-Pratt drain)
2. You must listen for 5 minutes over each quadrant before deciding that bowel sounds are absent. It is common for bowel sounds to be hypoactive for 24 hours or more following abdominal surgery.
3. 1 and 5; *Rationale:* The general survey includes assessment of vital signs, height and weight, general behavior, and appearance.
4. 3; *Rationale:* A lesion colored blue/black or variegated, nonuniform pigmentation or variations/multiple colors (tan, black) with areas of pink, white, gray, blue, or red may indicate a melanoma.
5. 4; *Rationale:* Crackles sound like crushing cellophane; rhonchi sound like blowing air through fluid with a straw.
6. 4; *Rationale:* S1 and S2 are normal components of the cardiac cycle and an expected physical assessment finding.
7. Correct order is 2, 3, 4, 1; *Rationale:* Percussion and palpation are completed after inspection and auscultation because of the risk for causing increased bowel sounds that could be interpreted as an abnormal finding.
8. 3; *Rationale:* The dorsum of the hand is most sensitive to temperature variations.
9. 2; *Rationale:* In a normal Get Up and Go Test, a patient does not use the arms to sit up from a chair or to sit back down.
10. Total 352 mL intake (3 ounces apples juice = 90 mL; ¼ carton milk = 63 mL; 6 ounces soda = 180 mL; and 8 ounces of ice (½ volume) = 120 mL).

CHAPTER 8

1. 4; *Rationale:* Performing procedure using appropriate steps minimizes contamination of the specimen, increases efficiency, and allows timely delivery to the laboratory.
2. 3; *Rationale:* Indicates understanding that a culture is for identification of the pathogenic microorganism and sensitivity identifies medications that are active against the microorganism.
3. 1; *Rationale:* The forearm is an appropriate alternate site, especially if blood sugars are not changing. The patient is having a routine check. Applying pressure to the puncture site might cause an abnormal reading because of the changes of cellular metabolism. Warm water increases blood flow to the area but does not address patient's discomfort. Placing the lancet firmly against the skin is not likely to reduce pain in fingers.
4. 4; *Rationale:* The median cubital vein is easier to puncture and less likely to rupture. The basilic and cephalic veins of the lower arm and hand are preferred for administering IV fluids. The antecubital vein is often less visible.
5. 4; *Rationale:* Pressure controls bleeding and allows for clot formation. Ice decreases circulation to area. Analgesia medication is for pain relief, not nasal bleeding. Antibiotic is used for an infection, not nasal bleeding. Hemoccult testing is used for assessment of stool for blood.
6. 3; *Rationale:* A repeat wound specimen is necessary to correctly identify pathogenic organism. Antibiotic therapy begins after results from the specimen. Monitoring a patient is not indicated as a result of specimen contamination. Water would cause drying of the wound.

7. 1; *Rationale:* Assessing Mrs. Henderson's understanding would allow reinforcement of the information and determine what action the nurse may need to take to ensure that all urine is collected for 24 hours. All urine needs to be collected for a full 24-hour period; not including urine results in an inaccurate report. Restarting the procedure is necessary, but the nurse must first determine the patient's ability to collect the specimen. Drinking water would be helpful for voiding but would not influence the patient's ability to collect the specimen.
8. 1, 3, 4; *Rationale:* The patient's blood sugar remains uncontrolled. To control his diabetes it is important for him to understand the need to be consistent and follow his personal regimen for blood sugars.
9. 3; *Rationale:* The absence of the radial pulse indicates absence of arterial blood flow, which can cause injury to the patient. Blood returns to the arterial system immediately, and in 60 seconds flow is normal.

CHAPTER 9

1. 2 and 4; *Rationale:* Cardiac catheterization poses a risk for blood loss and complications that require immediate cardiac surgery. Therefore it is important to have baseline information regarding the patient's hemoglobin and hematocrit (CBC). The PT provides a baseline to determine if Mr. Hall is at risk for postprocedure bleeding. The BUN, creatinine, and urine specific gravity are used to further assess Mr. Hall's dehydration status. Patients who are dehydrated or who have renal failure are at risk for impaired excretion of the contrast dye.
2. 3, 5; *Rationale*: Patients who have not given informed consent must wait until the physician fully explains the procedure. Sedatives impair decision making, and informed consent is obtained first.
3. 1 and 2; *Rationale:* Catheter site pain and loss of distal pulses can be caused by arterial bleeding from the arterial site. Anxiety, backache, and increased heart rate can be signs of internal bleeding and must be evaluated.
4. 1; *Rationale:* The patient with renal failure is not able to filter out the toxins from the contrast medium. The patient with one kidney may have complete renal function in the remaining kidney.
5. 1; *Rationale:* Sedation is the recommended anesthesia for pediatric patients requiring a bone marrow aspirate.
6. 3, 4, 2, 1; *Rationale:* Informed consent is verified before starting any procedure. For ease of transfer, position patient before administering sedation. Perform the "Time Out" before any invasive procedure or cutting an incision.
7. 1; *Rationale:* Assisting to help maintain the patient's side-lying position is the only appropriate option. Nos. 2 and 3 deal with assessment; assessment is always the responsibility of the nurse. Preparing a site and a sterile tray is also a nursing responsibility.
8. 3: *Rationale:* When fluid is removed from the abdominal cavity, the abdominal girth decreases. Removing abdominal ascetic fluid allows the lungs to further expand to meet oxygen needs. As this occurs, the respiratory rate declines.
9. 3 and 4; *Rationale:* Because sedation is part of the procedure, patient needs to have an empty stomach to reduce the risk of vomiting and aspiration. the patient is instructed not to drive or operate machinery for 24 hours after any sedation procedure. The patient is sedated and positioned by staff during the procedure. Bowel preparation occurs anywhere from 36 to 24 hours before the procedure to ensure an empty colon.
10. 1, 2, and 4; *Rationale:* 1, 2, and 4 are necessary evaluation measures to compare with baseline data to determine if the patient's condition worsens. The patient's status is unstable or likely to become unstable; and, although obtaining vital signs are part of a NAP's responsibility, delegating this to the NAP at this time is not appropriate.

CHAPTER 10

1. 2; *Rationale*: It is important to ask patient preferences before beginning procedure so the nurse knows what supplies to gather. Perform hand hygiene and don gloves before removing dentures. After upper and lower dentures are removed, hold dentures over emesis basin or lined sink to protect them in event they are dropped before brushing the dentures. Storing dentures would be the last step.
2. 2; *Rationale:* Mr. Kline becomes short of breath with any exertion. It would be best at this time to give a partial bath. A complete bath requires more time and movement. Tub bath and shower require more exertion and would not be appropriate at this time.
3. 1, 3, 5, 7; *Rationale*: To be safe, the bed must be elevated to working height. Tuck in the top sheet and spread at the foot of the bed and then make a modified mitered corner. To save steps, apply all bottom linen on one side of bed before moving to opposite side. Horizontal toe pleats are made on all beds. Gloves do not need to be worn except if drainage is present. Soiled linen should be placed in linen bag, not on the floor. Top covers need to be fanfolded to the end of the bed when the procedure is complete.
4. 3; *Rationale:* Follows the principle of cleansing from least contaminated to most contaminated. Leaving a foreskin retracted results in tightening of the foreskin around the shaft of the penis, which can lead to permanent urethral damage. Cleansing the perineum should proceed from the least to most contaminated; in this case from "front to back" or perineum to rectum. A patient with a Foley catheter needs more frequent perineal care because of the increased risk of infection.
5. 4; *Rationale*: The side-lying position because it is less likely that the patient will aspirate in this position since fluid would most likely pool in the mouth, where it can

be suctioned. Nos. 1, 2, and 3 place the patient at risk for aspiration.

6. 4; *Rationale:* Although bath bags are easy to use, quick, and promote comfort, the patient was concerned about not using a basin. No. 4 addresses that concern. Bath basins may be a reservoir and a way that harmful bacteria are spread.
7. 3; *Rationale*: Washing from distal to proximal promotes venous return to the right side of the heart. It does not enhance comfort, prevent skin irritation, or reduce swelling.
8. 1, 3; *Rationale***:** Using the razor at 45 degrees and shaving in the direction of hair growth facilitates shaving of facial hair. A warm, moist washcloth is used; and short downward strokes are recommended to facilitate shaving of facial hair.
9. 1; *Rationale***:** Eyes are first, using plain water without soap. Bathing then proceeds from top (face) to bottom so the most contaminated areas are last.
10. 4; *Rationale:* Individuals with diabetes have poor circulation. Cutting nails could cause trauma, impaired skin integrity, and infection. Always use nail clippers to trim nails straight across; clipping nails to fit the contour of the fingers could result in ingrown nails. Use an emery board to shape nails after being trimmed.

CHAPTER 11

1. 2; *Rationale:* Apply clean gloves when drainage is present. Turn off the aid volume before it prevents feedback (whistling) during removal. Grasping the device prevents accidentally dropping the aid. The brush supplied with the aid is used to dislodge any wax that is transferred from the ear canal to the aid. Wash the ear canal to remove any drainage or wax. Storing the aid in its storage case further reduces the risk of damage to the aid.
2. 1, 3; *Rationale:* Nos. 1 and 3 are safety concerns. The batteries are very toxic to children and pets when swallowed, and the child would need to be seen by a health care professional. The aids are small and present a choking hazard to the child. No. 2 teaches Mr. Arthur to have his grandchildren face him to increase his hearing clarity when the children are speaking but is not related to child safety. No. 4 offers him a way to show the children about the aid to address some of their curiosity.
3. 1; *Rationale:* Ear irrigations are contraindicated when a foreign matter such as a vegetable is present. Potentially the foreign object could absorb the solution and expand in the ear canal.
4. 2; *Rationale:* This position straightens the ear canal and facilitates entrance of the irrigant.
5. 2; *Rationale:* Holding the syringe correctly directs the irrigant into the ear canal without occluding the canal and damaging the internal ear structures.
6. 1; *Rationale:* An artificial eye cleaned too frequently can lead to irritation of the eye socket. However, it must be cleaned as often as necessary to prevent discomfort. The other answers are correct and indicate adequate teaching.
7. 3; *Rationale:* It is important to note if any inflammation or infection is present in the eye socket. An infection in this area needs immediate treatment to prevent further injury to the socket, which might require further surgery.
8. 1; *Rationale:* This is an urgent situation. The priority of care is to determine the level of injury and prevent further damage. The nurse must quickly assess the injured eye; determine the level of pain, which might indicate the need for pain relief; and prepare to irrigate the eye to flush out any remaining chemical and reduce further damage to the eye. Although teaching eye safety is important and needs to occur before discharge, it is not an immediate nursing action. The fact that the patient's wife ran water over the eyes to remove the chemical before coming to the emergency department was good; however, this action has no relevance to the nurse's immediate actions.
9. 3; *Rationale:* Eye care practices include providing artificial tears or moistures to lubricate and hydrate the eye. These artificial tears wash debris from the eye, moisten the cornea, and prevent microorganisms from adhering to the cornea.
10. 4; *Rationale:* It is the nurse's responsibility to further assess the patient's eyes before contacting the patient's health care provider. The NAP was instructed to notify the nurse for further assessment if drainage, redness, or irritation was present when performing eye care.

CHAPTER 12

1. 3; *Rationale*: The nurse would expect a pH 5.0 because of the continuous tube feeding that contains a basic solution. A pH of 3.0 and 4.0 would be expected if feedings were not being administered. A pH of 7.0 suggests that the tube is in the small intestine or tracheobronchial tree.
2. 3, 4; *Rationale*: Sterile water is indicated for irrigation when a patient is immunocompromised or critically ill and before and after the patient receives a medication via the tube. Sterile water is not necessary for routine irrigation, and pH values of gastric aspiration do not influence selection of irrigation fluid.
3. 1, 3; *Rationale:* A wet voice and coughing on food are two common signs of dysphagia that are predictive for the risk of aspiration. The patient may have difficulty smiling if there is facial nerve paralysis following the stroke. The ability to smile has not been associated with dysphagia. Aversion to food and change in taste are not predictors of aspiration.
4. 3; *Rationale*: Placing a patient upright at a 90-degree angle reduces the incidence of gastric reflux. Providing oral hygiene reduces the number of bacteria in the saliva that could be aspirated. Pulse oximetry may reveal oxygen desaturation in patients who have aspirated. Adding thickener to liquids reduces risk of aspiration.

5. 1; *Rationale:* The correct technique requires the nurse to first check tube placement and then irrigate. The procedure is done every 4 hours.
6. 1, 3, 4; *Rationale:* Unexpected outcomes of a tube feeding include aspiration, the retention of large residual volumes 250 mL or more, and clogging of a tube indicated by the inability to irrigate. Diarrhea, not constipation, is a symptom of tube-feeding intolerance. The ulcer on the naris is an unexpected outcome resulting from improper tube care, not the feeding.
7. 1 and 3; *Rationale:* Always wash hands before touching food and keep the refrigerator at 4.4° C (40° F). Discourage drinking unpasteurized milk, which might contain bacteria. Never use leftovers past 2 days.
8. 4; *Rationale:* A patient unable to chew is able to have a clear-liquid, full-liquid, or pureed diet. Full liquid is indicated if the patient cannot tolerate solid foods. However, the pureed diet provides the most nutrients of the three and is indicated when the patient's GI function is normal. Mechanical and high-fiber diets require chewing.
9. 2; *Rationale:* High-fiber foods such as fresh uncooked fruits and steamed vegetables are useful in relieving constipation. Just because the patient has dentures does not mean that he is unable to chew; thus a pureed diet would be inappropriate. There is no indication for a fat-modified diet, and a low-residue diet is low in fiber content.
10. 2; *Rationale:* When a patient is forced to remain supine, place in reverse Trendelenburg's position when administering a tube feeding.

CHAPTER 13

1. The patient will benefit from avoiding or reducing drug therapy; since she has incomplete pain relief with NSAIDs, she would be a good candidate for nonpharmacological alternatives.
2. The patient should take the NSAID before her pain increases in severity and before any activities that might aggravate her pain. If her pain increases, the nurse might recommend that she talk with her doctor about the safety of taking medication ATC.
3. 2; *Rationale*: If the dressing over a local analgesia infusion catheter becomes moist, it indicates that the tubing is either disconnected or displaced, resulting in leakage of medication onto the gauze. If an infection were present, drainage would likely be green or yellow in color. Normal drainage from a postoperative wound is serosanguineous at 48 hours. Excess perspiration would unlikely cause moistening of a dressing over the knee area.
4. 1, 3, and 4; *Rationale*: The nurse can ask a family member to describe patient behaviors, but she cannot assume that the family member will know the pain location. Pain is what a patient says it is, either verbally or nonverbally. A previous assessment is not necessarily current and reflective of the patient's present condition.
5. 4; *Rationale:* A massage can cause deep relaxation; thus sitting up quickly may cause temporary postural hypotension. Deep breathing relaxes the patient but does not affect muscle cramping or clotting. Holding one's breath and straining are Valsalva maneuvers.
6. Clinical case 3 is most at risk. *Rationale*: Respiratory depression is only clinically significant if there is a decrease in the rate *and* depth of respirations from the patient's baseline assessment. Also, sedation *always* occurs before respiratory depression. In case 3 the patient's rate and depth of respiration deteriorate, and sedation increases.
7. 1; *Rationale*: Bupivacaine (Marcaine) toxicity presents with hypotension, dizziness, tremor, severe itching, swelling of the skin or throat, irregular heartbeat, palpitations, confusion, ringing in the ears, muscle twitching, numbness around the mouth, metallic taste, and seizures.
8. 1, 4, and 5; *Rationale*: There is no indication that the catheter is disconnected since the dressing is dry and intact. Seeking a basal dose is not appropriate since the patient is oversedated and requires immediate treatment.
9. *P:* Precipitating/palliative factors; *Q:* Quality of pain; *R:* Region of pain or radiation; *S:* Severity; *T:* Timing; and *U*: How is pain affecting U (patient) regarding ADLs, work, relationships, and enjoyment of life.
10. 2, 4, 5; *Rationale:* Nonverbal indications of pain include guarding, diaphoresis, and irritability. The patient's respiratory rate would be slow during sleeping. He is lying in an anatomically correct position. An abnormal posture might indicate pain.

CHAPTER 14

1. 1, 2, 3, 4; *Rationale:* All of these are correct. The nurse initially observes the patient throughout the respiratory cycle. In this patient it is also important to obtain vital signs because these data will give the nurse information about the overall status of the patient. Auscultation provides information about lung expansion; the nurse also notes if the expansion is symmetrical. The chest tube is an intervention to improve lung expansion, and in this patient it is part of the respiratory assessment.
2. 2; *Rationale*: A Venturi mask is the only method of delivering an FiO_2 of 80% with the stated liters per minute. The nasal cannula delivers 44% at most, the partial rebreather must be set at a minimum of 8 L, and the nonrebreather must be set at a minimum of 6 L.
3. 1 and 4; *Rationale*: Assess for location of leak by clamping chest tube with two rubber-shod or toothless clamps close to the chest wall. If bubbling stops, an air leak is inside patient's thorax or at chest insertion site. If bubbling continues with the clamps near the chest wall, gradually move one clamp at a time down drainage tubing away from patient and toward suction control chamber. When bubbling stops, leak is in section of tubing or connection between the clamps. If the tube becomes kinked, tidaling will stop; but bubbling will not be noted unless there is a breach in a connection of the

system. The nurse should never disconnect the tubing unless hemostats are in place when changing the drainage system.

4. 4; *Rationale:* By dipping the catheter in normal saline before suctioning, the catheter is lubricated for easier insertion. A nurse should hyperoxygenate a patient with 100% oxygen, use a sterile catheter, and only activate suction when the catheter is being withdrawn from the ET tube to decrease risk of damage to tracheal mucosa.
5. 1, 2, 3; *Rationale*: The effects of hypoxia from suctioning can cause dysrhythmias, hemodynamic instability, and increased intracranial pressure, among other complications. A maximum of two suction passes is recommended to minimize effects of hypoxemia.
6. 2, 3; *Rationale:* Tracheostomy care and suctioning can be delegated to NAP if the tracheostomy is well established and not for an acutely ill patient. An NAP can attach a nasal cannula, if the RN previously adjusted oxygen flow rate and assessed the patient. Suctioning for any patient with an ET tube cannot be delegated to NAP.
7. 2, 3, 4; *Rationale*: Assess for clinical indicators for suctioning: coarse breath sounds, noisy breathing or adventitious breath sounds, weak cough, increased or decreased pulse, increased or decreased respirations, increased or decreased blood pressure, prolonged expiratory breath sounds, and decreased lung expansion. Secretions in the airway, decreased oxygen saturations or level of consciousness, anxiety, lethargy, unilateral breath sounds, and cyanosis may also indicate a need for suctioning. Wheezing indicates hyperactive airways and can be worsened by suctioning.
8. 1, 2; *Rationale:* Toothbrushes should be used every 8 hours to provide oral care for ventilated patients. Toothettes are not adequate to clean the dental plaque, but they may be used between brushing for moistening mucosa. Although increasing mobility in this population is challenging, such interventions as repositioning, sitting, or standing at the bedside or ambulation have decreased the risk of VAP.
9. 2, 3; *Rationale:* When caring for an intubated patient, nurses are encouraged to use positive verbal and nonverbal communication with direct eye contact and questions that only require yes or no responses. Alphabet charts, pen and paper, slates or chalkboards, or magnetic pen doodle boards are some common communication tools. Intubated patients do not have a hearing loss; thus speaking loudly does not help communication and may frustrate the patient even more. Families can speak to the patient, but the patient still needs a mechanism with which to reply.
10. 1; *Rationale:* Monitoring chest tube drainage and maintaining chest tube patency are the key priorities.

CHAPTER 15

1. 1 and 3; *Rationale*: Mr. Clark is in pain most likely related to his lacerations and fractures. Pain management is a priority at this time. To safely transfer the patient, three nurses are necessary because of the patient's weight. In addition, explaining to Mr. Clark the purpose of the CT scan helps elicit his cooperation. Mr. Clark is most likely fearful of movement because of his pain and uncertainty of his condition. Two nurses are insufficient for the transfer. The nurse may inform Mr. Clark that it is a physician's order, but the patient has the right to refuse treatment.
2. Logrolling; *Rationale:* Mr. Clark maintains proper alignment by moving all body parts at the same time, preventing tension or twisting of the spinal column.
3. 2; *Rationale:* Hypotension would result after prolonged bed rest. There is no indication that the patient is experiencing difficulty with proprioception. There is no indication that the patient has pathology to the CNS.
4. 2; *Rationale*: Because of the patient's weight and limited ability to bear weight, a bariatric transfer aid provides the best and safest technique to transfer this patient. A friction-reducing device is used when transferring a patient from a bed to stretcher. A three-person carry is inappropriate and not recommended any longer. No. 4 is incorrect because of patient's weight and limited weight bearing.
5. 2; *Rationale:* Logrolling and moving the patient as a unit prevents twisting and damage to the unstable spinal cord. The step-by-step method causes twisting and bending of the spine, resulting in further damage. The patient should remain nonweight bearing to prevent further damage to the injured spine; No. 4 is incorrect because there is risk of twisting and bending the spine during transfer.
6. 1; *Rationale:* The patient may be refusing to move because his pain is not under control. Nos. 2, 3, and 4 are important assessment data once the patient has agreed to transfer.
7. 4; *Rationale:* This allows the nurse to determine if the patient is experiencing symptoms of orthostatic hypotension such as dizziness. Place the transfer belt around the patient's waist after the patient is in a sitting position. The under-axilla method may cause injury to the patient and places undo stress on the patient's axilla area. Offer the patient his or her glasses after positioning in chair to prevent damage to eyeglasses.
8. 4; *Rationale:* A slide board is the most appropriate method to transfer this patient because the patient is unable to assist. If any one caregiver must lift more than 35 pounds, there is a risk of injury. Body mechanics alone are insufficient. A slide board is the most appropriate method.
9. The correct sequence is 7, 1, 4, 3, 2, 5, 6; *Rationale:* This sequence first positions the bed and wheelchair at equal height, with the wheelchair appropriately angled to the bed. The safety features of the wheelchair are used, and the patient is safely transferred to the wheelchair.
10. 2; *Rationale:* The 30-degree lateral position is designed to reduce pressure over bony prominences. The patient who has shortness of breath would benefit most from a

Fowler's position. The 30-degree lateral position does not prevent orthostatic hypotension. The patient with hemiplegia needs to be turned often side to side.

CHAPTER 16

1. 1,2; *Rationale:* Use of device on strong side provides more support; a dry surface prevents slipping and falls. A patient should walk while wearing firm shoes with nonslip sole. The elbow should remain flexed when using a cane.
2. 3; *Rationale*: Space activities to avoid exhaustion. Rest is needed between activities such as bathing and ambulation. An opioid could result in dizziness. A person should blow out when rising to a standing position.
3. 2; *Rationale*: Walking does not cost the older adults anything, and it is a safe means of exercise. A local fitness club and purchase of exercise equipment would be costly. A readers' club is an excellent social activity but does not involve exercise.
4. 3; *Rationale*: It is important to support joints to prevent damage or injury. The nurse does not inject analgesic; positioning is 2 cm (0.8 inch) below knee joint; patient is continuously assessed to ensure that he or she tolerates the CPM and is not left in severe pain.
5. 1, 3, 4; *Rational*: Pallor, nausea, and dizziness are all signs of orthostatic hypotension. Bradycardia is incorrect; tachycardia is actually a symptom. Irritability is not a classic sign of the condition.
6. 3; *Rationale*: Raising the arm above the head achieves 180-degree abduction.
7. 1; *Rationale:* The four-point gait provides most support and improves balance.
8. 2, 4, 5; *Rationale*: Avoid twisting to avoid injury. Using the arm and leg muscles protects the back; the arms and legs are stronger than the back. Patient assistance promotes ability and strength.
9. 2; *Rationale:* The success of a skin graft could be compromised by the application of elastic stockings to the site.
10. Correct sequence: 2, 4, 3, 1; *Rationale*: Allows patient to balance by providing wide base of support first.

CHAPTER 17

1. 2; *Rationale:* A plaster cast needs to breathe and should not be covered completely for any length of time. In addition, a fiberglass cast can sustain exposure to water without losing structural integrity, but a plaster cast will begin to crumble. Any sharp edges of a cast should be covered with tape or moleskin to prevent skin damage to adjacent tissues.
2. 2; *Rationale:* The first step involves appropriate positioning. Before using the saw, it is important to inform the child of what to expect from it to prevent anxiety and fear. Inspecting the skin determines if the skin is intact and can be washed. An enzyme wash assists in dissolving dead skin, and gentle manipulation of tissue prevents damaging delicate skin.
3. 2, 4; *Rationale:* Shaving is not necessary and may create micro nicks that could become inflamed under the traction apparatus. The boot should fit snugly to prevent slipping and ensure the traction pull but not be so tight that it leads to pressure on the tissues under the boot. The heel should sit properly in the boot without the need for padding. Padding can cause pressure to the heel. Adding weight slowly and gently avoids involuntary muscle spasms and pain. Neurovascular status should be assessed distal to the traction, primarily in the foot.
4. Every 2 hours; *Rationale*: Altered circulation, sensation, or motion indicates potential deficits that can occur quickly and result in permanent damage.
5. 5; *Rationale:* The symptoms indicate swelling of the tissues under the cast. Elevating the cast to promote venous return and decrease edema may relieve the symptoms. Lowering the cast or applying warm compresses would only aggravate the swelling and increase the edema. A window is used when there is a specific pressure point, not generalized edema. An analgesic could mask the pain and would not relieve the swelling. Because neurovascular damage can occur quickly, it is imperative to notify the physician if elevation does not work. The physician will likely order bivalving the cast, and the nurse would need to gather the appropriate equipment to perform this procedure. In many agencies the nurse would perform this procedure.
6. 2; *Rationale*: A cotton T-shirt should be worn beneath the brace to protect the skin. Likewise, the brace should be inspected for anything that could damage the skin. Metal joints should only be cleaned with pipe cleaners and oiled weekly. Plastic parts would be damaged by ammonia and should be wiped with a damp cloth and dried thoroughly.
7. 4; *Rationale*: It is normal to expect a small amount of crusting from the serous (clear) drainage from pin sites. An ashen skin color may indicate circulatory problems but not an infection. Erythema (redness), warmth, and / or purulent drainage from the pin site indicates infection.
8. 2; *Rationale*: It is not within the scope of nursing to determine the amount of weight to be applied to traction or to manipulate traction pins. Pins should be stationary and not move. The nurse would not adjust a Steinmann pin but would notify the physician of any pin that moved. The pull of traction should be in a straight line, with the rope going over a pulley at a 90-degree angle. Weights can be moved so that they hang freely for the traction force to be engaged.
9. 3; *Rationale*: Patients can use an overhead trapeze to move in bed without disrupting the pull of the traction. Weights are never removed from skeletal traction because removal may damage the callus forming at the ends of the broken bones and delay healing. If weights are not hanging freely at the end of the bed, the pull of the

traction is affected. Proper alignment of the injured limb ensures proper pull of the traction.

10. 1; *Rationale*: Itching is expected but can be managed with medication. Scratching of any sort can lead to skin infection.

CHAPTER 18

1. 3; *Rationale:* Perineal hygiene minimizes skin irritation and removes microorganisms that can cause infection. There needs to be 2.5 to 5 cm (1 to 2 inches) of space between tip of the glans penis and the end of the catheter. Excess space may cause pooling of urine, causing excessive exposure to urine. Shaving the pubic area increases the risk for skin irritation. The condom should be secure but not tight. Application of tape is contraindicated because it could interfere with circulation, causing necrosis of the penis.
2. 2 is the correct sequence of steps for insertion of an indwelling urinary catheter.
3. 4; *Rationale:* Keeping the drainage tubing attached to the bed prevents it from pulling the catheter and preventing dependent loops that cause urine to not flow into the drainage bag. Catheters should only be irrigated when the patency of the catheter is threatened by occlusion. Routine irrigation interrupts the closed system, increasing risk for CAUTI. Routine catheter care involves washing with soap and water. Drainage bags should never be hung on a movable part of the bed where movement could pull on the catheter, causing trauma to the urethra and bladder.
4. 2, 3; *Rationale:* By allowing the balloon to drain by gravity, the development of creases or ridges in the balloon may be avoided and thus minimize trauma to the urethra during withdrawal. All patients who have a catheter removed should have their voiding monitored using a voiding record or bladder diary. The size syringe used to deflate the balloon is dictated by the size of the balloon. Catheters should be pulled out slowly and smoothly. Pulling fluid out of the balloon with force can cause the formation of creases or ridges in the balloon.
5. 1, 3, 4; *Rationale*: A new suprapubic catheter insertion site is a surgical incision and should be treated similarly to other incisions, including sterile dressing change and inspection of the site for signs of infection. To minimize trauma and increase comfort, the catheter should be anchored to the abdomen. Wiping the catheter toward the skin violates principals of asepsis. Tension to the catheter should be avoided in all circumstances to minimize discomfort and potential for damage to the bladder wall.
6. 2; *Rationale:* The most appropriate action would be to ensure that the catheter is not occluded.
7. 1; *Rationale:* A common cause of posturological surgery catheter occlusion is blood clots. This catheter has not been in long enough to be occluded by biofilm; decreased fluid intake or defective catheter is not likely causes.
8. 5,4,1,2,3; *Rationale*: These steps ensure that the patient is treated with respect and dignity.
9. 4; *Rationale:* 4 is the only selection that applies to open intermittent irrigation. No. 1 applies to closed intermittent irrigation, and No. 2 applies to closed continuous irrigation. Temporarily clamping the catheter (No. 3) is appropriate after a solution is instilled.

CHAPTER 19

1. 2; *Rationale:* Nasal trauma can cause a deviated septum, which makes passing the NG tube difficult. Assess patency of each naris to determine if a deviation is present before tube insertion. If the deviation is noted, placement of the tube through that naris is contraindicated; use the other naris.
2. 3; *Rationale:* The color and pH of the aspirate is consistent with acidic gastric secretions.
3. 2, 3; *Rationale:* Breathing slowly helps the patient relax. Lowering the container slows the instillation of the enema solution, which eases cramping. If the patient continues to cramp, the enema solution will be evacuated too soon, altering the effectiveness of the enema.
4. 2; *Rationale:* The oil retention enema is absorbed into the fecal mass, softening it for easier evacuation.
5. 4; *Rationale:* Functional constipation is characterized by straining and the sensation of incomplete evacuation. Absent bowel sounds usually are an indication of absent peristalsis, which is not associated with functional constipation. The presence of diarrhea and abdominal distention is associated with fecal impaction.
6. 1; *Rationale:* Reflex bradycardia occurs from the manipulation of the sacral branch of the vagus nerve. The vagus nerve is a parasympathetic nerve that once stimulated decreased heart rate.
7. 2; *Rationale:* This is the approximated distance from naris to stomach so that the tip of the tube enters the patient's stomach.
8. 1; *Rationale:* Over time the NG tube may rest along the stomach wall or is no longer patent because of abdominal secretions. Irrigation of the tube gently moves the tube away from the stomach lining and facilitates patency. Once the tube is patent, drainage of abdominal secretions occurs; and abdominal distention, discomfort, and nausea are relieved. If irrigation is not successful, the nurse should contact the health care provider.
9. 1, 2; *Rationale:* Abdominal distention results when abdominal secretions and gas accumulate. Decreased bowel sounds indicate a decrease in peristalsis, which causes secretions and gas to accumulate, causing further distention. If these occur following NG tube removal, the tube may need to be replaced.
10. 3, 4; *Rationale*: The blue pigtail is an air vent, which prevents suctioning of gastric mucosa at the distal end of the NG tube. This air vent is never be clamped, irrigated, or attached to suction.

CHAPTER 20

1. 1; *Rationale*: The stoma should be red and moist and protruding above the skin level. Stents would be present in a urostomy, not an ileostomy.
2. 2; *Rationale*: The pouch is not emptied on a schedule but when it is ⅓ to ½ full. Changing the pouch should be done on a schedule to avoid unexpected leakage. The frequency of change should be every 3 to 7 days.
3. 3; *Rationale*: After colon removal the bowel movement will never be formed but will have a thin or thick liquid consistency.
4. 3; *Rationale*: Site marking before surgery helps to ensure that the patient will have a well-placed stoma that is easy to see and is not in an abdominal crease or fold. This will make care of the ostomy easier and a reliable pouching system easier to achieve.
5. 1; *Rationale*: Catheterizing the stoma is the best way to avoid contamination of the specimen.
6. The correct sequence is 5, 4, 1, 6, 3, 2.
7. 1, 6, 7; *Rationale*: The pouch should be emptied when it is ⅓ to ½ full and changed on a schedule that meets the patient's needs and provides a reliable seal on the pouch. Self-care is expected unless there are limitations posed by disability unrelated to the ostomy. Peristomal skin should be intact and free of pain or itching. The pouches are waterproof and disposable.
8. 4; *Rationale*: Postoperative edema in the stoma and distention in the abdomen will decrease in the first 4 to 6 weeks after surgery; then the stoma size will be stable.
9. 3; *Rationale:* Family support is more important to adjustment to the body image change that occurs with an ostomy than age, level of education, or manual dexterity.
10. 2; *Rationale*: It is normal to be distressed when there is a body image change, and a process of grieving occurs. Allowing the patient to express these feelings is helpful to the patient.

CHAPTER 21

1. 3; *Rationale:* Medication should be given 1 hour before physical therapy for peak effectiveness to minimize discomfort during the treatment.
2. 3; *Rationale:* The medication order lacks the route of administration and possible start time.
3. Medication, dose, patient, route, time, and documentation. All of the six rights must be followed to ensure safe medication administration.
4. 3; *Rationale*: Polypharmacy. This amount of medications for one medical problem needs further evaluation.
5. 2; *Rationale:* The nurse needs to clarify medication orders that do not follow safe medication order guidelines.
6. 3; *Rationale:* 1 tbsp = 15 mL (see Table 21-4).
7. 4; *Rationale:*

$$\text{Tablets} = \frac{1\ \text{tablet}}{250\ \text{mg}} \times \frac{500\ \text{mg}}{1} \times \frac{500}{250} = 2\ \text{tablets}$$

8. 2; *Rationale:* The rest of the patients are stable; thus treating the pain in this situation is the priority.
9. 1, 2; *Rationale:* Larger print and a dispensing system can ensure safe medication administration to the older adult. Large-print pamphlets are also available.
10. 1; *Rationale:* One of the 2009 patient safety goals includes a "read back" to verify any verbal or telephone orders.

CHAPTER 22

1. 4; *Rationale:* A cream should be spread evenly over the skin surface, using long, even strokes that follow the direction of hair growth to ensure proper absorption.
2. The patient should take a preadministration measurement and retake the blood pressure 30 to 60 minutes after taking the medication to determine patient's baseline blood pressure and response to the medication.
3. 2, 6; *Rationale:* The mouthpiece should not be inserted beyond the raised lip on the mouthpiece. When taking two medications prescribed at the same time, the patient should wait 2 to 5 minutes before taking the second medication.
4. 4; *Rationale:* It is important to remove any medication residue before applying a new patch. This ensures a consistent dosage delivery. When giving a transdermal patch, always rotate the application site. A patient should never cut a patch in half because there is no way to determine dosage. If the patient becomes oversedated, the health care provider should be notified. Always remove a patch before applying the next dose.
5. 3; *Rationale:* Rectal suppositories are contraindicated in patients with rectal surgery or active rectal bleeding. A suppository can be given for hemorrhoids; however, extra lubricant is helpful for insertion. A suppository is often used for treatment of fever. The presence of diarrhea is often an indication for a suppository and does not contraindicate use in this situation.
6. 4; *Rationale:* a DPI is breath activated; there is no need to coordinate puffs with inhalation.
7. 2; *Rationale:* A 5-year-old child receives an ear medication the same way as an adult receives it. The nurse straightens the ear canal by pulling the pinna upward and outward.
8. When administering a medication through a feeding tube, always flush the tubing with 15-30 mL of water after each medication. After the last medication flush the tubing with 30 to 60 mL of water.
9. 2, 4; *Rationale*: No. 2 is the correct position for a rectal suppository insertion, and No. 4 is the correct distance for inserting a rectal suppository. Steps 1 and 3 are correct for a vaginal suppository insertion.
10. The first two steps include (1) checking accuracy and completeness of MAR with health care provider's written

medication order, including patient's name, drug name, form (foam, jelly, cream, tablet, suppository, or irrigating solution), route, dosage, and time of administration; and (2) reviewing pertinent information related to medication, including action, purpose, normal dose, side effects, and nursing implications.

CHAPTER 23

1. *Answer:* The nurse needs to know the following: the drug classification, effect, and nursing implications related to heparin therapy; the patient's current diet, OTC, herbal supplements, and medications to ensure that there is no increased risk of bleeding; and the safe medication dose, which must be compared to the order before administration. The nurse needs to calculate how many milliliters to draw from the vial and if he or she needs a filter needle.
2. *Answer:* The nurse needs to assess the rate per minute to administer and the IV compatibility of the medication. She also needs to assess the patency of the IV and the condition of the IV site.
3. 4; *Rationale:* Medication is drawn from the vial first to prevent contamination of the vial with medication from the ampule.
4. 2; *Rationale:* An induration of greater than 10 mm in a healthy individual indicates TB exposure and requires follow-up.
5. 1; *Rationale:* Symptoms indicate paresthesia and should not be present after an IM injection.
6. *Match:* 1, b; 2, c; 3, a
7. 4; *Rationale:* This is an appropriate size needle for administering a subcutaneous medication.
8. 2; *Rationale:* The nurse should calculate how much medication will be used for the injection while considering the route. This should be done before the diluent and powder are mixed.
9. 1; *Rationale:* Stop the infusion. The IV line is infiltrated, and the site needs to be changed.
10. 1; *Rationale:* Assessing the IV site is the nursing priority; medication cannot be given into a problem IV site.

CHAPTER 24

1. 1, 2, 4; *Rationale:* These are important descriptors that provide information about the wound. Over time the results of a wound assessment help identify how well the wound is healing (pp. 586-587). Information about the moist dressing application does not provide wound assessment information.
2. 2, 4, 6, 7; *Rationale:* The objective of using wound irrigation on this wound is to help clean out the beige drainage and soften the yellow slough tissue. Using a 19-gauge Angio catheter with a 35-mL syringe provides the necessary amount of pressure to clean the wound. Because of the amount of pressure, there may be some splashing from the wound; thus protective garments are advised. The volume of irrigant is high, and it will run out of the wound; using a collection device will collect the wound irrigation runoff. Leaving the gauze in does not give the nurse a clear view of the wound and does not allow the irrigation to reach the wound tissue. Administering the wound irrigant in either No. 3 or 5 will not allow the necessary irrigant pressure to cleanse the wound.
3. 2; *Rationale*: Because Mr. Garcia's wound was contaminated by the ruptured appendix, his surgeon left the wound open to heal by secondary intention. This allows a moist wound dressing to wick any drainage from the wound and support wound healing. A wound healing by primary intention would have the wound edges approximated.
4. 1, 3, 4; *Rationale:* The location, dimensions, and tissue type are some of the wound assessment parameters that help to determine wound healing progress. The estimate of the wound healing progress is not an objective assessment parameter because the time toward healing depends on many factors that cannot be predicted. A healing ridge is only present in a wound healing by primary intention such as a surgical wound that was approximated with staples.
5. 2, 3; *Rationale*: The first intervention would be to gently milk the tubing from the insertion site to the collection device in case something is plugging the tubing. Next the nurse would check to see if the drainage is coming from around the tube rather than through it, as indicated by an increased amount of drainage on the gauze pad. She should do these before calling the surgeon because the Jackson-Pratt drain may only be plugged. It is not advisable to wait 8 hours before any intervention since you know that this patient had 100 mL of drainage only 8 hours ago. Jackson-Pratt drains are not irrigated routinely.
6. 3; *Rationale***:** The collection bulb should be below the insertion site to facilitate drainage. To prevent pulling of the tube at the insertion site, pin the bulb to the patient's gown. Never allow the bulb to become full because it becomes heavy as it pulls on the insertion site and the full bulb prevents further drainage collection. Never do anything to prevent drainage, and the insertion site should remain dry and clean with no lubrication to the site.
7. 2; *Rationale*: Start by explaining to patient what will happen. After applying gloves to protect patient's incision, determine if the healing ridge is present; if not, do not proceed. Remove staples and apply Steri-Strips.
8. 2; *Rationale*: The recommended amount of pressure to be used in NPWT is −75 to −125 mm Hg. Using more negative pressure can cause harm to the wound and pain to the patient.
9. 1, 3, 4; *Rationale*: Use pieces of the adhesive drape over the areas where air is leaking. The leak causes a break in the seal, and the suction is no longer effective. Patching maintains the airtight seal. Shave the skin before application. Hair can interfere with the seal of the adhesive

drape. Do not use adhesive remover because this can leave a residue, preventing a good seal. Many adhesive removers leave a film on the skin that is greasy and does not allow the adhesive drape to make a good seal. Patching the leaking area with gauze does not work because the gauze does not allow an airtight seal. If soap is used on the periwound area, it must be rinsed off thoroughly to obtain an adequate seal.

10. 2; *Rationale*: The Steri-Strips provide support to the wound by distributing tension across the wound.

CHAPTER 25

1. 2 and 3; *Rationale:* Moisture barrier ointment is applied to areas that will be in contact with the stool. A thick layer prevents the liquid stool from contacting the skin. If the amount of fecal incontinence is high and the consistency is watery to slightly pasty, the use of a fecal incontinence collector can keep the stool from contacting the skin. Talcum powder absorbs moisture and holds the moisture to the skin and should not be used in areas of fecal incontinence. The use of towels under the patient is not indicated because the towels remain moist and damage the patient's skin.
2. 4; *Rationale*: The base of the wound must be visible to determine the true depth of the wound. Until the necrotic tissue is removed, the stage cannot be determined.
3. 1, 2; *Rationale:* The patient with the surgical wound most likely has an infection that delays wound healing as the inflammatory phase of wound healing is prolonged. A steroid such as cortisol also delays the inflammatory phase of wound healing. Vitamin C and a moist dressing are factors that promote wound healing.
4. 2, 4; *Rationale:* Mrs. Gibbs is at risk for pressure ulcers at the mouth or lips because of the endotracheal tube location. All patients have the risk of pressure ulcers over bony prominences, but Mrs. Gibb's risk is greater posteriorly because of her weight and difficulty turning. The pillows remove the risk of heel ulcers, and the IV site is not subject to pressure. There is no tube exiting the patient's nose.
5. 2; *Rationale*: A moist saline gauze dressing provides a moist environment to the wound and wicks away excessive drainage, facilitating healing.
6. 2; *Rationale:* A hydrocolloid dressing interacts with the moist wound base and forms a gel over the wound to support moist wound healing.
7. 3; *Rationale*: Explain the purpose of the dressing change to the patient before application. Position him in a way that provides easy access to wound for cleansing. Once cleansed, the entire wound can be visualized and measured to determine the correct size of hydrocolloid dressing (as the dressing should extend at least 2.5 cm (1 inch) beyond the wound edge. The dressing adheres best is gently pressed to the skin.
8. 3; *Rationale:* All four patients have some risk factors for developing a pressure ulcer. However, the 50-year-old patient has more factors, three, placing him at risk: poor circulation from diabetes, limited mobility from his postoperative status, and presence of diaphoresis.
9. 3; *Rationale:* The category of frictional shear should be added.

CHAPTER 26

1. c, b, g, a, e, f, d; *Rationale:* Using any other order would contaminate the dressing change and increase the patient risk for a wound infection.
2. 2,3,4; *Rationale:* Hydrogel dressings are nonadherent and easy to remove. The hydrogel gauze can be easily packed into a wound and any dead space. This type of dressing is appropriate for Mr. Alberts who has 2 cm of tunneling not visible in the wound bed. The hydrogel dressings have absorptive properties and are designed to hydrate wounds. They do not have antimicrobial properties.
3. 1; *Rationale:* A transparent dressing is a clear, adherent, nonabsorptive polyurethane moisture- and vapor-permeable dressing that can be used to manage superficial, minimally draining wounds. A transparent dressing would be inappropriate for a deep draining wound.
4. 3; *Rationale*: A dressing should remove exudate, but it is important not to dry out the wound. Tissue growth takes place best in a moist, warm environment.
5. 2; *Rationale:* It is important for the NAP to observe the patient's ventilation, determined by the ability to deep breathe and cough. This should be reported to the nurse. The length of time a binder has been applied does not indicate the patient's tolerance. The patient's heart rate does not reveal if the binder is too tight and does not measure local circulation. The condition of the wound is an important observation but does not pertain to the patient's tolerance of the binder.
6. 2; *Rationale:* Unlike bacterial infections, colonization is a chronic state in which low levels of bacteria exist in the wound but do not interfere with wound healing. Colonized wounds do need to be monitored for signs of bacterial overgrowth that may lead to infection.
7. 2,4; *Rationale:* A binder applied too tightly can cause skin breakdown where the binder is rubbing against skin that is unprotected by a dressing. It can also restrict comfortable full chest expansion, thereby adversely affecting respiratory status. A pulling sensation while ambulating indicates a binder that is too loose and needs to be adjusted.
8. 2,3; *Rationale*: Moist-to-dry and hydrocolloid gels both have debriding properties. A transparent dressing is appropriate for superficial, minimally draining wounds and does not have debriding capability. A dry dressing should never be used for debriding because it is likely to cause injury to new tissue.
9. 2; *Rationale*: A foam dressing is appropriate for moderate-to-heavy amounts of exudate. It generally needs to be changed daily to prevent maceration of periwound skin

once the foam has reached it absorption capacity. It is not appropriate for dry wounds or any wounds with tunneling.

10. 2; *Rationale*: When removing a dry dressing, moisten it first. Once it loosens, remove it gently. Never pull a dry dressing that adheres to a wound because this can injure the wound edges. The nurse always removes a single layer of gauze at a time to be sure that she does not disrupt underlying drains. Irrigating a wound before applying a dressing will not determine if the dressing sticks or not.

CHAPTER 27

1. 2; *Rationale*: Fill the bag and empty it to be sure that it has no leaks. This prevents maceration from unnecessary moisture.
2. 2; *Rationale*: Chilling is an undesirable effect of the administration of cold therapy. It is appropriate to discontinue the treatment to allow the patient to warm and resume it at a later time when appropriate covering for the patient can be provided to maintain warmth.
3. 1,2,4; *Rationale*: Reduction of pain, edema, and need for analgesics are all potential desired outcomes of cold therapy.
4. 2; *Rationale:* A patient with a preexisting condition that impairs circulation would be at greater risk for injury because of the vasoconstrictive action of cold applications.
5. 1; *Rationale*: Moisture in combination with heat increases the risk of developing macerated skin.
6. 2; *Rationale:* Use of microwaves to heat compresses places the patient at risk from injury because of the uneven heating that occurs. In addition, placing objects such as moist towels into a microwave may be a violation of safety and fire regulations of the facility.
7. Moist heated compresses.
8. Chilled, mottled, or bluish; *Rationale:* Mottled, reddened, or bluish purple skin are indications of prolonged exposure to cold.
9. 3; *Rationale*: Frequent assessment of the area receiving heat therapy must be done to prevent breakdown of the skin.

CHAPTER 28

1. g, c, a, f, d, e, b; *Rationale:* Medication must be removed from refrigerator before infusion. Cold IV fluids can cause arrhythmias and bubbles in tubing. Closing roller clamp prevents fluid from leaking from tubing. Removing spike from old IV tubing maintains sterility and prevents tubing from running dry. Inserting spike into new IV bag ensures no break in therapy and maintains sterility. Air in tubing can cause emboli and be fatal to patient. Regulating flow rate ensures that correct rate of fluid is given. Labeling bag provides for accuracy when assessing right patient right medication; ensures that fluid is running on time.
2. 2; *Rationale:* The IV bag has only been hanging for 30 minutes and is ¾ empty at a rate of 83 mL/hr, which would place patient at risk for fluid overload. Signs and symptoms indicate fluid overload.
3. 1, 3; *Rationale:* IV fluid should continue, but at a slower rate. Placing patient in High fowler's will improve her breathing. Kinks in IV tubing would cause fluid to decrease flow rate or not infuse at all; therefore patient would not experience fluid overload. IV device should not be removed in the event diuretics need to be given,
4. 4; *Rationale:* Signs and symptoms of phlebitis do not include respiratory, cardiac or GI presentations, but they do include the local symptoms of erythema and pain.
5. 2; *Rationale:* If a transfusion reaction is suspected based on an elevated temperature, pulse, or complaints of itching or presences of hives, the priority nursing intervention is to STOP the blood transfusion but maintain IV access.
6. 4; *Rationale:* Based on INS standards of practice, the smallest device and smallest gauge possible to give the prescribed therapy should be used.
7. 4; *Rationale:* According to the INS, optimal tip placement for a central line is the SVC. A PICC is placed in the arm via the antecubital fossa or upper arm; therefore it would be advanced to the SVC.
8. 4; *Rationale:* Based on calculations:

$$\frac{100}{60} \times \frac{10}{1} = 16.667; \text{ round to } 17 \text{ gtts/min.}$$

9. 2 (False); *Rationale:* Partial PN can be administered through either a peripheral device or a central venous device since the osmolarity is less then 600 mOsm/L. Total PN must be given through a central device because the osmolarity is greater than 600 mOsm/L.

CHAPTER 29

1. 4, 5; *Rationale:* Identification of the correct patient, surgical site, and procedure occurs immediately before moving to procedure area, and a "Time-Out" is performed before starting the procedure. This also occurs during any patient hand-off.
2. 1, 2, 4, 5; *Rationale*: Although family contact information is important, it is not a requirement for the procedural checklist.
3. 2; *Rationale*: Site marking should include the patient and is an important element required by The Joint Commission Universal Protocol.
4. 2; *Rationale*: Patient education is not a skill that can be delegated to the NAP.
5. 3; *Rationale*: The surgeon is ultimately responsible for obtaining informed consent. The nurse should verify the patient's understanding and be sure patient's signature is complete before signing the consent form as a witness.
6. 2; *Rationale*: It is important for the patient to be in the correct position to allow for increased lung expansion.

7. 1, 2; *Rationale*: Surgeon should be notified immediately to evaluate bleeding source and possible respiratory depression.
8. 2; *Rationale*: Small amounts of drainage are normal. Marking the amount allows nurse to evaluate progression of drainage.
9. 2; *Rationale*: Elevating head of bed allows for lung expansion and prevention of aspiration.

CHAPTER 30

1. 2; *Rationale*: Patient needs to be assessed as soon as possible. Alerting co-workers of equipment needed expedites interventions after the initial assessment has been completed.
2. 4; *Rationale*: The sequence for basic CPR is to check responsiveness, check for a pulse, begin compressions, provide 2 breaths, and attach AED.
3. 2; *Rationale*: According to the American Heart Association 2010 CPR guidelines, begin CPR immediately after the shock to provide immediate perfusion to the heart after shock.
4. 1; *Rationale*: Head tilt–chin lift provides the best technique to open a nontraumatic airway.
5. 1; *Rationale:* Patient has a better than 80% chance of survival if the first shock is delivered in less than 3 minutes inside a hospital. For every minute of delay after the first 3 minutes, the chance of survival drops by 10% per minute.
6. 3; *Rationale:* In performing chest compressions, fractured ribs may lacerate the liver or puncture the lung.
7. 4; *Rationale*: Oral airway should only be inserted in unconscious patients because of the vomiting risk.
8. 1; *Rationale*: Once an advanced airway is in place, breaths should be delivered at a rate of 8 to 10 per minute to avoid hyperventilation.
9. 3; *Rationale:* To provide more continuous perfusion to the body, chest compressions to ventilation rate should be 30:2.

CHAPTER 31

1. 2; *Rationale*: The nurse recognizes that both Mr. and Mrs. Robinson are suffering and having a difficult time making health care decisions. An extended discussion with someone from the health care team will help them more fully and carefully explore their feelings. The goal is not to support one person more than another but rather to help them understand the other person's feelings and wishes so their relationship remains strong in this difficult time.
2. 2, 5; *Rationale*: Members from a multidisciplinary team help address any symptoms that decrease a patient's quality of life. Patients of any age or diagnosis can receive palliative care in any setting. Options 1 and 4 apply to hospice care, a form of palliative care for people who likely only have 6 months or less to live. Option 3 refers to palliative care in the home setting. Palliative care occurs in all health care settings.
3. 4, 5; *Rationale:* An advance directive can be a written document, or a person can appoint a durable power of attorney for health care to make decisions when the patient is no longer able. A person preparing an advance directive should share it with his or her health care providers and family members and place it in his or her medical record. An advance directive provides an opportunity for a person to ask for certain care interventions (effective pain management) or refuse other interventions (artificial food or water), although some states have differing policies regarding the use of advance directives.
4. 4; *Rationale*: There may be a time when an ethical matter should go to an ethics committee or the whole health care team needs to be involved. However, the nurse should first nonjudgmentally listen to the family member and gather more information. Sometimes a clarification helps the person deliberate. Talking also helps validate the person's concerns. The nurse might report the family member's concern, with the added information, to the health care team.
5. 1, 4; *Rationale*: When a patient is not able to give information, the nurse often relies on observation and the input of people who know him or her. If a patient in hospice care wants to eat favorite foods, those foods are offered to enhance his or her sense of well-being. A person cannot prepare an advance directive for someone else.
6. 4; *Rationale*: The most therapeutic response would not scold, shame, minimize, or explain away the wife's fears and uncertainty about her ability. Answer 4 opens the door for further conversation to help the nurse offer caregiver education, validate the wife's feelings, and help her address practical problems.
7. 2, 4, 5; *Rationale*: The patient's behaviors most likely indicate a grief response in which she is experiencing strong emotional or spiritual symptoms of fear or hopelessness. The assessments that further the nurse's understanding of what the patient is facing (treatment plan) and knowing those who usually support her and her emotional and spiritual state yield the most helpful information.
8. 1, 3, and 4; *Rationale*: Pain medications may not provide relief for a number of reasons that should be validated. The patient's disease progression or type of pain may be changing, or the patient may perceive pain more intensely because of an emotional or spiritual reason. To doubt the patient's description of his or her pain relief will likely not provide the patient with the best patient-centered care.
9. 1; *Rationale*: In most instances support the activity that helps a patient maintain some control and participation in meaningful activities. Answer 1 best accomplishes that goal.

10. 2; *Rationale:* It is best to elevate the head of the bed as soon as possible after death to prevent pooling of blood in the face and discoloration. Before beginning body preparations, ask if family members would like to participate. Don protective barriers as needed and proceed from dirty to clean tasks, replacing soaked dressings, bathing, and placing the patient in a clean gown.

CHAPTER 32

1. 1, 2, 4; *Rationale:* Pot handles should be turned inward and heaters set below 120° F (49° C). A stove lock is a good safety measure to prevent burns of small children. Smoking is a risk factor for burns; therefore encourage client to stop smoking by offering access to classes.
2. 3; *Rationale:* Area rugs are trip hazards. A cane is an appropriate assistive device, and shoes should have thin soles with traction. Diuretics are better scheduled early in day to avoid client getting up in middle of night for bathroom, which increases risk of falls.
3. 2; *Rationale:* Discharge planning begins with admission to a health care facility and is modified as client's condition changes.
4. 3; *Rationale:* Having a client describe his or her own level of health requires the client to describe his or her health abilities. Assessment should be performed in a quiet place, without distractions, over a short period of time. Do not limit assessment to caregivers.
5. 1, 3; *Rationale:* Allowing wandering in a safe place reduces the risk of the client leaving home. Locks and electronic alarms are necessary to reduce wandering. Signs give clues to guide clients to desired locations. Restraints are not appropriate and increase client's agitation.
6. 3; *Rationale*: A pill dispenser helps a client self-administer medications as scheduled. The other three options are important for medication safety but do not directly affect administration.
7. 1, 5; *Rationale:* Color coding is a safe way to distinguish drugs to be given at the same time. Keeping medications in an easy-to-open container makes it easier for clients with dexterity problems to self-administer. Nos. 2 and 4 are for storage. Never place needles in a plastic bag. Storage techniques are important to review since different medications are stored in different ways.
8. 4; *Rationale*: Ensures safe disposal of medical waste.
9. 3; *Rationale:* Firearms are the second leading cause of death in 10- to 24-year-olds. Guns need to be secured and kept in a locked cabinet to avoid injury.

APPENDIX B

Abbreviations and Equivalents

ABBREVIATIONS FOR CONVERSION USING HOUSEHOLD MEASURES

1 drop (gtt) = 1 minim
1 teaspoon (1 tsp) = 5 mL
3 tsp = 1 tablespoon (tbsp)
1 cup = 8 oz
16 oz = 1 pound (lb)

STANDARD EQUIVALENTS, ABBREVIATIONS, AND CONVERSIONS

1000 mg = 1 g
1000 mL = 1 liter (L)
2.2 lb = 1 kilogram (kg) = 1000 g
1 tsp = 5 mL
1 dr = 4 mL
mEq: milliequivalent
mcg: microgram

SYMBOLS

/	Per
≤	Equal to or less than
≥	Equal to or more than
≅	Approximately equal to
+/–, ±	Plus or minus
♂	Male
♀	Female
1°	Primary; first degree
2°	Secondary; second degree
3°	Tertiary; third degree
↑	Up; increase
↓	Down; decrease

ABBREVIATIONS

ā: before
abd: abdomen
ABGs: arterial blood gases
ac: before meals
ad lib: as desired
ADH: antidiuretic hormone
ADLs: activities of daily living
AFB: acid-fast bacillus (related to tuberculosis)
AIDS: acquired immunodeficiency syndrome
ALL: acute lymphoblastic leukemia
AMB: ambulatory
AP (and lateral chest): anterior and posterior
ASA: aspirin
ASHD: arteriosclerotic heart disease
ax: axillary
BE: barium enema
bid: twice a day
BM: bowel movement
BP: blood pressure
BPH: benign prostatic hypertrophy
BR: bed rest
BRP: bathroom privileges
BSE: breast self-examination
BSI: body substance isolation
BUN: blood urea nitrogen
bx: biopsy
c̄: with
C&S: culture and sensitivity
CA: cancer
CABG: coronary artery bypass graft
CAD: coronary artery disease
cap: capsule
CBC: complete blood count
CBI: continuous bladder irrigation
CBR: complete bed rest
CC: chief complaint
CDC: Centers for Disease Control and Prevention
CHF: congestive heart failure
Cl: chloride
CN: cranial nerve
CNS: central nervous system
c/o: complains of
CO_2: carbon dioxide
COPD: chronic obstructive pulmonary disease
CPM: continuous passive motion
CPR: cardiopulmonary resuscitation
CSF: cerebrospinal fluid
CT: computed tomography
CVA: cerebrovascular accident (stroke)
CVP: central venous pressure
D5NS, D_5NS: 5% dextrose in 0.9% (normal) saline
DAT: diet as tolerated
DM: diabetes mellitus
DNR: do not resuscitate

DSD: dry sterile dressing
DTR: deep tendon reflex
DVT: deep venous thrombosis
dx: diagnosis
EC: enteric coated
ECG, EKG: electrocardiogram
elix: elixir
ER: extended release
ESR: erythrocyte sedimentation rate
ESRD: end-stage renal disease
ET: enterostomal therapist
FUO: fever of unknown origin
fx: fracture
g: gram
GI: gastrointestinal
gtt: drops
GU: genitourinary
Hb, Hgb: hemoglobin
HBV: hepatitis B virus
HCO_3^-: bicarbonate
Hct: hematocrit
HCV: hepatitis C virus
HEPA: high-efficiency air
HIV: human immunodeficiency virus
h/o: history of
HOB: head of bed
HR: heart rate
hs: at bedtime
HTN: hypertension
I&O: intake and output
ICP: intracranial pressure
ICU: intensive care unit
IDDM: insulin-dependent diabetes mellitus
IM: intramuscular
IPPB: intermittent positive-pressure breathing
IV: intravenous
JVD: jugular vein distention
K: potassium
KUB: kidney, ureter, bladder
KVO: keep vein open (run IV very slowly)
LLQ: left lower quadrant
LMP: last menstrual period
LOC: level of consciousness
LR: lactated Ringer's solution
lytes: electrolytes
MAP: mean arterial pressure
MCHC: mean corpuscular hemoglobin concentration
MCV: mean corpuscular volume
MI: myocardial infarction
N: nitrogen
Na: sodium
NaCl: sodium chloride
neg: negative
NG: nasogastric
NPO: nothing by mouth
NS: normal saline
NSAIDs: nonsteroidal antiinflammatory drugs
O_2: oxygen
OOB: out of bed
OR: operating room
OT: occupational therapy
OTC: over-the-counter (medicine available without prescription)
P: pulse
PACU: postanesthesia care unit
pc: after meals
PCA: patient-controlled analgesia
PE: pulmonary embolism
PID: pelvic inflammatory disease
PMH: past medical history
PMI: point of maximal impulse
PO: by mouth
postop: after surgery
preop: before surgery
prn: as needed
pt: patient
PT: physical therapy
PT: prothrombin time
PTT: partial thromboplastin time
PVD: peripheral vascular disease
q: each
q_h (fill in the number of hours), e.g. q3h: every 3 hours
qs: sufficient quantity
R: respirations
RA: rheumatoid arthritis
RBC: red blood cells
R/O: rule out (eliminate possibility of a condition)
ROM: range of motion
ROS: review of systems
r/t: related to
RUQ: right upper quadrant
Rx: treatment
$\bar{s}$: without
sl (SL): sublingual
SOB: shortness of breath
sp gr: specific gravity
SR: sustained release
STAT: immediately
STD: sexually transmitted disease
supp: suppository
susp: suspension
sx: symptoms, signs
T: temperature
T&C: type and crossmatch
Tab: tablet
TB: tuberculosis
TCDB: turn, cough, deep breathe
tid: three times a day
TPN: total parenteral nutrition
TPR: temperature, pulse, respirations
TURP: transurethral resection of prostate
UA: urinalysis
up ad: up as desired
URI: upper respiratory infection

US: ultrasound
UTI: urinary tract infection
VS: vital signs
VTBI: volume to be infused
WBC: white blood cell
WC: wheelchair
WNL: within normal limits
wt: weight

OFFICIAL "DO NOT USE" LIST*

DO NOT USE	POTENTIAL PROBLEM	USE INSTEAD
U (unit)	Mistaken for "0" (zero), the number "4" (four), or "cc"	Write "unit"
IU (International Unit)	Mistaken for IV (intravenous) or the number 10 (ten)	Write "International Unit"
Q.D., QD, q.d., qd (daily) Q.O.D, QOD, q.o.d., qod (every other day)	Mistaken for each other Period after the Q mistaken for "I" and the "O" mistaken for "I"	Write "daily" Write "every other day"
Trailing zero (X.0 mg)† Lack of leading zero (.X mg)	Decimal point is missing	Write X mg Write 0.X mg
MS MSO_4 and $MgSO_4$	Can mean morphine sulphate or magnesium sulphate Confused for one another	Write "morphine sulphate" Write "magnesium sulphate"

Official "Do Not Use" List, Joint Commission on Accreditation of Healthcare Organizations, December 29th, 2009, www.jointcommission.org, accessed May 7, 2010.

*Applies to all orders and all medication-related documentation that is handwritten (including free-text computer entry) or on preprinted forms.

†**Exception**: A "trailing zero" may be used only where required to demonstrate the level of precision of the value being reported such as for laboratory results, imaging studies that report size of lesions, or catheter/tube sizes. It may not be used in medication orders or other medical-related documentation.

ADDITIONAL ABBREVIATIONS, ACRONYMS, AND SYMBOLS *(for possible future inclusion in the Official "Do Not Use" List)*

DO NOT USE	POTENTIAL PROBLEM	USE INSTEAD
> (greater than) < (less than)	Misinterpreted as the number "&" (seven) or the letter "L" Confused for one another	Write "greater than" Write "less than"
Abbreviations for drug names	Misinterpreted due to similar abbreviations for multiple drugs	Write drug names in full
Apothecary units	Unfamiliar to many practitioners Confused with metric units	Write drug names in full
@	Mistaken for the number "2" (two)	Write "at"
cc	Mistaken for U (units) when written poorly	Write "mL" or "milliliters"
µg	Mistaken for mg (milligrams) resulting in one thousand-fold overdose	Write "mcg" or "micrograms"

Official "Do Not Use" List, Joint Commission on Accreditation of Heathcare Organizations, December 29th, 2009, www.jointcommission.org, accessed May 7th, 2010.

INDEX

f indicates illustrations, *t* indicates tables, and b indicates boxes.

INDEX OF SKILLS